FEMALE UROLOGY, UROGYNECOLOGY, AND VOIDING DYSFUNCTION

FEMALE UROLOGY, UROGYNECOLOGY, AND VOIDING DYSFUNCTION

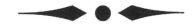

EDITED BY

SANDIP P. VASAVADA, M.D.
CLEVELAND CLINIC FOUNDATION,
CLEVELAND, OHIO, U.S.A

RODNEY A. APPELL, M.D.
BAYLOR COLLEGE OF MEDICINE,
HOUSTON, TEXAS, U.S.A.

PETER K. SAND, M.D.
NORTHWESTERN UNIVERSITY,
EVANSTON, ILLINOIS, U.S.A.

SHLOMO RAZ, M.D.
DAVID GEFFEN SCHOOL OF MEDICINE AT UCLA,
LOS ANGELES, CALIFORNIA, U.S.A.

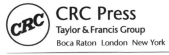

CRC Press
Taylor & Francis Group
Boca Raton London New York

CRC Press is an imprint of the
Taylor & Francis Group, an informa business

CRC Press
Taylor & Francis Group
6000 Broken Sound Parkway NW, Suite 300
Boca Raton, FL 33487-2742

First issued in paperback 2019

© 2005 by Taylor & Francis Group, LLC
CRC Press is an imprint of Taylor & Francis Group, an Informa business

No claim to original U.S. Government works

ISBN-13: 978-0-8247-5426-6 (hbk)
ISBN-13: 978-0-367-39333-5 (pbk)

Visit the Taylor & Francis Web site at
http://www.taylorandfrancis.com

and the CRC Press Web site at
http://www.crcpress.com

Preface

There has been a convergence of the sub-specialties of female urology and urogynecology over the last several years. This development has resulted in improved care for women, as we have had to "escalate" our own knowledge and abilities. Recently, we have even seen fellowship training transcend towards this multidisciplinary goal by the creation of joint accredited fellowship programs in female urology and urogynecology. These programs have as their primary aim to create the thought leaders of tomorrow in women's health by creating a unique group of physicians who see the "whole" patient and can treat them accordingly. It is evident that there is a strong need for more subspecialization in the field with the aging population and prevalence of incontinence and pelvic floor disorders that is present worldwide. This book speaks to the combined nature of our practices that has emanated from this approach.

We have sought to have some of the top thought leaders and experts from around the world to contribute to this publication. Furthermore, these authors embody some of the exact principles, which establish our sub-specialties as being progressive and forward thinking in their approaches to the various disease processes and disorder that we treat. One of the prevailing undertones of our book speaks to the fact that there are many ways in which to treat any single disorder. We have, therefore, had several chapters written by physicians or subspecialists who may do things differently to present contradictory views. The purpose is more than to be controversial, but rather to give an entrance point for those wishing to advance the field and aim for the utopian dream of literal cures for incontinence and other women's disorders.

We all have much to learn in this area of urinary incontinence and pelvic floor disorders. It is our hope that this book will help to build on the currently existing framework and provide a platform towards better understanding of the disease processes that affect so many of our patients.

Sandip P. Vasavada, M.D.
Rodney A. Appell, M.D.
Peter K. Sand, M.D.
Shlomo Raz, M.D.

Introduction

Times have changed and so should our intellectual basis for the management of diseases and conditions. Once thought of as an anatomic structure containing disparate and unrelated viscera, the human pelvis is now appreciated as a functional syncytium as complex as any within the human body. The dysfunctions of urinary, genital, and gastrointestinal elements which constitute this complex functional–anatomic arrangement require comprehensive and inclusive management strategies.

None of us is capable of mastering the vagaries of function and structure of all the elements of the human pelvis and therefore it is requisite that expertise be drawn from collaborative fields of endeavor so that as complete a management schema as is possible be developed. Additionally, the very real superimposition of behavioral, vascular and neurologic dysfunctions further make the inclusive "team" approach concept a mandatory one. This textbook represents a superb example of the inclusive approach for management. The interaction between colorectal (and gastroenterologic), urogynecologic, and urologic specialists can and does produce the best possible outcome for individual patients as well as for entire populations of individuals.

The concept of pelvic medicine remains not only viable, but one that reflects the aforementioned global interaction and collaboration of similarly motivated specialists whose primary concern is the attainment of the best outcome possible for women severely afflicted by conditions which are disruptive and destructive to quality of life and, in some cases, to well being and life expectancy. This book should be viewed in the context of intellectual instruction and exchange which will make the pelvic medicine endeavor that much more successful from both the patient and medical standpoint. The editors of the authors of the text represent the best and their achievement should serve as a model for subsequent efforts in cross specialty collaboration and, possibly more importantly, harmony.

Roger Dmochowski, M.D., F.A.C.S.
Department of Urology
Vanderbilt University Medical Center
Nashville, Tennessee, U.S.A.

Introduction

Over the last 10 years, all of you who care for women in your practice have been impressed with the increasing call to provide services for urinary incontinence and pelvic organ prolapse. These pelvic floor disorders are becoming more prevalent within our practices as the number of women in the age groups most affected by these disorders increases. Also, women now coming into these age groups have a more proactive approach to their own health care than did their mothers and their sophistication and expectations demand optimal care.

It is estimated that the demand for pelvic floor disorders care will double in the next 25 years. This increasing demand combined with the remarkable growth in high quality research is both encouraging and intimidating. Intimidating in that as we learn more, we realize how much more we have to learn and encouraging as we watch great strides in both basic science and outcomes research take hold.

This text embraces one of the fundamental concepts that leaders within both female urology and urogynecology have come to understand—that women with pelvic floor disorders are best served by an approach that acknowledges the wisdom and experience of both of these developing subspecialties. Thus, these varied accounts by divergent authors give the reader the opportunity to consider these issues from many points of view. This will inevitably lead to a richness of understanding that a single doctrine could not provide.

As we face the challenge of training our residents, fellows and colleagues, we will come to appreciate this text as an excellent resource and frequent reference. These in depth discussions of both basic and complex components of *Female Urology, Urogynecology and Voiding Dysfunction* offer us an opportunity to both reflect and to look forward. As all involved in research and providing care in this growing field combine forces, the wisdom and philosophy embodied in this work will enable us to expand the foundation of physicians able to join in the process toward the ultimate goal of improving the quality of the care that these women receive.

Karl M. Luber, M.D.
University of California, San Diego
Southern California Permanente Medical Group
San Diego, California, U.S.A.

Contents

Contributors

Joseph B. Abdelmalak   Cleveland Clinic Foundation, Cleveland, Ohio, U.S.A.

Fernando Almeida*   University of California, Los Angeles, California, U.S.A.

Rodney A. Appell, M.D.   Head, Section of Female Urology and Voiding Dysfunction, F. Brantley Scott Chair. Professor of Urology and Gyneocology, Baylor College of Medicine, Houston, Texas, U.S.A.

Matthew D. Barber, M.D., M.H.S.   Section of Urogynecology, Pelvic Reconstruction Surgery, Cleveland Clinic Foundation, Cleveland, Ohio, U.S.A.

Jennifer R. Berman   Female Sexual Medicine Center, David Geffen School of Medicine at UCLA, Los Angeles, California, U.S.A.

Jerry G. Blaivas   Joan and Sanford Weil College of Medicine, Cornell University, New York, New York, U.S.A.

Dawn M. Bodell   Fellow, Tower Urology Institute for Continence, Los Angeles, California, U.S.A.

Timothy B. Boone, M.D., Ph.D.   Professor and Chairman, Scott Department of Urology, Baylor College of Medicine, Houston, Texas, U.S.A.

Linda Cardozo, M.D., F.R.C.O.G.   Professor of Urogynaecology, Department of Obstetrics and Gynaecology, King's College Hospital, London, England

R. Duane Cespedes, M.D.   Chairman, Department of Urology, Wilford Hall Medical Center, Lackland AFB, Texas, U.S.A.

***Current affiliation*: Senior Associate Consultant, Department of Urology, Mayo Clinic Scottsdale, Scottsdale, Arizona, U.S.A.

Craig V. Comiter   University of Arizona Health Sciences Center, Tucson, Arizona, U.S.A.

Jeffrey L. Cornella   Mayo Clinic Scottsdale, Scottsdale, Arizona, U.S.A.

Firouz Daneshgari   Director, Center for Female Pelvic Medicine and Reconstructive Surgery, The Cleveland Clinic Foundation, Cleveland, Ohio, U.S.A.

G. Willy Davila   Cleveland Clinic Florida, Weston, Florida, U.S.A.

Karyn Schlunt Eilber, M.D. [†]   Department of Urology, University of California, Los Angeles, California, U.S.A.

Paul M. Fine   Baylor College of Medicine, Houston, Texas, U.S.A.

Adam J. Flisser   Joan and Sanford Weil College of Medicine, Cornell University, New York, New York, U.S.A.

Sanjay Gandhi, M.D.   Research Fellow, Department of Obstetrics and Gynecology, Northwestern University, Evanston, Illinois, U.S.A.

John B. Gebhart   Mayo Clinic and Mayo Clinic College of Medicine, Rochester, Minnesota, U.S.A.

Gamal M. Ghoniem, M.D., F.A.C.S.   Head, Section of Voiding Dysfunction and Female Urology, Cleveland Clinic Florida and the Cleveland Clinic Foundation Health Sciences Center of OSU, Weston, Florida, U.S.A.

David A. Ginsberg   Assistant Professor of Urology, Department of Urology, University of Southern California School of Medicine, Los Angeles, California, U.S.A.

Roger P. Goldberg, M.D., M.P.H.   Director of Urogynecology Research, Evanston Continence Center, Northwestern University Medical School, Evanston, Illinois, U.S.A.

Howard B. Goldman, M.D.   Assistant Professor of Urology, Department of Urology and Reproductive Biology, University Hospitals of Cleveland, CASE School of Medicine, Cleveland, Ohio, U.S.A.

Matthew B. Gretzer   The Johns Hopkins Medical Institutions, Baltimore, Maryland, U.S.A.

Michael Gross   Fellow in Neurourology, Scott Department of Urology, Baylor College of Medicine, Houston, Texas, U.S.A.

Jennifer Gruenenfelder   University of Michigan, Ann Arbor, Michigan, U.S.A.

H. Roger Hadley, M.D.   Professor and Chief, Division of Urology, Loma Linda University, Loma Linda, California, U.S.A.

[†]*Current affiliation*: Assistant Attending, Department of Urology, Memorial Sloan-Kettering Cancer Center, New York, New York, U.S.A.

John C. Hairston, M.D.   Assistant Professor of Urology, Division of Urology, University of Texas Medical School at Houston, Houston, Texas, U.S.A.

Sender Herschorn   University of Toronto and Sunnybrook and Women's Health Sciences Centre, Toronto, Ontario, Canada

Adonis Hijaz   University of Toronto and Sunnybrook and Women's Health Sciences Centre, Toronto, Ontario, Canada

Tracy L. Hull, M.D.   Staff Surgeon, Department of Colon and Rectal Surgery, Cleveland Clinic Foundation, Cleveland, Ohio, U.S.A.

Nancy B. Itano[§]   University of California, Los Angeles, California, U.S.A.

Dallas Johnson   Baylor College of Medicine, Houston, Texas, U.S.A.

Mickey M. Karram, M.D.   Director Urogynecology, Professor OBGYN, Department of OBGYN, Good Samaritan Hospital, Cincinnati, Ohio, U.S.A.

Kathleen C. Kobashi, M.D.   Co-Director, Urology and Renal Transplantation, Continence Center, Virginia Mason Medical Center, Seattle, Washington, U.S.A.

Neeraj Kohli, M.D.   Associate Professor; Director, Division of Urogynecology, Brigham and Womens Hospital, Harvard University, Boston, Massachusetts, U.S.A.

Karl J. Kreder, M.D.   Professor and Clinical Vice Chair, Department of Urology, University of Iowa, Iowa City, Iowa, U.S.A.

Christina H. Kwon   Evanston Continence Center, Northwestern University, Evanston, Illinois, USA

Peter O. Kwong, M.D.   Fellow in Female Urology and Urinary Tract Reconstruction, Department of Surgery/Urology, University of Texas Health Science Center, Houston, Texas, U.S.A.

H. Henry Lai, M.D.   Resident, Scott Department of Urology, Baylor College of Medicine, Houston, Texas, U.S.A.

Gary E. Leach   Director, Tower Urology Institute for Continence, Los Angeles, Califonia, U.S.A.

Raymond A. Lee   Mayo Clinic and Mayo Clinic College of Medicine, Rochester, Minnesota, U.S.A.

Gary E. Lemack, M.D.   Associate Professor of Urology, Southwestern Medical Center, University of Texas, Dallas, Texas, U.S.A.

[§]*Current affiliation*: Senior Associate Consultant, Department of Urology, Mayo Clinic Scottsdale, Scottsdale, Arizona, U.S.A.

Mark S. Litwin, M.D., M.P.H.   Professor, Department of Urology, David Geffen School of Medicine at UCLA and UCLA School of Public Health, Los Angeles, California, U.S.A.

Vincent R. Lucente, M.D., M.B.A.¶   Pennsylvania State University, College of Medicine, Hershey, Pennsylvania, U.S.A.

James Chivian Lukban   Urogynerology Associates of Colorado, Denver, Colorado, U.S.A.

Thomas L. Lyons, M.S., M.D.   Director, Center for Women's Care and Reproductive Surgery, Atlanta, Georgia, U.S.A.

Shahar Madjar   Northern Michigan Urology at Bell, Bell Memorial Hospital, Marquette County, Michigan, U.S.A.

Marisa A. Mastropietro, M.D.**   Lehigh Valley Hospital, Allentown, Pennsylvania, U.S.A.

Edward J. McGuire   University of Michigan, Ann Arbor, Michigan, U.S.A.

John R. Miklos, M.D.   Director Urogynecology, Atlanta Urogynecology Associates, Atlanta, Georgia, U.S.A.

Elizabeth A. Miller   Duke University Medical Center, Durham, North Carolina, U.S.A.

Robert D. Moore, D.O.   Assistant Director Urogynecology, Atlanta Urogynecology Associates, Atlanta, Georgia, U.S.A.

Tristi W. Muir, M.D.   Assistant Chief, Female Pelvic Medicine and Reconstructive Surgery, Department of Obstetrics and Gynecology, Brooke Army Medical Center, Fort Sam Houston, Texas, U.S.A.

Minda Neimark   Cleveland Clinic Florida, Weston, Florida, U.S.A.

Diane K. Newman   University of Pennsylvania Medical Center, Philadelphia, U.S.A.

Victor W. Nitti   New York University School of Medicine, New York, U.S.A.

Keith J. O'Reilly††   Tripler Army Medical Center, Honolulu, Hawaii, U.S.A.

Donald R. Ostergard, M.D.   University of California, Irvine, and Long Beach Memorial Medical Center, Long Beach, California, U.S.A.

Marie Fidela R. Paraiso   Cleveland Clinic Foundation, Cleveland, Ohio, U.S.A.

¶*Current affiliation*: Medical Director, Institute for Female Pelvic Medicine and Reconstructive Surgery, Allentown, Pennsylvania, U.S.A.
***Current affiliation*: Director of Gynecologic Services, Lincoln Hospital, Bronx, New York, U.S.A.
††*Current affiliation*: Department of Urology, Madigan Army Hospital, Tacoma, Washington, U.S.A.

David F. Penson, M.D., M.P.H.[§§]   Section of Urology, 112-UR, University of Washington School of Medicine, VA Puget Sound HCS, Seattle, Washington, U.S.A.

Shlomo Raz, M.D.   Professor, Department of Urology, David Geffen School of Medicine at UCLA, Los Angeles, California, U.S.A.

Raymond R. Rackley, M.D.   Co-Head, Section of Female Urology, Urological Institute, Cleveland Clinic Foundation, Cleveland, Ohio, U.S.A.

Martin B. Richman, M.D.   Department of Urology, Case Western Reserve University, University Hospitals of Cleveland, Cleveland, Ohio, U.S.A.

Dudley Robinson, M.D., M.R.C.O.G.   Sub-speciality Trainee—Urogynaecology, Department of Obstetrics and Gynaecology, King's College Hospital, London, England

Larissa V. Rodríguez, M.D.   Assistant Professor, Co-director of Division of Female Urology, Reconstructive Surgery and Urodynamics, Department of Urology, University of California, Los Angeles, California, U.S.A.

Nirit Rosenblum, M.D.[¶¶]   Department of Urology, University of California, Los Angeles, California, U.S.A.

Eric S. Rovner   Assistant Professor Urology, Department of Surgery, Division of Urology, University of Pennsylvania School of Medicine, Philadelphia, Pennsylvania, U.S.A.

Christopher Saigal, M.D., M.P.H.   Assistant Professor, Department of Urology, David Geffen School of Medicine at UCLA, Los Angeles, California, U.S.A.

Peter K. Sand, M.D.   Professor, Department of Obstetrics and Gynecology, Evanston Continence Center, Northwestern University, Evanston, Illinois, U.S.A.

Harriette M. Scarpero   New York University School of Medicine, New York, U.S.A.

Jeffrey L. Segal, M.D.   Clinical Instructor OBGYN, Fellow Urogynecology, Department of OBGYN, Good Samaritan Hospital, Cincinnati, Ohio, U.S.A.

Patrick J. Shenot   Thomas Jefferson University, Philadelphia, Pennsylvania, U.S.A.

John P. Stein   Department of Urology, University of Southern California, Los Angeles, California, U.S.A.

Steven Swift, M.D.   Associate Professor, Department of Obstetrics and Gynecology, Medical University of South Carolina, Charleston, South Carolina, U.S.A.

[§§]*Current affiliation*: Associate Professor Urology and Preventive Medicine, Keck School of Medicine, University of Southern California, Los Angeles, Califonia, U.S.A.
[¶¶]*Current affiliation*: Assistant Professor, Department of Urology, NYU School of Medicine, New York, New York, U.S.A.

Marie-Blanche Tchetgen   Cleveland Clinic Foundation, Cleveland, Ohio, U.S.A.

Richard Vanlangendonck, M.D.   Director of Minimally Invasive Surgery, Department of Urology, Ochsner Clinic Foundation, New Orleans, Louisiana, U.S.A.

Sandip P. Vasavada, M.D.   Co-Head, Section of Female Urology, Urological Institute, Cleveland Clinic Foundation, Cleveland, Ohio, U.S.A.

Stacey J. Wallach, M.D.***   University of California, Irvine, and Long Beach Memorial Medical Center, Long Beach, California, U.S.A.

Kathleen E. Walsh   Female Sexual Medicine Center, David Geffen School of Medicine at UCLA, Los Angeles, California, U.S.A.

Mark D. Walters, M.D.   Head, Section of Urogynecology and Reconstructive Pelvic Surgery, Department of Obstetrics and Gynecology, Cleveland Clinic Foundation, Cleveland, Ohio, U.S.A.

George D. Webster   Duke University Medical Center, Durham, North Carolina, U.S.A.

O. Lenaine Westney, M.D.   Assistant Professor, Department of Surgery/Urology, University of Texas Health Science Center, Houston, Texas, U.S.A.

Alan J. Wein   Chair, Division of Urology, Department of Surgery, University of Pennsylvania School of Medicine, Philadelphia, Pennsylvania, U.S.A.

Kristene E. Whitmore   Graduate Hospital, Philadelphia, Pennsylvania, U.S.A.

Tracey Small Wilson   University of Texas Southwestern Medical Center, Dallas, Texas, U.S.A.

J. Christian Winters, M.D.   Director of Female Urology, Department of Urology, Ochsner Clinic Foundation, New Orleans, Louisiana, U.S.A.

E. James Wright   The Johns Hopkins Medical Institutions, Baltimore, Maryland, U.S.A.

Philippe E. Zimmern, M.D.   Professor of Urology, Southwestern Medical Center, University of Texas, Dallas, Texas, U.S.A.

****Current affiliation*: Assistant Professor, Department of Obstetrics and Gynecology, University of California, Sacramento, California, U.S.A.

1

Anatomy of Pelvic Support

Nirit Rosenblum,* Karyn S. Eilber,† Larissa V. Rodríguez, and Shlomo Raz
University of California, Los Angeles, California, U.S.A.

I. INTRODUCTION

Female pelvic anatomy is a complex combination of muscles, ligaments, nerves, and blood vessels that act dynamically to provide support for the urethra, bladder, uterus, and rectum. An understanding of normal mechanisms of pelvic support are essential in the evaluation of women with voiding complaints, urinary incontinence, and bowel dysfunction related to pelvic floor relaxation. Thus, the treatment of female urinary incontinence often involves recognition and treatment of concurrent pelvic pathophysiology such as cystocele, uterine prolapse, enterocele, rectocele, and perineal laxity. Identification of the various components of pelvic floor dysfunction is aided by diagnostic tools such as video urodynamics and magnetic resonance imaging of the pelvis. This chapter will focus on normal female pelvic anatomy, including the supporting structures relevant to voiding dysfunction and incontinence, as well as the pathophysiology of pelvic floor relaxation, with a description of the various components of pelvic organ prolapse.

II. PELVIC SUPPORTING STRUCTURES

A. Bone

Passive support of the pelvic floor is provided by the bony structures, which act as anchors for the important muscular and fascial structures comprising the pelvic floor. The pubic rami, ischial spines, and sacrum represent the anchoring points of the true bony pelvis, which is made up of pubis, ilium, ischium, sacrum, and coccyx (1). The pelvic floor is diamond-shaped with the pubic symphysis and sacrum at the anterior and posterior apices while the ischial spines serve as lateral anchors. The pelvic floor can be further subdivided into anterior and posterior compartments by drawing a line between the two ischial spines.

B. Ligaments

The sacrospinous ligaments span the posterior portion of the pelvic floor, from the ischial spines to the anterolateral aspect of the sacrum and coccyx. The coccygeus muscle is found between the

Current affiliation: NYU School of Medicine, New York, New York, U.S.A.
†*Current affiliation*: Memorial Sloan-Kettering Cancer Center, New York, New York, U.S.A.

ischial spines and the lateral aspect of the sacrum and coccyx, overlying the sacrospinous ligament and is an important landmark in vaginal surgery. Above the coccygeus muscle lies the sciatic nerve and its plexus, while the pudendal nerve and vessels lie lateral (Alcock's canal). Medially, the sacrospinous ligament fuses with the sacrotuberous ligament (2). Anteriorly, the tendinous arc, a curvilinear condensation of pelvic fascia arising from the obturator internus muscle, runs between the ischial spines and the lower portion of the pubic symphysis. This crucial structure provides a musculofascial origin for the majority of the anterior pelvic diaphragm, allowing its attachment to the bony pelvis. The arcus tendinous flanks the urethra and bladder neck anteriorly and rectum posteriorly, providing lateral attachment of the pelvic diaphragm and its ligaments (1).

The perineal body is a tendinous structure located in the midline of the perineum between the anus and the vaginal introitus, which provides a central point of fixation for the transverse perineal musculature (3). This anchoring site provides a second level of pelvic support to the posterior vaginal wall and rectum, incorporating the levator ani and transverse perineal musculature as well as the external anal sphincter.

C. Musculature

The striated musculature comprising the pelvic floor acts as a supporting structure for the visceral contents of the abdominopelvic cavity as well as a dynamic organ involved in maintenance of urinary and fecal continence. The pelvic diaphragm is composed of the levator ani and coccygeus muscles. The levator ani muscle group and its fascia provide the most critical support for the pelvic viscera, acting as the true muscular pelvic floor. The levator ani group is composed of the pubococcygeus, ischiococcygeus, and iliococcygeus, named according to their origin from the pelvic sidewall (4). This broad sheet of muscular tissue extends from the undersurface of the pubic symphysis to the pelvic surface of the ischial spines, taking origin from the tendinous arc laterally. The anterior muscle group, primarily made up of pubococcygeus (puborectalis) with its overlying endopelvic fascia, directly attaches to the bladder, urethra, vagina, uterus, and rectum, actively contributing to visceral control (Fig. 1). This important muscular support mechanism is crucial during times of suddenly increased intra-abdominal pressure (1).

The posterior muscle group consists of the posterior portion of the levator ani and the coccygeus muscle. Their points of origin include the more posterior portions of the tendinous arc and the ischial spines. The two sides fuse in the midline posterior to the rectum and attach to the coccyx. This plate of horizontal musculature spans from the rectal hiatus to the coccyx and allows maintenance of the normal vaginal and uterine axis. The upper vagina and uterine cervix lie on this horizontal plane created by the levator plate. This posterior muscle group is active at rest and contracts further during rectus abdominis contraction, maintaining proper vaginal axis (1).

Midline apertures in the levator ani group, collectively referred to as the levator hiatus, allow passage of the urethra, vagina, and rectum. Adjacent fascial attachments provide support to these pelvic viscera as they exit the pelvis, fashioning a "hammock" of horizontal support (5). The bladder, proximal vagina, and rectum rest on the levator floor and become coapted against it during periods of increased intra-abdominal pressure. Resting tone of the levator muscle, as well as reflex and voluntary contraction, acts to pull the vagina and rectum forward, thereby preventing incontinence of both urine and stool. These active mechanisms of pelvic floor support maintain both urinary and fecal continence.

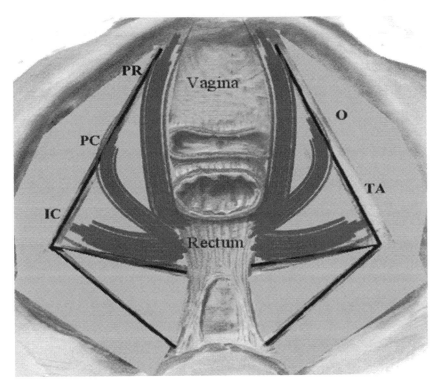

Figure 1   Schematic diagram of the striated musculature of the pelvic floor. PR, puborectalis; PC, pubococcygeus; IC, iliococcygeus; O, obturator muscle; TA, tendinous arc of the obturator muscle.

III. ANTERIOR VAGINAL SUPPORT

The fascia overlying the pelvic floor musculature plays a critical role in pelvic support. The abdominal portion of the fascia is referred to as *endopelvic fascia* and represents a continuation of the abdominal transversalis fascia (1). The levator ani muscle is covered superiorly and inferiorly by a fascial layer (Fig. 2). The two fascial layers split at the levator hiatus to cover the pelvic organs that traverse it. The superior or intra-abdominal segment (endopelvic fascia) and the inferior or vaginal side of the levator fascia together constitute the pubocervical fascia in the classical anatomic descriptions. This levator fascia is divided into discrete areas of specialization, depending on the associated organ it supports. The specialization of levator fascia around the urethra, the pubourethral ligament, represents a fusion of the periurethral fascia and endopelvic fascia attaching to the tendinous arc. The levator fascia associated with the bladder, the vesicopelvic ligament or fascia, represents the fusion of perivesical and endopelvic fascia attached to the tendinous arc. Such condensations of the endopelvic fascia create "ligamentous" structures that support the pelvic viscera, such as the pubourethral ligaments, urethropelvic ligaments, pubocervical fascia, and cardinal and uterosacral ligaments (Fig. 3). These represent discrete supportive structures that are part of a continuum of connective tissue surrounding the pelvic organs and serve as important surgical and physiologic landmarks. An understanding of their individual contribution to pelvic visceral support is essential in reconstructive surgery. Therefore, these four fascial structures will be discussed in detail as a basis for understanding the pathophysiology of pelvic organ prolapse.

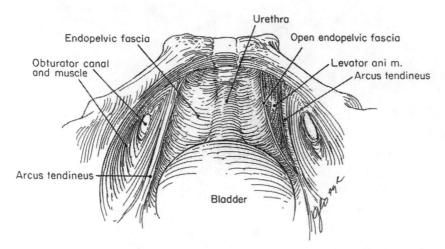

Figure 2 Schematic diagram of the pelvic floor, specifically the levator ani musculature and its fascial condensations. The endopelvic fascia represents the abdominal side of the levator fascia. The arcus tendineus represents the insertion of the levator muscle into the obturator muscle of the lateral pelvic side wall.

A.   Pubourethral Ligaments

The pubourethral ligaments are a condensation of levator fascia connecting the inner surface of the inferior pubis to the midportion of the urethra. They provide support and stability to the urethra and its associated anterior vaginal wall. These ligaments divide the urethra into proximal and distal halves; the proximal or intra-abdominal portion is responsible for passive or involuntary continence. The striated external urethral sphincter is located just distal to the pubourethral ligaments so that the midurethra becomes primarily responsible for active or

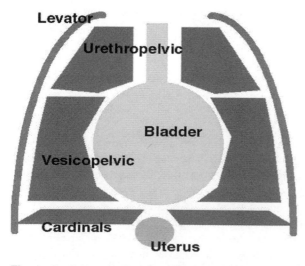

Figure 3 Schematic diagram of the levator muscle fascia viewed from the vaginal side, with specifically named condensations which form supportive ligamentous structures for the urethra, bladder, and uterus.

voluntary continence. The distal one-third of urethra is simply a conduit and does not significantly change continence when damaged or resected. Weakening or detachment of the pubourethral ligament causes separation of the urethra from the inferior ramus of the pubic symphysis. This pathologic process has an unclear role in continence.

B. Urethropelvic Ligaments

The urethropelvic ligaments are composed of a two-layer condensation of levator fascia, which provides the most important anatomic support of the bladder neck and proximal urethra to the lateral pelvic wall (Fig. 4). The first layer is known as the periurethral fascia (vaginal side) and is located immediately beneath the vaginal epithelium, apparent as a glistening white layer surrounding the urethra. The second layer of the urethropelvic ligament consists of the levator fascia covering the abdominal side of the urethra (endopelvic fascia), which fuses with the periurethral fascia. The two layers attach as a unit to the tendinous arc of the obturator fascia along the pelvic sidewall (Fig. 5). These lateral fusions of the levator and periurethral fascia provide important, elastic musculofascial support to the bladder outlet, thereby maintaining passive continence in women. Voluntary or reflex contractions of the levator or obturator musculature increase the tensile forces across these ligaments, increasing outlet resistance and continence. Thus, these ligamentous structures are critically important in the surgical correction of stress incontinence.

C. Pubocervical Fascia (Vesicopelvic Ligament)

The pubocervical fascia is a continuous sheet of connective tissue support from pubic symphysis to cervix, including the periurethral, perivesical, and endopelvic fascia, which fuse to support the bladder to the lateral pelvic wall (Fig. 6). It is formed by the fusion of fascia from the bladder wall and anterior vaginal wall in the region of the bladder base. It is continuous distally with the periurethral fascia and proximally with the uterine cervix and cardinal ligament complex. This fascial condensation, sometimes referred to as the vesicopelvic ligament, fuses laterally with the

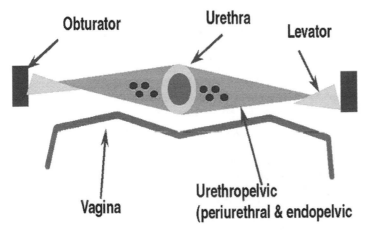

Figure 4 Schematic diagram demonstrating the urethropelvic ligaments, a two-layer condensation of levator fascia which envelops the urethra and surrounding neurovascular structures and attaches to the lateral side wall.

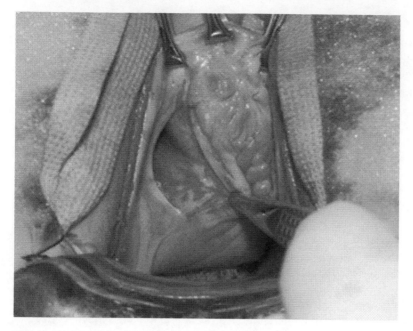

Figure 5 Intraoperative photograph of the urethropelvic ligament, as it attaches laterally to the tendinous arc.

endopelvic fascia, attaching to the pelvic sidewall at the tendinous arc and supporting the bladder base and anterior vaginal wall (Fig. 7). Attenuation of this lateral bladder support results in a lateral cystocele defect (paravaginal).

IV. UTERINE AND VAGINAL VAULT SUPPORT

The cardinal ligaments are thick, triangular condensations of pelvic fascia that originate from the region of the greater sciatic foramen. They insert into the lateral aspects of a fascial ring encircling the uterine cervix and isthmus as well as the adjacent vaginal wall, providing important uterine and apical vaginal support. In addition, the cardinal ligaments are an important mechanism of support for the bladder base and can be seen extending to the perivesical fascia. It is often difficult to differentiate the two structures surgically, and sharp dissection is required. These ligaments contain numerous blood vessels branching from the hypogastrics that supply the uterus and upper vagina (1). The cardinal ligaments fuse posteriorly with the uterosacral ligaments (sacrouterine), which stabilize the uterus, cervix, and upper vagina posteriorly toward the sacrum. They originate from the second, third, and fourth sacral vertebrae and insert into the posterolateral aspect of the pericervical fascia and lateral vaginal fornices (6). The fascial unit comprising cardinal ligaments, uterosacral ligaments, and pubocervical fascia spreads out posterolaterally on each side of the vaginal apex, uterus, and cervix to the pelvis (7).

The broad ligaments provide additional uterine support and are located more superiorly, covered by anterior and posterior sheets of peritoneum. They attach the lateral walls of the uterine body to the pelvic sidewall and contain the Fallopian tubes, round and ovarian ligaments, and uterine and ovarian vessels.

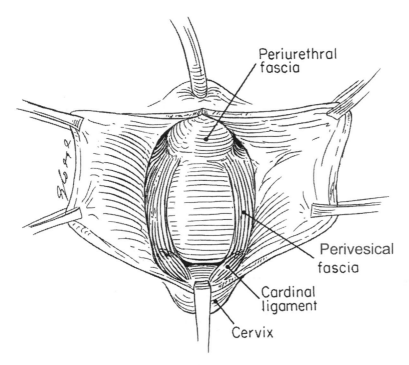

Figure 6   Schematic diagram of the vaginal fascial condensations from the pubic symphysis to the cervix, including the periurethral fascia, perivesical fascia, and cardinal ligaments. This continuous sheet of fascial support is also known as the pubocervical fascia.

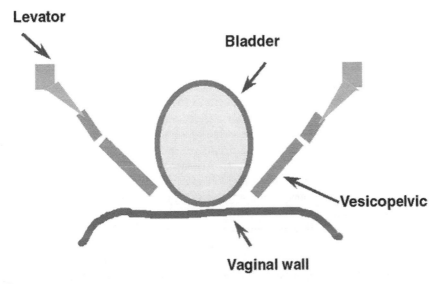

Figure 7   Schematic diagram of the vesicopelvic ligament, the fascial condensation providing lateral support to the bladder base and anterior vaginal wall.

V. POSTERIOR VAGINAL AND PERINEAL SUPPORT

A. Rectovaginal Septum

The rectovaginal septum represents a fascial extension of the peritoneal cul-de-sac between the vaginal apex and the anterior rectal wall. This septum comprises two distinct layers, the posterior vaginal fascia and the prerectal fascia, which fuse distally at their insertion into the perineal body. More proximally, these fascial layers fuse with the cardinal-uterosacral complex to provide support for the posterior vaginal apex. The proximal posterior vagina and intrapelvic rectum are supported by the pubococcygeus portion of the levator ani group, which inserts into the midline raphe between the vagina and rectum.

B. Perineum

The perineal body, a tendinous structure located between the anus and vagina in the midline, provides a central point of musculofascial insertion. This acts as an additional level of pelvic support, which is elastic in nature, thereby allowing significant distortion and recoil during childbirth and intercourse (1). Two paired superficial transverse perineal muscles run on each side of the perineal body to the ischial tuberosities laterally, with a similar deeper pair of transverse perineal muscles found more superiorly. Voluntary contraction of these transverse perineal muscles causes lateral vaginal compression as well as stability of the perineum during acute increases in intra-abdominal pressure.

The perineum can be conceptually divided into anterior and posterior triangular compartments by drawing a line between the two ischial tuberosities. The anterior urogenital triangle in the female contains the clitoris, urethra, and vaginal vestibule in the midline. The ischiocavernosus muscles cover the clitoral crura at their attachments to the pubis. The bulbo-cavernosus muscles run on each side of the vaginal vestibule beneath the labia between the clitoris and the perineal body. The anal canal is found in the center of the posterior anal triangle. The external anal sphincter is composed of two layers of fibers, the deeper layer completely encircling the anal canal and fusing with the pubococcygeus-puborectal muscles superiorly.

VI. PATHOPHYSIOLOGY OF PELVIC FLOOR DYSFUNCTION

Disruption of the normal supporting structures of the pelvis can occur secondary to numerous processes. Congenital defects are rare and will usually present in early childhood. Iatrogenic or traumatic injury as well as heavy physical labor may cause various degrees of pelvic floor relaxation. Furthermore, nulliparous women may experience pelvic floor dysfunction related to postmenopausal tissue atrophy (8). Neuromuscular damage of the pelvic floor can be caused by chronic constipation with straining, childbirth, and pelvic organ prolapse. Such denervation injury leads to levator ani and coccygeal muscular atrophy and dysfunction, contributing to pelvic floor relaxation and urinary and fecal incontinence (9).

Deficiency of pelvic support is most commonly related to childbirth or hysterectomy. Aging is associated with both loss of tissue elasticity and neuronal mass, additional factors contributing to loss of pelvic support. Genitourinary and bowel manifestations of pelvic floor relaxation do not routinely occur immediately following childbirth, but often present soon after menopause, when the hormonal milieu changes. This adds further evidence to the importance of dynamic changes in pelvic musculature and connective tissue following hormonal alterations, which contribute to loss of pelvic support. The initial symptom associated with pelvic floor dysfunction in women is usually stress urinary incontinence. However, bowel, urinary, and sexual functions are all significantly affected by loss of pelvic support. Bladder outlet resistance is compromised, allowing intravesical pressures to exceed those of the urethra and bladder neck and leading to urinary incontinence. Thus, the mechanisms of maintaining bladder outlet resistance in women are an important and integral component of pelvic floor dysfunction.

A. Mechanisms of Urethral Continence in Women

Bladder outlet resistance in women is attained by several factors working together to provide continence at rest and during stress maneuvers. Urethral anatomy, including functional length and elastic closure, is an important determinant of continence. In addition, activity of the muscular pelvic floor with its associated connective-tissue elements helps to maintain outlet resistance during times of increased intra-abdominal pressure. The anatomic position of the urethra is another factor contributing to continence. Each of these entities will be discussed separately in order to provide a basis for understanding the pathophysiology of pelvic floor relaxation.

B. Urethral Length

The distance between internal meatus and external urethral meatus in a female determines anatomic length. Congenital anomalies and traumatic injuries may result in significant urethral loss with subsequent incontinence. Functional urethral length is determined by urethral pressure profilometry where the total urethral length is assessed by urethral pressure exceeding bladder pressures (10). The clinical utility of urethral length has not been consistently proven. Funneling of the bladder neck and proximal urethra during straining cystography is seen in up to 50% of continent women (11). Furthermore, surgical incision of the bladder neck and Y-V plasty do not cause incontinence in women with otherwise normal outlets. In addition, resection of the distal one-third of the urethra does not produce incontinence. However, despite these observations, a critical length of healthy urethra is necessary to provide the coaptation for passive continence and continence during increases in abdominal pressure. Bladder neck suspensions may restore functional urethral length, thereby improving continence.

C. Urethral Closure

The urethra is made up of three functional anatomic components that result in an elastic, dynamic conduit with mucosal coaptation. The urethral mucosa is a transitional epithelium with numerous infoldings that allow distensibility and closure with excellent coaptation. Beneath the mucosa is a spongy tissue made up of vascular networks analogous to the corpus spongiosum in the male. Surrounding the spongy tissue is a thin musculofascial envelope, the periurethral fascia, which appears as a glistening white membrane. These three components create a coaptive seal.

Urethral closure is also affected by surrounding connective tissue structures. The puborethral ligaments provide stability to the midurethra, especially during increases in intra-abdominal pressure. In addition, the tensile forces of the urethropelvic ligaments along with the adjacent levator musculature facilitate compression of the proximal and midurethra. Finally, the striated musculature of the midurethral complex adds resting tone to the urethra, further effecting closure. Surrounding the sphincteric unit is skeletal musculature that provides an important additional mechanism for urethral closure. The striated musculature provides resting urethral tone as well as an involuntary reflex contraction in response to stress that increases coaptation. Furthermore, voluntary contraction also helps to prevent loss of urine by improving urethral closure. These mechanisms increase urethral resistance, as measured by leak point pressures, but may not directly affect urethral pressures.

D. Pelvic Floor Activity During Increased Intra-Abdominal Pressure

Female continence is maintained during increases in intra-abdominal pressure by several distinct mechanisms. Abdominal pressure is passively transmitted to the proximal urethra followed by an active contraction of the striated external sphincter musculature (12). Furthermore, the suburethral supportive layer, made up of periurethral fascia, anterior vaginal wall, and levator ani muscles, provides a firm backboard against which the urethra is compressed rapidly during increases in intra-abdominal pressure (13). Both the levator musculature and the urogenital diaphragm undergo reflex contraction, resulting in increased midurethral pressure. Furthermore, voluntary contraction of the levator and obturator muscles increases tension on the urethropelvic ligaments. These factors act in concert to promote urethral continence during changes in position and abdominal pressure.

E. Anatomic Position

Both the bladder neck and the urethra are normally maintained in a high retropubic position relative to the more dependent bladder base, creating a valvular effect. The bladder neck and urethra are supported by a musculofascial layer that suspends these structures from the pubic bone and pelvic sidewalls, thereby preventing their descent during increases in intra-abdominal pressures (14). A limited degree of bladder base rotation against a well-supported urethra occurs with increased abdominal pressures, further creating a valvular effect between these two structures (5). Furthermore, direct transmission of intra-abdominal forces to a well-supported proximal urethra increases its resistance and promotes coaptation (15).

This complex set of compensatory mechanisms in a normal healthy woman allows maintenance of sufficient outlet resistance to promote continence, especially during episodes of abdominal stress such as coughing, sneezing, walking, and straining. Any process that results in deterioration of these mechanisms can result in incontinence. Urethral function can be compromised by atrophy of its spongy tissue secondary to menopausal hormonal deficiency, altered neuromuscular function, or intrinsic damage from surgery, radiation, or trauma. In addition, a weakening of the levator musculature impairs the compensatory increases in midurethral pressures during stress. Although these physiologic changes can adversely impact on continence, the most common etiology of impaired outlet resistance in women is the loss of anatomic support of the bladder neck and urethra. Relaxation of the pelvic floor as well as weakening of the urethropelvic ligaments and midurethral complex produces significant posterior and downward rotation of the urethra and bladder neck (Fig. 8).

This anatomic repositioning of the urethra and bladder neck to a more dependent pelvic position eliminates the valvular effect. Sudden increases in intra-abdominal forces facilitate funneling and opening of a poorly supported bladder outlet. The extra-abdominal location of the poorly supported proximal urethra and the loss of the backboard of strong normal support of the urethropelvic ligaments do not allow effective transmission of abdominal forces. Although such anatomic changes can lead to incontinence, urethral hypermobility does not always correlate with incontinence. Many asymptomatic women with urethral hypermobility on physical examination do not report urinary incontinence. Thus, the anatomic position of the urethra alone does not correlate with the degree of incontinence. A component of intrinsic sphincter deficiency must be present along with these anatomic changes to create incontinence.

The factors responsible for pelvic floor relaxation rarely affect isolated anatomic areas. Thus, stress urinary incontinence resulting from urethral and bladder neck hypermobility is often accompanied by associated defects of pelvic support. The identification of these concomitant defects is crucial to planning effective therapy, with restoration of pelvic support, anatomic vaginal axis, and outlet resistance. Defects in pelvic support can be organized

URETHRAL PROLAPSE

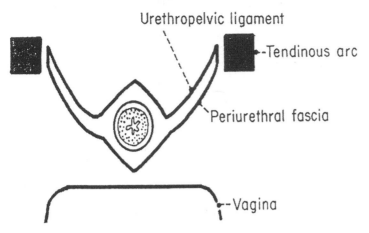

Urethropelvic ligament

-Tendinous arc

Periurethral fascia

--Vagina

Figure 8 Schematic diagram demonstrating weakness of the urethropelvic ligament, allowing posterior and downward rotation of the urethra.

according to their effects on various pelvic organs and structures, in order to allow a more systematic approach to treatment planning (5). The vaginal compartment contains a confluence of urinary, genital, and bowel organs. The goal of pelvic reconstructive surgery is to restore both anatomy and function. However, the restoration of anatomy does not always correlate with restoration of function.

VII. ANTERIOR VAGINAL WALL PROLAPSE

A. Bladder Neck and Urethra

Bladder neck hypermobility associated with stress incontinence most commonly results from attenuation of the urethropelvic ligaments or their attachment to the pelvic sidewall at the level of the tendinous arch of the obturator fascia. Furthermore, intrinsic sphincter deficiency (ISD) in addition to hypermobility gives way to incontinence. Normally, loss of anatomic position can be compensated for by the balance of forces that maintain continence: urethral length, urethral closure, and changes in urethral function that take place during episodes of stress (the valvular effect, increased urethral resistance secondary to levator contraction, and the transmission of intra-abdominal forces). Failure of these compensatory mechanisms will lead to stress incontinence.

Recently, more attention has been given to midurethral function as an etiologic factor in the development of stress incontinence. Normally, the bladder neck acts as the primary mechanism of continence. However, with intrinsic sphincter deficiency, the midurethral complex becomes the main compensatory mechanism maintaining continence. Much of our current armamentarium for curing stress incontinence is aimed at improving mid to distal urethral function and competence (i.e., transvaginal tape or sling). Although it is unclear how such methods correct incontinence in this segment of the urethra, we do know that anatomy and hypermobility have not necessarily been corrected.

In patients with stress incontinence and urethral hypermobility, there is rotational descent of the bladder neck and urethra under the pubic symphysis. The bladder neck funnels with Valsalva maneuvers, facilitating the loss of urine. However, the degree of rotational descent does not correlate with the degree of incontinence. The urethra rotates beyond the pubourethral ligament, often with separation of the midurethral complex from the inferior pubic ramus. The significance of this anatomic finding is unclear, but it is thought to play a role in midurethral function. Videourodynamic evaluation confirms separation of the midportion of the urethra from its normal attachment to the underside of the symphysis pubis as well as bladder neck and urethral hypermobility in women with stress incontinence and loss of pelvic support. Based on these findings we have altered our surgical approach in treating stress incontinence, by focusing on the midurethral complex during attempts at restoring support.

Although restoration of both anatomic position and underlying support are critical in the treatment of stress incontinence, it is important to recognize that the majority of women with bladder neck hypermobility do not experience significant incontinence. Intrinsic urethral function contributes significantly to continence and may be the determining factor in compensating for loss of bladder neck and urethral support. Therefore, women with stress incontinence and bladder outlet hypermobility must have some component of intrinsic urethral dysfunction. Anatomic support alone is not sufficient to achieve continence if urethral resistance remains inadequate.

B.   Intrinsic Urethral Dysfunction

The plasticity of the highly efficient mucosal seal mechanism found in the urethra allows perfect continence. Infolding and deformity of the inner mucosal layer create a seal mechanism and provide a leak-proof mechanism. Minimal extraurethral forces are necessary for continence if this inner layer is intact. The intrinsic urethral tissues are affected by trophic hormonal influences. Thus, the lack of estrogen following menopause may lead to thinning and flattening of the urethral epithelium as well as atrophy of the spongy vascular tissue, which is replaced by fibrous tissue. Additional factors, which may impair the ability of the urethra to achieve or maintain a perfect seal, include numerous surgical procedures, pelvic trauma, radiation therapy, and neurogenic disease.

Incontinence related to the bladder outlet was previously categorized into anatomic incontinence, due to inadequate support of the bladder neck and urethra, and intrinsic sphincter dysfunction, due to inadequacy of urethral resistance. However, this differentiation is no longer important because we now recognize that every woman with stress incontinence has a component of ISD. Thus, surgical therapy is aimed not only at correcting the anatomical defect but also at restoring coaptation and urethral closure (16). With compromise of intrinsic urethral function, stress incontinence may result despite adequate pelvic support. Thus, simple suspension of the bladder neck or urethra will be insufficient in restoring continence, and treatment must be aimed at restoring urethral coaptation and compression as well as anatomic support. Such treatments include sling procedures, injection of urethral bulking agents, or implantation of artificial sphincter devices.

C.   Cystocele

Loss of bladder neck and urethral support represents only one component of anterior vaginal wall prolapse. A significant number of women with stress incontinence will also have a cystocele, which may require surgical correction as well. A cystocele is defined as descent of the bladder base below the inferior ramus of the symphysis pubis, either at rest or with straining (17). Several systems of classification are in use that grade cystoceles based on degree of descent. We utilize a system of cystocele grading that includes four degrees of anterior vaginal wall prolapse. Grades I and II cystourethroceles are described as a mild to moderate degree of anterior vaginal wall hypermobility during straining, usually <2 cm. As a solitary entity, these are usually asymptomatic unless associated with significant bladder neck and urethral hypermobility, leading to stress incontinence. A grade III cystourethrocele is described as descent of the bladder base and anterior vaginal wall to the introitus during straining, while a grade IV cystourethrocele is descent of the bladder base and anterior vaginal wall beyond the introitus at rest. These higher degrees of cystocele are more frequently symptomatic, with complaints of dyspareunia, a sensation of a painful or painless vaginal bulge, recurrent urinary tract infections, nonspecific back pain, renal failure, and difficulty walking. Importantly, retention of urine may occur secondary to kinking at the level of the bladder neck, especially if the urethra has been fixed by previous surgery (17). Many patients will describe the need to manually reduce the cystocele in order to facilitate voiding. Silent hydroureteronephrosis can develop as a result of ureteral obstruction, often confounded by a patient's delay in seeking treatment.

Anterior vaginal wall support defects are further categorized by location of the primary anatomic defect. Weakness or disruption of the lateral attachments of the vesicopelvic or cardinal ligaments to the pelvic sidewall, at the level of the tendinous arch of the obturator, causes lateral cystocele defects. These lateral defects account for 70–80% of all anterior vaginal wall prolapse (17). Central cystocele defects result from attenuation of the vesicopelvic fascia in the midline, allowing herniation of the bladder base into the vagina (5) (Fig. 9). Isolated central cystoceles account for 5–15% of all cystocele defects (17). Commonly, the two support defects occur in conjunction and are often found in women with high-grade prolapse, such as grade IV cystoceles (Fig. 10). Both the lateral and the central defects must be corrected at the time of surgical repair in order to restore anatomic position and prevent progression or recurrence of the cystocele defect.

The anterior vaginal wall is supported in a rectangular configuration by the cardinal-sacrouterine ligament complex combined with the periurethral fascia and vesicopelvic ligaments. The superior aspect of the rectangle is the periurethral fascia, the lateral walls are the vesicopelvic ligaments, and the inferior aspect (base) is made up of the cardinal ligaments. The fibers of the pubocervical fascia fuse bilaterally with the anterior aspect of the cardinal

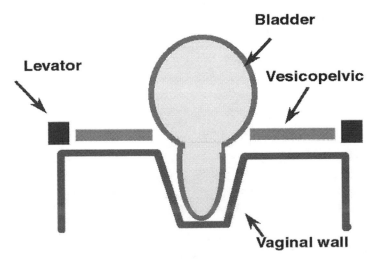

Figure 9   Schematic diagram of a central defect cystocele, resulting from attenuation of the vesicopelvic fascia in the midline.

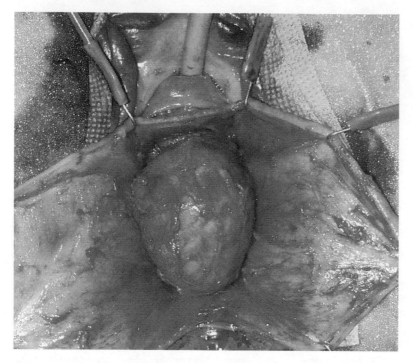

Figure 10   Intraoperative photograph of high-grade cystocele following dissection of the perivesical fascia from the overlying vaginal wall.

ligaments. Thus, in women with good uterine support as a result of strong cardinal ligaments, the base of this rectangle will be short and centrally located. On the other hand, in cases of uterine prolapse or significant laxity of the cardinal-sacrouterine ligament complex following hysterectomy, there will be elongation and separation of the rectangular base and widening of the levator hiatus. These defects in support allow formation of a central cystocele defect (5). Thus, the first maneuver during surgical correction of a cystocele involves reapproximation of the cardinal and uterosacral ligaments to the midline, essentially narrowing the base of the rectangle to prevent further cystocele progression.

VIII.   VAGINAL VAULT PROLAPSE

A.   Uterus and Vaginal Vault

The most critical supporting structures of the uterus and vaginal vault are the sacrouterine and cardinal ligament complex. Relaxation of these structures results not only in anterior vaginal wall prolapse, but also in vault and uterine prolapse as well as enterocele formation. Uterine prolapse is described as uterine descent at rest or with straining and is further classified in a manner similar to cystocele grading, as previously described. Grade I uterine prolapse is described as minimal mobility, grade II as uterine descent to the level of the midvagina with straining, grade III as descent to the vaginal introitus with straining, and grade IV, or procidentia, as prolapse through the introitus. Grades I and II uterine prolapse are often asymptomatic, but when symptomatic present with back pain aggravated by standing. More severe grades of uterine prolapse are associated with a vaginal mass, pelvic pain, dyspareunia, urinary retention, and incontinence (17).

Initially, weakness of the sacrouterine ligaments allows anterior movement of the cervix, compromising the position of the uterus over the horizontal levator plate. The uterine axis gradually changes, leading to retroversion with the corpus falling backward. Abdominal pressures are transmitted to the anterior surface of the uterus, causing progression of uterine prolapse (17). Following hysterectomy, deficient sacrouterine and cardinal ligamentous support may result in prolapse of the vaginal dome and cuff. Uterine prolapse rarely occurs as an isolated defect of pelvic support and is treated either by uterine suspension procedures or by hysterectomy, with treatment of the accompanying defects in pelvic support. Vault prolapse or eversion requires fixation of the apex to the sacrum, sacrospinous ligament or ileococcygeus muscle, often in conjunction with repair of anterior and posterior vaginal wall defects (18).

B. Enterocele

An enterocele is defined as a herniation of peritoneum and its contents at the level of the vaginal apex. Enteroceles occur in the upper, posterior portion of the vagina in association with the cul-de-sac of Douglas. Most enteroceles are acquired following hysterectomy, caused by separation of the cardinal-sacrouterine complex and described as a "pulsion" defect at the vaginal dome (19). Enteroceles are classically divided into four types: *Congenital enteroceles* result from failure of fusion of the layers of peritoneum at the level of the rectovaginal septum and are not associated with cystocele or rectocele. *Traction enteroceles* occur when prolapse of the vaginal vault or uterus pulls the peritoneum in a caudal direction. *Pulsion enteroceles* form as a result of chronic pressure exerted on the vaginal vault. This force creates a hernia sac and pushes the vaginal vault caudally, causing a sliding herniation of the vault and anterior vaginal wall along the surface of the rectum. Pulsion enteroceles are very rarely associated with uterine prolapse. *Iatrogenic enteroceles* form following a surgically induced change in the vaginal axis, where the cul-de-sac of Douglas is left unprotected. Classically, this type of enterocele is seen after colposuspension, with an incidence of 26.7% following Burch colposuspension (17).

Furthermore, enteroceles can be classified based on associated anatomic findings at the time of examination, in order to guide the course of treatment. *Simple enteroceles* exist without concomitant vault prolapse, and the vaginal cuff is well supported. In addition, no cystocele or rectocele is present. *Complex enteroceles* are associated with vault or uterine prolapse, with poor support of the vaginal cuff. Prolapse may include the anterior vaginal wall (cystocele) or the posterior vaginal wall (rectocele) (17). In patients with complex enteroceles there are two discrete defects: separation of the prerectal from the perivesical fascia, and descent of the vault due to weakness of the sacrouterine and cardinal ligaments. Both of these defects must be addressed during vault prolapse repair.

In general, enteroceles are minimally symptomatic until descent reaches the level of the hymen. The patient may complain of a sensation of fullness in the perineal area or sensation of a vaginal bulge. Dyspareunia, vaginal discomfort, and low back pain accentuated in the upright position are also common. In rare instances, complications of bowel obstruction may be seen. Concomitant cystocele and/or rectocele may produce bowel and bladder symptoms (17). Diagnosis of an enterocele is made by physical examination, often with observation of a vaginal mass bulging through the introitus. Bimanual rectovaginal examination during straining may reveal an impulse of the peritoneal sac against the examining fingertip. Furthermore, thickness of the proximal rectovaginal septum may be appreciated. Radiographic imaging can be utilized to confirm the suspected diagnosis of an enterocele. Plain film radiography may reveal bowel gas within a prolapsing mass below the pubic symphysis. A voiding cystourethrogram during straining will exclude the bladder as the source of a mass (17). Magnetic resonance imaging of the pelvis during both a relaxed and straining state can elucidate the presence of an enterocele. Fat, small intestine, fluid, and bowel gas can be identified within a protruding vaginal mass well below the pubococcygeal line (20). Enterocele repair commonly involves repair of concomitant pelvic prolapse defects as well as resuspension of the vaginal vault.

IX. POSTERIOR VAGINAL WALL PROLAPSE AND PERINEUM

Two distinct levels of musculofascial support, the pelvic floor (the pubococcygeal portion of the levator ani musculature) and the perineum, make up the posterior vaginal wall in addition to the prerectal and pararectal fasciae. The perineum is made up of the bulbocavernosus muscle, the superficial and deep transverse perineal muscles, the external anal sphincter, and the central tendon of the perineum (21,22) (Fig. 11). In the normal upright female, the proximal two-thirds of the vagina is 110° from the horizontal plane compared with the distal one-third. The transition from proximal to distal vagina occurs at the point where the vagina crosses the pelvic floor, influenced by the degree of support of the levator musculature and urogenital diaphragm. Thus, the proximal half of the vagina is oriented horizontally, lying over the levator plate (Fig. 12). Levator contraction pulls the vagina forward and increases the angulation between proximal and distal posterior vagina. Changes in intra-abdominal pressure tend to further close and support the posterior vaginal wall, thereby preventing prolapse. When the posterior vaginal wall axis is altered, i.e., following bladder neck suspension, intra-abdominal

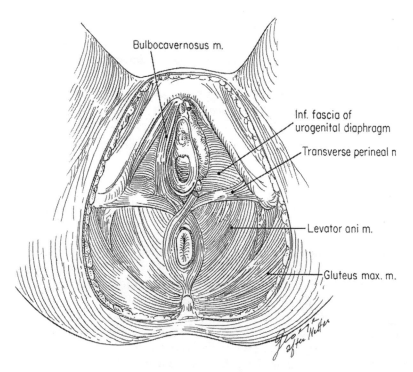

Figure 11   Schematic diagram of perineal musculature, providing support to posterior vaginal wall and rectum.

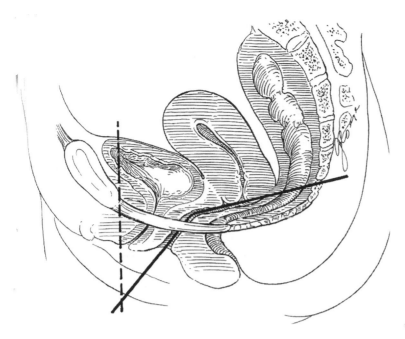

Figure 12 Schematic diagram representing a sagittal view of the pelvis with a normal vaginal axis. The proximal portion of the vagina lies horizontally, resting on the levator plate, providing support for the uterus, rectum, and bladder base.

forces tend to push the posterior vaginal wall forward, increasing the tendency for rectocele formation. The levator musculature and the perineal body support the distal aspect of the vagina (17).

Damage to or relaxation of the levator musculature results in widening and elongation of the levator hiatus and disappearance of the normal proximal vaginal axis. The posterior vaginal wall becomes flattened, and intra-abdominal forces will tend to make the posterior vaginal wall prolapse forward (17). There are several components of posterior vaginal wall support to take into consideration: the presence of a rectocele; separation of the levator hiatus; relaxation and widening of the introitus; and relaxation and herniation of the perineum. In addition, damage to the perineal support mechanisms results in further widening of the vaginal introitus, with an increase in the distance between the urethra and the posterior fourchette. Perineal tears may also be present in varying degrees, the most severe form being direct continuity between the posterior vaginal wall and underlying rectum. The result of these anatomic changes is the development of a rectocele, possibly a posterior and high enterocele and perineal laxity.

The importance of the rectovaginal septum as a supporting structure for the rectum has been emphasized by Richardson (23). Milley and Nichols described this layer of fascia after performing both surgical and cadaveric dissections. This fascial layer envelops the posterior vaginal wall, merging into the uterosacral ligaments and adhering to the cul-de-sac peritoneum. Distally, it merges into the perineal body fusing with the fibers of the deep transverse perineal muscle. Laterally, this fascial layer fuses with the iliococcygeus and pubococcygeus muscles just below the arcus tendineus (23). The rectovaginal septum acts to separate the rectal compartment from the urogenital compartment.

A. Rectocele

A rectocele is described as intravaginal herniation of the rectum through an attenuated rectovaginal septum. In addition, defects in the prerectal and pararectal fasciae are also associated with rectocele formation. Isolated breaks in the rectovaginal septum facilitate rectocele formation. Generally, there are several areas along the rectovaginal septum where breaks are commonly found. The most common site is a transverse separation immediately above the attachment of this septum to the perineal body, resulting in a low rectocele (seen just inside the introitus). A midline vertical defect is equally common and most likely represents a poorly repaired or poorly healed episiotomy. Rarely, one can see lateral separation on one side (23).

Symptoms of rectocele are often related to bowel function and sexual intercourse; they include a sensation of fullness in the vagina, a mass bulging through the introitus, difficulty with rectal evacuation, constipation, the need for manual reduction to improve bowel emptying, and interference with intercourse (17).

The diagnosis of a posterior vaginal wall support defect is made by physical examination. A rectocele manifests as a bulge extending from the posterior vaginal wall, which can be better identified by placing a half-speculum anteriorly to support the anterior vaginal wall and bladder during straining maneuvers. Bimanual rectovaginal examination reveals significant attenuation of the rectovaginal septum. In addition, loss of the normal right-angle configuration between the proximal and distal vaginal segments is exhibited. Similar to enteroceles, rectoceles can be diagnosed radiographically by the presence of bowel gas below the inferior pubic ramus on plain radiography or by magnetic resonance imaging of the pelvis during relaxed and straining conditions (Fig. 13).

It is rare to find an isolated posterior wall defect, or rectocele. One must identify associated defects in pelvic floor support prior to planning surgical correction. Perineal tears are commonly seen in conjunction with severe rectoceles in multiparous women. Type I defects have an intact, but thin, perineum with a defect in the anterior muscle fibers of the external anal sphincter, the puborectalis muscle and perirectal fascia, and the transverse perineal muscles. Type II defects result in total loss of the perineal body secondary to obstetric trauma. Type III defects present with a rectovaginal fistula in the lower rectovaginal wall following a history of obstetric trauma. In type IV defects, a fistula is present in the bottom third of the vaginal wall with an intact perineum. This usually results from a partially healed fourth-degree laceration during delivery. These defects in the perineum, with resultant widening of the levator hiatus, may lead to progressive loss of control of both gas and feces (24). Further discussion of external anal sphincter defects as well as perineal herniation is found in subsequent sections.

B. Perineal Laxity

Perineal herniation or laxity results most commonly from obstetric trauma, with attenuation of the central tendon of the perineum. The discrete anatomic defect results in an increase in the distance from the posterior fourchette to the anus as well as an outward convexity of the perineum during straining. In addition, perineal laxity contributes further to widening of the vaginal introitus. This defect in perineal support can be seen either with or without a concomitant rectocele. Symptoms or signs specifically associated with perineal body defects can include incontinence of stool, incontinence of flatus, or severe constipation requiring perineal pressure to facilitate defecation. In general, this is a relatively rare condition and is often associated with a severe degree of posterior vaginal wall prolapse.

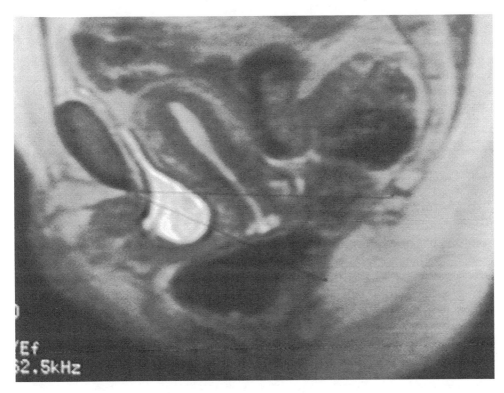

Figure 13 Magnetic resonance imaging of the pelvis in a sagittal plane during straining. A large, dark structure is seen below the both the pubococcygeal line and puborectalis muscular sling, representing a high-grade rectocele.

C. Anal Sphincter

Damage to the external anal sphincter can also result from obstetric trauma, such as grade IV perineal tear involving the rectum and/or anus or injury to the central tendon of the perineum as previously mentioned. Furthermore, anal sphincter laxity or defects can be a result of neurologic injury. This defect will lead to fecal incontinence, incontinence of flatus, poor sphincter tone on physical examination, and a palpable anatomic defect in the external anal sphincter. This defect is often present when signs of perineal laxity are found in addition to high-grade pelvic prolapse. Reconstruction of the anal sphincter involves transperineal plication of the levator ani musculature and the external anal sphincter as well as reapproximation of the transverse perineal musculature to the external anal sphincter.

X. CONCLUSIONS

A complete and thorough understanding of pelvic floor anatomy provides a basis for the goals of vaginal and pelvic reconstructive surgery. First, identification of all pelvic floor pathology and organ prolapse is necessary to plan a definitive therapeutic approach to reconstruction. Diagnostic imaging of pelvic prolapse is a useful adjunct to physical examination, specifically haste sequence magnetic resonance imaging during relaxed and strained states. Concurrent pelvic organ pathology, including ovarian and uterine abnormalities as well as hydronephrosis, can be identified and subsequently addressed at the time of surgical intervention. Repair of all elements of pelvic floor prolapse must be achieved with special emphasis given to restoration of vaginal axis. The normal posterior curvature of the proximal vagina must be restored to allow intra-abdominal forces to cause vaginal coaptation and prevent subsequent or recurrent organ prolapse. This goal of reconstructive surgery cannot be overemphasized.

REFERENCES

1. Klutke CG, Siegel CL. Functional female pelvic anatomy. Urol Clin North Am 1995; 22:487–498.
2. De Lancey JO. Surgical anatomy of the female pelvis. In: Rock JA, Thompson JD, eds. Te Linde's Operative Gynecology. Philadelphia: Lippincott-Raven, 1997:63–93.
3. Tanagho EA. Anatomy of the lower urinary tract. In: Walsh PC, Retik AB, Stamey TA, Vaughan ED, eds. Campbell's Urology. Philadelphia: W.B. Saunders, 1992:40–69.
4. Redman JF. Surgical anatomy of the female genitourinary system. In: Buchsbaum HJ, Schmidt JD, eds. Gynecologic and Obstetric Urology. Philadelphia: W.B. Saunders, 1993:25–60.
5. Raz S, Little NA, Juma S. Female urology. In: Walsh PC, Retik AB, Stamey TA, Vaughan ED, eds. Campbell's Urology. Philadelphia: W.B. Saunders, 1992:2782–2829.
6. De Lancey JOL, Richardson AC. Anatomy of genital support. In: Hurt WG, ed. Urogynecologic Surgery. Gaithersburg, IL; Rockville, MD: Aspen Publishers, 1992:19–33.
7. Baden WF, Walker T. The anatomy of uterovaginal support. In: Baden WF, Walker T, eds. Vaginal Defects. Philadelphia: Lippincott, 1992:25–50.
8. Stanton SL. Vaginal prolapse. In: Raz S, ed. Female Urology. Philadelphia: W.B. Saunders, 1983:229–240.
9. Strohbehn K. Normal pelvic floor anatomy. Obstet Gyn Clin North Am 1998; 25:683–705.
10. Bruskewitz R. Urethral pressure profile in female lower urinary tract dysfunction. In: Raz S, ed. Female Urology. Philadelphia: W.B. Saunders, 1983:112–122.
11. Versi E, Cardozo LD, Studd JWW, Brincat M, O'Dowd TM, Cooper DJ. Internal urinary sphincter in maintenance of female continence. B M J 1986; 292:166–167.
12. Steers WD. Physiology and pharmacology of the bladder and urethra. In: Walsh PC, Retik AB, Vaughan ED, Wein AJ, eds. Campbell's Urology. Philadelphia: W.B. Saunders, 1998:870–915.
13. Wein AJ. Pathophysiology and categorization of voiding dysfunction. In: Walsh PC, Retik AB, Vaughan ED, Wein AJ, eds. Campbell's Urology. Philadelphia: W.B. Saunders, 1998:917–926.
14. Blaivas JG, Romanzi LJ, Heritz DM. Urinary incontinence: pathophysiology, evaluation, treatment overview, and nonsurgical management. In: Walsh PC, Retik AB, Vaughan ED, Wein AJ, eds. Campbell's Urology. Philadelphia: W.B. Saunders, 1998:1007–1043.
15. Enhorning G. Simultaneous recording of intravesical and intraurethral pressure. Acta Chir Scand 1961; 276:3.
16. Raz S, Siegel AL, Short JL, Snyder JA. Vaginal wall sling. J Urol 1989; 141:43–46.
17. Raz S, Stothers L, Chopra A. Vaginal reconstructive surgery for incontinence and prolapse. In: Walsh PC, Retik AB, Vaughan ED, Wein AJ, eds. Campbell's Urology. Philadelphia: W.B. Saunders, 1998:1059–1094.
18. Raz S. The anatomy of pelvic support and stress incontinence. In: Raz S, ed. Atlas of Transvaginal Surgery. Philadelphia: W.B. Saunders, 1992:1–22.
19. Zacharin RF. Pulsion enterocele: review of the functional anatomy of the pelvic floor. Obstet Gynecol 1980; 55:135–140.
20. Rodriguez LV, Raz S. Diagnostic imaging of pelvic floor dysfunction. Curr Opin Urol 2001; 11:423–428.

21. Huisman AB. Aspects of the anatomy of the female urethra with special relation to urinary continence. Contrib Gynecol Obstet 1983; 10:1–31.
22. Joseph J. Female genital structure and function. The bones, joints, and ligaments of the female pelvis. In: Phillip E, Barnes J, Newton M, eds. Scientific Foundations of Obstetrics and Gynecology. Chicago: Year Book, 1986:86–94.
23. Richardson AC. The rectovaginal septum revisited: its relationship to rectocele and its importance in rectocele repair. Clin Obstet Gynecol 1993; 36:976–983.
24. Wiskind AK, Thompson JD. Fecal incontinence and rectovaginal fistulas. In: Rock JA, Thompson JD, eds. Te Linde's Operative Gynecology. Philadelphia: Lippincott-Raven, 1997:1207–1236.

2
Neurophysiology of Micturition

Gamal M. Ghoniem
Cleveland Clinic Florida and the Cleveland
Clinic Foundation Health Sciences Center of OSU, Weston, Florida, U.S.A.

John C. Hairston
University of Texas Medical School at Houston, Houston, Texas, U.S.A.

I. INTRODUCTION

The lower urinary tract has two essential functions: the low-pressure storage of urine in a continent reservoir, and the timely expulsion of stored urine in a coordinated, efficient, and complete fashion. These two mutually exclusive functions are ultimately determined by the activity of the smooth and striated musculature of the bladder, urethra, and external urethral sphincter under the control of various neural circuits in the brain and spinal cord. Although a result of complex interplay between both the central and peripheral nervous systems, these functions are also influenced by several anatomic factors such as integrity of the pelvic floor support and dynamic relationship of the bladder and its outlet to various points in the bony pelvis and adjacent organs during voiding. In addition, as our understanding of lower urinary tract neurophysiology grows, so grows the list of neurotransmitters and receptors identified as having a role in voiding function and dysfunction. Voiding dysfunction can occur as a result of neurologic disease or injury, disturbance of anatomical relationships within the pelvis and urinary organs, or as an unwanted, often unrecognized pharmacologic effect of medical therapy for other diseases. Voiding dysfunction also occurs as a result of normal aging and is affected by changes in the viscoelastic properties of the bladder wall. As with other neurologic systems, innervation of the lower urinary tract is not static; it changes in response to disease and aging. This phenomenon is known as neural plasticity. More often than not, the etiology of voiding dysfunction is multifactorial, so a fundamental understanding of the neuroanatomy and neurophysiologic mechanisms of the lower urinary tract is essential.

II. PROPERTIES OF DETRUSOR MUSCLE AND BLADDER WALL

A. Excitation-Contraction Coupling

The process of force generation of muscle in response to ligand binding has been termed excitation-contraction coupling. It is a very complex process that results from molecular changes induced by a neurotransmitter crossing the postsynaptic cleft. The details of these intricate events are beyond the scope of this chapter and best left to a major physiology text, but the central concepts can be summarized as follows.

Smooth muscle cell morphology differs from that of striated muscle in that the major contractile protein in smooth muscle is actin, whereas myosin predominates in striated muscle. Nevertheless, force is ultimately generated by interaction of these two myofilaments. Cardiac muscle and striated muscle have been studied to a much larger extent than smooth muscle, but much of what we know about smooth-muscle physiology comes from the fields of gastroenterology and obstetrics. The molecular events leading to smooth-muscle contraction are shown in Figure 1. The first step in this process is smooth-muscle cell excitation by either ligand binding (neurotransmitter with its associated receptor) or membrane depolarization. This leads to an increase in free cytosolic calcium. Free cytosolic calcium ion levels are usually <0.1 μM. Total intracellular calcium concentrations are much higher, indicating a considerable pool of stored calcium. The increase in cytosolic calcium may come from influx across the cell membrane of extracellular calcium through specific voltage-sensitive channels or via release of intracellular stores. The release of intracellular stores can be triggered by second messengers such as inositol trisphosphate (IP3), cyclic AMP, or guanosine triphosphate (GTP). The excess of free cytosolic calcium binds with calmodulin, altering this molecule and allowing it to bind to the enzyme myosin light-chain kinase. Myosin light-chain kinase causes phosphorylation of the myosin light chain, which then interacts with actin, causing a conformational change of these proteins and allowing them to slide over each other, thus shortening the muscle. Adenosine triphosphate (ATP) is a necessary cofactor for this step. This process can be repeated over and over as long as there is a stimulus for contraction.

The process of muscle relaxation also depends highly on ATP. A significant amount of energy is expended by certain ATP-dependent pumps (ATPases) as they act to pump calcium (often against tremendous gradients) out of the cell or into storage sites thus allowing calcium homeostasis and cell repolarization.

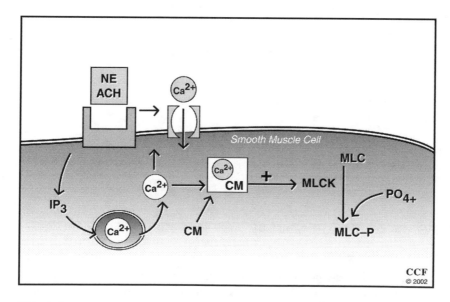

Figure 1

B. Compliance

The ability of the bladder to accommodate increasing volumes of urine at low pressures is termed bladder compliance. In mathematical terms, it is measured as a change in unit volume per change in pressure ($C = \Delta V / \Delta P$). A bladder that can hold large volumes of urine at low pressures is "highly" compliant. At physiologic rates of filling (< 10 mL/min), bladder pressure rarely rises above 10 cm H_2O up to a capacity of 400–500 cc. This phenomenon is unique to the bladder as an organ if one considers that bladder smooth muscle must undergo a 100–200% displacement in slack length to create this kind of compliance. The vena cava, in contrast, need only undergo 25–50% displacement to produce significant changes in vessel diameter (1). Compliance is a product of both the neuromechanical and viscoelastic properties of the bladder wall. The fact that even acutely denervated bladders maintain adequate compliance underscores the importance of the passive viscoelastic properties in maintaining adequate bladder compliance. The human bladder wall is composed of detrusor smooth muscle interspersed with islands of connective tissue or extracellular matrix (ECM). The ECM is composed of proteins such as collagen, proteoglycans, elastin, and many other molecules that are now being identified. Because bladder muscle does not have a "skeleton" on which to exert force, these ECM proteins are extremely important with regard to energy transmission. They are also crucial to compliance, and any alteration in the composition of the ECM can result in decreased compliance. Such alterations can occur with chronic inflammation, injury, obstruction, or chronic denervation and typically result in increased collagen content and fibrosis. There is no agreement yet on the definition of abnormal compliance values. Ghoniem suggested that a value of < 10 mL/cm H_2O is severely impaired compliance and dangerous to the upper urinary tracts, 10–20 mL/cm H_2O is moderately impaired and > 20 mL/cm H_2O is normal.

III. LOWER URINARY TRACT INNERVATION

The pelvic and hypogastric nerves supply the bladder and urethra with efferent parasympathetic and sympathetic neurons, and both convey afferent (sensory) neurons from these organs to the spinal cord. The storage phase of micturition is controlled primarily by sympathetic, and voiding phase by parasympathetic, vesicourethral innervation. The somatic innervation is important mainly in regard to the musculature of the pelvic floor and the external or striated urethral sphincter (EUS), and is supplied via efferents in the pudendal nerve (2–4).

A. Parasympathetic Supply

The parasympathetic efferent supply is classically described as originating in the intermediolateral region of the gray matter of the spinal cord segments S 2–4 and emerges as preganglionic fibers in the ventral roots and exits as the pelvic nerve. This nerve courses deep in the pelvis on each side of the rectum as three or four trunks in human. Bilaterally, at a variable distance from the bladder and urethra, the pelvic and hypogastric nerves meet and branch to form the pelvic plexus, sometimes known as the inferior hypogastric plexus, or plexus of Frankenhauser. This is a plexus of freely interconnected nerves in the pelvic fascia that is lateral to the rectum, internal genitalia, and lower urinary organs. Divergent branches of this plexus innervate these pelvic organs. The hypogastric and pelvic nerves also carry afferent autonomic nerve impulses to synapses in the dorsal column of the lumbosacral spinal cord (2,3).

B. Sympathetic Supply

The sympathetic innervation to the lower urinary tract originates in the intermediolateral nuclei of the thoracolumbar spinal cord in segments from T11 through L2 or L3. They traverse the lumbar sympathetic ganglion and join the presacral nerve (superior hypogastric plexus). The hypogastric plexus lies anterolateral to the great vessels at the level of third lumbar to first sacral vertebrae and gives rise to the left and right hypogastric nerves which are really elongated nerve plexuses. These nerve plexuses join the pelvic nerves to form the plexuses of Frankenhauser, from which they spread out to innervate the pelvic organs (5).

As demonstrated by Gilepsie, two nerve bundles extended from the inferior hypogastric plexus (plexus of Frankenhauser), each accompanied by artery derived from the vaginal artery (6). The first bundle (vesicoureteric plexus) parallels the inferior border of the ureter until it reaches the cardinal ligament, from where, some fibers supply the dorsum of the bladder, while the remaining nerve fibers continue to parallel the ureter to pierce the bladder at the level of the interureteric ridge of the trigone. The destruction of this plexus (vesicoureteric plexus) was found effective in the treatment of women with hypersensitive bladder disorders. The second nerve bundle passes downward to the junction of the urethra with the anterior wall of the vagina. However, more anatomical dissections are needed for this area.

Classically, the autonomic nervous system has been regarded as a two-neuron system composed of two neuron models; preganglionic and postganglionic neurons. Elbadawi has nicely reviewed the anatomic aspects of the contemporary modifications of classical autonomic nervous system (7–11). He stated that the muscular innervation of the lower urinary tract is derived exclusively from postganglionic neurons of what is called the urogenital short neuron system. Although paraganglia and preganglia exist, actual innervation predominantly emanates from peripheral ganglia that are at a short distance from, adjacent to, or within the organs they innervate, thus the name short. The ganglia are composed of three cell types: cholinergic principal neurons, adrenergic principal neurons, and small intensely fluorescent (SIF) cells. The SIF cells are thought to play an important role in modulation of interganglionic vasomotor function and ganglionic transmission. In addition, there are complex intraganglionic networks of cholinergic and adrenergic fibers. Thus, there is a wide variety of modulating synaptic relays. In addition, postganglionic neurons do not necessarily terminate in the peripheral end organ, but many actually terminate within the ganglia of some systems. Increasing scientific work is revealing that the neural control of the lower urinary tract is more complex than had previously been thought.

C. Somatic Supply

The somatic supply arises from motorneurons in the anterior horn of S2, S3, and S4, clustered in an area known as Onuf's nucleus. There are contradictory views of the neural supply of the striated sphincter. The EUS is composed of an extramural and intramural component that differ physiologically and will be discussed later. However, most authors agree that the striated sphincter, including both components, is innervated only through motor end plates, implying purely somatic innervation, through there may be differences in opinions regarding the actual nerve trunks carrying these fibers (4,12). In a recent neuroanatomical study, Hollabaugh et al. described an intrapelvic branch of the pudendal nerve that joins the pelvic nerve branch at the level of the proximal urethral sphincter (13). The morphologic evidence of autonomic innervation of the striated sphincter has not been definitively demonstrated in other species or in human. However, Elbadawi and Atta (11) reported that there is evidence for triple innervation (somatic plus cholinergic and adrenergic autonomic) of the intramural striated sphincter of the male cat. This finding is supported by electrophysiologic studies (14). These conclusions are applicable only to the intramural portion of the striated sphincter, and other authors' conclusions regarding the intramural component may have been erroneously drawn from specimens from the adjacent extramural component.

IV. NEUROTRANSMISSION AND RECEPTORS

A. General

In both the parasympathetic and sympathetic systems, the preganglionic neurotransmitter is acetylcholine, which affects nicotinic cholinergic receptors. The primary postganglionic parasympathetic neurotransmitter is also acetylcholine, which affects muscarinic cholinergic receptors, while the postganglionic sympathetic neurotransmitter is a catecholamine, norepinephrine, which affects the adrenergic receptors. Newer scientific data are supporting the existence of many other neurotransmitters and receptors responsible for lower urinary tract function. These include ATP, nitric oxide (NO), dopamine, serotonin, glutamine, gamma amino butyric acid (GABA), various neuropeptides, and prostanoids. Representative parasympathetic and sympathetic nerve terminals are depicted in Figures 2 and 3.

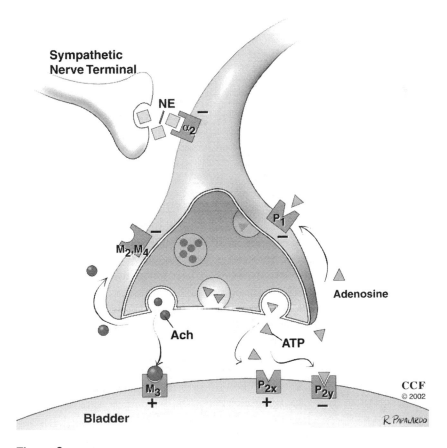

Figure 2

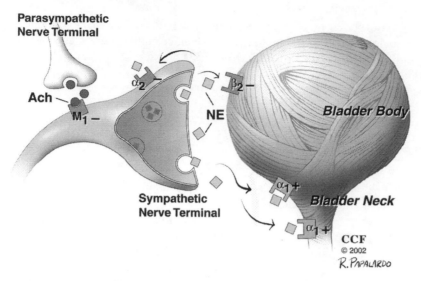

Figure 3

B. Cholinergic Mechanisms

The voiding phase of the micturition cycle is primarily controlled by the parasympathetic nervous system. Stimulation of the pelvic nerves produces a strong, sustained bladder contraction that leads to bladder emptying. Cholinergic receptors are ubiquitous throughout the bladder body but scarce at the region of the bladder neck and the ventral part of the urethra. They are absent in an area called the superficial trigonal muscle. The human bladder has two muscarinic cholinergic receptor subtypes, M2 and M3. M2 receptors predominate immuno-histochemically (~80% overall), but functional studies show that bladder contractions are mediated primarily by M3 receptors through hydrolysis of phosphoinositol and the resultant release of intracellular calcium (15,16). M1, M2, and M4 receptors are also present prejunctionally on nerve terminals in the bladder and are thought to play a modulating role through amplification (M1) and inhibition (M2 and M4) of acetylcholine release (17,18). Drugs with anticholinergic properties such as propantheline, dicyclomine, imipramine, and oxybutynin have been used for many years to suppress overactive detrusor contractions. The usefulness of these medicines, however, has been somewhat limited owing to their lack of specificity with regard to mucscarinic receptors. Muscarinic receptors are also present extensively in salivary glands, bowel, and the accommodation apparatus of the eye, with M3 receptors predominating in the salivary glands. As a result, the use of standard antimuscarinic drugs often leads to intolerable side effects such as dry mouth, constipation and visual disturbances.

Newer, more selective muscarinic antagonists are being developed. Tolterodine, a competitive antagonist that binds all receptor subtypes, was shown in clinical studies to be equal in efficacy to oxybutynin in reducing micturition frequency and urge incontinence episodes while having a lower incidence of dry mouth (19). The apparent bladder selectivity of these newer agents may be due to several factors. The action of these drugs on prejunctional muscarinic receptors may play a larger role than initially thought. In addition, heterogeneity of the M3 receptor population has been postulated. In fact, radioligand-binding studies showed tolterodine and oxybutynin to have similar affinities for M3 receptors in the bladder, but oxybutynin had an eightfold higher affinity for parotid gland M3 receptors. These types of sensitivity differences have also been detected with other M3-selective antagonists, darifenacin and zamifenacin (15,20).

Botulinum toxin, now commonly used for treatment of skeletal muscle spasticity, inhibits acetylcholine release from cholinergic nerve terminals. It has been used successfully in the treatment of detrusor-sphincter dyssynergia in spinal cord-injured men by injecting it into the external sphincter to lower outlet resistance (21). It is also showing promise as a treatment for bladder hyperreflexia and possibly overactive bladder. Injection of the toxin into detrusor muscle has been effective in suppressing contractions in these patient populations, and further studies are eagerly awaited (22).

Bethanechol chloride, a cholinergic agonist, has been used rather commonly to enhance voiding, and this seems theoretically sound. Although cholinergic agonists may raise baseline bladder pressure, the use of such agents does not appear to be clinically useful in promoting bladder emptying (23–25). There are several reasons for this. Cholinergic agonists appear to cause a reflex sympathetic urethral constriction, prohibiting coordinated voiding (26). Furthermore, cholinergic activation leads to a feedback mechanism via the aforementioned prejunctional M2 and M4 receptors, inhibiting further acetylcholine release. Finally, bethanechol is poorly absorbed from the gastrointestinal tract, necessitating subcutaneous administration or prohibitively high oral doses to achieve pharmacologic effect.

C. Adrenergic Mechanisms

The adrenergic receptors (α and β) have different distributions in the lower urinary tract. The α receptors are distributed mainly in the urethra and bladder neck. They are further subclassified into $\alpha1$ (postsynaptic) and $\alpha2$ (presynaptic) receptors. Stimulation of $\alpha1$ receptors regulates vasoconstriction and smooth muscle contraction, whereas stimulation of $\alpha2$ receptors inhibits the release of norepinephrine from nerve terminals through a negative feedback mechanism. Several subtypes of the $\alpha1$ receptor have been identified. Studies have shown that $\alpha1$ receptors in the urethras of humans are of the $\alpha1a$ subtype (27,28). In addition, radioligand binding has suggested the majority of α receptors in female animals are $\alpha2$, whereas $\alpha1$ receptors predominate in the male (29).

Phentolamine and phenoxybenzamine are both nonspecific α-adrenergic antagonists and are not routinely used in the treatment of voiding disorders. Prazosin, doxazosin, and terazosin are relatively selective antagonists of $\alpha1$ receptor sites and are commonly used in the treatment of outlet obstruction in males secondary to benign prostatic hyperplasia because of their relaxing effect on prostatic smooth muscle. The use of these agents is somewhat limited by cardiovascular side effects owing to the presence of $\alpha1$ receptors throughout the vascular tree. Tamsulosin, an $\alpha1a$-selective antagonist, targets urethral smooth muscle with a decreased incidence of cardiovascular side effects such as postural hypotension. Although sometimes used to treat female bladder outlet obstruction, the efficacy of these drugs in this capacity has not been definitively established, chiefly owing to a lack of standardized criteria to define this entity in women. Any lack of efficacy may also be explained by the deficiency of $\alpha1$ receptors in the female urethra. α-Stimulating drugs such as phenylpropranolamine and ephedrine will increase the tone of urethra and bladder neck by stimulating smooth muscle contraction at these sites. In fact, over-the-counter cold medications and decongestants are a common cause of urinary retention in elderly males. It is also for this reason that these drugs have been used in the pharmacologic treatment of stress incontinence in women (30).

There have been conflicting animal studies regarding the role of α receptors in the spinal cord, with data to support both inhibitory and facilitative influences. Some studies have indicated an excitatory role for $\alpha1$ receptors at both the end-organ level and in the spinal cord. These effects include the release of NO, the enhancement of acetylcholine release (α1a), and direct excitatory effects on bladder smooth muscle (α1b/α1d) (31,32). This last postjunctional excitatory effect is hardly present in younger animals but becomes prominent in older animals, supporting the concept of neural plasticity and change of adrenergic receptor expression over time. In addition, the intrathecal administration of doxazosin (α1 antagonist) has been shown to suppress bladder hyperactivity and decrease the amplitude of bladder contractions in rats (33). This effect was more pronounced in the setting of chronic bladder outlet obstruction, again suggesting the plastic nature of neural control of the diseased bladder. There is other evidence to support age-related changes in lower urinary tract adrenergic receptor expression, an intriguing concept that may hold promise for future research.

β-Adrenergic receptors in the urinary tract (β2) tend to cluster in the bladder body, as opposed to the bladder base and neck. They appear to modulate smooth-muscle relaxation; β stimulants, e.g., terbutaline, cause bladder relaxation and may contribute to urinary retention when given in high doses for premature labor. Unfortunately, β agonists do not appear to be clinically useful in treating detrusor instability (DI) (34).

The role of the sympathetic nervous system in the lower urinary tract is a matter of dispute. However, many authors advocate its major role in the lower urinary tract. The sympathetic nervous system acts primarily to facilitate the filling and/or storage phase of micturition and does so by three mechanisms: (a) increasing accommodation by stimulation of β-adrenergic receptors in the bladder body; (b) increasing outlet resistance by stimulation of the predominantly α-adrenergic receptors in the bladder base and proximal urethra and by causing an increase in activity of striated muscle of the pelvic floor ("guarding reflex"); and (c) inhibiting bladder contractility by means of a blocking effect on parasympathetic ganglionic transmission (35,36). Edvardsen postulated a spinal reflex in the cat—with afferents in the pelvic nerves and efferents in the hypogastric nerves—causing bladder relaxation during filling and therefore an increased volume threshold for micturition (37,38). Consistent with this hypothesis is the fact that in the cat β-adrenergic blockade or surgical sympathectomy has been reported to increase bladder activity, decrease bladder capacity, and produce a shift to the left of the accommodation limb of the cystometric curve (39,40).

D. Nonadrenergic, Noncholinergic Mechanisms

The fact that not all bladder contractile activity can be blocked by atropine even with massive doses (the phenomenon of atropine resistance) has led to the postulation of nonadrenergic, noncholinergic (NANC) neurotransmitter system, which is responsible for part of the neurotransmission in the bladder. Experimental studies on bladder muscles have shown that the bladder contraction is biphasic. Only the contraction of the second phase can be blocked by atropine; not the first phase. ATP and other substances are responsible for the contraction of the first phase (41,42). More recently, numerous substances have been shown to play a role in regulation of the lower urinary tract. These substances acting as neurotransmitters or neuromodulators, include an extensive list, e.g., opioids, vasoactive intestinal polypeptide (VIP), serotonin, dopamine, glutamic acid, GABA, ATP, and prostaglandins (F2, E, E2). Many of these substances exhibit both inhibitory and facilitative influence on the micturition cycle at the spinal cord level and higher. These developments have significant potential implications for the future development of drugs affecting nervous control mechanisms in the urinary tract and elsewhere (43,44). However, the role of NANC mechanisms in the contractile activation of the human bladder is still disputed. In normal human detrusor, atropine was found to cause >95% inhibition of electrically evoked contraction (45). In detrusor strips from patients with a diagnosis of unstable bladder or from patients with benign prostatic hyperplasia, atropine resistance was found in up to 65% (46). These apparently conflicting data may be explained by differences in the tissues investigated. Ghoniem found a significant atropine-resistant component to the electrically induced detrusor contraction of meningomyelocele patients undergoing augmentation cystoplasty, which was absent in normal bladders of patients undergoing ureteral reimplantation (47). Most probably, normal human detrusor muscle exhibits little atropine resistance while abnormal detrusor exhibits high atropine resistance, making study of NANC mechanisms more attractive in disease states. There is much research being done in this regard, and these studies are eagerly awaited.

E. Purinergic Mechanisms

Purinergic receptors are classified as P1 and P2 based on their affinity for either adenosine or ATP respectively. ATP-sensitive P2 receptors can be subclassified into P2X and P2Y receptor families based on whether the mechanism is ion channel gated (P2X) or G-protein coupled (P2Y). The P2X family can be further subclassified into seven subtypes ($P2X_1$, $P2X_2$, etc.). Levin suggested that purinergic stimulation initiates a bladder contraction (first phase) whereas cholinergic stimulation leads to sustained bladder emptying (48). Chancellor showed that ATP generated a more forceful smooth muscle contraction than a cholinergic agonist, a finding that was corroborated by Sneddon, who showed that purinergic mediated contraction is more forceful in neonates (49,50). Theobald demonstrated a greater rise in bladder pressure in cats treated with purinergic agonists versus cholinergic agonists (51). These findings have not been consistent, however, as others have shown decreased bladder emptying with purinergic agonists (52). Animal studies have implied the presence of multiple types of purinergic (P2X and P2Y) receptors in the bladder and that the response of detrusor muscle to purinergic stimulation is itself biphasic depending on the receptor stimulated (P2X, fast response; P2Y, slow, sustained response) (53). $P2X_1$ receptors have been shown to be dominant in rat detrusor and vascular smooth muscle (54). O'Reilly and coworkers studied P2X receptors and their role in idiopathic DI in human females. They found that $P2X_2$ receptors were increased and other P2X subtypes were decreased in women with idiopathic DI, again demonstrating the trend toward atropine resistance in abnormal bladders (55). These data hold promise as the search for novel approaches to the treatment of overactive bladder and other bladder disorders continues.

It is likely that purinergic mechanisms also play an excitatory role at higher sites, including parasympathetic ganglia and afferent nerve terminals in dorsal root ganglia. $P2X_3$ receptors have been identified in neurons in dorsal root ganglia in addition to subepithelial afferent nerves plexuses in the bladder and ureteral wall (54,56). Intravesical administration of ATP activates bladder afferent fibers and desensitization of these afferents with suramin, a purinergic antagonist, decreased reflex bladder activity (57,58). Afferent activity induced by bladder distention was reduced in $P2X_3$ knockout mice (53). These data argue that purinergic mechanisms play a sensory role in the lower urinary tract as well and could provide potential targets for therapy of disorders such as sensory urgency and interstitial cystitis.

F. Dopaminergic Mechanisms

Central dopaminergic pathways appear to exhibit both inhibitory and excitatory influences on micturition, based on the site and receptor type stimulated. D1 or D1-like receptors mediate inhibition whereas D2 or D2-like receptors mediate excitatory reflexes. Activation of D1 receptors in the substantia nigra causes suppression of reflex bladder activity in cats (59). Bladder hyperreflexia produced in monkeys through destruction of these pathways (inducing Parkinson-like motor symptoms) was also suppressed using a D1-like agonist in one study (60).

From a clinical standpoint, however, treatment in humans with standard anti-Parkinsonian medications does not appear to correlate well with improvement in bladder symptoms or urodynamic findings (61). These patients often require treatment with anticholinergics to control bladder hyperreflexia, underscoring the complex nature of voiding dysfunction.

The diversity of dopaminergic influence on micturition is demonstrated by the fact that stimulation of D2-like receptors in animals in both the pontine micturition center (PMC) and in the spinal cord can induce bladder hyperactivity (62,63). It is likely that central dopaminergic pathways play a significant role in micturition, but the translational value of current basic science knowledge to the clinical arena has yet to be realized.

G.   Serotonergic Mechanisms

It is possible that serotonin (5HT) has an impact on neural control of the lower urinary tract at both the central and peripheral levels, although the degree of this impact is still largely unknown. This uncertainty is a product of the multiple receptors that have been identified coupled with the lack of specific drugs with which to target them. There have been at least seven different 5HT receptors identified ($5HT_1$, $5HT_2$, etc.). Nonetheless, immunohistochemical studies have identified 5HT-containing neurons in the pelvic ganglia. Similarly, 5HT-containing neurons in the raphe nucleus of the caudal brainstem project to the dorsal horn in addition to the autonomic and sphincter motor nuclei in the lumbosacral cord. In cats, activation of these 5HT neurons in the cord inhibits reflex bladder activity and decreases firing of sacral efferents to the bladder (62,64). Administration of 5HT antagonists in animals blocks these effects and causes a decreased functional bladder capacity indicating that descending serotonergic pathways cause tonic inhibition of the afferent limb of the micturition reflex (65). Of interest is the possible role of serotonergic pathways in enuresis or overactive bladder. Tricyclic antidepressants are often used in the treatment of nocturnal enuresis. The efficacy of these agents may be explained by decreased 5HT reuptake, increasing levels available for suppression of reflex detrusor activity. Is has also been shown that the incidence of overactive bladder and urge incontinence is greater in individuals with depression, a condition associated with low levels of 5HT.

Peripherally, 5HT has been shown to induce bladder contractions as well as facilitate acetylcholine release from nerve terminals in the bladder via activation of prejunctional receptors (66,67). Anatomically, the sympathetic autonomic nuclei and sphincter motor nuclei receive serotonergic input, and there is evidence to show that sphincter reflexes are facilitated by activation of 5HT receptors as in the case of duloxetine, a combined 5HT and norepinephrine reuptake inhibitor (68,69).

H.   Glutaminergic Mechanisms

Glutamic acid or glutamate plays an important role as a facilatory transmitter in the central pathways controlling micturition. It is present in visceral afferents in the dorsal horn of the lumbosacral cord, spinal interneurons, and the descending pathway from the PMC to the sacral parasympathetic plexus (70,71). Glutamate appears to facilitate bladder function at all of these levels via either NMDA (N-methyl-D-aspartate) or AMPA (α-amino-3-hydroxy-5-methyl-4-isoxazoleproprionic acid) receptors. NDMA antagonists depress reflex bladder activity and sphincter electromyographic activity in anesthetized animals as well as animals with cord transection at the midthoracic level (72). This indicates that the spinal reflex pathways controlling micturition rely on glutaminergic transmitter mechanisms. Studies also indicate that differences in bladder and external sphincter sensitivity to glutaminergic suppression may be explained by differing receptor expression at each site. In situ hybridization studies have revealed high messenger RNA for AMPA receptor subunits GluR-A and GluR-B in sacral parasympathetic preganglionic neurons, but not NR2 NMDA receptor subunits. Conversely, high levels of messenger RNA for all four AMPA receptor subunits (GluR-A thru D) as well as the NR1 NMDA subunit are expressed in the motorneurons of the EUS (53).

I. GABA Inhibitory Mechanisms

GABA is a well-known inhibitory transmitter in the central nervous system. It appears to influence micturition at both spinal and supraspinal sites via both GABA-A and GABA-B receptors. In animal studies, injection of a GABA-A agonist into the PMC suppressed reflex bladder activity and intrathecal administration of either GABA-A or GABA-B antagonists increased bladder capacity and decreased voiding pressure (73).

V. SENSORY INNERVATION

Afferent nerve fibers have been demonstrated in the pelvic, pudendal, and hypogastric nerves (74). In the cat, the afferents subserving the sensation of distension (and active therefore in evoking micturition) are more prominent in muscularis propria layer and are distributed evenly to all regions of the bladder, but the afferents subserving the sensations of pain and conscious touch are more prominent in the submucosa in the regions of trigone and anterior bladder neck. Both pelvic and hypogastric afferent pathways carry nociceptive afferents, whereas afferent pathways from the striated sphincter and from the urethra transmit sensations of temperature, pain, wall distension (urethra), urine passage, and travel in the pudendal nerve (74).

Anatomical and electrophysiological studies have shown that sacral afferent fibers projecting from the bladder to the spinal cord are either myelinated (A-delta with fast conduction up to 30 m/sec) or unmyelinated (C-fibers with slow conduction 0.3 m/sec) (75,76). Figure 4 represents a schematic of sensory pathways. A large body of evidence suggests that substance P (SP) and other tachykinins are likely to be involved in afferent neurotransmission in the lower urinary tract via vanilloid receptor (VR1). Exposure of bladder mucosa to the neurotoxin capsaicin, the pungent ingredient in hot pepper, causes the release of SP and produces smooth muscle contraction that can be blocked by SP antagonists and the neurotoxin tetrodoxin. Systemic use of capsaicin produces either partial or complete denervation of capsaicin-sensitive afferents, depending on the dose, species, and the age of experimental animal (77). In rats, intravesical administration of capsaicin causes neuroanatomic or functional changes that prevent bladder afferents from transmitting nociceptive input (78). In humans, capsaicin-sensitive nerves have been postulated. A concentration-dependent reduction in first sensation and bladder capacity occurs following acute administration of intravesical capsaicin. It causes desensitization of C-fiber sensory afferents inducing reversible suppression of sensory neuron activity. These pharmacological data support the use of capsaicin or other neurotoxins to treat painful bladder disorders (79).

Resiniferatoxin (RTX), a substance isolated from the cactus plant *Euphorbia resinifera*, is 1000 times more potent than capsaicin. In contrast, however, RTX has weaker initial excitatory effects than capsaicin on bladder afferents thus eliciting less discomfort. This agent holds significant promise as an alternative to capsaicin in the treatment of both painful bladder disorders as well as detrusor hyperreflexia (80,81).

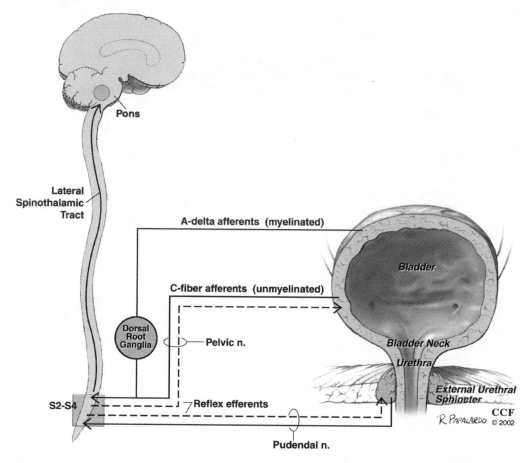

Figure 4

VI. PHYSIOLOGY OF THE EXTERNAL URETHRAL SPHINCTER (EUS)

There are two types of muscle fibers in the striated sphincter or EUS. The first one is the strongly reactive fast-twitch muscle fibers, and the second is the weekly reactive slow-twitch muscle fibers. Speed of contraction seems to correlate with histochemical reaction for ATP. Resistance to fatigue is directly related to the intensity of oxidative enzyme staining in the same fibers. Slow-twitch fibers are high in oxidative enzyme activity and relatively fatigue resistant. Fast-twitch fibers may be fatigable or relatively fatigue resistant (82).

The entire intramural (intrinsic) striated sphincter is composed of slow-twitch fibers, whereas the extramural (extrinsic) component consists of both slow-twitch and fast-twitch fibers. Telealogically, this would be convenient because the intramural striated component would then consist of specialized fibers functionally capable of maintaining tension over prolonged time periods without fatigue. The structure of the extramural component might be related to a role played by this muscle in activity supporting the pelvic viscera and that the slow-twitch fibers are responsible for (background activity) during electromyographic recording. The fast-twitch population of the extramural component is functionally associated with rapid, forceful muscle contraction. It is these fibers then that are recruited to increase the force and speed of contraction of the levator ani during those events that might otherwise cause stress incontinence by raising intra-abdominal pressure (83). However, Bazeed and colleagues, studying the dog, reported a different fiber distribution in the intramural component of the striated sphincter (84). They found that the slow-twitch fatigue resistant fibers are only 35%, fast-twitch fatigue-resistant 20%, and fast-twitch fatigable fibers 45% of the intramural striated sphincter. The fast-twitch fibers (fatigable) can convert to slow-twitch fibers by physiotherapy (e.g., electrical stimulation). This is also a theoretical advantage of pelvic floor exercises and behavioral modifications. Some authors explain the success of these therapies for the treatment of urinary incontinence on the basis of changes in the oxidative characteristics of striated muscle. However, other authors have shown that these types of therapies more successfully treat urge incontinence rather than stress incontinence, raising doubt as to the validity of alterations in muscle morphology (85).

VII. CENTRAL NERVOUS CONNECTIONS OF THE LOWER URINARY TRACT

It has yet to be resolved whether voiding is the result of a segmental reflex arc that is facilitated and inhibited by supraspinal neurologic pathways, or a long routed reflex that is integrated at higher nervous system levels (86,87). However, in the cat, it appears that the most fundamental micturition reflex is a spinal reflex occurring largely in the sacral micturition center (SMC) at S 2–4 (88). The spinal cord itself has complex patterns of facilitation and inhibition that take place among the ascending and descending pathways at the spinal cord level. Above the level of the cord, the PMC is located. It is the most important facilitative motor center for micturition, and it is believed that this center serves as the final common pathway for all bladder motor neurons. The region is known as Barrington's center and is present in the anterior pons. The cerebellum serves as a major center for coordinating pelvic floor relaxation and force of detrusor contraction. There are extensive cerebellar interconnections with the brainstem reflex centers (87,89).

Above this level, the basal ganglia exert inhibitory function on detrusor contractility. Consequently, detrusor hyperactivity is frequently seen in Parkinson's disease. The cerebral cortex, particularly the frontal lobes and genu of the corpus callosum, exerts primarily inhibitory influences on the micturition reflex. Thus, facilitative influences that release inhibition occur in the upper cortex and permit the anterior PMC to send efferent impulses through the spinal cord allowing a sacral micturition reflex to occur with resultant bladder emptying. Any lesion in these centers can produce a disturbance in bladder function characterized by a reflex coordinated contraction with complete emptying (87,89). A simplified overview of micturition reflexes is shown in Figures 5 and 6.

A. Bradley's Loop Concept

Bradley et al. described a concept of neurological control of the lower urinary tract in the cat (90). This concept described four loops and circuits that are interconnected by axons, and their integrated output contributes to the determination of the threshold of the detrusor reflex and coordinated synchronized opening of the urethra and relaxation of the urinary bladder. Most of the micturition reflex requires a balanced contribution by all four loops.

Loop I: Cerebral-Brainstem Circuit

This loop consists of pathways to and from the frontal lobes to the pontine mesencephalic reticular formation, with contribution from the thalamic nuclei in the basal ganglia and cerebellum. This loop coordinates volitional control of micturition. It matures during infancy, and may account for voluntary control over the micturition reflex in the childhood. This loop integrity can be demonstrated during cystometry by asking the patient to voluntarily suppress detrusor contraction. Interruption of this circuit severs the micturition reflex from volitional control, e.g., in brain tumor, trauma, cerebrovascular disease (91).

Loop II: The Brainstem Sacral Loop

This loop consists of pathways from the brainstem (pontine-mesencephalic reticular formation) to the sacral micturition area. Additionally, sensory afferents from the bladder musculature travel directly in the spinothalamic tract to the brainstem without synapsing in the sacral micturition area. These sensory afferent fibers are responsible for the normal sensation of desire to micturate. Loop II is responsible for the occurrence of a coordinated detrusor reflex of adequate duration to produce total evacuation of the intravesical content. Partial interruption of loop II, as in spinal cord injury, results in detrusor reflex of low threshold and the presence of postvoiding residual urine. While abrupt and complete interruption (in spinal shock) produce areflexia and urinary retention. With recovery, uninhibited detrusor reflex contractions appear in the cystogram (92,93).

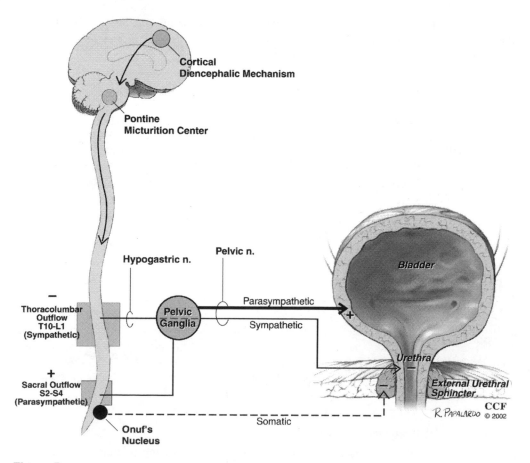

Figure 5

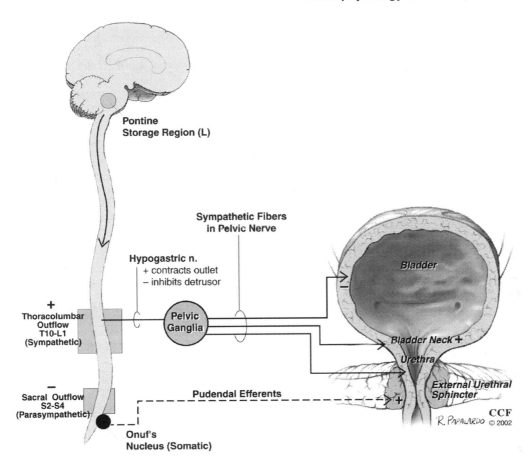

Figure 6

Loop III: Vesical-Sacral Sphincter Loop

This loop consists of the detrusor nuclei and pudendal nuclei in the gray matter of the sacral spinal cord with their neurons. Sensory afferents in the detrusor muscle travel the detrusor nucleus and influence the closely located pudendal motor nucleus. Pudendal motor neurons terminate in the striated muscular component of the urethral sphincter. Loop III provides the circuit for coordination of detrusor and urethral muscular activity during voiding. Dysfunction of this loop will be manifested in electromyographic recording as either detrusor sphincter dyssynergia or uninhibited sphincter relaxation (94).

Loop IV: Cerebral-Sacral Loop

This loop consists of two components: (a) supraspinal and (b) segmental innervation of the peripheral striated muscle. The supraspinal component consists of sensory pathways originating from muscle spindles and tendon organs in the pelvic floor musculature. These axons course through the posterior column and synapse in the thalamus, to reach the pudendal area of the sensorimotor cortex. From there, the motor fibers originate and travel to terminate by synapsing on motor neurons on the pudendal nucleus in the spinal cord. The segmental portion of the loop consists of sensory axons arising from the muscle spindles and tendon organs, which end by synapsing on pudendal motor neurons. The pudendal neurons give origin to efferent axons to innervate the pelvic floor musculature and to regulate the sensitivity of spindle stretch receptors. Electromyographic evidence of voluntary contraction of the external sphincter demonstrate an intact loop IV (90,95).

B.   Integral Theory of Voiding Reflexes

Mahoney et al. described another concept of micturition as a reflex event that occurs largely in the peripheral autonomic nervous system, permitted to do so by the central nervous system (96). They proposed 12 reflexes operating among bladder, urethra, brainstem micturition center, and spinal cord micturition center. These reflexes could be grouped into four groups according to their function.

1.   Storage-Favoring Reflexes (Four Reflexes)

a.   Sympathetic-Detrusor Inhibition Reflex (SDIR).   The afferent is the pelvic nerve; the efferent is the hypogastric nerve. This reflex is activated by bladder wall stretch during filling and its function is to inhibit detrusor contraction.

b.   Sympathetic Sphincter Constrictor Reflex (SSCR).   This reflex consists of the same stimulus and pathway as SDIR, but the target organ is the smooth muscle component of the urethral sphincter. It produces an increase in the tone of the sphincter during bladder filling. Together, these two reflexes comprise the "sympathetic stabilizing reflexes" favoring continence of urine (97).

c.   Perineodetrusor Inhibitory Reflex (PDIR).   Stimulation of the stretch receptors of the perineum and pelvic floor muscles produces impulses that travel through pudendal nerve afferents to the SMC. Efferent impulses travel via the pelvic nerve, and the function is inhibition of the detrusor contraction.

d.   Urethrosphincteric Guarding Reflex (USGR).   The stimulus is an increase in mural tension in the trigone and bladder neck during filling or escape of urine into proximal urethra. The afferent limb is via the pelvic nerve to the SMC, and the efferent is via the pudendal nerve to the striated component of the external urethral sphincter producing contraction.

2.   Initiation of Micturition Reflexes (Two Reflexes)

a.   Perineobulbar Detrusor Facilitative Reflex (PBDFR).   The stimulus is the voluntary contraction of the diaphragm and abdominal wall muscles with simultaneous relaxation of the pelvic floor muscles. The impulse travels through the pudendal nerve and other somatic nerves cranially to the brainstem and brain cortex, which in turn produce stimulation of the SMC.

b.   Detrusodetrusor Facilitative Reflex (DDFR).   An increase in detrusor mural tension produces an impulse that travels via the pelvic nerve to the PMC. The PMC sends facilitative impulses via the lateral reticulospinal tract to the SMC. From here, stimulatory impulses are sent to the detrusor muscle via pelvic nerve efferents producing a detrusor contraction.

3.   Intramicturition Reflexes (Five Reflexes)

These reflexes are concerned with maintaining a strong detrusor contraction with synchronous relaxation of the sphincter during the voiding phase to provide complete and efficient emptying of the bladder.

a.   Detrusourethal Inhibitory Reflex (DUIR).   The impulse from the detrusor stretch receptors travels via the pelvic nerve to the SMRC producing stimulation, then via the pelvic nerve again to the bladder neck and smooth muscle component of the external urethral sphincter producing relaxation.

  b. Detrusosphincteric Inhibitory Reflex (DSIR). An inhibitory impulse via the pelvic nerves to the "pudendal nucleus" producing relaxation of the striated component of the external urethral sphincter is generated in response to a stimulus from the stretch receptors in the detrusor muscle.

  c. Urethrodetrusor Facilitative Reflexes (UDFR). Both of these reflexes originate in the proximal urethra and produce detrusor contractions via efferents from the SMC. There are two reflex pathways proposed, one with a brainstem component and one without. Both may act to cause a detrusor contraction in response to the presence of urine in the proximal urethra.

  d. Urethrosphincteric Inhibitory Reflex (USIR). This reflex has both its afferent and efferent limbs in the pudendal nerves. It is responsible for the prompt synchronous relaxation of the external sphincter at the onset of micturition and is additive to the effect of the DSIR in this regard.

4. Micturition Cessation Reflex (One Reflex)

  a. Perineobulbar Detrusor Inhibitory Reflex (PBDIR). At the end of micturition, inhibitory impulses from the stretch receptors in the perineum and pelvic muscles travel to the brainstem. Efferent inhibitory impulses are then sent to the SMC, thus reestablishing the storage reflexes (Group I).

VIII. SUMMARY

Much controversy still abounds regarding the exact processes of the micturition cycle, but most experts would agree that it involves two relatively discrete phases: (a) bladder filling and storage, and (b) bladder emptying. From a clinical standpoint, most disorders of voiding can be categorized into a failure of either one of these discrete processes, although quite often there is a combination of the two. While some of the basic concepts of pathways and neural circuits have been around for decades, our understanding of the details of these pathways and circuits has grown tremendously in the past several years. With the advent of functional MRI and PET scanning, as well as the continued discovery of new neurotransmitters and receptors, this knowledge base will continue to develop allowing more effective diagnosis and treatment of voiding dysfunction well into the future.

REFERENCES

1. Zderic SA, Levin RM, Wein AJ. Voiding function and dysfunction. In: Gillenwater JY, Grayhack JT, Howards SS, Duckett JW, eds. Adult and Pediatric Urology. 4th ed. Baltimore: Lippincott Williams & Wilkins, 2002.
2. Keith LM. Anatomy of the pelvis and perineum. In: Clinically Oriented Anatomy. 2nd ed. Baltimore: Williams & Wilkins, 1985:359–403.
3. Clemente C, ed. Gray's Anatomy of the Human Body. 30th American ed. Philadelphia: Lea & Febiger, 1985.
4. Romanes GJ. Muscles and fascia. In: Cunningham's Textbook of Anatomy. Oxford: Oxford University Press, 1972:360–364.
5. Mitchell BS. Morphology and neurochemistry of the pelvic, and paracervical ganglia. Histol Histopathol 1993; 8(4):761–773.

6. Gilepsie L. Destruction of the vesicoureteric plexus for the treatment of hypersensitive bladder disorders. Br J Urol 1994; 74:40.
7. Elbadawi A. Neuromorphologic basis of vesicouretheral function. I. Histochemistry, ultastructure and function of intrinsic nerves of the bladder and urethra. Neurourol Urodyn 1982; 1:3.
8. Elbadawi A. Autonomic muscular innervation of the vesical outlet and its role in micturition. In: Hinman FJ, ed. Benign Prostatic Hypertrophy. Berlin: Springer-Verlag, 1983:330–348.
9. Elbadawi A. Ultrastructure of vesicourethral innervation. II. Postganglionic axoaxonal synapses in intrinsic innervation of the vesicourethral lissosphincter. A new structural and functional concept in micturition. J Urol 1984; 131:781.
10. Elbadawi A. Ultrastructure of vesicourethral innervation. III. Anoaxonal synapses between postganglionic cholinergic axons and probably SIF cell derived processes in the feline lissosphincter. J Urol 1985; 133:524.
11. Elbadawi A. Ultrastructure of vesicourethral innervation. IV. Evidence for somatomotor plus autonomic innervation of the male feline rhabdosphincter. Neurourol Urodyn 1985; 4:23.
12. Kakizaki H, Koyanagi T, Kato M. Sympathetic innervation of the male feline urethra rhabdosphincter. Neurosci Lett 1991; 129:165–167.
13. Hollabaugh RS, Steiner MS, Dmochowski RR. Neuroanatomy of the female continence complex: clinical implications. Urology 2001; 57(2):382–388.
14. Kakizaki H, Fraser MO, De Groat WC. Reflex pathways controlling urethral striated and smooth muscle function in the male rat. Am J Physiol 1997; 272(5 Pt 2):1647–1656.
15. Wang P, Luthin GR, Ruggieri MR. Muscarinic acetylcholine receptor subtypes mediating urinary bladder contractility and coupling to GTP binding proteins. J Pharmacol Exp Ther 1995; 273:959–956.
16. Hegde SS, Choppin A, Bonhaus D, Briaud S, Loeb M. Functional role of M2 and M3 muscarinic receptors in the urinary bladder of rats in vitro and in vivo. Br J Pharmacol 1997; 120:1409–1418.
17. Somogyi GT, De Groat WC. Functional, signal transduction mechanisms, and plasticity of presynaptic muscarinic receptors in the urinary bladder. Life Sci 1998; 64:411–418.
18. Tobin G, Sjogren C. Prejunctional facilitatory and inhibitory modulation of parasympathetic nerve transmission in the rabbit urinary bladder. J Auton Nerv Syst 1998; 68:153–156.
19. Hills CJ, Winter SA, Balfour JA. Tolterodine. Drugs 1998; 55:813–820.
20. Smith CM, Wallis RM. Characterization of [3H]darifenacin as a novel radioligand for the study of M3 receptors. J Recept Signal Transduct Res 1997; 17:177–184.
21. Dykstra DD, Sidi AA, Scott AB, Pagel JM, Goldish GD. Effects of botulinum A toxin on detrusor-sphincter dyssnergia in spinal cord patients. J Urol 1988; 139:919–922.
22. Stohrer M, Schurch B, Kramer G, Schmid D, Daul D, Hauri D. Botulinum A-toxin detrusor injections in the treatment of detrusor hyperreflexia. J Urol 2000; 163:244A. Abstract.
23. D'Agostino G, Kilbinger H, Chiari MC, Grana E. Presynaptic inhibitory muscarinic receptors modulating [3H]acetylcholine release in the rat urinary bladder. J Pharm Exp Ther 1986; 239:522.
24. Mattiasson A, Andersson KE, Elbadawi A. Interaction between adrenergic and cholinergic nerve terminals in the urinary bladder of rabbit, cat and man. J Urol 1987; 137:1017.
25. Alberts P. Classification of the presynaptic muscarinic receptor subtype that regulates 3H-acetylcholine secretion in the guinia pig urinary bladder in vitro. J Pharmacol Exp Ther 1995; 274:458–468.
26. Sogbein SK, Downie JW, Awad SA. Urethral response during bladder contraction induced by subcutaneous bethanechol chloride: elicitation of sympathetic reflex constriction. J Urol 1984; 131:791.
27. Testa R, Guarneri L, Ibba M. Characterization of the alpha-1 adrenoceptor subtypes in the prostate and prostatic urethra of rat, rabbit, dog and man. Eur J Pharmacol 1993; 249:307–315.
28. Chess-Williams R, Aston N, Couldwell C. Alpha-1A subtype mediates contraction of the rat urethra. J Auton Pharmacol 1994; 14:375–381.
29. Andersson KE. Pharmacology of lower urinary tract smooth muscle and penile erectile tissues. Pharmacol Rev 1993; 45:253–307.

30. Treatment of urinary incontinence. Urinary Incontinence in Adults. Clinical Practice Guideline. U.S. Department of Health and Human Services, Public Health Service, Agency for Health Care Policy and Research. March 1992:27–65.

31. De Groat WC, Yoshiyama M, Ramage AG, Yamamoto T, Somogyi GT. Modulation of voiding and storage reflexes by activation of alpha$_1$ adrenoceptors. Eur Urol 1999; 36(suppl 1):68–73.

32. Szell EA, Yamamoto T, De Groat WC, Somogyi GT. Smooth muscle and parasympathetic nerve terminals in the rat urinary bladder have different subtypes of α_1 adrenoceptors. Br J Pharmacol 2000; 130:1685–1691.

33. Ishizuka O, Persson K, Mattiasson A, Naylor A, Wyllie M, Andersson K. Micturition in conscious rats with and without bladder outlet obstruction: role of spinal alpha$_1$ adrenoceptors. Br J Pharmacol 1996; 117:962–966.

34. Castleden CM, Morgan B. The effect of beta-adrenoceptor agonists on urinary incontinence in the elderly. Br J Clin Pharmacol 1980; 10(6):619.

35. De Groat WC, Lalley PM. Reflex firing in lumbar sympathetic outflow to activation of vesical afferent fibers. J Physiol 1972; 226:289.

36. Blaivas JG, Labib KL, Bauer SB, Retik AB. A new approach to electromyography of the external urethral sphincter. J Urol 1977; 117:773.

37. Edvardsen P. Nervous control of urinary bladder in cats. I. The collecting phase. Acta Physiol Scand 1968; 72(1):157–171.

38. Edvardsen P. Sympathetic inhibition of the urinary bladder. Electroencephalogr Clin Neurophysiol 1968; 24(1):91.

39. Skehan AM, Downie JW, Awad SA. Control of detrusor stiffness in the chronic decentralized feline bladder. J Urol 1993; 149(5):1165–1173.

40. Skehan AM, Downie JW, Awad SA. The pathophysiology of contractile activity in the chronic decentralized feline bladder. J Urol 1993; 149(5):1156–1164.

41. Burnstock G. Dumsday B, Smythe A. Atropine-resistant excitation of the urinary bladder: possibility of transmission via nerves releasing a purine nucleotide. Br J Pharmacol 1972; 44:451.

42. Bolego C, Pinna C, Abbracchio MP, Cataberi F, Puglisi L. Br J Pharmacol 1995; 114:1557–1562.

43. Klarskov P, Gerstenberg T, Hald T. Vasoactive intestinal polypeptide influence on lower urinary tract smooth muscle from human and pig. J Urol 1984; 131:1000.

44. Cardozo LD, Stanton SL. A comparison between bromocriptine and indomethacin in the treatment of detrusor instability. J Urol 1980; 123:399–401.

45. Kinder RB, Mundy AR. Atropine blockade of nerve-mediated stimulation of the human detrusor. Br J Urol 1985; 57(4):418–421.

46. Bayliss M, Wu C, Newgreen D, Mundy AR, Fry CH. A quantitative study of atropine-resistant contractile responses in human detrusor smooth muscle, from stable, unstable and obstructed bladders. J Urol 1999; 162(5):1833–1839.

47. Ghoniem GM, Shoukry MS, Hassouna ME. Detrusor properties in myelomeningocele patients: in vitro study. J Urol 1998; 159:2193–2196.

48. Levin RM, Ruggieri MR, Wein AJ. Functional effects of the purinergic innervation of the rabbit urinary bladder. J Pharmacol Exp Ther 1986; 236:432.

49. Chancellor MB, Kaplan SA, Blaivas JG. The cholinergic and purinergic components of detrusor contractility in a whole rabbit bladder model. J Urol 1992; 148.906–909.

50. Sneddon P, McLees A. Purinergic and cholinergic contractions in adult and neonatal rabbit bladder. Eur J Pharmacol 1992; 214:7–12.

51. Theobald RJ. Purinergic and cholinergic components of bladder contractility and flow. Life Sci 1995; 56:445–454.

52. Igawa Y, Mattiasson A, Andersson KE. Functional importance of cholinergic and purinergic neurotransmission for micturition contraction in the normal unanesthetized rat. Br J Pharmacol 1993; 109:473–479.

53. De Groat WC, Yoshimura N. Pharmacology of the lower urinary tract. Annu Rev Pharmacol Toxicol 2001; 41:691–721.

54. Lee HY, Bardini M, Burnstock G. Distribution of P2X receptors in the urinary bladder and the ureter of the rat. J Urol 2000; 163:2002–2007.
55. O'Reilly MA, Kosaka AH, Knight GF, Chang TK, Ford A, Rymer JM, Popert R, Burnstock G, McMahon SB. P2X receptors and their role in female idiopathic detrusor instability. J Urol 2002; 167:157–164.
56. Ralevic V, Burnstock G. Receptors for purines and pyrimidines. Pharmacol Rev 1998; 50:413–492.
57. Namasivayam S, Eardley I, Morrison JFB. Purinergic sensory neurotransmission in the urinary bladder: an in vivo study in the rat. Br J Urol Int 1999; 84:854–860.
58. Dmitrieva N, Burnstock G, McMahon SB. ATP and 2-methyl thio ATP activate bladder reflexes and induce discharge of bladder sensory neurons. Soc Neurosci Abstr 1998; 24:2088.
59. Yoshimura N, Sasa M, Yoshida O, Takaori S. Dopamine D1 receptor-mediated inhibition of micturition reflex by central dopamine from the substantia nigra. Neurourol Urodyn 1992; 11:535–545.
60. Yoshimura N. Mizuta E, Kuno S, Sasa M, Yoshida O. The dopamine D1 receptor agonist SKF 38393 suppresses detrusor hyperreflexia in the monkey with Parkinsonism induced by 1-methyl-4-phenyl-1,2,3,6-tetrahydropyridine (MPTP). Neuropharmacology 1993; 32:315–321.
61. Araki I, Kitahara M, Oida T, Kuno S. Voiding dysfunction and Parkinson's disease: urodynamic abnormalities and urinary symptoms. J Urol 2000; 164:1640–1643.
62. De Groat WC, Booth AM, Yoshimura N. Neurophysiology of micturition and its modification in animal models of human disease. In: Maggi CA, ed. The Autonomic Nervous System. Vol 3. Nervous Control of the Urogenital System. London: Harwood, 1993:227–290.
63. Kuno S, De Groat WC, Yoshimura N. Dopaminergic mechanisms underlying bladder hyperactivity in rats with unilateral 6-hydroxydopamine (6-OHDA) lesion of the nigrostriatal pathway. Soc Neurosci Abstr 1999; 25:1686.
64. McMahon SB, Spillane K. Brain stem influences on the parasympathetic supply to the urinary bladder of the cat. Brain Res 1982; 234:237–249.
65. Steers WD, De Groat WC. Effects of m-chlorophenylpiperazine on penile and bladder function in rats. Am J Physiol Regul Integr Comp Physiol 1989; 257:R1441–R1449.
66. Andersson KE. Changes in bladder tone during filling: pharmacological aspects. Scand J Urol Nephrol Suppl 1999; 201:67–72.
67. Candura SM, Messori E, Franceschetti GP, D'Agostino G, Vicini D. Neural $5HT_4$ receptors in the human isolated detrusor muscle: effects of indole, benzimidazolone and substituted benzamide agonists and antagonists. Br J Pharmacol 1996; 118:1965–1970.
68. Espey MJ, Du HJ, Downie JW. Serotonergic modulation of spinal ascending activity and sacral reflex activity evoked by pelvic nerve stimulation in cats. Brain Res 1998; 798:101–108.
69. Danuser H, Thor KB. Spinal $5HT_2$ receptor-mediated facilitation of pudendal nerve reflexes in the anaesthetized cat. Br J Pharmacol 1996; 118:150–154.
70. Araki I, De Groat WC. Unitary excitatory synaptic currents in preganglionic neurons mediated by two distinct groups of interneurons in neonatal rat sacral parasympathetic nucleus. J Neurophysiol 1996; 76:215–226.
71. Matsumoto G, Hisamitsu T, De Groat WC. Non-NMDA glutaminergic excitatory transmission in the descending limb of the spinobulbospinal micturition reflex pathway in the rat. Brain Res 1995; 693:246–250.
72. Yoshiyama M, Roppolo JR, De Groat WC. Effects of LY215490, a competitive α-amino-3-hydoxy-5-methylisooxazole-4-propionic acid (AMPA) receptor antagonist, on the micturition reflex in the rat. J Pharmacol Exp Ther 1997; 280:894–904.
73. Kontani H, Kawabata Y, Koshiura R. In vivo effects of γ-aminobutyric acid on the urinary bladder contraction accompanying micturition. Jpn J Pharmacol 1987; 45:45–53.
74. McMahon SB. Sensory-motor integration in urinary bladder function. In: Cervero F, Morrison JFB, eds. Visceral Sensation. Amsterdam: Elsevier Science, 1986:245–283.
75. Hulsebosch CE, Coggeshall RE. An analysis of the axon populations in the nerves to the pelvic viscera in the rat. J Comp Neurol 1982; 211:1.
76. Yoshimura N, De Groat WC. Patch clamp analysis of afferent and efferent neurons that innervated the urinary bladder of the rat. Soc Neurosci Abstr 1992; 18(59.7):127. Abstract.

77. Maggi CA, Meli A. The sensory-efferent function of capsaicin-sensitive sensory neurons. Gen Pharmacol 1988; 19:1.

78. Chen C, Ma C, De Groat WC. Effects of capsaicin on micturition and associated reflexes in rats. Am J Physiol 1993; 265: R132–R138.

79. Fagerli J, Fraser MO, De Groat WC, Chancellor MB, Flood HD, Smith D, Jordan ML. Intravesical capsaicin for the treatment of interstitial cystitis: a pilot study. Can J Urol 1999; 6(2):737–744.

80. Avenilo A, Cruz F, Coimbra A. Intravesical resiniferatoxin desensitizes rat bladder sensory fibres without causing intense noxious excitation: a c-fos study. Eur J Pharmacol 1999; 378:17–22.

81. Park WH, Kim HG, Park BJ, Kim DY, Oh DJ, Lim YS. Comparison of the effects of intravesical capsaicin and resiniferatoxin for treatment of detrusor hyperreflexia in patients with spinal cord injury. Neurourol Urodyn 1999; 18:402. Abstract.

82. Gosling JA, Dixon JS. The structure and innervation of smooth muscle in the wall of the bladder neck and proximal urethra. Br J Urol 1975; 47:549–554.

83. Gosling JA, Dixon JS, Critchley OD, Thompson SA. A comparative study of the human external sphincter and periurethral levator ani muscles. Br J Urol 1981; 53:35–41.

84. Bazeed MA, Thuroff JW, Schmidt R, Tanagho EA. Histochemical study of the urethral striated musculature in the dog. J Urol 1982; 128:406.

85. Stein M, Discippio W, David M, Taub H. Biofeedback for the treatment of stress and urge incontinence. J Urol 1995; 153:641–643.

86. De Groat WC, Steers WD. Autonomic regulation of the urinary bladder and sexual organs. In: Lowey AD, Spyer KM, eds. Central Regulation of the Autonomic Functions. 1st ed. Oxford: Oxford University Press, 1990:313.

87. De Groat WC. Nervous control of the urinary bladder in the cat. Brain Res 1975; 87:201.

88. Bradley WE, Scott FB. Physiology of the urinary bladder. In: Harrison JH, Gittes RF, Pearlmutter AD. eds. Campbell's Urology, 4th ed. Philadelphia: W.B. Saunders, 1978:87–124.

89. Bradley WE, Rockswold GL, Timm GW, Scott FB. Neurology of micturition. J Urol 1976; 115:481–486.

90. Fowler CJ. Neurological disorders of micturition and their treatment. Brain 1999; 122(Pt 7):1213–1231.

91. Andrew J, Nathan PW. The cerebral control of micturition. Proc R Soc Med 1965; 58:553–555.

92. Bradley WE, Timm JW, Scott FB. Cystometry. V. Bladder sensation. Urology 1975; 6:654–658.

93. Bradley WE, Timm JW, Scott FB. Innervation of the detrusor muscle and urethra. Urol Clin North Am 1974; 1:3–27.

94. Bhatia NN. Neurophysiology of micturition. In: Ostergard DR, Bent AE, eds. Urogynecology and Urodynamics. Baltimore: Williams & Wilkins, 1991:31–54.

95. Mahoney DT, Laberte RO, Blais DJ. Integral storage and voiding reflexes: neurophysiological concept of continence and micturition. Urology 1977; 10:95–106.

3
Epidemiology of Female Urinary Incontinence

Christopher Saigal
David Geffen School of Medicine at UCLA, Los Angeles, California, U.S.A.

Mark S. Litwin
David Geffen School of Medicine at UCLA and UCLA School of Public Health, Los Angeles, California, U.S.A.

I. INTRODUCTION

Urinary incontinence, defined as the involuntary passage of urine per urethra, can be divided into four clinical entities, as defined by the Agency for Healthcare Research and Quality's clinical practice guidelines (1). These are stress incontinence, in which a rapid increase in intra-abdominal pressure causes urine leakage; urge incontinence, in which precipitous, uninhibited detrussor contractions result an urgent need to void and leakage of urine; mixed stress and urge incontinence; and overflow incontinence, in which chronic retention of urine results in passive loss of small amounts of urine as the bladder is filled beyond capacity.

Recent estimates of the societal costs attributable to urinary incontinence are as high as $26.3 billion (1995 dollars), in the over-65-year-old population alone (2). Others have estimated the current costs of urinary incontinence to be $16.3 billion (1995 dollars), with 76% of those costs attributable to female incontinence (3). In the latter study, for women, routine care comprised the majority of the cost (70%), although nursing-home admissions (14%) and treatment (9%) were also major contributors. Others have confirmed that urinary incontinence is a significant reason for nursing-home admissions, with incontinent women having twice the risk of admission as continent women (4). Given the burden of this condition on the health and economy of the nation, much work has been done to create a descriptive epidemiology of urinary incontinence.

II. RISK FACTORS

A. Age

Increasing age was accepted as one of the risk factors for urinary incontinence at the 1988 National Institutes of Health consensus panel on urinary incontinence (5). Several studies have since documented an increasing prevalence and severity of urinary incontinence with advanced age (6–9). This increased prevalence in elderly women may be due to age-related laxity of pelvic musculature and connective tissue supporting the urethra. Additionally, factors in the elderly such as impaired mobility and/or declining mental status can increase the risk of incontinent episodes. The elderly suffer from significant rates of fecal impaction and constipation, both clinically associated with urinary incontinence (10).

B. Heredity

Some researchers have questioned whether there is a genetic basis for the connective tissue atrophy and weakness that contribute to stress urinary incontinence. Mushkat and colleagues examined the prevalence of stress urinary incontinence in first-degree relatives of 259 female probands (11). As a control, they collected data on the first-degree relatives of 165 women (matched for age, parity, and weight) without stress urinary incontinence being seen in a gynecology clinic. Prevalence of stress urinary incontinence was almost three times higher (20.3% vs. 7.8%) in first-degree female relatives of women with stress urinary incontinence themselves. These data suggest that there may be familial transmission of traits that can lead to an increased incidence of stress urinary incontinence.

C. Obesity

Several studies have documented an increased risk for urinary incontinence in women with high body mass indices (BMIs). Estimates of odds ratios for urinary incontinence range from 1.5 (95% confidence interval, 1.15–1.95) in a study of women using a criteria for high BMI of $>26\,kg/m^2$ (12), to 3.0 (95% CI 1.8, 5.0) in a study examining those in the heaviest quartile of BMI (13). Several other studies have suggested a relationship between weight and incontinence (9,14,15). One prospective study of women undergoing a surgical procedure for obesity found a reduction in incontinence after weight loss (16).

D. Hysterectomy

Data on the risk hysterectomy confers on the development of subsequent urinary incontinence are conflicting. In one large, systematic review of the literature published from 1966 to 1997, Brown and colleagues constructed a summary estimate of the increased odds for development of urinary incontinence in women who undergo hysterectomy (17). They found that among women >60 years of age, those who had a history of hysterectomy had an odds ratio of 1.6 (95% CI 1.4–1.8) compared to those without such a history. There was not a similar increase in odds for women younger than 60. They concluded that urinary incontinence following hysterectomy might not be seen until many years after the procedure.

E. Pregnancy and Parity

Several studies suggest that parity is a risk factor for urinary incontinence (18–20). Investigators have documented incidence rates for urinary incontinence occurring after pregnancy as high as 26% at 6 months, although most women recover continence with time (21). Possible explanations for this relationship lie in pelvic floor denervation due to compression during pregnancy and delivery and stretching or tearing of pelvic floor connective tissue and musculature during pregnancy and delivery.

A Danish study which followed a cohort of 278 women for 5 years after delivering their first child found a 5-year prevalence of International Continence Society–defined stress urinary incontinence of 30%, and 5-year incidence of 19%. Use of vacuum extraction or episiotomy during delivery was found to increase the risk of stress urinary incontinence (22). Although in another analysis of this group of women, a second delivery did not increase the risk for stress urinary incontinence (23), others have found a linear relationship between number of deliveries and risk of stress urinary incontinence (13).

The relative effect of pregnancy itself versus the process of vaginal delivery on the development of urinary incontinence has been debated. One study addressed this issue with a comprehensive physical exam and medical history on 189 women being seen for menopausal symptoms in a gynecology clinic (24). Ninety-eight of the patients were found to have urinary incontinence, and multivariate analysis revealed that the risk of urinary incontinence was almost five times higher among women with at least one pregnancy than in women who had never been pregnant. The risk was 3.5 times higher among women who had had only cesarean sections than in women who had never been pregnant. These data suggest that pregnancy itself confers risk for urinary incontinence, and calls into question the use of cesarean section to mitigate this risk. However, in a prospective study of 595 nulliparous women undergoing first pregnancy, in whom continence status had been ascertained prior to pregnancy, the relative risk of urinary incontinence when a woman delivered vaginally versus via cesarean section was 2.8 (21).

F. Tobacco Use

Some evidence links stress urinary incontinence and urge incontinence with cigarette smoking in women. In a case control study, Bump and McClish examined 606 women with known smoking history (current, former, or never) and recorded the results of urodynamic tests for the 322 women who were incontinent. Urinary incontinence was significantly more prevalent in current and former smokers than in nonsmokers. The odds ratio for urodynamically proven stress urinary incontinence in current female smokers was 2.48 (95% CI 1.60–3.84), while the odds ratio for current female smokers with urodynamically proven urge incontinence was 1.89 (95% CI 1.19–3.02) (25). In further study of the urodynamic characteristics of stress urinary incontinence in smoking and nonsmoking women, Bump and McClish found that smokers were at increased risk despite having stronger urethral sphincters (26). They speculated that increased and more forceful coughing associated with smoking "likely promotes the earlier development of the anatomic and pressure transmission defects that allow genuine stress incontinence and overcomes any protective advantage of a stronger urethral sphincter." However, other work has not supported a link between smoking and urinary incontinence (15).

G. Race

Some evidence suggests that African-American women have a lower prevalence of urinary incontinence than Caucasian women. In a population-based study of elderly (>70 years old) noninstitutionalized Americans, 16% of African-American women reported an episode of urinary incontinence in the past year, versus 23% of Caucasian women, a statistically significant difference (27). In a population-based survey of 1922 health maintenance organization members, Thom found a significant association between Caucasian race and the reporting of an incontinent episode in the last year (odds ratio 1.8, 95% CI 1.2–2.8) (13).

In addition to racial variation in the prevalence of urinary incontinence in women, race appears to play a role in the distribution of types of incontinence in incontinent women. In a study of 200 consecutive patients with urinary incontinence who were subject to a comprehensive physical exam and urodynamic testing, significant differences were found in the distributions of stress urinary incontinence, urge incontinence, and mixed incontinence between African-American and Caucasian patients (28). Stress urinary incontinence was found in 27% of incontinent African-American women, versus 61% of incontinent Caucasian women. Urge incontinence was found in 56% of African-American women, versus 28% of Caucasian women. Similar results were obtained in a study by Graham and Mallet, who examined urodynamic findings in 183 African-American and 132 Caucasian women with urinary incontinence (29). African-American women had a significantly lower prevalence of stress urinary incontinence and higher prevalence of urge incontinence than Caucasian women. In stepwise logistic regression, race emerged as a stronger predictor of stress urinary incontinence than age, obesity, tobacco use, parity, and other risk factors.

These studies were not population based, as the women studied sought care for their condition. However, if these differences in the distribution of incontinence type reflect the population at large, the higher prevalence of urge incontinence in African-American women may make them a group well served by more intensive urodynamic evaluation of their incontinence. Research examining differences in distribution of the type of incontinence in Hispanic and Caucasian women has not uncovered significant differences with urodynamic evaluation (30).

III. PREVALENCE

Estimates of the prevalence of urinary incontinence in non-institutionalized adults vary considerably, from 2% to 55% (31). Variation in published prevalence and incidence rates for this condition may be related to the variety of definitions of incontinence employed in the population-based studies examining the issue. For some studies, urinary incontinence is defined as *any* involuntary loss of urine per urethra, regardless of frequency, while other studies use definitions with minimum frequency or volume criteria. Another source of variation in the estimates can be attributed to the different populations included in these studies. Urinary incontinence rates are higher in older women and in those confined to nursing homes; studies with a preponderance of either group of women may arrive at higher estimates for prevalence and incidence of the disease. Additionally, variation in response rates to surveys regarding urinary incontinence may produce different estimates of prevalence owing to response bias.

A. Urinary Incontinence in Younger Women

Although urinary incontinence is often perceived as a problem primarily of elderly women, evidence suggests that it has a significant impact on women as young as 18. In a study of 1250 women between the ages of 18 and 44, Turan found the prevalence of urinary incontinence to be 24% (32). In a population-based study of 436 Swedish women between the ages of 20 and 59, investigators followed subjects for 5 years, and administered a gynecologic exam and incontinence questionnaire at the beginning and end of the study. The prevalence of urinary incontinence in the population was 23.6% at baseline and 27.5% at follow-up (33). Similarly, in two large studies of active-duty female Army soldiers, the reported prevalence of urinary incontinence during exercise or work activity was ~33% (34,35). Fitzgerald and colleagues sent a urinary incontinence questionnaire to 2000 women who were randomly selected from a population of 4000 employed women (36). The response rate in this study was 57%. Defining urinary incontinence as "the accidental loss of urine at least monthly," including incontinence both with and without associated increased intra-abdominal pressure or urgency, they found a urinary incontinence prevalence rate of 17.6% in women <50 years old. In this study, fewer than half of affected women reported urinary incontinence as a problem to their health care provider, underscoring the consistent finding that urinary incontinence is an underreported and undertreated condition.

B. Urinary Incontinence in Older Women

In an effort to address the variation in reported estimates of the prevalence of urinary incontinence in older women, Thom et al. performed an extensive literature search and reviewed 90 articles relating to the issue (31). Of these, 21 met inclusion criteria (e.g., they were population based, not limited to institutionalized women, and reported in English). Study sizes ranged from 388 to 18,084 subjects. The median study response rate was 76%. Prevalence data were abstracted and combined, and calculations were made for the prevalence rates in several populations. The mean prevalence of urinary incontinence that occurred "ever" or "ever in the last year" in "older women" (50 years and older) was 34%. The mean prevalence of urinary incontinence occurring on a daily basis in older women was 14%. Thom found that in studies in which it was possible to distinguish between these types of incontinence the proportion of all urinary incontinence attributable to stress incontinence ranged from 30% to 80%.

C. Incidence

Fewer studies have addressed the issue of incidence of urinary incontinence. The overall incidence rate in the population-based study of 436 Swedish women described above (33) was 2.9% in these younger women, while the incidence of urinary incontinence occurring weekly or more was 0.5%. One study of continent middle-aged women found the incidence of urinary incontinence (occurring monthly) to be 8% at 3 years (37). Nygaard found a 3-year incidence rate of urinary incontinence of 28.6% in a community-based sample of rural elderly women. In his study, a significant number of women had remission of disease, although data were not adjusted for incontinence treatment (8). Another community-based investigation, "The Medical, Epidemiologic, and Social Aspects of Aging" study, found a 1-year incidence rate of 20% in women >60 years of age (38).

Urinary incontinence is a common and costly national health problem. Epidemiological data have identified risk factors for urinary incontinence, such as obesity and smoking, which might serve as targets for preventive health interventions. Other data from studies on race and its relationship to specific types of urinary incontinence may help physicians tailor diagnosis and treatment efforts. Data regarding the prevalence of the condition in both younger and older women serve to remind health care providers to be diligent in querying these patients regarding symptoms. Given the many successful therapeutic options open to women with urinary incontinence, an overlooked diagnosis represents a missed opportunity to improve health.

REFERENCES

1. Agency for Healthcare Research and Quality. Overview: Urinary Incontinence in Adults, Clinical Practice Guideline Update. 1996. http://www.ahrq.gov/clinic/ulovervw.htm
2. Wagner TH, Hu TW. Economic costs of urinary incontinence in 1995. Urology 1998; 51(3):355–361.
3. Wilson L, Brown JS, Shin GP, Luc KO, Subak LL. Annual direct cost of urinary incontinence. Obstet Gynecol 2001; 98(3):398–406.
4. Thom DH, Haan MN, Van den Eeden SK. Medically recognized urinary incontinence and risks of hospitalization, nursing home admission and mortality. Age Ageing 1997; 26(5):367–374.
5. National Institutes of Health. NIH Consensus Statement Online: Urinary Incontinence in Adults; 1988 Oct 3–5. http://odp.od.nih.gov/consensus/cons/071/071_statement.htm (date accessed September 2001).
6. Milsom IEP, Molander U. The influence of age, parity, oral contraception, hysterectomy and the menopause on the prevalence of urinary incontinence in women. J Urol 1993; 148:1459–1462.

7. JC B. Urinary incontinence in the community-analysis of a MORI poll. BMJ 1993; 306:832–834.
8. Nygaard IE, Lemke JH. Urinary incontinence in rural older women: prevalence, incidence and remission. J Am Geriatr Soc 1996; 44(9):1049–1054.
9. Schmidbauer J, Temml C, Schatzl G, Haidinger G, Madersbacher S. Risk factors for urinary incontinence in both sexes. Analysis of a health screening project. Eur Urol 2001; 39(5):565–570.
10. Cheater FM, Castleden CM. Epidemiology and classification of urinary incontinence. Baillieres Best Pract Res Clin Obstet Gynaecol 2000; 14(2):183–205.
11. Mushkat Y, Bukovsky I, Langer R. Female urinary stress incontinence—does it have familial prevalence? Am J Obstet Gynecol 1996; 174(2):617–619.
12. Sherburn M, Guthrie JR, Dudley EC, O'Connell HE, Dennerstein L. Is incontinence associated with menopause? Obstet Gynecol 2001; 98(4):628–633.
13. Thom DH, Van den Eeden SK, Brown JS. Evaluation of parturition and other reproductive variables as risk factors for urinary incontinence in later life. Obstet Gynecol 1997; 90(6):983–989.
14. Resnick NM. Geriatric incontinence. Urol Clin North Am 1996; 23(1):55–74.
15. Brown JS, Seeley DG, Fong J, Black DM, Ensrud KE, Grady D. Urinary incontinence in older women: who is at risk? Study of Osteoporotic Fractures Research Group. Obstet Gynecol 1996; 87(5 Pt 1):715–721.
16. Bump RSH, Fantl A, McClish D. Obestiy and lower urinary tract function in women: effect of surgically induced weight loss. Am J Obstet Gynecol 1992; 167:392–399.
17. Brown JS, Sawaya G, Thom DH, Grady D. Hysterectomy and urinary incontinence: a systematic review. Lancet 2000; 356(9229):535–539 (Comment In: Lancet. 2000 Dec 9;356(9246):2012-3 UI: 21013012 Comment In: Lancet. 2000 Oct 7;356(9237):1275 UI: 20523126.)
18. Foldspang AMS, Lam GW, Elving L. Parity as a correlated of adult female urinary incontinence prevalence. J Epidemiol Community Health 1992; 46:595.
19. Milson IEP, Molander U, Arvidsson L, Areksoug B. The influence of age, parity, oral contraception, hysterectomy and menopause on the prevalence of urinary incontinence in women. J Urol 1993; 149:1459.
20. Foldspang A, Mommsen S, Djurhuus JC. Prevalent urinary incontinence as a correlate of pregnancy, vaginal childbirth, and obstetric techniques. Amer J Public Health 1999; 89(2):209–212.
21. Farrell SA, Allen VM, Baskett TF. Parturition and urinary incontinence in primiparas. Obstet Gynecol 2001; 97(3):350–356.
22. Viktrup L, Lose G. The risk of stress incontinence 5 years after first delivery. Am J Obstet Gynecol 2001; 185(1):82–87.
23. Viktrup L, Lose G. Lower urinary tract symptoms 5 years after the first delivery. Int Urogynecol J Pelvic Floor Dysfunct 2000; 11(6):336–340.
24. Faúndes A, Guarisi T, Pinto-Neto AM. The risk of urinary incontinence of parous women who delivered only by cesarean section. Int J Gynaecol Obstet 2001; 72(1):41–46.
25. Bump RMD. Cigarette smoking and urinary incontinence in women. Am J Obstet Gynecol 1992; 167(5):1213–1218.
26. Bump R. Cigarette smoking and pure genuine stress incontinence of urine: a comparison of risk factors and determinants between smokers and nonsmokers. Am J Obstet Gynecol 1994; 170(2): 579–582.
27. Fultz NH, Herzog AR, Raghunathan TE, Wallace RB, Diokno AC. Prevalence and severity of urinary incontinence in older African American and Caucasian women. J Gerontol Ser A Biol Sci Med Sci 1999; 54(6):M299–M303.
28. Bump R. Racial comparisons and contrasts in urinary incontinence and pelvic organ prolapse. Obstet Gynecol 1993; 81(3):421–425.
29. Graham CA, Mallett VT. Race as a predictor of urinary incontinence and pelvic organ prolapse. Am J Obstet Gynecol 2001; 185(1):116–120.
30. Mattox TF, Bhatia NN. The prevalence of urinary incontinence or prolapse among white and Hispanic women. Am J Obstet Gynecol 1996; 174(2):646–648.
31. Thom D. Variation in estimates of urinary incontinence prevalence in the community: effects of differences in definition, population characteristics, and study type. J Am Geriatr Soc 1998; 46(4):473–480.

32. Turan C, Zorlu CG, Ekin M, Hancerlio N, Saraço F. Urinary incontinence in women of reproductive age. Gynecol Obstet Invest 1996; 41(2):132–134.
33. Samuelsson EC, Victor FT, Svärdsudd KF. Five-year incidence and remission rates of female urinary incontinence in a Swedish population less than 65 years old. Am J Obstet Gynecol 2000; 183(3):568–574.
34. Sherman RA, Davis GD, Wong MF. Behavioral treatment of exercise-induced urinary incontinence among female soldiers. Mil Med 1997; 162(10):690–694.
35. Davis G, Sherman R, Wong MF, McClure G, Perez R, Hibbert M. Urinary incontinence among female soldiers. Mil Med 1999; 164(3):182–187.
36. Fitzgerald ST, Palmer MH, Berry SJ, Hart K. Urinary incontinence. Impact on working women. Aaohn J 2000; 48(3):112–118.
37. Burgio K, Matthews K, Engel B. Prevalence, incidence and correlates of UI in healthy, middle-aged women. J Urol 1991; 146:1255–1259.
38. Herzog AR, Fultz NH. Prevalence and incidence of urinary incontinence in community-dwelling populations. J Am Geriatr Soc 1990; 38(3):273–281.

4

Quality-of-Life Issues in Incontinence

David F. Penson*
University of Washington, Seattle, Washington, U.S.A.

Mark S. Litwin
David Geffen School of Medicine at UCLA and UCLA School of Public Health, Los Angeles, California, U.S.A.

I. INTRODUCTION

Urinary incontinence is a common condition in older women (1). However, unlike other common medical conditions, such as coronary artery disease or cancer, one cannot measure the public health impact of urinary incontinence in terms of years of life lost or overall mortality. Nonetheless, there is little doubt that urinary incontinence has a considerable impact on patients' health, well-being, and overall quality of life. The problem facing clinicians and researchers alike is finding ways to measure outcomes objectively in women with this common condition.

Objective measures, such as urodynamic assessments and urinary pad tests, often used when studying urinary incontinence, may provide important clinical information during the diagnostic evaluation of urinary incontinence. However, they are not always meaningful to patients. For example, some women who report urinary leakage at home cannot reproduce their symptoms during urodynamic evaluation (2). Others may experience minimal leakage during pad testing but find even the smallest leak to be a problem (3). Finally, some patients may present with symptoms such as urgency or dysuria, which cannot be easily quantified with objective tests (4). These observations underscore the need to find ways to measure patient experience in urinary incontinence accurately, as the ultimate goal of treatment for this condition is to improve quality of life.

Advances in research methodology now allow reliable collection of meaningful data on patients' health-related quality of life (HRQOL). HRQOL includes both objective evaluation of functional status and patients' perceptions of their own health and its impact on their existence. In the past decade, several valid and reliable questionnaires have been developed that are specifically designed to measure HRQOL in urinary incontinence. These instruments can be used to quantify the qualitative, subjective outcomes, allowing us to capture the public health impact of urinary incontinence on women and better assess the effectiveness of existing therapies for this common condition.

**Current affiliation*: Keck School of Medicine, University of Southern California, Los Angeles, California, U.S.A.

The goal of this chapter is to provide background on HRQOL research as it applies to urinary incontinence and to present an overview of the existing instruments available for patients with urinary incontinence. In addition, we will summarize the literature on the impact of urinary incontinence on quality of life.

II. HEALTH-RELATED QUALITY-OF-LIFE RESEARCH

HRQOL encompasses a wide range of human experience, including the daily necessities of life, such as food and shelter, intrapersonal and interpersonal responses to illness, and activities associated with professional fulfillment and personal happiness (5). Most importantly, HRQOL involves patients' perceptions of their own health and ability to function in life. HRQOL is often confused with functional status (6). While functional status is an important dimension of HRQOL, other aspects of HRQOL, such as role function, vitality, mental health, and psychosocial interactions, are equally important.

Health-related quality of life is a patient-centered variable, measured using questionnaires or surveys (also known as instruments), which are administered directly to patients in an objective, nonjudgmental manner. The principles of psychometric test theory are used to design instruments that measure HRQOL in a reproducible, quantifiable manner (7). HRQOL instruments typically contain questions, or items, that are organized into scales. Each scale measures a different aspect, or domain, of HRQOL. Responses to the items in a given scale are tabulated to produce a numerical score within that domain, which can then be used for statistical testing. Numerical values typically range from 0 to 100, the higher numbers representing better outcomes.

Many health care providers mistakenly believe that they can accurately estimate a patient's quality of life during the clinical interaction, obviating the need for patient-centered data collection. In one study of 2252 men with localized prostate cancer, patients' self-assessment of urinary HRQOL was compared with physicians' assessment. While 97% of patients reported some impairment due to urinary incontinence, only 21% of physicians reported that their patients were impaired by this problem ($P < .0001$). Similar findings were noted when assessing impairment due to urinary frequency (97% of patients as opposed to 19% of physicians, $P < .0001$) or due to decreased stream (97% vs. 14%, $P < .0001$) (8). This study demonstrates the difficulty providers have when trying to assess their patients' quality of life and underscores the need to use patient-centered instruments when assessing this outcome.

HRQOL instruments may be general or disease specific. General HRQOL domains address the components of overall well-being, while disease-specific domains focus on the impact of particular organ dysfunctions that affect HRQOL (9). General HRQOL instruments typically address general health perceptions, sense of overall well-being, and function in the physical, emotional, and social domains. Disease-specific HRQOL instruments for patients with urinary incontinence focus on more directly relevant domains, such as urinary leakage, urgency, and lifestyle changes due to urinary problems or distress/anxiety caused by urinary dysfunction. When studying quality of life in urinary incontinence, it is important to measure both general and disease-specific domains to obtain a complete portrait of the patient's experience.

III. DEVELOPMENT AND EVALUATION OF NEW INSTRUMENTS

The development and validation of a new HRQOL instruments is a long and arduous process that should not be undertaken lightly. Therefore, it is always preferable to use established instruments when available. An added advantage of using existing HRQOL instruments is that it allows clinicians to compare their results to other, previously studied populations and assess their own outcomes.

When instruments are developed, they are first pilot tested to ensure that the target population can understand and complete them with ease. Pilot testing may reveal problems that might otherwise go unrecognized by researchers. For example, many commonly used medical terms are poorly understood by patients. This may result in missing data if patients leave questions blank. Furthermore, because many patients with urinary incontinence are older and may have poor eyesight, pilot testing often identifies easily corrected visual barriers such as type size and page layout. Pilot testing is a necessary and valuable phase of instrument development. Instruments are also evaluated for the two fundamental psychometric statistical properties of reliability and validity.

Reliability refers to how reproducible the scale is—in other words, what proportion of a patient's test score is true and what proportion is due to individual variation. Test-retest reliability is a measure of response stability over time. It is assessed by administering scales to patients at two separate time points, usually a short period apart. If too long an interval transpires, real change in the variable may artificially deflate test-retest reliability coefficients. The correlation coefficients between the two scores reflect the stability of responses. Internal consistency reliability is a measure of the similarity of an individual's responses across several items, indicating the homogeneity of a scale (7). The statistic used to quantify the internal consistency, or unidimensionality, of a scale is called Cronbach's coefficient alpha (10). Generally accepted standards dictate that reliability statistics measured by these two methods should exceed 0.70 (11).

Validity refers to how well the scale or instrument measures the attribute it is intended to measure. Validity provides evidence to support drawing inferences about HRQOL from the scale scores. Three types of validity are usually evaluated in scales and instruments. Content validity involves a nonquantitative assessment of the scope and completeness of a proposed scale (12). Although more superficial, it is always included in the early stages of instrument development. *Criterion validity* is a more quantitative approach to assessing the performance of scales and instruments. It requires the correlation of scales scores with other measurable health outcomes (predictive validity) and with results from other established tests (concurrent validity). For example, the predictive validity of a new HRQOL scale for physical function might be correlated with the number of subsequent physician visits or hospitalizations. Likewise, the concurrent validity of a new urinary function scale might be correlated with daily pad use in a urinary pad test. A new emotional HRQOL scale might be correlated with an established mental health index. Generally accepted standards dictate that validity statistics should exceed 0.70 (11).

Construct validity is the most valuable yet most difficult way of assessing a survey instrument. It is often determined only after years of experience with a survey instrument. It is a measure of how meaningful the scale or survey instrument is when in practical use. Often, it is not calculated as a quantifiable statistic. Rather, it is frequently seen as a Gestalt of how well a survey instrument performs in a multitude of settings and populations over a number of years. Construct validity requires much effort over many years of evaluation.

IV. HEALTH-RELATED QUALITY-OF-LIFE INSTRUMENTS AVAILABLE FOR USE IN URINARY INCONTINENCE

A. General HRQOL Instruments

Although there are over 50 established and published instruments designed to measure general HRQOL, few have been used in the specific setting of primary urinary incontinence. These include only the RAND 36-item Health Survey (SF-36), the Sickness Impact Profile (SIP), and the Nottingham Health Profile.

Many researchers feel that the SF-36 is the "gold standard" for measuring general HRQOL in medical research (6). Developed during the Medical Outcomes Study, a large study that examined health-related aspects of daily life in many different types of patients (13), it is a 36-item, self-administered instrument that takes < 10 min to complete and quantifies HRQOL in eight multi-item scales that address different health concepts: physical function, social function, bodily pain, emotional well-being, energy/fatigue, general health perceptions, and role limitation due to physical or emotional problems. Two summary scales, a physical health composite and a mental health composite, may also be calculated (14). Each of the eight individual scales is scored from 0 to 100, with higher scores corresponding to better outcomes. The composite scales are standardized to a population mean of 50 with a population standard deviation of 10. Importantly, the SF-36 has been used in prior studies of patients with urinary incontinence and has been shown to perform well in this patient group (15). There is also a shortened version of the SF-36, known as the SF-12, which can be used in place of the SF-36 if the researcher wishes to reduce the respondent burden. Although the results are not reported in eight distinct domains, as with the SF-36, the two summary domains generated in the SF-12 are still acceptable in many research settings.

The SIP is considerably longer (136 items) than the SF-36. However, the greater number of questions results in more domains—12—which may allow for a more comprehensive view of general HRQOL. Individual summary scores can be generated for each of these domains (16,17). The Nottingham Health Profile contains six domains comprising a total 38 items that the subject responds to with binary (yes/no) answers (18). It has been used primarily in the United Kingdom to measure general HRQOL in a number of disease processes (19–21). While not as widely used in the general population as the SF-36, both of the Nottingham Health Profile and the SIP have been successfully utilized to measure general HRQOL in women with incontinence (22,23). In a recent review of HRQOL instruments for use in incontinence, Corcos and colleagues (24) concluded that these three generic HRQOL instruments were not responsive to change in incontinent patients. This observation underscores the need for valid, reliable, and responsive disease-specific HRQOL instruments in incontinence.

B.   Disease-Specific HRQOL Instruments

There are now numerous HRQOL instruments designed specifically to look at the impact of both stress and urge incontinence on HRQOL. No one instrument has been demonstrated to be superior to another, and the choice of outcome measure should be based upon one's particular clinical or research goals. Most of these questionnaires are available in the public domain. Interested clinicians and researchers can therefore review the items in an instrument and select the established questionnaire that best suits their purposes.

The Incontinence Impact Questionnaire (IIQ) and the Urogenital Distress Inventory (UDI) are two of the most common questionnaires used to measure disease-specific HRQOL in urinary incontinence. Developed in the mid 1990s, the original versions of these questionnaires were relatively long (roughly 53 items combined) (25). The two questionnaires had the advantage of adequately capturing both dysfunction and bother due to urgency, frequency and incontinence, etc. The IIQ generates four domain subscores: physical activity, travel, social, and emotional. The IIQ and UDI were specifically designed for females with urinary incontinence and have been extensively tested in this population and shown to be valid and reliable. The IIQ has been shown to perform well in both English- and French-speaking women (26). In clinical practice, however, the questionnaires were cumbersome to complete, which limited their utility. This was remedied with the development of short-form versions of these questionnaires—the IIQ-7 and the UDI-6. Although the information obtained is not as detailed, it is adequate and still provides a relatively comprehensive measure of disease-specific HRQOL in women with urinary incontinence. In addition, the IIQ-7 and UDI-6 have been shown to be responsive to change. In a group of 55 women with pelvic organ prolapse, FitzGerald et al. (27) found that women who reported subjective continence following surgery for this condition also reported lower IIQ-7 and UDI-6 scores (better HRQOL) when compared to baseline. Finally, although not originally developed for men, the IIQ-7 and UDI-6 have since been used in a population of older men and have performed well (28,29).

The IIQ and UDI instruments have also been modified for use in various subsets of patients with specific forms of urinary dysfunction. Lubeck et al. (30) developed and validated modified versions of the IIQ and UDI specifically for use in patients with urge incontinence and overactive bladder, known as the Urge-Incontinence Impact Questionnaire (U-IIQ) and the Urge-Urinary Distress Inventory (U-UDI). The U-IIQ and the U-UDI are longer (42 items) than the IIQ-7 and UDI-6, but have the advantage of measuring the impact of urgency, frequency, and urge incontinence on HRQOL in much greater detail. HRQOL is measured in seven domains: severity of urge symptoms, and impact on travel, activities, feelings, physical activities, relationships, and sexual function. The instrument has good psychometric properties and appears to capture most of the psychosocial concerns of patients with overactive bladder. Similarly, Barber and colleagues (31) modified the IIQ and UDI instruments for use in women with pelvic floor disorders. The new instruments, known as the Pelvic Floor Distress Inventory (PFDI) and the Pelvic Floor Impact Questionnaire (PFIQ), contain six scales. The PFDI consists of 61 items and generates scores in three domains: distress due to urinary incontinence, distress due to colorectal-anal dysfunction; and distress due to pelvic organ prolapse. The PFIQ includes 93 items and measures life impact in the same three domains. While the new scales have been shown to have acceptable criterion validity, further use in the clinical and research setting is needed to determine if the total number of items on the PFIQ and PFDI will affect subject's willingness to complete the questionnaire.

The Bristol Female Lower Urinary Tract Symptoms (BFLUTS) instrument is a modified version of the ICS*male* survey questionnaire that was developed to measure lower urinary tract symptoms (LUTS) in males (32). To develop the BFLUTS, the majority of the items on voiding symptoms in the *ICSmale* questionnaire were replaced with items quantifying the frequency and extent of urinary incontinence. The new questionnaire contains 20 items that address urinary incontinence, voiding symptoms in the voiding and storage phase, sexual function, and other aspects of quality of life. The BFLUTS was shown to be valid and reliable in a population of 85 incontinent women from the United Kingdom. It has the advantage of capturing both function and bother in the urinary domains, which are both important components of HRQOL. Although the BFLUTS has not been formally validated in men, a modified version of the questionnaire has been administered to males and was shown to perform well (33).

Kelleher et al. developed a 21-item survey, known as the King's Health Questionnaire, to assess HRQOL in incontinent women (34). This questionnaire measures the domains of general health perception, incontinence impact, urinary symptoms, severity of disease, role limitations, physical limitations, social limitations, personal limitations, emotional problems, and sleep disturbances. It has been shown to be valid and reliable and correlates well with outcomes from the SF-36.

Black and colleagues (35) developed two instruments, a Symptom Severity Index (SSI) and a Symptom Impact Index (SII), to assess the impact of incontinence on women's HRQOL. They developed their instruments in a population of 442 women undergoing surgery for stress urinary incontinence. The new questionnaires have the advantage of being brief (eight items total), yet able to generate to distinct summary scores that show acceptable validity and reliability. Research is ongoing to assess the responsiveness of these instruments to change.

Patrick et al. (36) have developed the I-QOL, a 22-item questionnaire, that specifically examines HRQOL in three domains, avoidance and limiting behavior due to incontinence, social embarrassment, and psychosocial impact of incontinence. This instrument has the advantage of being developed and test in both sexes and has been cross-culturally adapted for use in numerous countries in various languages (37). As it does not capture urinary function well, it should be used with a functional scale, such as a voiding diary or the SSI.

The York Incontinence Perceptions Scale (YIPS) is a simple eight-item questionnaire that is specifically designed to capture a subject's psychosocial adjustments to urinary incontinence (38). This instrument, like most of the others described so far, tends to focus on stress incontinence, and is therefore of less utility when studying urge incontinence or overactive bladder. If the YIPS were to be used in this setting, it would need to be accompanied by other instruments that capture the impact of urgency and frequency on HRQOL. The 24-item Urge Impact Scale (URIS) (39) has the added advantage of examining urge incontinence in particular, although it doesn't specifically capture the impact of urgency or overactive bladder on HRQOL.

V. IMPACT OF URINARY INCONTINENCE ON GENERAL HEALTH-RELATED QUALITY OF LIFE

Although urinary incontinence is traditionally thought of as a condition that affects quality of life, there are few studies that quantify the impact of this health problem on general health-related quality of life. However, the studies that have been performed clearly demonstrate that this condition has a broad effect on quality of life. Using the Nottingham Health Profile, Grimby, et al. (40) measured general HRQOL in 120 elderly women (mean age 75.4 years) with urinary incontinence. As a comparison group, 313 age-matched women without urinary incontinence also completed the questionnaire. They found that incontinent women experienced greater emotional disturbance and social isolation than the age-matched controls. When they compared women with either stress or urge incontinence to the control group, they found that the women with urge incontinence had significantly greater emotional disturbance than the controls, while no differences were noted between women with stress incontinence and controls in this domain. Both groups (stress and urge incontinence) reported more social isolation than the controls. Direct comparisons between women with stress and urge incontinence were hindered by sample size issues. Although these data demonstrate that all types of urinary incontinence have a broad impact on women's daily lives and cause significant social isolation, they also underscore the fact that the quality-of-life impact of urge incontinence is uniquely different from that of stress incontinence.

In another study, Haggland et al. (41) used a population-based approach to assess the impact of stress and urge incontinence on HRQOL (as measured by the SF-36) in Surahammar, Sweden. HRQOL data were available in 596 women without incontinence, 440 women with stress incontinence, and 71 women with urge incontinence. Incontinent women, regardless of type, reported significantly lower general HRQOL scores in all eight domains of the SF-36. However, when stratified by type of incontinence, women with urge incontinence reported significantly worse general HRQOL in all domains even when compared to women with stress incontinence. The magnitude of difference in general HRQOL scores between women with stress, as opposed to urge, incontinence was particularly striking, 10–20 points lower in all domains, and underscores the clinical importance of these findings. Similarly, Hunskaar and Visnes used the Sickness Impact Profile to specifically compare women with urge incontinence to those with stress incontinence and found that the group with urge incontinence had significantly worse HRQOL in the sleep and social interaction domains of the SIP. In addition, they divided their cohort by age, comparing HRQOL in 36 incontinent women aged 40–60 years and 40 women age ≥70 years, while controlling for type of incontinence. Younger women had worse HRQOL than older women, particularly in the domains of emotional behavior and effect on recreation and pastimes. This study demonstrates that the effect of incontinence on general HRQOL is affected not only by the type of incontinence but also by the age of the patient.

Interestingly, it is not simply incontinent episodes that affect quality of life in urge incontinence. In a telephone study of overactive bladder (OAB), Liberman and colleagues administered the SF-36 to 483 subjects with OAB symptoms and 191 controls. After adjusting for age, sex, and use of medical care, subjects with incontinent OAB (n = 185) had worse HRQOL in the physical function, role-functional, bodily pain, health perceptions, social functioning, and mental health domains of the SF-36 when compared to controls. However, in the subgroup of patients with overactive bladder symptoms and no incontinence (n = 298), significantly lower HRQOL scores were still noted in the role-functioning, mental health, health perception, and bodily pain domains. The investigators further divided this population into continent OAB patients with frequency only (n = 175), urgency only (n = 80), and both frequency and urgency symptoms (n = 43). Of these three subgroups, only patients with continent OAB who experience both frequency and urgency have significant lower HRQOL scores than controls. This association was noted in all domains except for social function. This study, and others (42) indicate that, while much of the quality of life impact of urge incontinence is due to the actual leakage episodes, the combination of frequency and urgency symptoms, in and of itself, also affects quality of life.

It is also notable that urinary incontinence can have a significant impact on psychological health, which may in turn impact general HRQOL. In a study of 668 adults seen in 41 community primary care practices in North Carolina, 43% of patients who reported urinary incontinence also noted depressive symptoms, as opposed to 30% in patients without urinary incontinence. Furthermore, in the 230 subjects who reported urinary incontinence, lower domain scores in physical and mental health, life satisfaction, and the perception that incontinence interfered with daily life were significant predictors of depression (43). Other studies have found a similar relationship between urinary incontinence and depression and social isolation (44,45). In conclusion, urinary incontinence and lower urinary-tract symptoms appear to impact health-related quality of life extensively, affecting physical, psychological, and emotional domains to a greater degree than clinicians might expect.

VI. THE IMPACT OF INCONTINENCE TREATMENT ON HRQOL

Given the broad impact of urinary incontinence on health-related quality of life as described above, it is important that we document that treatment for urinary incontinence result in improved quality of life for our patients. Although the field of health-related quality-of-life research in urinary incontinence is still young, several authors have used validated HRQOL instruments to document that successful incontinence treatment results in improved quality of life.

A. Behaviorally Based and Other Noninvasive Interventions

A number of investigators have explored the impact of noninvasive approaches for urinary incontinence on health-related quality of life. These studies have all used validated instruments to demonstrate that quality of life in incontinent women can be improved with the use of behaviorally based or other non invasive interventions. For example, Bo and colleagues (46) randomized 59 women with stress incontinence to either pelvic floor muscle exercises or no intervention for a period of 6 months. General HRQOL was assessed using a modified version of an existing Norwegian quality-of-life instrument, while disease-specific HRQOL was assessed using the BFLUTS instrument. Although there were no differences in general HRQOL at the end of the trial, women in the behavioral intervention arm experienced a significant improvement in disease-specific HRQOL. In particular, patients in the pelvic floor exercise group had significantly fewer problems with interference with social life (4% vs. 41% in controls), fewer problems with interference with physical activity (44% vs. 79% in controls), less overall influence of incontinence with life (58% vs. 82% in controls), and less dissatisfaction if the subject had to spend the rest of her life with her current urinary symptoms (4% vs. 38% in controls). While the study could be criticized as having a placebo effect, as there is no way to blind patients to a behavioral intervention, it still demonstrates that women who use pelvic floor muscle exercises for urinary incontinence can expect to have improved disease-specific quality of life.

A number of studies have examined the impact of urinary control inserts on quality of life. Sand et al. (47) used the SF-36 to assess HRQOL in 63 women who used the Reliance urinary control insert. Fully 79% of patients reported that they were completed dry with this device. Importantly, patients reported significant improvement in the physical function domain of the SF-36. The SF-36 and the IIQ were used in another study that assessed the impact of a vaginal device (continence guard) on urinary incontinence and HRQOL. In this study of 55 women with stress incontinence, no differences were noted in the general domains of the SF-36, but significant improvements were seen in disease-specific HRQOL as measured by the IIQ. Other studies have noted similar findings (48). Taken as a whole, it appears that the behaviorally based or noninvasive therapies for urinary incontinence appear to have little impact on general HRQOL, but result in dramatic improvements in disease-specific HRQOL. Further research is needed to confirm or refute these preliminary observations.

B.   Medical Management of Urinary Incontinence

Medical therapy has an important role in the treatment of urge incontinence and overactive bladder. Prior to the introduction of disease-specific HRQOL questionnaires in the past 5 years, little information was available regarding the impact of these medications on the quality of life of patients with these conditions. However, the majority of recent randomized clinical trials of new agents for this condition include HRQOL, measured with validated instruments, as an important outcome measure.

For example, Dmochowski et al. (49) recently completed a double-blind randomized clinical trial (RCT) of the safety and efficacy of a transdermal oxybutynin patch in subjects with urge and mixed incontinence. There were three groups of patients receiving active agent of varying doses (n = 125–133), and one placebo group (n = 132). Outcomes included number of weekly incontinence episodes, adverse events, and changes in HRQOL, as measured by the IIQ. Patients in the highest dosing group (3.9 mg daily) reported improvement in all functional measures, such as number of weekly incontinence episodes and average daily urinary frequency, when compared to placebo but, importantly, also reported a significant improvement in disease-specific HRQOL, with a reduction in mean IIQ score from 144 at baseline to 89 at the end of the 3-month trial.

Similarly, Naglie et al. (50) performed an RCT to assess the efficacy of a calcium channel blocker, nimodipine, in detrusor instability and overactive bladder. Like the prior study, they assessed functional outcomes and HRQOL using the IIQ. Again, significant improvements in disease-specific HRQOL were noted in the active treatment arm of the study. Other authors have used the IIQ-7 (51) and the I-QOL instruments (52) to demonstrate the beneficial impact of effective medical therapies for urinary incontinence on quality of life. Given these prior studies, and the wide availability of disease-specific HRQOL instruments for urinary incontinence, it is safe to say that any future randomized clinical trial of new agents for this condition would be considered incomplete without the inclusion of HRQOL as an important endpoint.

C. Surgical Treatment of Urinary Incontinence

Health-related quality of life can and should be assessed following surgical therapy for urinary incontinence. Like other treatment modalities for this condition, there are few published studies to date that have used validated instruments to assess this outcome, but this number should increase in the coming years. To date, there have been studies assessing HRQOL following Burch colposuspension (53), pubovaginal sling procedures (54), and tension-free vaginal tape placement (55).

Bidmead et al. (53) assessed videourodynamic and HRQOL outcomes in 83 consecutive women who underwent the Burch procedure at a single institution. HRQOL was measured using the King's Health Questionnaire. Ninety-two percent of women were "objectively cured" according to videourodynamic testing. Accordingly, 95% of women reported improved HRQOL, although only 28% of women reported ≥50% improvement in HRQOL. This study demonstrates the importance of measuring both "objective" and "subjective" outcomes following surgical treatment for urinary incontinence, as patients who may be "objectively cured" may still experience minor decrements in quality of life that may be amendable to additional, nonsurgical therapy.

Morgan et al. (54) used a cross-sectional design to study the long-term efficacy of pubovaginal sling in 247 women who underwent this procedure in the mid-1990s. In addition to assessing efficacy, the investigators also measured HRQOL outcomes using the UDI-6 instrument. With a mean follow-up of 51 months, the overall objective continence rate was 88%, with 26% of patients who experienced urge incontinence preoperatively having persistent symptoms, and 7% of patients reporting de novo urge incontinence. Summary scores from the UDI-6, usually reported on a scale from 0 to 18 with lower scores being better quality of life, were transformed into a 0–100 scale. Ninety-two percent of patients reported transformed scores of <20 (implying good quality of life), closely mirroring the overall objective continence rate. Surprisingly, patients with de novo urge incontinence also reported reasonable HRQOL (mean score 24) while those with persistent urge incontinence reported significantly worse HRQOL (mean score 44). These results demonstrate that patients' expectations can play an important role in HRQOL outcomes, as patients with similar objective urge incontinence symptoms had differing HRQOL experiences, depending upon whether these symptoms were present preoperatively.

VII. CONCLUSIONS

As urinary incontinence is a highly prevalent condition that has a significant impact on quality of life, it is important that we measure this outcome when studying this incontinence. In the past decade, numerous valid and reliable HRQOL instruments have been developed for use in urinary incontinence. These instruments have been used in various patient populations and are readily available for use in both clinical and research settings. While the exact role of these questionnaires at the bedside is still evolving, it is clear that there is a pressing need for further research on the impact of various treatments for urinary incontinence on HRQOL. With information on how these treatments affect quality of life, we can better counsel our patients on which therapy is best for them and what to expect after treatment. This, in turn, will result in better outcomes and better care for incontinent patients.

REFERENCES

1. Diokno AC. Epidemiology and psychosocial aspects of incontinence. Urol Clin North Am 1995; 22:481–485.
2. FitzGerald MP, Brubaker L. Urinary incontinence symptom scores and urodynamic diagnoses. Neurourol Urodyn 2002; 21:30–35.
3. Harvey MA, Kristjansson B, Griffith D, Versi E. The incontinence impact questionnaire and the urogenital distress inventory: a revisit of their validity in women without a urodynamic diagnosis. Am J Obstet Gynecol 2001; 185:25–31.
4. Nager CW, Schulz JA, Stanton SL, Monga A. Correlation of urethral closure pressure, leak-point pressure and incontinence severity measures. Int Urogynecol J Pelvic Floor Dysfunct 2001; 12:395–400.
5. Patrick DL, Erickson P. Assessing health-related quality of life for clinical decision-making. In: Walker SR, Rosser RM, eds. Quality of Life Assessment: Key Issues in the 1990's. Dordrecht: Kluwer Academic Publishers, 1993.
6. Gill TM, Feinstein AR. A critical appraisal of the quality-of-life measurements. JAMA 1994; 272:619–626.
7. Tulsky DA. An introduction to test theory. Oncology 1990; 4:43–48.
8. Litwin MS, Lubeck DP, Henning JM, Carroll PR. Differences in urologist and patient assessments of health related quality of life in men with prostate cancer: results of the CaPSURE database. J Urol 1998; 159:1988–1992.
9. Patrick DL, Deyo RA. Generic and disease-specific measures in assessing health care status and quality of life. Med Care 1989; 27(suppl):S217–S232.
10. Cronbach LJ. Coefficient alpha and the internal structure of tests. Psychometrika 1951; 16:297–334.
11. Nunnally JC. Psychometric Theory. New York: McGraw-Hill, 1978.
12. Messick S. The once and future issues of validity: assessing the meaning and consequences of measurement. In: Wainer H, Braun HI, eds. Test Validity. Hillside, NJ: Lawrence Erlbaum Associates, 1988.
13. Stewart AL, Greenfield S, Hays RD. Functional status and well-being of patients with chronic conditions. Results from the medical outcomes study. JAMA 1989; 262:907–913.
14. Ware JE. SF-36 Health Survey: Manual and Interpretation Guide. Boston, MA: Health Institute, 1997.
15. Kutner NG, Schechtman KB, Ory MG, Baker DI. Older adults' perceptions of their health and functioning in relation to sleep disturbance, falling, and urinary incontinence. FICSIT Group. J Am Geriatr Soc 1994; 42:757–762.
16. Bergner M, Bobbitt RA, Carter WB, Gilson BS. The sickness impact profile: development and final revision of a health status measure. Med Care 1981; 19:787–805.
17. Bergner M, Bobbitt RA, Pollard WE, Martin DP, Gilson BS. The sickness impact profile: validation of a health status measure. Med Care 1976; 14:57–67.
18. Hunt SM, McEwen J, McKenna SP. Measuring health status: a new tool for clinicians and epidemiologists. J R Coll Gen Pract 1985; 35:185–188.
19. Thorpe AC, Cleary R, Coles J, Neal DE. Nottingham health profile measurement in the assessment of clinical outcome after prostatectomy. Northern regional prostate audit group. Br J Urol 1995; 76:446–450.
20. Hasan ST, Marshall C, Robson WA, Neal DE. Clinical outcome and quality of life following enterocystoplasty for idiopathic detrusor instability and neurogenic bladder dysfunction. Br J Urol 1995; 76:551–557.

21. Joly F, Brune D, Couette JE. Health-related quality of life and sequelae in patients treated with brachytherapy and external beam irradiation for localized prostate cancer. Ann Oncol 1998; 9:751–757.

22. Hunskaar S, Vinsnes A. The quality of life in women with urinary incontinence as measured by the sickness impact profile. J Am Geriatr Soc 1991; 39:378–382.

23. Grimby A, Milsom I, Molander U, Wiklund I, Ekelund P. The influence of urinary incontinence on the quality of life of elderly women. Age Ageing 1993; 22:82–89.

24. Corcos J, Beaulieu S, Donovan JL, Naughton M, Gotoh M. Quality of life assessment in men and women with urinary incontinence. J Urol 2002; 168:896–905.

25. Shumaker SA, Wyman JF, Uebersax JS, McClish D, Fantl JA. Health-related quality of life measures for women with urinary incontinence: the incontinence impact questionnaire and the urogenital distress inventory. Continence program in women (CPW) research group. Qual Life Res 1994; 3:291–306.

26. Beaulieu S, Collet JP, Tu LM, Macrammalla E, Wood-Dauphinee S, Corcos J. Performance of the incontinence impact questionnaire in Canada. Can J Urol 1999; 6:692–699.

27. FitzGerald MP, Kenton K, Shott S, Brubaker L. Responsiveness of quality of life measurements to change after reconstructive pelvic surgery. Am J Obstet Gynecol 2001; 185:20–24.

28. Moore KN, Jensen L. Testing of the incontinence impact questionnaire (IIQ-7) with men after radical prostatectomy. J Wound Ostomy Continence Nurs 2000; 27:304–312.

29. Robinson JP, Shea JA. Development and testing of a measure of health-related quality of life for men with urinary incontinence. J Am Geriatr Soc 2002; 50:935–945.

30. Lubeck DP, Prebil LA, Peeples P, Brown JS. A health related quality of life measure for use in patients with urge urinary incontinence: a validation study. Qual Life Res 1999; 8:337–344.

31. Barber MD, Kuchibhatla MN, Pieper CF, Bump RC. Psychometric evaluation of 2 comprehensive condition-specific quality of life instruments for women with pelvic floor disorders. Am J Obstet Gynecol 2001; 185:1388–1395.

32. Jackson S, Donovan J, Brookes S, Eckford S, Swithinbank L, Abrams P. The bristol female lower urinary tract symptoms questionnaire: development and psychometric testing. Br J Urol 1996; 77:805–812.

33. Temml C, Haidinger G, Schmidbauer J, Schatzl G, Madersbacher S. Urinary incontinence in both sexes: prevalence rates and impact on quality of life and sexual life. Neurourol Urodyn 2000; 19:259–271.

34. Kelleher CJ, Cardozo LD, Khullar V, Salvatore S. A new questionnaire to assess the quality of life of urinary incontinent women. Br J Obstet Gynaecol 1997; 104:1374–1379.

35. Black N, Griffiths J, Pope C. Development of a symptom severity index and a symptom impact index for stress incontinence in women. Neurourol Urodyn 1996; 15:630–640.

36. Patrick DL, Martin ML, Bushnell DM, Yalcin I, Wagner TH, Buesching DP. Quality of life of women with urinary incontinence: further development of the incontinence quality of life instrument (I-QOL). Urology 1999; 53:71–76.

37. Patrick DL, Martin ML, Bushnell DM, Marquis P, Andrejasich CM, Buesching DP. Cultural adaptation of a quality-of-life measure for urinary incontinence. Eur Urol 1999; 36:427–435.

38. Lee PS, Reid DW, Saltmarche A, Linton L. Measuring the psychosocial impact of urinary incontinence: the york incontinence perceptions scale (YIPS). J Am Geriatr Soc 1995; 43:1275–1278.

39. DuBeau CE, Kiely DK, Resnick NM. Quality of life impact of urge incontinence in older persons: a new measure and conceptual structure. J Am Geriatr Soc 1999; 47:989–994.

40. Grimby A, Milsom I, Molander U, Wiklund I, Ekelund P. The influence of urinary incontinence on the quality of life of elderly women. Age Ageing 1993; 22:82–89.

41. Hagglund D, Walker-Engstrom ML, Larsson G, Leppert J. Quality of life and seeking help in women with urinary incontinence. Acta Obstet Gynecol Scand 2001; 80:1051–1055.

42. O'Conor RM, Johannesson M, Hass SL, Kobelt-Nguyen G. Urge incontinence. Quality of life and patients' valuation of symptom reduction. Pharmacoeconomics 1998; 14:531–539.

43. Dugan E, Cohen SJ, Bland DR. The association of depressive symptoms and urinary incontinence among older adults. J Am Geriatr Soc 2000; 48:413–416.

44. Melville JL, Walker E, Katon W, Lentz G, Miller J, Fenner D. Prevalence of comorbid psychiatric illness and its impact on symptom perception, quality of life, and functional status in women with urinary incontinence. Am J Obstet Gynecol 2002; 187:80–87.

45. Fultz NH, Herzog AR. Self-reported social and emotional impact of urinary incontinence. J Am Geriatr Soc 2001; 49:892–899.

46. Bo K, Talseth T, Vinsnes A. Randomized controlled trial on the effect of pelvic floor muscle training on quality of life and sexual problems in genuine stress incontinent women. Acta Obstet Gynecol Scand 2000; 79:598–603.

47. Sand PK, Staskin D, Miller J. Effect of a urinary control insert on quality of life in incontinent women. Int Urogynecol J Pelvic Floor Dysfunct 1999; 10:100–105.

48. Versi E, Harvey MA. Efficacy of an external urethral device in women with genuine stress urinary incontinence. Int Urogynecol J Pelvic Floor Dysfunct 1998; 9:271–274.

49. Dmochowski RR, Davila GW, Zinner NR. Efficacy and safety of transdermal oxybutynin in patients with urge and mixed urinary incontinence. J Urol 2002; 168:580–586.

50. Naglie G, Radomski SB, Brymer C, Mathiasen K, O'Rourke K, Tomlinson G. A randomized, double-blind, placebo controlled crossover trial of nimodipine in older persons with detrusor instability and urge incontinence. J Urol 2002; 167:586–590.

51. Woodman PJ, Misko CA, Fischer JR. The use of short-form quality of life questionnaires to measure the impact of imipramine on women with urge incontinence. Int Urogynecol J Pelvic Floor Dysfunct 2001; 12:312–315; discussion 315–316.

52. Norton PA, Zinner NR, Yalcin I, Bump RC. Duloxetine versus placebo in the treatment of stress urinary incontinence. Am J Obstet Gynecol 2002; 187:40–48.

53. Bidmead J, Cardozo L, McLellan A, Khullar V, Kelleher C. A comparison of the objective and subjective outcomes of colposuspension for stress incontinence in women. Br J Obstet Gynaecol 2001; 108:408–413.

54. Morgan TO Jr, Westney OL, McGuire EJ. Pubovaginal sling: 4-year outcome analysis and quality of life assessment. J Urol 2000; 163:1845–1848.

55. Mukherjee K, Constantine G. Urinary stress incontinence in obese women: tension-free vaginal tape is the answer. Br J Urol Int 2001; 88:881–883.

5

Female Sexual Dysfunction

Kathleen E. Walsh and Jennifer R. Berman
Female Sexual Medicine Center, David Geffen School of Medicine at UCLA, Los Angeles, California, U.S.A.

I. INTRODUCTION

Sexuality is one of the most important quality-of-life issues in both men and women. Societal, religious, family, and individual belief systems can significantly influence an individual's sexuality. Female sexual dysfunction has been recognized as a common medical problem in all age groups. Basic science research in the anatomy and physiology of normal female sexual response and the pathophysiology of female sexual dysfunction has been limited. However, recent advances in understanding male sexual dysfunction and treatment options have facilitated interest in women's health issues and the study of female sexual dysfunction.

Sexual dysfunction is highly prevalent in both sexes, ranging from 25% to 63% of women and from 10% to 52% of men. Data from the National Health and Social Life Survey (NHSLS), a study of adult sexual behavior in the United States, found that sexual dysfunction (SD) is more prevalent in women (43%) than in men (31%). They also found an association between SD and various demographic characteristics, including age, education and race (1). In a study of 329 women, aged 18–73, a standardized sexual function questionnaire identified 38.1% with anxiety or inhibition during sexual activity, 16.3% lacked sexual pleasure, and 15.4% had difficulty achieving orgasm (2). A survey of 448 women over the age of 60 found that 12% of married women had difficulty with intercourse and 14% experienced pain with intercourse. Two-thirds of the women surveyed were sexually inactive. Sexual activity was strongly correlated with marital status (3).

In 1998, the American Foundation of Urologic Disease (AFUD) Consensus Panel classified female sexual dysfunction into 4 categories: desire, arousal, orgasmic, and sexual pain disorders (4).

1. *Hypoactive sexual desire disorder*: the persistent or recurring lack of sexual fantasies/ thoughts and/or receptivity to sexual activity
2. *Sexual arousal disorder*: the persistent or recurring inability to attain or maintain sufficient sexual excitement
3. *Orgasmic disorder*: the persistent or recurring difficulty, delay in, or absence or attaining orgasm following sufficient sexual stimulation and arousal
4. *Sexual pain disorders*: includes dyspareunia (genital pain with intercourse), vaginismus (involuntary muscle spasms of the outermost third of the vagina), and other (genital pain caused by noncoital sexual stimulation)

Pelvic floor disorders can also contribute to female sexual dysfunction. Disorders of the pelvic floor include incontinence, cystocele, rectocele, enterocele, and vaginal and uterine prolapse. It is estimated that 10–58% of adult women have symptoms of urinary incontinence (5). Studies have shown that urinary incontinence can be a significant contributing factor to female sexual dysfunction (6,7). Recent data have identified high rates of sexual dysfunction in patients with pelvic prolapse (8).

II. FEMALE SEXUAL RESPONSE CYCLE

The definition of sexual dysfunction has included both psychological and physiological components. Masters and Johnson first characterized the female sexual response cycle in 1966 (9). The cycle consisted of four consecutive phases: excitement, plateau, orgasmic, and resolution. Kaplan proposed a three-phase model in 1974, which included desire, arousal, and orgasm (10). Both of these cycles depict excitement or sexual desire as a spontaneous force that by itself stimulates sexual arousal. In contrast to these cycles, a five-phase model focusing on intimacy has been proposed by Basson (11) (Fig. 1). Basson suggests that for a large majority of women, the wish to enhance intimacy is the driving force of the female sexual response cycle. The cycle begins with basic intimacy needs, which may include mutuality, respect, and communication. When these needs are met, a woman will seek out and will be more receptive to sexual stimuli. The model hypothesizes a receptive type of desire, which stems from arousal and a woman's conscious choice of sexual stimuli. If there is an overall positive emotional and physical interaction, the woman's intimacy is enhanced and the cycle strengthened.

III. NEUROGENIC MEDIATORS OF THE FEMALE SEXUAL RESPONSE

The medial preoptic, anterior hypothalamic, and related limbic-hippocampal regions are areas within the central nervous system that are responsible for sexual arousal. Once stimulated, these regions will emit signals to both the sympathetic and parasympathetic nervous systems.

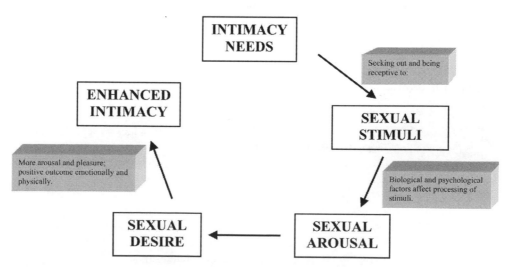

Figure 1   Alternative model of the female sexual response cycle.

A. Nonadrenergic/Noncholinergic Mediated Responses

Neuropeptide Y (NPY), vasoactive intestinal polypeptide (VIP), nitric oxide synthetase (NOS), cyclic gyanylate monophosphate (cGMP), and substance P have all been identified in human vaginal tissue nerve fibers (12,13). Recent studies suggest that nitric oxide (NO) and VIP are involved in altering vaginal relaxation and secretory processes (14,15). In organ bath analysis of rabbit clitoral cavernosal smooth muscle strips, enhanced relaxation was demonstrated in response to sodium nitroprusside and L-arginine (both NO donors). Using the same model, VIP was found to cause dose-dependent relaxation of clitoral and vaginal muscle (16). Phosphodiesterase type 5 (PDE5) has also been isolated in human clitoral, vestibular, and vaginal smooth muscle cultures (17,18). PDE5 is the enzyme responsible for degradation of cGMP and NO production. Sildenafil (Viagra), a PDE5 inhibitor, promotes intracellular cGMP synthesis and accumulation, thus allowing for enhanced relaxation of clitoral and vaginal smooth muscle (19).

B. Alpha-1-and Alpha-2-Adrenergic Responses

Alpha-adrenergic agents have been shown to be effective treatment for male erectile dysfunction. The adrenergic receptors associated with penile erection, libido, and erection are located in the male brain. Alpha-adrenergic mediators may also play a role in female sexual arousal (20). In preliminary organ chamber experiments using rabbit vaginal tissue, exogenous norepinephrine (alpha-1 and alpha-2 agonist) was found to cause dose-dependent contraction of vaginal smooth muscle. In addition, both alpha-1- (prazosin and tamsulosin) and alpha-2- (delequamine) selective antagonists inhibit smooth muscle contraction (21). These findings suggest that adrenergic nerves mediate contractile response. There also appears to be a difference in the quality of contractile responses in upper and lower vaginal segments, reflective of their different innervation and embryologic origin.

IV. HORMONAL INFLUENCE ON FEMALE SEXUAL FUNCTION AND RESPONSE

A. Testosterone

Only 1–2% of total testosterone circulates unbound. The remainder is bound by sex hormone–binding globulin (SHBG) or albumin. The nonbound (free) testosterone is biologically active. Within the central nervous system, testosterone has been shown to affect female sexual behavior (22,23). Low levels of testosterone are associated with decreased sexual arousal, libido, sexual responsiveness, genital sensation, and orgasm (24,25). Recent evidence suggests that testosterone may help promote the expression of endothelial NOS, the enzyme responsible for production of NO (26).

There is no direct regulator, stimulator, or feedback mechanism of androgen production in women. An increase in ovarian activity or adrenal activity has been shown to cause a rise in androgen production (27). Androgen deficiency in women can be caused by a number of factors including adrenal, pituitary, or ovarian surgery. Conditions such as hypopituitarism, adrenal insufficiency, anorexia nervosa, exercise-induced amenorrhea, and premature ovarian failure can also cause androgen deficiency. Lower androgen levels can occur in women taking exogenous corticosteroids and in women with chronic illness. Oral administration of hormones that elevate SHBG levels and reduce bioavailable androgens must also be considered to place women at risk of androgen deficiency. Increased levels of estradiol such as in the oral contraceptive pill or hormone replacement therapy (HRT) can increase SHBG, thus decreasing biologically available testosterone (28,29). Current commercial assays measuring total and free testosterone levels were developed to measure the much higher circulating concentrations in males.

B. Estrogen

Female sexual function is strongly influenced by estrogen. Both the neurological and vascular systems are affected by circulating levels of estrogen. In postmenopausal women, estrogen replacement was found to restore clitoral and vaginal vibration and pressure thresholds to levels to premenopausal levels (30). The vasoprotective and vasodilatory effects of estrogen have also been demonstrated. ERT has been shown to increase in vaginal, clitoral, and urethral arterial flow (31). Low estradiol levels are associated with thinning of mucosal epithelium, atrophy of vaginal wall smooth muscle, and an increase in vaginal pH. The less acidic environment within the vaginal canal can lead to vaginal infections, incontinence, urinary tract infections, and sexual dysfunction (32). Levels of estradiol <50 pg/mL have been directly correlated with increased sexual complaints (33).

Estrogen has also been shown to play a role in regulating vaginal and clitoral NOS (34). In animal models, aging and surgical castration are associated with decreased vaginal and clitoral NOS expression and apoptosis vaginal smooth muscle and mucosal epithelium. Estrogen replacement restored vaginal mucosal health, NO expression, and decreased vaginal cell death (35). These findings suggest that medications such as sildenafil (Viagra), which increases levels of NO, may have a role in the treatment of female sexual dysfunction, in particular sexual arousal disorder.

V. MEDICAL RISK FACTORS ASSOCIATED WITH SEXUAL DYSFUNCTION

Current evidence suggests that up to 80% of cases of sexual dysfunction have some organic component. Conditions associated with sexual dysfunction are listed in Table 1.

A. Vascular

Males and females can experience sexual dysfunction secondary to diabetes, cardiovascular disease, hypertension, peripheral vascular disease, and tobacco use (36,37). Diminished blood flow of the iliohypogastric/pudendal arterial bed leads to significant compromise of the vascular bed in both male and female genitalia (38,39). In females this is termed clitoral and vaginal vascular insufficiency syndromes (40). Sufficient blood flow is crucial for maintaining vascular and muscular integrity, both components integral in sexual arousal. Diminished blood flow can lead to vaginal wall and clitoral smooth muscle fibrosis that can result in symptoms of vaginal dryness and dyspareunia. Pelvic fractures, blunt trauma, surgical disruption, radiation, or chronic perineal pressure from bicycle riding can all lead to diminished vaginal and clitoral blood flow and sexual dysfunction.

B. Hormonal

In females, the most common causes of primary endocrine abnormalities are menopause, surgical or medical castration, premature ovarian failure, dysfunction of the hypothalamic/pituitary axis, and chronic birth control use. The percentage of women with a primary endocrine

Table 1   Medical Risk Factors Associated With Sexual Dysfunction

Vascular
    Diabetes mellitus
    Atherosclerosis
    Hypertension
    Lipid disorders
    Peripheral vascular disease

Hormonal
    Hypogonadism
    Hyperprolactinemia
    Hypo/hyperthyroidism

Neurogenic
    Spinal cord injury
    Multiple sclerosis

Musculogenic
    Pelvic floor muscle hyper/hypotonicity

Medications (see Table 2)

Psychogenic
    Depression
    Anxiety/obsession-compulsive disorder
    Social stressors
    Religious inhibitions
    Posttraumatic sexual experiences
    Dysfunctional attitudes about sex

Other
    Autoimmune disorders
    Renal disease (dialysis)
    Bowel disease (colostomy)
    Bladder disease (incontinence, cystitis)
    Skin disorders (contact dermatitis, eczema)

dysfunction responsible for their sexual dysfunction is unknown. Estrogen and testosterone play a significant role in regulating female sexual function.

There is a decline in both estrogen and testosterone levels with age, although the decline in testosterone is much less pronounced (28). A decrease in estrogen levels is associated with adverse neurovascular events affecting vaginal, clitoral, and urethral tissues. Low testosterone levels in females have been associated with a decline in sexual arousal, genital stimulation, libido, and orgasm. Therapy with combination estrogen-androgen compared with estrogen alone has shown to enhance libido, sexual desire and motivation, and overall sense of well-being (41).

C. Neurogenic

Neurogenic sexual dysfunction can occur in both men and women with spinal cord injury (SCI) or disease of the central or peripheral nervous system. In a study comparing premenopausal women with SCI, <50% of women with SCIs were able to achieve orgasm, compared with 100% of able-bodied women. They also reported that only 17% of women with complete lower motor neuron dysfunction affecting the S2–S5 spinal segments were able to achieve orgasm, compared with 59% of women with other levels of SCI. Time to orgasm was also significantly increased in women with SCIs (42). Women with complete upper motor neuron injuries affecting sacral spinal segments had difficulty achieving psychogenic lubrication (43). Focus group studies examining diabetes and female sexuality identified complaints of increased fatigue, vaginitis, decreased sexual desire, decreased vaginal lubrication, and an increased time to reach orgasm (44,45).

D. Musculogenic

The levator ani and perineal membrane make up the pelvic floor musculature that influences female responsiveness during sexual activity. The perineal membrane consists of the bulbocavernous and ischiocavernosus muscles. These muscles contract both voluntarily and involuntarily, intensifying sexual arousal and orgasm. The levator ani muscles are involved in modulating motor responses during vaginal receptivity and orgasm. Hypertonicity in the muscles can occur secondary to trauma (surgery, radiation, childbirth) and aging. This can cause vaginal hypoanesthsia, coital anorgasmia, or urinary incontinence during sexual intercourse or orgasm. Hypertonicity of the levator ani muscles can cause sexual pain disorders such as vaginismus that leads to dyspareunia.

E. Psychogenic

For many women who experience symptoms of sexual dysfunction, a combination of psychogenic and organic causes can be established. Psychogenic issues may include poor partner communication, performance anxiety, low self-esteem, social stressors, and religious inhibitions (46). Psychological disorders such as depression, posttraumatic sexual experiences, obsessive-compulsive disorder, or anxiety disorder can also have a significant impact on sexual function (47,48).

F. Medications

There are ~1.5 billion prescriptions written every year in the United States. One or more new prescriptions are written in over two-thirds of physician office visits (49). While many prescription medications have been implicated in causing sexual dysfunction, antihypertensive, antidepressant, and antipsychotic medications are the most frequently cited (50). Controlled research is limited for the majority of medications and substances believed to cause female SD. Many articles present only subjective evidence or case reports. The classes of medications most commonly associated with causing sexual dysfunction are listed in Table 2.

VI. EVALUATION OF THE FEMALE SEXUAL RESPONSE

A. Psychosocial/Psychosexual

Diagnosis of sexual dysfunction begins with sensitive and comprehensive questioning regarding sexual history. The Brief Index of Sexual Function in Women (BISF-W) is a validated 21-item, self-reported inventory of sexual interest, activity, satisfaction, and preference. This instrument can be used to differentiate among depressed, sexually dysfunctional, and healthy patients. This

Table 2   Common Classes of Medications With Sexual Side Effects

Class	Examples
Antihypertensive agents	α1 and 2 blockers (clonidine, reserpine, prasozin)
	β-blockers (metoprolol, propranolol)
	Calcium channel blockers (diltiazem, nifedipine)
	Diuretics (hydrochorothiazide)
Chemotherapeutic	Alkylating agents (busulfan, chlorambucil, cyclophosphamide)
Central nervous	Anticholinergics (diphenhydramine)
system agents	Anticonvulsants (carbamazepine, phenobarbital, phenytoin)
	Antidepressants (MOAIs, TCAs, SSRIs)[a]
	Antipsychotics (phenothiazines, butyrophenones)
	Narcotics (oxycodone)
	Sedatives/anxiolytics (benzodiazepines)
Agents that affect	Antiandrogens (cimetidine, spironolactone)
hormones	Antiestrogens (tamoxifen, raloxifene)
	Oral contraceptives

[a]MAOIs, monoamine oxidase inhibitors; TCAs, tricylcic antidepressants; SSRIs, selective serotonin reuptake inhibitors.

subjective report from the patient is crucial to understanding whether or not psychotherapy and/ or medical therapy is useful. Studies have shown that physicians are reluctant to address sexual topics. The physicians cited several reasons including awkwardness with sex language, fear of insulting the patient, feeling uncomfortable with the topic, and not knowing what questions to ask or how to ask them (51,52). Evidence suggests, however, that patients believe sexual function is an appropriate topic and are relieved when it is discussed with their physician (53). Patients may feel pressure to live up to an idealized standard of performance and have unrealistic expectations for themselves or their partner. Many men and women question where they fit on the continuum from normality to dysfunction. Open-ended and/or direct questioning can help guide the physician and patient to understanding the patient's sexual dysfunction.

B. Physical Exam

Every patient complaining of sexual dysfunction should undergo a thorough physical exam, including an external and internal gynecological exam. During the external gynecological exam, assessment of muscle tone, skin color, turgor and texture, and pubic hair distribution can identify conditions such as vaginismus, vulvar dystrophy, dermatitis, and atrophy. Examination of the posterior forchette and hymenal ring can help recognize episiotomy scars and possible strictures. The monomanual exam should include palpation of the rectovaginal surface, levator ani, and bladder/urethra in order to identify any rectal disease, levator ani myalgia, vaginismus, urethritis, cystitis, or urinary tract infections. Cervical motion tenderness may indicate infection or peritonitis. Palpation of the uterus and adnexa are included in the bimanual exam and assist in the identification of uterine retrogression, fibroids, adnexal masses/cysts, and possible endometriosis.

Finally, the speculum exam is utilized to evaluate for discharge, pH, vaginal mucosa, Papanicolaou smear, and prolapse. In females, vaginal pH, an indirect measurement of lubrication, can be measured using a digital pH probe. Decreased pulses, bruits, elevated blood pressure, and cool extremities are suggestive of vascular disease. Assessment should include a lipid profile and Doppler exams.

The suggested baseline hormonal profile includes follicle-stimulating hormone (FSH), luteinizing hormone (LH), total and free testosterone levels, SHBG, and estradiol and prolactin levels. Measurements of FSH and LH can assist in evaluating for primary versus secondary hypogonadism. High levels of FSH and LH are indicative of primary gonadal failure, and low or normal levels suggest hypothalamic or pituitary disease. Decreased levels of estrogen and testosterone have been associated with decreased libido, decreased sensation, vaginal dryness, dyspareunia, and decreased arousal. Hyperprolactemia can be seen in patients with decreased libido, galactorrhea, visual complaints, and headaches. Physical examination is positive for bitemporal hemianopsia. A CT or MRI may be needed to assess the pituitary gland.

Fatigue and cold intolerance are seen in patients with hypothyroidism. Examination for a possible goiter, myxedema, dry skin, and coarse hair is warranted. An increased TSH and decreased free T_4 are seen on laboratory tests. Hyperthyroidism can present with heat intolerance, weight loss, diaphoresis, and palpitations. Lid lag, exophthalamos, hyperreflexia, tremor, and tachycardia may be present on clinical exam. Laboratory values include a decreased TSH and an increased free T_4.

Cushing's syndrome is diagnosed on clinical exam by easy bruising, weight gain, truncal obesity, "moon face," "buffalo hump," and striae. An elevated overnight dexamethasone suppression test is needed for confirmation of clinical exam. Diabetic patients should be evaluated for peripheral neuropathy, retinopathy, and abnormal body mass index.

A thorough neurological exam is necessary in patients who have known or suspected SCI, nerve injury (prostate surgery, hysterectomy, childbirth), peripheral neuropathy, multiple sclerosis, or Parkinson's disease. The neurologic exam may uncover sensory or motor impairment that will account for residual urine (neuropathic bladder) or incontinence. Since the bladder and its sphincter are innervated by the second to fourth sacral segments. Somatic function of the sacral cord levels S_{2-4} is assessed by touching the perianal skin or placing a finger in the patient's rectum and noting contraction of the external anal sphincter muscles. This is termed the bulbocavernosus reflex.

VII. TREATMENT

In patients in whom an underlying medical condition has been diagnosed, treatment for correction or to control progression is appropriate. However, patients should be made aware that treatment of their condition does not guarantee the elimination of their sexual dysfunction. Consideration should be given to discontinuation of any medication suspected of contributing to sexual dysfunction or, if possible, switching to an alternative medication. For patients with a component of psychogenic dysfunction, referral to a psychologist or psychiatrist with expertise in sexual dysfunction may be beneficial.

A. Estrogen

Medical management of sexual dysfunction in women has focused on hormonal treatment. Both estrogen and testosterone are being used alone and in combination. In postmenopausal women, estrogen replacement has been found to improve clitoral and vaginal sensitivity, increase libido, restore vibratory and pressure thresholds, and decrease symptoms of vaginal dryness and pain during intercourse (33,54). Estrogen is available in several forms including oral pill, dermal patch, vaginal ring, and cream. The vaginal ring is a therapeutic option for women with breast cancer who are unable to take oral or transdermal estrogen.

Estrogen, especially when begun early in menopause, has been shown to be beneficial in the prevention and treatment of osteoporosis. ERT has also been shown to significantly reduce the risk for colon cancer, but not rectal cancers (55). Postmenopausal estrogen replacement, with or without progestin therapy, has a generally favorable impact on lipids, improves endothelial function, and has anti-inflammatory and antioxidant effects. However, the results of the Heart and Estrogen/Progestin Replacement Study (HERS) trial found no overall reduction in coronary events among women assigned to active hormone treatment. It is also suggested that there may be a transitory increase in coronary risk after starting hormone therapy in women with established coronary heart disease and a decreased risk thereafter (56). Prospective studies are under way to try to delineate how estrogen impacts Alzheimer's disease. Potential risks of HRT include gallbladder disease, thromboembolism, and breast cancer.

B. Testosterone

Testosterone supplementation has been shown to improve mood and well-being in naturally menopausal and surgical postmenopausal women (41,57,58). Women treated with testosterone and intramuscular E_2 were found to have improvements in sexual desire, fantasy, arousal, and orgasm (25,30,59). Decreased testosterone levels can be seen in women with premature ovarian failure and following natural, surgical or post-chemotherapy-induced menopause.

For replacement purposes, testosterone is available in lozenger pill form, sublingual, dermal patch, and cream. Oral methyltestosteronc is available in the United States either alone or in combination with estrogen (Estratest). In postmenopausal women who experience inhibited desire, dyspareunia, or lack of vaginal lubrication, testosterone can be prescribed in combination with estrogen. The transdermal testosterone patch is under clinical investigation. The patches contain 150 μg testosterone. Two patches are applied simultaneously twice a week. Preliminary results have been promising (60,61).

Testosterone topical cream has been approved for treatment of vaginal lichen planus. Topical preparations can be make in 1%, 2%, and 3% formulations and can be applied up to three times per week. Benefits from testosterone therapy include improved libido, increased vaginal and clitoral sensitivity, increased vaginal lubrication, and heightened arousal. Side effects of testosterone use that need to be monitored for in women include weight gain, clitoral enlargement, increased facial hair, and hypercholesterolemia. Measurement of testosterone levels before and after therapy, lipid panels (cholesterol, triglyceride, HDL, LDL), and liver function tests are recommended (62,63). Whether or not testosterone therapy in premenopausal women is beneficial is under investigation.

C. Investigational Medications/Devices

Secondary to the increase in both clinical and biological research in female sexual dysfunction, several new investigational medications and devices are now available. See Table 3.

VIII. SUMMARY

Female sexual dysfunction is a multicausal medical problem. Evaluation of the patient should include a comprehensive and collaborative effort between a physician and a psychologist.

Table 3 Investigational Medications

Treatment	Company	Ingredient	Already used for	Side effects
Alista (cream)	Vivus Inc.	Topical Alprostadil/ PGE 1	Sexual arousal disorder	Transient burning in men; in trials in women now
Androsorb (cream)	Novavax	Testosterone	Hormone booster for hypogonadal men	Early stages of clinical trial; may heighten libido in postmenopausal women
EROS-CTD	Urometrics	Clitoral therapy device	Arousal disorder	Increased sensation and blood flow to clitoris via gentle suction
Estratest (pill)	Solvay Pharm.	Estrogen-testosterone combination	HRT	Heightens libido in some women; side effects include acne and hair growth
Femprox (cream)	NexMed, Inc.	Blood vessel dilator	Sexual arousal disorder	Improves blood flow to genitals; enhances arousal
Intrinsa (patch)	Proctor & Gamble Watson Labs	Testosterone	Hypoactive sexual desire disorder	Increases sexual activity and pleasure
Livial (pill)	Organon	Synthetic steroid	Osteoporosis, HRT	Approved in Europe for menopause symptoms; improved mood and libido
Argimax	NitroMed	Yohimbine African tree bark fortified with L-Argine	Arousal disorder	Increases vaginal blood flow in postmenopausal women; may enhance arousal
Premarin or Estrace (cream)	Wyeth-Ayerst Warner Chilcott	Estrogen 17-β estradiol	Osteoporosis, vaginal atrophy, HRT	Vaginal dryness and discomfort; not for use in women with history of blood clots or breast or endometrial cancer
Steryl-Norleucine VIP (cream)	Senetek PLC	Synthetic version of VIP	Arousal disorder	Enhances vaginal lubrication, sensation, and genital engorgement
Testosterone (cream)	Off-label prescriptions from compounding pharmacies	Testosterone	New product	Not FDA approved; side effects include weight gain, hair growth, oily skin, enlarged clitoris

(continued)

Table 3.   Continued

Treatment	Company	Ingredient	Already used for	Side effects
Tostrelle (gel)	Cellegy	Testosterone	Hormone booster for hypogonadal men	Early study: testosterone levels in women on HRT jumped to levels of teenage girls
Uprima (pill)	Tap Pharm.	Apomorphine	Sexual arousal disorder and low desire	Targets the brain and stimulates the release of dopamine; side effects: nausea, vomiting, not yet FDA approved
Vagifem	Pharmacia Upjohn	Estrogen	Vaginal atrophy	Improves dryness and irritation; not absorbed systemically
Vasofem (pill)	Zonagen	Blood vessel dilator	Sexual arousal disorder	Increases blood flow to genitals
Viagra (pill)	Pfizer	Blood vessel dilator	Male erectile dysfunction and female sexual arousal disorder	Increases blood flow to genitals; enhances arousal
Levitra	Bayer	Blood vessel dilator, smooth muscle relaxer	Male erectile dysfunction and female sexual arousal disorder	Increases blood flow to genitals; enhances arousal

Although there are anatomic similarities between male and females, the complexity of female sexual dysfunction remains distinct from that of a man. The context in which a woman experiences her sexuality is equally as if not more important than the physiologic outcome she experiences. It is imperative that issues regarding how a woman views her sexuality be addressed before beginning medical therapy or determining treatment efficacies.

REFERENCES

1. Laumann EO, Paik A, Rosen RC. Sexual dysfunction in the United States: prevalence and predictors. JAMA 1999; 281:537–544.
2. Rosen RC, Taylor JF, Leiblum SR, Bachmann GA. Prevalence of sexual dysfunction in women: results of a survey study of 329 women in an outpatient gynecological clinic. J Sex Marital Ther 1993; 19:171–188.
3. Diokno AC, Greiff V. Sexuality in older women. Arch Intern Med 1990; 150:197–200.
4. Basson R, Berman J, Burnett A, Derogatis L, Ferguson D, Fourcroy J, Goldstein I, Graziottin A, Heiman J, Laan E, Leiblum S, Padma-Nathan H, Rosen R, Segraves K, Segraves RT, Shabsigh R, Sipski M, Wagner G, Whipple B. Report of the international consensus development conference on female sexual dysfunction: definitions and classifications. J Urol 2000; 183:888–893.

5. Mallett VT, Bump RC. The epidemiology of female pelvic floor dysfunction. Curr Opin Obstet Gynecol 1994; 6:308–312.
6. Bo K, Talseth T, Vinsnes A. Randomized controlled trial of the effect of pelvic floor muscle training on quality of life and sexual problems in genuine stress incontinent women. Acta Obstet Gynecol Scand 2000; 79:598–603.
7. Hilton P. Urinary incontinence during sexual intercourse: a common, but rarely volunteered, symptom. Br J Obstet Gynaecol 1988; 95(4):377–381.
8. Berman JR, Raz S. Sexual dysfunction in women with pelvic prolapse [Abstract A2]. In: Program for Female Sexual Function Forum, Boston, MA, October 2001.
9. Masters EH, Johnson VE. Human Sexual Response. Boston: Little Brown, 1966.
10. Kaplan HS. The New Sex Therapy. London: Bailliere Tindall, 1974.
11. Basson R. Using a different model for female sexual response to address women's problematic low sexual desire. J Sex Marital Ther 2001; 27(5):395–403.
12. Hoyle CH, Stones RW, Robson T, Whitley K, Burnstock G. Innervation of vasculature and microvasculature of human vagina by NOS and neuropeptide-containing nerves. J Anat 1996; 188:633–644.
13. Hsueh WA. Sexual dysfunction with aging and systemic hypertension. Am J Cardiol 1998; 61:18H–23H.
14. Burnett AL, Calvin DC, Silver RI, Peppas DS, Docimo SG. Immunohistochemical description of nitric oxide synthase isoforms in human clitoris. J Urol 1997; 158:75–78.
15. Helm G, Ottesen B, Fahrenkrug J. Vasoactive intestinal polypeptide in the human female reproductive tract: distribution and motor effects. Biol Reprod 1981; 25:227–234.
16. Berman JR. VIP neurotransmitter in organ bath analysis of rabbit clitoral cavernosal smooth muscle strips (unpublished data; in progress).
17. Park K, Moreland RB, Goldstein I, Atala A, Traish A. Characterization of phosphodiesterase activity in human clitoral corpus cavernosum smooth muscle cells in culture. Biochem Biophy Res Commun 1998; 249:612–617.
18. Traish A, Moreland RB, Huang YH, Kim NN, Berman J, Goldstein I. Development of human and rabbit vaginal smooth muscle cell cultures: effects of vasoactive agents on intracellular levels of cyclic nucleotides. Mol Cell Biol Res Commun 1999; (2):131–137.
19. Min K, Kim NN, McAuley I, Stankowicz M, Goldstein I, Traish AM. Sildenafil augments pelvic nerve-mediated female genital sexual arousal in the anesthetized rabbit. Int J Impot Res 2000; 12(suppl 3):S32–S39.
20. Meston CM, Heiman JR. Ephedrine-activated physiological sexual arousal in women. Arch Gen Psychiatry 1998; 55:652–666.
21. Berman JR. Alpha-1 (prazosin and tamsulosin) and alpha-2 (delequamine) selective antagonists inhibit smooth muscle contraction. (unpublished data; in progress).
22. Hutchison JB, Steimer TH. Preoptic formation of 17β oestradiol is influenced by behavioural stimuli in the dove. Brain Res 1985; 360:366–369.
23. Katz S, Morales AJ. Dehydroepiandrosterone (DHEA) and DHEA-sulphate (DHEAS) as therapeutic options in menopause. Semin Reprod Endocrinol 1998; 16:161–170.
24. Rako S. The Hormone of Desire: The Truth About Testosterone, Sexuality and Menopause. New York: Three Rivers Press, 1999.
25. Sherwin BB, Gelfand MM. Differential symptom response to parental estrogen and androgen in the surgical menopause. Am J Obstet Gynecol 1985; 151:153–160.
26. Marin R, Escrig A, Abreu P, Mas M. Androgen-dependent nitric oxide release in rat penis correlates with levels of constitutive nitric oxide synthase isoenzymes. Biol Reprod 1999; 61:1012–1016.
27. Rittmaster RS. Clinical relevance of testosterone and dihydrotestosterone metabolism in women. Am J Med 1995; 98(suppl 1A):17–21.
28. Burger HG, Dudley EC, Hopper JL. The endocrinology of menopausal transition: a cross-sectional study of population-based sample. J Clin Endocrinol Metab 1995; 80:3537–3547.
29. Davis SR, Burger HG. Androgens and the postmenopausal woman. J Clin Endocrinol Metab 1996; 81:2759–2764.

30. Sarrel P, Dobay B, Wiita B. Estrogen and estrogen-androgen replacement in postmenopausal women dissatifisfied with estrogen-only therapy. Sexual behavior and neuroendocrine response. J Reprod Med 1998 43(10):847–856.

31. Sarrel PM. Ovarian hormones and vaginal blood flow: using laser Doppler velocimetry to measure effects in a clinical trial of post-menopausal women. Int J Impot Res 1998; 10:S91–S93.

32. Caillouette JC, Sharp CF Jr, Zimmerman GJ, Roy S. Vaginal pH as a marker for bacterial pathogens and menopausal status. Am J Obstet Gynecol 1997; 176(6):1270–1275; discussion 1275–1277.

33. Sarrel PM. Sexuality and menopause. Obstet Gynecol 1990; 75(suppl 4):26S–30S.

34. Wyckoff MH, Chambliss KL, Mineo C, Yuhanna IS, Mendelsohn ME, Mumby SM, Shaul PW. Plasma membrane estrogen receptors are coupled to endothelial nitric-oxide synthase through Galpha(i). J Biol Chem 2001; 276:27071–27076.

35. Berman JR, McCarthy MM, Kyprianou N. Effect of estrogen withdrawal on nitric oxide synthase expression and apoptosis in the rat vagina. Urology 1998; 51:650–656.

36. Benet AE, Melman A. The epidemiology of erectile dysfunction. Urol Clin North Am 1995; 22:699–709.

37. Kaiser FE, Korenman SG. Impotence in diabetic men. Am J Med 1988; 85:147–152.

38. Morley JE, Korenman SG, Kaiser FE, Mooradian AD, Viosca SP. Relationship of penile brachial pressure index to myocardial infaction and cerebrovascular accidents in older men. Am J Med 1988; 84:445–448.

39. Park K, Goldstein I, Andry C, Siroky MB, Krane RJ, Azadzoi KM. Vasculogenic female sexual dysfunction: the hemodynamic basis for vaginal engorgement insufficiency and clitoral erectile insufficiency. Int J Impot Res 1997; 9(1):27–37.

40. Goldstein I, Berman JR. Vasculogenic female sexual dysfunction: vaginal engorgement and clitoral erectile insufficiency syndromes. Int J Impot Res 1998; 10(suppl 2):S84–S90; discussion S98–S101.

41. Sherwin BB, Gelfand MM, Brender W. Androgen enhances sexual motivation in females: a prospective, crossover study of sex steroid administration in the surgical menopause. Psychosom Med 1985; 47:339–351.

42. Sipski ML, Alexander CJ, Rosen RC. Sexual response in women with spinal cord injuries: implications for our understanding of the able-bodied. J Sex Marital Ther 1999; 25:11–22.

43. Sipski ML. Sexual response in women with spinal cord injury: neurologic pathways and recommendations for the use of electrical stimulation. J Spinal Cord Med 2001; 24(3):155–158.

44. Le Mone P. The physical effects of diabetes on sexuality in women. Diabetes Educ 1996; 22(4):361–366.

45. Sarkadi A, Rosenqvist U. Contradictions in the medical encounter: female sexual dysfunction in primary care contacts. Fam Pract 2001; 18(2):161–166.

46. Meston, CM. The psychophysiological assessment of female sexual function. J Sex Educ Ther 2000; 25(1): 6–16.

47. Aksaray G, Yelken B, Kaptanoglu C, Oflu S, Ozaltin M. Sexuality in women with obsessive compulsive disorder. J Sex Marital Ther 2001; 27(3):273–277.

48. Clayton AH. Recognition and assessment of sexual dysfunction associated with depression. J Clin Psychol 2001; 62(suppl 3):5–9.

49. Woosley RL, Flockhart D. A case for the development of Centers for Education and Research in Therapeutics (C.E.R.T.) Pharm Week 1995; 4(23):1 3.

50. Finger WW, Lund M, Slagle MA. Medications that may contribute to sexual disorders. A guide to assessment and treatment in family practice. J Fam Pract 1997; 44(1):33–43.

51. Lewis CE, Freeman HE. The sexual history-taking and counseling practice of primary care physicians. West J Med 1987; 147:165–167.

52. Risen CB. A guide to taking a sexual history. Psychiatr Clin North Am 1995; 18:39–53.

53. Ende J, Rockwell S, Glasgow M. The sexual history in general medicine practice. Arch Intern Med 1984; 144:558–561.

54. Collins A. Landgren BM. Reproductive health, use of estrogen and experience of symptoms in postmenopausal women: a population based study. Maturitas 1994; 20(2):101–111.

55. Burkman RT, Collins JA, Greene RA. Current perspectives on benefits and risks of hormone replacement therapy. Am J Obstet Gynecol 2001; 185(suppl 2):S13–S23.
56. Khurana PS, Khurana C, Hsia J. Hormone replacement therapy for prevention of coronary heart disease: current evidence. Curr Atheroscler Rep 2001; 5:399–403.
57. Montgomery JC, Appleby L, Brincat M, Versi E, Tapp A, Fenwick PB, Studd JW. Effect of oestrogen and testosterone implants on psychological disorders in the climacteric. Lancet 1987; 1:297–299.
58. Shifren JL, Braunstein GD, Simon JA, Casson PR, Buster JE, Redmond GP, Burki RE, Ginsburg ES, Rosen RC, Leiblum SR, Caramelli KE, Mazer NA. Transdermal testosterone treatment in women with impaired sexual function after oophorectomy. N EngL J Med 2000; 343:682–688.
59. Davis SR, Tran J. Testosterone influences libido and well being in women. Trends Endocrinol Metab 2001; 12:33–37.
60. Javanbakht M, Singh AB, Mazer NA, Beall G, Sinha-Hikim I, Shen R, Bhasin S. Pharmacokinetics of a novel testosterone matrix transdermal system in healthy, premenopausal women and women infected with the human immunodeficiency virus. J Clin Endocrinol Metab 2000; 85:2395–2401.
61. Mazer NA. New clinical applications of transdermal testosterone delivery in men and women. J Control Release 2000; 65:303–315.
62. Berman LA, Berman JR, Chhabra S, Goldstein I. Novel approaches to female sexual dysfunction. Expert Opin Invest Drugs 2001; 10(1):85–95.
63. Rako S. Testosterone supplemental therapy after hysterectomy with or without concomitant oophorectomy: estrogen alone is not enough. J Womens Health Gend Based Med 2000; 9:17–23.

6

Hormonal Influence on the Lower Urinary Tract

Dudley Robinson and Linda Cardozo
King's College Hospital, London, England

I. INTRODUCTION

The female genital and lower urinary tract share a common embryological origin, arising from the urogenital sinus. Both are sensitive to the effects of female sex steroid hormones. Estrogen is known to have an important role in the function of the lower urinary tract throughout adult life, with estrogen and progesterone receptors demonstrated in the vagina, urethra, bladder, and pelvic floor musculature (1–4). This is supported by the fact that estrogen defiency occurring following the menopause is known to cause atrophic changes within the urogenital tract (5) and is associated with urinary symptoms such as frequency, urgency, nocturia, incontinence, and recurrent infection. These may also coexist with symptoms of vaginal atrophy such as dyspareunia, itching, burning, and dryness. This chapter will review the role of estrogen and progesterone on lower urinary tract function in addition to assessing the role of estrogens in the management of lower urinary tract dysfunction.

II. ESTROGEN RECEPTORS AND HORMONAL FACTORS

The effects of the steroid hormone 17β-estradiol are mediated by ligand-activated transcription factors known as estrogen receptors. These are glycoproteins and share common features with both androgen and progesterone receptors and can be divided into several functional domains (6). The classic estrogen receptor (ERα) was first discovered by Jensen in 1958 and cloned from uterine tissue in 1986 (7), although it was not until 1996 that the second estrogen receptor (ERβ) was identified (8). The precise role of the two different receptors remains to be elucidated although ERα appears to play a major role in the regulation of reproduction whilst ERβ has a more minor role (9).

Estrogen receptors have been demonstrated throughout the lower urinary tract and are expressed in the squamous epithelium of the proximal and distal urethra, vagina, and trigone of the bladder (3,10), although not in the dome of the bladder, reflecting its different embryological origin. Pubococcygeus and the musculature of the pelvic floor have also been shown to be estrogen sensitive (11), although estrogen receptors have not yet been identified in the levator ani muscles (12).

The distribution of estrogen receptors throughout the urogenital tract has also been studied, with both α and β receptors being found in the vaginal walls and uterosacral ligaments of premenopausal women, although the latter were absent in the vaginal walls of postmenopausal women (13). In addition, α receptors are localized in the urethral sphincter and when sensitised by estrogens are thought to help maintain muscular tone (14).

In addition to estrogen receptors, both androgen and progesterone receptors are expressed in the lower urinary tract although their role is less clear. Progesterone receptors are expressed inconsistently, having been reported in the bladder, trigone, and vagina. Their presence may be dependent on estrogen status (5). While androgen receptors are present in both the bladder and urethra, their role has not yet been defined (15). Interestingly, estrogen receptors have also been identified in mast cells in women with interstitial cystitis (16,17) and in the male lower urinary tract (18).

More recently, the incidence of both estrogen and progesterone expression has been examined throughout the lower urinary tract in 90 women undergoing gynecological surgery; 33 were premenopausal, 26 postmenopausal without hormone replacement therapy (HRT), and 31 postmenopausal and taking HRT (19). Biopsies were taken from the bladder dome, trigone, proximal urethra, distal urethra, vagina, and vesicovaginal fascia adjacent to the bladder neck. Estrogen receptors were found to be consistently expressed in the squamous epithelia, although were absent in the urothelial tissues of the lower urinary tract of all women, irrespective of estrogen status. Progesterone receptor expression, however, showed more variability, being mostly subepithelial, and was significantly lower in postmenopausal women not taking oestrogen replacement therapy.

III. HORMONAL INFLUENCES ON LOWER URINARY TRACT SYMPTOMS

To maintain continence, the urethral pressure must remain higher than the intravesical pressure at all times except during micturition (20). Estrogens play an important role in the continence mechanism, with bladder and urethral function becoming less efficient with age (21). Elderly women have been found to have a reduced flow rate, increased urinary residuals, higher filling pressures, reduced bladder capacity, and lower maximum voiding pressures (22). Estrogens may affect continence by increasing urethral resistance, raising the sensory threshold of the bladder, or increasing α adrenoreceptor sensitivity in the urethral smooth muscle (23,24). In addition, exogenous estrogens have been shown to increase the number of intermediate and superficial cells in the vagina of postmenopausal women (25). These changes have also been demonstrated in the bladder and urethra (26).

More recently, a prospective observational study has been performed to assess cell proliferation rates throughout the tissues of the lower urinary tract (27). Fifty-nine women were studied of whom 23 were premenopausal, 20 were postmenopausal and not taking HRT, and 20 were postmenopausal and taking HRT. Biopsies were taken from the bladder dome, trigone, proximal urethra, distal urethra, vagina, and vesicovaginal fascia adjacent to the bladder neck. The squamous epithelium of oestrogen replete women was shown to exhibit greater levels of cellular proliferation than in those women who were estrogen deficient.

Cyclical variations in the levels of both estrogen and progesterone during the menstrual cycle have been shown to lead to changes in urodynamic variables and lower urinary tract symptoms, with 37% of women noticing a deterioration in symptoms prior to menstruation (28). Measurement of the urethral pressure profile in nulliparous premenopausal women shows there is an increase in functional urethral length midcycle' and early in the luteal phase corresponding to an increase in plasma estradiol (29). Furthermore, progestogens have been associated with an increase in irritative bladder symptoms (30,31) and urinary incontinence in those women taking combined hormone replacement therapy (32). The incidence of detrusor overactivity in the luteal phase of the menstrual cycle may be associated with raised plasma progesterone following ovulation, and progesterone has been shown to antagonize the inhibitory effect of estradiol on rat detrusor contractions (33). This may help to explain the increased prevalence of detrusor overactivity found in pregnancy (34).

The role of estrogen replacement therapy in the prevention of ischemic heart disease has recently been assessed in a 4-year randomized trial, the Heart and Estrogen/Progestin Replacement Study (35). In the study 55% of women reported at least one episode of urinary incontinence each week, and were randomly assigned to oral conjugated estrogen plus medroxyprogesterone acetate or placebo daily. Combined HRT was associated with worsening stress and urge urinary incontinence, although there was no significant difference in daytime frequency, nocturia, or number of urinary tract infections.

Finally, the role of estrogen therapy in the management of women with fecal incontinence has also been investigated in a prospective observational study using symptom questionnaires and anorectal physiological testing before and after 6 months of ERT. At follow-up, 25% of women were asymptomatic and a further 65% were improved in terms of flatus control, urgency, and fecal staining. In addition, anal resting pressures and voluntary squeeze increments were significantly increased following estrogen therapy, although there were no changes in pudendal nerve terminal latency. The authors conclude that estrogen replacement therapy may have a beneficial effect, although larger studies are needed to confirm these findings (36).

IV. HORMONAL INFLUENCES ON URINARY TRACT INFECTION

Urinary tract infection is also a common cause of urinary symptoms in women of all ages. This is a particular problem in the elderly, with a reported incidence of 20% in the community and >50% in institutionalized patients (37,38). Pathophysiological changes such as impairment of bladder emptying, poor perineal hygiene, and both fecal and urinary incontinence may partly account for the high prevalence observed. In addition, changes in the vaginal flora due to estrogen depletion lead to colonization with gram-negative bacilli which in addition to causing local irritive symptoms also act as uropathogens. These microbiological changes may be reversed with estrogen replacement following the menopause, offering a rationale for treatment and prophylaxis.

V. HORMONAL INFLUENCES ON LOWER URINARY TRACT FUNCTION

A. Neurological Control

Sex hormones are known to influence the central neurological control of micturition, although their exact role in the micturition pathway has yet to be elucidated. Estrogen receptors have been demonstrated in the cerebral cortex, limbic system, hippocampus, and cerebellum (39,40), while androgen receptors have been demonstrated in the pontine micturition centre and the preoptic area of the hypothalamus (41).

B. Bladder Function

Estrogen receptors, although absent in the transitional epithelium at the dome of the bladder, are present in the areas of the trigone that have undergone squamous metaplasia (10). Estrogen is known to have a direct effect on detrusor function through modifications in muscarinic receptors (42,43) and by inhibition of movement of extracellular calcium ions into muscle cells (44). Consequently, estradiol has been shown to reduce the amplitude and frequency of spontaneous rhythmic detrusor contractions (45), and there is also evidence that it may increase the sensory threshold of the bladder in some women (46).

C. Urethra

Estrogen receptors have been demonstrated in the squamous epithelium of both the proximal and distal urethra (10), and estrogen has been shown to improve the maturation index of urethral squamous epithelium (47). It has been suggested that estrogen increases urethral closure pressure and improves pressure transmission to the proximal urethra, both promoting continence (48–51). Additionally, estrogens have been shown to cause vasodilatation in the systemic and cerebral circulation, and these changes are also seen in the urethra (52–54).

   The vascular pulsations seen on urethral pressure profilometry secondary to blood flow in the urethral submucosa and urethral sphincter have been shown to increase in size following estrogen administration (55), while the effect is lost following estrogen withdrawal at the menopause. The urethral vascular bed is thought to account for around a third of the urethral closure pressure, and estrogen replacement therapy in postmenopausal women with stress incontinence has been shown to increase the number of periurethral vessels (56).

D. Collagen

Estrogen are known to have an effect on collagen synthesis, and they have been shown to have a direct effect on collagen metabolism in the lower genital tract (57). Changes found in women with urogenital atrophy may represent an alteration in systemic collagenase activity (58), and genuine stress incontinence and urogenital prolapse have been associated with a reduction in both vaginal and periurethral collagen (59–61). Furthermore, there is a reduction in skin collagen content following the menopause (62), with rectus muscle fascia being shown to become less elastic with increasing age, resulting in a lower energy requirement to cause irreversible damage (63). Changes in collagen content have also been identified, the hydroxyproline content in connective tissue from women with stress incontinence being 40% lower than in continent controls (64).

VI. LOWER URINARY TRACT SYMPTOMS

A. Urinary Incontinence

The prevalence of urinary incontinence is known to increase with age, affecting 15–35% of community dwelling women over the age of 60 years (65) and other studies reporting a prevalence of 49% in women over 65 years (66). In addition, rates of 50% have been reported in elderly nursing-home residents (67). A recent cross-sectional population prevalence survey of 146 women aged 15–97 years found that 46% experienced symptoms of pelvic-floor dysfunction defined as stress or urge incontinence, flatus or fecal incontinence, symptomatic prolapse, or previous pelvic-floor surgery (68).

   Little work has been done to examine the incidence of urinary incontinence, although a study in New Zealand of women over the age of 65 years found 10% of the originally continent developed urinary incontinence in the 3-year study period (69).

Epidemiological studies have implicated estrogen deficiency in the etiology of lower urinary tract symptoms, with 70% of women relating the onset of urinary incontinence to their final menstrual period (5). Lower urinary tract symptoms have been shown to be common in postmenopausal women attending a menopause clinic, with 20% complaining of severe urgency and almost 50% complaining of stress incontinence (70). Urge incontinence in particular is more prevalent following the menopause, and the prevalence would appear to rise with increasing years of estrogen deficiency (71). There is, however, conflicting evidence regarding the role of estrogen withdrawal at the time of the menopause. Some studies have shown a peak incidence in perimenopausal women (72,73), while other evidence suggests that many women develop incontinence at least 10 years prior to the cessation of menstruation, with significantly more premenopausal women than postmenopausal women being affected (74).

B. Urogenital Atrophy

Urogenital atrophy is a manifestation of estrogen withdrawal following the menopause, and symptoms may appear for the first time more than 10 years after the last menstrual period (75). In addition, increasing life expectancy has led to an increasingly elderly population, and it is now common for women to spend a third of their lives in the estrogen-deficient postmenopausal state (76), with the average age of the menopause being 50 years (77).

Postmenopausal women comprise 15% of the population in industrialised countries, with a predicted growth rate of 1.5% over the next 20 years. Overall, in the developed world 8% of the total population have been estimated to have urogenital symptoms (78), this representing 200 million women in the United States alone.

It has been estimated that 10–40% of all postmenopausal women are symptomatic (79), although only 25% are thought to seek medical help. In addition, two out of three women report vaginal symptoms associated with urogenital atrophy by the age of 75 years (80). However, the prevalence of symptomatic urogenital atrophy is difficult to estimate since many women accept the changes as being an inevitable consequence of the aging process and thus do not seek help leading to considerable under reporting.

A study assessing the prevalence of urogenital symptoms in 2157 Dutch women has been recently reported (81). Overall, 27% of women complained of vaginal dryness, soreness, and dyspareunia, while the prevalence of urinary symptoms such as leakage and recurrent infections was 36%. When considering severity, almost 50% reported moderate to severe discomfort, although only a third had received medical intervention. Interestingly, women who had previously had a hysterectomy reported moderate to severe discomfort more often than those who had not.

The prevalence of urogenital atrophy and urogenital prolapse has also been examined in a population of 285 women attending a menopause clinic (82). Overall, 51% of women were found to have anterior vaginal wall prolapse, 27% posterior vaginal prolapse, and 20% apical prolapse. In addition, 34% of women were noted to have urogenital atrophy, 40% complaining of dyspareunia. While urogenital atrophy and symptoms of dyspareunia were related to menopausal age, the prevalence of prolapse showed no association.

However, while urogenital atrophy is an inevitable consequence of the menopause, women may not always be symptomatic. A recent study of 69 women attending a gynecology clinic were asked to fill out a symptom questionnaire prior to examination and undergoing vaginal cytology (83). Urogenital symptoms were found to be relatively low and were poorly correlated with age and physical examination findings although not with vaginal cytological maturation index. Women who were taking estrogen replacement therapy had higher symptom scores and physical examination scores.

From this evidence it would appear that urogenital atrophy is a universal consequence of the menopause, although elderly women may be minimally symptomatic. Hence, treatment should not be the only indication for replacement therapy.

VII.   MANAGEMENT OF LOWER URINARY DYSFUNCTION

A.   Estrogens in the Management of Incontinence

Estrogen preparations have been used for many years in the treatment of urinary incontinence (84,85), although their precise role remains controversial. Many of the studies performed have been uncontrolled observational series examining the use of a wide range of different preparations, doses, and routes of administration. The inconsistent use of progestogens to provide endometrial protection is a further confounding factor, making interpretation of the results difficult. To clarify the situation a meta-analysis from the Hormones and Urogenital Therapy (HUT) committee has been reported (86). Of 166 articles identified that were published in English between 1969 and 1992, only six were controlled trials and 17 were uncontrolled series. Meta-analysis found an overall significant effect of estrogen therapy on subjective improvement in all subjects and for subjects with urodynamic stress incontinence alone. Subjective improvement rates with estrogen therapy in randomized controlled trials ranged from 64% to 75%, although placebo groups also reported an improvement of 10–56%. In uncontrolled series subjective improvement rates were 8–89%, with subjects with urodynamic stress incontinence showing improvement of 34–73%. However, when assessing objective fluid loss, there was no significant effect. Maximum urethral closure pressure was found to increase significantly with estrogen therapy, although this outcome was influenced by a single study showing a large effect (87).

B.   Estrogens in the Management of Stress Incontinence

In addition to the studies included in the HUT meta-analysis, several authors have also investigated the role of estrogen therapy in the management of urodynamic stress incontinence only (Table 1). Oral estrogens have been reported to increase the maximum urethral pressures and lead to symptomatic improvement in 65–70% of women (88,89), although other work has not confirmed this (90,91). More recently, two placebo-controlled studies have been performed examining the use of oral estrogens in the treatment of urodynamic stress incontinence in postmenopausal women. Neither conjugated equine estrogens and medroxyprogesterone (92)

Table 1   Summary of Randomized Controlled Trials Assessing the Use of Estrogens in the Management of Urinary Incontinence

Study	Year	Type of incontinence	Estrogen	Route
Henalla et al. (87)	1989	Stress incontinence	Conjugated estrogen	Vaginal
Hilton et al. (96)	1990	Stress incontinence	Conjugated estrogen	Vaginal
Beisland et al. (95)	1984	Stress incontinence	Estriol	Vaginal
Judge (120)	1969	Mixed incontinence	Quinestradol	Oral
Kinn and Lindskog (121)	1988	Stress incontinence	Estriol	Oral
Samsioe et al. (97)	1985	Mixed incontinence	Estriol	Oral
Walter et al. (91)	1978	Urge incontinence	Estradiol and estriol	Oral
Walter et al. (122)	1990	Stress incontinence	Estriol	Oral
Wilson et al. (90)	1987	Stress incontinence	Piperazine estrone sulfate	Oral

nor unopposed estradiol valerate (93) showed a significant difference in either subjective or objective outcomes. Furthermore, a review of eight controlled and 14 uncontrolled prospective trials concluded that estrogen therapy was not an efficacious treatment for stress incontinence but may be useful for symptoms of urgency and frequency (94).

From the available evidence estrogen does not appear to be an effective treatment for stress incontinence, although it may have a synergistic role in combination therapy. Two placebo-controlled studies have examined the use of oral and vaginal estrogens with the α-adrenergic agonist phenylpropanolamine used separately and in combination. Both studies found that combination therapy was superior to either drug given alone, although while there was subjective improvement in all groups (95), there was only objective improvement in the combination therapy group (96). This may offer an alternative conservative treatment for women who have mild urodynamic stress incontinence.

Estrogens have been used in the treatment of urinary urgency and urge incontinence for many years, although there have been few controlled trials to confirm their efficacy (Table 1). A double-blind placebo controlled crossover study using oral estriol in 34 postmenopausal women produced subjective improvement in eight women with mixed incontinence and 12 with urge incontinence (97). However, a double-blind multicenter study of the use of estriol (3 mg/d) in postmenopausal women complaining of urgency has failed to confirm these findings (98), showing both subjective and objective improvement but not significantly better than placebo. Estriol is a naturally occurring weak estrogen that has little effect on the endometrium and does not prevent osteoporosis although it has been used in the treatment of urogenital atrophy. Consequently, it is possible that either the dosage or route of administration in this study was not appropriate in the treatment of urinary symptoms, and higher systemic levels may be required.

The use of sustained release 17β-estradiol vaginal tablets (Vagifem, Novo Nordisk) has also been examined in postmenopausal women with urgency and urge incontinence or a urodynamic diagnosis of sensory urgency or detrusor overactivity. These vaginal tablets have been shown to be well absorbed from the vagina and to induce maturation of the vaginal epithelium within 14 days (99). However, following a 6-month course of treatment, the only significant difference between active and placebo groups was an improvement in the symptom of urgency in those women with a urodynamic diagnosis of sensory urgency (100). A further double-blind, randomized, placebo-controlled trial of vaginal 17β-estradiol vaginal tablets has shown lower urinary tract symptoms of frequency, urgency, urge, and stress incontinence to be significantly improved, although no objective urodynamic assessment was performed (101). In both of these studies the subjective improvement in symptoms may simply represent local estrogenic effects reversing urogenital atrophy rather than a direct effect on bladder function.

More recently a randomized, parallel-group, controlled trial has been reported comparing the estradiol-releasing vaginal ring (Estring, Pharmacia, Uppsala, Sweden) with estriol vaginal pessaries in the treatment of postmenopausal women with bothersome lower urinary tract symptoms (102). Low-dose vaginally administered estradiol and estriol were found to be equally efficacious in alleviating lower urinary tract symptoms of urge incontinence (58% vs. 58%), stress incontinence (53% vs. 59%), and nocturia (51% vs. 54%), although the vaginal ring was found to have greater patient acceptability.

To try to clarify the role of estrogen therapy in the management of women with urge incontinence, a meta-analysis of the use of estrogen in women with symptoms of "overactive bladder" has been reported by the HUT committee (103). In a review of 10 randomized placebo-controlled trials, estrogen was found to be superior to placebo when considering symptoms of urge incontinence, frequency, and nocturia, although vaginal estrogen administration was found to be superior for symptoms of urgency. In those taking estrogens there was also a significant increase in first sensation and bladder capacity as compared to placebo.

C.   Estrogens in the Management of Recurrent Urinary Tract Infection

Estrogen therapy has been shown to increase vaginal pH and reverse the microbiological changes that occur in the vagina following the menopause (104). Initial small uncontrolled studies using oral or vaginal estrogens in the treatment of recurrent urinary tract infection appeared to give promising results (105,106), although unfortunately this has not been supported by larger randomized trials. Several studies have been performed examining the use of oral and vaginal estrogens although these have had mixed results (Table 2).

Kjaergaard and colleagues (107) compared vaginal estriol tablets with placebo in 21 postmenopausal women over a 5-month period and found no significant difference between the two groups. However, a subsequent randomized, double-blind, placebo-controlled study assessing the use of estriol vaginal cream in 93 postmenopausal women during an 8-month period did reveal a significant effect (108).

Kirkengen randomized 40 postmenopausal women to receive either placebo or oral estriol and found that although initially both groups had a significantly decreased incidence of recurrent infections, after 12 weeks estriol was shown to be significantly more effective (109). However, these findings were not confirmed subsequently in a trial of 72 postmenopausal women with recurrent urinary tract infections randomized to oral estriol or placebo. Following a 6-month treatment period and a further 6-month follow-up estriol was found to be no more effective than placebo (110).

More recently a randomized, open, parallel-group study assessing the use of an estradiol-releasing silicone vaginal ring (Estring; Pharmacia, Uppsala, Sweden) in postmenopausal women with recurrent infections has been performed which showed the cumulative likelihood of remaining infection free was 45% in the active group and 20% in the placebo group (111). Estring was also shown to decrease the number of recurrences per year and to prolong the interval between infection episodes.

D.   Estrogens in the Management of Urogenital Atrophy

Symptoms of urogenital atrophy do not occur until the levels of endogenous estrogen are lower than that required to promote endometrial proliferation (112). Consequently, it is possible to use a low dose of estrogen replacement therapy in order to alleviate urogenital symptoms while avoiding the risk of endometrial proliferation and removing the necessity of providing endometrial protection with progestogens (113). The dose of estradiol commonly used in systemic estrogen replacement is usually $25-100$ µg, although studies investigating the use of estrogens in the management of urogenital symptoms have shown that $8-10$ µg of vaginal estradiol is effective (114). Thus, only $10-30\%$ of the dose used to treat vasomotor symptoms may be effective in the management of urogenital symptoms. Since $10-25\%$ of women receiving systemic HRT still experience the symptoms of urogenital atrophy (115), low-dose local preparations may have an additional beneficial effect.

A recent review of estrogen therapy in the management of urogenital atrophy has been performed by the HUT committee (116). Ten randomized trials and 54 uncontrolled series were examined from 1969 to 1995 assessing 24 different treatment regimens. Meta-analysis of 10 placebo-controlled trials confirmed the significant effect of estrogens in the management of urogenital atrophy (Table 3).

The route of administration was assessed, and oral, vaginal, and parenteral (transcutaneous patches and subcutaneous implants) were compared. Overall, the vaginal route of administration was found to correlate with better symptom relief, greater improvement in cytological findings, and higher serum estradiol levels.

Table 2 Summary of Randomized Controlled Trials Assessing the Use of Estrogens in the Management of Recurrent Lower Urinary Tract

Study	Study group	Type of estrogen	Route of delivery	Duration of therapy	Results
Kjaergaard et al. 1990 (107)	21 postmenopausal women with recurrent cystitis 10 active group 11 placebo	Estradiol	Vaginal tablets	5 months	Number of positive cultures not statistically different between the two groups.
Kirkengen et al. 1992 (109)	40 postmenopausal women with recurrent UTIs 20 active group 20 placebo	Estriol	Oral	12 weeks	Both estriol and placebo significantly reduced the incidence of UTIs ($P < .05$). After 12 weeks estriol was significantly more effective than placebo ($P < .05$).
Raz and Stamm 1993 (108)	93 postmenopausal women with recurrent UTIs 50 active group 43 placebo	Estriol	Vaginal cream	8 months	Significant reduction in the incidence of UTIs in the group given estriol compared to placebo ($P < .001$).
Cardozo et al. 1998 (110)	72 postmenopausal women with recurrent UTIs 36 active group 36 placebo	Estriol	Oral	6-month treatment period with a further 6 months follow-up	Reduction in urinary symptoms and incidence of UTIs in both groups. Estriol no better than placebo.
Eriksen 1999 (111)	108 women with recurrent UTIs 53 active group 55 no treatment	Estradiol	Estring	36 weeks for the active group 36 weeks or until first recurrence for the controls	Cumulative likelihood of remaining free of infection was 45% in active group and 20% in control group ($P = .008$).

Table 3 Summary of Randomized Controlled Trials Assessing the Use of Estrogens in Urogenital Atrophy

Study	Year	Estrogen	Route
Bellatoni et al. (123)	1991	Estradiol	Transdermal
Campbell et al. (124)	1977	Conjugated estrogen	Oral
Campbell et al. (124)	1977	Conjugated estrogen	Oral
Erikson and Ramussen (101)	1992	Estradiol	Pessary
Felding et al. (125)	1992	Estradiol	Pessary
Foidart et al. (126)	1991	Estriol	Vaginal cream
Laufer et al. (127)	1983	Estradiol	Transdermal
Mettler and Olsen (113)	1991	Estradiol	Pessary
Molander et al. (128)	1990	Estriol	Oral
Raz and Stamm (108)	1993	Estriol	Vaginal cream
Van der Linden et al. (129)	1993	Estriol	Oral

With regard to the type of estrogen preparation estradiol was found to be most effective in reducing patient symptoms, although conjugated estrogens produced the most cytological change and the greatest increase in serum levels of estradiol and estrone.

Finally, the effect of different dosages was examined. Low-dose vaginal estradiol was found to be the most efficacious according to symptom relief, although oral estriol was also effective. Estriol had no effect on the serum levels of estradiol or estrone, while vaginal estriol had minimal effect. Vaginal estradiol was found to have a small effect on serum estrogen, although not as great as systemic preparations. In conclusion, it would appear that estrogen is efficacious in the treatment of urogenital atrophy, and low-dose vaginal preparations are as effective as systemic therapy.

More recently, the use of a continuous low dose estradiol-releasing silicone vaginal ring (Estring; Pharmacia, Uppsala, Sweden) releasing estradiol $5-10$ $\mu g/24$ h has been investigated in postmenopausal women with symptomatic urogenital atrophy (111). There was a significant effect on symptoms of vaginal dryness, pruritis vulvae, dyspareunia, and urinary urgency with improvement being reported in $>90\%$ of women in an uncontrolled study; the maturation of vaginal epithelium was also significantly improved. The patient acceptability was high, and while the maturation of vaginal epithelium was significantly improved, there was no effect on endometrial proliferation.

These findings were supported by a 1-year multicenter study of Estring in postmenopausal women with urogenital atrophy that found subjective and objective improvement in 90% of patients up to 1 year. However, there was a 20% withdrawal rate with 7% of women reporting vaginal irritation, two having vaginal ulceration, and three complaining of vaginal bleeding although there were no cases of endometrial proliferation (117). Long-term safety has been confirmed by a 10-year review of the use of the estradiol ring delivery system that has found its safety, efficacy, and acceptability to be comparable to other forms of vaginal administration (118). A comparative study of safety and efficacy of Estring with conjugated equine estrogen vaginal cream in 194 postmenopausal women complaining of urogenital atrophy found no significant difference in vaginal dryness, dyspareunia, or resolution of atrophic signs between the two treatment groups. Furthermore, there were similar improvement in the vaginal mucosal maturation index and a reduction in pH in both groups, with the vaginal ring being found to be preferable to the cream (119).

VIII.   CONCLUSIONS

Estrogens are known to have an important physiological effect on the female lower genital tract throughout adult life, leading to symptomatic, histological, and functional changes. Urogenital atrophy is the manifestation of estrogen withdrawal following the menopause, presenting with vaginal and/or urinary symptoms. The use of estrogen replacement therapy has been examined in the management of lower urinary tract symptoms as well as in the treatment of urogenital atrophy, although only recently has it been subjected to randomized placebo-controlled trials and meta-analysis.

Estrogen therapy alone has been shown to have little effect in the management of urodynamic stress incontinence, although when used in combination with an α-adrenergic agonists it may lead to an improvement in urinary leakage. When considering the irritive symptoms of urinary urgency, frequency, and urge incontinence, estrogen therapy may be of benefit, although this may simply represent reversal of urogenital atrophy rather than a direct effect on the lower urinary tract. The role of estrogen replacement therapy in the management of women with recurrent lower urinary tract infection remains to be determined although there is now some evidence that vaginal administration may be efficacious. Finally, low-dose vaginal estrogens have been shown to be have a role in the treatment of urogenital atrophy in postmenopausal women and would appear to be as effective as systemic preparations.

REFERENCES

1.   Cardozo LD. Role of oestrogens in the treatment of female urinary incontinence. J Am Geriatr Soc 1990; 38:326–328.
2.   Iosif S, Batra S, Ek A, Astedt B. Oestrogens receptors in the human female lower urinary tract. Am J Obstet Gynecol 1981; 141:817–820.
3.   Batra SC, Fossil CS. Female urethra, a target for oestrogen action. J Urol 1983; 129:418–420.
4.   Batra SC, Iosif LS. Progesterone receptors in the female urinary tract. J Urol 1987; 138:130–134.
5.   Iosif C, Bekassy Z. Prevalence of genitourinary symptoms in the late menopause. Acta Obstet Gynaecol Scand 1984; 63:257–260.
6.   Beato M, Herrich P, Schutz G. Steroid hormone receptors: many actors in search of a plot. Cell 1995; 83:851–857.
7.   Green S, Walter P, Kumar V. Human oestrogen receptor cDNA: sequence, expression and homology to v-erbA. Nature 1986; 320:134–139.
8.   Kuiper G, Enmark E, Pelto-Huikko M, Nilsson S, Gustafsson J-A. Cloning of a novel oestrogen receptor expressed in rat prostate and ovary. Proc Natl Acad Sci USA 1996; 93:5925–5930.
9.   Warner M, Nilsson S, Gustafsson JA. The oestrogen receptor family. Curr Opin Obstet Gynecol 1999; 11:249–254.
10.   Blakeman PJ, Hilton P, Bulmer JN. Mapping oestrogen and progesterone receptors throughout the female lower urinary tract. Neurourol Urodyn 1996; 15:324–325.
11.   Ingelman-Sundberg A, Rosen J, Gustafsson SA. Cytosol oestrogen receptors in urogenital tissues in stress incontinent women. Acta Obstet Gynecol Scand 1981; 60:585–586.
12.   Bernstein IT. The pelvic floor muscles: muscle thickness in healthy and urinary-incontinent women measured by perineal ultasonography with reference to the effect of pelvic floor training. Oestrogen receptor studies. Neurourol Urodyn 1997; 16(4):237–275.
13.   Chen GD, Oliver RH, Leung BS, Lin LY, Yeh J. Oestrogen receptor α and β expression in the vaginal walls and uterosacral ligaments of premenopausal and postmenopausal women. Fertil Steril 1999; 71(6):1099–1102.
14.   Screiter F, Fuchs P, Stockamp K. Oestrogenic sensitivity of α receptors in the urethral musculature. Urol Int 1976; 31:13–19.

15. Blakeman PJ, Hilton P, Bulmer JN. Androgen receptors in the female lower urinary tract. Int Urogynaecol J 1997; 8:S54.
16. Pang X, Cotreau-Bibbo MM, Sant GR, Theoharides TC. Bladder mast cell expression of high affinity oestrogen receptors in receptors in patients with interstitial cystitis. Br J Urol 1995; 75:154–161.
17. Letourneau R, Pang X, Sant GR, Theoharides TC. Intragranular activation of bladder mast cells and their association with nerve processes in interstitial cystitis. Br J Urol 1996; 77:41–54.
18. Bodker A, Balsev E, Juul BR. Oestrogen receptors in the human male bladder, prostatic urethra and prostate. Scand J Urol Nephrol 1995; 29:161–165.
19. Blakeman PJ, Hilton P, Bulmer JN. Oestrogen and progesterone receptor expression in the female lower urinary tract, with reference to oestrogen status. Br J Urol Int 2000; 86:32–38.
20. Abrams P, Blaivas JG, Stanton SL. The standardisation of terminology of lower urinary tract dysfunction. Br J Obstet Gynaecol 1990; 97:1–16.
21. Rud T, Anderson KE, Asmussen M. Factors maintaining the urethral pressure in women. Invest Urol 1980; 17:343–347.
22. Malone-Lee J. Urodynamic measurement and urinary incontinence in the elderly. In: Brocklehurst JC, ed. Managing and Measuring Incontinence. Proceedings of the Geriatric Workshop on Incontinence, July 1988.
23. Versi E, Cardozo LD. Oestrogens and lower urinary tract function. In: Studd JWW, Whitehead MI, eds. The Menopause. Oxford: Blackwell Scientific Publications, 1988:76–84.
24. Kinn AC, Lindskog M. Oestrogens and phenylpropanolamine in combination for stress incontinence. Urology 1988; 32:273–280.
25. Smith PJB. The effect of oestrogens on bladder function in the female. In: Campbell S, ed. The Management of the Menopause and Postmenopausal Years. Carnforth: MTP, 1976:291–298.
26. Samsioe G, Jansson I, Mellstrom D, Svandborg A. Occurance, nature and treatment of urinary incontinence in a 70 year old female population. Maturitas 1985; 7:335–342.
27. Blakeman PJ, Hilton P, Bulmer JN. Cellular proliferation in the female lower urinary tract with reference to oestrogen status. Br J Obstet Gynaecol 1996; 8:813–816.
28. Hextall A, Bidmead J, Cardozo L, Hooper R. Hormonal influences on the human female lower urinary tract: a prospective evaluation of the effects of the menstrual cycle on symptomatology and the results of urodynamic investigation. Neurourol Urodyn 1999; 18(4):282–283.
29. Van Geelen JM, Doesburg WH, Thomas CMG. Urodynamic studies in the normal menstrual cycle: the relationship between hormonal changes during the menstrual cycle and the urethral pressure profile. Am J Obstet Gynaecol 1981; 141:384–392.
30. Burton G, Cardozo LD, Abdalla H, Kirkland A, Studd JWW. The hormonal effects on the lower urinary tract in 282 women with premature ovarian failure. Neurourol Urodyn 1992; 10:318–319.
31. Cutner A, Burton G, Cardozo LD, Wise BG, Abbot D, Studd JWW. Does progesterone cause an irritable bladder? Int Urogynaecol J 1993; 4:259–261.
32. Benness C, Gangar K, Cardozo LD, Cutner A. Do progestogens exacerbate urinary incontinence in women on HRT? Neurourol Urodyn 1991; 10:316–318.
33. Elliot RA, Castleden CM. Effect of progestagens and oestrogens on the contractile response of rat detrusor muscle to electrical field stimulation. Clin Sci 1994; 87:342.
34. Cutner A. The urinary tract in pregnancy. MD thesis, University of London, 1993.
35. Grady D, Brown JS, Vittinghoff E, Applegate W, Varner E, Synder T. Postmenopausal hormones and incontinence: the Heart and Estrogen/Progestin Replacement Study. Obstet Gynaecol 2001; 97:116–120.
36. Donnelly V, O'Connell PR, O'Herlihy C. The influence of hormonal replacement on faecal incontinence in post menopausal women. Br J Obstet Gynaecol 1997; 104:311–315.
37. Sandford JP. Urinary tract symptoms and infection. Annu Rev Med 1975; 26:485–505.
38. Boscia JA, Kaye D. Assymptomatic bacteria in the elderly. Infect Dis Clin North Am 1987; 1:893–903.
39. Maggi A, Perez J. Role of female gonadal hormones in the CNS. Life Sci 1985; 37:893–906.
40. Smith SS, Berg G, Hammar M, eds. The Modern Management of the Menopause. Hormones, Mood and Neurobiology—A Summary. Carnforth, UK: Parthenon Publishing, 1993:204.

41. Block EFM, Holstege G. Androgen receptor immunoreactive neurones in the hypothalamic preoptic area project to the pontine micturition centre in the male cat. Neurourol Urodyn 1998; 17(4):404–405.

42. Shapiro E. Effect of oestrogens on the weight and muscarinic receptor density of the rabbit bladder and urethra J Urol 1986; 135:1084–1087.

43. Batra S, Anderson KE. Oestrogen induced changes in muscarinic receptor density and contractile responses in the female rat urinary bladder. Acta Physiol Scand 1989; 137:135–141.

44. Elliott RA, Castleden CM, Miodrag A, Kirwan P. The direct effects of diethylstilboestrol and nifedipine on the contractile responses of isolated human and rat detrusor muscles. Eur J Clin Pharmacol 1992; 43:149–155.

45. Shenfield OZ, Blackmore PF, Morgan CW, Schlossberg SM, Jordan GH, Ratz PH. Rapid effects of oestriol and progesterone on tone and spontaneous rhythmic contractions of the rabbit bladder. Neurourol Urodyn 1998; 17(4):408–409.

46. Fantl JA, Wyman JF, Anderson RL. Post menopausal urinary incontinence. comparison between non-oestrogen and oestrogen supplemented women. Obstet Gynaecol 1988; 71:823–828.

47. Bergman A, Karram MM, Bhatia NN. Changes in urethral cytology following oestrogen administration. Gynaecol Obstet Invest 1990; 29:211–213.

48. Rud T. The effects of oestrogens and gestogens on the urethral pressure profile in urinary continent and stress incontinent women. Acta Obstet Gynaecol Scand 1980; 59:365–370.

49. Hilton P, Stanton SL. The use of intravaginal oestrogen cream in genuine stress incontinence. Br J Obstet Gynaecol 1983; 90:940–944.

50. Bhatia NN, Bergman, A, Karram MM. Effects of oestrogen on urethral function in women with urinary incontinence. Am J Obstet Gynecol 1989; 160:176–180.

51. Karram MM, Yeko TR, Sauer MV. Urodynamic changes following hormone replacement therapy in women with premature ovarian failure. Obstet Gynaecol 1989; 74:208–211.

52. Ganger KF, Vyas S, Whitehead RW. Pulsitility index in the internal carotid artery in relation to transdermal oestradiol and time since the menopause. Lancet 1991; 338:839–842.

53. Jackson S, Vyas S. A double blind, placebo controlled study of postmenopausal oestrogen replacement therapy and carotid artery pulsatility index. Br J Obstet Gynaecol 1998; 105(4):408–412.

54. Penotti M, Farina M, Sironi L. Long term effects of postmenopausal hormone replacement therapy on pulsatility index of the internal carotid and middle cerebral arteries. Menopause 1997; 4(2):101–104.

55. Versi E, Cardozo LD. Urethral instability: diagnosis based on variations in the maximum urethral pressure in normal climateric women. Neurourol Urodyn 1986; 5:535–541.

56. Girao MJ, Jarmy-Di Bella ZI, Sartori MG, Baracat EC, Lima GR. Doppler velocimetry parameters of periurethral vessels in postmenopausal incontinent women receiving oestrogen replacement. Int Urogynaecol 2001; 12:241–246.

57. Falconer C, Ekman-Ordeberg G, Ulmsten U. Changes in paraurethral connective tissue at menopause are counteracted oestrogen. Mauturitas 1996; 24:197–204.

58. Kushner L, Chen Y, Desautel M, Moak S, Greenwald R, Badlani G. Collagenase activity is elevated in conditioned media from fibroblasts of women with pelvic floor weakening. Int Urogynaecol 1999; 10(S1):34.

59. Jackson S, Avery N, Shepherd A. The effect of oestradiol on vaginal collagen in postmenopausal women with stress urinary incontinence. Nurourol Urodyn 1996; 15:327–328.

60. James M, Avery N, Jackson S, Bailey A, Abrams P. The pathophysiological changes of vaginal skin tissue in women with stress urinary incontinence: a controlled trial. Int Urogynaecol 1999; 10(S1):35.

61. James M, Avery N, Jackson S, Bailey A, Abrams P. The biochemical profile of vaginal tissue in women with genitourinary prolapse: a controlled trial. Neurourol Urodyn 1999; 18(4):284–285.

62. Brincat M, Moniz CF, Studd JWW. Long term effects of the menopause and sex hormones on skin thickness. Br J Obstet Gynaecol 1985; 92:256–259.

63. Landon CR, Smith ARB, Crofts CE, Trowbridge EA. Biochemical properties of connective tissue in women with stress incontinence of urine. Neurourol Urodynam 1989; 8:369–370.

64. Ulmsten U, Ekman G, Giertz G. Different biochemical composition of connective tissue in continent and stress incontinent women. Acta Obstet Gynaecol Scand 1987; 66:455.
65. Diokno AC, Brook BM, Brown MB. Prevalence of urinary incontinence and other ueological symptoms in the non-institutionalised elderly. J Urol 1986; 136:1022.
66. Yarnell J, Voyle G, Richards C, Stephenson T. The prevalence and severity of urinary incontinence in women. J Epidemiol Community Health 1981; 35:71–74.
67. Ouslander JG. Urinary incontinence in nursing homes. J Am Geriatr Soc 1990; 38:289–291.
68. MacLennan AH, Taylor AW, Wilson AW, Wilson D. The prevalence of pelvic floor disorders and their relationship to gender, age, parity, and mode of delivery. Br J Obstet Gynaecol 2000; 107:1460–1470.
69. Kok AL, Voorhorst FJ, Burger CW, Van Houten P, Kenemans P, Jannsens J. Urinary and faecal incontinence in community residing elderly women. Age Ageing 1992; 21:211.
70. Cardozo LD, Tapp A, Versi E, Samsioe G, Bonne Erickson P. The lower urinary tract in peri- and postmenopausal women. In: The Urogenital Defiency Syndrome. Bagsverd, Denmark: Novo Industri AS, 1987:10–17.
71. Kondo A, Kato K, Saito M. Prevalence of hand washing incontinence in females in comparison with stress and urge incontinence. Neurourol Urodyn 1990; 9:330–331.
72. Thomas TM, Plymat KR, Blannin J. Prevalence of urinary incontinence. BMJ 1980; 281:1243–1245.
73. Jolleys JV. Reported prevalence of urinary incontinence in a general practice. BMJ 1988; 296:1300–1302.
74. Burgio KL, Matthews KA, Engel B. Prevalence, incidence and correlates of urinary incontinence in healthy, middle aged women. J Urol 1991; 146:1255–1259.
75. Iosif CS. Effects of protracted administration of oestrol on the lower genitourinary tract in postmenopausal women. Acta Obstet Gynaecol Scand 1992; 251:115–120.
76. American National Institute of Health Population Figures. U.S. Treasury Dep. NIH. 1991.
77. Research on the menopause in the 1990's. Report or a WHO Scientific Group. In: WHO Technical Report Series 866. Geneva: WHO, 1994.
78. Barlow D, Samsioe G, Van Greelan H. Prevalence of urinary problems in European countries. Maturitas 1997; 27:239–248.
79. Greendale GA, Judd JL. The menopause: health implications and clinical management. J Am Geriatr Soc 1993; 41:426–436.
80. Samsioe G, Jansson I, Mellstrom D, Svanborg A. The occurrence, nature and treatment of urinary incontinence in a 70 year old population. Mauturitas 1985; 7:335–343.
81. Van Geelen JM, Van de Weijer PH, Arnolds HT. Urogenital symptoms and resulting discomfort in non-institutionalised Dutch women aged 50–75 years. Int Urogynecol J Pelvic Floor Dysfunct 2000; 11(1):9–14.
82. Versi E, Harvey MA, Cardozo L, Brincat M, Studd JW. Urogenital prolapse and atrophy at menopause: a prevalence study. Int Urogynaecol J Pelvic Dysfunct 2001; 12(2):107–110.
83. Davila GW, Karapanagiotou I, Woodhouse S, Singh A, Huber K, Zimberg S, Seiler J. Are women with urogenital artophy syymptomatic? Obstet Gynaecol 2001; 97(4 suppl 1):S48.
84. Salmon UL, Walter RI, Gast SH. The use of oestrogen in the treatment of dysuria and incontinence in postmenopausal women. Am J Obstet Gynaecol 1941; 14:23–31.
85. Youngblood VH, Tomlin EM, Davis JB. Senile urethritis in women. J Urol 1957; 78:150–152.
86. Fantl JA, Cardozo LD, McClish DK, HUT. Committee. Oestrogen therapy in the management of incontinence in postmenopausal women: a meta-analysis. First report of the Hormones and Urogenital Therapy Committee. Obstet Gynaecol 1994; 83:12–18.
87. Henalla SM, Hutchins CJ, Robinson P, Macivar J. Non-operative methods in the treatment of female genuine stress incontinence of urine. Br J Obstet Gynaecol 1989; 9:222–225.
88. Caine M, Raz S. The role of female hormones in stress incontinence. In: Proceedings of the 16th Congress of the International Society of Urology, Amsterdam, Netherlands.
89. Rud T. The effects of oestrogen and gestagens on the urethral pressure profile in urinary continent and stress incontinent women. Acta Obstet Gynaecol Scand 1980; 59:265–270.

90. Wilson PD, Faragher B, Butler B, Bullock D, Robinson EL, Brown ADG. Treatment with oral piperazine oestrone sulphate for genuine stress incontinence in postmenopausal women. Br J Obstet Gynaecol 1987; 94:568–574.

91. Walter S, Wolf H, Barlebo H, Jansen H. Urinary incontinence in postmenopausal women treated with oestrogens: a double-blind clinical trial. Urology 1978; 33:135–143.

92. Fantl JA, Bump RC, Robinson D. Efficacy of oestrogen supplementation in the treatment of urinary incontinence. Obstet Gynaecol 1996; 88:745–749.

93. Jackson S, Shepherd A, Brookes S, Abrams P. The effect of oestrogen supplementation on post-menopausal urinary stress incontinence: a double-blind, placebo controlled trial. Br J Obstet Gynaecol 1999; 106:711–718.

94. Sultana CJ, Walters MD. Oestrogen and urinary incontinence in women. Maturitas 1995; 20:129–138.

95. Beisland HO, Fossberg E, Moer A. Urethral insufficiency in post-menopausal females: treatment with phenylpropanolamine and oestriol scparately and in combination. Urol Int 1984; 39:211–216.

96. Hilton P, Tweddel AL, Mayne C. Oral and intravaginal oestrogens alone and in combination with alpha adrenergic stimulation in genuine stress incontinence. Int Urogynecol J 1990; 12:80–86.

97. Samsicoe G, Jansson I, Mellstrom D, Svanberg A. Urinary incontinence in 75 year old women. Effects of oestriol. Acta Obstet Gynaecol Scand 1985; 93:57.

98. Cardozo LD, Rekers H, Tapp A. Oestriol in the treatment of postmenopausal urgency: a multicentre study. Maturitas 1993; 18:47–53.

99. Nilsson K, Heimer G. Low does oestradiol in the treatment of urogenital oestrogen deficiency—a pharmacokinetic and pharamacodynamic study. Maturitas 1992; 15:121–127.

100. Benncss C, Wise BG, Cutner A, Cardozo LD. Does low does vaginal oestradiol improve frequency and urgency in postmenopausal women. Int Urogynecol J 1992; 3(2):281.

101. Eriksen PS, Rasmussen H. Low does 17β-oestradiol tablets in the treatment of atrophic vaginitis: a double-blind placebo controlled study. Eur J Obstet Gynaecol Reprod Biol 1992; 44:137–144.

102. Lose G, Englev E. Oestradiol-releasing vaginal ring versus oestriol vaginal pessaries in the treatment of bothersome lower tract symptoms. Br J Obstet Gynaecol 2000; 107:1029–1034.

103. HUT Committee, 2001. Unpublished.

104. Brandberg A, Mellstrom D, Samsioe G. Low dose oral oestriol treatment in elderly women with urogenital infections. Acta Obstet Gynaecol Scand 1987; 140:33–38.

105. Parsons CL, Schmidt JD. Control of recurrent urinary tract infections in postmenopausal women. J Urol 1982; 128:1224–1226.

106. Privette M, Cade R, Peterson J. Prevention of recurrent urinary tract infections in postmenopausal women. Nephron 1988; 50:24–27.

107. Kjaergaard B, Walter S, Knudsen A. Treatment with low dose vaginal oestradiol in postmenopausal women. A double blind controlled trial. Ugeskar Laeger 1990; 152:658–659.

108. Raz R, Stamm WE. A controlled trial of intravaginal oestriol in postmenopausal women with recurrent urinary tract infections. N Engl J Med 1993; 329:753–756.

109. Kirkengen AL, Anderson P, Gjersoe E. Oestriol in the prophylactic treatment of recurrent urinary tract infections in postmenopausal women. Scand J Prim Health Care 1992; 10:142.

110. Cardozo LD, Benness C, Abbott D. Low dose oestrogen prophylaxis for recurrent urinary tract infections in elderly women. Br J Obstet Gynaecol 1998; 105:403–407.

111. Eriksen B. A randomised, open, parallel-group study on the preventitive effect of an oestradiol-releasing vaginal ring (Estring) on recurrent urinary tract infections in postmenopausal women. Am J Obstet Gynecol 1999; 180:1072–1079.

112. Samicore G. Urogenital ageing—a hidden problem. Am J Obstet Gynecol 1998; 178(5):S245–S249.

113. Mettler L, Olsen PG. Long term treatment of atrophic vaginitis with low dose oestradiol vaginal tablets. Maturitas 1991; 14:23–31.

114. Smith P, Heimer G, Lindskog, Ulmsten U. Oestradiol releasing vaginal ring for treatment of postmenopausal urogenital atrophy. Mauturitas 1993; 16:145–154.

115. Smith RJN, Studd JWW. Recent advances in hormone replacement therapy. Br J Hosp Med 1993; 49:799–809.

116. Cardozo LD, Bachmann G, McClish D, Fonda D, Birgerson L. Meta-analysis of oestrogen therapy in the management of urogenital atrophy in postmenopausal women: second report of the Hormones and Urogenital Therapy committee. Obstet Gynaecol 1998; 92:722–727.

117. Henriksson L, Stjernquist M, Boquist L, Cedergren I, Selinus I. A one-year multicentre study of efficacy and safety of a continuous, low dose, oestradiol-releasing vaginal ring. (Estring) in postmenopausal women with symptoms and signs of urogenital aging. Am J Obstet Gynaecol 1996; 174:85–92.

118. Bachmann G. Oestradiol-releasing vaginal ring delivery system for urogential atrophy. Experience over the last decade. J Reprod Med 1998; 43:991–998.

119. Ayton RA, Darling GM, Murkies AL. A comparative study of safety and efficacy of low dose oestradiol released from a vaginal ring compared with conjugated equine oestrogen vaginal cream in the treatment of postmenopausal vaginal atrophy. Br J Obstet Gynaecol 1996; 103:351–358.

120. Judge TG. The use of quinestradol in elderly incontinent women: a preliminary report. Gerontol Clin 1969; 11:159–164.

121. Kinn AC, Lindskog M. Oestrogens and phenylpropanolamine in combination for stress incontinence in postmenopausal women. Urology 1988; 32:273–280.

122. Walter S, Kjaergaard B, Lose G, Anderson JT, Heisterberg L, Jakobson H. Stress urinary incontinence in postmenopausal women treated with oral oestrogen (oestriol) and an α-adrenoceptor stimulating agent (phenylpropanolamine): a randomised double-blind placebo-controlled study. Int Urogynaecol J 1990; 1:74–79.

123. Bellatoni MF, Harman SM, Cullins VE, Engelhardt SM, Blackman MR. Transdermal oestradiol with oral progestin: biological and clinical effects in younger and older postmenopausal women. J Gerontol 1991; 46:M216–M222.

124. Campbell S, Whitehead M, Oestrogen therapy and the menopausal syndrome. Clin Obstet Gynaecol 1977; 4:31–47.

125. Felding C, Mikkelse AL, Chausen HV, Loft A, Larson LG. Preoperative treatment with oestradiol in women scheduled for vaginal operations for genital proplapse. A randomised double blind trial. Maturitas 1992; 15:241–249.

126. Foidart JM, Vervliet J, Buytaert P. Efficacy of sustained release vaginal formulation of oestriol in alleviating urogenital and systemic climeteric complaints. Maturitas 1991; 13:99–107.

127. Laufer LR, Defazio JL, Lu JKH. Oestrogen replacement therapy by transdermal oestradiol administration. Am J Obstet Gynaecol 1983; 146:533–540.

128. Molander U, Milson I, Ekelund P, Mellstrom D. An epidemiological study of urinary incontinence and related urogenital symptoms in elderly women. Maturitas 1990; 12:51–60.

129. Van der Linden MCGJ, Gerretsen G, Brandhurst MS, Doms ECM, Kremer CME, Doesburg WH. The effects of oestriol on the cytology of urethra and vagina in postmenopausal women with genitourinary symptoms. Eur J Obstet Gynaecol Repord Biol 1993; 51:29–33.

7

Obstetric Issues and the Female Pelvis

Roger P. Goldberg and Peter K. Sand
Northwestern University, Evanston, U.S.A.

I. BACKGROUND

Urinary incontinence, anal incontinence, pelvic organ prolapse, and sexual dysfunction—the major disorders of the female pelvic floor—are associated with a substantial public health burden. And for many women, pregnancy, labor, and delivery represent the most important physiological events predisposing to these conditions. Although many aspects of obstetrical pelvic floor injury have yet to be fully understood, our knowledge of etiological mechanisms and epidemiological risk factors has markedly expanded over the past several years. This chapter will explore the effects of pregnancy and childbirth on the pelvic floor, and the impact of obstetrical events on these prevalent postreproductive disorders.

II. PELVIC FLOOR DURING PREGNANCY, LABOR, AND DELIVERY

A. Evolutionary Strains and Anatomic Adaptations

From an evolutionary standpoint, certain anatomic trends have produced a maternal pelvic floor that is highly vulnerable to injury during pregnancy and childbirth. One factor was the increasing size of the newborn cranium to accommodate an enlarging brain, resulting in disproportion with the maternal pelvic outlet. With enhanced nutrition resulting in larger offspring, the maternal-fetal disproportion further increased. This trend was magnified by changes in locomotion and posture, as the upright bipedal stance (first adopted by the Australopithecines) shifted the pelvic outlet directly beneath the abdominopelvic contents. The female pelvis became increasingly foreshortened in the anterior-posterior plane, and laterally, more anterior and prominent ischial spines presented a further obstacle to delivery (1). The maternal pelvic floor can be viewed as an evolutionary response to these anatomical selection pressures—a transformation of vertically oriented "tail-wagging" muscles into a horizontal platform supporting the abdominopelvic organs. In the normal female pelvis, the major foundation consists of the paired levator ani muscles (2,3), whose position is maintained by endopelvic connective tissue and tone is preserved by nerves arising from the lumbosacral roots. All of these components—muscular anatomy, connective tissue supports, and nerve supply—are exposed to acute physical strains during childbirth, and also chronic wear and tear resulting from intraperitoneal forces. Pelvic floor dysfunction, in its various forms, can be viewed as a consequence of these conflicting demands.

During pregnancy and delivery, both maternal and fetal adaptations serve to mitigate the full impact of anatomical strains on the maternal pelvis. On the fetal side, "molding" results in reduction of the fetal head circumference. On the maternal side, estrogen-mediated smooth muscle hypertrophy, connective tissue relaxation, and increased lubrication result in an accentuation of vaginal length, skin thickness, and soft tissue compliance. Relaxin may be responsible for a variety of connective tissue changes within the bony pelvis, including increased mobility of the sacroiliac joint and pubic symphysis (4–6). Animal models have demonstrated relaxin-mediated collagen reorganization in the pubic symphysis (7). After the return of the nongravid hormonal milieu during the postpartum period, normal rigidity of the bony pelvis is resumed.

Despite these and other compensatory adaptations, the potential for injury to the pelvic floor cannot be avoided even for "normal" childbirth. For nulliparas the first stage of labor may involve tissue compression for 20 or more. The second stage of labor, though substantially shorter, involves pressures between the fetal head and vaginal wall averaging 100 mm Hg and reaching as high as 230 mm Hg. As a benchmark for comparison, consider that compressive forces of only 20–80 mm Hg will cause blood perfusion to cease in the setting of orthopedic compartment syndrome, leading to permanent tissue damage if sustained. Unsurprisingly, obstetrical forces up to three times that intensity within the maternal pelvis, applied over many hours, may often result in physical sequelae.

B. Perineum and Anal Sphincter

In the nulliparous female the bulbocavernosis muscles, transverse perineal muscles, and anterior portion of the external anal musculature contribute to normal introital tone and anal sphincter pressure. Attenuation, widening or descent of the perineum after childbirth—whether resulting from episiotomy or a spontaneous injury—may result in bulging or laxity near the vagina and rectum, loss of vaginal sensation during intercourse, and/or anal incontinence. Perineal lacerations involving the anal sphincter have been reported in ~10% of first vaginal deliveries, and 0.3% of subsequent births (8). Apart from the presence or absence of perineal laceration, descent of the perineal plane relative the ischial tuberosities is common following vaginal delivery and appears to correlate with anal sphincter dysfunction (9), but has the potential for resolving to the normal antenatal position in some women. Excessive descent of the perineal body during voluntary straining may represent a marker for persistent neuromuscular dysfunction after childbirth (10). However, the degree of perineal trauma evident after delivery has not been shown to accurately predict subsequent pelvic floor symptoms (11). One prospective study (12), using anal manometry in primiparous women prenatally and at 4–6 weeks postnatally, found vaginal delivery to be associated with significantly reduced squeeze pressure (SP: prenatal 269 cmH$_2$O vs. postnatal 204 cmH$_2$O; $P = .004$). Cesarean section was not associated with any significant change in anal pressures. Thus, normal vaginal deliveries with no evidence of sphincter injury are associated with a significant effect on postpartum anal function.

External anal sphincter lacerations complicate up to 20% of vaginal deliveries (13) and represent a major risk factor for reduced squeeze pressure (14) and anal incontinence, which will be subsequently reported in 4–50% of cases (8,15–20). Incontinence of flatus is reported six times more often by women who experienced anal sphincter injury during delivery (15). Vaginal delivery is independently associated with anal incontinence (21), and the risk is increased with prolonged labor, operative vaginal delivery, and episiotomy (22). Although in the absence of a visible anal sphincter injury the incidence of subsequent anal incontinence is <3%, a normal perineum on clinical examination does not exclude underlying anal sphincter damage (23).

Postpartum endoanal ultrasound has demonstrated external anal sphincter defects in 20–53% of women after normal vaginal delivery (24–28).

Unfortunately, even a complete repair of visible anal sphincter lacerations, at the time of delivery, may be associated with suboptimal long-term results. According to postpartum ultrasonography, external anal sphincter separations can be detected in 11–85% of cases after primary obstetrical repair of a sphincter injury (14,29). Among women with anal incontinence and a past history of repaired episiotomy or perineal laceration, up to 95% may have persistent external or internal anal sphincter defects visible by transanal ultrasound (30). Sixty-five percent of residual defects in this study were found in the mid or upper anal canal, suggesting an important role for internal anal sphincter injuries. The internal anal sphincter extends an additional 12 mm cranial to the external sphincter margin, is prone to disruption with severe perineal lacerations, and may be commonly overlooked during primary obstetrical repair (31). Using transanal ultrasonography, Sultan et al. (32) demonstrated internal anal sphincter lacerations in 17% of primiparas experiencing no visible perineal injury at the time of delivery. Posterior anal sphincter injuries, though far less common than anterior injuries, may also escape notice during perineal repair.

Finally, neurological injury to the anal sphincter may play a role. Prolonged motor latencies may persist in the internal (upper) anal sphincter, for up to 5 months after vaginal delivery (33). Denervation of the internal anal sphincter system after vaginal delivery may persist even after the restoration of anal squeeze pressures, and may be associated with later development of fecal incontinence. Some surgeons advocate overlapping sphincteroplasty rather than end-to-end sphincter repair for the primary management of third- to fourth-degree perineal lacerations (34). Long-term outcomes following overlapping external anal sphincter repair are still being evaluated; however, recent case series have reported failure rates exceeding 50%, and the potential for decreased efficacy over time (35,36). Success rates appear to be lower among individuals with demonstrably abnormal pudendal nerve function preoperatively (16% vs. 62%) (37). Because of the limitations associated with the surgical repair of severe perineal injuries, primary prevention of obstetrical trauma should be regarded as the most effective approach for reducing the incidence of postreproductive perineal and anal sphincter dysfunction.

C. Effects of Episiotomy

Episiotomies were introduced from Europe during the early 1900s and have subsequently become the most common obstetrical operation. In the United States, 1.2 million are performed each year, with midline episiotomy performed in up to 60% of vaginal deliveries (13). In decades past, the routine use of episiotomy was thought to provide an array of maternal benefits including preservation of pelvic muscle tone and sexual function, improved perineal healing, and a reduced risk of anal sphincter injury. Since then, however, a steadily growing number of observational studies support the conclusion that episiotomies increase rather than decrease the risk of pelvic floor dysfunction.

Rectal injuries appear to be more often associated with than prevented by episiotomies, with the risk of anal sphincter laceration increasing by 1–11%. Midline episiotomy in particular has been associated with a sharply elevated risk of severe lacerations into the vagina, perineum, and rectum, in primiparous women (38–40). Mediolateral episiotomies confer only a 1–2% likelihood of anal or rectal injury, but may be associated with a greater risk of postpartum and sexual pain. During second, third, or later deliveries, an even higher proportion of severe perineal injuries are preceded by episiotomy, though the absolute incidence is decreased in comparison to a first delivery.

Episiotomies appear to be associated with slower recovery of pelvic floor muscle strength compared with an intact perineum after delivery and also spontaneous perineal lacerations (41,39). One Argentine study randomized >2000 women to undergo episiotomy either "routinely" or "selectively" if a significant perineal injury appeared to be imminent, and found pain and healing complications to be more common within the routine episiotomy group (42). Another randomized trial of selective episiotomy found that multiparous women in the selective group more often gave birth with an intact perineum (31% vs. 19%) (43). Nearly all perineal lacerations involving the anal sphincter were associated with midline episiotomy (46/47 in primiparous women and 6/6 among multiparous women). No differences were found between groups with respect to postpartum perineal pain, antepartum, and 3-month postpartum EMG perineometry, and urinary and pelvic floor symptoms. The authors concluded that restriction of episiotomy use among multiparous women results in significantly less perineal injury. With respect to anal incontinence, one retrospective cohort study (44) found midline episiotomy to be associated with an elevated risk of fecal incontinence at 3 (odds ratio 5.5) and 6 (3.7) months postpartum compared with women with an intact perineum. Compared with women with a spontaneous laceration in this cohort, episiotomy tripled the risk of fecal incontinence at 3 months (95% confidence interval 1.3–7.9) and 6 months (0.7–11.2) postpartum, and doubled the risk of flatal incontinence at 3 months (1.3–3.4) and 6 months (1.2–3.7) postpartum.

The effects of episiotomy on sexual function have not been definitively established. One study demonstrated that at 3 months postpartum, sexual satisfaction appears to be highest among women without perineal injury, and lowest among women with an episiotomy that had extended during birth (39). A more recent study also found highest satisfaction among women with an intact perineum during delivery, but no difference between those who had undergone episiotomy or spontaneous perineal laceration (45).

In summary, although selective episiotomies maintain a valid role in obstetrical management room, the scientific evidence does not support their routine use. A Cochrane report (46) concluded that the practice of routine episiotomy increases the overall risk of maternal trauma and complications during vaginal delivery. Even during forceps or vacuum-assisted delivery, previously regarded as an absolute indication for episiotomy, the selective use of episiotomy has become increasingly common (47,48). The American College of Obstetricians and Gynecologists (ACOG) formally stated in March 2000 that routine episiotomy should not be considered a part of current obstetrical practice.

D. Levator Ani Muscles and Childbirth

The levator muscles represent the most important foundation of pelvic floor support, a broad muscular complex counteracting the constant downward force of the pelvic and abdominal organs. The iliococcygeous components form a shelflike barrier across the urogenital hiatus—supporting the uterus, vagina, bladder, and other pelvic organs, and allowing the pelvic viscera to compress against a muscular floor rather than prolapsing through the urogenital hiatus with increased intra-abdominal pressure. The pubococcygeous and puborectalis muscles encircle the anal and urethral sphincters in the manner of a sling, augmenting intrinsic smooth muscle tone and maintaining tonic and phasic pressures. When intra-abdominal pressure is increased, reflex contraction of these muscular components contributes to urethral and anal sphincter tone, promoting continence.

Injuries to the levator ani muscles and their nerve supply may, in many instances, represent the seminal obstetrical events ultimately leading to pelvic prolapse or urinary incontinence. Several forms of trauma to the levator ani may occur. Direct injury may include attenuation of the musculature, detachment of individual muscle components from their insertion points along the pelvic sidewalls, or both. Indirect changes may involve generalized atrophy of the levator muscles resulting from pudendal neuropathy. Finally, diminished basal tone of the levator muscles may result in widening of the urogenital hiatus and descent of the levator plate from its horizontal position, thus orienting the pelvic viscera more directly over the widened urogenital hiatus (49) and shifting the burden of their support to connective tissues and ligaments. With cumulative intra-abdominal stress over time, weakening of these "secondary" endopelvic connective tissue supports may lead to pelvic organ prolapse (50) years after the initial neuromuscular insult.

Diminished levator ani function after childbirth is common, but the severity of change varies according to the timing of postpartum assessment. Sampselle et al. (51) evaluated pelvic floor muscle strength using digital palpation before deliver and again at 3 months postpartum in a small cohort of primiparous women. Diminished levator strength was found to be associated with the onset of urinary stress incontinence. Peschers et al. (52) evaluated levator ani function before and after childbirth using intravaginal perineometry, and found that pelvic muscle strength was significantly reduced 3–8 days postpartum following vaginal birth, but not after cesarean delivery, and returned to normal values within 2 months for most women. Allen and Hosker (53), using perineometry, also demonstrated a significant and persistent reduction in pelvic floor contraction strength. Prolonged EMG motor duration was associated with urinary incontinence postpartum, and appeared to be more likely after a long second stage of labor or vaginal delivery of a macrosomic baby.

E. Pudendal Nerve and Neuropathic Changes

The majority of the important pelvic floor support structures, including the levator ani and sphincter muscles, receive their innervation from S2–S4 anterior sacral nerve roots with motor branches coursing along the cranial surface of the pelvic floor. The pudendal nerve, arising from these same nerve roots, supplies the external anal and urethral sphincter, and perineum. Compression and stretching of the pudendal during childbirth appears to be a major risk factor associated with diminished levator muscle function afterwards. With delayed conduction, the slinglike components of the levator complex, such as the pubococcygeous muscle, may fail to reflexively contract and elevate sphincter pressure during a cough or sneeze. Basal tone of the shelflike levator plate and perineal body, as previously mentioned, may also diminish as a result of neuropathic changes.

The pudendal nerve and its three branches supply most of the anatomic structures helping to maintain pelvic support and continence—including the perineum and vagina, levator muscle complex, and anus. Stretching and compression of the pudendal nerve appears to be particularly vulnerable as the fetus descends past the ischial spine in the midpelvis. Apart from the pudendal nerve, a recent cadaveric study by Barber et al. (54) suggested that the levator ani musculature may receive substantial innervation from independent "levator nerve" components arising from the lumbosacral nerve roots. In 1986, Snooks and Swash (55) reported that partially reversible pudendal nerve injury occurs commonly with vaginal birth. Pudendal nerve terminal motor latency measurements indicate decreased conduction in women with vaginal birth compared with nulliparous controls, an effect that appears to be prevented by cesarean delivery (114). The likelihood of nerve injury is increased by forceps delivery, multiparity, increased duration of the second stage of labor, third-degree perineal tear, and macrosomia (53,56). Pelvic floor neuromuscular function can also be measured by concentric needle electromyography or single-fiber electromyography, providing a quantitative measure of pelvic floor denervation. Denervation changes within the pubococcygeous and striated anal sphincter muscles have been observed following 42–80% of vaginal deliveries (55). While some degree of reinnervation by surrounding nerves will frequently occur, loss of muscle function is common. Evidence of denervation injury appears to increase with parity, and can be demonstrated 5–6 years after delivery (57,58). Cesarean delivery appears to effectively prevent denervation injuries when performed electively, but does not confer full protection if performed after the onset of labor.

For many women, pelvic neuropathy will have no clinical consequences; for others, these nerve injuries initiate a pathophysiologic cascade eventually leading to incontinence, prolapse, and pelvic floor dysfunction. Women with stress incontinence have delayed pudendal conduction relative to controls on motor latency testing. Increased pudendal nerve terminal motor latency has been associated with genuine urinary stress incontinence. (59,60) and lower maximal urethral closure pressure (60) compared to asymptomatic controls. However, electromyography of the urethral sphincter has not demonstrated increased denervation among stress-incontinent subjects (61) and has also failed to correlate sphincter denervation with a reduction in urethral closure pressures (62). Smith et al. (63) showed that partial denervation of the pelvic floor after childbirth is associated with both genital prolapse and urinary incontinence. A 5-year follow-up by Snooks et al. (58) demonstrated that denervation-reinnervation patterns on electromyography may become more pronounced over time, and indicate higher risks of urinary and fecal incontinence. Others have found anal incontinence to be associated with pelvic floor neuropathy in 75–80% of cases (64,65). Among multiparas, levator denervation appears to be more common among those with prolapse, according to histological and electromyelographic study, occurring in up 50% of women with symptomatic pelvic organ prolapse (66,67). To what extent these changes to the levator ani musculature represent a direct cause of pelvic organ prolapse, or its consequence, is not fully certain. In summary, pelvic floor neuropathy is a common repercussion of childbirth—less often recognized than vaginal and perineal injury, but arguably more significant with respect to the etiology of subsequent pelvic floor dysfunction. Our understanding of the mechanisms of neuromuscular injury, and its repercussions, continues to evolve.

F. Connective Tissues, Ligaments, and Bony Pelvis

Some element of injury to the connective tissues of the pelvic floor is inevitable during childbirth. And in the etiology of pelvic floor disorders after childbirth, endopelvic connective tissue injuries have an established role (68). Investigations into the etiology and treatment of pelvic organ prolapse have sought to identify "site-specific" breaks and detachments of the endopelvic connective tissue from their anatomical insertion sites, as the origins for pelvic organ prolapse (69). These include paravaginal defects in the anterior vaginal compartment, site-specific defects in the rectovaginal (Denonvillier's) fascia, and ligamentous/fascial detachments of the vaginal apex. Attenuation injuries to the endopelvic connective tissue during childbirth may account for a variety of other forms of prolapse, including central cystoceles, rectoceles, and uterine prolapse resulting from laxity of the uterosacral ligaments.

Bony pelvic anatomy may have an important relationship to the progress of childbirth, the physical ease or difficulty encountered during childbirth, and the amount of pressure, stretch, and potential injury to the soft-tissue structures of the pelvic floor. Among the pelvic shapes described in the 1930s, the "gynecoid" pelvis is most common among women, and also best suited for childbirth owing to its generous anterior-posterior and lateral dimensions with a wide pubic arch. "Android" features present a greater challenge for vaginal delivery and may exist to some degree in up to 24% of women undergoing x-ray pelvimetry before labor (70). The relatively narrow pubic arch, prominent ischial spines, and anterior-posterior foreshortening resulting from the protuberant sacrum create a heart-shaped passageway. The "anthropoid" pelvis resembles a narrow oval, restricted laterally by convergent sidewalls and prominent spines. "Platypoid" pelvises resemble a horizontal oval, and are the least commmon shape in the female population.

Although it remains unclear which specific bony pelvic features signal a higher risk of pelvic floor injury, certain shapes would seem, at least in theory, to be of potential significance. For instance, a narrow pubic arch (android, anthropoid) may indicate less anterior space for the fetal vertex, and thus a greater likelihood of posterior injury to the perineum and anal sphincter. A wide pubic arch (gynecoid, platypoid) or prominent coccyx may force the fetal head from posterior to anterior, increasing the risk of compression injury to the bladder and urethra. Finally, in the case of a narrow midpelvic region due to prominent ischial spines or convergent pelvic sidewalls (anthropoid), the pudendal nerves may be exposed to an increased risk of compression near Alcock's canal. However, these potential "pelvic factors" in maternal injury have not been scientifically evaluated. Spinal anatomy may also influence the risk of pelvic prolapse according to one case control study of 92 women. When compared with patients with a normal curvature, patients with an abnormal spinal curvature were 3.2 times more likely to have development of pelvic organ prolapse (71). A loss of lumbar lordosis appeared to be the most significant risk factor in the development of pelvic organ prolapse. Another matched observational study of bony pelvic anatomy concurred that women with advanced uterovaginal prolapse have less lumbar lordosis and a pelvic inlet that is oriented less vertically than women without prolapse (72). The impact of specific pelvic shapes on postreproductive pelvic floor dysfunction, and the proper role of pelvic anatomy assessment in obstetrical decision making, warrants future investigation.

III. OBSTETRICAL CORRELATES OF URINARY INCONTINENCE

The symptom of stress urinary incontinence occurs in 32–85% of pregnant women, peaking in the third trimester (73–75). Francis showed an intrapartum prevalence of 85% in multiparas and 53% in nulliparas, with nearly half of these patients noting some degree of incontinence before the observed pregnancy. Several other investigators have observed that stress incontinence, arising with pregnancy and childbirth, may often fail to resolve. Stanton et al. (76) prospectively studies 181 women in the third trimester and through the puerperium. Of the 83 nulliparas, 38% had stress incontinence during the third trimester and 6% had persistent postpartum incontinence. Among 98 multiparas, 10% had stress incontinence symptoms prior to pregnancy, 42% had stress incontinence in the third trimester, and 11% had persistent postpartum incontinence. Meyer et al. (77) examined 149 women during pregnancy, and again at 9 weeks postpartum. The rates of stress urinary incontinence were 31% and 7%, respectively, meaning that 22% of patients with stress incontinence during pregnancy had persistence after delivery.

Several investigators have observed that mode delivery may have a profound impact on the persistence of incontinence for the long term. Viktrup et al. (73) prospectively studied urinary incontinence symptoms before, during, and after pregnancy in 305 primiparous women. The multivariate analysis identified the length of second stage, fetal head circumference, episiotomy, and birth weight as risk factors for postpartum stress incontinence, whereas cesarean section was protective against incontinence. Among women with stress incontinence during pregnancy, 21 of 167 women (13%) had persistent incontinence postpartum compared to none of the 35 delivered by cesarean ($P < .05$). At 3 months postpartum, only 4% of these women had persistent stress incontinence complaints; after 1 year, only 3% still had stress incontinence. In subsequent pregnancies, however, it appears that these patients are at greater risk for more severe incontinence with earlier onset and persistence beyond the puerperium. And in a 5-year follow-up study, Viktrup and Lose (78) questioned 278 of the 305 women (91%) comprising their original cohort, and found a 30% prevalence of stress incontinence. Nineteen percent of women who were not incontinent in the original trial developed stress incontinence in the ensuing 5 years. Again, cesarean section was found to significantly decrease the risk of stress incontinence. The proper role of elective cesarean delivery, for preventing urinary incontinence, remains uncertain. Iosif and Ingemarsson (1) showed that stress urinary incontinence does occur following elective cesarean delivery, but to a much lesser degree than after vaginal birth. Among 204 of 264 women who had undergone an elective cesarean section 1–6 years earlier, 4.7% had persistent stress urinary incontinence after primary cesarean section, and 4.1% after a second cesarean section.

Several mechanisms may contribute to the relationship among pregnancy, childbirth, and urinary incontinence. An increased prevalence of urethral hypermobility is one important change (79,80) known to be associated with genuine stress urinary incontinence. Peschers and colleagues (81) studied the anatomic effects of vaginal delivery and found that bladder neck support was significantly weaker after vaginal delivery than following cesarean section ($P < .001$) or compared to a group of 25 nulliparous controls ($P < .001$). They also found that bladder neck descent during Valsalva was significantly increased after vaginal delivery compared to cesarean section in both primiparous and multiparous women ($P < .001$). Diminished intrinsic urethral function, immediately after childbirth or later on also plays an important role in the development of genuine stress incontinence (82). Van Geelen et al. (83) demonstrated an association between vaginal delivery and decreased urethral closure pressure and functional length; the absence of these changes after cesarean delivery highlights the importance of birth mode rather than only pregnancy. Meyer et al. (77), in a prospective study of 149 women, found similar changes in functional urethral length, and intravaginal and intra-anal pressure, 9 weeks after vaginal delivery compared to antepartum values. None of these changes were found in the 33 women who had delivered by cesarean. As previously mentioned, vaginal delivery can produce neurological changes in the pelvic floor, adversely affecting pudendal nerve conduction velocity, vaginal contraction strength, and urethral closure pressure. Presumably, these alterations may account for persistent or new-onset genuine stress incontinence in women after vaginal delivery. After cesarean section, these pathophysiological changes are far less pronounced.

Whether or not pelvic floor damage leading to persistent stress urinary incontinence is cumulative for multiparous women—"from delivery to delivery"—has been controversial. Mallett et al. (84) demonstrated that absolute parity and further childbearing did not further influence pelvic floor neurophysiology, and concluded that most pudendal nerve damage occurs during the first vaginal delivery. Hojberg et al. (85) studied 1781 primiparas at 16 weeks' gestation and showed an odds ratio of 5.7 for stress incontinence after vaginal delivery compared to 1.3 with cesarean delivery. Within their cohort, the first vaginal delivery was a major risk factor for developing urinary incontinence; subsequent deliveries did not increase the risk significantly. However, other population-based observational studies and prospective trial have shown strong associations between vaginal delivery and increasing parity with stress incontinence. Persson et al. (86) studies 10,074 women in Sweden having surgery for stress incontinence and found a strong association with stress incontinence and parity, and also that the odds ratio of prior cesarean section versus vaginal delivery was 0.21. Moller et al. (87) studie 502 women with lower urinary tract symptoms and 742 controls. They found an association of parity and stress incontinence with an odds ratio of 2.2 after one vaginal delivery, 3.9 after a second vaginal delivery, and 4.5 after a third delivery. Marshall et al. (88) studied 7771 women early in the pueperium and found a strong association between parity and stress incontinence. A 1989 consensus conference of the National Institutes of Health identified parity as an established risk factor for urinary incontinence (89).

IV. PREVENTION OF OBSTETRICAL PELVIC FLOOR INJURY

From the standpoint of pelvic injury a great number of obstetrical complications of previous generations are now fully preventable. Obstetrical fistulae, for instance, are today exceedingly rare due to the recognition and prevention of obstructed labor. Unfortunately, the more commonplace pelvic floor disorders—urinary incontinence, anal incontinence, and pelvic prolapse—remain largely overlooked.

It could be argued that pelvic floor disorders are natural consequences of childbirth just as skin cancer is a natural consequence of sun exposure. Both are associated with identifiable risk factors, both can affect quality of life greatly, and both, in many cases, are preventable. During and after pregnancy, strategies for reducing the risk of subsequent pelvic floor dysfunction should be considered.

A. During Pregnancy

1. Pelvic Floor Exercises, Perineal Massage, and General Health

Daily pelvic floor exercises may consist of 20–30 daily repetitions throughout pregnancy. Increased muscle "reserve" before delivery may help to decrease the risk of injury during childbirth and accelerate healing afterward. Improved muscular tone, and awareness of muscular location, may enhance the patient's ability to voluntarily relax the pelvic floor musculature during labor and delivery. Two controlled trials of antenatal pelvic floor exercises have demonstrated reduced urinary stress incontinence postpartum, but no discernible differences in pelvic muscle strength according to perineometry (90,91). Prenatal pelvic floor exercises may reduce the likelihood of incontinence symptoms after delivery (90).

Perineal massage represents another strategy for the prevention of obstetrical injury, which involves gentle stretching of the lubricated perineum in preparation for delivery. The protective effects of perineal massage remain a subject of debate, with some investigators concluding no benefit when performed only during labor (92). However, two studies of perineal massage begun during the third trimester have reported a decreased risk of perineal laceration. One found that among women aged 30 or older, massage increased the chances of an intact perineum by 12%. Another study, involving over 1500 women, found that for those without a previous vaginal birth, 3 weeks of perineal massage routine increased the likelihood of an intact perineum by 9% (93). A follow-up analysis (94) 1 year later reported on subsequent symptoms within the same cohort; among women with a previous vaginal birth, perineal massage reduced the odds of perineal pain at 3 months postpartum from 94% to 86%. For women without a previous vaginal birth, no differences were found between the two groups.

Maintaining a moderate exercise routine during pregnancy, and optimal body weight, may reduce the strain of pregnancy and childbirth on the pelvic floor. One study demonstrated that although transient urinary incontinence during pregnancy improving postpartum is common, *persistent* leakage is more likely among women gaining more weight before delivery. Excess body weight has been identified as a risk factor for postpartum stress urinary incontinence and urgency (95), with a body mass index >30 conferring an elevated risk (96). A reasonable target for weight gain is ~2–4 pounds during the first trimester and 1 pound per week thereafter, translating into 25–35 pounds for a full-term pregnancy. For women who are overweight before pregnancy, significantly less weight gain is acceptable. Exercise during pregnancy should be tailored to specific consideration, including changes in posture, balance, and coordination; altered respiratory patterns; increased joint and ligament mobility due to relaxin; and increased vulnerability of the pelvic floor beneath the gravid uterus.

Finally, preventing constipation is an important cornerstone for minimizing pelvic floor strain during pregnancy, as gastrointestinal motility decreases owing to the effects of progesterone and iron supplementation. Maintaining regular bowel movements, with proper consistency, helps to reduce straining with defecation and thus reduces stress on the pelvic floor supports. Dietary fiber should be accompanied by adequate hydration, regular exercise, and stool softeners.

2.   Predicting Pelvic Floor Injury: Maternal and Fetal Factors

Predicting the ease or difficulty of childbirth, and forecasting which women are at highest risk for pelvic floor dysfunction, has challenged physicians and midwives for centuries. In the 1940s, for instance, some obstetricians maintained that a large number of abdominal striae indicated an increased risk of pelvic injury. More recently, double-jointed fingers and distensible skin have been implicated as markers for generalized connective tissue disorders predisposing to pelvic floor dysfunction. Specific demographic factors may have an impact on the risk of pelvic floor injury. One report of >50,000 women, from the University of Miami, found maternal age might relate to be predictive of severe lacerations involving the anal sphincter or rectum; older women during their first delivery were found to be most at risk, especially with delivery of a large baby (97). Within a cohort to African mothers, women <150 cm tall were more likely to experience cephalopelvic disproportion leading to a failed labor. Short stature (<10th centile) within this group was associated with a twofold risk of cesarean delivery, and 15 times the usual risk of requiring forceps or vacuum assistance. Urethral and bladder neck hypermobility, defined by transvaginal ultrasound before delivery, has also been associated with an elevated risk of postpartum incontinence (98).

Fetal head engagement may influence the relationship between childbirth and the pelvic floor. For nulliparous women, engagement before the onset of labor is regarded as an indicator of good maternal-fetal "fit." Conversely, a lack of fetal head engagement at term may reflect cephalopelvic disproportion and higher risk for arrest of labor. One study assessed >1200 women carrying their first pregnancy, demonstrating that the risk of cesarean section nearly tripled if fetal head engagement had not yet occurred at the start of active labor (99). Another study found that lack of fetal head engagement was associated with both a longer second stage of labor and an elevated risk of cesarean, from 6.9% to 27%. Other studies have reported equal success at achieving vaginal delivery even if the fetal head is floating above the pelvic inlet. The relationship of fetal engagement to the maternal pelvic floor, and postreproductive body, remains uncertain. If an unengaged fetus portends a longer labor, more physical effort, or greater odds of an operative delivery, it could represent a risk factor for subsequent pelvic floor dysfunction.

Pelvimetry during pregnancy or labor has been used to help determine the most important features of the bony pelvis. Unfortunately, pelvimetry—whether performed clinically or with radiological imaging—has not been found to reliably predict the course of labor and delivery, or obstetrical pelvic injury. Forecasting pelvic floor injuries and postreproductive problems based on pelvic shape remains a medical area posing more questions than answers.

B.   During Labor and Delivery

During the second stage of labor, many elements of childbirth are viewed as inevitable. But in fact, a number of important decisions may have implications for subsequent pelvic floor function. Recognizing modifiable risk factors for pelvic floor injury is an important aspect of routine obstetrical care.

1. Pushing Positions and Techniques

Whereas some women will be instructed to push immediately after reaching "full" cervical dilatation, others will be advised to wait until feeling the strong urge created by fetal descent, and still others are encouraged to wait until the urge is unbearable. Determining the most appropriate technique and time parameters for second stage from the standpoint of the maternal pelvic floor—and the relative impact of "active" versus "passive" laboring—remains an area of women's health warranting attention. "Full dilatation," after all, refers exclusively to the cervix; from the standpoint of the major pelvic floor supports, an enormous degree of tissue dilatation has yet to occur for most women. It has been suggested that premature active pushing before full cervical dilatation may create sever stress against the pelvic floor, by advancing the cervix and its surrounding attachments ahead of the fetal vertex (100).

Lithotomy is the most common position used by women choosing regional analgesia, with the lower extremities held fully flexed and abducted during each contraction. Although some practitioners suspect that the "uphill" orientation of this pushing style may increase the difficulty of delivery, specific disadvantages for pelvic floor function have not been proven. Squatting is purported to increase the diameter of the pelvic outlet compared with the lying-down position, and help to shift the tail bone posteriorly. Studies have shown reduced rates of forceps delivery and perineal lacerations compared with semirecumbent position (101). One study of 300 women (102) showed squatting to be associated with a decreased risk of perineal laceration and episiotomy. The effects of squatting on the deeper pelvic floor supports are unknown.

Other, less common delivery positions may have a positive or negative impact on the pelvic floor. Sitting has been associated with more rapid delivery; however, studies evaluating birthing chairs have shown perineal swelling and labial lacerations to be more likely, and blood loss increased. Lateral positioning ("side lying") may be useful for multiparous women with an already relaxed introitus, by improving control over the speed of fetal expulsion at the end of second stage, and thereby helping to avoid perineal injury caused by a precipitous delivery. Upright positioning has been advocated as a means to shorten the duration of labor and reduce the need for forceps or vacuum assistance. Randomized trials have found the upright position to be associated with lower rates of perineal injury, postpartum pain, and risk of undergoing episiotomy compared with lithotomy (103). A Cochrane analysis concluded similar benefits of upright or lateral, compared with supine, positioning (104). The upright, sitting, and squatting positions should be avoided if significant perineal swelling develops. Finally, the "hands and knees" position may help to correct fetal malposition—for instance, rotation from occiput posterior, which has been associated with higher rates of anal sphincter injury (105). This position may also help to shift the pressure of the fetal vertex from posterior to anterior, if an imminent perineal injury appears likely. Management of the "final push," at the time of fetal crowning, may occasionally take on significance to pelvic floor injury, with shallow breathing and pelvic relaxation, rather than straining, allowing the fetal head to ease gradually past the introitus. There is evidence that the common hands-on approach, including counterpressure against the fetal head and "guarding" of the perineum with the practitioner's second hand, may be of little benefit to preventing perineal injury (106). Hyperflexion of the lower extremities may increase the risk of a sudden laceration as the fetal head rapidly distends the perineum, and should therefore be avoided in most cases.

2. Second-Stage Labor Strategies

Directed Valsalva pushing starting at full cervical dilatation is the most common second-stage labor strategy, its advocates arguing that the duration of labor grows too long in the absence of a constant maternal expulsive effort, introducing more stress for the baby and a greater likelihood of maternal neuromuscular injury. Critics of active pushing, on the other hand, maintain that it shortens labor and delivery less than is often assumed while increasing maternal exhaustion, stressing the pelvic floor supports, and possibly increasing the risk for pelvic injury. Among primigravid women, active pushing for >1 h has been shown to confer an increased risk of pudendal neuropathy and denervation injury; however, prolonging the passive (nonpushing) second stage may not increase the risk of injury.

"Delayed" pushing involves resisting the urge to push, while allowing the fetus to passively descend past the pelvic supports. One 1998 randomized controlled trial of delayed pushing demonstrated a nonsignificant trend with fewer instrumental vaginal deliveries. More recently, a multicenter study (107) conducted at 12 different sites throughout Canada, Switzerland, and the United States evaluated a delayed pushing strategy among 1862 nulliparous women, all with epidural analgesia, randomized to either immediate pushing at full dilatation or delayed pushing for up to 2 h before pushing. "Difficult deliveries" were less likely in the delayed pushing group, and forceps assistance was less often necessary. The benefits of delayed pushing were greatest for women whose fetus was at a high station, or in the occiput posterior position, when full cervical dilatation was determined. Notably, the 41% episiotomy rate in this study may limit the external validity of its conclusions. A more recent randomized controlled trial of delayed pushing found no increase in adverse events, despite prolongation of second stage of up to 4.9 h (108). "Physiologic" (or "spontaneous") pushing is similar to the delayed pushing approach, entailing the delay of expulsive efforts until the onset of an overwhelming physical urge. A 1999 survey compared spontaneous to directed pushing and found that advanced perineal lacerations were less likely, and an intact perineum more likely, in the "spontaneous pushing" group (109). A randomized trial of 350 women in Denmark found no differences between women "actively" or "spontaneously" pushing, with respect to perineal injury or duration of labor (110). A shorter active (pushing) phase and less maternal fatigue have also been cited as potential benefits (111).

The effects of pushing styles on pelvic floor function are largely unknown. Increased terminal nerve motor latency may be associated with a longer pushing stage. One study (112) evaluated the effect of pushing time on anal function, comparing primiparous women with a second stage shorter than 2 h to those with a second stage exceeding $3\frac{1}{2}$ h. The "long labor" group had a significantly higher rate of new-onset flatal incontinence (73% vs. 44%). Finally, in some cases a prolonged active second stage may predispose to maternal exhaustion. If this results in a greater likelihood of operative delivery by forceps or vacuum, the increased risk for pelvic floor injury resulting from these interventions should be recognized.

3. Impact of Operative Vaginal Delivery: Forceps and Vacuum

Eighty years ago, episiotomies and forceps were routine elements of childbirth and were advocated, until recently, as a means to avoid pelvic injury and provide a more "controlled" delivery. However, the majority of existing research has debunked this viewpoint, and today it is widely accepted that operative delivery tends to increase rather than decrease the risk of perineal injury, and often has a negative impact on other pelvic floor structures (113). Although vacuum and forceps procedures retain a valuable role in obstetrical care, they should not be routinely performed.

Forceps delivery markedly increases the risk of third- and fourth-degree lacerations (114) and also pelvic neuropathy—perhaps not surprising, since the average force of forceps against the surrounding pelvic tissues has been estimated at 75 psi. Up to 80% of women who undergo forceps delivery will have anal sphincter injuries detectable by transanal ultrasound

(25). Forceps also confer an elevated risk of urinary incontinence. Within one cohort, the odds of stress incontinence 7 years after childbirth were shown to be 10 times higher among women with a previous forceps delivery (115). A prospective study evaluating the incidence of new-onset urinary incontinence after forceps and vacuum delivery compared with spontaneous vaginal delivery found that in primiparous women, urinary incontinence after forceps delivery is more likely to persist compared with spontaneous vaginal or vacuum delivery (116). At 6 months postpartum, the relative risk of urinary incontinence after forceps has been estimated as 1.5 compared to spontaneous vaginal delivery (117). Women after forceps delivery have significantly weaker levator and anal strength than those who had a spontaneous vaginal birth (118).

Vacuum-assisted deliveries accounted for almost 6% of all deliveries in 1995. Although vacuum application is not appropriate for all operative deliveries, there is evidence to suggest that, compared with forceps, vacuum delivery is generally associated with lower rates of pelvic trauma (119–121). Studies randomizing operative deliveries to either forceps or vacuum have demonstrated lower rates of severe perineal lacerations, and anal injury, for the latter (122). One 1999 study randomized women undergoing operative delivery to one of these two instruments, and found that anal sphincter injury was significantly more common after forceps (79% vs. 40%). Anal incontinence was also more common after forceps delivery (32% vs. 16%). The incidence of occult anal sphincter injury is also increased after forceps, compared with vacuum delivery (123). A Cochrane report concluded that vacuum delivery is associated with significantly less risk of perineal injury compared with forceps (124).

4. Physical Effects of Macrosomia

Macrosomia is associated with a variety of potential fetal problems, including birth trauma, shoulder dystocia, and lower Apgar scores. However, it is important not to overlook the potential maternal complications including higher rates of spontaneous perineal injury and episiotomies, increased nerve damage detected by EMG (53), an increased risk of perineal injuries involving the anorectum (40,125–127), pudendal nerve injury (128), and significantly weaker anal squeeze pressures postpartum (129). Vaginal delivery of one or more babies weighing at least 4000 g raises the risk of long-term stress incontinence (130). Larger infants have been linked to a 60% increase in the risk of an episiotomy at delivery (131). Newborn head circumference has been demonstrated as an independent risk factor for third-degree perineal injury during childbirth (132).

5. Multiple Pregnancy and Childbirth: Effects on the Pelvic Floor

The effects of multiple gestation on pelvic floor injury, and postreproductive problems such as incontinence, prolapse, and sexual dysfunction, were recently investigated (133). Among 733 mothers of multiples, with a mean age of 40 years, substantial rates of pelvic floor symptoms were reported, including urinary stress incontinence by 45%, flatal incontinence by 28%, fecal soiling among 12%, and fecal incontinence by 9.6%. A subanalysis of obstetrical risk factors found that avoiding vaginal delivery resulted in a 50% reduction in the risk of urinary incontinence, even after controlling for age, total parity, and body mass index. As the prevalence of multiple gestation continues to increase in the modern obstetrical landscape, the risk factors influencing the maternal pelvic floor, and the most rational strategies for the prevention of significant injuries, need to be more precisely defined.

6.   Other Factors: Fetal Position and Analgesia

Fetal position may also have prognostic significance for the effects of labor and delivery on the pelvic floor. The occiput posterior fetal position, for instance, has been long associated with childbirth that is more prolonged, and sometimes more painful, based on anecdotal experience. One study from Ireland (134) validated these observations, analyzing a large number of deliveries and comparing babies descending in the posterior and anterior positions. Occiput posterior deliveries were associated with less favorable outcomes, including an increased incidence of anal sphincter injuries, and higher rates of delivery by cesarean and forceps. Fewer than half of occiput posterior deliveries ended in a spontaneous vaginal birth. Another study found similar results, including higher rates of perineal injury and episiotomy (135).

The effects of epidural analgesia on the maternal pelvis have also been investigated. Some investigators claim that epidurals may help to relax the pelvic floor musculature, facilitating a smoother and less traumatic delivery. Others express concern that by producing a sensory blockade, epidurals may increase the risk for stalled labor, leading to higher rates of forceps or cesarean delivery and thus greater risks for pelvic floor injury. The potential effects of epidurals on perineal injury were evaluated in a 1995 retrospective analysis (136). Within this sample of nulliparous women, severe perineal lacerations occurred in 16% of women receiving epidurals versus only 9.7% in women without one. Further analysis of this cohort, however, indicated that this difference was the result of more frequent episiotomy and operative (forceps and vacuum) assistance within the epidural group. Thus, avoiding these interventions whenever possible— rather than avoiding the epidural per se—appeared to be the important principle for preventing obstetrical pelvic floor injury. Other studies examining the effect of epidurals on pelvic floor injury (137) have found no differences with respect to intrapartum trauma.

V.   ELECTIVE CESAREAN DELIVERY FOR PROTECTING THE PELVIC FLOOR

Opinions and attitudes regarding the appropriate use of cesarean section for the prevention of pelvic injury vary widely. According to a 1996 survey of obstetricians published in the Lancet (138), 31% of female obstetricians report that if faced with a normal full-term pregnancy, they would personally select cesarean over vaginal delivery. Remarkably, 80% of these individuals cited concern over perineal injury as the main rationale. Another survey of female gynecologists reported, somewhat more modestly, that 16% would personally choose cesarean delivery for delivery of their own full-term, nonmacrosomic infant; most respondents, again, cited a desire to prevent incontinence and pelvic prolapse. A survey of 135 midwives, in contrast, found that only 6% would choose cesarean to protect their pelvic floor. Whether this reflects the fact that midwives provide care only to women before and during childbirth—and not years later, when the majority of pelvic floor symptoms arise—is an unexplored question.

Medically, it is important to emphasize that pregnancy itself may for some women be enough to cause pelvic floor injury with the route of delivery playing only a minor role. Nonetheless, cesarean birth clearly appears to reduce the likelihood of multiple pelvic floor disorders. Pelvic nerve and muscle functions are generally protected by cesarean delivery (128), the timing of intervention largely determining the degree of protection. When cesareans were performed before the onset of their first labor, pudendal nerve injury is effectively prevented (139). Yet the same study found that cesareans performed after the onset of labor resulted in rates of nerve injury similar to vaginal birth. The most protective cesareans appear to be those performed before the onset of a woman's first labor.

Stress urinary incontinence is less common after cesarean compared with vaginal birth, though it is not fully eliminated (117,140,141). After a first vaginal delivery, the risk of incontinence is increased up to 2.8 times compared with cesarean section (117). Among women with a history of multiple gestation, delivery by cesarean-only confers a 50% reduction in the risk of stress urinary incontinence after controlling for age, parity, and body mass index (133). A randomized trial of vaginal versus cesarean delivery, for breech presentation, revealed a significantly lower rate of urinary incontinence at 3 months postpartum in the cesarean group (142).

Anal sphincter lacerations can follow cesarean deliveries performed late in labor (143) but are nearly nonexistent after cesareans that are performed before the onset of labor. And yet since anal incontinence is a relatively uncommon outcome, it remains uncertain under which circumstances an elective cesarean delivery would be an appropriate consideration for preventing anal injury. As mentioned, certain fetal position including "occiput posterior" may represent another potential high-risk group, since the risk for anal and perineal trauma is significantly increased (135).

The broader application of "elective cesarean at term," in the absence of specific risk factors, is a topic fraught with controversy. Even if the likelihood of postreproductive pelvic floor dysfunction could be decreased for some women, it would be essential to factor the broad medical impact and costs that would be required to achieve this narrow gain. Cesarean is by no means always in the best interest of mother or baby. Therefore, despite the fact that up to 31% of British female obstetricians would consider a cesarean delivery for themselves in order to prevent pelvic floor injury, most societies remain appropriately ambivalent regarding each woman's "right to choose" cesarean birth. The full scope of issues regarding elective cesarean delivery is well beyond the scope of this chapter, but will undoubtedly gain increasing attention.

VI. POSTPARTUM ISSUES

Despite the remarkable level of stress endured by the pelvic floor during labor and delivery, little attention is devoted to its recuperation afterward. Immediately postpartum, strategies for pelvic floor recuperation should be reviewed. Perineal care may include ice packs and lower-extremity elevation to counteract swelling. Proper perineal hygiene is also important to avoid infection and early suture breakdown. Lotions, ointments, and direct scrubbing of the perineal area should be avoided. Breastfeeding may contribute to pelvic floor symptoms during the postpartum period, as hypoestrogenic changes throughout the vagina and lower urinary tract result in diminished urethral function, and occasionally increased severity of stress and urge incontinence. Estrogen-dependent symptoms will improve after the cessation of breastfeeding, as normal ovarian function resumes.

Rehabilitation for the deeper pelvic floor should include pelvic floor exercises, resumed during the immediate postpartum period. An appropriate postpartum Kegel exercise routine may consist of two to five daily sessions of 10–20 slow levator contractions for up to 10 sec. Exercising in the recumbent position may help to minimize caudal traction on the pelvic floor supports before full involution of the uterine fundus. Strengthening the perineal and levator musculature will help to improve vaginal tone and restore the ability to "brace" the pelvic floor muscles during increased intra-abdominal pressure, a reflex that can be otherwise lost after childbirth. Several studies have demonstrated the potential efficacy of postpartum pelvic floor exercises in preventing incontinence and other pelvic floor symptoms (144). One study of 268 women, 3 months after their first delivery, demonstrated reduction in the rate of stress incontinence from 33% to 19% (145). Morkved and Bo demonstrated that postpartum urinary incontinence could be reduced by 8 weeks of structured group training combined with home exercises three time weekly, and that benefits are still present at 1 year postpartum (146,147). Supervised pelvic floor rehabilitation was also evaluated in a New Zealand study (148), randomly assigning women with postpartum urinary incontinence to either "intensive" pelvic exercises with personal instruction and multiple daily workouts, or "simple instruction." At 1 year, the intensive group had less urinary incontinence, fecal incontinence, anxiety, and depression. However, their improvement remained for only as long as the exercises were continued. Trials randomizing women to either a structured pelvic floor exercise program or routine postpartum care have demonstrated modest reductions in the rate of stress incontinence with the structured treatment (149,150). When pelvic floor exercises are combined with with biofeedback and electrostimulation, one study demonstrated a reduction in stress incontinence for 19% of women, significantly $>2\%$ in the placebo group ($p = .002$) (151).

Proper bowel and bladder habits should be emphasized after childbirth. After episiotomy or spontaneous perineal laceration, constipation and straining should be avoided to protect suture integrity, and to minimize stress against the pelvic floor muscles. For multiparas with descent of the perineal body, perineal branches of the pudendal nerve may be particularly prone to cumulative stretch injury during straining efforts. Pudendal nerve terminal motor latencies and descent of the perineum on straining are significantly associated in patients with fecal incontinence (152); the cause-effect of this relationship is not fully understood. Dietary fiber and stool softeners, along with occasional laxatives or suppositories, should be used as needed. Finally, returning to exercise and physical activity after childbirth should take into consideration the vulnerability of pelvic floor supports, with limited weight bearing to reduce abdominopelvic straining. "Bracing" the pelvic floor during sudden physical stress may be useful for reducing leakage episode and safeguarding the pelvic floor supports.

VII. AFTER PELVIC FLOOR INJURY: MANAGING THE NEXT PREGNANCY

After childbirth has resulted in pelvic floor dysfunction, appropriate guidelines for managing the next pregnancy and delivery are often unclear. Perineal injuries represent one concern; although they are most common during a woman's first vaginal birth, "repeat" injuries can occur during subsequent deliveries. Women with a history of severe perineal laceration during their first delivery are up to 3.4 times likely to suffer a repeat injury in their next delivery (153). The same study indicated the highest risk among women undergoing forceps, vacuum, or repeat episiotomy in their second delivery—around one in five in this group—suffered a second severe perineal injury. Perineal massage during pregnancy and labor, attention to fetal size and position, and avoiding episiotomy and operative delivery whenever possible, appear to be the most effective strategies whether it is a woman's first childbirth or a subsequent one (154).

For pelvic prolapse following childbirth, there is no evidence suggesting that operative intervention should be routinely considered. Pudendal nerve injury can accumulation with later deliveries and presumably "set the stage" for the progression of prolapse, but it is unclear whether specific obstetrical interventions can help to counteract the progression of these changes. Patients should focus on symptom relief, consider the use of a pessary, and avoid strenuous activity until later in pregnancy. By 18–20 weeks, as the gravid uterus rises above the pelvic brim, prolapse symptoms will often improve for the remainder of pregnancy. Likewise, there is no clear evidence to support the use of elective cesarean section for parous women already affected by urinary incontinence. After previous stress incontinence surgery, elective cesarean for subsequent deliveries has been suggested to reduce the risk of recurrence (155), but controlled trials are lacking. The risks and benefits need to be strongly considered for each individual.

The management of childbirth after anal sphincter injuries represents another area of debate. Ultrasonography demonstrates that occult anal sphincter injuries can occur during second deliveries (156) and that the risk of anal incontinence increases, particularly among women with a sphincter defect diagnosed after the first delivery (157). Thus, although the first childbirth appears to be most important, postobstetrical pelvic floor injury can accumulate, with subsequent deliveries potentially causing new symptoms to arise, old ones to recur, or existing ones to worsen. A 1999 study (158) observed a cohort of Irish women experiencing some degree of fecal incontinence after their first vaginal birth. Nearly all of those who remained symptomatic at the time of their next pregnancy noticed that symptoms became more severe following that next second pregnancy, the second birth still led to recurrence 40% of the time. Pudendal nerve latency was significantly longer after second delivery in this cohort, a finding corroborated by other studies (159).

Strategies for preventing repeat injury vary widely, with some experts suggesting that event women with postpartum anal incontinence should be offered cesarean delivery since a loss of bowel control is arguably one of childbirth's most distressing repercussions. According to survey data, up to 71% of colorectal surgeons would advise women with previous anal injuries to deliver by cesarean, versus only 22% of obstetricians. Because a broad strategy of cesarean delivery is not feasible, the identification of risk factors for injury is important. For instance, in the setting of macrosomia diagnosed by prenatal ultrasound, elective cesarean delivery may represent a sound strategy both medically and economically for the prevention of anal incontinence. The use of episiotomy in the setting of a previously repaired anal sphincter is another area of debate—recommended by only 1% of colorectal surgeons, compared with up to 30% of obstetricians. Future research will hopefully result in a broader consensus regarding the best preventive obstetrical approach.

VIII. CONCLUSIONS

Pelvic floor dysfunction among postreproductive women has emerged as a major area of interest in the realm of clinical practice and research. Our awareness of the numerous underlying pathophysiologic mechanisms continues to increase, including neuropathic change and anatomic alterations to muscular and connective tissue anatomy. A variety of procedures and events during labor and delivery, including episiotomy and operative delivery, may have implications for pelvic function afterward. These and other obstetrical practices should be weighed against their potential long-term effects on the maternal pelvic floor. As future research further clarifies the most significant determinants of obstetrical pelvic floor injury, efforts at prevention will undoubtedly improve.

REFERENCES

1. Abitbol MM. Evolution of the ischial spine and of the pelvic floor in the Hominoidea. Am J Phys Anthropol 1988; 75(1):53–67.
2. DeLancey JOL. Anatomy and biomechanics of genital prolapse. Clin Obstet Gynecol 1993; 36:897–909.
3. Wall LL. The muscles of the pelvic floor. Clin Obstet Gynecol 1993; 36:910–925.

4. Abramson D, Roberts S, Wilson P. Relaxation of the pelvic joints in pregnancy. Surg Gynecol Obstet 1934; 58:595–613.
5. Calguneri M, Bird H, Wright V. Changes in joint laxity occurring during pregnancy. Ann Rheum Dis 1982; 41:126–128.
6. Thomas H. Relaxation of the symphysis pubsis in pregnancy. JAMA 1936; 106:1364–1366.
7. Samuel CS. Effects of relaxin, pregnancy and parturition on collagen metabolism in the rat public symphysis. J Endocrinol 1998; 159(1):117–25.
8. Eason E, Labrecque M, Marcoux S, Mondor M. Anal incontinence after children. Can Med Assoc J 2002; 166(3):326–330.
9. Henry MM, Parks AG, Swash M. The pelvic floor musculature in the descending perineum syndrome. Br J Surg 1982; 69:470–472.
10. Snooks SJ, Swash M, Mathers SE, Henry MM. Effect of vaginal delivery on the pelvic floor: a 5-year follow-up. Br J Surg 1990; 77:1358–1360.
11. Pregazzi R, Sartore A, Bortoli P, Grimaldi E, Ricci G, Guaschino S. Immediate postpartum perineal examination as a predictor of puerperal pelvic floor dysfunction. Obstet Gynecol 2002; 99(4):581–584.
12. Rieger N, Schloithe A, Saccone G, Wattchow D. The effect of a normal vaginal delivery on anal function. Acta Obstet Gynaecol Scand 1997; 76(8):769–772.
13. Thacker SB, Banta HD. Benefits and risks of episiotomy: an interpretative review of the English language literature 1860–1980. Obstet Gynecol Surv 1983; 38:322–338.
14. Williams AB, Bartram CI, Halligan S, Spencer JA, Nicholls RJ, Kmiot WA. Anal sphincter damage after vaginal delivery using three-dimensional endosonography. Obstet Gynecol 2001; 97(5 Pt 1): 770–775.
15. Crawford LA, Quint EH, Pearl ML, DeLancey JOL. Incontinence following rupture of the anal sphincter during delivery. Obstet Gynecol 1993; 82:527–531.
16. Bek KM, Laurberg S. Risks of anal incontinence from subsequent vaginal delivery after a complete obstetric anal sphincter tear. Br J Obstet Gynaecol 1992; 99:724–726.
17. Go PMNYH, Dunselman GAL. Anatomic and functional results of surgical repair after total perineal rupture at delivery. Surg Gynecol Obstet 1988; 166:121–124.
18. Sorenson M, Bondesen H, Istre O, Vilmann P. Perineal rupture following vaginal delivery: long-term consequences. Acta Obstet Gynaecol Scand 1988; 67:315–318.
19. Faltin DL, Sangalli MR, Roche B, Lucia F, Boulvain M, Weil A. Does a second delivery increase the risk of anal incontinence? Br J Obstet Gyaecol 2001; 108:684–688.
20. Fornell EK, Berg G, Hallbook O, Matthiesen LS, Sjodadhal R. Clinical consequences of anal sphincter rupture during vaginal delivery. J Am Coll Surg 1996; 183:553–558.
21. MacArthur C, Bick DE, Keighly MR. Faecal incontinence after childbirth. Br J Obstet Gynaecol 1997; 104:46–50.
22. Groutz A, Fait G, Lessing JB, David MP, Wolman I, Jaffa A, Gordon D. Incidence and obstetric risk factors of postpartum anal incontinence. Scand J Gastroenterol 1999; 34(3):315–318.
23. Frudinger A, Bartram CI, Sepncer JAD, Kamm MA. Perineal examination as a predictor of underlying external anal sphincter damage. Br J Obstet Gynaecol 1997; 104:1009–1013.
24. Burnett SJ, Spence-Jones C, Speakman CT, Kamm MA, Hdson CN, Bartram CI. Unsuspected sphincter damage following childbirth revealed by anal endosonography. Br J Radiol 1991; 64:225–227.
25. Sultan AH, Kamm MA, Hudson CN, Thomas JM, Bartram CI. Anal sphincter disruption during vaginal delivery. N Engl J Med 1993: 329:1905–1911.
26. Rieger N, Schloithe A, Saccone G, Wattchow D. A prospective study of anal sphincter injury due to childbirth. Scand J Gastroenterol 1998; 33:950–955.
27. Canpbell DM, Behan M, Donnelly VS, O'Herlihy C, O'Connell PR. Endosonographic assessment of postpartum anal sphincter injury using a 120 degree sector scanner. Clin Radiol 1996; 51:559–561.
28. Zetterstrom J, Mellgren A, Jensen LL, Wong WD, Kim DG, Lowry AC, Madoff RD, Congilosi SM. Effect of delivery on anal sphincter morphology and function. Dis Colon Rectum 1999; 42(10):1253–1260.
29. Sultan AH, Kamm MA, Hudson CN, Bartram CI. Third degree obstetric anal sphincter tears: risk factors and outcome of primary repair. BMJ 1994; 308(6933):887–891.

30. Deen KI, Kumar D, Williams JG, Olliff J, Keighley MR. The prevalence of anal sphincter defects in faecal incontinence: a prospective endosonic study. Gut 1993; 34(5):685–688.

31. DeLancey JOL, Toglia MR, Perucchini D. Internal and external anal sphincter anatomy as it relates to midline obstetric lacerations. Obstet Gynecol 1997; 90:924–927.

32. Sultan AH, Kamm MA, Hudson CN, Thomas JM, Bartram CI. Anal sphincter disruption during vaginal delivery. N Engl J Med 1993; 329:1905–1911.

33. Sato T, Konishi F, Minakami H, Nakatsubo N, Kanazawa K, Sato I, Itoh K, Nagai H. Pelvic floor disturbance after childbirth: vaginal delivery damages the upper levels of sphincter innervation. Dis Colon Rectum 2001; 44(8):1155–1161.

34. Sultan AH, Monga AK, Kumar D, Stanton SL. Primary repair of obstetric anal sphincter rupture using the overlap technique. Br J Obstet Gynaecol 1999; 106:318–323.

35. Halverson AL, Hull TL. Long-term outcome of overlapping anal sphincter repair. Dis Colon Rectum 2002; 45(3):345–348.

36. Malouf AJ, Norton CS, Engel AF, Nicholls RJ, Kamm MA. Long-term results of overlapping anterior anal-sphincter repair for obstetric trauma. Lancet 2000; 355(9200):260–265.

37. Gilliland R, Altomare DF, Moreira H Jr, Oliveira L, Gilliland JE, Wexner SD. Pudendal neuropathy is predictive of failure following anterior overlapping sphincteroplasty. Dis Colon Rectum 1998; 41(12):1516–1522.

38. Shiono P, Klebanoff MA, Carey JC. Midline episiotomies: more harm than good? Obstet Gynecol 1990; 75:765–770.

39. Klein MC, Gauthier RJ, Robbins JM, Kaczoroswki J, Jorgensen SH, Franco ED. Relationship of episiotomy to perineal trauma and morbidity, sexual dysfunction, and pelvic floor relaxation. Am J Obstet Gynecol 1994; 171:591–598.

40. Green JR, SooHoo SL. Factors associated with rectal injury in spontaneous deliveries. Obstet Gynecol 1989; 73:732–738.

41. Rockner G, Jonasson A, Olund A. The effect of mediolateral episiotomy at delivery on pelvic floor muscle strength evaluated with vaginal cones. Acta Obstet Gynecol Scand 1991; 70:51–54.

42. Argentine Episiotomy Trial Collaborative Group. Routine vs. selective episiotomy: a randomized controlled trial. Lancet 1993; 342(8886–8887):1517–1518.

43. Klein MC, Gauthier RJ, Jorgensen SH, Robbins JM, Kaczorowski J, Johnson B, Corriveau M, Westreich R, Waghorn K, Gelfand MM. Does episiotomy prevent perineal trauma and pelvic floor relaxation? Online J Curr Clin Trials 1992; Doc. No. 10..

44. Signorello LB, Harlow BL, Chekos AK, Repke JT. Midline episiotomy and anal incontinence: retrospective cohort study. BMJ 2000; 320(7227):86–90.

45. Signorello LB, Harlow BL, Chekos AK, Repke JT. Postpartum sexual functioning and its relationship to perineal trauma: a retrospective cohort study of primiparous women. Am J Obstet Gynecol 2001; 184(5):881–888.

46. Carroli G, Belizan J. Episiotomy for vaginal birth. Cochrance Database Syst Rev 2000;(2):CD000081.

47. Combs CA, Robertson PA, Laros RK. Risk Cochrance Database Syst Rev 2000;(2):CD000081-degree and fourth-degree perineal lacerations in forceps and vacuum deliveries. Am J Obstet Gynecol 1990; 163:100–104.

48. Helwigh JT, Thorp JM, Bowes WA. Does midline episiotomy increase the risk of third- and fourth-degree lacerations in operative vaginal deliveries? Obstet Gynecol 1993; 82:276–279.

49. Berglas B, Rubin IC. Study of the supportive structures of the uterus by levator myography. Surg Gynecol Obstet 1953; 97:677–692.

50. Delancey JOL. Anatomy and biomechanics of genital prolapse. Clin Obstet Gynecol 1993; 36:897–909.

51. Sampselle CM, Miller JM, Mims BL, DeLancey JOL, Ashton-Miller JA, Antonakos CL. Effect of pelvic muscle exercise on transient incontinence during pregnancy and after birth. Obstet Gynecol 1988; 91:406–412.

52. Peschers UM, Schaer GN, DeLancey JO, Schuessler B. Levator ani function before and after childbirth. Br J Obstet Gynaecol 1997; 104:1004–1008.

53. Allen RE, Hosker GL, Smith ARB, Warrell DW. Pelvic floor damage in childbirth: a neurophysiological study. Br J Obstet Gynaecol 1990;97:770–779.
54. Barber MD, Bremer RE, Thor KB, Dolber PC, Kuehl TJ, Coates KW. Innervation of the female levator ani muscles. Am J Obstet Gynecol 2002; 187(1):64–71.
55. Snooks SJ, Swash M, Setchell M, Henry MM. Injury to innervation of pelvic floor sphincter musculature in childbirth. Lancet 1984; ii:546–550.
56. Snooks SJ, Swash M, Henry MM, Setchell M. Risk factors in childbirth causing damage to the pelvic floor innervation. Int J Colorectal Dis 1986; 1(1):20–24.
57. Mallett VT, Hosker G, Smith ARB, Warrell DW. Pelvic floor damage and childbirth; a neurophysiologic follow-up study. Neurourol Urodyn 1993; 12:357–358.
58. Snooks SJ, Swash M, Mathers SE, Henry MM. Effect of vaginal delivery on the pelvic floor: a 5-year follow-up. Br J Surg 1990; 77:1358–1360.
59. Snooks SJ, Barnes PR, Swash M. Damage to the innervation of the voluntary anal and periurethral sphincter musculature in continence: an electrophysiological study. J Neurol Neurosurg Psychiatry 1984; 47:1269–1273.
60. Smith AR, Hosker GL, Warrell DW. The role of pudendal nerve damage in the aetiology of genuine stress incontinence in women. Br J Obstet Gynaecol 1989; 96(1):29–32.
61. Barnick CGW, Cardozo LD. Denervation and re-innervation of the urethral sphincter in the aetiology of genuine stress urinary incontinence: An electromyographic study. Br J Obstet Gynaecol 1992; 80:906–911.
62. Barnick CGW, Cardozo LD. A comparison of bioelectrical and mechanical activity of the female urethra. Br J Obstet Gynaecol 1993; 100:754–757.
63. Smith ARB, Hosker GL, Warrell DW. The role of partial denervation of the pelvic floor in the aetiology of genitourinary prolapse and stress incontinence of urine. A neurophysiological study. Br J Obstet Gynaecol 1989; 96:24–28.
64. Snooks SJ, Henry MM, Swash M. Faecal incontinence due to external anal sphincter division in childbirth is associated with damage to the innervation of the pelvic floor musculature; a double pathology. Br J Obstet Gynaecol 1985; 92: 824–828.
65. Snooks SJ, Swash M, Setchell M, Henry MM. Injury to innervation of pelvic floor sphincter musculature in childbirth. Lancet 1984; ii:546–550.
66. Gilpin SA, Gosling JA, Smith ARB, Warrell DW. The pathogenesis of genitourinary prolapse and stress incontinence of urine: a histological and histochemical study. Br J Obstet Gynaecol 1989; 96:15–23.
67. Sharf B, Zilberman A, Sharf M, Mitrani A. Electromyogram of pelvic floor muscles in genital prolapse. Int J Gynaecol Obstet 1976; 14:2–4.
68. Norton PA. Pelvic floor disorders: the role of fascia and ligaments. Clin Obstet Gynecol 1993; 36:926–301.
69. Richardson AC, Lyon JB, Williams NL. A new look at pelvic relaxation. Am J Obstet Gynecol 1976; 126:568–571.
70. Abitbol MM. The shapes of the female pelvis. Contributing factors. J Repord Med 1996; 41(4):242–250.
71. Mattox TF, Lucente V, McIntyre P, Miklos JR, Tomezsko J. Abnormal spinal curvature and its relationship to pelvic organ prolapse. Am J Obstet Gynecol 2000; 183(6):1381–1384.
72. Nguyen JK, Lind LR, Choe Jy, McKindsey F, Sinow R, Bhatia NN. Lumbosacral spine and pelvic inlet changes associated with pelvic organ prolapse. Obstet Gynecol 2000; 95(3):332–336.
73. Viktrup L, Lose G, Rolff M, Barfoed K. The symptom of stress incontinence caused by pregnancy or delivery in primiparas. Obstet Gynecol 1992; 79:945–949.
74. Francis WJA. The onset of stress incontinence. J Obstet Gynaecol Br Emp 1960; 67:899–903.
75. Marshall K, Thompson KA, Walsh DM, Baxter GD. Incidence of urinary incontinence and constipation during pregnancy and postpartum: survey of current findings at the Rotunda Lying-in Hospital. Br J Obstet Gynaecol 1998; 105:400–402.
76. Stanton SL, Kerr-Wilson R, Harris VG. The incidence of urological symptoms in normal pregnancy, Br J Obstet Gynaecol 1980; 87:897–900.

77. Meyer S, Schreyer A, DeGrandi P, Hohlfeld P. The effects of birth on urinary continence mechanisms and other pelvic floor characteristics. Obstet Gynecol 1998; 92:613–618.

78. Viktrup L, Lose G. The risk of stress incontinence 5 years after first delivery. Am J Obstet Gynecol 2001; 185:82–87.

79. Bergman A, McCarthy TA, Ballard CA, Yanai J. Role of the Q-tip in evaluating stress urinary incontinence. J Reprod Med 1987; 32:273–275.

80. Peschers U, Schar G, Anthuber C, Schussler B. Postpartal pelvic floor damage: is connective tissue impairment more important than neuromuscular changes? Neurourol Urodyn 1993; 12:376–377.

81. Peschers U, Schaer G, Anthuber C, Delancey JOL, Schuessler B. Changes in vesical neck mobility following vaginal delivery, Obstet Gynecol 1996; 88:1001–1006.

82. Tapp A, Cardozo L, Versi E, Montgomery J, Studd J. The effect of vaginal delivery on the urethral sphincter. Br Obstet Gynaecol 1988; 95:142–145.

83. Van Geelen JM, Lemmens WAJG, Eskes TKAB, Martin CB. The urethral pressure profile in pregnancy and after delivery in healthy nulliparous women. Am J Obstet Gynecol 1982; 144:636–649.

84. Mallett V, Hosker G, Smith ARB, Warrell D. Pelvic floor damage and childbirth: a neurophysiologic follow up study. Neurourol Urodyn 1994; 13:357–358.

85. Hojberg KE, Salvig JD, Winslow NA, Lose G, Secher NJ. Urinary incontinence: prevalence and risk factors at 16 weeks of gestation. Br J Obstet Gynaecol 1999; 106:842–850.

86. Persson J, Wolner-Hanssen PAL, Rydhstroem. Obstetric risk factors for stress urinary incontinence: a population-based study. Obstet Gynecol 2000; 96:440–445.

87. Moller LA, Lose G, Jorgensen T. Risk factors for lower urinary tract symptoms in women 40 to 60 years of age. Obstet Gynecol 2000; 96:446–451.

88. Marshall K, Thompson KA, Walsh DM, Baxter GD. Incidence of urinary incontinence and constipation during pregnancy and postpartum: survey of current findings at the Rotunda Lying-in Hospital. Br J Obstet Gynaecol 1998; 105:400–402.

89. Rowe JW. NIH consensus development panel: urinary incontinence in adults. JAMA 1989; 261:2685–2690.

90. Sampselle CM, Miller JM, Mims BL, Delancey JO, Ashton-Miller JA, Antonakos CL. Effect of pelvic muscle exercise on transient incontience during pregnancy and after birth. Obstet Gynecol 1998; 91(3):406–412.

91. Reilly ET, Freeman RM, Waterfield MR, Waterfield AE, Steggles P, Pedlar F. Prevention of postpartum stress incontinence in primigravidae with increased bladder neck mobility: a randomised controlled trial of antenatal pelvic floor exercises. Br J Obstet Gynaecol 2002; 109(1):68–76.

92. Stamp G, Kruzins G, Crowther C. Perineal massage in labour and prevention of perineal trauma: randomised controlled trial. BMJ 2001; 322(7297):1277–1280.

93. Labrecque M, Eason E, Marcoux S, Lemieux F, Pinault JJ, Feldman P, Laperriere L. Randomized controlled trial of prevention of perineal trauma by perineal massage during pregnancy. Am J Obstet Gynecol 1999; 180(3 Pt 1):593–600.

94. Labrecque M, Eason E, Marcoux S. Randomized trial of perineal massage during pregnancy: perineal symptoms three months after delivery. Am J Obstet Gynecol 2000; 182(1 Pt 1):76–80.

95. Rasmussen KL, Krue S, Johansson LE, Knudsen HJ, Agger AO. Obesity as a predictor of postpartum urinary symptoms. Acta Obstet Gynaecol Scand 1997; 76(4):359–362.

96. Elia G, Dye TD, Scariati PD. Body mass index and urinary symptoms in women. Int Urogynecol J Pelvic Floor Dysfunct 2001; 12(6)366–369.

97. Angioli R, Gomez-Marin O, Cantuaria G, O'sullivan MJ. Severe perineal lacerations during vaginal delivery: the University of Miami experience. Am J Obstet Gynecol 2000; 182(5):1083–1085.

98. King JK, Freeman RM. Is antenatal bladder neck mobility a risk factor for postpartum stress incontinence? Br J Obstet Gynaecol 1998; 105(12):1300–1307.

99. Roshanfekr D, Blakemore KJ, Lee J, Hueppchen NA, Witter FR. Station at onset of active labor in nulliparous patients and risk of cesarean delivery. Obstet Gynecol 1999; 93(3):329–331.

100. Nichols DH. In: Vaginal Surgery. 4th ed. Baltimore: Williams & Wilkins, 1996: 49.

101. Gardosi J, Hutson N, B-Lynch C. Randomised, controlled trial of squatting in the second stage of labour. Lancet 1989; 2(8654):74–77.

102. Golay J, Vedam S, Sorger L. The squatting position for the second stage of labor: effects on labor and on maternal and fetal well-being. Birth 1993; 20:73–78.

103. De Jong PR, Johanson RB, Baxen P, Adrians VD, Van der Westhuisen S, Jones PW. Randomised trial comparing the upright and supine positions for the second stage of labour. Br J Obstet Gynaecol 1997; 104(5):567–571.

104. Gupta JK, Nikodem VC. Woman's position during second stage of labour. Cochrane Database Syst Rev 2000; (2):CD002006.

105. Combs CA, Robertson PA, Laros RK. Risk factors for third-degree and fourth-degree perineal lacerations in forceps and vacuum deliveries. Am J Obstet Gynecol 1990; 163:100–104.

106. Mayerhofer K, Bodner-Adler B, Bodner K, Rabl M, Kaider A, Wagenbichler P, Joura EA, Husslein P. Traditional care of the perineum during birth. A prospective, randomized, multicenter study of 1,076 women. J Reprod Med 2002; 47(6):477–482.

107. Fraser WD, Marcoux S, Krauss I, Douglas J, Goulet C, Boulvain M. Multicenter, randomized, controlled trial of delayed pushing for nulliparous women in the second stage of labor with continuous epidural analgesia. The PEOPLE (Pushing Early or Pushing Late with Epidural) Study Group. Am J Obstet Gynecol 2000; 182(5):1165–1172.

108. Hansen SL, Clark SL, Foster JC. Active pushing versus passive fetal descent in the second stage of labor: a randomized controlled trial. Obstet Gynecol 2002; 99(1):29–34.

109. Sampselle CM, Hines S. Spontaneous pushing during birth. Relationship to perineal outcomes. J Nur Midwifery 1999; 44(1):36–39.

110. Parnell C, Langhoff-Roos J, Iversen R, Damgaard P. Pushing method in the expulsive phase of labor. A randomized trial. Acta Obstet Gynaecol Scand 1993; 72(1):31–35.

111. Hansen SL, Clark SL, Foster JC. Active pushing versus passive fetal descent in the second stage of labor: a randomized controlled trial. Obstet Gynecol 2002; 99(1):29–34.

112. Janni W, Schiessl B, Peschers U, Huber S, Strobl B, Hantschmann P, Uhlmann N, Dimpfl T, Rammel G, Kainer F. The prognostic impact of a prolonged second stage of labor on maternal and fetal outcome. Acta Obstet Gynaecol Scand 2002; 81(3):214–221.

113. Combs CA, Robertson PA, Laros RK. Risk factors for third-degree and fourth-degree perineal lacerations in forceps and vacuum deliveries. Am J Obstet Gynecol 1990; 163:100–104.

114. Donnelly V, Fynes M, Campbell D, Johnson H, O'Connell PR, O'Herlihy C. Obstetric events leading to anal sphincter damage. Obstet Gynecol 1998; 92(6):955–961.

115. Van Kessel K, Reed S, Newton K Meier A, Lentz G. The second stage of labor and stress urinary incontinence. Am J Obstet Gynecol 2001; 184(7):1571–1575.

116. Arya LA, Jackson ND, Myers DL, Verma A. Risk of new-onset urinary incontinence after forceps and vacuum delivery in primiparous women. Am J Obstet Gynecol 2001; 185(6):1318–1323.

117. Farrell SA, Allen VM, Baskett TF. Parturition and urinary incontinence in primiparas. Obstet Gynecol 2001; 97(3):350–356.

118. Meyer S, Hohlfield P, Achtari C, Russolo A, De Grandi P. Birth trauma: short and long term effects of forceps delivery compared with spontaneous delivery on various pelvic floor. Br J Obstet Gynaecol 2000; 107(11):1360–1365.

119. Combs CA, Robertson PA Laros RK Jr. Risk factors for third-degree and fourth-degree perineal lacerations in forceps and vacuum deliveries. Am J Obstet Gynecol 1990; 163(1 Pt 1): 100–104.

120. Sultan AH, Kamm MA, Bartram CI, Hudson CN. Anal sphincter trauma during instrumental delivery. Int J Gynaecol Obstet 1993; 43(3):263–270.

121. Wen SW, Liu S, Kramer MS, Marcoux S, Ohlsson A, Sauve R, Liston R. Comparison of maternal and infant outcomes between vacuum extraction and forceps deliveries. Am J Epidemiol 2001; 153(2):103–107.

122. Bofill JA, Rust OA, Schorr SJ, Brown RC, Martin RW, Martin JN Jr, Morrison JC. A randomized prospective trial of the obstetric forceps versus the M-cup vacuum extractor. Am J Obstet Gynecol 1996; 175(5):1325–1330.

123. Sultan AH, Johanson RB, Carter JE. Occult anal sphincter trauma following randomized forceps and vacuum delivery. Int J Gynaecol Obstet 1998; 61(2):113–119.

124. Johanson RB, Menon BK. Vacuum extraction versus forceps for assisted vaginal delivery. Cochrane Database Syst Rev 2000; (2):CD000224.
125. Jander C, Lyrenas S. Third and fourth degree perineal tears. Predictor factors in a referral hospital. Acta Obstet Gynaecol Scand 2001; 80(3):229–234.
126. Handa VL, Danielsen BH, Gilbert WM. Obstetric anal sphincter lacerations. Obstet Gynecol 2001; 98(2):225–230.
127. Riskin-Mashiah S, O'Brian Smith E, Wilkins IA. Risk factors for severe perineal tear: can we do better? Am J Perinatol 2002; 19(5):225–234.
128. Snooks SJ, Swash M, Henry MM, Sretchell M. Risk factors in childbirth causing damage to the pelvic floor innervation. Int J Colorectal Dis 1986; 1:20–24.
129. Meyer S, Schreyer A, De Grandi P, Hohlfeld P. The effects of birth on urinary continence mechanisms and other pelvic-floor characteristics. Obstet Gynecol 1998; 92(4 Pt 1):613–618.
130. Groutz A, Gordon D, Keidar R, Lessing JB, Wolman I, David MP, Chen B. Stress urinary incontinence: prevalence among nulliparous compared with primiparous and grand multiparous premenopausal women. Neurourol Urodyn 1999; 18(5):419–425.
131. Robinson JN, Norwitz ER, Cohen AP, Lieberman E. Predictors of episiotomy use at first spontaneous vaginal delivery. Obstet Gynecol 2000; 96(2):214–218.
132. Bodner K, Bodner-Adler B, Wagenbichler P, Kaider A, Leodolter S, Husslein P, Mayerhofer K. Perineal lacerations during spontaneous vaginal delivery. Wien Klin Wochenschr 2001; 113(19):743–746.
133. Goldberg RP, Kwon C, Gandhi S, Atkuru LV, Sorensen M, Sand PK. Urinary incontinence among 'mothers of multiples': the protective effect of cesarean delivery.
134. Fitzpatrick M, McQuillan K, O'Herlihy C. Influence of persistent occiput posterior position on delivery outcome. Obstet Gynecol 2001; 98(6):1027–1031.
135. Pearl ML, Roberts JM, Laros RK, Hurd WW. Vaginal delivery from the persistent occiput posterior position. Influence on maternal and neonatal morbidity. J Reprod Med 1993; 38(12):955–961.
136. Robinson JN, Norwitz ER, Cohen AP, McElrath TF, Lieberman ES. Epidural analgesia and third- or fourth-degree lacerations in nulliparas. Obstet Gynecol 1999; 94(2):259–262.
137. Walker MP, Farine D, Rolbin SH, Ritchie JW. Epidural anesthesia, episiotomy, and obstetric laceration. Obstet Gynecol 1991; 77(5):668–671.
138. Al-Mufti R, McCarthy A, Fisk NM. Obstetricians personal choice and mode of delivery. Lancet 1996; 347–544.
139. Sultan AH, Kamm MA, Hudson CN. Pudendal nerve damage during labour: prospective study before and after childbirth. Br J Obstet Gynaecol 1994; 101(1):22–28.
140. Viktrup L, Lose G, Rolff M, Barfoed K. The symptom of stress incontinence caused by pregnancy or delivery in primiparas. Obstet Gynecol 1992; 79:945–949.
141. Faundes A, Guarisi T, Pinto-Neto AM. The risk of urinary incontinence of parous women who delivered only by cesarean section. Int J Gynaecol Obstet 2001; 72(1):41–46.
142. Hannah ME, Hannah WJ, Hodnett ED, Chalmers B, Kung R, Willan A, Amankwah K, Cheng M, Helewa M, Hewson S, Saigal S, Whyte H, Gafni A, Term Breech Trial 3-Month Follow-up Collaborative Group. Outcomes at 3 months after planned cesarean vs planned vaginal delivery for breech presentation at term: the international randomized Term Breech Trial. JAMA 2002; 287(14):1822–1831.
143. Fynes M, Donnelly VS, O'Connell PR, O'Herlihy C. Cesarean delivery and anal sphincter injury. Obstet Gynecol 1998; 92(4 Pt 1):496–500.
144. Meyer S, Hohlfeld P, Achtari C, De Grandi P. Pelvic floor education after vaginal delivery. Obstet Gynecol 2001; 97(5 Pt 1):673–677.
145. Reilly ET, Freeman RM, Waterfield MR, Waterfield AE, Steggles P, Pedlar F. Prevention of postpartum stress incontinence in primigravidae with increased bladder neck mobility: a randomised controlled trial of antenatal pelvic floor exercises. Br J Obstet Gynaecol 2002; 109(1):68–76.
146. Morkved S, Bo K. The effect of post-natal exercises to strengthen the pelvic floor muscles. Acta Obstet Gynaecol Scand 1996; 75(4):382–385.

147. Morkved S, Bo K. Effect of postpartum pelvic floor muscle training in prevention and treatment of urinary incontinence: a one-year follow up. Br J Obstet Gynaecol 2000; 107(8):1022–1028.

148. Wilson PD, Herbison GP. A randomized controlled trial of pelvic floor muscle exercises to treat postnatal urinary incontinence. Int Urogynecol J Pelvic Floor Dysfunct 1998; 9(5):257–264.

149. Chiarelli P, Cockburn J. Promoting urinary continence in women after delivery: randomised controlled trial. BMJ 2002; 324(7348):1227–1228.

150. Morkved S, Bo K. The effect of post-natal exercises to strengthen the pelvic floor muscles. Acta Obstet Gynaecol Scand 1996; 75(4):382–385.

151. Meyer S, Hohlfeld P, Achtari C, De Grandi P. Pelvic floor education after vaginal delivery. Obstet Gynecol 2001; 97:673–677.

152. Laurberg S, Swash M, Snooks SJ, Henry MM. Neurologic cause of idiopathic incontinence. Arch Neurol 1988; 45(11):1250–1253.

153. Payne TN, Carey JC, Rayburn WF. Prior third- or fourth-degree perineal tears and recurrence risks. Int J Gynaecol Obstet 1999; 64(1):55–57.

154. Peleg D, Kennedy CM, Merrill D, Zlatnik FJ. Risk of repetition of a severe perineal laceration. Obstet Gynecol 1999; 93(6):1021–1024.

155. Casper FW, Linn JF, Black P. Obstetrical management following incontinence surgery. J Obstet Gynaecol Res 1999; 25(1):51–53.

156. Abramowitz L, Sobhani I, Ganansia R, Vuagnat A, Benifla JL, Darai E, Madelenat P, Mignon M. Are sphincter defects the cause of anal incontinence after vaginal delivery? Results of a prospective study. Dis Colon Rectum 2000; 43(5):590–596.

157. Faltin DL, Sangalli MR, Roche B, Floris L, Boulvain M, Weil A. Does a second delivery increase the risk of anal incontinence? Br J Obstet Gynaecol 2001; 108(7):684–688.

158. Fynes M, Donnelly V, Behan M, O'Connell PR, O'Herlihy C. Effect of second vaginal delivery on anorectal physiology and faecal continence: a prospective study. Lancet 1999; 354(9183):983–986.

159. Tetzschner T, Sorensen M, Jonsson L, Lose G, Christiansen J. Delivery and pudendal nerve function. Acta Obstet Gynaecol Scand 1997; 76(4):324–331.

8

History and Physical Examination in Pelvic Floor Disorders

Sanjay Gandhi and Peter K. Sand
Northwestern University, Evanston, Illinois, U.S.A.

I. INTRODUCTION

Women with a pelvic floor disorder may present with a symptom, a previously identified physical sign, or a previously identified diagnosis. A clinician must take each of these and start a comprehensive inquiry into the patient's medical history and constellation of symptoms. Further evaluation includes a focused general examination and a comprehensive genitourinary examination.

Most evaluations will focus on pelvic organ prolapse and on urinary and fecal incontinence, but clinicians specializing in pelvic floor medicine will see a diverse range of problems. Knowledge of urology, gynecology, gastroenterology, and neurology is crucial in conducting an appropriate evaluation. A consistent methodology to evaluate patients with urogenital tract symptoms is most important in establishing the underlying etiology of the patient's pelvic floor disorder. Effective treatment of pelvic floor disorders depends on an accurate diagnosis and an understanding of the patient's expectations of treatment.

The history, physical examination, and simple office testing may establish a preliminary diagnosis on which a clinician may begin treatment or may serve as an excellent screening tool to determine which individuals require further evaluation. If a complex or recurrent problem is present, surgery is planned, or the patient's symptoms do not improve with initial treatment, specialized tests such as complex urodynamics should be employed to definitively establish diagnoses. Urogenital, gastrointestinal, musculoskeletal, neurologic, and endocrinologic factors may affect pelvic floor disorders, and a comprehensive history and physical examination begins the process of evaluating these conditions. Other, more specific criteria to select patients for further evaluation of urinary incontinence are listed in Table 1.

II. HISTORY

The history is an essential part of the evaluation of every female with a pelvic floor disorder. No urogenital tract symptom is pathognomonic for an underlying condition. While the history is limited in its specificity and is only the first step of the diagnostic inquiry into the patient's disorder, it defines the problem by identifying the symptoms that must be explained by the

Table 1   Criteria for Further Testing

1. Uncertain diagnosis and inability to develop a reasonable treatment plan based on the basic evaluation. Uncertainty in diagnosis may occur when there is lack of correlation between symptoms and clinical findings
2. Failure to respond to the patient's satisfaction to an adequate therapeutic trial, and the patient is interested in pursuing further therapy
3. Surgical intervention planned
4. Hematuria without infection
5. Presence of any of the following conditions:
    Recurrent symptomatic UTI
    Persistent symptoms of difficult bladder emptying
    History of prior incontinence operation or radical pelvic surgery
    Significant genital prolapse
    Retention
    Neurological condition (e.g., multiple sclerosis or spinal cord lesions/injury)

Source: Ref. 54.

evaluation. The clinician must evaluate information gathered from the patient history to selectively choose which diagnostic tests will reveal a condition's etiology.

A concise history may be obtained using premailed questionnaires providing the patient time to consider her symptoms, past medical history, and family history and reconfirm them. Bowel and bladder diaries or other chronological records of symptoms recorded at home may provide further clarification of the patient's symptoms. An office interview supplements this initial history and should include an assessment of symptoms, risk factors for disease, and a general medical and social history.

Most authors have found a medical history to be inadequate in establishing an accurate etiology of incontinence (1–6), with only a few exceptions. Farrar et al. concluded that history alone was accurate in establishing a diagnosis. Two of 56 women (3.6%) with stress incontinence symptoms alone and 89% of the 110 women with symptoms of urge incontinence were found to have detrusor overactivity on cystometry (7). Hastie and Moisey (8) also concluded that a history of pure stress incontinence was 100% accurate in establishing the diagnosis of genuine stress incontinence. In contrast, Jensen and colleagues (9) in a meta-analysis of thousands of patients found that reliance on history alone to identify genuine stress incontinence resulted in a misdiagnosis in 25% of patients. Patient history was an even less accurate predictor of detrusor overactivity, with a misdiagnosis in 45% of patients with a history of urge loss (9). In addition, advanced pelvic prolapse may mask underlying incontinence unless the pelvic prolapse is reduced (10–12). Ghoneim and colleagues (12) found in a small cohort of women that reducing the prolapse by a vaginal pack during urodynamic testing demonstrated stress incontinence in 69% of women who were otherwise asymptomatic. Based on these studies, a clinician cannot depend on a patient's symptoms to accurately reflect the underlying disorder. While the patient's history will not be diagnostic, a complete assessment of symptoms will serve as an outline to guide the clinician's evaluation.

III. SYMPTOMS

Symptoms are the subjective indicator of disease or change in condition as perceived by the patient, her caregiver, or partner and may lead her to seek help from health care professionals (13). They are categorized separately from signs, conditions, and urodynamic observations (13).

Anatomic, physiologic, and pathologic factors within the lower urogenital tract as well as nongenitourinary factors or conditions may result in pelvic floor disorders with a variety of acute or chronic symptoms. Recurrent symptoms may represent acute exacerbations of chronic disease. Women seeking care of a pelvic floor medicine specialist may present with symptoms of disease in the lower or upper urinary tract, in the gynecologic or gastrointestinal organs, or in the musculoskeletal or neurological system. Therefore, only a comprehensive review of systems will assure the clinician that all aspects of the disease process are being assessed.

A. Systemic Manifestations

Systemic manifestations of urogenital tract disorders include fever and weight loss. While simple acute cystitis typically does not cause a fever, acute pyelonephritis in adults typically causes high fevers with rigors and costovertebral angle tenderness. In children, simply the presence of fever should prompt the clinician to perform a bacteriologic evaluation of the urine, as often no other localizing signs or symptoms of a renal infection may be present. Renal infection may also present differently with recurrent fevers in the absence of other urinary tract symptoms or with no fevers at all. Chronic pyelonephritis may only present with general malaise. While infection is the typical cause of fevers, renal cell carcinoma may present with fevers.

Weight loss and general malaise are nonspecific symptoms that may prompt one to consider urogenital tract pathology such as advanced stages of cancer or renal insufficiency due to obstruction or infection.

B. Incontinence

The most common symptom of pelvic floor dysfunction is urinary incontinence—the involuntary leakage of urine. Urinary incontinence should be described by type, frequency, severity, precipitating factors, and impact on hygiene and on a patient's social activities. The clinician should understand the measures a patient uses to contain the leakage. Finally, it is crucial for the clinician to assess the impact of the incontinence on a patient's quality of life and on her caregivers. Understanding a partner, caregiver, or patient's expectations of treatment is crucial to rendering effective care. The original ICS definition of incontinence—"Urinary incontinence is the involuntary loss of urine that is a social or hygienic problem"—relates the complaint of incontinence to quality of life issues. Whether or not the individual or their caregiver seeks or desires help because of urinary incontinence should be known prior to beginning an evaluation.

1. Stress Urinary Incontinence

The symptom of stress urinary incontinence is the involuntary loss of urine during coughing, sneezing, laughing, or other physical activities that increase intra-abdominal pressure. Stress incontinence, the sign, is the observation of involuntary leakage from the urethra with exertion, coughing, or sneezing. Urodynamic stress incontinence, the condition, is defined as the involuntary loss of urine during an increase in intra-abdominal pressure in the absence of a detrusor contraction. This occurs when the bladder pressure exceeds the urethral pressure because of decreased transmission of intra-abdominal pressure to the urethra. This is usually secondary to urethral hypermobility. The decrease in transmission of intra-abdominal pressure to the urethra relative to the bladder is referred to as a *deficient extrinsic continence mechanism*.

Incontinence can also occur secondary to deficient intrinsic urethral sphincteric function. The smooth muscle, skeletal muscle, periurethral vasculature, and intrinsic urethral fibrous tissue all contribute to the resting urethral resistance or tone. Intrinsic sphincteric deficiency is the condition where the urethral sphincter is unable to generate enough resistance to retain urine in the bladder. Intrinsic urethral function can be measured urodynamically by calculating the resting urethral closure pressure. The leak point pressure is also used by some investigators to measure both the extrinsic and intrinsic continence mechanisms. Although increased age and multiparity are thought to increase the risk of stress incontinence, we know that even in nulliparous women with a well-supported urethra and an intact sphincter (normal urethral pressures), urinary incontinence may be present in as many as 50% of women (14,15). In elite female athletes, urinary loss may be present in up to 52% during their sport (16,17).

2. Urge Urinary Incontinence

The symptom of urge urinary incontinence is the involuntary loss of urine accompanied by or immediately preceded by a sudden compelling desire to pass urine, which is difficult to deter (i.e., urgency). Women with urge incontinence often demonstrate, on urodynamics, involuntary detrusor contractions, or detrusor overactivity. The prevalence of detrusor overactivity appears to increase with age.

3. Mixed Urinary Incontinence

Women with symptoms of both urge and stress urinary incontinence are said to have mixed urinary incontinence. Often one symptom is more bothersome than the other, and the clinician should attempt to make this differentiation.

C. Pain

A patient may feel local pain near the involved organ. Acute pyelonephritis manifests with pain in the costovertebral angle and the flank. In contrast, the spatial displacement of pain sensation from the point of stimulation is known as referred pain. Convergence of many sensory inputs to a single pain transmission neuron in the spinal cord underlies the phenomenon of referred pain.

   The brain has no way of knowing the source of the pain and mistakenly projects the pain sensation to a site distant from the original point of stimulation in the diseased organ (18). Ureteral colic is a classic symptom with referred pain. In women, ureteral calculi may result in pain felt in the vulva or inner thigh. Inflammation of the bladder trigone as seen in acute cystitis often results in terminal dysuria felt at the urethral meatus.

1. Renal Pain

Renal pain or colic is typically felt in the area lateral to the sacrospinalis muscle and below the 12th rib. This pain may spread along the subcostal area around to the umbilicus or lower abdomen (19). Such pain is typical in conditions that cause acute distension of the renal capsule such as acute pyelonephritis or acute ureteral obstruction from urolithiasis. Many conditions, however, are painless as they progress slowly without capsular distension including neoplasia, chronic pyelonephritis, staghorn calculi, polycystic kidney disease, and hydronephrosis from chronic ureteral obstruction (as seen in cervical cancer, massive fibroid tumors, or severe pelvic organ prolapse).

2. Pseudorenal Pain (Radiculitis)

Musculoskeletal derangements of the thoracic spine may irritate costal nerves, causing pain that mimics renal pain. Lifting of a heavy object, trauma to the flank, or a sudden fall may precipitate such pain. Relief of this pain by changes in position and movement of the spine differentiates it from true renal colic (19).

3. Ureteral Pain

Acute obstruction by calculi or blood clots typically results in ureteral pain. Renal capsular distension causes back pain, and ureteral muscle spasm elicits severe colicky pain from the costovertebral angle down toward the lower anterior abdominal quadrant along the course of the ureter. Stones in the midportion of the ureter on the right side may simulate appendicitis with referred pain to McBurney's point, while on the left, ureteral pain may resemble diverticulitis. A stone at the ureteral orifice may cause inflammation and edema in the bladder, producing lower urinary symptoms such as urgency and frequency. Finally, if the calculus is small, it may not even cause pain.

4. Vesical Pain

Overdistension of the bladder from acute retention causes severe suprapubic or retropubic pain. Chronic retention from bladder outlet obstruction or an acontractile bladder typically does not result in significant vesical pain even though the bladder may reach the level of the umbilicus. Interstitial cystitis or bladder ulceration caused by tuberculosis or schistosomiasis infection may cause suprapubic pain or discomfort when the bladder fills even to small volumes. Because these conditions often result in diminished bladder capacities, voiding results in significant relief of their suprapubic discomfort. Associated symptoms include urgency and frequency. Detrusor overactivity, which also causes urgency and frequency, does not commonly cause bladder pain. As stated earlier, bladder infection often results in referred pain to the distal urethra.

D.   Abdominal and Gastrointestinal Symptoms of Urogynecolgic Disease

Gastrointestinal symptoms often accompany renal and ureteral disease. The gastrointestinal and genitourinary systems share common autonomic and sensory innervations. Afferent stimuli from the renal capsule may, by reflex, alter the tone of smooth muscle in the enteric tract leading to gastrointestinal manifestations of renal disease. Enlargement of the kidneys may abut or displace intraperitoneal organs (e.g., stomach, colon, liver, gallbladder), causing gastrointestinal symptoms while inflammation may result in peritoneal irritation that results in muscle rigidity and rebound tenderness on abdominal examination. Abdominal pain, distension, nausea, and vomiting secondary to renointestinal reflexes are all common accompanying symptoms of acute pyelonephritis and ureteral colic. The connection between severe pelvic organ prolapse and abdominopelvic symptoms is less clear. Although anecdotally a large enterocele may lead to peritoneal irritation that may produce abdominal pain and gastrointestinal distress, Heit and Culligan (20) recently reported that pelvic organ prolapse was not associated with pelvic pain when controlling for patient age and prior prolapse surgery.

E.   Dyspareunia and Vulvodynia

Dyspareunia is pain in the pelvic area during or after intercourse. It occurs with vaginal penetration—either at the introitus or deep in the vagina. Differentiation between locations of pain with intercourse may point to distinct etiologies. Pain with deep penetration may suggest endometriosis, vaginal infection, or interstitial cystitis, while pain with initial intromission is more suggestive of vestibulitis, urethrotrigonitis, or vulvodynia.

Vulvodynia is chronic vulvar pain. It may be present constantly, intermittently, or only with intromission during intercourse. Activities that cause friction or pressure on the vulva aggravate the allodynic symptoms. Wearing tight pantyhose or jeans may elicit vulvar pain. Urine-soaked pads, excessive perspiration, and allergens may cause inflammation of the small vestibular glands and epithelium (i.e., vestibulitis) with secondary vulvodynia.

F. Medical and Social History

There are many medical conditions that may cause or aggravate urinary incontinence. The clinician should exclude these when evaluating a woman with urinary incontinence. One should take a medical, neurological, and genitourinary history including a detailed exploration of symptoms. The medications and supplements used by the patient should be carefully reviewed. The history should also include information on previous surgery, trauma, radiation therapy, use of hormone replacement, past medical history, and current active medical conditions. Information on previous urogynecologic treatments and assessment of their impact on current symptoms may be helpful. Other associated pelvic floor dysfunction involving bowel or sexual function is important to identify as these conditions may be interrelated with the patient's lower urinary tract symptomatology and may have been previously unrecognized. Correction of some reversible causes of urinary incontinence may resolve or improve their incontinence (Table 2) (21). Medications can often impact urinary symptoms such as incontinence or retention (Table 3).

Assessment should include psychosocial and environmental questions. An understanding of how a patient's problem impacts her daily living is crucial to providing appropriate and timely treatment. While pelvic prolapse may directly cause pain or discomfort and thus impact well-being, incontinence has broad psychological effects that may prevent an otherwise functional or healthy woman from leaving her home. An understanding of a patient's environmental conditions at home may help identify individuals with incontinence who are at risk for falls or fractures (22). Urinary symptoms can often force the elderly to hastily move to the toilet in less than ideal circumstances. A questionnaire can serve as a screening tool for psychosocial and environmental conditions that impact the patient's quality of life.

Knowledge of the amount and types of pads, briefs, and protective devices may provide insight into the extent of debilitation caused by a patient's incontinence. In elderly individuals, a mental status evaluation and assessment of physical mobility is important. An understanding of a patient's access to toilets, especially at night, when the elderly may be at greater risk of falls and

Table 2   Reversible Causes of Incontinence

DIAPPERS

Delirium or confusion
Infection, urinary tract
Atrophic genital tract changes (vaginitis or urethritis)
Pharmaceutical agents (see Table 3).
Psychologic
Excess urine production (excess fluid intake, volume overload,
     metabolic such as hyperglycemia or hypercalcemia)
Restricted mobility (chronic illness, injury, or restraint)
Stool impaction

Table 3 Drugs That May Affect Lower Urinary Tract

Class of drugs	Side effect	Impact on lower urinary tract function
Psychotropic agents		
Antidepressants	Anticholinergic, sedation	Urinary retention
Antipsychotics	Anticholinergic, sedation	Urinary retention
Sedatives/hypnotics	Sedation, muscle relaxation, confusion	Urinary retention
Alcohol	Sedation, impaired mobility	Diuresis, frequency
Caffeine		Urgency, frequency
Diuretics		Polyuria, urgency, frequency
Narcotics	Sedation, delirium	Urinary retention, fecal impaction
ACE inhibitors	Cough	Aggravate preexisting stress incontinence
Calcium-channel blockers		Urinary retention, overflow incontinence
Anticholinergic		Urinary retention, overflow incontinence
Alpha-adrenergic agonists	Increased urethral tone	Urinary retention
Alpha-adrenergic blockers	Decreased urethral tone	Stress incontinence
Beta-adrenergic agonists	Inhibited detrusor function	Urinary retention

injuries, of their living arrangements, and of the involvement of caregivers will help the clinician plan an individualized treatment plan.

Signs of lower urinary tract dysfunction are observed by the physician to verify symptoms and quantify them. Observations from bladder diaries, pad tests, and validated questionnaires are examples of other instruments used to confirm and quantify symptoms.

IV. QUESTIONNAIRES

Filling out a standardized questionnaire at home before coming into the office may help patients clarify and enhance their understanding of their symptoms. This gives patients time to delineate their symptoms, increase the accuracy of their answers, and obtain information from other family members if needed. It also speeds up their office evaluation.

Various validated questionnaires are useful not only to quantify the severity of symptoms and their impact on quality of life, but to provide quantitative data for use in research studies and outcomes analysis. Generalized health-related quality-of-life (HRQOL) instruments enable researchers to compare groups with different diseases. However, condition-specific instruments best allow the clinician to assess the impact of urogenital symptoms on a particular woman. Table 4 presents a list of some of the numerous validated questionnaires that have been developed for collecting and reporting subjective information about pelvic floor disorders in women. Unfortunately, no single instrument has emerged as the preferred one since questionnaires vary widely, depending on their intended purpose and target population (23). Choosing the appropriate questionnaire—one that is comprehensive yet easy for patient to complete—may be challenging. These questionnaires may be modified to meet the needs of a specific clinician or practice and may be included in a general information packet.

Table 4 Validated Questionnaires

Generalized	Medical Outcomes Survey Short Form-36 (SF-36) (55)
Condition-specific	
Urinary incontinence	Incontinence Impact Questionnaire (IIQ) (56)
	Urinary Distress Inventor (UDI) (56)
	IIQ-7 and UDI-6 (57)
	Incontinence Quality of Life Measure (I-QOL) (58)
	King's Health Questionnaire (59)
	Bristol Female Lower Urinary Tract Symptom Questionnaire (60)
	York Incontinence Perception Scale (YIPS) (61)
	Medical Epidemiologic and Social Aspects of Aging (MESA) Urinary Incontinence Questionnaire (UIQ)
Sexual dysfunction	Pelvic Organ Prolapse/Urinary Incontinence Sexual Questionnaire (PISQ) (62), PISQ-12
Pelvic organ prolapse	Pelvic Floor Dysfunction Inventory (PFDI) (63)
Defecatory dysfunction	Fecal Incontinence Quality of Life Scale (64)
	Pelvic Floor Dysfunction Inventory (PFDI) (63)
Interstitial cystitis	Interstitial Cystitis Symptom Index (ICSI) and Interstitial Cystitis Problem Index (ICPI) (65)

A. Bladder Diary

Bladder diaries assist in providing quantitative data on urinary frequency, voiding intervals, the volume of continent voids, and the number of incontinent episodes. They also enable the clinician to better understand triggers of incontinence such as coughing, exercises, Valsalva, or strenuous activity. Bladder diaries (Fig. 1) help to accurately assess fluid intake patterns, including the consumption of caffeine-containing fluids. The diary may help to establish voiding patterns that can help clinicians select appropriate behavioral interventions, and may also serve as a baseline of symptom severity for assessment of treatment efficacy. Seven-day bladder diaries have been found to correlate well with actual symptoms and incontinence severity (24). In addition, while filling out a diary may be tedious, the process of filling out a diary may in itself be a form of bladder training, resulting in an improvement in incontinence symptoms.

B. Physical Examination

The physical examination attempts to identify neurological deficits, defects in pelvic support, pelvic pathology, infection, estrogen deficiency, tenderness, and other urogenital problems. One must employ a methodical approach to the evaluation of the urogenital tract for pathology. In addition, a systematic general physical and neurological examination may also reveal other causes (e.g., cardiac, endocrine) of urogynecologic symptoms.

1. Neurological Examination

The screening neurological examination should include an evaluation of mental status, gait, and the lumbosacral nerves. A complete evaluation of the lumbosacral nerve roots includes testing of deep tendon reflexes, sensation (Fig. 2), and strength in the lower extremities as well as the bulbocavernosus and clitoral sacral reflexes (Fig. 3). Isolated deficits are often not a cause of urogenital symptoms, and a comprehensive neurological examination may seem to be of low

Your Daily Bladder Diary

This diary will help you and your health care team. Bladder diaries help show the causes of bladder control trouble. The "Example" line (below) will show you how to use the diary.

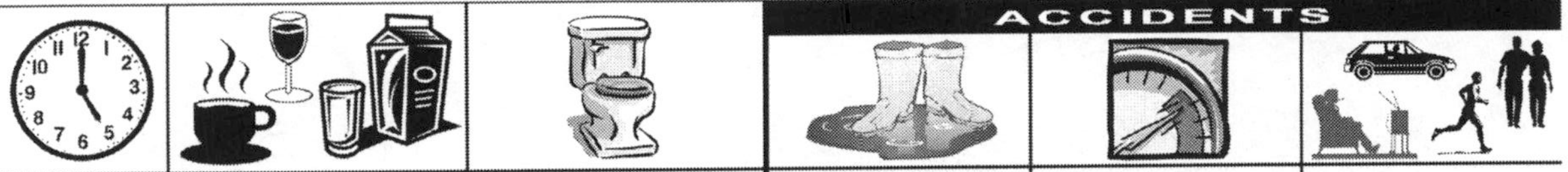

ACCIDENTS

Time	Drinks		Urine		Accidental Leaks sm med lg	Did you feel a strong urge to go?	What were you doing at the time? Sneezing, exercising, driving, lifting, etc.
	What Kind?	How Many?	How many times?	How Much? sm med lg			
Example	Coffee	2 cups	//	☐ ☒ ☐	☐ ☒ ☐	☒ Yes ☐ No	Running
6-7 am				☐ ☐ ☐	☐ ☐ ☐	☐ Yes ☐ No	
7-8 am				☐ ☐ ☐	☐ ☐ ☐	☐ Yes ☐ No	
8-9 am				☐ ☐ ☐	☐ ☐ ☐	☐ Yes ☐ No	
9-10 am				☐ ☐ ☐	☐ ☐ ☐	☐ Yes ☐ No	
10-11 am				☐ ☐ ☐	☐ ☐ ☐	☐ Yes ☐ No	
11-12 noon				☐ ☐ ☐	☐ ☐ ☐	☐ Yes ☐ No	
12-1 pm				☐ ☐ ☐	☐ ☐ ☐	☐ Yes ☐ No	
1-2 pm				☐ ☐ ☐	☐ ☐ ☐	☐ Yes ☐ No	
2-3 pm				☐ ☐ ☐	☐ ☐ ☐	☐ Yes ☐ No	
3-4 pm				☐ ☐ ☐	☐ ☐ ☐	☐ Yes ☐ No	
4-5 pm				☐ ☐ ☐	☐ ☐ ☐	☐ Yes ☐ No	
5-6 pm				☐ ☐ ☐	☐ ☐ ☐	☐ Yes ☐ No	
6-7 pm				☐ ☐ ☐	☐ ☐ ☐	☐ Yes ☐ No	

Your Name: _____   Date: _____

Figure 1   Bladder Diary.

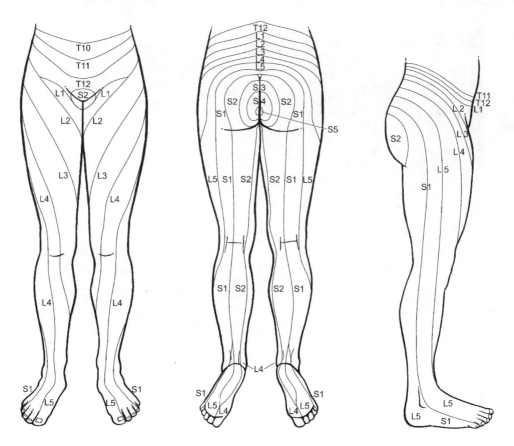

Figure 2 Sensory dermatomes.

yield (Table 5). However, simple observations (e.g., deep tendon hyperreflexia, intention tremor, or the presence of altered mental status) may identify women with predisposing functional impairments (e.g., dementia, Parkinson's disease, spinal cord disease, or previous strokes) that explain their urinary symptoms. Urinary retention and/or incontinence may be the first sign of multiple sclerosis in an otherwise healthy woman (25).

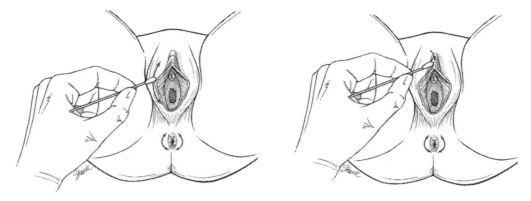

Figure 3 Examination of bulbocavernosus and clitoral reflexes.

Table 5 Significance of Abnormal Findings on Neurologic Testing

Examination	Neurological level	Significance of findings
Sensory testing around knee (light touch, pin prick)	L2-S2 and peripheral nerves	Mapping altered sensations to follow either dermatome or a peripheral nerve distribution determines level of injury
Deep tendon reflexes	Upper and lower motor neurons	Hyperreflexia—UMN lesion Absent—LMN lesion
Babinski	Corticospinal tracts	Fanning and dorsiflexion; interruption of tracts
Muscle strength:		Neuropathy or simply muscular weakness
Flexion extension knees	(L3-L5)	
Flexion hips	(L4-L5)	
Extension hips	(L2-L3)	
Plantarflexion ankles	(S1-S2)	
Dorsiflexion ankles	(L4-L5)	
Gait	Cerebellum	Cerebellar lesion: stroke or tumor
Bulbocavernosus/anal wink	L5-S5 and pudendal nerve	Pudendal neuropathy or other sacral nerve injury (66)

Source: Ref. 34.

2. General Examination

All women presenting for evaluation of pelvic floor dysfunction should undergo age-appropriate routine health checks and cancer screening according to the U.S. Preventive Services Task Force (26–28). Pulmonary and cardiovascular examination may identify individuals with chronic cough or those in need of diuretics for fluid overload. The back is examined for vertebral or flank tenderness or paraspinal muscle spasm.

Masses, ascites, and organomegaly can influence intra-abdominal pressure and impact urinary tract function. Visual inspection of the abdomen will reveal any scars from surgeries unexplained by the patient's history or unusual distention of the abdomen. In addition to palpating the abdomen to assess for hepatosplenomegaly, masses, distention, and tenderness, a Valsalva maneuver and cough will reveal any hernias. Palpation of the inguinal area may reveal lymphadenopathy.

3. Gynecologic Examination

Inspection of the external genitalia will reveal any lesions or skin changes. "Rashes" may indicate chronic irritation from urine or feces. Whitish skin changes, erythema, or loss of normal architecture of the vulva may indicate hypoestrogenism or vulvar dystrophies. In women with introital dyspareunia or vulvodynia, a careful examination of the vagina and vestibule to Hart's line is important. Hart's line is the mucocutaneous junction where the outer vestibule meets the squamous epithelium of the labia minora. A Q-tip and a pain scale may be used to elicit point tenderness in this area. Asking the patient to rate the pain on a scale of 0 to 5 will enable the clinician to identify the exact location of the pain and the point of maximal tenderness. Speculum examination should include an inspection of the cervix or vaginal cuff and notations of any lesions, discharge, inflammation, or atrophy.

Several gynecologic surgeons have attempted to develop classification systems to categorize pelvic organ prolapse over the years. Figure 4 provides a comparison of major

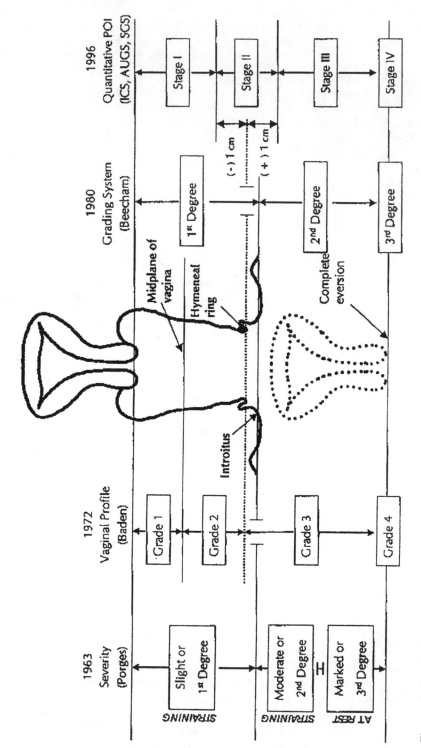

Figure 4 Comparison of pelvic organ classification systems.

prolapse classification systems. In 1996, the American Urogynecologic Society and the Society of Gynecologic Surgeons adopted the International Continence Society's Pelvic Organ Prolapse Quantification (POP-Q) system (29). The system has been demonstrated to be learned easily and performed quickly with highly reproducible findings between and within observers (30). However, the classification lacks sensitivity to detect anterior and posterior wall prolapse in the upper vaginal vault and may confuse redundant suburethral vaginal tissue or urethral hypermobility with significant cystoceles. In addition, women with pelvic organ prolapse experience symptoms that do not necessarily correlate with compartment-specific defects identified by the POP-Q classification system (31). While many research centers have adopted this system in favor of the Baden Half Way system, widespread use of the POP-Q system by all practitioners that perform pelvic examinations is hampered by its relative complexity. Although limitations of the POP-Q system exist, it is a sensitive measure of change in pelvic prolapse in an individual patient. A uniform system of describing prolapse is necessary to facilitate collaborative communications and research.

C. POP-Q

The POP-Q system of assessing pelvic support unlike other prolapse grading systems quantifies descent of the vaginal wall rather than speculating on what is on the other side of the vaginal epithelium. It avoids specific labels such as cystocele, rectocele, or enterocele recognizing, for example, that an anterior wall defect may not be the result of a cystocele. Table 6 and Figure 5 describe the different points used in the POP-Q system for describing prolapse, and Figure 6 shows the grid used to record the findings. Table 7 lists the stages of pelvic organ prolapse that

Table 6 POP-Q Points of Reference

Point	Definition
Points A	3 cm proximal to or above the hymen in the midline, values from -3 cm (no prolapse) to $+3$ cm (maximal prolapse)
Aa	Anterior, corresponds to location of the urethrovesical junction
Ba	Posterior
Points B	Lowest extent of the segment of the vagina between point A and the apex of the vagina, values from -3 cm to TVL location not fixed If point A protrudes the most (situation in most women without severe prolapse), then point B = point A
Ba	Anterior
Bp	Posterior
C	Most distal part of the cervix or in women after hysterectomy, the vaginal cuff
D	Posterior fornix Omitted after hysterectomy
GH (genital hiatus)	Distance (cm) from middle of the external urethral meatus to the posterior midline hymen
PB (perineal body)	Distance (cm) from the posterior midline hymen to the midanal opening
TVL (total vaginal length)	Greatest depth of vagina (cm) when prolapse is fully reduced Avoid excessive pressure or stretching

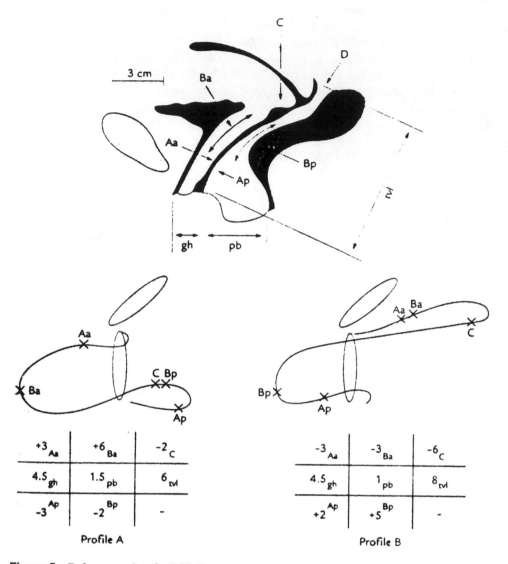

Figure 5   Reference points for POP-Q measurements.

are assigned based on the POP-Q examination when the full extent of the prolapse has been demonstrated.

Performing a systematic pelvic examination enables the practitioner to consistently assess patients and follow their progress longitudinally. We separate the speculum and place the lower blade in posteriorly and hold a ruler or calibrated Q-tip 3 cm away from the urethral meatus. While pulling the speculum blade posteriorly, we ask the patient to perform a Valsalva maneuver and measure the descent of point Aa. At this time, the most dependent part of any anterior wall prolapse is also measured (Ba). By inspecting the vaginal rugae of the anterior wall, one may gain a hint of whether lateral and or central defects have caused anterior vaginal wall prolapse. If the vaginal rugae appear to be prominent in the midline, it may be indicative of a paravaginal defect. Direct assessment of the support of anterior lateral vaginal sulcus is used as a more definitive marker of diagnosing a paravaginal defect unilaterally or bilaterally. This may be

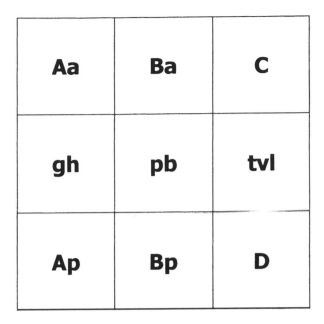

Aa	Ba	C
gh	pb	tvl
Ap	Bp	D

Figure 6 Grid for recording prolapse measurements.

assessed during the speculum exam with the aid of ring forceps or a Baden defect analyzer elevating the anteriorlateral vaginal sulcus to the level of the arcus tendineous and observing if normal anterior vaginal wall support is restored. This may result in artifact and misdiagnosis if the opened instrument is elevated above the level of the arcus tendineus.

In one study, while the sensitivity of the clinical assessment of paravaginal defects in comparison with the operative confirmation of the defects was 92%, the specificity of 53% was poor (32). We prefer a simpler, more consistent alternative to performing this assessment that can avoid any potential over correction artifact. We take both halves of a Grave's speculum and insert them bilaterally along the lateral vaginal walls in the vertical axis. If the cystocele is resolved completely, it is probably secondary to a unilateral or bilateral paravaginal defect. Removing each blade with the other in place will elucidate whether it is a bilateral or unilateral paravaginal defect. If the anterior vaginal wall descent is not completely corrected, it probably

Table 7 Staging of Pelvic Organ Prolapse Based on the POP-Q Examination

Stage	Description
0	No descensus of pelvic structures during straining (Aa, Ap, Ba, Bp $= -3$ and C or D $\leq -([tvl - 2])$
I	The leading surface of the prolapse does not descend below 1 cm above the hymenal ring (i.e., prolapse is not stage 0 and all points are < -1)
II	The leading edge of the prolapse extends into the region from 1 cm proximal to the hymen to 1 cm distal to the hymen (i.e., most distal point is ≥ -1 but $\leq +1$)
III	The leading edge of the prolapse extends 1 cm beyond the hymen, but there is not complete vaginal eversion (i.e., most distal point is $> +1$ but $< +[tvl-2]$)
IV	Essentially complete eversion (i.e., most distal point is $\geq +[tvl-2]$)

represents a combination of central and paravaginal defects. This method is relatively quick and may avoid the common overdiagnosis of paravaginal defects.

By rotating the speculum blade 180° and reinserting it along the anterior vaginal wall, the clinician can inspect the posterior wall and uterine or vaginal apex mobility. Digital examination will help to measure vaginal length (TVL) as well as descent of the apex (C and/or D). Finally, external examination will give measurements of the genital hiatus (GH) and perineal body (PB).

On bimanual examination, initial palpation of the posterior fourchette to assess for tenderness at the introitus and palpation of the posterior vaginal wall and deeper pelvic musculature to assess for tenderness or spasm of the levator ani muscle may help to identify sources of dyspareunia. Palpation of the urethra and bladder neck may reveal tenderness or masses that should be further evaluated with urethroscopy and cystoscopy. Routine assessment of contour, size, and abnormalities of the pelvic organs is performed focusing on the presence of pelvic tenderness or masses. Rectovaginal examination helps to assess the anal sphincter tone, possible sphincter defects, fecal impaction, the presence of occult blood or rectal lesions, and subtle distal rectoceles.

Asking the patient to contract her levator ani muscles during this examination will help the clinician assess her ability to contract the muscles, the strength of the contraction, and the duration of the contraction. The pelvic muscles have been considered integral to continence since Kegel (33) observed that women with urinary incontinence experienced symptomatic improvement by improving the strength of these muscles. The pubococcygeous and puborectalis components of the levator ani form a hammock beneath the rectum and insert superiorly and laterally upon the pubic rami. Contraction of these muscles, especially during strenuous physical activity, compresses the rectum, vagina, and urethra, maintaining flatal, fecal, and urinary continence (34). Although the utility of this assessment may be questioned, it is useful to grade levator strength to better implement behavioral interventions such as pelvic floor muscle exercises, biofeedback, or electrical stimulation. Many patients will have no ability to contract their levator ani. Pelvic floor exercises without "biofeedback" in those women would be futile. Various techniques to assess levator ani tone (35–42) have been studied, although no single technique is widely accepted. The modified Oxford scale is presented in Table 8 (39). Given the lack of a standardized scale, the clinician should adopt a single scale and consistently use it to preserve internal consistency.

4.   Measuring Urethral Hypermobility: Q-tip Test

If we believe that the underlying pathophysiology of most stress urinary incontinence (previously identified as genuine stress incontinence) involves urethral hypermobility, then some assessment of urethral mobility should be made. The Q-tip test is an excellent test to document quantitatively the presence of urethral hypermobility (43,44). It was originally designed to take the place of the bead chain cystourethrogram in the evaluation of the urethral

Table 8   Modified Oxford Scale for Measuring Pelvic Muscle Strength

Number	Definition
0	No palpable muscle contraction
1	Flicker
2	Weak pelvic contraction
3	Moderate contraction with an element of lift
4	Good contraction with lift and holding power
5	Strong squeeze with good lift gripping examining hand

axis. Although the determination of urethral hypermobility is a poor predictor of the etiology of a patient's urinary incontinence (45–47), it has been included in the urogynecologic examination to assess urethrovesical junction support. To perform the test, a sterile cotton applicator soaked in 2% Xylocaine jelly is inserted into the urethra, and withdrawn slowly until slight resistance indicates that the tip is at the bladder neck. A goniometer or compass (Fig. 7) provides a measurement of the resting angle from the horizontal. The patient is then asked to repetitively cough and perform Valsalva maneuvers while the maximum straining angle is measured (Fig. 8). If the cotton tip is not in the bladder, the angle will be underestimated. A straining angle $\geq 30^\circ$ has been arbitrarily suggested to indicate significant bladder neck mobility. Few normative data are available regarding these measurements and factors during testing that may affect measurements.

Walters and Diaz (48) reported that asymptomatic women with a mean parity of two and mean age of 32 had an average maximum straining angle of 54°. Although this was less than the straining angle of 73° seen in a group of symptomatic women, there was considerable overlap between groups (48). Fedorkow and colleagues (49) performed a receiver-operator characteristic analysis and found the optimal diagnostic cutoff point for stress urinary incontinence to be $\geq 40^\circ$ from the horizontal. At this cutoff, 84% of patients with genuine stress incontinence would have a positive test. Thus, an arbitrary cutoff of 30° in parous women may be too low.

Handa and colleagues (50) noted that 71% of women diagnosed with urethral hypermobility in the supine position did not have urethral hypermobility in the standing position. This observation brings into question the reproducibility of the Q-tip test. Despite this information, the test is still used by many in making decisions in selecting treatments for stress incontinence primarily because the absence of a positive Q-tip test in someone diagnosed with

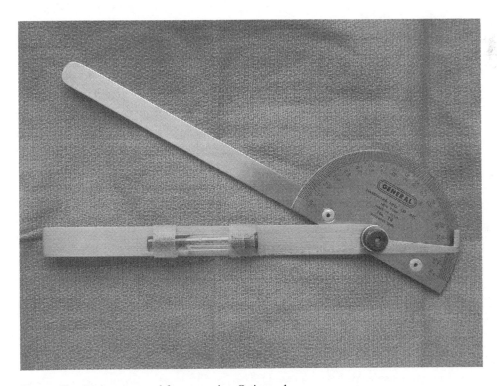

Figure 7   Goniometer used for measuring Q-tip angle.

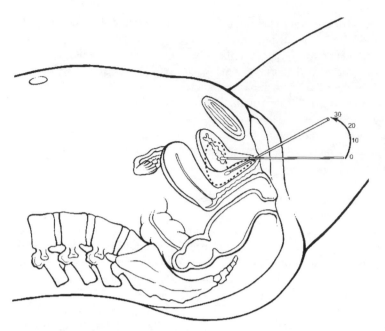

Figure 8   Demonstration of resting and straining angles during the Q-tip test.

stress incontinence is important. Bergman and colleagues (51), using a Q-tip test cut-off point of ≥35°, found a 50% failure rate in women with stress incontinence and negative Q-tip tests who underwent Pereyra operations and a 55% failure rate for women who had Burch procedures.

By asking the patient to cough at this time, one can perform a supine empty stress test as a screen for a low pressure urethra or a low leak point pressure (52,53). This simple test has been identified as a very specific and reasonably sensitive test to assess for intrinsic sphincteric deficiency.

Finally, we repeat a vaginal examination while the patient bears down in the standing position to reassess for the sign of stress incontinence and for increased genital prolapse with gravity. Occasionally, pelvic organ descent may only be evident with the help of gravity.

V. CONCLUSIONS

A careful history and physical examination will guide the clinician in further evaluation of the patient's symptoms or allow them to begin empiric treatment in uncomplicated pelvic floor disorders.

REFERENCES

1. Haylen BT, Sutherst JR, Frazer MI. Is the investigation of most stress incontinence really necessary? Br J Urol 1989; 64:147–149.
2. Cundiff GW, Harris RL, Coates KW, Bump RC. Clinical predictors of urinary incontinence in women. Am J Obstet Gynecol 1997; 177:262–266; discussion 266–267.
3. Sand PK, Hill RC, Ostergard DR. Incontinence history as a predictor of detrusor stability. Obstet Gynecol 1988; 71:257–260.

4. Cardozo LD, Stanton SL. Genuine stress incontinence and detrusor instability—a review of 200 patients. Br J Obstet Gynaecol 1980; 87:184–190.

5. Glezerman M, Glasner M, Rikover M, Tauber E, Bar-Ziv J, Insler V. Evaluation of reliability of history in women complaining of urinary stress incontinence. Eur J Obstet Gynecol Reprod Biol 1986; 21:159–164.

6. Ouslander J, Staskin D, Raz S, Su HL, Hepps K. Clinical versus urodynamic diagnosis in an incontinent geriatric female population. J Urol 1987; 137:68–71.

7. Farrar DJ, Whiteside CG, Osborne JL, Turner-Warwick RT. A urodynamic analysis of micturition symptoms in the female. Surg Gynecol Obstet 1975; 141:875–881.

8. Hastie KJ, Moisey CU. Are urodynamics necessary in female patients presenting with stress incontinence? Br J Urol 1989; 63:155–156.

9. Jensen JK, Nielsen FR Jr, Ostergard DR. The role of patient history in the diagnosis of urinary incontinence. Obstet Gynecol 1994; 83:904–910.

10. Fianu S, Kjaeldgaard A, Larsson B. Preoperative screen for latent stress incontinence in women with cystocele. Neurourol Urodyn 1985, 4:3–7.

11. Bergman A, Koonings PP, Ballard CA. Predicting postoperative urinary incontinence development in women undergoing operation for genitourinary prolapse. Am J Obstet Gynecol 1988; 158:1171–1175.

12. Ghoniem GM, Walters F, Lewis V. The value of the vaginal pack test in large cystoceles. J Urol 1994; 152:931–934.

13. Abrams P, Cardozo L, Fall M. The standardisation of terminology of lower urinary tract function: report from the Standardisation Subcommittee of the International Continence Society. Am J Obstet Gynecol 2002; 187:116–126.

14. Bo K, Stien R, Kulseng-Hanssen S, Kristofferson M. Clinical and urodynamic assessment of nulliparous young women with and without stress incontinence symptoms: a case-control study. Obstet Gynecol 1994; 84:1028–1032.

15. Wolin LH. Stress incontinence in young, healthy nulliparous female subjects. J Urol 1969; 101:545–549.

16. Thyssen HH, Clevin L, Olesen S, Lose G. Urinary incontinence in elite female athletes and dancers. Int Urogynecol J Pelvic Floor Dysfunct 2002; 13:15–17.

17. Nygaard IE, Thompson FL, Svengalis SL, Albright JP. Urinary incontinence in elite nulliparous athletes. Obstet Gynecol 1994; 84:183–187.

18. Fauci. Harrison's Principles of Internal Medicine.

19. McAninch J. Symptoms of Disorders of the Genitourinary Tract in General Urology.

20. Heit M, Culligan P, Rosenquist C, Shott S. Is pelvic organ prolapse a cause of pelvic or low back pain? Obstet Gynecol 2002; 99:23–28.

21. Resnick NM, Yalla SV. Management of urinary incontinence in the elderly. N Engl J Med 1985; 313:800–805.

22. Brown JS, Vittinghoff E, Wyman JF. Urinary incontinence: does it increase risk for falls and fractures? Study of Osteoporotic Fractures Research Group. J Am Geriatr Soc 2000; 48:721–725.

23. Graham CW, Dmochowski RR. Questionnaires for women with urinary symptoms. Neurourol Urodyn 2002; 21:473–481.

24. Wyman JF, Choi SC, Harkins SW, Wilson MS, Fantl JA. The urinary diary in evaluation of incontinent women: a test-retest analysis. Obstet Gynecol 1988; 71:812–817.

25. Beck RP, Warren KG, Whitman P. Urodynamic studies in female patients with multiple sclerosis. Am J Obstet Gynecol 1981; 139:273–276.

26. Calonge N. New USPSTF guidelines: integrating into clinical practice. US Preventive Services Task Force. Am J Prev Med 2001; 20:7–9.

27. Berg AO, Allan JD. Introducing the third US Preventive Services Task Force. Am J Prev Med 2001; 20:3–4.

28. Franco EL, Duarte-Franco E, Rohan TE. Evidence-based policy recommendations on cancer screening and prevention. Cancer Detect Prev 2002; 26:350–361.

29. Bump RC, Mattiasson A, Bo K. The standardization of terminology of female pelvic organ prolapse and pelvic floor dysfunction. Am J Obstet Gynecol 1996; 175:10–17.

30. Hall AF, Theofrastous JP, Cundiff GW. Interobserver and intraobserver reliability of the proposed International Continence Society, Society of Gynecologic Surgeons, and American Urogynecologic Society pelvic organ prolapse classification system. Am J Obstet Gynecol 1996; 175:1467–1470; discussion 1470–1471.

31. Ellerkmann RM, Cundiff GW, Melick CF, Nihira MA, Leffler K, Bent AE. Correlation of symptoms with location and severity of pelvic organ prolapse. Am J Obstet Gynecol 2001; 185:1332–1337; discussion 1337–1338.

32. Barber MD, Cundiff GW, Weidner AC, Coates KW, Bump RC, Addison WA. Accuracy of clinical assessment of paravaginal defects in women with anterior vaginal wall prolapse. Am J Obstet Gynecol 1999; 181:87–90.

33. Kegel A. The physiologic treatment of urinary stress incontinence. J Urol 1950; 63:808–814.

34. Theofrastous JP, Swift SE. The clinical evaluation of pelvic floor dysfunction. Obstet Gynecol Clin North Am 1998; 25:783–804.

35. Sampselle CM, Brink CA, Wells TJ. Digital measurement of pelvic muscle strength in childbearing women. Nurs Res 1989; 38:134–138.

36. Sampselle CM, DeLancey JO. The urine stream interruption test and pelvic muscle function. Nurs Res 1992; 41:73–77.

37. Sampselle CM. Using a stopwatch to assess pelvic muscle strength in the urine stream interruption test. Nurse Pract 1993; 18:14–16, 18–20.

38. Brink CA, Sampselle CM, Wells TJ, Diokno AC, Gillis GL. A digital test for pelvic muscle strength in older women with urinary incontinence. Nurs Res 1989; 38:196–199.

39. Laycock J. Pelvic muscle exercises: physiotherapy for the pelvic floor. Urol Nurs 1994; 14:136–140.

40. Toglia MR, DeLancey JO. Anal incontinence and the obstetrician-gynecologist. Obstet Gynecol 1994; 84:731–740.

41. Peschers UM, Gingelmaier A, Jundt K, Leib B, Dimpfl T. Evaluation of pelvic floor muscle strength using four different techniques. Int Urogynecol J Pelvic Floor Dysfunct 2001; 12:27–30.

42. Isherwood PJ, Rane A. Comparative assessment of pelvic floor strength using a perineometer and digital examination. Br J Obstet Gynaecol 2000; 107:1007–1011.

43. Crystle CD, Charme LS, Copeland WE. Q-tip test in stress urinary incontinence. Obstet Gynecol 1971; 38:313–315.

44. Karram MM, Bhatia NN. The Q-tip test: standardization of the technique and its interpretation in women with urinary incontinence. Obstet Gynecol 1988; 71:807–811.

45. Bergman A, McCarthy TA, Ballard CA, Yanai J. Role of the Q-tip test in evaluating stress urinary incontinence. J Reprod Med 1987; 32:273–275.

46. Montz FJ, Stanton SL. Q-Tip test in female urinary incontinence. Obstet Gynecol 1986; 67:258–260.

47. Fantl JA, Hurt WG, Bump RC, Dunn LJ, Choi SC. Urethral axis and sphincteric function. Am J Obstet Gynecol 1986; 155:554–558.

48. Walters MD, Diaz K. Q-tip test: a study of continent and incontinent women. Obstet Gynecol 1987; 70:208–211.

49. Fedorkow DM, Sand PK, Retzky SS, Johnson DC. The cotton swab test. Receiver-operating characteristic curves. J Reprod Med 1995; 40:42–46.

50. Handa VL, Jensen JK, Ostergard DR. The effect of patient position on proximal urethral mobility. Obstet Gynecol 1995; 86:273–276.

51. Bergman A, Koonings PP, Ballard CA. Negative Q-tip test as a risk factor for failed incontinence surgery in women. J Reprod Med 1989; 34:193–197.

52. Lobel RW, Sand PK. The empty supine stress test as a predictor of intrinsic urethral sphincter dysfunction. Obstet Gynecol 1996; 88:128–132.

53. McLennan MT, Bent AE. Supine empty stress test as a predictor of low Valsalva leak point pressure. Neurourol Urodyn 1998; 17:121–127.

54. Fantl JA, Newman DK, Colling J. Urinary incontinence in adults: acute and chronic management. Clinical Practice Guideline, No. 2, 1996 Update. Rockville, MD: U.S. Department of Health and

Human Services. Public Health Service, Agency for Health Care Policy and Research, March 1996 (vol. AHCPR Publication No. 96-0682).

55. Ware JE Jr, Sherbourne CD. The MOS 36-item short-form health survey (SF-36). I. Conceptual framework and item selection. Med Care 1992; 30:473–483.

56. Shumaker SA, Wyman JF, Uebersax JS, McClish D, Fantl JA. Health-related quality of life measures for women with urinary incontinence: the Incontinence Impact Questionnaire and the Urogenital Distress Inventory. Continence Program in Women (CPW) Research Group. Qual Life Res 1994; 3:291–306.

57. Uebersax JS, Wyman JF, Shumaker SA, McClish DK, Fantl JA. Short forms to assess life quality and symptom distress for urinary incontinence in women: the Incontinence Impact Questionnaire and the Urogenital Distress Inventory. Continence Program for Women Research Group. Neurourol Urodyn 1995; 14:131–139.

58. Wagner TH, Patrick DL, Bavendam TG, Martin ML, Buesching DP. Quality of life of persons with urinary incontinence: development of a new measure. Urology 1996; 47:67–71; discussion 71–72.

59. Kelleher CJ, Cardozo LD, Khullar V, Salvatore S. A new questionnaire to assess the quality of life of urinary incontinent women. Br J Obstet Gynaecol 1997; 104:1374–1349.

60. Jackson S, Donovan J, Brookes S, Eckford S, Swithinbank L, Abrams P. The Bristol female lower urinary tract symptoms questionnaire: development and psychometric testing. Br J Urol 1996; 77:805–812.

61. Lee PS, Reid DW, Saltmarche A, Linton L. Measuring the psychosocial impact of urinary incontinence: the York Incontinence Perceptions Scale (YIPS). J Am Geriatr Soc 1995; 43:1275–1278.

62. Rogers RG, Kammerer-Doak D, Villarreal A, Coates K, Qualls C. A new instrument to measure sexual function in women with urinary incontinence or pelvic organ prolapse. Am J Obstet Gynecol 2001; 184:552–558.

63. Barber MD, Kuchibhatla MN, Pieper CF, Bump RC. Psychometric evaluation of 2 comprehensive condition-specific quality of life instruments for women with pelvic floor disorders. Am J Obstet Gynecol 2001; 185:1388–1395.

64. Rockwood TH, Church JM, Fleshman JW. Fecal Incontinence Quality of Life Scale: quality of life instrument for patients with fecal incontinence. Dis Colon Rectum 2000; 43:9–16; discussion 16–17.

65. O'Leary MP, Sant GR, Fowler FJ Jr, Whitmore KE, Spolarich-Kroll J. The interstitial cystitis symptom index and problem index. Urology 1997; 49:58–63.

66. Blaivas JG, Zayed AA, Labib KB. The bulbocavernosus reflex in urology: a prospective study of 299 patients. J Urol 1981;126:197–199.

9

Urodynamic Assessment: Urethral Pressure Profilometry and PTR

Stacey J. Wallach* and Donald R. Ostergard
University of California, Irvine, and Long Beach Memorial Medical Center, Long Beach, California, U.S.A.

I. INTRODUCTION

For a person to be continent, the pressure in the urethra must exceed the pressure in the detrusor at all times. If bladder pressure should overcome urethral pressure, urine loss may result. Researchers have devised different tests to assess the relationship between urethral and bladder pressure. Their goal is to differentiate between patients with urinary incontinence based solely on an anatomic loss of urethral support, from patients with a loss of ability to maintain urethral pressure due to an incompetent urethral sphincter. Both urethral pressure profilometry and leak point pressure look at urethral resistance to voiding. However, urethral pressure profiles are static measurements along the length of the urethra thought to represent the intrinsic sphincter mechanism, while leak point pressures are dynamic tests of the amount of pressure it takes to overcome urethral resistance (1).

The female urethra is 3–4 cm in length and is composed of a longitudinal layer of smooth muscle surrounded by a circular layer of smooth muscle. These smooth muscle layers are, in turn, encompassed by a circular sphincter of striated muscle. Lying beneath the urethral mucosa is a vascular plexus that helps to produce a hermetic seal (2). The striated muscle, the vascular bed, and the smooth muscle and connective tissue together generate the intrinsic urethral pressure. Ulmsten et al. showed that each component is responsible for about a third of the intraurethral pressure (3). Extrinsic factors can further augment urethral pressure. According to DeLancey, the urethra itself lies on a hammock formed by the anterior vaginal wall (4). By contracting the pelvic diaphragm, the urethra is compressed against the vagina further augmenting urethral pressures.

II. HISTORY

In 1923, Victor Bonney (5) became the first person to measure urethral pressures. He used a manometer to determine the pressure required to retrograde infuse fluid into the urethra. Since

---

**Current affiliation*: University of California, Sacramento, California, U.S.A.

that time, various methods to gauge urethral pressure have been devised. In 1940, Barnes (6) used a fluid-filled balloon connected to a pressure transducer to evaluate the urethra's resistance to distension. In 1957, Lapides and colleagues (7) used a water manometer to quantify urethral wall pressure at specific segments along the urethra.

A. Perfusion Catheters

Brown and Wickham (8) perfected the fluid perfusion technique developed by Toews (9) to create an accurate and reproducible urethral pressure profile. A double- or triple-lumen catheter allowed simultaneous recording of bladder and urethral pressure. Multiple circumferential side holes minimized rotational error. A pump infused fluid at a constant rate of 2 mL/min while a mechanical puller withdrew the catheter 1–2 mm every second. The transducer measured the pressure of the fluid required to lift the wall of the urethra off the side holes. Later on, other researchers tried carbon dioxide gas as a perfusion medium but this was found to be less accurate (10). (see Fig. 1).

B. Membrane Catheters

The accuracy of perfusion catheters depended on the ability of the urethra to create a seal around the catheter. This shortcoming was remedied with the introduction of membrane catheters in the 1970s. These catheters had a cylindrical balloon or membrane over the infusion holes thus preventing the loss of infusion media. They were more accurate but harder to use (11). All air bubbles needed to be eliminated for accurate readings. The catheter was calibrated to

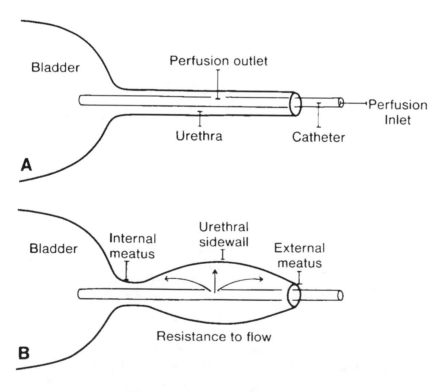

Figure 1   Perfusion catheter. (A) Before perfusion; (B) during infusion. The catheter measures resistance to flow of the perfusion media. (From Ref. 66, p. 124.)

atmospheric pressure prior to insertion. The urethral pressure measured represented the average pressure over the length of the membrane.

C. Microtransducer Catheters

All of the above methods were adequate for recording resting urethral pressure profiles but lacked the ability to accurately measure rapid changes in pressure such as what happens during a cough. In 1973, Millar and Baker (12) developed the microtip transducer. These catheters had a pressure-sensitive piezoelectric unit mounted at the catheter tip and one mounted 6 cm proximal. They were highly sensitive and very accurate and could record dynamic changes in intra-vesicular pressure and urethral pressure simultaneously. On the downside, they were expensive, extremely fragile, and prone to rotational error since the transducer was unidirectional. In reality, the microtransducer measures a unidirectional force (not pressure) from contact of the piezoelectric unit with the urethral wall (13).

D. Fiberoptic Catheters

Ten years after Millar and Baker (12) developed microtip transducers, Kyarstein and coworkers adapted fiberoptic catheters for urodynamics (14). Fiberoptic catheters were more durable than microtip catheters, did not require orientation, and, like microtip catheters, were able to record dynamic changes in pressure. These catheters were marketed as a reliable and inexpensive way for the average gynecologist/urologist to perform urodynamics. Fiberoptic catheters came in both disposable and reusable forms. However, they tended to record lower than microtip catheters, potentially leading to overdiagnosis of low-pressure urethras (15,16). Some fiberoptic catheters also lacked the ability to record bladder pressure and urethral pressure simultaneously, leaving them vulnerable to error should a bladder contraction occur during the urethral closure pressure profile.

III. TECHNIQUE

The resting urethral pressure profile is performed with the patient in the sitting position with a full bladder, often immediately after the cystometrogram. As with the cystometrogram, the patient sits in a urodynamic chair. Surface electrodes are placed on either side of the anal sphincter to measure pelvic floor muscle activity. The catheters are calibrated prior to insertion. In the past, the transducers were zeroed at the level of the bladder, but this is no longer necessary with some of the newer catheters. Any prolapse is reduced, with care taken not to apply pressure on the urethra.

The intra-abdominal catheter is inserted into the vagina or rectum and secured. Then the urethral meatus is cleaned and the dual-tipped microtransducer catheter is inserted into the bladder. Before beginning the test, any residual urine is drained and the patient is filled with warm saline to maximum bladder capacity. By convention, the dual-tipped catheter is oriented with the transducer facing 9 o'clock and attached to the mechanical puller device. The mechanical puller is set to withdraw the catheter at a rate between 1 and 2 mm/sec. Orienting the catheter toward 12 o'clock will spuriously elevate urethral pressure, whereas orienting it toward 6 o'clock tends to record lower values (17,18). At the start of the procedure, both transducers on the dual-tipped catheter begin inside the bladder. Therefore, the pressure recorded in the bladder channel should equal the initial pressure recorded in the urethral channel.

Once the patient is at maximum bladder capacity, the puller is turned on and the patient is asked to cough to ensure the catheters are recording equally. The catheter is slowly drawn through the urethra by the puller mechanism. The proximal transducer measuring intraurethral pressure will note a progressive increase in pressure from the bladder neck to the midurethra followed by a progressive decrease in pressure to zero as the transducer is pulled past the urethral meatus to outside atmospheric pressure (Fig. 2) This test is repeated to ensure reproducibility, and the results are averaged.

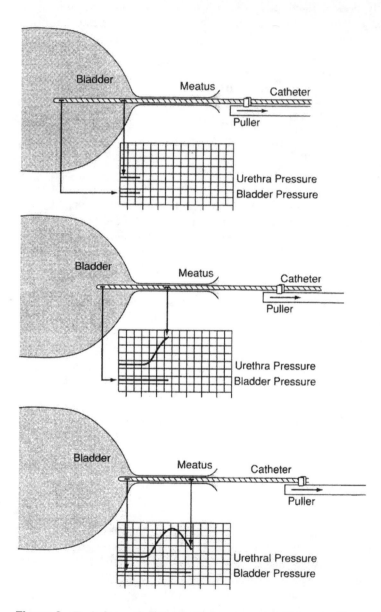

Figure 2   Technique of static urethral pressure profilometry. The study begins with both microtip transducers in the bladder (top), as the catheter is withdrawn through the urethra the proximal transducer records urethral pressure. The urethral pressure increases to maximal urethral pressure near the midurethra (middle), then decreases again (bottom) to zero as the proximal transducer is pulled out of the external meatus to atmospheric pressure. (From Ref. 67, p. 83.)

IV. DEFINITIONS

Ideally, when performing a urethral closure pressure profile, six channels are recorded simultaneously—EMG, intravesical pressure, intraabdominal pressure, intraurethral pressure, true detrusor pressure, and urethral closure pressure (Fig. 3). Like true detrusor pressure, urethral closure pressure is a subtracted channel created by deducting intravesical pressure from intraurethral pressure. Thus, the urethral pressure profile differs from the urethral closure pressure profile in that the latter has bladder pressure already subtracted. Rarely, the withdrawal of the catheter through the urethra can cause a detrusor contraction. If bladder pressure is not measured simultaneously with urethral pressure, one may erroneously label the urethral closure pressure as inadequate.

The urethral closure pressure profile (UCPP) graphically represents the pressure in the urethra throughout its anatomic length. The maximal urethral closure pressure (MUCP) is the highest amount of pressure attained in the urethra. Thus, the MUCP is the highest point on the urethral closure pressure profile curve (Fig. 4). Anatomically, this point correlates to the area of

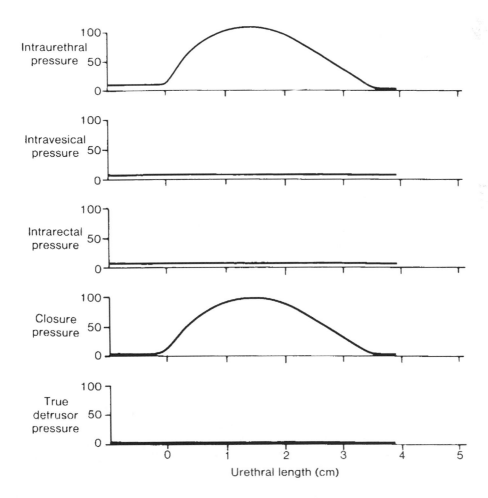

Figure 3 The static urethral closure pressure profile in the normal female. Intravesical pressure, intraurethral pressure, and intrarectal pressure are measured simultaneously. The detrusor pressure channel and urethral closure pressure channel are subtracted channels. (From Ref. 66, p. 127.)

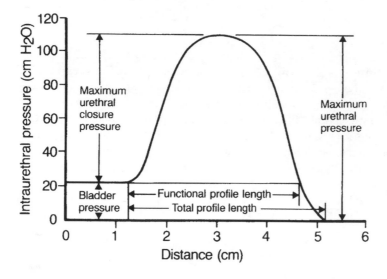

Figure 4   The static urethral pressure profile with ICS recommended nomenclature in the normal female. (From Ref. 66, p. 646.)

the midurethra where the striated and smooth muscle sphincters overlap. Since the mechanical puller device withdraws the transducer at a set rate, various distances can be calculated. The length from the external urethral meatus to the point of maximum urethral pressure can be determined based on the amount of time it takes the catheter to move from the point of MUCP to the urethral meatus.

Functional urethral length and total urethral length can also be measured. Functional urethral length is the length of the urethra along which urethral pressure exceeds bladder pressure. Total urethral length includes the additional length needed to reach atmospheric pressure, but this parameter has not been found to have clinical importance. Investigators have also looked at the area under the urethral closure pressure curve termed the continence area (Fig. 5). This area can be thought of as representing the intrinsic continence mechanism. The space between the urethral closure pressure curve and the zero axis represents the patient's "margin to leakage," or the pressure that must be overcome to cause equalization and urine loss.

Both the amount of fluid in the bladder and the patient's position during the test can alter the results of the urethral pressure profile (19–21). The closure profile of a stress-incontinent patient with a half-full bladder may still show positive pressure with a cough; thus, the patient may not leak. This same person with stress at maximum bladder capacity may lose urine because bladder pressure overcomes urethral pressure. A more upright position creates a larger hydrostatic pressure, which leads to increased activation of urethral and pelvic floor skeletal muscle. This results in higher urethral closure pressures and longer functional urethral lengths. In the continent patient, there is a 25–70% increase in the maximum urethral closure pressure with standing. This increase is seen primarily in the mid to distal urethra corresponding to the striated sphincter. The patient with genuine stress incontinence has a weakness in her compensatory ability to augment urethral closure pressures by increasing activity of the striated urethral sphincter. For this reason, urethral closure pressures decrease in the stress-incontinent patient as the patient assumes a more upright position (22,23).

In addition, other factors may influence urethral closure pressures and functional urethral length. Incontinent patients have lower maximum urethral closure pressures and shorter

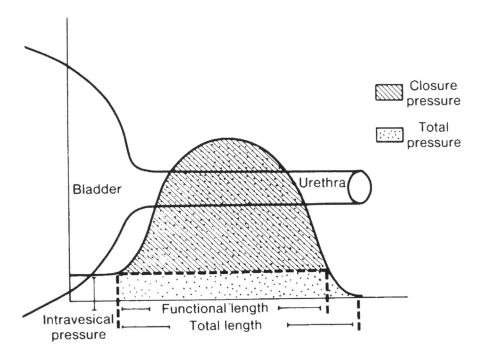

Figure 5 The static urethral pressure profile in the normal female comparing urethral closure pressure to total urethral pressure. (From Ref. 66, p. 128.)

functional urethral lengths than continent controls, although there is considerable overlap (24,25). Maximum urethral closure pressure and functional urethral length decrease after menopause (26–28). Both of these parameters increase with the administration of estrogen to postmenopausal women (29,30). Other medications, such as phenylpropanolamine and norephedrine, also increase maximal urethral closure pressure (31,32). On the other hand, various surgeries, e.g., radical hysterectomy, abdominalperineal resection, and internal urethrotomy, have been shown to decrease urethral closure pressure and urethral length (33–36).

A. Low Pressure Urethra

In fact, researchers noted that patients who failed previous incontinence procedures were at a higher risk of a subsequent failure (37). McGuire was the first to document that these patients had maximum urethral closure pressures <20 cmH$_2$O (38,39). Later on, Sand et al showed that patients with genuine stress incontinence (GSI) and low urethral closure pressures preoperatively were at a higher risk of failure (54% vs. 18% at 3-month follow-up) from a Burch procedure (40). Other researchers concurred with their findings (41,42). Thus, the low-pressure urethra is defined as one in which the maximal urethral closure pressure is ≤ 20 cmH$_2$O. This low-pressure urethra is considered to be associated with intrinsic sphincter deficiency.

Since patients with low-pressure urethras are at higher risk of surgical failure from traditional retropubic suspension procedures, it is important to diagnose these patients preoperatively. A suburethral sling is the current procedure of choice for these patients with low-pressure urethras. Certain clues in the patient's history may suggest that further evaluation is necessary to rule out a low-pressure urethra. These include patients with previous failed

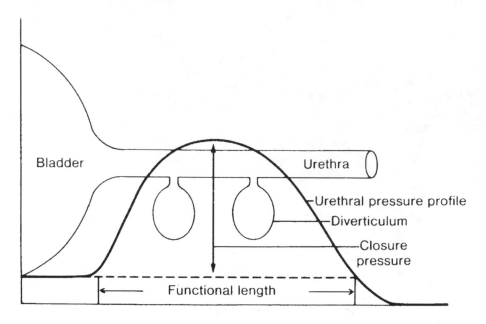

Figure 6   The static urethral pressure profile superimposed onto a urethra with two diverticulum, one proximal and one distal to the point of maximal urethral pressure. (From Ref. 66, p. 365.)

incontinence procedures, supine urine loss with an empty bladder, urine loss with a change in position, presence of a meningomyelocele (43), previous pelvic radiation (44), history of extensive pelvic surgery such as a radical hysterectomy (33), low anterior resection or abdominalperineal resection (35), or age >50 (45).

B.   Double-Peaked UCPPs

The urethral closure pressure profile may also help in detecting urethral kinking, a urethral stricture, diverticulum, or fistula. If a sudden rapid elevation in urethral pressure is visualized during the urethral closure pressure profile, the examiner should be on alert for urethral kinking from a large prolapse or a urethral stricture (46,47). The opposite holds true for a urethral diverticulum or fistula. As the catheter moves over the diverticular ostia or fistula opening, a sudden drop in pressure will occur owing to the absence of the urethral wall. The urethral pressure profile may have a double-peaked or biphasic appearance. Bhatia and coworkers used the urethral closure pressure profile to determine the location of the urethral diverticulum in relationship to the point of maximal urethral pressure (48) (Fig. 6). If the diverticular opening is distal to the peak closure pressure, a Spence procedure can be performed. However, when the diverticular ostia is proximal to the point of maximal closure pressure, a diverticulectomy should be performed since a Spence procedure may result in genuine stress incontinence.

V.   AUGMENTED UCPP

The augmented urethral closure profile reflects the patient's ability to contract her periurethral and levator ani muscles. This suggests an intact motor pathway from the brain down the spinal cord and out the efferent motor neurons. Patients with motor lesions above the level of the sacral spinal cord cannot control the striated sphincter. These patients lack the ability to relax their external sphincter during voiding, called detrusor sphincter dyssynergia (49).

The study is performed in the same manner as the resting urethral closure pressure profile except that the patient is asked to contract the muscles around her urethra as if she is holding her urine while the catheter is withdrawn. Once this is accomplished, the same procedure is performed again with the patient squeezing her rectum while the catheter is withdrawn. With both of these procedures, the maximal urethral closure pressure and functional urethral length should increase if the patient is able to contract her muscles. These tests are analogous to performing a Kegel's maneuver and are thus dependent on the patient's understanding the actions requested. Augmented urethral profiles have not been shown to have prognostic value for women undergoing surgery (50).

VI. DYNAMIC UCPP

The dynamic or stress urethral closure pressure profiles reflect the patient's ability to maintain continence in the face of increases in intraabdominal pressure. In the continent patient, increases in intra-abdominal pressure should be transmitted to both the bladder and proximal/midurethra. (Pressure is not transmitted to the distal urethra because it is below the urogenital diaphragm.) In patients with genuine stress incontinence, the dynamic urethral closure pressure profile equalizes and urine loss occurs in the absence of a detrusor contraction.

There are two types of dynamic urethral closure pressure profiles, the Valsalva profile and the cough profile. With the Valsalva profile, the patient is asked to give a maximal Valsalva effort as the catheter is withdrawn through the urethra. The cough profile is performed in the same manner except that the patient is asked to cough every 2–3 sec as the catheter is withdrawn (Fig. 7). In both of these tests, the urethral meatus is observed for urine loss. As with static urethral pressure profiles, dynamic urethral pressure profiles are performed at maximum bladder capacity in the sitting position, as patients may be continent at lower bladder volumes.

In the continent patient, positive pressure is transmitted to the proximal urethra with each cough. This can be seen as small spikes along the top of the urethral closure pressure profile and represent a negative test. In patients with genuine stress incontinence, less pressure maybe transmitted to the urethra with coughing than the bladder. This represents a failure in the extrinsic continence mechanism, allowing bladder pressure to overcome urethral pressure and urine loss to occur. For the cough urethral pressure profile to be considered positive, the cough spikes must cross the zero axis. When this happens, the pressure in the urethra equalizes with bladder pressure.

The functional urethral length is divided into four quarters. Investigators calculate pressure transmission ratios in each quartile by comparing the amount of pressure transmitted to the bladder to the amount of pressure transmitted to the urethra. The pressure transmission ratio is defined as the change in urethral pressure divided by the change in intravesical pressure multiplied by a hundred (Fig. 8). Thus, values >100% imply positive pressure transmission (the urethral pressure spike exceeds the bladder pressure spike), whereas values <100% suggest that more pressure is transmitted to the bladder than the urethra.

As a group, patients with genuine stress incontinence have lower pressure transmission ratios than continent controls (25,51). However, marked overlap exists between pressure transmission ratios in continent and incontinent women, making it difficult to set cutoff values (52,53). That said, most patients with genuine stress incontinence have pressure transmission ratios <90% (51). Pressure transmission ratios may be useful in excluding genuine stress incontinence, but they lack the sensitivity to diagnose it (low sensitivity, high specificity) (54,55).

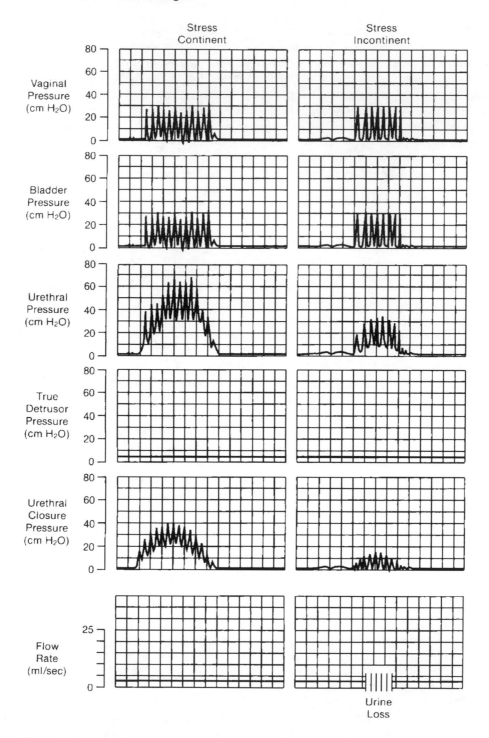

Figure 7   The cough urethral pressure profile in the continent female (left) and incontinent female (right). The curve on the left shows good pressure transmission with the space under the curve representing this patient's "margin to leakage." The curve on the right equalizes with each cough and the patient leaks urine. (From Ref. 67, p. 84.)

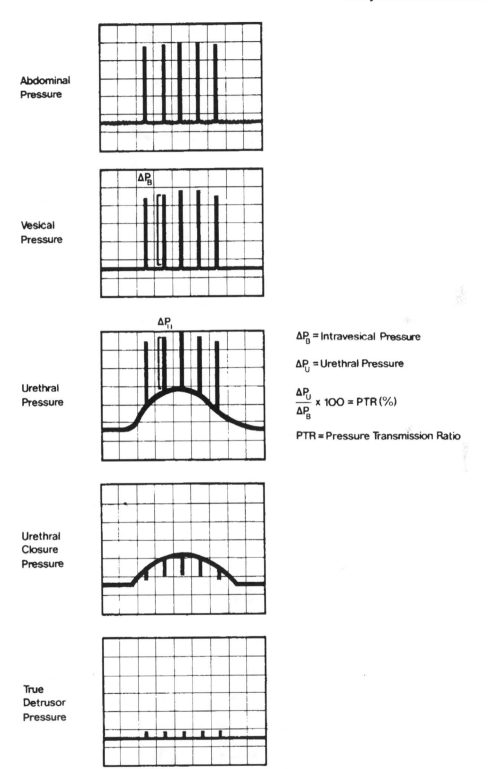

ΔP_B = Intravesical Pressure

ΔP_U = Urethral Pressure

$$\frac{\Delta P_U}{\Delta P_B} \times 100 = PTR\,(\%)$$

PTR = Pressure Transmission Ratio

Figure 8   Calculation of pressure transmission ratios during a cough urethral pressure profile. (From Ref. 68.)

No difference in pressure transmission ratios has been demonstrated between patients with genuine stress incontinence and those with low urethral closure pressures (56).

Pressure transmission ratios increase after retropubic urethropexies and traditional slings (57–61). The improved pressure transmission is theorized to be due to prevention of rotational descent of the urethra (62,63). However, since pressure transmission ratios also increase after the tension-free vaginal tape procedure, bladder neck support may not be the entire cause for improved transmission ratios (64). Constantinou and colleagues showed that the urethral pressure spike in continent patients precedes the intravesical pressure spike by several hundred milliseconds (65). This relationship is lost in stress-incontinent women even after surgical correction. Thus, there may be an active component to continence as well as the passive transmission of pressure. The urethra may contract closing the bladder neck prior to the increase in bladder pressure.

VII. MICTURITION UCPP

The micturition urethral closure pressure profile is used to detect outlet obstruction and its location. The catheter is slowly withdrawn through the urethra as the patient voids. This study is used primarily in men to look for obstruction at the bladder neck from a hypertrophied prostate. In the case of obstruction in women, the distal urethra is a more common site. Causes for obstruction in women vary from a urethral stricture, which can result from instrumentation, to urethral kinking from a large prolapse.

VIII. ANCILLARY TESTS

A. Bulbocavernosus Reflex

The bulbocavernosus reflex is elicited by tapping the clitoris with a cotton swab. This results in contraction of the bulbocavernosus and ischiocavernosus muscles. With a microtip transducer in the urethra, the bulbocavernosus reflex is detected as a brisk increase in urethral pressure. This reflex depends on the integrity of the pudendal nerve and the sacral spinal cord.

B. Anal Sphincter Reflex

The anal sphincter reflex can also be visualized with a pressure catheter in the urethra. The skin next to the anus is stroked with a Q-tip, eliciting the reflex. An intact reflex indicates normal function of L5–S2.

REFERENCES

1. Kohli N, Karram MM. Urodynamic evaluation for female urinary incontinence. Clin Obstet Gynecol 1998; 41:672–690.
2. DeLancey JO. Anatomy of the female bladder and urethra. In: Ostergard DR, Bent AE, eds. Urogynecology and Urodynamics Theory and Practice. Baltimore: Williams & Wilkins, 1996:5.
3. Rud T, Andersson KE, Asmussen M, Hunting A, Ulmsten U. Factors maintaining the intraurethral pressure in women. Invest Urol 1980; 17:343–347.
4. DeLancey JOL. Structural support of the urethra as it relates to stress urinary incontinence: the hammock hypothesis. Am J Obstet Gynecol 1994; 170:1713–1720.

5. Bonney V. On diurnal incontinence of urine in women. J Obstet Gynaecol Br Emp 1923; 30:358–365.
6. Barnes AC. A method for evaluating the stress of urinary incontinence. Am J Obstet Gynecol 1940; 40:381–390.
7. Lapides J, Ajemian EP, Stewart BH. Further observations on the kinetics of the urethrovesical sphincter. J Urol 1960; 84:86–94.
8. Brown M, Wickham JEA. The urethral pressure profile. Br J Urol 1969; 41:211–217.
9. Toews H. Intraurethral and intravesical pressure in normal and stress incontinent women. Obstet Gynecol 1967; 29:613–624.
10. Gleason DM, Bottaccini MR, Reilly RJ. Comparison of cystourethrograms and urethral profiles with gas and water media. Urology 1977; 9:155–160.
11. Schmidt RR, Witherow R, Tanagho EA. Recording urethral pressure profile: comparison of methods and clinical implications. Urology 1977; 10:390–397.
12. Millar HD, Baker LE. Stable ultraminiature catheter-tip pressure transducer. Med Biol Eng 1973; 11:86–91.
13. Schafer W. Regarding differences in urethral pressure recordings: contributions from stiffness and weight of the recording catheter. Neurourol Urodyn 1986; 5:119–120.
14. Kvarstein B, Aase O, Hansen T, Dobloug P. A new method with fiberoptic transducers used for simultaneous recording of intravesical and urethral pressure during physiological filling and voiding phases. J Urol 1983; 130:504–506.
15. Elser DM, London W, Fantl JA, McBride MA, Beck RP. A comparison of urethral profilometry using microtip and fiberoptic catheters. Int Urogynecol J Pelvic Floor Dysfunct 1999; 10:371–374.
16. Culligan PJ, Goldberg RP, Blackhurst DW, Sasso K, Koduri S, Sand PK. Comparison of microtransducer and fiberoptic catheters for urodynamic studies. Obstet Gynecol 2001; 98:253–257.
17. Anderson RS, Shepherd Am, Feneley RC. Microtransducer urethral profile methodology: variations caused by transducer orientation. J Urol 1983; 130:727–728.
18. Masuda H, Yamada T, Nagamatsu H, Nagahama K, Kawakami S, Watanabe T, Negishi T, Morita T. Study of directional differences on static and stress urethral pressure profiles of female urethra. Nippon Himyokika Gakkai Zasshi 1997; 88:40–45.
19. Jensen JK. Urodynamic evaluation. In: Ostergard DR, Bent AE, eds. Urogynecology and Urodynamics Theory and Practice. 4th ed. Baltimore: Williams and Wilkins, 1996:129–130.
20. Abrams PH. Perfusion urethral profilometry. Urol Clin North Am 1979; 6:103–110.
21. Sorensen S. Urethral pressure variations in healthy and incontinent women. Neurourol Urodyn 1992; 11:549–591.
22. Tanagho EA, Stoller ML. Urodynamics: cystometry and urethral closure pressure profile. In: Ostergard DR, Bent AD, eds. Urogynecology and Urodynamics Theory and Practice. 3rd ed. Baltimore: Williams and Wilkins, 1991:134.
23. Bhatia NN. Neurourology and urodynamics: sphincter electromyography and electrophysiological testing. In: Ostergard DR, Bent AD, eds. Urogynecology and Urodynamics Theory and Practice. 3rd ed. Baltimore: Williams and Wilkins, 1991:156–157.
24. Tanagho AE. Urodynamics of female urinary incontinence with emphasis on stress incontinence. J Urol 1979; 122:200–203.
25. Hilton P, Stanton SL. Urethral pressure measurements by microtransducer: the results in symptom-free women and in those with genuine stress incontinence. Br J Obstet Gynaecol 1983; 90:919–933.
26. Rud T. Urethral pressure profile in continent women from childhood to old age. Acta Obstet Gyneacol Scand 1980; 59:331–335.
27. Tanagho AE, Miller ER. Functional considerations of urethral sphincteric dynamics. J Urol 1973; 109:2273–2278.
28. Asmussen M. Intraurethral pressure recordings. Scand J Urol Nephrol 1976; 10:1–6.
29. Rud T. The effects of estrogens and gestagens on the urethral pressure profile in urinary continent and stress incontinent women. Acta Obstet Gynaecol Scand 1980; 59:265–270.
30. Hilton P, Stanton SL. The use of intravaginal oestrogen cream in genuine stress incontinence. Br J Obstet Gynaecol 1983; 90:940–944.

31. Beisland HO, Fossberg E, Moer A, Sander S. Urethral sphincteric insufficiency in postmenopausal females: treatment with phenylpropanolamine and estriol separately and in combination. A urodynamic and clinical evaluation. Urol Int 1984; 39:211–216.

32. Ek A, Andersson KE, Ulmsten U. The effects of norephedrine and bethanechol on the human urethral closure pressure profile. Scand J Urol Nephrol 1978; 12:97–104.

33. Sasaki H, Yoshida T, Noda K, Yachiku S, Minami K, Kaneko S. Urethral pressure profiles following radical hysterectomy. Obstet Gynecol 1982; 59:101–104.

34. Farquharson DI, Shingleton HM, Orr JW, Hatch KD, Hester S, Soong SJ. The short-term effect of radical hysterectomy on urethral and bladder function. Br J Obstet Gynaecol 1987; 94:351–357.

35. Zanolla R, Campo B, Ordesi G, Martino G. Bladder urethral dysfunction after abdominoperineal resection of the rectum for ano-rectal cancer. Tumori 1984; 70:555–559.

36. Kessler R, Constantinou CE. Internal urethrotomy in girls and its impact on the urethral intrinsic and extrinsic continence mechanisms. J Urol 1986; 136:1248–1253.

37. Stanton SL, Cardozo L, Williams JE, Ritchie D, Allan V. Clinical and urodynamic features of failed incontinence surgery in the female. Obstet Gynecol 1978; 51:515–520.

38. McGuire EJ, Lytton B, Pepe V, Kohorn EI. Stress urinary incontinence. Obstet Gynecol 1976; 47:255–264.

39. McGuire EJ. Urodynamic findings in patients after failure of stress incontinence operations. Prog Clin Biol Res 1981; 78:351–356.

40. Sand PK, Bowen LW, Panganiban R, Ostergard DR. The low pressure urethra as a factor in failed retropubic urethropexy. Obstet Gynecol 1987; 69:399–402.

41. Bowen LW, Sand PK, Ostergard DR. Unsuccessful Burch retropubic urethropexy: a case controlled urodynamic study. Am J Obstet Gynecol 1989; 160:451–458.

42. Koonings PP, Bergman A, Ballard CA. Low urethral pressure and stress urinary incontinence in women: risk factor for failed retropubic surgical procedure. Urology 1990; 16:245–248.

43. McGuire EJ, Woodside JR, Borden TA, Weiss RM. Prognostic value of urodynamic testing in myelodysplastic patients. J Urol 1981; 126:205–209.

44. Parkin DE, Davis JA, Symonds RP. Urodynamic findings following radiotherapy for cervical carcinoma. Br J Urol 1988; 61:213–217.

45. Horbach NS, Ostergard DR. Predicting intrinsic sphincter dysfunction in women with stress urinary incontinence. Obstet Gynecol 1994; 84:188–192.

46. Richardson DA, Bent AE, Ostergard DR. The effect of uterovaginal prolapse on urethrovesical pressure dynamics. Am J Obstet Gynecol 1982; 146:901–905.

47. Højsgaard A. The urethral pressure profile in female patients with meatal stenosis. Scand J Urol Nephrol 1976; 10:97–99.

48. Bhatia NN, McCarthy TA, Ostergard DR. Urethral pressure profiles of women with diverticula. Obstet Gynecol 1981; 58:375–378.

49. Steele GS, Sullivan MP, Yalla SV. Urethral pressure profilometry: vesicourethral pressure measurements under resting and voiding conditions. In: Nitti VW, ed. Practical Urodynamics. Philadelphia: W.B. Saunders, 1998:113.

50. Sand PK, Bowen LW, Ostergard DR. The prognostic significance of augmentation of urethral closure pressure and functional urethral length. Int J Gynaecol Obstet 1990; 33:135–139.

51. Bump RC, Copeland WE, Hurt WG, Fantl JA. Dynamic urethral pressure/profilometry pressure transmission ratio determinations in stress-incontinent and stress-continent subjects. Am J Obstet Gynecol 1988; 159:749–755.

52. Rosenzweig BA, Bhatia NN, Nelson AL. Dynamic urethral pressure profilometry pressure transmission ratios: what do the numbers really mean? Obstet Gynecol 1991; 77:586–590.

53. Lose G, Thind P, Colstrup H. The value of pressure transmission ratio in the diagnosis of stress incontinence. Neurourol Urodyn 1990; 9:323–324.

54. Richardson DA. Value of the cough pressure profile in the evaluation of patients with stress incontinence. Am J Obstet Gynecol 1986; 155:808–811.

55. Hanzal E, Berger E, Koelbl H. Reliability of the urethral closure pressure profile during stress in the diagnosis of genuine stress incontinence. Br J Urol 1991; 68:369–371.

56. Summitt RL, Sipes DR, Bent AE, Ostergard DR. Evaluation of pressure transmission ratios in women with genuine stress incontinence and low urethral pressure: a comparative study. Obstet Gynecol 1994; 83:984–988.

57. Faysal MH, Constantinou CE, Rother LF, Govan DE. The impact of bladder neck suspension on the resting and stress urethral pressure profile: a prospective study comparing controls with incontinent patients preoperatively and postoperatively. J Urol 1981; 125:55–60.

58. Hilton P, Stanton SL. A clinical and urodynamic assessment of the Burch colposuspension for genuine stress incontinence. Br J Obstet Gynaecol 1983; 90:934–939.

59. Weil A, Reyes H, Bischoff P, Rottenberg RD, Krauer F. Modifications of the urethral rest and stress profiles after different types of surgery for urinary stress incontinence. Br J Obstet Gynaecol 1984; 91:46–55.

60. Beck RP, McCormmick S, Nordstrom L. Intraurethral-intravesical cough-pressure spike differences in 267 patients surgically cured of genuine stress incontinence of urine. Obstet Gynecol 1988; 72:302–306.

61. Baker KR, Drutz HP. Retropubic colpourethropexy: clinical and urodynamic evaluation in 289 cases. Int Urogyncol J 1991; 2:196–200.

62. Bunne G, Obrink A. Influence of pubococcygeal repair on urethral closure pressure at stress. Acta Obstet Gynaecol Scand 1978; 57:355–359.

63. Barbic M, Kralj B. Effect of intra-abdominal position of the bladder neck and stability of its supporting structures on pressure transmission ratio after colposuspension. Int Urogynecol J Pelvic Floor Dysfunct 2000; 11:97–102.

64. Mutone N, Mastropietro M, Brizendine E, Hale D. Effect of tension-free vaginal tape procedure on urodynamic continence indices. Obstet Gynecol 2001; 98:638–645.

65. Constantinou CE, Govan DE. Spatial distribution and timing of transmitted and reflexly generated urethral pressures in healthy women. J Urol 1982; 127:964–969.

66. Ostergard DR, Bent AD, eds. Urogynecology and Urodynamics Theory and Practice, 4th ed. Baltimore: Williams & Wilkins, 1996.

67. Walters MD, Karram MM, eds. Urogynecology and Reconstructive Pelvic Surgery, 2nd ed. St. Louis: Mosby, 1999.

68. Karram MM. Urodynamics. In: Benson JT, ed. Female pelvic floor disorders: Investigation and management. New York: Norton Medical Books, 1992.

10
Leak Point Pressures

Shahar Madjar
Northern Michigan Urology at Bell, Bell Memorial Hospital, Marquette County, Michigan, U.S.A.

Rodney A. Appell
Baylor College of Medicine, Houston, Texas, U.S.A.

I. INTRODUCTION

The concept of leak point pressure (LPP) determination was introduced by McGuire et al. (1). The first LPP to be defined was the detrusor or bladder leak point pressure (DLPP) and was correlated with an increased risk of upper tract deterioration in children with meningomyelocele (1). The definition of abdominal LPP (ALPP) was to follow (2), and it was used to categorize patients into either anatomical or intrinsic sphincteric deficiency (ISD), the two types of stress urinary incontinence. ALPPs can be further divided to ALPP measured during Valsalva maneuver (VLPP) and ALPP measured during cough (CLPP). There is lack of standardization of how LPPs are measured. Different entities of LPP and a great variation in the techniques used to measure each of these entities have led to considerable confusion among professionals. The clinical applicability of these tests is therefore still controversial, and interpretation of results is difficult. The definitions of LPP, the techniques used for their measurement, and their clinical applicability are described and discussed.

II. DEFINITIONS

The following definitions were made by the Standardization Committee of the International Continence Society (ICS) and approved at the 28th annual meeting of the society in Jerusalem (3).

Detrusor leak point pressure is the lowest value of detrusor pressure at which leakage is observed in the absence of abdominal strain or a detrusor contraction. It is described as a static or passive test to assess the storage function and detrusor compliance, particularly in patients with neurogenic lower tract dysfunction.

Abdominal leak point pressure is the lowest of the intentional or actively increased intravesical pressure that provokes urinary leakage in the absence of detrusor contraction. Increased abdominal pressure can be induced by coughing (CLPP) or by a Valsalva maneuver

(VLPP). ALPP is a dynamic test used to assess the severity and the type (anatomical vs. ISD) of stress urinary incontinence.

The pressure measured in the bladder (P_{ves}) is equal to the abdominal pressure plus the pressure produced by the detrusor itself ($P_{ves} = P_{abd} + P_{det}$). ALPP is defined as an intravesical pressure measurement at a time where no detrusor contraction appears (change in $P_{det} = 0$). Therefore, the change in pressure measured at the bladder will be equal to that measured in the abdomen ($P_{ves} = P_{abd}$). ALPP can thus be determined with no pressure measurement probe in the bladder. This may allow for a true measurement of ALPP without interference of a urethral catheter partially obstructing the bladder outlet.

III. ABDOMINAL LEAK POINT PRESSURE

A. Technique

Various techniques have been described to measure LPPs. These variations affect the actual readings of LPP values. It is therefore recommended by the ICS that the location and access of pressure sensors, position of the patient, the method by which the bladder is filled (diuresis or catheter), and the volume at which the measurement is performed (both absolute and in relation to maximum cystometric capacity) be specified. The mode of leak detection (e.g., direct or fluoroscopic observation), the catheters used, and the measuring equipment for pressure measurement should also be reported.

ALPP measurement is usually performed during urodynamic testing after cystometrography with an intraurethral catheter. Rectal or vaginal pressure sensors can be alternatively used to prevent interference of the urethral catheter with urinary leakage. The bladder is filled to 200 mL, 250 mL, 50% of maximum cystometric capacity, or another predetermined fixed volume. The patient is then asked to gradually increase his/her intra-abdominal pressure (in the case of VLPP measurement) or to cough several times with increasing strength (CLPP). Some laboratories use CLPP only when Valsalva maneuver has failed to produce leakage. The lowest abdominal or vesical pressure at which leakage occurs is recorded and interpreted as ALPP. Leakage can be detected using visual recording (4–6), video or fluoroscopy (1,7,8), or electric conductance (9–11).

B. Study Conditions

Several factors have been described as influencing ALPP measurement and interpretation. The following are variations and modifications in the technique used to measure ALPP and their effect on ALPP values.

1. Catheter

VLPP measured by a urethral catheter was found to be higher than that measured with a rectal catheter (12). This may result from the catheter's partially occluding the bladder outlet. Catheter size also affects LPP results, with larger-diameter catheters correlating with higher VLPP measurement (4, 13). In a recent report by Bump et al., VLPP measurements were significantly higher when an 8Fr catheter was used compared with a 3Fr catheter (4).

2. Bladder Volume

VLPP is correlated with bladder volume in the majority of clinical studies. Theofrastous (14) reported on 120 women with genuine stress urinary incontinence who underwent serial VLPP determinations at bladder volumes of 100, 200, and 300 mL, and at maximum cystometric capacity. Thirty-three women had leakage starting at a vesical volume of 100 mL, 18 at 200 mL, 19 at 300 mL, and 17 had leakage only at maximum cystometric capacity. The mean first positive VLPPs were significantly higher than VLPPs at maximum capacity in all groups. It was concluded that VLPP in women with stress urinary incontinence decreases significantly with bladder filling. This was supported by the findings reported by Faerber and Vashi (15). Still others found no correlation between bladder volumes (150, 300, maximal cystometric capacity) and VLPP (16).

3. Cough Versus Valsalva Leak Point Pressures

Both Valsalva maneuver and cough have been used to provoke leakage in the determination of ALPP. Peschers et al. (17) reported on their evaluation in 59 incontinent women: CLPP was found to be significantly higher than VLPP (112.5 $\pm$ 46.9 cm water vs. 58.9 $\pm$ 27.6, $P < .0001$). While CLPP was negative in two women only, VLPP was negative in 24 of 59 women evaluated (40.1%). If intrinsic sphincter deficiency (ISD) was defined as a leak point pressure of 65 cm water, 16.9% of women fulfilled this criterion using the CLPP compared to 35.6% when VLPP is used. Therefore, coughing and Valsalva maneuver result in a different classification of stress urinary incontinence into ISD and anatomical stress incontinence. A similar correlation between CLPP and VLPP values was reported by Bump et al. (4).

4. Interpretation of Results

One of the debates concerning interpretation and the clinical applicability of VLPP measurements is how they should be read. Should only the increase in intravesical pressure (P_{ves}) over baseline resting P_{ves} (**ΔVLPP**) be accepted in the interpretation of the urodynamic tracing or should the total increase in P_{ves} (**VLPP$_{tot}$**), meaning the resting baseline P_{ves} + the increase in P_{ves} during Valsalva, be accepted in the interpretation of urodynamic tracing? Madjar et al. (18) studied 264 female patients who had undergone an anti-incontinence procedure. Baseline P_{abd} varied between 10 and 55 cmH$_2$O (mean = 32.7 $\pm$ 8.8) and was significantly correlated with patient's weight ($P < .001$) and patient's body mass index ($P < .001$). Higher VLPP$_{tot}$ significantly correlated with decreased age ($P = .004$), less severe incontinence ($P = .004$), higher peak Valsalva pressure ($P < .0001$), and the ability to increase abdominal pressure for a longer period of time (time to peak P_{abd} during Valsalva). VLPP$_{tot}$ and ΔVLPP had similar statistical correlation with all the clinical variables examined, and neither could predict the outcome of any anti-incontinence surgery. Using a VLPP of 60 cmH$_2$O as a cutoff to differentiate severe ISD from anatomical incontinence, 211 (67.4%) of the patients would be categorized as having ISD according to their ΔVLPP, compared with only 106 (40.1%) using the VLPP$_{tot}$. Looking at VLPP$_{tot}$ and ΔVLPP will therefore result in a different categorization of the type of incontinence in at least 25% of patients.

5. Alternatives to ALPP Measurement

Supine stress tests at empty bladder and at 200 mL were suggested as alternatives to the VLPP measurement by McLennan (19) and Hsu et al. (20), respectively. McLennan reported on 179 patients with a history of genuine stress incontinence confirmed with urodynamic testing. All patients had a supine stress test performed after voiding. Residual urine determinations were all <100 cc. A vesical Valsalva leak point pressure determination (cough and strain) was performed during multichannel urodynamics with 150 cc in the bladder. A statistically significant relationship between a low leak point pressure and a positive supine empty stress test ($P < .000$) was found. The supine empty stress test had a sensitivity of 79% and a specificity of 62.5% for the detection of a low leak point pressure. The negative predictive value was high at 90%.

Hsu et al. (20) reported on their experience with a supine stress test performed at a bladder volume of 200 mL. Cough and Valsalva maneuvers were performed after bladder filling to 200 mL with sterile normal saline solution by gravity. Efflux of the bladder solution from the meatus coinciding with the cough or Valsalva maneuver was defined as a positive clinical test. ISD was defined as an ALPP of <100 cmH$_2$O, and the supine stress test had 93.5% sensitivity, 90.0% specificity, 96.7% positive predictive value, and 81.8% negative predictive value for detecting ISD. It was concluded that the supine stress test is easy, quick, and inexpensive, and a positive test is a reliable predictor of ISD.

IV. CLINICAL APPLICATION

A. Female Stress Urinary Incontinence

Urethral pressure measurements, such as maximal urethral closing pressure, have been frequently and extensively used to assess urethral sphincteric deficiency (21–23). Despite a great deal of evidence to the contrary, maximal urethral pressure measurements have been considered by many to be closely related to continence function. This theory was challenged by McGuire et al. (2), who in 1993 reported on results comparing MUCP with ALPP. One hundred twenty-five women were divided into three types of stress urinary incontinence according to their proximal urethral closing pressure and the degree of rotational descent of the urethra (no rotation, $\leq 45°$ rotation, and $>45°$ rotation). Patients with low abdominal leak point pressure (<60 cmH$_2$O) had more severe incontinence, with 75% of them having type 3 incontinence (low urethral pressure, no urethral hypermobility). Patients with high ALPP (>90 cmH$_2$O) showed a lesser degree of incontinence and were classified as having only types 1 or 2 of incontinence (high urethral pressure and minimal or gross hypermobility, respectively). The middle group (ALPP 60–89 cmH$_2$O) had either type 2 or type 3 stress urinary incontinence. ALPPs were therefore correlated with the type of incontinence. However, abdominal pressures required to cause stress incontinence were unrelated to maximum urethral pressure, which indicates that maximum urethral pressure has little relationship with urethral resistance to abdominal pressure. This correlation between low ALPP values and ISD has been confirmed by others (24–26).

The value of distinguishing between ISD and anatomical incontinence is based primarily on different treatment modalities allocated for different types of incontinence. Traditionally, sling procedures, injectable bulking agents, and artificial urinary sphincters have been used for the treatment of ISD, while other treatment modalities, such as suspension procedures, have been used for the treatment of anatomical incontinence. This concept has recently been challenged. A considerable overlap exists between these entities (27,28). Moreover, treatments such as sling procedures, which were traditionally used for the treatment for ISD, are reported to be as effective for anatomical incontinence (29). In light of these facts, the true value of ALPP determinations and the categorization of patients into anatomic and ISD types of incontinence are still to be determined.

B. Postprostatectomy Incontinence

VLPP has been extensively used as a research tool in studies on the pathophysiology of postprostatectomy incontinence. Desautel et al. (30) report their findings in 39 (35 radical, 4 TURP and radiation) patients referred for evaluation of incontinence after prostatectomy.

Sphincteric damage was found to be the sole cause of urinary incontinence in 23 patients (59%) and a major contributor in 14 others (36%). Twenty-seven patients (69%) had VLPP <103 cmH$_2$O (mean $= 55$) with a urethral urodynamic catheter in place. An additional 10 (26%) had VLPP <150 cmH$_2$O (mean $= 63$) upon removal of the catheter. VLPP is suggested as an indication of the severity of sphincteric damage. The importance of removing the urodynamic catheter during measurement of the VLPP was emphasized. Bladder dysfunction characterized by detrusor instability and/or decreased bladder compliance was seen in 15 patients (39%). Thus, in this group of patients, incontinence was mainly due to sphincteric damage. The severity of incontinence was correlated with VLPP values.

Winters et al. (31) reported similar results in 92 patients with incontinence at least 1 year after prostatectomy (65 patients [71%] after radical prostatectomy [RP] and 27 patients [29%] after transurethral resection of the prostate or TURP). Valsalva leak point pressures (VLPP) were measured in the absence of a bladder contraction at a 150-mL volume and at 50-mL increments thereafter until maximum functional capacity was reached. The predominant urodynamic finding was sphincteric incompetence, as VLPPs were obtained in 85 patients (92%) and ranged from 12 to 120 cmH$_2$O. Detrusor overactivity was a common finding and occurred in 34 patients (37%); however, it was found to be the sole cause of incontinence in only three patients (3.3%). There was no statistically significant difference in the incidence of sphincteric incompetence after RP or TURP; however, TURP patients had a higher incidence of detrusor overactivity, which was statistically significant ($P = .019$). No correlation was found between the severity of incontinence (measured by preoperative pad usage) and VLPP. It was concluded that, although bladder dysfunction may be contributing problem in patients with post-prostatectomy incontinence, it is rarely the only mechanism for this disorder. Since bladder dysfunction may coexist or be the sole cause of postprostatectomy incontinence, urodynamic studies are important to define the exact cause(s) of incontinence after prostatectomy.

Gudziak et al. (32) examined the relationship between maximum urethral pressure, which was measured at the level of the membranous urethra, or extrinsic urethral sphincter function, and abdominal leak point pressure in 27 men with postprostatectomy incontinence. No correlation was found between maximum urethral and abdominal leak point pressures. Extrinsic urethral sphincter function was normal in all patients, while all patients but one had evidence of ISD. It is suggested that postprostatectomy stress incontinence is caused by sphincter dysfunction due to ISD and is not correlated with extrinsic sphincteric function, or maximal urethral pressure.

C. Urinary Diversion

Leak point pressure was used as part of the evaluation of bilateral hydroureteronephrosis following ileal conduit urinary diversion by Knapp et al. (33) A conduit urodynamic study was used to evaluate conduit function with a triple-lumen urodynamic catheter to simultaneously measure conduit pressure proximal and distal to the fascia during filling under fluoroscopy. In four control patients with normal upper tracts, conduit leak point pressures ranged from 5 to 20 cmH$_2$O. Abnormalities were found in five of six patients with bilateral hydroureterone-phrosis. These included functional stomal stenosis in two patients, an atonic loop in one patient, segmental obstruction in one patient, and a high-pressure, noncompliant distal segment in one patient. It is concluded that loop urodynamics can serve as a useful tool in the evaluation of postoperative bilateral hydronephrosis. Leak point pressures were also used to evaluate the postoperative continence status in women who had undergone modified nerve sparing radical cystectomy and creation of an ileal orthotopic neobladder (34).

Intraoperative use of LPP measurements have been attempted to adjust the continence mechanism and thus insure adequate continence after cutaneous urinary diversion (35). Intraoperative LPP was measured before detubularization using a simple standing column manometer and arterial line tubing. Whenever leakage occurred at pressure $<75-80 \, cmH_2O$, the continence mechanism was adjusted and LPP measurement was repeated to ensure adequate continence. Seventy-seven patients participated in the study. Adjustment of the continence mechanism was required in 32 of the 41 patients in whom the native appendicocolic junction was used and in all 36 patients in whom the tapered ileum and ileocecal valve were used. After adjustment, all patients attained leak pressures $>80 \, cmH_2O$. With a follow-up period of 30–100 months, all 77 patients were continent on an intermittent catheterization program and none has required revision of the continence mechanism.

Leak point pressures have been also used to evaluate operative success of incontinent ileovesicostomies in tetraplegic patients (36). Postoperative urodynamics demonstrated subjects ($n = 7$) to have a mean stomal leak point pressure of $7.7 \, cmH_2O$ (range 5–10). In follow-up of 12–15 months, no patient demonstrated calculus formation, hydronephrosis, autonomic dysreflexia, or worsening renal function.

V. DETRUSOR LEAK POINT PRESSURE

A. Technique

For DLPP determination, the bladder is first emptied. Bladder filling is performed at $60 \, mL/min$ in adults and at up to $20 \, mL/min$ in children. Bladder pressure is measured while the urethral meatus is observed for leakage. The study is completed once a P_{det} of $40 \, cmH_2O$ is reached, leakage is observed, a detrusor contraction occurs, or the maximum volume recovered at a few episodes of intermittent catheterization is reached (37).

B. Clinical Application

In 1981 McGuire et al. (1) reported the clinical progress of 42 myelodysplastic patients studied urodynamically and followed for a mean of 7.1 years. DLPP was $40 \, cmH_2O$ or less in 20 patients and $>40 \, cmH_2O$ in 22 patients. No patient in the low-pressure group had vesicoureteral reflux, and only two patients showed ureteral dilatation on excretory urography. In contrast, of the patients in the higher-pressure group 15 (68%) showed vesicoureteral reflux, and 18 (81%) showed ureteral dilatation on excretory urography. Thus, a striking relationship between intravesical pressure at the time of urethral leakage and the clinical course in this group of myelodysplastic patients was demonstrated.

A new modification of the technique used to measure detrusor leak point pressure in patients with myelodysplasia was later introduced by Combs and Horowitz (38). DLPP is measured during standard multichannel urodynamics. Once leakage occurs, DLPP is recorded and the catheter is removed. With the cessation of leakage, the catheter is reinserted and detrusor pressure is again noted. This cycle is repeated several times, and the average difference is noted. Fifty-four patients in whom leakage occurred were included in this study. Three groups of patients were identified: (a) (20 patients)—detrusor leak point pressure >40 and $<40 \, cmH_2O$ with the catheter in and out, respectively; (b) (29 patients)—detrusor leak point pressure consistently $<40 \, cmH_2O$ with the catheter in and out; and (c) (five patients)—detrusor leak point pressure consistently $>40 \, cmH_2O$ with the catheter in and out. All patients in group (b) had normal upper tracts. Although detrusor leak point pressure was $>40 \, cmH_2O$ using standard measurement techniques in both groups (a) and (c), upper-tract changes were demonstrated in

40% of patients in group (c) but only in 5% of patients in group (a). This modification is suggested as a more accurate measurement of DLPP and a better means of identifying patients at increased risk for renal deterioration. The main critique of this study is the low number of participants in group (c), making comparison between groups (a) and (c) difficult.

Kim et al. (39) have demonstrated that DLPP of 40 cmH$_2$O is also useful in the case of transurethral resection of the external sphincter in patients with spinal cord injury and detrusor-external sphincter-dyssynergia (DSD). DLPP was retrospectively analyzed in 55 spinal cord injury patients who had undergone transurethral resection of the external sphincter. Patients with DLPP >40 cmH$_2$O had a significantly higher incidence of upper-tract damage ($P = .021$) and persistent DSD ($P = .00008$). DLPP >40 cmH$_2$O is therefore suggested as a valid indicator of failure of transurethral resection of the external sphincter procedure.

DLPP has been widely used in other instances as a outcome measure of various operative procedures to treat neurogenic bladder such as external sphincterotomy (40), external sphincter dilatation (41), and combination therapy of intermittent catheterization and oral anticholinergic medications (42).

VI. CONCLUSIONS

Both ALPP and DLPP have been extensively studied. DLPP is a valuable tool in identifying patients at increased risk for upper-tract deterioration. ALPP is used to determine the severity of stress urinary incontinence and to categorize patients with stress urinary incontinence into anatomical and ISD types of incontinence. The clinical value of ALPP will be determined by standardization of technique and interpretation. Future determination of the need to categorize patients into ISD and anatomical types of stress urinary incontinence will also have an impact on the clinical value of ALPP.

REFERENCES

1. McGuire EJ, Woodside JR, Borden TA, Weiss RM. Prognostic value of urodynamic testing in myelodysplastic patients. J Urol 1981; 126:205.
2. McGuire EJ, Fitzpatrick CC, Wan J, Bloom D, Sanvordenker J, Ritchey M, Gormley EA. Clinical assessment of urethral sphincter function. J Urol 1993; 150:1452.
3. Stohrer M, Goepel M, Kondo A, Kramer G, Madersbacher H, Millard R, Rossier A, Wyndaele JJ. The standardization of terminology in neurogenic lower urinary tract dysfunction: with suggestions for diagnostic procedures. International Continence Society Standardization Committee. Neurourol Urodyn 1999; 18:139.
4. Bump RC, Elser DM, Theofrastous JP, McClish DK. Valsalva leak point pressures in women with genuine stress incontinence: reproducibility, effect of catheter caliber, and correlations with other measures of urethral resistance. Continence Program for Women Research Group. Am J Obstet Gynecol 1995; 173:551.
5. Sultana CJ. Urethral closure pressure and leak-point pressure in incontinent women. Obstet Gynecol 1995; 86:839.
6. Van Venrooij GE, Blok C, van Riel MP, Coolsaet BL. Relative urethral leakage pressure versus maximum urethral closure pressure. The reliability of the measurement of urethral competence with the new tube-foil sleeve catheter in patients. J Urol 1985; 134:592.
7. Hernandez RD, Hurwitz RS, Foote JE, Zimmern PE, Leach GE. Nonsurgical management of threatened upper urinary tracts and incontinence in children with myelomeningocele. J Urol 1994; 152:1582.
8. McGuire EJ. Urodynamic evaluation of stress incontinence. Urol Clin North Am 1995; 22:551.

9. Plevnik S, Vrtacnik P, Janez J. Detection of fluid entry into the urethra by electric impedance measurement: electric fluid bridge test. Clin Phys Physiol Meas 1983; 4:309.

10. Plevnik S, Brown M, Sutherst JR, Vrtacnik P. Tracking of fluid in urethra by simultaneous electric impedance measurement at three sites. Urol Int 1983; 38:29.

11. Sutherst J, Brown M. The fluid bridge test for urethral incompetence. A comparison of results in women with incontinence and women with normal urinary control. Acta Obstet Gynaecol Scand 1983; 62:271.

12. Payne CK, Raz S, Babiarz JW. The Valsalva leak point pressure in evaluation of stress urinary incontinence. Technical aspects of measurements. J Urol 1994; 151:478 [Abstract].

13. Decter RM, Harpster L. Pitfalls in determination of leak point pressure. J Urol 1992; 148:588.

14. Theofrastous JP, Cundiff GW, Harris RL, Bump RC. The effect of vesical volume on Valsalva leak-point pressures in women with genuine stress urinary incontinence. Obstet Gynecol 1996; 87:711.

15. Faerber GJ, Vashi AR. Variations in Valsalva leak point pressure with increasing vesical volume. J Urol 1998; 159:1909.

16. Petrou SP, Kollmorgen TA. Valsalva leak point pressure and bladder volume. Neurourol Urodyn 1998; 17:3.

17. Peschers UM, Jundt K, Dimpfl T. Differences between cough and Valsalva leak-point pressure in stress incontinent women. Neurourol Urodyn 2000; 19:677.

18. Madjar S, Balzarro M, Appell RA, Tchetgen MB, Nelson D. Baseline abdominal pressure and Valsalva leak point pressures—correlation with clinical and urodynamic data. Neurourol Urodyn 2003; 22:2–6.

19. McLennan MT, Bent AE. Supine empty stress test as a predictor of low Valsalva leak point pressure. Neurourol Urodyn 1998; 17:121.

20. Hsu TH, Rackley RR, Appell RA. The supine stress test: a simple method to detect intrinsic urethral sphincter dysfunction. J Urol 1999; 162:460.

21. Awad SA, Bryniak SR, Lowe PJ, Bruce AW, Twiddy DA. Urethral pressure profile in female stress incontinence. J Urol 1978; 120:475.

22. Brown M, Wickham JE. The urethral pressure profile. Br J Urol 1969; 41:211.

23. Hilton P, Stanton SL. Urethral pressure measurement by microtransducer: the results in symptom-free women and in those with genuine stress incontinence. Br J Obstet Gynaecol 1983; 90:919.

24. Bump RC, Coates KW, Cundiff GW, Harris RL, Weidner AC. Diagnosing intrinsic sphincteric deficiency: comparing urethral closure pressure, urethral axis, and Valsalva leak point pressures. Am J Obstet Gynaecol 1997; 177:303.

25. Haab F, Zimmern PE, Leach GE. Female stress urinary incontinence due to intrinsic sphincteric deficiency: recognition and management. J Urol 1996; 156:3.

26. Nitti VW, Combs AJ. Correlation of Valsalva leak point pressure with subjective degree of stress urinary incontinence in women. J Urol 1996; 155:281.

27. Dietz HP, Herbison P, Clarke B. The predictive value of hypermobility and urethral closure pressure in the diagnosis of female stress urinary incontinence. Neurourol Urodyn 2001; 20:490.

28. Madjar S, Balzarro M, Appell RA. Urethral hypermobility and intrinsic sphincteric deficiency—separate entities or coexisting factors in women with stress urinary incontinence. J Urol 2002 [Abstract].

29. Zaragoza MR. Expanded indications for the pubovaginal sling: treatment of type 2 or 3 stress incontinence. J Urol 1996; 156:1620.

30. Desautel MG, Kapoor R, Badlani GH. Sphincteric incontinence: the primary cause of post-prostatectomy incontinence in patients with prostate cancer. Neurourol Urodyn 1997; 16:153.

31. Winters JC, Appell RA, Rackley RR. Urodynamic findings in postprostatectomy incontinence. Neurourol Urodyn 1998; 17:493.

32. Gudziak MR, McGuire EJ, Gormley EA. Urodynamic assessment of urethral sphincter function in post-prostatectomy incontinence. J Urol 1996; 156:1131.

33. Knapp PM Jr, Konnak JW, McGuire EJ, Savastano JA. Urodynamic evaluation of ileal conduit function. J Urol 1987; 137:929.

34. Aboseif SR, Borirakchanyavat S, Lue TF, Carroll PR. Continence mechanism of the ileal neobladder in women: a urodynamics study. World J Urol 1998; 16:400.

35. Bissada NK, Marshall I. Leak point pressure use for intraoperative adjustment of the continence mechanism in patients undergoing continent cutaneous urinary diversion. Urology 1998; 52:790.
36. Mutchnik SE, Hinson JL, Nickell KG, Boone TB. Ileovesicostomy as an alternative form of bladder management in tetraplegic patients. Urology 1997; 49:353.
37. McGuire EJ, Cespedes RD, O'Connell HE. Leak-point pressures. Urol Clin North Am 1996; 23:253.
38. Combs AJ, Horowitz M. A new technique for assessing detrusor leak point pressure in patients with spina bifida. J Urol 1996; 156:757.
39. Kim YH, Kattan MW, Boone TB. Bladder leak point pressure: the measure for sphincterotomy success in spinal cord injured patients with external detrusor-sphincter dyssynergia. J Urol 1998; 159:493.
40. Juma S, Mostafavi M, Joseph A. Sphincterotomy: long-term complications and warning signs. Neurourol Urodyn 1995; 14:33.
41. Park JM, McGuire EJ, Koo HP, Schwartz AC, Garwood CK, Bloom DA. External urethral sphincter dilation for the management of high risk myelomeningocele: 15-year experience. J Urol 2001; 165:2383.
42. Pannek J, Diederichs W, Botel U. Urodynamically controlled management of spinal cord injury in children. Neurourol Urodyn 1997; 16:285.

11
Videourodynamics

Jennifer Gruenenfelder and Edward J. McGuire
University of Michigan, Ann Arbor, Michigan, U.S.A.

I. INTRODUCTION

The patient with complaints of urinary incontinence or urinary retention cannot be diagnosed reliably on the basis of history and physical alone. Urodynamics is an attempt to measure bladder and urethral function objectively. Videourodynamics adds anatomic detail to these measurements with the addition of a fluoroscopy unit, which allows real time imaging of the bladder and urethra during filling and voiding. The information obtained is useful for both the diagnosis and prognosis of urologic disease.

Urologic disease may result from a number of different etiologies. Neurologic diseases are associated with bladder and urethral dysfunction, and generalizations can be made about the type of dysfunction based upon the type of disease and the level of the lesion. These inferences are not reliable. For example, among patients with spinal cord injury, we assume the following: Cervical injury is associated with detrusor external sphincter dyssynergia (DESD); thoracic injury is associated with detrusor hyperreflexia (DH) and DESD; and lumbar and sacral injuries are associated with detrusor areflexia (DA). Kaplan et al. (1) showed that although these generalizations are largely true. There are statistically significant numbers of patients with cervical injury who have DA and patients with sacral injury with DESD. Patients with thoracic and lumbar lesions had even greater variation in their urodynamic findings in the same study. This study shows clearly why individual patients require urodynamic testing rather than making treatment plans based on assumptions about dysfunction from the level of the lesion. Chancellor et al. (2) showed that even patients with incomplete injuries to the thoracolumbar spine often have occult neurogenic bladder dysfunction, including 41% of patients with ASIA E impairment (otherwise completely neurologically intact).

Similarly, one cannot infer bladder dysfunction based on MRI findings of the anatomical lesion of multiple sclerosis (3). The patterns of dysfunction in patients with neurogenic bladder dysfunction caused by MS change over time, which means that urodynamics has a role not only in initial diagnosis but also in managing patients with multiple sclerosis as it progresses (4). Clearly, urodynamic monitoring is also important for diagnosis and prognosis of the neurogenic bladder associated with myelodysplasia (5–7). It is from this patient population that we have drawn many of our assumptions about the long-term prognosis of patients with poorly managed neurogenic bladders.

The use of urodynamics is not limited to investigating the urologic manifestations of neurologic disease. Its role has been delineated in the diagnosis of diseases of otherwise healthy patients such as stress incontinence (8,9), benign prostatic hyperplasia (10,11), diabetic cystopathy (12), vesicoureteral reflux (13,14), and incontinence resulting from surgical or radiation injury (15–18). Thus, videourodynamics is an important tool in the diagnosis and treatment of patients with a wide range of urological complaints. This chapter will describe the basics of videourodynamics with some clinical applications to demonstrate its utility.

II. CYSTOMETROGRAM

The cystometrogram (CMG) is a measurement of bladder pressure during filling. A catheter with a pressure transducer in its tip is placed into the bladder. There are a number of catheters available. We prefer a triple-lumen catheter with pressure transducers placed to measure the bladder and urethral pressure simultaneously (19–21). A rectal balloon with a pressure transducer is also placed. The bladder is filled with saline, contrast dye, or carbon dioxide at variable fill rates. We prefer a liquid infusion because leakage is more obvious and because the gas can be irritating to the bladder wall (22). P_{ves} is the measure of the bladder pressure during filling. P_{abd} is the abdominal pressure measured by the rectal catheter. P_{det} is the difference, $P_{ves}-P_{abd}$, and it is thought to be a measure of pure detrusor pressure. Although the subtracted difference may give a more accurate measurement of pure detrusor function, many investigators feel that P_{ves} is sufficient clinical information, particularly in patients with high spinal cord lesions who are unlikely to generate high abdominal pressures (23,24). We fill at a flow rate of 50 cc/min. The rate of filling should be slower in patients with detrusor hyperactivity and in children.

The patients are asked to note the first sensation and the point at which they would normally void. Sensation is thus a tool in measuring bladder function. First sensation, first desire to void, and strong desire to void are reproducible, and there is a normal pattern to them that likely corresponds with physiology (25). Delayed sensation can be seen in many disease processes (12,17,26,27). Early sensation may indicate sensory urgency or interstitial cystitis, although it often occurs simply as an artifact of filling the bladder with solution colder than body temperature.

Capacity is the volume the patient is able to tolerate before he needs to void. This is partially a subjective measurement as it also reflects bladder sensation. Typically the awake bladder capacity is measured, although CMG can also be performed on patients receiving general anesthesia. Functional bladder capacity is more accurately measured with a careful voiding diary. Bladder capacity should be estimated prior to performing urodynamics, particularly in children (28).

Compliance is a measure of the change in pressure as the volume changes, which is expressed by the equation $C = \Delta V/\Delta P_{det}$. Normal bladders have a high compliance; in other words, they allow storage of a large volume of fluid with minimal changes in pressure. Low-compliance bladders, in contrast, register large changes in P_{det} over small changes in volume. The expression of a ratio does not give an accurate picture of the change over time, and other methods such as calculating the slope of the compliance curve or integrating the area under the curve have been proposed as more methodical means of making the calculation (29). In practice, most clinicians look at the slope of the detrusor pressure curve during filling (flat vs. steep) without making formal calculations. Figure 1 demonstrates a study of a patient with low bladder compliance which was improved with treatment. Low compliance is a marker of disease, and it prognosticates deterioration of upper tract morphology and diminished renal function (30,31).

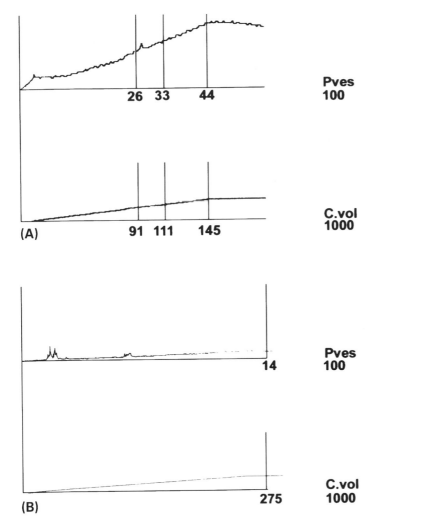

Figure 1   This study demonstrates changes in compliance. A 60-year-old female with a history of a radical hysterectomy and radiation for cervical cancer presented to the hospital with bilateral hydronephrosis and elevated creatinine. A Foley catheter was placed. Her creatinine returned to baseline values, and the hydronephrosis resolved. (A) Abnormal compliance. She was placed on ditropan, imipramine, and intermittent self-catheterization. (B) The study done ~2 months later; the abnormal compliance has resolved.

Leak point pressures are another important variable in the CMG. There are two leak point pressures of clinical significance: detrusor leak point pressure (DLPP), and abdominal leak point pressure (ALPP). DLPP is the measure of P_{det} required to induce leakage across the urethra when the bladder is the main expulsive force, and it is an important measurement in patients with neurogenic bladders. ALPP, in contrast, measures the resistance of the urethra to short increases in P_{abd} induced by cough or Valsalva maneuvers.

DLPP is an important prognosticator of kidney function. Studies conducted on myelodysplastic children correlated DLPP with the probability of upper tract damage. It was shown that patients with DLPP > 40 cmH$_2$O will develop upper tract damage (5,7,31). Thus, compliance is an important factor, but outlet resistance also contributes to safe bladder function.

An abnormally compliant bladder that leaks at low pressures is not a dangerous bladder. Conversely, in patients with poor compliance but high outlet resistance, damage will occur (5,32). Figure 2 illustrates two examples of patients with neurogenic bladders and different detrusor leak point pressures. Children who are maintained at low bladder pressures do not develop upper tract damage, but they may not be continent. Efforts to lower outlet resistance will

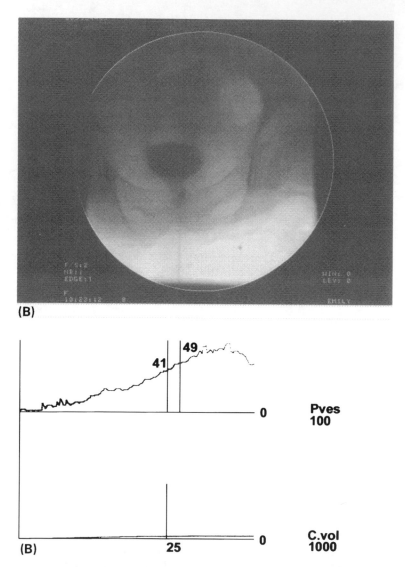

Figure 2   These examples compare patients with abnormal compliance and different outlet resistance. (A, B) A 61-year-old male with a T4 spinal cord injury (SCI) who underwent an ileal loop 38 years prior to this imaging who sought an undiversion. (A) The image obtained on fluoroscopy. Note the small bladder size and the open bladder neck. (B) Shows the tracing, which demonstrates a low capacity bladder and markedly abnormal compliance. His DLPP is 43 cmH$_2$O. In contrast, (C) shows a 46-year-old with a T12 SCI (Asia D) who presented to a urologist complaining of leakage of urine. Initial urodynamics revealed ISD felt to be of neurological origin. The patient was treated with an artificial urinary sphincter (AUS), and the reservoir is visible. He subsequently complained of persistent leakage, and this urodynamics study shows a low volume, poorly compliant bladder with a high DLPP. (D) The tracing.

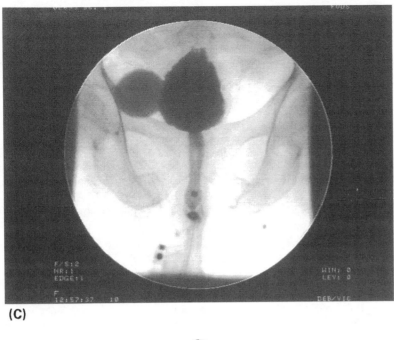

(C)

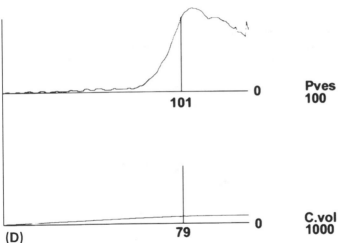

(D)

Figure 2 Continued.

result in an improvement in compliance in this neurogenic population (33). These clinical discoveries are corroborated by laboratory investigations documenting the effects of hydrostatic pressure in bladder smooth muscle cells (34). Treatments in the neurogenic population should be aimed at lowering DLPP by increasing capacity, improving compliance, and lowering outlet resistance.

ALPP is the leak point pressure that measures resistance of the urethra to short increases in abdominal pressure induced by cough or Valsalva maneuvers. This is the more important variable in the patient complaining of leakage who does not have underlying neurological disease. The standardized measurement is obtained by filling the bladder at a medium fill rate to 200 cc. The transducer is placed at a level even with the symphysis, and the patient is asked to strain or cough repetitively until leakage is induced (33). ALPPs <65 cmH$_2$O are indicative of intrinsic sphincter deficiency. Leakage at pressures 100–150 cmH$_2$O is more characteristic of urethral hypermobility, although it helps to verify this with videourodynamics (33). Figure 3 demonstrates each of these conditions. These variables are less helpful in the presence of genital prolapse, which tends to dissipate the pressure (35). ALPP is also useful to determine the etiology of postprostatectomy incontinence (16). Figure 4 shows patients with incontinence following treatment for prostate cancer.

During the course of filling short increases in P$_{ves}$ that may or may not be associated with leakage are evidence of detrusor instability, also called detrusor hyperreflexia in patients with known neurological diagnoses. Figure 5 illustrates this condition. Detrusor instability is the urodynamic manifestation of urge incontinence, although many patients with urge incontinence will not have urodynamic evidence of detrusor instability (36–38). Urge and stress incontinence cannot be reliably distinguished by history and physical alone (8,39). Patients with a history of urge incontinence with demonstrable detrusor instability are said to have motor urge incontinence. If patients are symptomatic but have no evidence of bladder contraction on the CMG, they are said to have sensory urgency (36).

The patient is asked to void when he feels full. Voiding pressure is measured, and the flow is recorded in cc/sec. Q$_{max}$ denotes the highest flow rate recorded in the study. The normal values for men and women are 20–25 cc/sec and 25–30 cc/sec, respectively. Because bladder pressure and abdominal pressure can be measured simultaneously, it is

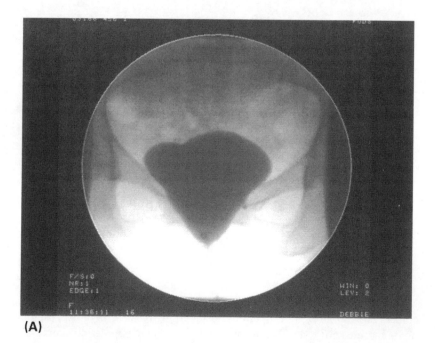

(A)

Figure 3   These are two examples of the uses of ALPP. (A) Study of a 47-year-old female who complains of incontinence. The photograph depicts urethral hypermobility and a cystocele. (B) The tracing, and she does not leak until she reaches a pressure of 144 cmH$_2$O during a cough. In contrast, (C) shows the videourodynamics of a 55-year-old female who had a bladder suspension 6 years prior subsequently treated with collagen and carbon particle injections. This photograph illustrates intrinsic sphincter deficiency. She has an open bladder neck at rest. The carbon particles can still be seen lateral to the urethra. (D) The tracing; and P$_{ves}$ is 39 cmH$_2$O when she leaks.

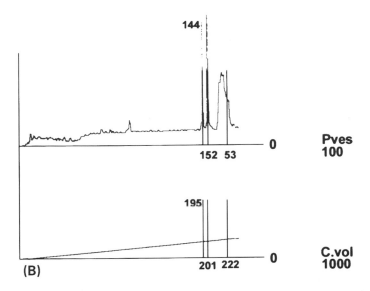

(B)

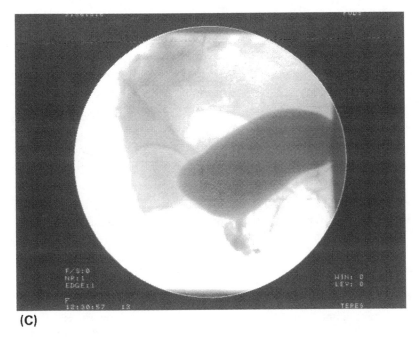

(C)

Figure 3 Continued.

possible to differentiate patients with poor flow caused by bladder outlet obstruction from patients with poor flow caused by poorly contracting bladders. Free flow studies and symptomatology are not as reliable measures of BOO. Figure 6 illustrates the urodynamics of a patient with bladder outlet obstruction (BOO). The most widely used measurement of BOO is the Abrams-Griffiths nomogram, which plots maximal flow rate against detrusor pressure at the time of flow. The resulting plot can divide patients into obstructed, nonobstructed, and equivocal (40). Nomograms for obstruction in women have been published but are not as widely used or as well validated (41). This discrepancy reflects that women have fewer

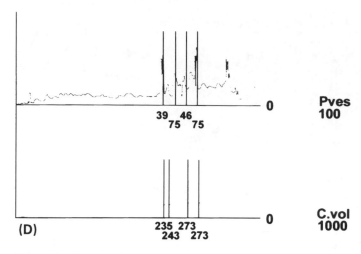

Figure 3 Continued.

pathological conditions that cause obstruction, and indeed prior anti-incontinence surgery is now the leading cause (42).

The electromyogram (EMG) is recorded during the filling and voiding phases of the urodynamics procedure. This is a measurement of depolarization of the sphincter muscle membrane. It can be recorded using either needle electrodes or surface electrodes (anal plug, vaginal, catheter mounted, or skin patch). The needle electrode perhaps gives more accurate measurements as it can measure individual motor units; however, needle electrodes are considerably more uncomfortable for the patient. A baseline measurement of spontaneous potentials should be recorded. The patient should then be asked to contract the perineal muscles to record maximal firing potential. EMGs can be used to measure integrity of perineal innervation, but they are more commonly used to measure the coordination of voiding (43).

The first phase of voiding should be cessation of the electrical activity of the sphincter. If the EMG shows an increase in perineal muscle activity at the onset of voiding, the patient is diagnosed with DESD. These patients are at an increased risk of upper-tract damage from high voiding pressures (44). Figure 7 illustrates the typical videourodynamics appearance of DESD. Learned voiding dysfunction (nonneurogenic neurogenic bladder, or Hinman's syndrome) is diagnosed when this pattern is seen in a patient with no other neurological findings (45–47). DESD patients historically were treated with sphincterotomy, but it has been shown that they have similar outcomes when treated with intermittent self-catheterization (ISC) for management of their bladder dysfunction (44). More recently, urodynamic data following sphincterotomy revealed that these patients often have incomplete surgeries resulting in persistently elevated bladder pressures, and these elevations can cause upper-tract damage (48). Patients with learned voiding dysfunction can be treated with ISC or bladder retraining combined with medications (49).

III. VIDEOURODYNAMICS

Videourodynamics improves upon the information obtained from a CMG with the addition of fluoroscopy. The bladder is filled with contrast dye during the CMG, and thus information about

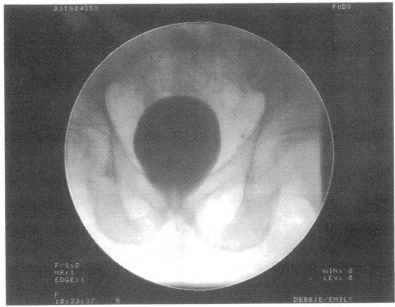

(A)

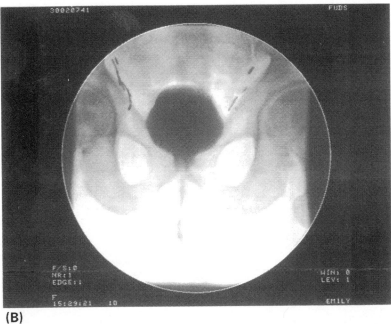

(B)

Figure 4   These are two examples of incontinence following a radical prostatectomy. (A) The first has the typical open bladder neck of postprostatectomy incontinence, and his leak point pressure is 39 cmH$_2$O. (B) The second patient has the typical open bladder neck, but a much higher pressure was reached before he leaked. The image shows that he had a urethral stricture that needed to be treated prior to treatment of his incontinence from the prostatectomy.

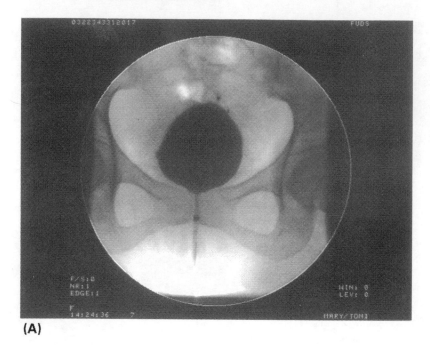

(A)

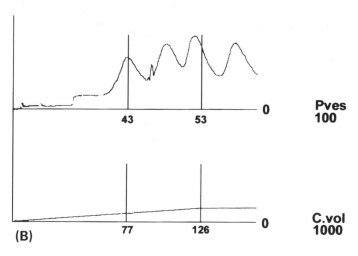

(B)

Figure 5   This is the study of a 37-year-old female recently diagnosed with multiple sclerosis who complains of urge incontinence and difficulty voiding. (A) Her bladder during filling. The wire above her bladder in this photograph is a nerve stimulator. The bladder neck opens slightly with each contraction. (B) The typical tracing of detrusor hyperreflexia.

structure and function can be gleaned during the test. It is important prior to the initiation of the study, which is more expensive than conventional CMG, to determine if this imaging will yield additional information. It does have the advantage of minimizing some of the artifacts of conventional CMG. Anatomic images can be captured on videotape and correlated specifically with the CMG during filling and voiding. The addition of video is most useful for the assessment of incontinence, neurogenic bladder, and bladder outlet obstruction. It can also be used in preparation for reconstructive procedures and to assess reservoirs or augmented bladders. We

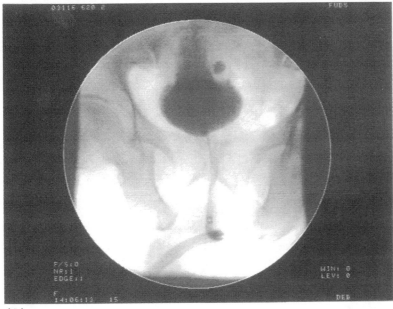

(A)

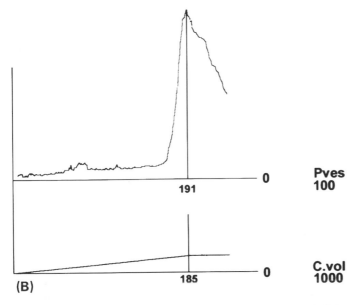

(B)

Figure 6 This 60-year-old male with atrial fibrillation and diabetes presented in urinary retention. Physical exam revealed a large prostate estimated at 110 g by subsequent ultrasound. Because of the possibility of diabetic cystopathy causing his retention, urodynamics was performed. (A) A trabeculated bladder with several diverticula. (B) A maximum pressure of 191 cmH$_2$O when the patient attempted to void, although no urine flowed from his bladder. He was subsequently treated with an open prostatectomy, and he now voids to completion.

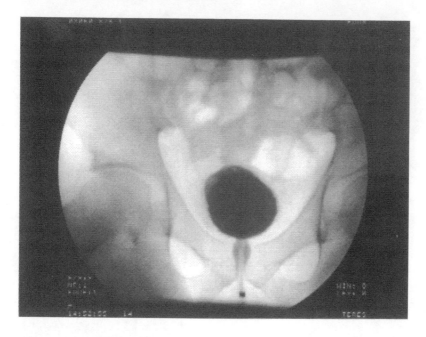

Figure 7   This 57-year-old male with multiple sclerosis presented with an inability to void. In this photograph of the voiding phase, his bladder neck is open, but the contraction of the external sphincter keeps the urine from passing through the urethra. He has a trabeculated bladder. Voiding pressure is high.

further use videourodynamics to assess ureters prior to reconstruction. What follows is a description of the methods and uses of videourodynamics.

A.   Equipment and Technique

The typical videourodynamics unit consists of a fluoroscopic unit, a television monitor with videotape capabilities, a multichannel recorder, a system for filling the bladder, and transducers. Almost any type of fluoroscopy unit can be used, and generally the patient is exposed to less than a minute of fluoroscopy. Although we have a dedicated fluoroscopic unit in our clinic, the same information could be obtained from bringing standard CMG equipment to the fluoroscopy suite of any hospital.

We favor a triple lumen 10F catheter. The most distal port is the largest, and it is used for infusion of contrast. The next most distal port measures the intravesical pressure, and the third port measures the pressure at the uretha. The catheter position is checked by fluoroscopy and verified when the port measuring urethral pressure gives a pressure tracing that is not identical to the bladder pressure measurements. We then infuse at a fill rate of 50 cc/min.

We do not routinely use a rectal balloon to monitor rectal pressure. We feel that the addition of this measurement is not helpful. It adds to the stress of the overall test. Rectal pressure measurements have been advocated as a way of separating increases in abdominal pressure from detrusor instability, but we feel that the same information can be obtained from watching the urethral pressure measurements, which are continuous, and from noting if the bladder neck opens or remains closed and if there is leakage during increases in vesical pressure. It has also been argued that the use of a rectal catheter allows the clinician to distinguish between obstructed and unobstructed flow. We feel that the combination of flow rate, the appearance of the bladder neck on video, and the measurement of total pressure is sufficient to make that diagnosis, as flow characteristics are determined more by urethral resistance than by the source of pressure, whether it is abdominal straining or elevated detrusor pressure. Similarly, we do not perform EMG during videourodynamics. It is most useful in the diagnosis of DESD, but we feel that the appearance of DESD on video combined with the expected elevations of vesical pressure are sufficient to make this diagnosis.

B. Stress Incontinence

Stress incontinence is a diagnosis clearly aided by the use of videourodynamics. The classification of incontinence historically relied upon radiographic findings (50,51). Stress urinary incontinence is currently defined as type 1, 2, or 3, depending on the presence or absence and degree of urethral and bladder descent (52). Figures 8–11 illustrate each of these types of incontinence. Figure 12 illustrates how videourodynamics may help clarify the type of leakage in an incontinent patient. Fluoroscopy allows for better visualization of a hypermobile urethra during strain compared to physical exam alone. Patients with significant cystocele and uterine descensus may have falsely elevated ALPP, which makes a diagnosis of the type of incontinence by CMG alone more difficult. Reduction of the prolapse manually or with a pessary is helpful to obtain a more accurate diagnosis, and this is helpful in planning treatment (35). Lack of stress incontinence symptoms in patients with cystoceles is an unreliable indicator of what their voiding may be like after surgical repair of the cystocele. It is therefore helpful to characterize their anatomy with videourodynamics (53). At this point it is unclear what percentage of patients with no symptoms of stress incontinence will be symptomatic following a repair of the prolapse, and it is also unclear if performing the videourodynamics with a pessary helps predict that population. The CARE study is addressing that question, and it is hoped that they will have some early data by 2004.

C. Vesicoureteral Reflux

Videourodynamics is useful for the determination of vesicoureteral reflux. This has several implications. The first is in the treatment of children with vesicoureteral reflux and no underlying neuropathy. Dysfunctional voiding has been implicated both as a cause of vesicoureteral reflux and a reason that surgery fails to correct it (54). Prospective videourodynamic studies have shown that patients with bladder instability and reflux managed nonoperatively with anticholinergics do as well as patients who are treated surgically (14). Thus, determination of the cause of reflux is important in deciding upon a course of therapy. The second use is in patients with neurogenic bladders. The presence of reflux has been shown to alter the reliability of the CMG in examining compliance and capacity (13), which clearly influences treatment decisions. Figure 13 shows an example of a patient with a neurogenic bladder and reflux. The elimination of reflux in patients being treated to alter their capacity and compliance has been shown to be a reliable marker of improvement (55,56).

D. Ureteral Obstruction

Videourodynamics can also be helpful in the measurement of ureteral obstruction. When a patient presents with hydronephrosis, it must be ascertained if the collecting system is merely dilated or truly obstructed. Diuresis scintigraphy and the Whitaker test are the two commonest methods of answering this question. The Whitaker test is performed by through a percutaneous nephrostomy tube. A pressure transducer is placed in the percutaneous nephrostomy tube and in

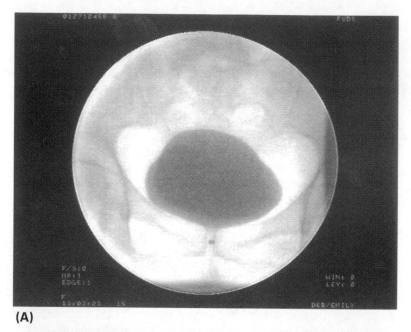

(A)

(B)

Figure 8   This is an example of type 1 incontinence. (A) The vesical neck closed at rest. (B) The descent, not more than 2 cm, during stress. She had an ALPP of 125 cmH$_2$O.

the bladder. The renal pelvis is then infused at a rate of 10 cc/min. The difference in pressure between the bladder and the renal pelvis is calculated. If the difference in pressure is <13 cmH$_2$O, the system is considered normal. Higher values are consistent with obstruction, and some investigators differentiate mild, moderate, and severe obstruction based on those values (57). Although diuresis scintigraphy has the advantage of being less invasive and is thus

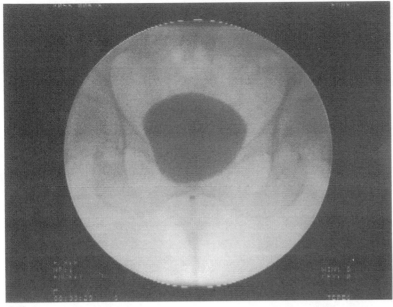

(A)

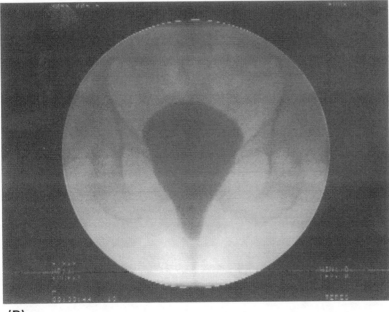

(B)

Figure 9   This figure demonstrates type 2A stress incontinence. (A) The bladder at rest, with the vesical neck closed and above the inferior margin of the pubic symphysis. (B) During stress the vesical neck and proximal urethra open and descend >2 cm.

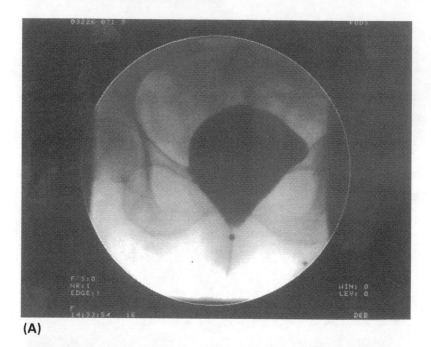

(A)

(B)

Figure 10 This patient illustrates type 2B incontinence. (A) A vesical neck closed at rest but located below the margin of the pubic symphysis. (B) When she coughs or Valsalvas, there is significant descent, although there does not have to be any descent be classified as type 2B. P_{ves} was 91 cmH$_2$O when she leaked.

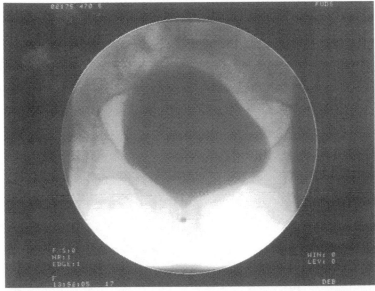

(A)

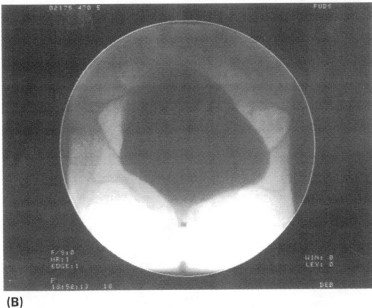

(B)

Figure 11 This is an examples of type 3 incontinence or intrinsic sphincter deficiency. (A) The bladder neck open at rest. (B) Leakage during at a leak point pressure <45 cmH$_2$O.

the preferred first test (58–61), the Whitaker test offers the advantage of imaging the anatomic point of obstruction when done with fluoroscopy in addition to giving functional information about the kidney. Figure 14 illustrates the use of the test. It has also been observed that positional changes can influence the results of the Whitaker test. Because such positional variations may be relevant clinically, it is important to consider the Whitaker test in diagnosis for patients with abnormal anatomy or intermittent symptoms (62).

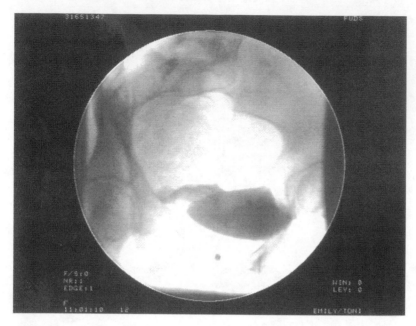

Figure 12 A 49-year-old female underwent a total vaginal hysterectomy ~2 months prior to this study. She complained of incontinence. Fluoroscopy revealed extravasation of contrast into the vagina consistent with a vesicovaginal fistula. The patient had normal compliance and no evidence of urethral hypermobility or leakage.

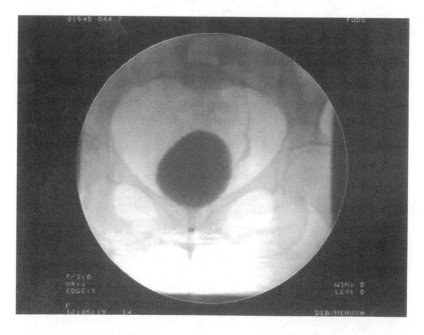

Figure 13 This is the bladder of a 22-year-old patient with myelodysplasia who had a small capacity, trabeculated bladder with poor compliance, reflux, and an open bladder neck at rest. Although the initiation of anticholinergic therapy corrected the compliance and the reflux, she subsequently required a pubovaginal sling for her intrinsic sphincter deficiency.

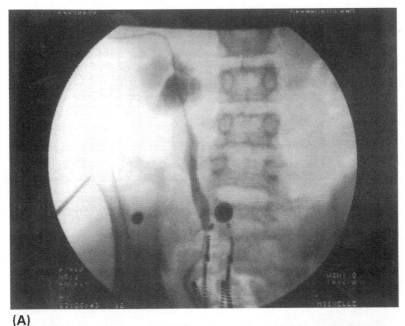

(A)

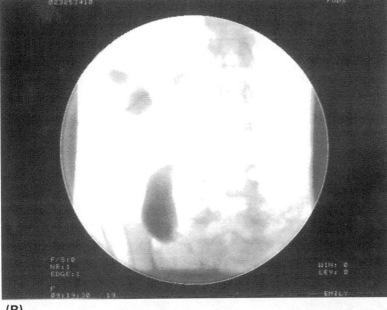

(B)

Figure 14 (A) The Whitaker test of a 17-year-old male who presented initially with a ureteropelvic junction obstruction diagnosed after a CT was done for abdominal trauma. He was treated with a ureterocalicostomy. His hydronephrosis did not improve. Contrast 50 cc was instilled through his percutaneous nephrostomy tube. Neither the bladder pressure nor the renal pelvis pressure exceeded 10 cmH$_2$O. (B) The Whitaker test of a 34-year-old female patient with myelodysplasia treated initially with a vesicostomy at birth, followed by an ileal loop at puberty. She subsequently had an undiversion with a neobladder and an AUS. She was referred because of bilateral hydronephrosis, and her renal scan was inconclusive. Whitaker test showed rapid appearance of contrast in the bladder; the highest pressure difference between the bladder and the renal pelvis was 2 cmH$_2$O.

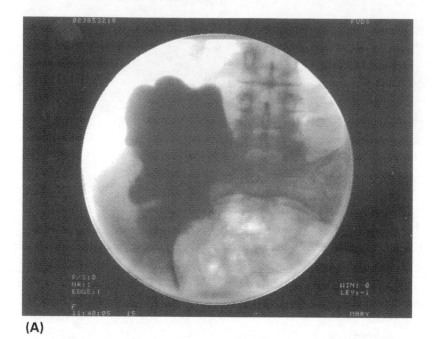

(A)

(B)

Figure 15   (A) Study of a 68-year-old female who complained of leakage from her stoma following a cystectomy with Indiana pouch. Fluoroscopic urodynamics showed that her compliance is normal, but she has phasic contraction of the bowel segments, during which time she leaked. (B, C) Fluoroscopy images of a 57-year-old male with a neobladder who presented in urinary retention. Videourodynamics revealed bilateral reflux, high voiding pressures, and a stricture at the anastamotic ring.

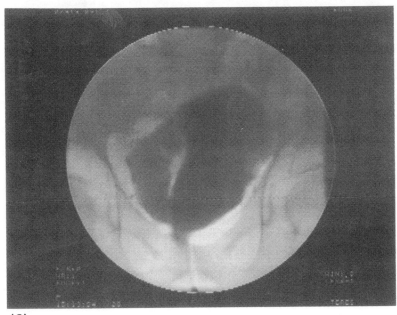

(C)

Figure 15   Continued.

E. Urinary Diversions

Videourodynamics is useful in the evaluation of patients who have had urinary diversions for malignancy and for neurogenic bladders. Ileal conduits are the most common incontinent urinary diversions. It is not unusual to have bilateral hydronephrosis following this procedure, but the etiology of the dilatation needs to be elucidated. Patients with refluxing ureteral anastamoses may get chronic dilatation of the urinary tract, but hydronephrosis may also arise from stomal stenosis, ureteroileal anastamosis, or a poorly compliant loop. Knapp et al. used urodynamics to study patients with ileal loops and bilateral hydronephrosis compared to patients with normal upper tracts and ileal loops, and they found significant differences in these patient groups (63).

Urodynamics is also helpful in patients with neobladders performed for diversions in patients with bladder cancer or neurogenic bladder. It has been used as an investigative tool to compare the methods of bladder substitution. Lin et al. (64) compared patients with gastric neobladders to patients with small-bowel or ileocecal substitution. They found greater incontinence with lower capacity and worse compliance in the gastric neobladders. Thus, we see that the use of videourodynamics offers a means of comparing new procedures to accepted standards of care for urinary diversion. Santucci (59) compared orthotopic neobladders to stomal urinary reservoirs with urodynamics, and this type of comparative analysis is certainly useful in the preoperative counseling of patients.

Videourodynamics also allows for the post operative assessment of patients who complain of incontinence or enuresis following diversion, as illustrated in Figure 15. Ordorica (60) investigated patients with continent colonic urinary reservoirs. Urodynamics allowed the diagnosis of incompetent outlet or high-pressure intestinal contraction of the reservoir as treatable causes of intractable incontinence and showed the causes of difficult catheterization (66,67). El Bahnasawy (62) showed that enuretic patient with orthotopic neobladders had higher pressure and postvoid residuals and lower maximum flow and compliance in patients with incontinence (68). Porru and Usai similarly used urodynamics to evaluate incontinence in their neobladder patients (69,70). Similarly, videourodynamics enables monitoring of patients with ileovesicostomy to show that the reservoirs continue to leak at low pressures that are safe for the upper tracts (71–73). These studies show that videourodynamics is essential in the diagnosis of the incontinent or enuretic patient following urinary diversion.

IV. CONCLUSIONS

Videourodynamics combines the functional information obtained with the CMG and flow studies with the anatomical information that can only be obtained using fluoroscopy. The use of urodynamics is clearly essential in the diagnosis and long-term follow-up of patients who have neurogenic bladders. It is also important in the treatment of patients who present with incontinence either initially or as the consequence of another surgical procedure. A primer of urodynamics is beyond the scope of this chapter, but we have attempted to show some of the uses of this valuable tool.

REFERENCES

1. Kaplan SA, Chancellor MB, Blaivas JG. Bladder and sphincter behavior in patients with spinal cord lesions. J Urol 1991; 146(1):113–117.
2. Watanabe T. High incidence of occult neurogenic bladder dysfunction in neurologically intact patients with thoracolumbar spinal injuries. J Urol 1998; 159(3):965–968.
3. Kim YH. The correlation of urodynamic findings with cranial magnetic resonance imaging findings in multiple sclerosis. J Urol 1998; 159(3):972–976.
4. Ciancio SJ. Urodynamic pattern changes in multiple sclerosis. Urology 2001; 57(2):239–245.
5. McGuire EJ. Prognostic value of urodynamic testing in myelodysplastic patients. J Urol 1981; 126(2):205–209.
6. Amundsen C. Do urinary symptoms correlate with urodynamic findings? J Urol 1999; 161(6):1871–1874.
7. McGuire EJ, Cespedes RD. Proper diagnosis: a must before surgery for stress incontinence. J Endourol 1996; 10(3):201–205.
8. McGuire EJ. The role of urodynamic investigation in the assessment of benign prostatic hypertrophy. J Urol 1992; 148(4):1133–1136.
9. Abrams P. Objective evaluation of bladder outlet obstruction. Br J Urol 1995; 76(suppl 1):11–15.
10. Kaplan SA, Te AE, Blaivas JG. Urodynamic findings in patients with diabetic cystopathy. J Urol 1995; 153(2):342–344.
11. Bomalaski MD, Bloom DA. Urodynamics and massive vesicoureteral reflux. J Urol 1997; 158(3 Pt 2):1236–1238.
12. Willemsen J, Nijman RJ. Vesicoureteral reflux and videourodynamic studies: results of a prospective study. Urology 2000; 55(6):939–943.
13. Morgan JL, O'Connell HE, McGuire EJ. Is intrinsic sphincter deficiency a complication of simple hysterectomy? J Urol 2000; 164(3 Pt 1):767–769.
14. Gudziak MR, McGuire EJ, Gormley EA. Urodynamic assessment of urethral sphincter function in post-prostatectomy incontinence. J Urol 1996; 156(3):1131–1134; discussion 1134–1135.
15. McGuire EJ. Urodynamic evaluation after abdominal-perineal resection and lumbar intervertebral disk herniation. Urology 1975; 6(1):63–70.
16. Cespedes RD. Long-term followup of incontinence and obstruction after salvage cryosurgical ablation of the prostate: results in 143 patients. J Urol 1997; 157(1):237–240.

17. Belville WD. Fiberoptic microtransducer pressure technology: urodynamic implications. Neurourol Urodyn 1993; 12(2):171–178.

18. Woodside JR, McGuire EJ. A simple inexpensive urodynamic catheter. J Urol 1979; 122(6):788–789.

19. Woodside JR, McGuire EJ. Clinical evaluation of new urodynamic catheter. Urology 1985; 26(1):95–96.

20. Watanabe T, Rivas DA, Chancellor MB. Urodynamics of spinal cord injury. Urol Clin North Am 1996; 23(3):459–473.

21. Chancellor MB, Blaivas JG. Diagnostic evaluation of incontinence in patients with neurological disorders. Comp Ther 1991; 17(2):37–43.

22. Chancellor MB, Kiilholma P. Urodynamic evaluation of patients following spinal cord injury. Semin Urol 1992; 10(2):83–94.

23. Wyndaele JJ. The normal pattern of perception of bladder filling during cystometry studied in 38 young healthy volunteers. J Urol 1998; 160(2):479–481.

24. Wyndaele JJ. Studies of bladder sensitivity in patients with myelodysplasia. Paraplegia 1992; 30(5):333–335.

25. Zoubek J. The late occurrence of urinary tract damage in patients successfully treated by radiotherapy for cervical carcinoma. J Urol 1989; 141(6):1347–1349.

26. Kaefer M. Estimating normal bladder capacity in children. J Urol 1997; 158(6):2261–2264.

27. Dmochowski R. Cystometry. Urol Clin North Am 1996; 23(2):243–252.

28. Ghoniem GM. Bladder compliance in meningomyelocele children. J Urol 1989; 141(6):1404–1406.

29. Ghoniem GM. The value of leak pressure and bladder compliance in the urodynamic evaluation of meningomyelocele patients. J Urol 1990; 144(6):1440–1442.

30. McGuire EJ, Woodside JR, Borden TA. Upper urinary tract deterioration in patients with myelodysplasia and detrusor hypertonia: a followup study. J Urol 1983; 129(4):823–826.

31. McGuire EJ, Cespedes RD, O'Connell HE. Leak-point pressures. Urol Clin North Am 1996; 23(2):253–262.

32. Haberstroh KM. The effects of sustained hydrostatic pressure on select bladder smooth muscle cell functions. J Urol 1999; 162(6):2114–2118.

33. Romanzi LJ, Chaikin DC, Blaivas JG. The effect of genital prolapse on voiding. J Urol 1999; 161(2):581–586.

34. Swami SK, Abrams P. Urge incontinence. Urol Clin North Am 1996; 23(3):417–425.

35. James M. Pure stress leakage symptomatology: is it safe to discount detrusor instability? Br J Obstet Gynaecol 1999; 106(12):1255–1258.

36. Lim CS, Abrams P. The Abrams-Griffiths nomogram. World J Urol 1995; 13(1):34–39.

37. Blaivas JG, Groutz A. Bladder outlet obstruction nomogram for women with lower urinary tract symptomatology. Neurourol Urodyn 2000; 19(5):553–564.

38. Groutz A, Blaivas JG, Chaikin DC. Bladder outlet obstruction in women: definition and characteristics. Neurourol Urodyn 2000; 19(3):213–220.

39. Siroky MB. Electromyography of the perineal floor. Urol Clin North Am 1996; 23(2):299–307.

40. Groutz A. Learned voiding dysfunction (non-neurogenic, neurogenic bladder) among adults. Neurourol Urodyn 2001; 20(3):259–268.

41. Phillips E, Uehling DT. Hinman syndrome: a vicious cycle. Urology 1993; 42(3):317–319; discussion 319–320.

42. Hinman F Jr. Nonneurogenic neurogenic bladder (the Hinman syndrome)—15 years later. J Urol 1986; 136(4):769–777.

43. McGuire EJ, Brady S. Detrusor-sphincter dyssynergia. J Urol 1979; 121(6):774–777.

44. Kim YH, Kattan MW, Boone TB. Bladder leak point ressure: the measure for sphincterotomy success in spinal cord injured patients with external detrusor-sphincter dyssynergia. J Urol 1998; 159(2):493–496; discussion 496–497.

45. Allen TD. The non-neurogenic neurogenic bladder. J Urol 1977; 117(2):232–238.

46. Blaivas JG, Olsson CA. Stress incontinence: classification and surgical approach. J Urol 1988; 139(4):727–731.

47. Gardy M. Stress incontinence and cystoceles. J Urol 1991; 145(6):1211–1213.
48. Greenfield SP, Wan J. The relationship between dysfunctional voiding and congenital vesicoureteral reflux. Curr Opin Urol 2000; 10(6):607–610.
49. Agarwal SK. Urodynamic correlates of resolution of reflux in meningomyelocele patients. J Urol 1997; 158(2):580–582.
50. Flood HD. Outcome of reflux in children with myelodysplasia managed by bladder pressure monitoring. J Urol 1994; 152(5 Pt 1):1574–1577.
51. Pfister RC, Papanicolaou N, Yoder IC. Diagnostic morphologic and urodynamic antegrade pyelography. Radiol Clin North Am 1986; 24(4):561–571.
52. Lupton EW. A comparison of diuresis renography, the Whitaker test and renal pelvic morphology in idiopathic hydronephrosis. Br J Urol 1985; 57(2):119–123.
53. Hay AM. A comparison between diuresis renography and the Whitaker test in 64 kidneys. Br J Urol 1984; 56(6):561–564.
54. Senac MO Jr, Miller JH, Stanley P. Evaluation of obstructive uropathy in children: radionuclide renography vs. the Whitaker test. AJR 1984; 143(1):11–15.
55. Jakobsen H. Sensitivity of ^{131}I-hippuran diuresis renography and pressure flow study (Whitaker test) in upper urinary tract obstruction. Urol Int 1988; 43(2):89–92.
56. Ellis JH. Positional variation in the Whitaker test. Radiology 1995; 197(1):253–255.
57. Knapp PM Jr. Urodynamic evaluation of ileal conduit function. J Urol 1987; 137(5):929–932.
58. Lin DW. Urodynamic evaluation and long-term results of the orthotopic gastric neobladder in men. J Urol 2000; 164(2):356–359.
59. Santucci RA. Continence and urodynamic parameters of continent urinary reservoirs: comparison of gastric, ileal, ileocolic, right colon, and sigmoid segments. Urology 1999; 54(2):252–257.
60. Ordorica RC. Evaluation and management of mechanical dysfunction in continent colonic urinary reservoirs. J Urol 2000; 163(6):1679–1684.
61. Masel JL. Evaluation of flap valve as an alternative continence mechanism in the Florida pouch. Urology 1999; 53(3):506–509.
62. El Bahnasawy MS. Nocturnal enuresis in men with an orthotopic ileal reservoir: urodynamic evaluation. J Urol 2000; 164(1):10–13.
63. Porru D. Behaviour and urodynamic properties of orthotopic ileal bladder substitute after radical cystectomy. Urol Int 1994; 53(1):30–33.
64. Porru D, Usai E. Orthotopic ileal bladder substitute after radical cystectomy: urodynamic features. Neurourol Urodyn 1994; 13(3):255–260.
65. Rivas DA, Karasick S, Chancellor MB. Cutaneous ileocystostomy (a bladder chimney) for the treatment of severe neurogenic vesical dysfunction. Paraplegia 1995; 33(9):530–535.
66. Mutchnik SE. Ileovesicostomy as an alternative form of bladder management in tetraplegic patients. Urology 1997; 49(3):353–357.
67. Leng WW. Long-term outcome of incontinent ileovesicostomy management of severe lower urinary tract dysfunction. J Urol 1999; 161(6):1803–1806.

12

Pharmacologic and Surgical Management of Detrusor Instability

H. Henry Lai, Michael Gross, Timothy B. Boone, and Rodney A. Appell
Baylor College of Medicine, Houston, Texas, U.S.A.

I. INTRODUCTION

Overactive bladder (OAB) is characterized by the urinary symptoms of frequency, urgency, and urge incontinence as a result of involuntary detrusor contractions during bladder filling. Such contractions are predominantly under the control of the parasympathetic nervous system. Acetylcholine released from the parasympathetic nerve endings activates the M_3 muscarinic receptors on the detrusor smooth muscles and modulates bladder contractility. Antimuscarinic agents inhibit the binding of acetylcholine to the muscarinic receptors and suppress involuntary detrusor contraction (1). Immediate-release oxybutynin was the gold standard in pharmacologic treatment of OAB for almost three decades. Its antimuscarinic (M_3) activity is nonselective for the urinary bladder, resulting in significant systemic side effects, particularly dry mouth, that limit its clinical utility (2,3). Even though alternative routes of administration of oxybutynin, such as intravesical instillation (4–6), intravesical implant (7), and rectal suppository (8), are available, oral agents remain the mainstay in treatment of OAB. Newer pharmacologic agents, e.g., tolterodine, and modified drug delivery mechanisms for oxybutynin (e.g., extended-release oxybutynin) have revolutionized the treatment of OAB (4,5).

New drugs are always compared not only to placebo but also to immediate-release oxybutynin, because of its long history and established efficacy (6). Originally identified in the 1960s as a potential treatment for gastrointestinal hypermobility, oxybutynin was found to be effective in inhibiting involuntary bladder contractions. It is a receptor subtype–specific antagonist that binds with higher affinity to the M_3 muscarinic receptors than to the other receptor subtypes (M_1, M_2, M_4, and M_5). Oxybutynin also has direct spasmolytic (musculo-tropic) and local anesthetic effects on the detrusor.

Even though the clinical efficacy of immediate-release oxybutynin is well documented, dose-related antimuscarinic side effects are frequent. Dry mouth is the most common and bothersome complaint, followed by constipation, blurred vision, dry eyes, urinary retention, and drowsiness. These systemic side effects occur because oxybutynin is not targeted specifically to the lower urinary tract. It also inhibits M_3 receptors in the salivary glands, which mediate salivary secretion, and M_3 receptors in the intestines, which regulate bowel peristalsis. Clinically, immediate-release oxybutynin appears more potent in causing dry mouth than in inhibiting detrusor instability. This adverse effect is often severe enough to cause poor patient compliance, suboptimal dosing, and even drug discontinuation. Only 18–22% of patients treated with immediate-release oxybutynin remained on the medication after 6 months due to intolerable side effects (9,10). Since OAB is a chronic debilitating condition requiring long-term treatment, it is important that pharmacologic therapy be not only effective but also well tolerated. The challenge has been to develop antimuscarinic agents that are as effective as immediate-release oxybutynin but without the side effect loads.

II. TOLTERODINE

Tolterodine (Detrol) was the first drug developed specifically for the treatment of OAB. It is a competitive muscarinic antagonist that exhibits similar affinities for muscarinic receptor subtypes $M_1–M_5$. Unlike immediate-release oxybutynin, which is a receptor subtype–specific agent (for M_3), tolterodine may be a more target-specific drug that possesses stronger selectivity for the urinary bladder than for the salivary glands. In an anesthetized cat model (but only six cats), tolterodine appeared more potent in inhibiting detrusor instability than salivation. This is in contrast to immediate-release oxybutynin, which exhibited the opposite tissue-selective profile (11,12). In a pilot study with healthy volunteers, tolterodine was well tolerated and exhibited greater objective and subjective antimuscarinic effects on detrusor function than on salivation (13). However, in another study on the effects on salivary volume, at 2 h following tolterodine (2 mg) or immediate-release oxybutynin in healthy volunteers, there was less suppression of salivary volume with immediate-release oxybutynin. However, there was a complete return to normal by 10 h in the volunteers taking tolterodine, and those taking immediate-release oxybutynin took longer to regain their respective salivary volume. In addition, another group taking extended-release oxybutynin (10 mg) had a constant salivary volume that was only slightly below that of those who were given placebo (14). The precise mechanism responsible for any bladder-selective property of tolterodine remains to be elucidated. Whether this is related to the differential affinities of the muscarinic receptors in salivary glands and those in detrusor muscles for tolterodine and for immediate-release oxybutynin or its metabolites remains to be confirmed in the human (4).

The recommended dosage of tolterodine is 2 mg BID based on Phase II dose-ranging studies. No dose adjustment is necessary on the basis of metabolic phenotype (cytochrome P_{450} "extensive" vs. "poor" metabolizers) (15). Obviously, as the dosage of tolterodine increases, clinical response improves, but tolerability declines. At a dosage of 2 mg BID, the incidence of adverse effects, including dry mouth, is similar to that found with placebo, but clinical efficacy is comparable to that of immediate-release oxybutynin. A lower dose (1 mg BID) results in less favorable improvements in maximum cystometric capacity and volume at first contraction in urodynamic tests. A higher dose (4 mg BID) quadruples postvoid residual volume (from 48 mL to 163 mL) and may increase the risk of urinary retention (15,16). The rate of dry mouth also approaches 56% at the higher dose (12). Ultimately, the recommended dosage of tolterodine was set at 2 mg BID with the aim of achieving efficacy similar to that of immediate-release oxybutynin but without the same side-effect burden. The half-life of tolterodine is ~4 h. Progression to peak therapeutic action is rapid. In Phase I clinical trials with healthy volunteers, tolterodine exerted a marked inhibitory effect on bladder function within 2 h after a single oral dose (13,17). However, clinically noticeable decreases in voiding frequency and incontinence episodes do not occur immediately when behavioral aspects of patients are taken into account. Modification of voiding habits is a gradual process, and it takes a period of time for the patient to trust the enhanced control that he or she begins to experience from the medication. Patients achieve ~70% of the maximum effects within 2 weeks of treatment initiation (18,19). Optimal relief of OAB symptoms is achieved after 8 weeks of treatment (6,18,20). Clinical response is sustained for at least a year in patients who are compliant and continue to take the medication (8).

A.   Tolerability of Tolterodine over Immediate-Release Oxybutynin

The tolerability of tolterodine over immediate-release oxybutynin has been demonstrated by numerous Phase III clinical trials. Most of these were prospective, randomized, multicenter, placebo-controlled, parallel-group, double-blind studies that directly compared tolterodine to immediate-release oxybutynin and placebo in patients who had urodynamically confirmed and/or clinically significant bladder overactivity (18,21,22). Many of these trials were 12 weeks in duration and virtually identical in study design, a feature that permitted data pooling and meta-analysis to include over 1000 patients, increasing statistical power (23,24).

Phase III randomized trials have consistently demonstrated comparable objective and subjective efficacy between tolterodine and immediate-release oxybutynin. Tolterodine reduced the micturition frequency by 17–21%, reduced urge incontinence episodes by 47%, and increased mean volume per micturition (which is a surrogate measurement of bladder capacity) by 21–27% (18,21). Improvements in voiding diary variables were comparable between patients who were randomized to receive 2 mg BID of tolterodine and those receiving 5 mg TID a day of immediate-release oxybutynin (see Table 1), with the exception that immediate-release oxybutynin appeared to more effective in relieving urge urinary incontinence than tolterodine in one study 71% vs. 47%, respectively (18). These objective improvements in voiding diary parameters were clinically relevant to the patient, as they translated into subjective improvements in the patient's perception of bladder symptoms. When asked to rate their symptoms on an analog scale, 52% of tolterodine patients reported an improvement in symptom scores after 12 weeks of treatment, compared with 50% and 39% of patients taking oxybutynin and placebo, respectively (23).

Despite comparable efficacy at their recommended doses, tolterodine was better tolerated than immediate-release oxybutynin. Dry mouth was still the most common adverse effect (18,21,23). However, with tolterodine, there was a lower incidence of dry mouth, and, as assessed by patients on an analog scale, there was a lower intensity of dry mouth when it occurred. Half as many patients experienced dry mouth in the tolterodine arm (30–50%) as in the oxybutynin group (69–87%). Most patients with dry mouth in the tolterodine arm reported it to be mild, whereas most patients in the immediate-release oxybutynin group reported it as moderate or severe (see Table 1). In studies that permitted dose reduction to prevent drug discontinuation, the frequency and intensity of dry mouth remained higher among patients who reduced their oxybutynin dosage from 5 mg TID to 2.5 mg TID (due to adverse effects), compared with those who remained on the regular dose of tolterodine (2 mg BID) (18).

Fewer patients in the tolterodine arm withdrew from the study (6–8% vs. 17–21% in the oxybutynin arm) or reduced their dosage (7–8% vs. 23–32% in oxybutynin) as a result of adverse effects (18,21,23). The equivalent clinical efficacy and superior tolerability of tolterodine compared to immediate-release oxybutynin translate into higher patient compliance and fewer treatment withdrawals or dosage reductions. Tolterodine overcomes the current limitations of immediate-release oxybutynin and offers a therapeutic advantage in terms of improved tolerability. There are suggestions that tolterodine improves overall quality of life (QOL) as measured by the Medical Outcomes Study 36 (MOS-36) 36-item short-form (SF-36) instrument of OAB patients to a greater extent than oxybutynin or placebo, even though at this time, no disease-specific QOL tool has been developed for patients with OAB (25).

In clinical practice, immediate-release oxybutynin is commonly started at a lower initial dose of 2.5 mg TID and then titrated up to 5 mg TID to achieve a balance between efficacy and

Table 1   Tolterodine (Detrol) Versus Immediate-Release Oxybutynin

Outcome	Study	Tolterodine	Oxybutynin	Placebo	Comments
Frequency of micturition	Abrams et al. (18)	−21%	−19.5%	−10.5%	Tolterodine and immediate-release oxybutynin demonstrated comparable efficacy.
	Drutz et al. (21)	−17%	−17%	−9%	
Number of urge incontinence episodes	Abrams et al.	−47%	−71%	−19%	
	Drutz et al.	−46%	−52%	−27%	
Volume per micturition	Abrams et al.	+27%	+31%	+7%	
	Drutz et al.	+21%	+34%	+8%	
Percent of patients with side effects	Abrams et al.	89%	97%	81%	Tolterodine exhibited tolerability superior to that of immediate-release oxybutynin.
	Drutz et al.	78%	90%	75%	
	Appell et al. (23)	75%	93%	78%	
Percent of patients with dry mouth	Abrams et al.	50%	86%	21%	
	Drutz et al.	30%	69%	15%	
	Appell et al.	40%	78%	40%	
Percent of patients with moderate to severe dry mouth	Abrams et al.	14%	51%	(not reported)	
	Drutz et al.	9%	44%	(not reported)	
	Appell et al.	17%	60%	6%	
Percent of patients who withdrew due to side effects	Abrams et al.	8%	17%	12%	
	Drutz et al.	6%	21%	7%	
	Appell et al.	8%	20%	5%	
Percent of patients who reduced dosage due to side effects	Abrams et al.	8%	32%	2%	
	Drutz et al.	7%	23%	4%	
	Appell et al.	9%	32%	4%	

tolerability (26–28). A study was therefore performed to compare tolterodine with immediate-release oxybutynin using an upward titration protocol (started at 2.5 mg, then increased to 5 mg TID after 2 weeks) in patients >50 years of age to determine whether tolterodine was better tolerated than immediate-release oxybutynin in that clinical scenario. Not surprisingly, despite the upward titration strategy, tolterodine still exhibited comparable efficacy and superior tolerability to those of immediate-release oxybutynin (20).

The long-term tolerability of tolterodine was demonstrated by open-label studies, even though randomized trials that directly compare long-term adverse effects of tolterodine to those of immediate-release oxybutynin are lacking. Only 9% and 15% of tolterodine patients withdrew from open-label studies owing to side effects at 9 months and 12 months, respectively. Another 13% and 23% opted for dose reduction at the end of 9 months and 12 months, respectively (29,30). This is in contrast to immediate-release oxybutynin; only 18% of OAB patients remained on this therapy after 6 months owing to intolerable side effects (2,10). Retrospective analysis of a filled prescription pharmacy database also confirmed that more OAB patients remained on tolterodine therapy than on immediate-release oxybutynin after 6 months of treatment (9). A poor response to oxybutynin in the past does not preclude patients from being able to tolerate long-term treatment with tolterodine. In fact, tolterodine was well tolerated in

89% of patients who had previously found oxybutynin to be unacceptable. There is no evidence that antimuscarinic side effects worsened over time with long-term use (29).

B. Safety

When clinical trials of tolterodine first began, there was concern over the cardiac safety of the medication, since it is closely related to terodiline, a drug that was removed from the market in the 1980s because of concerns over arrhythmias and acute cardiac events. In almost every tolterodine study, patients were very closely monitored and evaluated with respect to EKG changes and potential adverse cardiac events. Other than a slight dose-dependent increase in heart rate (3–12 beats per minute) (15,31,32), and a corresponding shortening in uncorrected QT interval, which one would expect from the antimuscarinic activity of tolterodine, no clinically relevant changes in corrected QT intervals or EKG morphology were apparent (32). No serious adverse cardiac event attributed directly to tolterodine use has been documented in any of more than a few dozen well-conducted clinical trials.

Overall, CNS side effects are rare (19,33). Unlike immediate-release oxybutynin and its major metabolite (N-desethyloxybutynin), which cross the blood-brain barrier and theoretically may cause CNS adverse effects such as somnolence and cognitive impairment (34), tolterodine has lower lipophilicity and therefore probably less penetration into the CNS (35,36), but it must be remembered that tertiary amines all pass through the blood-brain barrier and both oxybutynin and tolterodine are tertiary amines. Although tolterodine caused fewer disturbances on quantitative-topographic EEG than oxybutynin in healthy volunteers (37) and the reported incidence of somnolence in patients treated with immediate-release oxybutynin was 11.9%, in patients on tolterodine, it was 3.0% (38). This must be taken in the context that clinical problems have not been demonstrated in patients on extended-release oxybutynin, which may, again, mean that CNS problems, if any, on oxybutynin may relate to metabolites of oxybutynin and not the parent compound.

Tolterodine has no deleterious effects on blood pressure or on hematologic or biochemical laboratory values during long-term treatment (29). It is safe and well tolerated in the elderly over 65 years of age (20,39). No cardiac arrhythmias were noted in a study that exclusively recruited patients over 65 years of age (39). Although based on limited numbers of subjects, with short follow-ups, another study found that tolterodine (0.1 mg/kg/d in two divided doses) appeared to be safe in pediatric meningomyelocele patients with detrusor hyperreflexia (40).

III. EXTENDED-RELEASE OXYBUTYNIN

An extended-release formulation of oxybutynin (Ditropan XL) was released in 1999 (38). This once-a-day formulation uses a patented oral osmotic (OROS) drug delivery system to slowly release a controlled amount of oxybutynin into the gastrointestinal tract over a 24-h period. Physically, extended-release oxybutynin resembles a conventional tablet, but it consists of two core compartments: a drug layer containing the active ingredient (oxybutynin), and a push layer containing osmotically active compounds. Both are wholly surrounded by a semipermeable membrane with a laser-drilled hole on the drug side. Water in the gastrointestinal tract enters the tablet and mixes with the oxybutynin to form a suspension. Water also enters the push layer through the semipermeable membrane via osmosis. The push layer expands and pushes the suspended drug out of the orifice into the gastrointestinal tract for absorption.

Aside from the convenience of once-daily administration, extended-release oxybutynin eliminates the three times daily peak-to-trough serum concentration fluctuation associated with immediate-release oxybutynin. Such marked variation in oxybutynin level is thought to contribute to the intolerable dose-dependent side effects of the drug. Studies with adult volunteers have shown a smoother peak-to-trough fluctuation of plasma concentration with each dosing of extended-release oxybutynin. Plasma level rises slowly over 4–6 h and remains fairly constant over the 24-h dosing interval (41,42). Steady-state concentration is reached by day 3 of administration. In addition, the peak serum concentration of oxybutynin in the extended-release formulation is 2.5 times lower than that of the conventional formulation (41). Lower peak value and more stable serum concentration are the pharmacokinetic hallmarks of extended-release oxybutynin.

Oxybutynin is metabolized by the cytochrome P_{450} enzyme system in the liver and the small intestinal wall ("first-pass" metabolism). The primary metabolite, N-desethyloxybutynin, is largely responsible for systemic side effects, particularly dry mouth and CNS effects (41–43). There is evidence that although oxybutynin and N-desethyloxybutynin have similar effects on the detrusor, N-desethyloxybutynin is more potent in the salivary glands and causes more severe dry mouth than the parent compound. Immediate-release oxybutynin, like most other oral medications, is absorbed primarily in the small intestine and drains into the portal system. It undergoes extensive first-pass metabolism in the upper gastrointestinal tract, producing high serum levels of N-desethyloxybutynin, which causes intolerable side effects. In contrast, extended-release oxybutynin is protected inside a nondisintegrating OROS capsule. It is released at a steady rate for 24 h, spending only 3–5 h in the upper gastrointestinal tract. Most of it is released in the colon, where first-pass metabolism is much less extensive than in the small bowel (44,45). As a result, first-pass metabolism is proportionally reduced, the serum ratio of N-desethyloxybutynin to oxybutynin is reduced, and less severe dry mouth may be experienced (42). This hypothesis is supported by a pilot study that showed that mean bioavailability was higher for oxybutynin (153%) and lower for N-desethyloxybutynin (69%) in extended-release oxybutynin than with immediate-release oxybutynin (41).

A.   Improved Tolerability over Immediate-Release Oxybutynin

More stable serum concentration together with less first-pass metabolism may explain the improved tolerability of extended-release oxybutynin over immediate-release oxybutynin. Extended-release oxybutynin caused less suppression of saliva output and less severe dry mouth than immediate-release oxybutynin in healthy adult volunteers (41,42). Whereas patients taking extended-release oxybutynin and immediate-release oxybutynin had similar reductions in urge incontinence (83% and 76–87%, respectively) and total incontinence episodes (80–81% and 75–86%, respectively), indicating equivalent clinical efficacy (43,46), the incidence and severity of dry mouth were lower in the extended-release oxybutynin group (see Table 2). Dry mouth of any severity was reported by 68% and 87% of patients in the extended-release oxybutynin and immediate-release oxybutynin groups, respectively ($P = .04$) (43). Moderate or severe dry mouth occurred in 25% and 46%, respectively ($P = .03$). Dry mouth was still the most common side effect of the extended-release formulation (68%), followed by somnolence (38%), constipation (30%), and blurred vision (28%). With the exception of dry mouth, extended-release oxybutynin and immediate-release oxybutynin were comparable in terms of the rates of systemic side effects.

In one open-label study, 7.8% of OAB patients discontinued extended-release oxybutynin at the end of 12 weeks because of adverse effects (47). Notably, neither the comparative (43,46) nor the open-label studies (47) had a placebo arm, so the extent of placebo effects cannot be ascertained. Whether the more favorable side-effect profile of extended-release oxybutynin translates into higher patient compliance and fewer treatment withdrawals or dosage reductions remains to be studied in placebo-controlled trials. For patients whose bladder symptoms have

Table 2 Extended-Release Oxybutynin Versus Immediate-Release Oxybutynin

Outcome	Study	Extended-release oxybutynin	Immediate-release oxybutynin	Comments
Number of urge incontinence episodes	Anderson et al.(43)[a] Versi et al.(46)	−84% −83%	−88% −76%	Extended-release and immediate-release oxybutynin demonstrated equivalent efficacy.
Percent of patients achieving total continence	Anderson et al.	41%	40%	
Percent of patients with side effects	Anderson et al.	87%	94%	Extended-release oxybutynin is better tolerated than immediate-release oxybutynin.
Percent of patients with dry mouth	Anderson et al. Versi et al.	68% 48%	87% 59%	
Percent of patients with moderate to severe dry mouth	Anderson et al. Versi et al.	25% 4% (at 5 mg/d) 9% (at 10 mg/d) 19% (at 15 mg/d) 40% (at 20 mg/d)	46% 7% (at 5 mg/d) 26% (at 10 mg/d) 39% (at 15 mg/d) 45% (at 20 mg/d)	
Percent of patients who withdrew due to side effects	Anderson et al. Versi et al.	15% 3%	13% 6%	

[a]Dosage up to 30 mg/d was allowed in the extended-release randomized arm.

been stabilized on immediate-release oxybutynin, switching to extended-release oxybutynin reduces the side effects without compromising clinical efficacy (48).

Maximum clinical benefit is achieved by week 4 and is sustained through 12 weeks of maintenance therapy. The optimal dosage appears to be between 5 and 15 mg daily. In one trial, 70.8% of participants chose a maintenance dose of 5–15 mg, while 17% used a dose of 25–30 mg daily. Although the latter doses are higher than the maximum recommended dose, only 5.4% of these patients discontinued treatment owing to antimuscarinic side effects (47). Up to 30 mg/d of extended-release oxybutynin has been used safely in controlled studies (43). Extended-release oxybutynin may provide important therapeutic options for motivated patients who require a higher dose to achieve optimal relief of OAB symptoms without experiencing excessive side effects (e.g., neurogenic bladder).

B. Safety and Efficacy in the Elderly

Extended-release oxybutynin appears to be safe in the elderly. In a long-term, open-label, community-based study, there was a very low incidence of CNS side effects, including changes in mental acuity and memory (49). Over 50% of patients in that community-based study were over 65 years of age. The drug demonstrated comparable efficacy across all age groups. In a different open-label study evaluating urge incontinence, nearly equal numbers of patients older and younger than 65 years achieved complete urinary continence (46). In addition, the rates of dry mouth were similar. These results are important, since urge urinary incontinence is not only prevalent among the elderly (affecting 12–38% over age 60)(50) but is also the second leading cause of patient admissions to nursing homes (51).

C. Long-Term Tolerability and Compliance

Historically, only 18–22% of patients remained on long-term (>6 months) treatment with immediate-release oxybutynin (9,10), in contrast to the case with extended-release oxybutynin; 60% of patients remained on the latter drug at 12 months, at doses of 15 mg or less (49). Overall QOL is improved with long-term treatment of extended-release oxybutynin, as sleep disturbance is reduced and incontinence impact questionnaire scores are lowered. Of patients taking extended-release oxybutynin, 80% reported that the medication worked well or very well, and 88% were pleased or extremely pleased with the results. Only 16% of patients discontinued therapy owing to adverse effects over the 12-month study period; the majority of these did so by 3 months.

One prospective, randomized, double-blind, parallel-controlled study directly compared extended-release oxybutynin (10 mg/d) to tolterodine (2 mg BID) (52). Extended-release oxybutynin appeared to be more effective than tolterodine in reducing voiding frequency (26.9% vs. 21.9%), urge incontinence episodes (76.2% vs. 67.6%), and total incontinence episodes (75.2% vs. 65.6%). The incidence of dry mouth (28.1% with extended-release oxybutynin vs. 33.2% with tolterodine), the severity of dry mouth (moderate to severe: 10.2% vs. 10.9%), and rates of treatment discontinuation due to side effects (7.6% vs. 7.8%) showed no statistically significant difference.

IV. EXTENDED-RELEASE TOLTERODINE

An extended-release, once-daily formulation of tolterodine (Detrol LA) is now available (53). It uses a different extended-release technology from the OROS system. It has been found that gastric pH may affect the bioavailability of the drug and that if extended-release tolterodine is taken with antacids, the drug is released too soon, and the effective time of the medication may be shortened and the tolerability reduced (6). In contrast, the drug metabolism and bioavailability of extended-release oxybutynin are not affected by dietary intake of antacids. Pharmacokinetic studies in healthy volunteers suggested that the extended-release formulation of tolterodine has a smoother peak-to-trough concentration profile than immediate-release tolterodine (54).

In the largest placebo-controlled study ever conducted in patients with OAB (more than 1500 patients), extended-release tolterodine (4 mg/d) demonstrated efficacy and tolerability superior to those of immediate-release tolterodine (2 mg BID). Both extended-release and immediate-release tolterodine significantly reduced number of incontinence episodes, voiding frequency, and pad use compared to placebo (55). Notably, the extended-release formulation was reported to be 18% more effective than regular tolterodine in reducing the median number of incontinence episodes ($P < .05$). The physiological explanation for improved efficacy is not clear; the difference may be related to statistical variations induced in the performance of the analysis. For example, when the same statistics are based on the means rather than the median reduction of overactive bladder symptoms, there is no statistical difference between extended-release tolterodine (4 mg/d) and immediate-release tolterodine (2 mg BID).

The most common adverse effect was dry mouth. Aside from this, all other systemic side effects were seen with similar frequency in the treatment groups and the placebo group. In the extended-release arm, 23% of patients experienced dry mouth, of whom 1.8% reported severity that interfered significantly with patient's usual functioning (55). Patients taking extended-release tolterodine had a 23% lower incidence of dry mouth than those taking regular tolterodine ($P < .02$), even though the rates of drug withdrawal (5%) were similar between the two groups at the end of 12 weeks. Extended-release tolterodine was reported to be more effective in reducing urge incontinence and better tolerated than the immediate-release formulation.

Head-to-head comparative studies between extended-release tolterodine and extended-release oxybutynin are under way but have yet to be published. Both extended-release tolterodine and extended-release oxybutynin offer therapeutic advantages over immediate-release forms of these drugs, but it remains uncertain if either drug is better than the other in terms of efficacy, tolerability, and compliance.

V. SURGICAL MANAGEMENT FOR DETRUSOR INSTABILITY

When medical therapy fails, surgical intervention from electrical stimulation done as an office procedure to extensive procedures like augmentation or urinary diversion may be needed. Any surgical intervention should be tailored to the patient with consideration of the degree of his/her discomfort, underlying pathology, general health, and, obviously, the patient's own motivation.

A. Hydrodistension

Hydrodistension for irritative bladder symptoms was introduced in 1930 and was shown to reduce pain, urgency, frequency, and to increase bladder capacity (56,57). The mechanism of action is unclear. It has been suggested that hydrodistension leads to ischemic or mechanical damage to submucosal nerve plexuses and stretch receptors thus leading to attenuation of pain, frequency, and increase in bladder volume (58). This theory has been supported by axonal degeneration seen in animal bladders after hydrodistension (59). Other suggested theories are reduced proliferation rate of urothelial cells, reduced epidermal growth factors, and increased urinary antiproliferative growth factor (59,60). A defect in bladder surface mucin may exist in patients with interstitial cystitis in comparison to controls (61). In vitro and in vivo studies have demonstrated that hydrodistension leads to increased urothelial excretion of substances such as heparin-binding epidermal growth factor and glycoprotein-51 component of bladder surface mucin and decreased excretion of antiproliferative growth factors (62).

Even though hydrodistension is a commonly used procedure, the best regimen and the optimal frequency of treatments are still unknown. Two techniques that are used are the simple hydraulic filling and the Helmstein intravesical balloon hydrodistension (63). In most cases hydrodistension is done under regional or general anesthesia. In the simple hydraulic procedure the bladder is filled with either sterile water or saline at 80 cmH$_2$O until filling stops or until there is leakage around the cystoscope. The bladder is drained after a few minutes. Some physicians drain the bladder and refill it two or three times (62). For the Helmstein intravesical balloon hydrodistension, the patient is under regional anesthesia. A catheter with a pressure transducer is inserted into the bladder and the patient is taken to the recovery room. The intravesical pressure is monitored for 3 h, and whenever the pressure goes below the midsystolic diastolic pressure, more saline is applied to the catheter's balloon. This procedure is especially useful for low-capacity bladders. Most patients will require repeated procedures. The method of treatment and the definitions of response are not standardized, and the therapeutic efficacy of hydrodistension is therefore difficult to evaluate, but the reported success rates range from 18% to 77%. Complications range from 5% to 10% with hematuria, dysuria, urinary retention, and bladder perforation being the most common (62,64–66). The degree and duration of relief that will be obtained in a given patient are unpredictable, but in most cases the procedure offers only a temporary relief.

B. Ingelman-Sundberg Bladder Denervation Technique

Ingelman-Sunderg reported his transvaginal peripheral bladder denervation in 1959 (67). In his preliminary series he studied 32 women with detrusor instability, and reported an 88% success rate and a 70% cure rate. The procedure is considered to be most efficacious for patients with detrusor instability. Patients with neurogenic bladders, poor compliance, and interstitial cystitis gain less from the procedure. The assumption is that the procedure causes partial sensory denervation of the trigonal area. The original procedure required extensive dissection of the cervix and the bladder pedicals bilaterally with dissection of terminal pelvic nerve branches. Since then the procedure has been modified with dissection limited to the bladder neck and the subtrigonal area. Use of transvaginal local anesthesia in order to predict therapeutic outcome has achieved favorable results (68). Transvaginal local anesthesia may be achieved with 5–15 cc of 0.25% bupivacaine injected in the undersurface of the trigone. Resolution of symptoms for several hours indicates that the patient may benefit from the procedure.

The procedure is performed under local or regional anesthesia. The patient is put in lithotomy position, and a Foley catheter is inserted. The subtrigonal area is infiltrated with normal saline, and an inverted U-shaped incision is made over the anterior vaginal wall with the apex slightly proximal to the bladder neck. The vaginal mucosa and the pubocervical fascia are transected off the underlying surface of the bladder. The transection at this level causes partial denervation of the bladder. The vaginal flap is closed, and a vaginal pack is left for a few hours. The operation can be performed in ~15–30 min and may be done in an outpatient setting. Other studies that employed the Ingelman-Sundberg technique showed long-term success rates of 50–72% (69,70). Cespedes et al., selecting patients according to their response to transvaginal local anesthesia, demonstrated a cure rate of 64% (68). Cure was regarded as complete resolution of urge incontinence (UI). About 70% of these women still required some medications after the procedure. In 34% there was only temporary or no response. The most frequent complication after the procedure was urinary retention that was self-limited.

C. Transvesical Phenol Injections

Subtrigonal injections of 6% phenol for the treatment of bladder instability were reported in 1969 (71). Injection of these materials causes neurolysis of terminal pelvic nerve branches as they enter the trigone. Approximately 10–20 cc of the material is injected through a cystoscope in the submucosal level, bilaterally half-way between the bladder neck and each ureteral orifice. The procedure requires either general or regional anesthesia. This treatment modality has yielded mixed results, with some investigators reporting success rates as high as 82–90% (72,73) while others report poor success rates of 14–19% (74–76). Some studies attempted to identify subcategories of patients who were most likely to benefit from this procedure. Blackford et al. reported a success rate of 82% in women over the age of 55 years and <14% in women younger than that (72). In other studies patients with multiple sclerosis appeared to benefit most from this procedure (72,77). To improve patient selection Madjar et al. used a transvaginal bupivacaine injection (0.25%) on the assumption that patients who respond to the local anesthetic will later respond to the subtrigonal phenol injection. In their study 23 of 42 patients (54.7%) responded to the bupivacaine injection. Of all the patients who responded to the phenol injections, 26% had symptomatic relief that lasted >3 months. In most cases relief of symptoms is temporary and lasts from a few weeks to several months. Severe complications, such as vesicovaginal fistulas, excoriation of the vaginal wall, and even the need for urinary diversion, were reported in 25–40% in two series (73,78). However, in these patients the phenol was mixed in a nonaqueous, glycerol solution which retained the phenol in the perivesical fat for a longer period of time. Because of the high complication rate, many physicians consider previous pelvic surgery or pelvic irradiation to be contraindications for this treatment. The high risk for impotence in males is also a relative contraindication for injection.

D. Cystolysis

The theory underlying cystolysis is that adverse effects can be avoided by affecting only the terminal nerve fibers entering the bladder. The technique of cystolysis is to divide the superior vesical vessels and the ascending branches of the inferior vesical vessels in the posterior aspect of the bladder. The dissection is made down to the level of the trigone. Hunner in 1918 described a procedure of freeing the bladder from its surrounding tissue in order to alleviate irritative symptoms. He reported long-term success of 73% in 19 patients who underwent the procedure. These results were not reproduced in other studies that followed. Worth et al. reported that of 10 patients who had cystolysis, three were cured while the other seven had partial or no improvement (79). A 7-year follow-up showed that the three patients who were cured had no further symptoms (80). The procedure has been performed laparoscopically with similar results (81). Albers et al. reported long-term follow-up in 11 patients of whom one was cured, four had a partial response, and seven did not respond at all (82). Because there is disruption of sensory and motor fibers during the procedure, most patients lose some of their detrusor contraction ability, and in the Freiha report all patients augmented their detrusor contraction by straining after the procedure (83). Because of the inconsistent results, cystolysis is rarely employed at this time.

E. Percutaneous Neuromodulation

Electrical stimulation (ES) for the treatment of urinary incontinence has evolved over the past 40 years. In 1963 Caldwell experimented with implantation of an electrode in the periurethral area with the result that 50% of patients were cured or improved of their incontinence (84,85). Since then, various techniques have emerged but the response rate has not changed significantly. Although the mechanism of action of ES has been investigated in animal models, the mechanism of action remains unclear in humans. Several theories have been proposed to explain the effect of ES.

1. More than 100 years ago Griffith demonstrated relaxation of detrusor muscle in response to activation of the pudendal nerve (86). In humans it was shown that sensory input through the pudendal nerve inhibits detrusor activity (87). Thus, pudendal nerve stimulation and enhancement of external sphincter tone may serve to control bladder overactivity and facilitate urine storage.

2. Stimulation of afferent sacral nerves in either the pelvis or lower extremities increases the inhibitory stimuli to the efferent pelvic nerve and reduces detrusor contractility (88). The assumption is that at low bladder volumes there is stimulation of the hypogastric nerve through activation of sympathetic fibers, and at maximal bladder volume direct stimulation of the pudendal nerve nuclei in the spinal cord. Another theory is that there is supraspinal inhibition of the detrusor (89–91).

3. The bladder responds to neural stimulation initially with rapid contraction followed by slow, longer-lasting relaxation. With recurrent, repetitive stimuli there are decay and downregulation of the bladder's response, thus reducing the detrusor's over activity.

F. The Stoller Afferent Nerve Stimulator

The Stoller afferent nerve stimulator (SANS; UroSurge, Coralville, IA) utilizes the peroneal nerve for transcutaneous access to the S3 spinal cord region. Originally, McGuire reported the first study with ES of the posterior tibial nerve on 1983 (92). Of 22 patients with UI, 55% were cured and 32% improved.

Peripheral nerve stimulation is performed by insertion of a 34-gauge needle three fingerbreadths (~4 cm) cephalad to the medial malleolus. The needle is advanced at a 30° angle toward the ankle. A ground electrogram pad is placed on the same side, and the needle is connected to the SANS device, a 9-V AC monopolar generator. Pudendal nerve reflex stimulation at the frequency of 35–40 Hz improves reinnervation and conversion of fast-twitch into slow-twitch fibers. Stimulation of the detrusor muscle by 2–10 Hz leads to reflex inhibition. The SANS device is programmed to utilize both of these effects by generating a stimulus at the frequency of 20 Hz. The stimulation is 0.5–10 mA with a fixed pulse length of 200 μsec. Proper stimulation is recognized by great toe flexion or by fanning or flexion of the other digits.

In most cases the stimulation is applied for 30 min with repeated sessions that vary in different protocols. Klingler et al. (93) with a protocol of treatments four times a week for 12 weeks in a group of 15 patients (11 women, four men) with a mean follow-up of 10.9 months demonstrated reduction in pelvic discomfort in all patients. On the basis of patient complaints of urgency and frequency, 46.7% of patients were defined as cured, 20% as improved, and 33.3% as nonresponders. Urodynamic evidence of bladder instability was eliminated in 76.9%. In all patients maximal capacity of the bladder was increased, and there was an increase in the volume associated with first sensation and first desire to void. There was a statistically significant difference in the daytime and nighttime frequencies before and after the treatment ($P = .002$). Patients with prolonged a history of interstitial cystitis and those with a structural abnormality in the bladder wall did not seem to benefit from the treatment. No side effects or complications were observed except transient hematomas at the puncture site.

Govier et al. (94) used the same SANS device on a group of 53 patients. More than 90% of the patients were women. Needle placement, amperage, stimulus frequency, and stimulus duration were the same as in the previous study. The treatment protocol was for 12 weekly sessions of 30 min duration each. Eighty-nine percent of participants completed the 12-week study. Of the 53 patients, 71% were either cured or improved and were started on a long-term treatment. The patients had on average a 25% reduction in mean daytime and 21% reduction of mean nighttime frequency, with a 35% reduction of average UI events. There was a statistically significant improvement in the QOL and pain measurement indexes. Three adverse events were noted: throbbing pain in the puncture site, right foot pain, and stomach discomfort. During the study one patient was found to have cardiomyopathy, but it was not believed to be related to the percutaneous procedure. The effect of the SANS device lasted after cessation of the initial stimulation session. Proper selection of the stimulation site is very simple, and some suggest that the patients themselves can perform future stimulations. The SANS was approved by the FDA in February 2001.

G.   Sacral Neuromodulation

Sacral nerve stimulation stemmed from research focusing on the effect of the voiding reflex, the influence of sacral nerves on the voiding pattern, and central inhibitory control on micturition (95,96). It is thought that sacral nerve stimulation induces a reflex inhibitory effect on the detrusor through afferent and efferent fibers in the sacral nerves (97). As previously stated the first attempt of neuromodulation through sacral ES was carried out in the 1960s by Caldwell (95). About two decades later the technique has gained popularity for various lower urinary tract dysfunctions, and especially for uninhibited bladder contractions (98–101). All candidates are evaluated for response to sacral nerve stimulation. The goal of the first stage is to identify a percutaneous localization of the sacral nerve, which provides the best neuroanatomical response.

To localize the S3 foramen the sacral area needs to be sterilely prepared and draped. The sciatic notches can be palpated either uni- or bilaterally. The S3 foramen can be found one finger off the midline at the level of the sciatic notch. Local anesthetic is injected into the skin and the subcutaneous fat with a 2-inch 22-gauge needle all the way down to the sacrum. Injection of the local anesthetic to the foramina canal does not cause loss of motor response. Probing the relevant area with a 21-gauge needle identifies the foramen. Once the foramen is identified, the margins of the opening needs to be outlined. The nerve passes at the superior medial aspect of the foramen (97). The response is indicated by flexion of the ipsilateral great toe and contraction of the levator ani muscles. To facilitate the recognition of the stimulatory effect, two electrodes can be positioned in the urethra and the anal canal. These electrodes record excitation of the external urethral sphincter and the pelvic floor, respectively. Later, the electrode is firmly secured and a trial of continuous stimulation is undertaken for a period of 3–7 days. During this time the stimuli are 210 μsec, frequency 10 Hz, and amplitude ranging from 0.5 to 10 V, self-managed and adjusted by the patient. Patients who respond favorably and demonstrate a 50% reduction in their incontinent episodes are candidates for surgical implantation of the stimulator.

A prospective multicenter randomized study was carried out from December 1993 to September 1999 utilizing the InterStim System (Medtronic Inc., Minneapolis, MN) (102). A group of 96 patients (85 females, 11 males) were evaluated with an average follow-up time of 30.8 months. Baseline assessment included (a) medical and urological history, (b) urodynamic testing, and (c) a 3-day voiding diary. Patients' voiding diaries served as the primary outcome measure. Seventeen of the 96 patients did not benefit from the device, and in 11 of them the device was explanted. Twenty-six patients were defined as cured and had no episodes of UI. Thirty-six had a significant improvement. With the average follow-up of 30.8 months, there were a statistically significant reduction of leaking episodes, a decrease in the severity of the leaking episodes, and a decrease in use of diapers or other absorbent pads ($P < .0001$).

Concomitantly, statistically significant effects were an increase in average volume per void, an increase in maximal voided volume, improved urine stream, improved sensation of "emptying" postvoid, decreased number of voids per day, and reduced pelvic discomfort. The majority of patients who had a successful clinical outcome at 6 months demonstrated a sustained beneficial effect later on. Adverse effects were pain at the pulse generator site that in most cases was because of interference with a bony structure or belt line, infection, pain at lead site, and lead migration. Baseline demographic parameters including age and gender were not predictive of clinical outcome. While these results are encouraging, it should be emphasized that ~50% of patients do not respond to the test stimulation. Seventeen percent to 20% of those who initially have a favorable response will proceed with implantation later, but will not benefit from the device, and some of them will require an additional procedure to remove the stimulator. All in all, about one-third of patients will have a long-term response to the treatment.

H. Detrusor Myectomy

Spontaneously formed bladder diverticuli are seen frequently in patients with neurogenic bladders and in patients with long standing bladder outlet obstruction. The observation of this phenomenon led Cartwright and Snow in 1989 to suggest deliberate removal of the detrusor muscle in order to create a wide-mouthed iatrogenic diverticulum (103,104). The goal of the procedure is to increase bladder capacity, reduce bladder storage pressure, attenuate the amplitude of the uninhibited bladder contractions, and thus reduce episodes of urinary urgency, urge incontinence, and frequency. The procedure was termed "autoaugmentation" in contrast to "augmentation," which applied to use of gastrointestinal tissue to augment the bladder. Autoaugmentation was designed to avoid the inherent problems encountered when applying small or large bowel to the genitourinary tract. The procedure is performed under general or regional anesthesia, and the bladder is exposed extraperitoneally after filling by gravity via a transurethral catheter. Indigo Carmine or Methylene Blue mixed with saline may improve the view and aid in defining the dissection level. The peritoneum is displaced cephalad, and $\sim$25% of the detrusor muscle at the bladder's dome is removed by blunt and sharp dissection, exposing the underlying bulging urothelium. Cartwright recommends doing this part of the dissection with a two-channel urodynamic catheter to ensure a 30–50% increase in the bladder's volume under 20–40 cmH$_2$O. Mucosal tears may be repaired by figure of eight 6/0 absorbable sutures. The raised detrusor flaps may be anchored to the psoas muscle, although they are more often than not resected (105–108).

Swami et al. (107) recommended making a small peritoneal incision so that the great omentum may be pulled over and attached to the bladder's anterior wall to prevent inflammatory reaction and fibrosis. In their experience, patients who had an omental flap had less perivesical fibrosis if another intervention was required, whereas patients who had no omental flap were found to have the mucosa firmly adherent to the retropubic area when undergoing a subsequent procedure. Other techniques employ demucosalized, colonic, gastric, and sigmoid tissue to cover the urothelial diverticulum (109–111). Some physicians prefer not to cover the myectomized area, assuming the procedure will reduce overall compliance (106). After the procedure a catheter is left in place for 2–7 days. Before removal of the catheter a cystogram is performed. Cartwright (103) recommends periodically distending the bladder 1 week after the procedure in order to prevent contraction. However, most recent studies have not employed this technique. After removal of the catheter the patient is instructed to do timed voiding, and postvoid residuals are checked. If the patient is unable to void, he or she is instructed to perform clean intermittent catheterization (CIC) q3h during the day and q4h at night. Although satisfactory results have been achieved with laparoscopic autoaugmentation, only a limited number of patients have undergone the procedure (112–114). Autoaugmentation may be appropriate for patients with moderately reduced bladder capacity in need of a bladder augmentation no more than 50% of their original volume. The reported success rates of the procedure reach 80% (105,107,115). Swami et al. (107) reported an overall success rate of 63%, with a 70% success rate for patients with idiopathic instability and a 50% success rate for those with neuropathic instability. These results are inferior to the results obtained by enterocystoplasty; however, the morbidity and complication rates are lower. Leng et al. (108) compared the outcomes of two groups, 32 who had enterocystoplasty and 37 who had detrusor myectomy, and concluded that these two techniques offered comparable results. However, the enterocystoplasty group had a better outcome and needed fewer revisions than the myectomy group. The complications rate in the enterocystoplasty group and the detrusor myectomy group were 20% and 3%, respectively. Leng et al. (108) emphasized that detrusor myectomy had minimal morbidity and did not preclude subsequent bowel augmentation if subsequently required. Complications reported after autoaugmentation are urinary retention and bladder perforation. Urinary retention requiring CIC is observed in <15% of patients with no underlying urological deficit (107). The risk for bladder perforation is higher in patients who are required to perform CIC, especially in the early postoperative period.

I. Enterocystoplasty

The favorite, and still most commonly used technique for increasing bladder capacity and compliance is the enterocystoplasty. Goodwin introduced enterocystoplasty in 1958 (116). The goal of enterocystoplasty is to create a reservoir that will maintain low pressure and thus prevent upper urinary tract deterioration. The low-pressure compliant system buffers the increase in intravesical pressure secondary to uninhibited contractions and ameliorates the sensation of urgency. Comorbidities such as vesicoureteral reflux and bladder outlet incompetence may be treated concomitantly. The augmented bladder should hold sufficient volume to be comfortable for at least 4 h. On the other hand, the augmentation should be to a volume that will enable adequate drainage of the bladder. The augmentation creates a spherical shape, so the bladder's volume is determined by its radius according to the formula $V = 4/3R^3$. This formula can be employed when calculating the additional volume that is needed for augmenting the bladder and the length of bowel that is required (117). Various segments of bowel may be used for enterocystoplasty. Each segment of bowel has its own advantages and disadvantages. No matter which segment of bowel is chosen for the enterocystoplasty, several key points need to be remembered:

1. *The chosen segment of bowel needs to be detubularized.*
2. No nonabsorbable sutures should be applied to the intraluminal surface of the augment.
3. The segment of bowel chosen needs to have a sufficient mesentery to reach the true pelvis and be sewn to the bladder which has been divided either sagitally or transversely (118,119).
4. When the procedure is concluded, a cystostomy tube should be left through the wall of the native bladder and a drain should be left near the anastomotic site.

1. Choice of Bowel Segments

a. Ileum.   When ileum is chosen, a segment 15 cm proximal to the ileocecal valve is isolated. The total segment needs to be 20–40 cm long and may be formed into a U-shaped patch after it is detubularized. If a larger augmentation is needed the patch can be formed into an "S" or W-shaped patch. The configuration of the ileum to the desired shape may be achieved by a running 3-0 absorbable suture or by using absorbable staples. The patch is anastamosed to the bladder with a 3-0 running absorbable suture.

b. Cecum.   Cecocystoplasties have been performed since the early 1950s. In the last decade they were replaced by either ileocystoplasty or ileocecocystoplasty. In ileocecocystoplasty a segment of ileum and cecum of equivalent length are mobilized and transected. After detubularization through the ileocecal valve, the bowel is anastamosed to itself and then as a patch on the bivalved bladder. In the Mainz ileocecocystoplasty a segment of ileum twice the length of the cecum is isolated and anastamosed to itself in a U-shape and later to the cecum to create a bigger patch. If needed, a tubularized segment of ileum may be kept as a chimney serving for reanastomosis of the ureters.

c. Sigmoid.   Sigmoidcystoplasty is employed most often in cases in which the mesentery of the small bowel is too short and makes the anastomosis to the bivalved bladder impossible. A 15 to 20-cm length of sigmoid colon is mobilized and resected. The sigmoid is opened on its antimesenteric side and is formed to either a U-shape or an S-shape. Another technique is to close the two ends of the resected sigmoid and to open the antimesenteric side and then anastomose it to the bivalved bladder (120).

d. Stomach.   Two techniques are available for performing gastrocystoplasty. The first is to use the antrum with the blood supply of the left gastroepiploic artery. The gastric pedicle is passed through a window in the transverse mesocolon and mesentery of the distal ileum. The stomach is reanstomosed by a Billroth I gastroduodenostomy. The second technique is to use the gastric body which is mobilized on either the right or left gastroepiploic vessels. A segment of 10–20 cm of the greater curvature is mobilized and transected in a wedge shape that should not reach the lesser curvature in order to avoid injury to the vagus nerve. Because of the abundance of acid-secreting cells in the stomach, patients who undergo a gastrocystoplasty are more likely to suffer later with dysuria and other irritative symptoms.

In most cases the bowel patch can be anastamosed to a bivalved bladder. In certain instances, when the major complaint is pelvic pain associated with interstitial cystitis, some physicians perform a supratrigonal cystectomy. It has been reported that leaving the trigone results in persistent complaints of pelvic discomfort (121). It should be noted, however, that in some patients, complaints persisted even after complete cystectomy (122). Success rates of enterocystoplasty vary considerably and range from 25% to 95% (118,119,122–127). The wide range reflects the fact in many series a number of the patients who were treated had interstitial cystitis. These patients, as a rule, gained less from the procedure. Another reason for the wide discrepancy is the inconsistency in defining and measuring success. In some of the studies success rates vary considerably depending on the authors' definitions of success and the patients' view of the outcome (126). The complication rate after enterocystoplasty may be considerable. Flood et al. (127) report of 116 patients with early and late complication rates of 22% and 44%, respectively, and found the following:

2. Early Complications

Bowel obstruction—prolonged ileus after entercystoplasty—is infrequent and occurs in ~3% of patients. In other reports in which prolonged ileus was regarded as >5 days, 10% of the patients had prolonged ileus. However, at least some of these patients had some neurologic deficiency (128). The segment of bowel that is used does not impact the duration of the ileus.

Fistula—may occur in ~15% of patients. The most common site for leakage is the anastomotic suture line between the bladder and the augment. Other possible sites may be the suprapubic tube puncture site and the urethra in cases of concomitant sphincteric weakness. In most cases the leakage ceases by itself with proper drainage. Only 1–2% require an additional procedure to obliterate the fistula (127).

Wound infection—as with other clean contaminated procedures, the wound infection rate is 3–5%.

3. Late Complications

Diarrhea and bowel dysfunction may develop in 10–16% of patients after enterocystoplasty. Patients may complain of increased bowel frequency and fecal incontinence. The removal of the ileocecal valve is likely to cause diarrhea and may decrease transit time along the gastrointestinal tract and cause bacterial backflow into the ileum and malabsorbtion of fat, B_{12}, and bile salts (129,130). Because vitamin B_{12} is absorbed exclusively in the ileum, resection of the distal ileum may result in B_{12} deficiency, and subsequent megaloblastic anemia and neurologic impairment. Therefore, the use of the distal 10–20 cm of the ileum should be avoided, if possible. Because body stores of B_{12} are significant, deficiency may not be apparent for as long as 5 years. B_{12} levels should be monitored, and supplements should be given to ileocystoplasty patients if levels decline.

Bladder compliance following augmentation should be monitored because even detubularized segments of colon and ileum may cause peristaltic contractions and raise the bladder pressure to >40 cmH$_2$O (131). Colonic segments are more prone than small bowel to cause significant contractions (132).

Other metabolic alterations may also occur. In patients who undergo enterocystoplasty, acid is reabsorbed from the urine by the intestinal segments, which results in increased chloride and decreased bicarbonate in the serum (133). In patients with normal renal function, frank acidosis does not occur, but a continuous loss of bony buffers may lead to bone demineralization (134). Bicarbonate supplementions may be required. Use of gastric segments may cause hypokalemic hypochloremic metabolic alkalosis but may be the only option for patients with renal deficiency (135). Another unique side effect associated with use of gastric mucosa is the hematuria dysuria syndrome. The syndrome may affect up to 35% of the patients. H_2 blockers and hydrogen ion pump blockers may attenuate such symptoms.

Increased risk of adenocarcinoma in the urinary tract was observed in ureterosigmoido-stomies. The teratogenic compound is thought to be made up of nitrosocompounds that result from the mixture of feces and urine. Nitrosocompounds are also observed in bladder substitutions and bladder augmentations. Another factor that can increase production of nitro-socompounds is the inflammatory reaction at the anastomotic site that produces cellular proliferation and increased formation of free radicals. Tumor development occurs regardless of the segment of bowel utilized (136–138). There is a latency period until bladder neoplasms develop; therefore annual surveillance with cytology and/or cystoscopy should start 5–10 years after formation of the augmentation.

Bladder and kidney calculi formation of bladder stones occurs in 8–50% (137,138). Most stones are struvite and are the result of inadequate bladder drainage, retention of mucus, and infection associated with urea-splitting organisms. Struvite stones have not been noted in gastrocystoplasties. Formation of stones may be decreased by proper bladder emptying, adequate bladder irrigation, and eradication of urea-splitting bacteria. About 6% of the patients form kidney stones as result of reflux of contaminated urine and mucus to the upper collecting system. Bacteriuria is a common phenomenon after bladder augmentation, especially if there is a need for CIC. Treatment of the isolated bacteria should be applied only if the patient is symptomatic or when positive cultures show urea splitting organisms that may predispose the patient to bladder calculi. The incidence of post augmentation UTIs is 4–13% (127,139). The gastrointestinal segment used for augmentation continues to produce mucus, which may impede the bladder's drainage and may be a nidus for stone formation. Colonic segments produce the largest amount of mucus, and gastric segments produce the least. Inflammatory responses to UTI in the augmented bladder increase mucus formation. To prevent mucus buildup, routine bladder irrigation is recommended. Instillation of N-acetylcysteine into the bladder may help dissolve the mucus (140). N-acetylcysteine is not approved for this purpose by the Food and Drug Administration.

Bladder perforations have been reported in numerous studies with an incidence of 3–9% (127,139,141). Some of the perforations were attributed to improper technique or noncompliance with CIC. However, some of the perforations were regarded as "spontaneous" in patients who were not catheterizing at all. Spontaneous perforations may be the result of a chronic inflammatory process in the bladder, intestinal ischemia, or uncontrolled increased intravesical pressure. Any patient with an enterocystoplasty who exhibits signs of peritonitis should be suspected to have a bladder perforation. Urinary retention that necessitates CIC occurs in as many as 50% of patients (123,127,142). The rate of retention correlates with the underlying pathology and the ratio of the bowel's surface area to the entire augmented bladder. All patients need to be informed that they might need to do CIC after the operation and to learn how to perform it prior to the operation.

J. Urinary Diversion

There is almost no indication for performing urinary diversion in patients with OAB, in the absence of a neurogenic cause. In case of unremitting pain such as in IC or irradiated bladders a supratrigonal cystectomy should suffice. Diversion may be justified in a subcategory of patients with "end-stage" bladders combined with severe sphincteric damage or pelvic pain. Description of the various diversion options is beyond the scope of this chapter.

REFERENCES

1. Andersson KE. Current concepts in the treatment of disorders of micturition. Drugs 1988; 35(4):477–494.

2. Yarker YE, Goa KL, Fitton A. Oxybutynin: a review of its pharmacodynamic and pharmacokinetic properties, and its therapeutic use in detrusor instability. Drugs Aging 1995; 6(3):243–262.

3. Ouslander JG, Blaustein J, Conner A, Orzeck S, Yong CL. Pharmacokinetics and clinical effects of oxybutynin in geriatric patients. J Urol 1988; 140(1):47–50.

4. Rovner ES, Wein AJ. Modern pharmacotherapy of urge urinary incontinence in the USA: tolterodine and oxybutynin. BJU Int 2000; 86(suppl 2):44–54.

5. Dmochowski RR, Appell RA. Advancements in pharmacological management of the overactive bladder. Urology 2000; 56(suppl 6A):41–49.

6. Appell RA. Recent clinical studies of new pharmacological agents and their efficacy in the treatment of incontinence. Rev Urol 2001; 3(suppl 1):S15–S18.

7. Chancellor MB. Future trends in the treatment of urinary incontinence. Rev Urol 2001; 3(suppl 1): S27–S34.

8. Chancellor M, Freedman S, Mitcheson HA. Tolterodine, an effective and well tolerated treatment for urge incontinence and other overactive bladder symptoms. Clin Drug Invest 2000; 19:83–91.

9. Lawrence M, Guay DR, Benson SR, Anderson MJ. Immediate-release oxybutynin versus tolterodine in detrusor overactivity: a population analysis. Pharmacotherapy 2000; 20(4):470–475.

10. Kelleher CJ, Cardozo LD, Khullar V, Salvatore S. A new questionnaire to assess the quality of life of urinary incontinent women. Br J Obstet Gynaecol 1997; 104(12):1374–1379.

11. Nilvebrant L, Andersson KE, Gillberg PG, Stahl M, Sparf B. Tolterodine—a new bladder-selective antimuscarinic agent. Eur J Pharmacol 1997; 327(2–3):195–207.

12. Nilvebrant L, Hallen B, Larsson G. Tolterodine—a new bladder selective muscarinic receptor antagonist: preclinical pharmacological and clinical data. Life Sci 1997; 60(13–14):1129–1136.

13. Stahl MM, Eckstrom B, Spraf B, Mattiasson A, Andersson KE. Urodynamic and other effects of tolterodine: a novel antimuscarinic drug for the treatment of detrusor overactivity. Neurol Urodyn 1995; 14(6):647–655.

14. Chancellor MB, Appell RA, Sathyan G, Gupta SK. A comparison of the effects on saliva output of oxybutynin chloride and tolterodine tartrate. Clin Ther 2001; 23(5):735–760.

15. Larsson G, Hallen B, Nilvebrant L. Tolterodine in the treatment of overactive bladder: analysis of the pooled Phase II efficacy and safety data. Urology 1999; 53(5):990–998.

16. Rentzhog L, Stanton SL, Cardozo L, Nelson E, Fall M, Abrams P. Efficacy and safety of tolterodine in patients with detrusor instability: a dose-ranging study. B J Urol 1998; 81(1):42–48.

17. Brynne N, Stahl MMS, Hallen B, Edlund PO, Palmer L, Hoglund P, Gabrielsson J. Pharmacokinetics and pharmacodynamics of tolterodine in man. A new drug for the treatment of urinary bladder overactivity. Int J Clin Pharmacol Ther 1997; 35(7):287–295.

18. Abrams P, Freeman R, Anderstrom C, Mattiasson A. Tolterodine, a new antimuscarinic agent: as effective but better tolerated than oxybutynin in patients with overactive bladder. Br J Urol 1998; 81(6):801–810.

19. Millard R, Tuttle J, Moore K, Susset J, Clark B, Dwyer P, Davis BE. Clinical efficacy and safety of tolterodine compared to placebo in detrusor overactivity. J Urol 1999; 161(5):1551–1555.

20. Malone-Lee J, Shaffu B, Anand C, Powell C. Tolterodine: superior tolerability than and comparable efficacy to oxybutynin in individuals 50 years old or older with overactive bladder: a randomized controlled trial. J Urol 2001; 165(5):1452–1456.

21. Drutz H, Appell RA, Gleason D, Klimberg I, Radomski S. Clinical efficacy and safety of tolterodine compared to oxybutynin and placebo in patients with overactive bladder. Int Urogynecol J Pelvic Floor Dysfunct 1999; 10(5):283–289.

22. Hills CJ, Winter SA, Balfour JA. Tolterodine. Drugs 1998; 55(6):813–820.

23. Appell RA. Clinical efficacy and safety of tolterodine in the treatment of overactive bladder: a pooled analysis. Urology 1997; 50(suppl 6A):90–96.

24. Harvey M-A, Baker K, Wells GA. Tolterodine versus oxybutynin in the treatment of urge urinary incontinence: a meta-analysis. Am J Obstet Gynecol 2001; 185(1):56–61.

25. Ware JE, Sherbourne CD. The MOS 36-item short-form health survey (SF-36): conceptual framework and item selection. Med Care 1992; 30(6):473–483.

26. Moore KH, Hay DM, Imrie AE, Watson A, Goldstein M. Oxybutynin chloride (3 mg) in the treatment of women with idiopathic detrusor instability. Br J Urol 1990; 66(5):479–485.

27. Malone-Lee J, Lubel D, Szonyi G. Lower dose oxybutynin for the unstable bladder. Br Med J 1992; 304(6833):1053.

28. Szonyi G, Collas DM, Ding YY, Malone-Lee JG. Oxybutynin with bladder retraining for detrusor instability in elderly people: a randomized controlled trial. Age Ageing 1995; 24(4):287–291.

29. Appell RA, Abrams A, Drutz HP, Van Kerrebroeck PE, Millard R, Wein A. Treatment of overactive bladder: long-term tolerability and efficacy of tolterodine. World J Urol 2001; 19(2):141–147.

30. Abrams P, Malone-Lee J, Jacquetin B, Wyndaele JJ, Tammela T, Jonas U, Wein A. Twelve-month treatment of overactive bladder: efficacy and tolerability of tolterodine. Drugs Aging 2001:18(7):551–560.

31. Hallen B, Nordgren L, Landelius J. Tolterodine and terodiline—ECG safety profiles [abstract]. Presented at 27th Annual Meeting of the International Continence Society; September 1997; Yokohama, Japan.

32. Van Kerrebroeck PE, Amarenco G, Thuroff JW, Madersbacher HG, Lock MT, Messelink EJ, Soler JM. Dose-ranging study of tolterodine in patients with detrusor hyperreflexia. Neurourol Urodyn 1998; 17(5):499–512.

33. Malavaud B, Bagheri H, Senard JM, Sarramon JP. Visual hallucination at the onset of tolterodine treatment in a patient with a high-level spinal cord injury. BJU Int 1999; 84(9):1109.

34. Katz IR, Sands LP, Bilker W, DiFilippo S, Boyce A, D'Angelo K. Identification of medications that cause cognitive impairment in older people: the case of oxybutynin chloride. J Am Geriatr Soc 1998; 46(1):8–13.

35. Nilvebrant L, Pahlman I, D' Argy R. Tolterodine and its metabolites show very low penetration into the central nervous system [abstract]. Presented at 29th Annual Meeting of the International Continence Society; August 22–26, 1999; Denver, CO.

36. Pahlman I, D' Argy R, Nilvebrant L. Tissue distribution of tolterodine, a muscarinic receptor antagonist, and transfer into fetus and milk in mice. Arzneimittelforschung 2001; 51(2):125–133.

37. Todorova A, Vonderheid-Guth B, Dimpfel W. Effects of tolterodine, trospium chloride, and oxybutynin on the central nervous system. J Clin Pharmacol 2001; 41(6):636–644.

38. Ditropan XL product information. Available at: http://www.ditropanxl.com. Accessed 4/3/2002.

39. Malone-Lee JG, Walsh JB, Mongourd MF. Tolterodine: a safe and effective treatment for older patients with overactive bladder. J Am Geriatr Soc 2001; 49(6):700–705.

40. Goessl C, Sauter T, Michael T, Berge B, Staehler M, Miller K. Efficacy and tolerability of tolterodine in children with detrusor hyperreflexia. Urology 2000; 55(3):414–418.

41. Gupta SK, Sathyan G. Pharmacokinetics of an oral once-a-day controlled release oxybutynin formulation compared with immediate-release oxybutynin. J Clin Pharmacol 1999; 39(3):289–296.

42. Sathyan G, Chancellor MB, Gupta SK. Effect of OROS controlled release delivery on the pharmacokinetics and pharmacodynamics of oxybutynin chloride. Br J Clin Pharmacol 2001; 52(4):409–417.

43. Anderson RU, Mobley D, Blank B, Saltzstein D, Susset J, Brown JS. Once daily controlled versus immediate release oxybutynin chloride for urge urinary incontinence. J Urol 1999; 161(6):1809–1812.

44. Ilett KF, Tee LBG, Reeves PT, Minchin RF. Metabolism of drugs and other xenobiotics in the gut lumen and wall. Pharmacol Ther 1990; 46(1):67–93.

45. Paine MF, Khaighi M, Fisher JM, Shen DD, Kunze KL, Marsh CL, Perkins JD, Thummel KE. Characterization of interintestinal variations in human CYP3A-dependent metabolism. J Pharmacol Exp Ther 1997; 283(3):1552–1562.

46. Versi E, Appell RA, Mobley D, Patton W, Saltzstein D. Dry mouth with conventional and controlled-release oxybutynin in urinary incontinence. Obstet Gynecol 2000; 95(5):718–721.

47. Gleason DM, Susset J, White C, Munoz DR, Sand PK. Evaluation of a new once-daily formulation of oxybutynin in the treatment of urinary urge incontinence. Urology 1999; 54(3):420–423.

48. Birns J, Lukkari E, Malone-Lee JG. A randomized controlled trial comparing the efficacy of controlled release oxybutynin tablets (10 mg once daily) with conventional oxybutynin tablets (5 mg

twice daily) in patients whose symptoms were stabilized on 5 mg twice daily of oxybutynin. BJU Int 2000; 85(7):793–798.

49. Appell RA, Diokno A, Antoci J. One-year, prospective, open-label trial of controlled-release oxybutynin for overactive bladder in a community-based population [abstract]. Neurourol Urodyn 2000; 19:526. Abstract 117.

50. Thomas TM, Plymat KR, Blannun J, Meade TW. Prevalence of urinary incontinence. BMJ 1980; 281(6250):1243–1245.

51. Chamberlain TM, Stephenson DW, Appell RA. Urinary incontinence in the long-term care patient. Consul Pharm 1990; 5:173.

52. Appell RA, Sand P, Domchowski R, Anderson R, Zinner N, Lama D, Roach M, Miklos J, Saltzstein D, Boone T, Staskin DR, Albrecht D. Overactive Bladder: Judging Effective Control and Treatment Study Group. Prospective randomized controlled trial of extended-release oxybutynin chloride and tolterodine tartrate in the treatment of overactive bladder: results of the OBJECT study. Mayo Clin Proc 2001; 76(4):358–363.

53. Detrol LA physician package insert. Available at: http://www.pharmacia.com. Accessed 4/3/2002.

54. Olsson B, Szamosi J. Multiple dose pharmacokinetics of a new once daily extended release tolterodine formulation versus immediate release tolterodine. Clin Pharmacokinet 2001; 40(3):227–235.

55. Van Kerrebroeck P, Kreder K, Jonas U, Zinner N, Wein A; Tolterodine Study Group. Tolterodine once-daily: superior efficacy and tolerability in the treatment of overactive bladder. Urology 2001; 57(3):414–421

56. Bumpus H. Interstitial cystitis: its treatment by overdistention of the bladder. Med Clin North Am 1930, 1495.

57. Hanno PM, Wein AJ. Interstitial cystitis. J Urol 1987; 138: 595–596.

58. Hanno PM, Wein AJ. Conservative therapy of interstitial cystitis. Semin Urol 1991; 9:143–147.

59. Sehn J. The ultrastructural effect of prolonged distension on the neuromuscular apparatus of the bladder (MSc thesis). Oxford: University of Oxford, 1976.

60. Keay S, Zhang C, Marvel R, Chai T. Antiproliferative factor, heparin-binding epidermal growth factor-like growth factor, and epidermal growth factor: sensitive and specific urine markers for interstitial cystitis. Urology 2001; 57:104.

61. Rofeim O, Shupp-Byrne D, Mulholland GS, Moldwin RM. The effects of hydrodistention on bladder surface mucin. Urology 2001; 57:130.

62. Chai TC, Zhang CO, Shoenfelt JL, Johnson HW Jr, Warren JW, Keay S. Bladder stretch alters urinary heparin-binding epidermal growth factor and antiproliferative factor in patients with interstitial cystitis. J Urol 2000; 163:1440–1444.

63. Dunn M, Ramsden PD, Roberts JB, Smith JC, Smith PJ. Interstitial cystitis, treated by prolonged bladder distension. Br J Urol 1977; 49:641–645.

64. Ramsden PD, Smith JC, Dunn M, Ardran GM. Distension therapy for the unstable bladder: later results including an assessment of repeat distensions. Br J Urol 1976; 48:623–629.

65. Jorgensen L, Mortensen SO, Colstrup H, Andersen JT. Bladder distension in the management of detrusor instability. Scand J Urol Nephrol 1985; 19:101–104.

66. Pengelly AW, Stephenson TP, Milroy EJ, Whiteside CG, Turner-Warwick R. Results of prolonged bladder distension as treatment for detrusor instability. Br J Urol 1978; 50:243–245.

67. Ingelman-Sundberg A. Partial denervation of the bladder. A new operation for the treatment of urge incontinence and similar conditions in women. Acta Obstet Gynaecol Scand 1959; 38:487.

68. Cespedes RD, Cross CA, McGuire EJ. Modified Ingelman–Sundberg bladder denervation procedure for intractable urge incontinence. J Urol 1996; 156:1744–1747.

69. Warrell DW. Vaginal denervation of the bladder nerve supply. Urol Int 1977; 32: 114–116.

70. Hodgkinson CP, Drukker BH. Infravesical nerve resection for detrusor dyssynergia. The Ingelman–Sundberg operation. Acta Obstet Gynaecol Scand 1977; 56:401–408.

71. Susset JG, Pinheiro J, Otton P, Brindle F, Bertrand G. Selective phenolization and neurotomy in the treatment of neurogenic bladder dysfunction due to an incomplete central lesion. J Urol Nephrol (Paris) 1969; 75:12(suppl):502 (In French).

72. Blackford HN, Murray K, Stephenson TP, Mundy AR. Results of transvesical infiltration of the pelvic plexuses with phenol in 116 patients. Br J Urol 1984; 56:647–649.

73. Harris RG, Constantinou CE, Stamey TA. Extravesical subtrigonal injection of 50 per cent ethanol for detrusor instability. J Urol 1988; 140:116.

74. Ramsay IN, Clancy S, Hilton P. Subtrigonal phenol injections in the treatment of idiopathic detrusor instability in the female—a long-term urodynamic follow-up, Br J Urol 1992; 69:363–365.

75. McInerney PD, Vanner TF, Matenhelia S, Stephenson TP. Assessment of the long-term results of subtrigonal phenolisation. Br J Urol 1991; 67:586–587.

76. Chapple CR, Hampson SJ, Turner-Warwick RT, Worth PH. Subtrigonal phenol injection. How safe and effective is it?. Br J Urol 1991; 68:483–486.

77. Madjar S, Smith ND, Balzarro M, Appell A. Bupivacaine injections prior to subtrigonal phenolization: preliminary results. Presented at the 22nd Annual Meeting of the Society for Urodynamics and Female Urology, Annaheim, CA, 2001.

78 Bennani S. Evaluation of sub-trigonal injections in the treatment of the hyperactive bladder. Ann Urol 1994; 28:13–19.

79. Worth PH, Turner-Warwick R. The treatment of interstitial cystitis by cystolysis with observations on cystoplasty. Br J Urol 1973; 45:65–71.

80. Worth PH. The treatment of interstitial cystitis by cystolysis with observations on cystoplasty. A review after 7 years. Br J Urol 1980; 52:232.

81. Lucas MG, Thomas DG. Endoscopic bladder transection for detrusor instability. Br J Urol 1987; 59:526–528.

82. Albers DD, Geyer JR. Long-term results of cystolysis (supratrigonal denervation) of the bladder for intractable interstitial cystitis. J Urol 1988; 139:1205–1206.

83. Freiha FS, Stamey TA. Cystolysis: a procedure for the selective denervation of the bladder. J Urol 1980; 123:360–363.

84. Caldwell K. The electrical control of sphincter incompetence. Lancet 1963; ii:174–175.

85. Caldwell KP. The Treatment of Incontinence by Electronic Implants. London: Royal College of Surgeons of England, 1967.

86. Griffiths J. Observation on the urinary bladder and urethra. Part 2. The nerves. Part 3. Physiological. J Anat Physiol 1895; 29/61:254–261.

87. Vodusek DB, Libby J. Detrusor inhibition induced by stimulation of pudendal nerve afferents. Neurourol Urodyn 1986; 5:381–384.

88. Zvara P, Sahi S, Hassouna M. An animal model for the neuromodulation of neurogenic bladder dysfunction. Br J Urol 1988; 82:267–271.

89. Lindstrom S, Fall M, Carlsson CA, Erlandson BE. The neurophysiological basis of bladder inhibition in response to intravaginal electrical stimulation. J Urol 1983; 129:405–410.

90. Fall M, Lindstrom S. Electrical stimulation. A physiologic approach to the treatment of urinary incontinence. Urol Clin North Am 1991; 18:393–407.

91. Janez J, Plevnik S, Suhel P. Urethral and bladder responses to anal electrical stimulation. J Urol 1979; 122:192–194.

92. McGuire EJ, Zhang SC, Horwinski ER, Lytton B. Treatment of motor and sensory detrusor instability by electrical stimulation. J Urol 1983; 129:78–79.

93. Klingler HC, Pycha A, Schmidbauer J, Marberger M. Use of peripheral neuromodulation of the S3 region for treatment of detrusor overactivity: a urodynamic-based study. Urology 2000; 56:766–771.

94. Govier FE, Litwiller S, Nitti V, Kreder KJ Jr, Rosenblatt P. Percutaneous afferent neuromodulation for the refractory overactive bladder: results of a multicenter study. J Urol 2001; 165:1193–1198.

95. Bradley WE, Timm GW, Chou SN. A decade of experience with electronic simulation of the micturition reflex. Urol Int 1971; 26:283–302.

96. Juenemann KP, Lue TF, Schmidt RA, Tanagho EA. Clinical significance of sacral and pudendal nerve anatomy. J Urol 1988; 139:74–80.

97. Schmidt RA, Senn E, Tanagho EA. Functional evaluation of sacral nerve root integrity. Report of a technique. Urology 1990; 35:388–392.

98. Schmidt RA. Treatment of unstable bladder. Urology 1991; 37:28–32.

99. Koldewijn EL, Rosier PF, Meuleman EJ, Koster AM, Debruyne FM, Van Kerrebroeck PE. Predictors of success with neuromodulation in lower urinary tract dysfunction: results of trial stimulation in 100 patients. J Urol 1994; 152:2071–2075.

100. Bosch JL, Groen, J. Sacral (S3) segmental nerve stimulation as a treatment for urge incontinence in patients with detrusor instability: results of chronic electrical stimulation using an implantable neural prosthesis. J Urol 1995; 154:504–507.

101. Chartier-Kastler E, Richard F, Denys P, Perrigot M, Bussel B, Chatelain C. S3 sacral neuromodulation in patients with chronic refractory miction disorders. Presse Med 1997; 26:466–467 (In French).

102. Janknegt RA, Hassouna MM, Siegel SW, Schmidt RA, Gajewski JB, Rivas DA, Elhilali MM, Milam DC, van Kerrebroeck PE, Dijkema HE, Lycklama a Nyeholt AA, Fall M, Jonas U, Catanzaro F, Fowler CJ, Oleson KA. Long-term effectiveness of sacral nerve stimulation for refractory urge incontinence. Eur Urol 2001; 39:101–106.

103. Cartwright PC, Snow BW. Bladder autoaugmentation: partial detrusor excision to augment the bladder without use of bowel. J Urol 1989; 142:1050–1053.

104. Cartwright PC, Snow BW. Bladder autoaugmentation: early clinical experience. J Urol 1989; 142:505–508.

105. Stohrer M, Kramer G, Goepel M, Lochner-Ernst D, Kruse D, Rubben H. Bladder autoaugmentation in adult patients with neurogenic voiding dysfunction. Spinal Cord 1997; 35:456–462.

106. Stohrer M, Goepel M, Kramer G, Lochner-Ernst D, Rubben H. Detrusor myectomy (autoaugmentation) in the treatment of hyper- reflexive low compliance bladder. Urologe A 1999; 38:30–37 (In German).

107. Swami KS, Feneley RC, Hammonds JC, Abrams P. Detrusor myectomy for detrusor overactivity: a minimum 1-year follow-up. Br J Urol 1998; 81:68–72.

108. Leng WW, Blalock HJ, Fredriksson WH, English SF, McGuire EJ. Enterocystoplasty or detrusor myectomy? Comparison of indications and outcomes for bladder augmentation. J Urol 1999; 161:758–763.

109. Dewan PA, Stefanek W. Autoaugmentation gastrocystoplasty: early clinical results. Br J Urol 1994; 74:460–464.

110. Lima SV, Araujo LA, Vilar FO, Kummer CL, Lima EC. Nonsecretory sigmoid cystoplasty: experimental and clinical results. J Urol 1995; 153:651–654.

111. Gonzalez R, Buson H, Reid C, Reinberg Y. Seromuscular colocystoplasty lined with urothelium: experience with 16 patients. Urology 1995; 45:124–129.

112. Ehrlich RM, Gershman A. Laparoscopic seromyotomy (auto-augmentation) for non-neurogenic neurogenic bladder in a child: initial case report. Urology 1993; 42:175–178.

113. McDougall EM, Clayman RV, Figenshau RS, Pearle MS. Laparoscopic retropubic auto-augmentation of the bladder. J Urol 1995; 153:123–126.

114. Siracusano S, Trombetta C, Liguori G, De Giorgi G, D' Aloia G, Di Benedetto P, Belgrano E. Laparoscopic bladder auto-augmentation in an incomplete traumatic spinal cord injury. Spinal Cord 2000; 38:59–61.

115. Kennelly MJ, Gormley EA, McGuire EJ. Early clinical experience with adult bladder auto-augmentation. J Urol 1994; 152:303–306.

116. Goodwin WE, Winter CC. Results of ileocystoplasty. J Urol 1958; 80:461–466.

117. Koff SA. The shape of intestinal segments used for reconstruction. J Urol 1988; 94:201–203.

118. Kockelbergh RC, Tan JB, Bates CP, Bishop MC, Dunn M, Lemberger RJ. Clam enterocystoplasty in general urological practice. Br J Urol 1991; 68:38–41.

119. Kay R, Straffon R. Augmentation cystoplasty. Urol Clin North Am 1986; 13:295–305.

120. Mitchell ME, Rink RC. Urinary diversion and undiversion. Urol Clin North Am 1985; 12:111–122.

121. Christmas TJ, Holmes SA, Hendry WF. Bladder replacement by ileocystoplasty: the final treatment for interstitial cystitis. Br J Urol 1996; 78:69–73.

122. Baskin LS, Tanagho EA. Pelvic pain without pelvic organs. J Urol 1992; 147:683–686.

123. Mundy AR, Stephenson TP. "Clam" ileocystoplasty for the treatment of refractory urge incontinence. Br J Urol 1985; 57:641–646.

124. Goldwasser B, Webster GD. Augmentation and substitution enterocystoplasty. J Urol 1986; 135:215–224.
125. Luangkhot R, Peng BC, Blaivas JG. Ileocecocystoplasty for the management of refractory neurogenic bladder: surgical technique and urodynamic findings. J Urol 1991; 146:1340–1344.
126. Awad SA, Al-Zahrani HM, Gajewski JB, Bourque-Kehoe AA. Long-term results and complications of augmentation ileocystoplasty for idiopathic urge incontinence in women. Br J Urol 1998; 81:569–573.
127. Flood HD, Malhotra SJ, O'Connell HE, Ritchey MJ, Bloom DA, McGuire EJ. Long-term results and complications using augmentation cystoplasty in reconstructive urology. Neurourol Urodyn 1995; 14:297–309.
128. Rink RC, Adams MC. Complications of augmentation in children and comparison of gastrointestinal segments. AUA Update Ser 1995; 14:122–128.
129. King L. Cystoplasty in children. In: King LR, Webster GD, eds. Bladder Reconstruction and Continent Urinary Diversion. 2nd ed. St. Louis: Mosby Year Book, 1991:115–125.
130. Wood GA, Heathcote PS, Nicol DL. Bowel motility after enterocystoplasty. Br J Urol 1998; 81:565–568.
131. Sidi AA, Reinberg Y, Gonzalez R. Influence of intestinal segment and configuration on the outcome of augmentation enterocystoplasty. J Urol 1986; 136:1201–1204.
132. Goldwasser B, Barrett DM, Webster GD, Kramer SA. Cystometric properties of ileum and right colon after bladder augmentation, substitution or replacement. J Urol 1987; 138:1007–1008.
133. Mitchell ME, Piser JA. Intestinocystoplasty and total bladder replacement in children and young adults: followup in 129 cases. J Urol 1987; 138:579–584.
134. Koch MO, McDougal WS, Hall MC, Hill DE, Braren HV, Donofrio MN. Long-term metabolic effects of urinary diversion: a comparison of myelomeningocele patients managed by clean intermittent catheterization and urinary diversion. J Urol 1992; 147:1343–1347.
135. Ganesan GS, Adams MC. Use of stomach for the reconstructionof the lower urinary tract in patientswith compromised renal function. In: American Academy of Pediatrics, Urology Section Meeting, New Orleans, 1991.
136. Filmer RB, Spencer JR. Malignancies in bladder augmentations and intestinal conduits. J Urol 1990; 143:671–678.
137. Golomb J, Klutke CG, Lewin KJ, Goodwin WE, deKernion JB, Raz S. Bladder neoplasms associated with augmentation cystoplasty: report of 2 cases and literature review. J Urol 1989; 142:377–380.
138. Spencer JR, Filmer RB. Malignancy associated with urinary tract reconstruction using enteric segments. Cancer Treat Res 1992; 59:75–87.
139. Hollensbe DW, Rink RC. Comparison of different gastrointestinal segments for bladder augmentation. In: American Urological Association Meeting, Washington DC, 1992.
140. Gillon G, Mundy AR. The dissolution of urinary mucus after cystoplasty. Br J Urol 1989; 63:372–374.
141. Elder JS, Snyder HM, Hulbert WC, Duckett JW. Perforation of the augmented bladder in patients undergoing clean intermittent catheterisation. J Urol 1988; 140:1159–1162.
142. Nurse DE, McCrae P, Stephenson TP, Mundy AR. The problems of substitution cystoplasty. Br J Urol 1988; 61:423–426.

13

Pharmacologic Management of Urinary Incontinence

Alan J. Wein and Eric S. Rovner
University of Pennsylvania, School of Medicine, Philadelphia, Pennsylvania, U.S.A.

I. INTRODUCTION

There are multiple mechanisms, some proven in concept but others more theoretical, through which a pharmacologic effect could facilitate bladder filling/urine storage. These include peripheral and central motor (efferent) and sensory (afferent) sites of action. Clinical uropharmacology of the lower urinary tract is based primarily on an appreciation of the innervation and receptor content of the bladder, the bladder outlet, and their related anatomic structures. The drugs or classes of drugs used for therapy of lower urinary dysfunctions were, in general, developed originally for their actions on other organ systems whose functions are controlled or affected by innervation or drug receptor interaction. The targets of pharmacologic intervention in the bladder body, base, or outlet include specific nerve terminals that alter the release a variety of neurotransmitters, receptors and receptor subtypes, cellular second-messenger systems, and ion channels. Peripheral nerves and ganglia, spinal cord, and supraspinal areas are also sites of action of some agents to be discussed.

Despite disagreements on various details of neurophysiology, neuropharmacology, and neuromorphology, all "experts" undoubtedly would agree that, for the purposes of explanation and teaching, normal bladder filling and urine storage can be categorized as requiring the following: (a) accommodation of increasing volumes of urine at a low intravesical pressure and with appropriate sensation; (b) a bladder outlet that is closed at rest and remains so during increases in intraabdominal pressure; and (c) absence of involuntary bladder contractions. All types of therapy for storage disorders, regardless of whether the etiology is neurogenic or nonneurogenic, can be classified within a functional scheme derived from this simple concept. Using this classification, this presentation will summarize current thought regarding the efficacy of various types of drug therapy for incontinence in the female, borrowing liberally from similar prior presentations (1–8). As an apology to others in the field whose works are not specifically cited, it should be noted that references have generally been chosen because of their informational or review content and not because of originality or initial publication on a particular subject.

215

II. UROSELECTIVITY

Because autonomic innervation and receptor content are ubiquitous throughout the human body's organ systems, there are no agents in clinical use that are purely selective for action on the lower urinary tract. Thus, the majority of side effects attributed to drugs facilitating bladder storage or emptying are the collateral effects on organ systems that share some of the same neurophysiologic or neuropharmacologic characteristics as the lower urinary tract. In general, drug therapy for all lower urinary tract dysfunction is hindered by a lack of uroselectivity (9). This concept describes a lack of selectivity of a drug for the lower urinary tract and is responsible for a given agent's systemic side effects. Many of the drugs described in this chapter are highly effective agents in treating voiding dysfunction provided that the drug is administered in sufficient quantity. However, dose dependent systemic adverse effects can often limit the physician's ability to maximally exploit a given drug's therapeutic effects. Escalating dosages often lead to increasing collateral effects on other organ systems. This often impairs reaching the optimal dosage of the agent with resultant implications for an individual patient's quality of life. Nevertheless, improvements in uroselectivity can be approached in a number of ways: receptor selectivity; organ selectivity; and alterations in drug delivery, metabolism, and distribution. Receptor selectivity may be of little use unless the receptor is not expressed or operative in other organs or pathways or unless a receptor subtype exists that is specific for the organ being treated or its neurologic connections. Organ specificity, however, is indeed the Holy Grail of drug therapy. The ideal organ-selective drug for the lower urinary tract would exert its desirable effects only on the bladder and/or urethra, thus eliminating collateral effects elsewhere in the body. Theoretically, the concept of organ specificity is very attractive but practically and clinically it is very difficult to achieve. Alternate drug delivery systems may be helpful by increasing the target concentration of an agent (intravesical therapy, e.g.) or by changing the metabolism of a drug to lower the concentration of a metabolite particularly productive of side effects. Certain drugs or their metabolites may be prevented from gaining access to a potentially troublesome site of activity (through the blood brain barrier, e.g.) either by virtue of their innate characteristics or by alteration. Given our current state of imperfection in this area, it is important to distinguish potential laboratory from real clinical effects, both beneficial and adverse, and it would be especially useful to construct a "therapeutic index" for each agent in clinical use, one that integrates its therapeutic and undesirable effects and requirements.

III. THERAPY TO DECREASE DETRUSOR CONTRACTILITY OR INCREASE BLADDER CAPACITY

A. Relatively Pure Anticholinergic Agents

Most of the neurohumoral stimulus for physiologic bladder contraction is from acetylcholine (ACh)-induced stimulation of postganglionic parasympathetic muscarinic cholinergic receptor sites on bladder smooth muscle. Atropine and atropinelike agents inhibit normal and involuntary bladder contractions (IVC) of any etiology (10,11). Generally, volume to the first IVC increases, the amplitude of the IVC decreases, and the total bladder capacity increases (12). However, although the volume and pressure thresholds at which IVC is elicited may increase, the "warning time" (the time between the perception that an IVC is about to occur and its occurrence) and the ability to suppress the IVC do not increase. Therefore, to optimally suppress urgency and incontinence, pharmacologic therapy must be combined with behavioral modification. Anticholinergic agents do not significantly alter bladder compliance in normal individuals or in those with detrusor overactivity in whom the initial slope of the filling curve on cystometry is normal prior to the IVC (5). The effect of pure antimuscarinics in patients who exhibit only decreased compliance has not been well studied.

Andersson points out that, while it is widely accepted that there is no sacral parasympathetic outflow to the bladder during filling, antimuscarinic drugs increase and anticholinesterase inhibitors decrease bladder capacity (13). Antimuscarinic drugs seem to affect the sensation of urgency during filling, suggesting ongoing ACh-mediated stimulation of detrusor tone. If this is the case, agents that inhibit ACh release or activity should contribute to bladder relaxation or maintenance of low bladder tone during filling, with a consequent decrease in filling and storage symptomatology unrelated to the occurrence of an IVC. Outlet resistance does not seem to be clinically affected by anticholinergic agents.

The designations M_1 through M_5 are used to describe the pharmacologic and molecular subtypes of muscarinic ACh receptors (14). Human urinary bladder smooth muscle contains a mixed population of M_2 and M_3 subtypes, with a predominance of M_2 receptors (80% of the total muscarinic receptor population) (15). While the minor population of M_3 receptors is believed to be primarily responsible for mediating bladder contraction, experimental evidence suggests that M_2 receptors are also involved in bladder contractility in some species and in certain types of LUT dysfunction (7,15–17). As alluded to earlier, the clinical utility of available antimuscarinic agents is limited by a lack of selectivity that is responsible for the classic peripheral anticholinergic side effects. Although M_3-selective agents have the potential to eliminate some of these side effects, the M_3 receptors in lower urinary tract tissues appear identical to those elsewhere in the body (14). There may, however, be some heterogeneity among M_3 receptors, prompting many pharmaceutical companies to search for the "ideal" antimuscarinic that would be relatively specific for the muscarinic receptors that regulate bladder contractility.

The potential side effects of all antimuscarinic agents include inhibition of salivary secretions, blockade of the sphincter muscles of the iris and the ciliary muscle of the lens to cholinergic stimulation, tachycardia, drowsiness, cognitive dysfunction, inhibition of gut motility, and inhibition of sweat gland activity. Agents that possess ganglionic blocking activity may also cause orthostatic hypotension and erectile dysfunction at the high doses generally required for manifestation of nicotinic activity. In general, antimuscarinic agents are contraindicated in patients with narrow-angle glaucoma and should be used with caution in patients with significant bladder outlet obstruction. Detailed efficacy and tolerability data for several antimuscarinics are reviewed below.

1. Atropine sulfate (DL-hyoscyamine)

This agent is rarely used to treat OAB because of its adverse systemic effects (7). The pharmacologically active portion of the racemic mixture of atropine is L-hyoscyamine. This agent and hyoscyamine sulfate are reported to produce anticholinergic actions and side effects similar to other belladonna alkaloids. Hyoscyamine sulfate is also available in a sublingual formulation. The formulation offers a theoretical advantage, but controlled studies of its effects on bladder hyperactivity are lacking (7).

2. Propantheline Bromide

This is a nonselective antimuscarinic that, as a quaternary ammonium compound, has a low and varying biological availability (11). The usual adult dose is 15–30 mg every 4–6 h, but often titration is necessary and higher doses are required. Few evaluable data on the drug's effectiveness in treating bladder overactivity are available. The Agency for Health Care Policy and Research (AHCPR) Urinary Incontinence Guideline Panel reviewed five randomized controlled trials (RCTs) of propantheline (18). Of the total number of patients enrolled, 82%

were female. Reports of cure ranged from 0% to 5% (all figures refer to percent effect on drug minus percent effect on placebo), reductions in urge incontinence ranged from 0% to 53%, side effects ranged from 0% to 50%, and dropouts ranged from 0% to 9%. Controlled randomized trials were also reviewed by Thüroff et al. (19) who reported a positive but variable response.

3. Tolterodine Tartrate

This agent was developed specifically for treatment of overactive bladder. It is not receptor specific, but it and its primary metabolite have selectivity for the bladder over salivary gland selectivity in some experimental models (20,21). Clinically it seems to have a favorable side effect-profile not only with respect to dry mouth but with bowel and CNS effects as well (15).

A number of clinical trials have evaluated the efficacy and tolerability of tolterodine. Stahl and colleagues first studied the effect of a single 6.4-mg dose on bladder and salivary function and found that its inhibitory effect on bladder function persisted up to 5 h (22). Stimulated salivation, however, was inhibited only near the time of peak serum levels. At 5 h after administration, the effects on the bladder were maintained, but no significant effects on salivation were detected. Appell reported on a pooled analysis of 1120 patients in whom tolterodine (1 or 2 mg BID) was compared with immediate release oxybutynin (5 mg 3 TID) or placebo (23). Compared with placebo, both active drugs significantly decreased the number of incontinent episodes and micturitions occurring in 24 h and increased the volume voided per micturition. Mean episodes of urge urinary incontinence decreased from 40% to 60% compared to baseline, and frequency of urination decreased by ~20%. The 2-mg dose of tolterodine and the 5 mg (TID) dose of oxybutynin were equally efficacious, but tolerance was significantly better with tolterodine when adverse events such as dry mouth (frequency and intensity), dose reductions, and patient withdrawals were considered.

Chancellor and associates conducted a large double-blind study comparing tolterodine (2 mg BID) with placebo (24). Tolterodine reduced urge incontinence episodes and also produced significant reductions in micturition frequency and pad use compared with placebo. Of tolterodine treated patients, 2% reported severe dry mouth and 10% reported moderate dry mouth compared with 0% and 2%, respectively, of placebo patients. Mild dry mouth was reported by 18% of drug-treated patients and by 6% of placebo-treated patients. Constipation was reported by 7% of tolterodine recipients and 4% of placebo recipients. The profile and frequency of other adverse events in the two treatment groups were similar. CNS adverse events were not significantly different between the tolterodine and placebo groups. Several other studies have reported similar findings with respect to tolterodine's efficacy and tolerability (25,26).

Tolterodine is now available in a once-daily formulation. The approval of this formulation was based on a large-scale trial that compared the effects of this agent with placebo and the twice-daily formulation (27). In this study, the median number of urge incontinence episodes in patients receiving the once-daily formulation, the twice-daily formulation, and placebo were reduced by 71%, 60%, and 33% respectively. Both preparations were statistically superior to placebo, and the once-daily was statistically more effective than the twice-daily using this outcome indicator. Statistically significant improvement in all other micturition diary variables was recorded for both formulations over placebo. The incidence of dry mouth was 23% for once-daily tolterodine, 30% for twice-daily tolterodine, and 8% for placebo.

4. Trospium Chloride

This is a quaternary ammonium non-receptor-selective antimuscarinic with low biologic availability (19) and with minimal CNS penetration (28). In one study, trospium was as effective as oxybutynin in patients with hyperreflexia due to spinal cord injury, but had fewer adverse effects (29). Summarized data from published and unpublished RCTs showed an average of 43% (range 33–54%) of 113 patients reported systemic anticholinergic side effects, described as "generally mild" (29). This agent is currently undergoing trials in the United States.

5. Darifenacin

Darifenacin is a highly selective M_3 receptor antagonist with selectivity in some animal models for the urinary bladder over the salivary gland (30), but the clinical importance of this finding has not been established (7). In a small placebo-controlled study, published only in abstract form, a single 10-mg dose showed improvement in urodynamic parameters in patients with overactive bladder, although significant reductions in salivary flow were also apparent (31). No effects on salivation occurred at a dose of 2.5 mg, but this dose was no more effective than placebo as measured by urodynamic parameters. In a randomized, double-blind trial of 25 patients with detrusor instability, the effects of darifenacin 15 mg and 30 mg OD and oxybutynin 5 mg TID on ambulatory urodynamic monitoring and salivary flow were compared (32). The two drugs had similar urodynamic efficacy, but oxybutynin reduced salivary flow significantly more than darifenacin. Darifenacin is currently in Phase III evaluation in the United States and elsewhere.

B. Anticholinergic Agents with "Mixed" Actions

In addition to their antimuscarinic properties, this group of drugs induce multiple in vitro actions, including an independent "musculotropic" or "antispasmodic" action directly on smooth muscle. This effect occurs at a site that is metabolically distal to the cholinergic or other contractile receptor mechanism and is possibly related to calcium channel blockade. These drugs may also possess some local anesthetic properties, which, like the direct musculotropic relaxant effects, may only be relevant when given intravesically. When administered orally, the clinical relevance of these actions as compared to their well-recognized antimuscarinic properties is unclear, as these other effects only become apparent at much higher concentrations than their antimuscarinic actions (11,15). Thus their clinical effects when administered orally, likely occur solely through muscarinic blockade. If, however, any of these agents exerted a clinically significant direct inhibitory effect independent of their antimuscarinic action, there would be a therapeutic rationale for combination therapy with a relatively pure anticholinergic agent.

1. Oxybutynin Chloride

This agent is a potent muscarinic receptor antagonist, with some degree of selectivity for M_3 and M_1 receptors. In human tissues, it has a higher affinity for muscarinic receptors in the parotid gland than it does for those in the bladder (15).

Oxybutynin was originally developed to treat gastrointestinal hypermotility disorders. In vitro, its direct, smooth muscle relaxant effects are 500 times weaker than its antimuscarinic effects (11). This agent is a well-absorbed tertiary amine that undergoes an extensive first-pass (liver) metabolism (19). The pharmacologic properties of its active metabolite (N-desethyl oxybutynin) are similar to those of the parent compound, but the active metabolite occurs at concentrations six times higher. The major metabolite is also thought to cause the majority of adverse effects seen with this agent. Reducing the extent of first-pass metabolism by intravesical administration, GI absorption outside the portal system, transdermal, or rectal administration are potential avenues to improve tolerability.

Initial reports documented the agent's success in depressing detrusor overactivity in patients with neurogenic bladder dysfunction; subsequent reports have documented its success in inhibiting other types of bladder hyperactivity as well (10). Oxybutynin's side effects are antimuscarinic and are dose related. An additional theoretical consideration is its physiochemical composition that might permit relatively greater penetration into the CNS through the blood-brain barrier. This may account for some of the reports of adverse CNS effects seen with this agent, especially in the geriatric population (33,34). The recommended oral adult dose of the immediate release formulation is 5 mg three or four times daily.

The AHCPR Urinary Incontinence Guideline Panel reviewed six randomized clinical trials (RCTs); 90% of the patients were female (18). Reports of cure ranged from 28% to 44%, reductions in urge incontinence from 9% to 56%, side effects from 2% to 66%, and dropouts from 3% to 45%. In a review of 15 RCTs of 476 patients treated with oxybutynin, Thüroff et al. (19) reported a mean decrease in incontinence of 52% and a mean reduction in frequency of micturitions for 24 hours of 33%. The overall "subjective improvement" rate was 74% (range 61–100%). Side effects were reported by a mean of 70% (range 17–93%) of patients.

Once-daily formulations of oxybutynin have been developed. Oxybutynin ER or XL uses an innovative osmotic drug delivery system to release the drug at a controlled rate over 24 h. This formulation overcomes the marked peak-to-trough fluctuations in plasma levels of both the drug and its major metabolite, which occurs with immediate-release oxybutynin (35). A trend toward a lower incidence of dry mouth with XL was attributed to reduced first pass metabolism and to the maintenance of lower and less-fluctuating plasma levels of drugs. Clinical trials on XL have concentrated primarily on comparing this drug with immediate-release oxybutynin. Anderson et al. reported on a multicenter, randomized, double-blind study on 105 patients with urge incontinence, or mixed incontinence with a clinically significant urge component. All had been prior positive responders to IR oxybutynin (36). Urge urinary incontinence episodes were the primary efficacy parameter. The number of weekly urge incontinence episodes decreased from 27.4 to 4.8 after XL and from 23.4 to 3.1 after IR oxybutynin, and total incontinence episodes decreased from a mean of 29.3 to 6 and from 26.3 to 3.8, respectively. Since only patients who had previously responded to treatment with oxybutynin were selected for treatment, these figures are not likely representative of what can be expected in clinical practice in an untreated, naive patient population. Dry mouth of any severity was reported by 68% and 87% of the controlled and immediate-release groups, respectively, and moderate or severe dry mouth occurred in 25% and 46%, respectively. Curiously, as voiding frequency was measured in both groups, a statistically greater percent increase was seen in the XL patients (54%) than in the IR patients (17%). The reason for the increase in urinary frequency seen in this study is unclear and is at odds with nearly all other antimuscarinic studies in which urinary frequency was measured as an outcome parameter. Another controlled study comparing efficacy and safety of controlled-release oxybutynin with conventional immediate-release oxybutynin included 226 patients with urge incontinence (37). They were known to respond to anticholinergic therapy and had seven or more urge incontinence episodes per week. Reductions in urge urinary incontinence episodes from baseline to the end of treatment were 18.6 to 2.9 per week (83% mean decrease) and 19.8 to 4.4 per week (76% mean decrease) in the XL and IR oxybutynin groups (difference nonsignificant), respectively. The incidence of dry mouth increased with dose in both groups, but there was no statistically significant difference in dry mouth rates between the groups: 47.7% and 59.1% for the XL and IR, respectively. However, a significantly lower proportion of patients taking XL had moderate to severe dry mouth or any dry mouth compared with those taking IR oxybutynin.

Other administration forms of oxybutynin have been introduced. Rectal administration (38,39) was reported to have fewer adverse effects than the conventional tablets, as was a transdermal preparation (40). Intravesical administration has also been successful in reducing systemic adverse effects while maintaining clinical improvement (41,42).

2. Comparing Oxybutynin and Tolterodine

A comparison of the efficacy and tolerability profiles of the two once-daily preparations would be of interest. To date, however, there have been no reported head-to-head studies, and inferences from existing studies are complicated by differences in enrolled patient populations and methodologies. Both tolterodine IR and oxybutynin XL have been compared to oxybutynin IR. Oxybutynin XL was shown to have equivalent efficacy to IR. Tolterodine IR and oxybutynin IR have also demonstrated equivalent efficacy. Tolterodine LA has not yet been directly compared to any of the oxybutynin formulations in a clinical study, but has been shown to be 18% more effective than tolterodine IR using median episodes of urge incontinence as an outcome indicator (27).

One study has been completed that compared oxybutynin XL with tolterodine IR (43). Of 378 patients enrolled, 332 completed the 12-week study. Compared to baseline, weekly urge incontinence episodes per week were reduced (25.6 to 6.1 vs. 24.1 to 7.8, oxybutynin XL and tolterodine IR groups, respectively) as was urinary frequency (91.8 to 67.1 vs. 91.6 to 71.5 episodes per week). Although there was a statistically significant difference between the two drugs favoring oxybutynin in both of these outcome parameters, the overall clinical significance of these differences (e.g., a difference of 1.7 urge incontinent episodes per week) is unclear. Furthermore, like other oxybutynin XL controlled studies (36,37,43,44), there are some potential issues regarding the study design. Results were analyzed on a completer basis, which assesses the response rate in only those patients who completed the study. Secondly, statistical methods employed for analysis of the final data employed parametric analysis when the assumption of a normal distribution was unclear. Notably, however, adverse events including overall dry mouth (28.1% vs. 33.2% for oxybutynin XL vs. tolterodine IR, respectively) and constipation (7% vs. 6.2%, respectively) were not significantly different between the two groups. One small pharmacological study has been conducted which compared once daily tolterodine and oxybutynin (45). A double-blind, randomized, four-way crossover study compared oxybutynin XL 15 and 25 mg versus tolterodine LA 6 mg. XL treatment resulted in a linear dose-dependent increase in bladder capacity and a linear dose-dependent decrease in salivation. By extrapolation, LA 6 mg had the same effect on bladder capacity as a 20-mg dose of XL and the same effect on salivation as a 10-mg dosage.

3. Dicyclomine Hydrochloride

This agent is reported to possess a direct relaxant effect on smooth muscle in addition to an antimuscarinic action. However, it is not widely used to treat OAB. The International Consultation on Incontinence (Committee on Pharmacology) (7) rated this drug as effective based on pharmacologic and physiologic evidence, but clinical evidence from good-quality randomized control trials was lacking (15). The ICI failed to recommend dicyclomine for use.

4. Flavoxate Hydrochloride

This compound was originally thought to be a weak anticholinergic agent but, in addition, to possess a direct inhibitory action. Andersson and colleagues (7) cite references showing it has no anticholinergic effect but does have moderate calcium antagonist activity, local anesthetic properties, and the ability to inhibit phosphodiesterase (15). Overall, favorable clinical effects have been reported in some series of patients with frequency, urgency, and incontinence and in patients with urodynamically documented detrusor hyperreflexia (46). However, Briggs and colleagues reported essentially no effect on neurogenic detrusor overactivity in an elderly population (47). A similar conclusion was reached by Chapple and associates in a double-blind, placebo controlled, crossover study of idiopathic detrusor overactivity (48). Reported side effects are few. The drug failed to achieve a "recommended" assessment by the ICI, which noted that cogent evidence of pharmacologic or physiologic efficacy (or both) was lacking for this agent as well as evidence for its efficacy from good quality randomized controlled trials (48).

C. Potassium Channel Openers

These agents efficiently relax various types of smooth muscle (including detrusor smooth muscle) by increasing potassium efflux, which results in membrane hyperpolarization. This hyperpolarization reduces the probability that ion channels (primarily calcium) involved in membrane depolarization will open, with subsequent relaxation or inhibition of contraction (7,49). Potassium channel openers reduce spontaneous contractions as well as contractions induced by carbachol and electrical stimulation.

Pinacidil and cromakalim, first-generation adenosine triphosphate (ATP)-sensitive potassium channel openers, have been used clinically. Evidence from preliminary trials did not support further efforts to pursue these drugs as treatment for detrusor overactivity (50,51), perhaps because they were found to be up to 200 times more potent as inhibitors of vascular smooth muscle preparations than detrusor muscle (7). However, attempts continue to develop a bladder-selective potassium channel opener.

D. Calcium Antagonists

The role of calcium as a messenger in linking extracellular stimuli to the intracellular environment is well established, including its involvement in excitation-contraction coupling in striated, cardiac, and smooth muscle (7,49,52). The dependence of contractile activity on changes in cytosolic calcium varies from tissue to tissue, as do the characteristics of the calcium channels involved. However, interference with calcium inflow or intracellular release is potentially a very potent mechanism for inducing bladder smooth muscle relaxation. These results have prompted support for the view that combined muscarinic receptor and calcium channel blockade might offer a more effective way to treat bladder overactivity than using either type of agent alone.

Andersson conclude that available information does not currently support the use of oral calcium antagonists as an effective treatment for detrusor overactivity (49). A bladder-specific membrane calcium channel is not known to exist, and no agent blocks intracellular calcium release only in bladder smooth muscle cells. Intravesical therapy could theoretically prove useful, however.

E. Prostaglandin Antagonists

Prostaglandins are ubiquitous compounds that may potentially have a role in excitatory neurotransmission to the bladder, in the development of bladder contractility or tension occurring during filling, in the emptying contractile response of bladder smooth muscle to neural stimulation, and even in the maintenance of urethral tone during the storage phase of micturition, as well as in the release of this tone during the emptying phase (52–54). Multiple mechanisms exist whereby prostaglandin synthesis inhibitors might decrease bladder contractility in response to various stimuli. However, no compelling clinical evidence supports their use in the treatment of detrusor overactivity (52).

F. β-Adrenergic Agonists

Because β-adrenergic receptors are present in human bladder muscle, researchers have attempted to increase bladder capacity with β-adrenergic stimulation. Such stimulation can cause significant increases in the capacity of animal bladders, which contain a moderate density of β-adrenergic receptors (54,55). However, the International Consultation on Incontinence Committee on Pharmacology did not recommend this group of agents because there was no evidence of clinical effectiveness (54).

Recently, a β3-adrenergic receptor was identified and was shown to exist in human detrusor smooth muscle (56,57). The presence of this receptor may explain the β-adrenergic responses of detrusor muscle heretofore labeled atypical. Work is ongoing in this area.

G. α-Adrenergic Antagonists

At first glance, there seems to be no role for α-adrenergic antagonists to decrease detrusor contractility or increase bladder capacity since these have minimal, of any, contractile effects on human detrusor smooth muscle from normal individuals (7). However, the peripheral contribution of such receptors to bladder overactivity can change in neurologic disease or injury and as a result of bladder outlet obstruction or other causes. It is also possible that certain excitatory aspects of the micturition reflex may involve central α1-adrenergic receptors (49).

α-Adrenergic blocking agents have been used to treat bladder and outlet abnormalities in patients with so-called autonomous bladders (58). These include voiding dysfunction resulting from myelodysplasia, sacral spinal cord or infrasacral neural injury, and radical pelvic surgery. Decreased bladder compliance is often a clinical problem in such patients, and this, along with a fixed urethral sphincter tone, results in the paradoxical occurrence of both storage and emptying failure. Norlen summarized the evidence for the success of α-adrenolytic treatment in these patients (58). Most would agree that the success has been moderate at best. Whether the effects on detrusor overactivity are central or peripheral (or both) have yet to be definitively to be definitively settled.

H. Tricyclic Antidepressants

Many clinicians believe that tricyclic antidepressants (particularly imipramine hydrochloride) are useful agents for facilitating urine storage because they decrease bladder contractility and increase outlet resistance (59). These agents have been the subject of numerous pharmacologic investigations to determine the mechanisms of action responsible for their varied effects (60,61). Most data are from attempts to explain the antidepressant properties of these agents and therefore are primarily from CNS tissue. The results, conclusions, and speculations inferred from the data are extremely interesting, but it is unknown whether they have relevance for the lower urinary tract.

All of these agents possess varying degrees of at least three major pharmacologic actions: they have central and peripheral anticholinergic effects at some, but not all, sites; they block the active transport system in the presynaptic nerve ending, which is responsible for the reuptake of the released amine neurotransmitters norepinephrine and serotonin; and they are sedatives, an action that occurs presumably on a central basis, but may be related to antihistaminic properties. Imipramine and doxepin are the most commonly prescribed tricyclics for detrusor overactivity; data on their efficacy and tolerability for this indication are reviewed below.

1. Imipramine

While this agent has prominent systemic anticholinergic effects, it has only A weak anti-muscarinic effect on bladder smooth muscle (62). It does, however, exert a strong direct inhibitory effect—which is neither anticholinergic nor adrenergic—on bladder smooth muscle (63,64). The exact mechanism by which imipramine inhibits bladder activity is unknown. Recently, it has been postulated that these effects may be due to increased serotonin activity (due to reuptake blockade) in the central nervous system. This may involve a direct inhibition of normal excitatory pathways or a depression of afferent ascending neural activity (49,65).

Clinically, imipramine has been shown to be effective in decreasing bladder contractility and in increasing outlet resistance (66,67). The AHCPR combined results for imipramine and doxepin, citing only three randomized clinical trials and an unknown percentage of female patients (18). Percent cures were listed as 31%, percent reduction in urge incontinence as 20–77%, and percent side effects as 0–70%.

Our usual daily adult dosage for voiding dysfunction is 25–75 mg once daily (possible because of the drug's long half-life). We begin with the lowest dose and increase it by 25-mg increments every 7–10 days if necessary, exercising extra caution in the elderly with respect to any dose >50 mg. In our own experience, the effects of imipramine on the lower urinary tract are often additive to those of the atropinelike agents. Consequently, combining imipramine with an antimuscarinic or an antispasmodic is sometimes especially useful for decreasing bladder contractility. When imipramine is used in conjunction with an atropinelike agent, the anticholinergic side effects of the drugs may also be additive. When used in the larger doses employed for antidepressant effect, the most frequent side effects of imipramine are anticholinergic. However, though uncommon, serious other side effects can occur, including CNS effects, postural hypotension, cardiac toxicity, weakness, and fatigue (60,61).

Consultation with the internist or cardiologist is always helpful in questionable situations. Use is definitely contraindicated in patients receiving monamine oxidase inhibitors. All those contemplating the use of imipramine or other tricyclics (doxepin, e.g.) should be thoroughly familiar with the potential side effects and relative precautions.

I. Decreasing Sensory Input

Decreasing afferent input would be an ideal treatment for sensory disorders and for overactivity in a bladder with relatively normal elastic and viscoelastic properties in which the sensory afferents constitute the first limb in an abnormal micturition reflex. Maggi has written extensively about this type of treatment, specifically with reference to the properties of capsaicin (68,69).

Capsaicin

An irritant and algesiogenic compound obtained from hot red peppers, capsaicin has highly selective effects on a subset of mammalian sensory neurons, including polymodal receptors and warm thermoreceptors (70). It activates polymodal nociceptive neurons by opening a cation-selective ion channel, allowing an influx of calcium and sodium ions that depolarize neuronal pain fibers (71,72). This ion channel is known as vanilloid-receptor subtype 1 (VR1). Repeated administration of capsaicin desensitizes and inactivates sensory neurons by several mechanisms. Systemic and topical capsaicin produces a reversible antinociceptive and anti-inflammatory action after an initially undesirable algesic effect. Local or topical application blocks C-fiber conduction and inactivates neuropeptide release from peripheral nerve endings, accounting for local antinociception and reduction of neurogenic inflammation. With local administration (intravesical), the obvious potential advantage of capsaicin is a lack of systemic side effects. The actions are highly specific when the drug is applied locally, the compound affects primarily small-diameter nociceptive afferents, leaving the sensations of touch and pressure unchanged, although heat (not cold) perception may be reduced. Motor fibers are not affected. The effects are reversible, although it is not known whether initial levels of sensitivity are regained.

DeRidder and Baert, in an excellent review article (73), summarized trials to that date as detailed by DeSeze and colleagues (74). Eighty-four percent had "some improvement" in their symptoms. The largest single series had been reported by DeRidder et al. (75); of 49 patients with multiple sclerosis, in 27% results were termed excellent, and in 55%, improved. DeRidder and Baert (73) also cite double blind trials using either placebo or the vehicle (30% ethanol in saline), showing clearly that it is indeed the capsaicin that produces the positive result.

2. Resiniferatoxin (RTX)

This is the principal active ingredient in the drug euphorbium, the air-dried latex of the cactuslike plant *Euphorbia resinifera*, which is chemically related to the phorbol esters (73,76). RTX is likewise a vanilloid, and is, in fact, an ultrapotent (1000X) analog of capsaicin, but with minimal initial excitatory effect. RTX may induce desensitization in concentrations that are so low that no noxious effects are elicited (76). A summary of trials with resiniferatoxin is reported by DeRitter and Baert (73). These trials used concentrations ranging anywhere from 0.01 μmol/L to 1 μmol/L, dissolved in either 10% ethanol or saline. The largest open study comprised 27 patients with multiple sclerosis and involuntary bladder contractions. A concentration of 0.5–1 μmol/L in 10% ethanol was used. Twenty-one of 27 patients responded positively, mean bladder capacity increasing after 1 month from 208 to 467 mL and the mean urine loss for 24 h decreasing from 163 to 23 mL. Further randomized placebo controlled studies are ongoing.

Neither capsaicin nor RTX is approved for clinical use in the United States. However, the intravesical use of such agents has the potential to significantly contribute to the treatment of bladder overactivity in patients with neurogenic and other types of lower urinary tract dysfunction. Theoretically, activities affected by these agents should include only those subserved by small unmyelinated afferent C fibers. A micturition reflex stimulated via myelinated Aδ afferent fibers should not, theoretically, be affected by capsaicinlike agents.

IV. THERAPY TO INCREASE OUTLET RESISTANCE

A. α-Adrenergic Agonists

The bladder neck and proximal urethra contain a preponderance of α_1-receptor sites, which, when stimulated, produce smooth muscle contraction. The static infusion urethral pressure profile is altered by such stimulation, which produces an increase in maximum urethral pressure (MUP) and maximum urethral closure pressure (MUCP). Various orally administered pharmacologic agents are available that produce α-adrenergic stimulation. Generally, outlet resistance is increased to a variable degree by such an action. Potential side effects of all of these agents include blood pressure elevation, anxiety, and insomnia from stimulation of the CNS; headache; tremor; weakness; palpitations; cardiac arrhythmias; and respiratory difficulties. They should be used with caution in patients with hypertension, cardiovascular disease, or hyperthyroidism (5).

B. Ephedrine, Pseudoephedrine

Ephedrine is a noncatecholamine sympathomimetic agent that enhances release of nor-epinephrine from sympathetic neurons and directly stimulates both α- and β-adrenergic receptors. The oral adult dosage is 25–50 mg QID. Some tachyphylaxis develops to its peripheral actions, probably as a result of depletion of norepinephrine stores. Pseudoephedrine, a stereoisomer of ephedrine, is used for similar indications with similar precautions. The adult dosage is 30–60 mg QID, and the 30-mg dose form is available in the United States without prescription (Sudafed, others). Diokno and Taub (77) reported a "good to excellent" result in 27 of 38 patients with sphincteric incontinence treated with ephedrine sulfate. Beneficial effects were most often achieved in those with minimal to moderate wetting, and little benefit was achieved in patients with severe stress incontinence. In past years similar results had been reported in the literature with the use of these agents; however, in retrospect, these results are somewhat inconsistent with current opinion and show the value of accurate objective outcome indicators and double-blind placebo-controlled studies.

C. Phenylpropanolamine (PPA)

PPA has classically been reported to share the pharmacologic properties of ephedrine and be approximately equal in peripheral potency while causing less central stimulation. It is available in 25- and 50-mg tablets and 75-mg time-release capsules and is a component of numerous proprietary mixtures, some marketed for the treatment of nasal and sinus congestion (usually in combination with an H_1 antihistamine) and some marketed as appetite suppressants. Using doses of 50 mg TID, Awad and associates (78) claimed that 11 of 13 females and 6 of 7 males with stress incontinence were significantly improved after 4 weeks of therapy. MUCP increased from a mean of 47 cmH_2O to 72 cmH_2O in patients with an empty bladder and from 43 cmH_2O to 58 cmH_2O in patients with a full bladder. Using a capsule (Ornade) that then contained 50 mg of PPA, 8 mg of chlorpheniramine (an antihistamine), and 2 mg of isopropamide (an antimuscarinic), Stewart and associates (79) reported that, of 77 women with stress urinary incontinence, 18 were completely cured with one sustained release capsule taken BID. Twenty-eight patients were "much better," six were "slightly better," and 25 were no better. In 11 men with postprostatectomy stress incontinence, the numbers in the corresponding categories were 1, 2, 1, and 7. The formulation of Ornade has now been changed, and each capsule of drug contains 75 mg PPA and 12 mg chlorpheniramine.

The AHCPR Guideline (18) reports eight randomized controlled trials with PPA, 50 mg BID, for stress urinary incontinence in females. Percent cures (all figures refer to percent effect on drug minus percent effect on placebo) are listed as 0–14, percent reduction in incontinence as 19–60, and percent side effects and percent dropouts as 5–33 and 0–4.3, respectively.

There are potential complications of PPA, especially hypertension. Most recently the FDA has asked manufacturers to voluntarily stop selling PPA-containing drugs and replace the ingredient with a safer alternative (80). This request, which, it was hinted, may be replaced by a ban, was based on a study reported by Kernan and coworkers (81) in the New England Journal of Medicine. They compared 702 adults younger than 50 years old with subarachnoid or intracerebral hemorrhage to 1376 controls, reporting the risk of hemorrhagic stroke to be 16 times higher in women who had been taking PPA as an appetite suppressant and three times higher in women who had taken the drug for <24 h as a cold remedy. This last finding was not statistically significant. PPA was reported not to be associated with an increased risk of stroke in men. In commenting on this article, Abramowicz and Zuccotti (82) writing in the Medical Letter, noted that no case control studies were available on the safety of phenylephrine, ephedrine, or pseudoephedrine but did relate that case reports have associated ephedra alkaloids with hypertension, stroke, seizures, and death. Their article concluded, "Phenylpropanolamine may not be the only alpha-adrenergic agonist that can cause serious adverse effects when taken systemically in over-the-counter products marketed for nasal congestion or weight loss." Thus, extreme caution must be exercised in choosing patients, especially women, for α-adrenergic agonist therapy. We currently do not recommend this.

D. Imipramine; Duloxetine

The actions of imipramine have already been discussed in the section on inhibiting bladder contractility. On a theoretical basis, an increase in urethral resistance might be expected if indeed an enhanced α-adrenergic effect is produced at this level because of an inhibition of norepinephrine reuptake. Many clinicians have noted improvement in patients who were treated with imipramine primarily for reasons related to bladder hyperactivity, but who had, in addition, some component of sphincteric incontinence. Gilja and coworkers (83) reported a study of 30 women with stress incontinence treated with 75 mg imipramine daily for 4 weeks. Twenty-one women subjectively reported continence. Mean MUCP for the group increased from 34.06 mmHg to 48.23 mmHg. In an open study Lin and colleagues (84) reported that 25 mg imipramine TID for 3 months resulted in a 35% cure rate by pad test in 40 women with stress incontinence. In an additional 25%, there was a 50% or more improvement. Success seemed to correlate with a higher urethral closure pressure.

Duloxetine, a combined serotonin and norepinephrine reuptake inhibitor, under conditions of "bladder irritation," enhances external urethral sphincter activity in the cat through serotonergic and α_1-adrenergic mechanisms, probably at a central level. It also produces a centrally mediated increase in bladder capacity through a serotonergic mechanism (85). Duloxetine is currently undergoing clinical trials in the United States.

E. Summary

Although some clinicians have reported spectacular cure and improvement rates with α-adrenergic agonists and agents that produce an α-adrenergic effect in the outlet of patients with sphincteric urinary incontinence, our own experience coincides with those who report that treatment with such agents often produces satisfactory or some improvement in mild cases, but rarely total dryness in cases of severe or even moderate stress incontinence. Such therapy, when utilized, should always be employed in conjunction with pelvic floor physiotherapy/biofeedback to achieve optimal results.

V. ESTROGENS FOR URINARY INCONTINENCE

In the postmenopausal female, on a statistical basis, the prevalence of lower urinary tract symptoms, including incontinence, and urinary tract infection are increased. Estrogen levels have obviously declined. The question is whether these phenomena are causally related. If so, estrogen supplementation would be a rational therapy for incontinence. The role of estrogen therapy in the treatment of bladder overactivity and stress incontinence has remained controversial. Unfortunately, most reported studies are observational and not randomized, blinded, or controlled. The situation is further complicated by the fact that a number of different types of estrogen have been used with varying doses, routes of administration, and treatment duration—some with progestational agents and some without. Some authorities even seem to advocate opposite positions on this question in different articles. If estrogen has a role in treating LUTS in the postmenopausal female, it is most likely through one or more of the following mechanisms: (a) raising the sensory threshold of the bladder and/or urethra; (b) increasing the α-adrenoceptor sensitivity in urethral smooth muscle; (c) increasing urethral resistance by (b) or by another mechanism; (d) correcting underlying urogenital atrophy.

Both Hextall (86) and Andersson (28) have carefully reviewed the relevant literature on this subject and offered what we feel are valid summaries. Our inferences from their reports regarding the success of estrogen usage in the treatment of various LUTS in the postmenopausal female is as follows: stress incontinence—probably not; urge incontinence—probably not; urgency and frequency—maybe; urinary tract infections—yes, especially with a vaginal preparation.

REFERENCES

1. Wein AJ. Pharmacological agents for the treatment of urinary incontinence due to overactive bladder. Invest Drugs 2001; 10:65–83.
2. Rovner ES, Wein AJ. Pharmacologic treatment for non-BPH induced voiding dysfunction: facilitation of bladder emptying, Part I. AUA Update Series. AUA Update Series 17. Houston, TX: American Urological Association, 1998:258–265.
3. Rovner ES, Wein AJ. Pharmacologic treatment for non-BPH induced voiding dysfunction: facilitation of urine storage, Part II. AUA Update Series. AUA Update Series 17. Houston, TX: American Urological Association, 1998:266–272.
4. Wein AJ, Rovner ES. Pharmacologic management of the overactive bladder. Contem Urol 2001; 6:22–35.
5. Wein AJ. Neuromuscular dysfunction of the lower urinary tract and its management. In: Walsh PC, Retik A, Vaughan ED Jr, eds. Campbell's Urology. Philadelphia: W.B. Saunders, 2002.
6. Wein AJ. Pathophysiology and categorization of voiding dysfunction. In: Walsh PC, Retik A, Vaughan ED Jr, eds. Campbell's Urology. Philadelphia: W.B. Saunders, 2002.
7. Andersson K-E, Appell R, Cardozo L. Pharmacological treatment of urinary incontinence. In: Abrams P, Khoury S, Wein AJ, eds. Incontinence. Plymouth, UK: Heath Publication, 1999:447–486.
8. Andersson K-E, Appell R, Cardozo L. The pharmacological treatment of urinary incontinence. BJU Int 1999; 84:923–947.
9. Andersson K-E. The concept of uroselectivity. Eur Urol 1998; 33:7–11.
10. Andersson K-E. Current concepts in the treatment of disorders of micturition. Drugs 1988; 35:477–494.
11. Andersson K-E. Advances in the pharmacological control of the bladder. Exp Physiol 1999; 84:195–213.
12. Jensen D Jr. Pharmacological studies of the uninhibited neurogenic bladder. II. The influence of cholinergic excitatory and inhibitory drugs on the cystometrogram of neurological patients with normal and uninhibited neurogenic bladder. Acta Neurol Scand 1981; 64:175–195.
13. Andersson K-E. Changes in bladder tone during filling: pharmacological aspsects. Scand J Urol Nephrol 1999; 201:67–72; Discussion 76–99.
14. Caulfield MP, Birdsall NJ. International union of pharmacology XVII. Classification of muscarinic acetylcholine receptors. Pharmacol Rev 1998; 50:279–290.
15. Chapple C. Muscarinic receptor antagonists in the treatment of overactive bladder. Urology 2000; 55(suppl 5A):33–46.
16. Braverman A, Legos J, Young W. M_2 receptors in genitourinary smooth muscle pathology. Life Sci 1999; 64:432.
17. Braverman AS, Ruggieri MR, Pontari MA. The M_2 muscarinic receptor subtype mediates cholinergic bladder contractions in patients with neurogenic bladder dysfunction. J Urol 2001; 165:36.

18. Agency for Health Care Policy and Research: Urinary Incontinence Guideline Panel. Urinary Incontinence in Adults: Clinical Practice Guidelines (AHCPR publication #92-0038). Rockville, MD: Public Health Service, U.S. Department of Health & Human Services, 1992.

19. Thüroff J, Abrams P, Chartier-Kasher E. Medical treatment and medical side effects in urinary incontinence in the elderly. World J Urol 1998; 16:548–561.

20. Nilvebrant L, Sundquist S, Gilberg PG. Tolterodine is not subtype (M_1–M_5) selective but exhibits functional bladder selectivity in vivo. Neurourol Urodyn 1996; 15:310–311.

21. Nilvebrant L, Andersson K-E, Gilberg PG. Tolterodine—a new bladder-selective antimuscarinic agent. Eur J Pharmacol 1997; 327:195–207.

22. Stahl MM, Ekstrom B, Sparf B. Urodynamic and other effects of tolterodine: a novel antimuscarinic drug for the treatment of detrusor overactivity. Neurourol Urodyn 1995; 14:647–655.

23. Appell R. Clinical efficacy and safety of tolterodine in the treatment of ovracrtive bladder: a pooled analysis. Urology 1997; 50:90–99.

24. Chancellor M, Freedman S. Tolterodine, an effective and well tolerated treatment for urge incontinence and other overactive bladder symptoms. Clin Drug Invest 2000; 19:83–91.

25. VanKerrebroeck PH, Serment G, Deker E. Clinical efficacy and safety of tolterodine. Neurourol Urodyn 1997; 16:478–479.

26. Drutz HP, Appell RA, Gleason D. Clinical efficacy and safety of tolterodine compared to oxybutynin and placebo in patients with overactive bladder. Int Urogynecol J Pelvic Floor Dysfunc 1999; 10:283–289.

27. VanKerrebroeck PH, Kreder KJU. Tolterodine—once daily: superior efficacy and tolerability in the treatment of the overactive bladder. Urology 2001; 57:414–421.

28. Andersson K-E, Appell R, Awad S. Pharmacological treatment of urinary incontinence, in Abrams P, Khoury S, Cardozo L. eds. Incontinence. Plymouth, UK: Heath Publications, 2002.

29. Madersbacher H, Stöhrer M, Richter R. Trospium chloride versus oxybutynin: a randomized double blind multicentre trial in the treatment of detrusor hyperreflexia. Br J Urol 1995; 75:452–456.

30. Wallis RM, Napier CM. Muscarinic antagonists in development for disorders of smooth muscle function. Life Sci 1999; 64:395–401.

31. Rosario DJ, Cutinha PR, Chapple CR. The effects of single dose darifenacin on cystometric parameters and salivary flow in patients with urge incontinence secondary to detrusor instability. Eur Urol 1996; 30:240.

32. Mundy, AR, Abrams, P, Chapple, CR. Darifenacin, the first selective M_3 antagonist for overactive bladder: comparison with oxybutynin on ambulatory urodynamic monitoring and salivary flow. International Continence Society, 2001.

33. Katz IR, Sands LP, Bilker W. Identification of medications that cause cognitive impairment in older people: the case of oxybutynin chloride. J Am Geriatric Soc 1998; 46:8–12.

34. Todorova A, Vonderheid-Guth B, Dimpfel W. Effects of tolterodine, trospium chloride, and oxybutynin on the central nervous system. J Clin Pharmacol 2001; 41:636–641.

35. Gupta SK, Sathyan G. Pharmacokinetics of an oral once a day controlled release oxybutynin formulation compared with immediate release oxybutynin. J Clin Pharmacol 1999; 39:289–296.

36. Anderson RU, Mobley D, Blank B. Once daily controlled versus immediate release oxybutynin chloride for urge incontinence. J Urol 1999; 161:1809–1814.

37. Versi E, Appell R, Mobley D. Dry mouth with conventional and controlled-release oxybutynin in urinary incontinence. Obstet Gynecol 2000; 95:18–24.

38. Collas D, Malone-Lee JG. The pharmacokinetic properties of rectal oxybutynin—a possible alternative to intravesical administration. Neurourol Urodyn 1997; 16:346–350.

39. Winkler HA, Sand PK. Treatment of detrusor instability with oxybutynin rectal suppositories. Int Urogynecol J Pelvic Floor Dysfunc 1998; 9:100–104.

40. Davila GW, Daugherty CA, Sanders SW. A short term, multicenter, randomized, double-blind dose titration study of the efficacy and anticholinergic side effects of transdermal compared to immediate release oral oxybutynin treatment of patients with urge urinary incontinence. J Urol 2001; 166:140–145.

41. Brendler CB, Radebaugh LC, Mohler JL. Topical oxybutynin chloride for relaxation of dysfunctional bladders. J Urol 1989; 141:1350–1352.

42. O'Flynn KJ, Thomas DG. Intravesical instillation of oxybutynin hydrochlorixe for detrusor hyperreflexia. Br J Urol 1993; 723:566–570.

43. Appell RA, Sand P, Dmochowski R. Prospective randomized controlled trial of extended release oxybutynin chloride and tolterodine tartrate in the treatment of overactive bladder. Results of the OBJECT study. Mayo Clinic Proc 2001; 76:358–363.

44. Gleason DM, Susset J, White C. Evaluation of a once daily formulation of oxybutynin for the treatment of urinary urge incontinence. Ditropan XL Study Group. Urology 1999; 54:420–423.

45. Chapple C. Tolterodine once daily: selectivity for the bladder over effects on salivation compared to Ditropan XL. J Urol 2001; 165:253–257.

46. Jonas U, Petri E, Kissel J. Effect of flavoxate on uninhibited detrusor muscle. Eur Urol 1979; 5:106–109.

47. Briggs RS, Castleden CM, Asher MJ. The effect of flavoxate on uninhibited detrusor contractions and urinary incontinence in the elderly. J Urol 1980; 123:665–666.

48. Chapple CR, Parkhouse H, Gardener C. Double-blind placebo controlled crossover study of flavoxate in the treatment of idiopathic detrusor instability. Br J Urol 1990; 66:491–494.

49. Andersson K-E. Treatment of overactive bladder: other drug mechanisms. Urology 2000; 55:51–57; Discussion 76–99.

50. Fovaeus M, Andersson K-E, Hedlung H. The action of pinacidil in the isolated human bladder. J Urol 1989; 141:637–640.

51. Nurse DE, Restorick JM, Mundy AR. The effect of cromakalin on the normal and hyperreflexic human detrusor muscle. Br J Urol 1991; 68:27–31.

52. Andersson K-E. Pharmacology of lower urinary tract smooth muscles and penile erectile tissues. Pharmacol Rev 1993; 45:253–308.

53. Andersson K-E. Pathways for relaxation of detrusor smooth muscle. In: Baskin LL, Hayward SW, eds. Advances in Bladder Research. New York: Kluwer Academic/Plenum Publishers, 1999:241–252.

54. Zderic SA, Levin RM, Wein AJ. Voiding function: relevant anatomy, physiology, pharmacology, and molecular aspects. In: Gillenwater J, Grayhack J, Howards S, et al eds. Adult and Pediatric Urology. Chicago: Mosby-Year Book, 1995:1159–1219.

55. Levin RM, Wein AJ. Quantitative analysis of alpha and beta adrenergic receptor densities in the lower urinary tract of the dog and the rabbit. Invest Urol 1979; 17:75–77.

56. Igawa Y, Yamazaki Y, Takeda H. Functional and molecular biological evidence for a possible beta$_3$-adrenoceptor in the human detrusor muscle. Br J Pharmacol 1999; 126:819–825.

57. Takeda M, Obara K, Mizusawa T. Evidence for β_3-adrenoceptor subtypes in relaxation of the human urinary bladder detrusor: analysis by molecular biological and pharmacological methods. J Pharmacol Exp Ther 1999; 288:1367–1373.

58. Norlen L. Influence of the sympathetic nervous system on the lower urinary tract and its clinical implications. Neurourol Urodyn 1982; 1:129–133.

59. Wein AJ. Pharmacology of incontinence. Urol Clin North Am 1995; 22:557–577.

60. Baldessarini RJ. Drugs and the treatment of psychiatric disorders: depression and mania. In: Hardman JG, Limbird LE, Molinoff PB, et al eds. Goodman and Gilman's The Pharmacological Basis of Therapeutics. New York: McGraw-Hill Health Professions Division, 1996:431–461

61. Richelson E. Pharmacology of antidepressants—characteristics of the ideal drug. Mayo Clin Proc 1994; 69:1069–1081.

62. Levin RM, Staskin DR, Wein AJ. Analysis of the anticholinergic and musculotropic effects of desmethylimipramine on the rabbit urinary bladder. Urol Res 1983; 11:259–262.

63. Olubadewo J. The effect of imipramine on rat detrusor muscle contractility. Arch Int Pharmacodyn Ther 1980; 245:84–94.

64. Levin RM, Wein AJ. Comparative effects of five tricyclic compounds on the rabbit uirnary bladder. Neurourol Urodyn 1984; 3:127–135.

65. Espy MJ, Du HJ, Downie JW. Serotonergic modulation of spinal ascending activity and sacral reflex activity evoked by pelvic nerve stimulation in cats. Brain Res. 1998; 798:101–108.

66. Cole AT, Fried FA. Favorable experiences with imipramine in the treatment of neurogenic bladder. J Urol 1972; 107:44–45.

67. Castleden CM, George CF, Renwick AG. Imipramine—a possible alternative to current therapy for urinary incontinence in the elderly. J Urol 1981; 125:318–320.
68. Maggi CA, Barbanti G, Santicioli P. Cystometric evidence that capsaicin sensitive nerves modulate the afferent branch of micturition reflex in humans. J Urol 1989; 142:150–154.
69. Maggi CA. Capsaicin and primary afferent neurons: from basic science to humantherapy? J Auton Nerv Syst 1993; 33:1–14.
70. Dray A. Mechanism of action of capsaicin-like molecules onsensory neurons. Life Sci 1992; 51:1759–1765.
71. Caterina JJ, Schumacher MA, Tominaga M. The capsaicin receptor: a heat-activated ion channel in the pain pathway. Nature 1997; 389:816–824.
72. Caterina MJ, Rosen TA, Tominaga M. A capsaicin-receptor homologue with a high threshold for noxious heat. Nature 1999; 398:436–441.
73. DeRidder D, Baert L. Vanilloids and the overactive bladder. BJU Int 2000; 86:172–180.
74. DeSeze M, Wiart L, Ferriere J. Intravesical instillation of capsaicin in urology: a review of the literature. Eur Urol 1999; 36:267–277.
75. DeRidder D, Chanderamini VA, Dasgupta P. Intravesical capsaicin as a treatment for refractory detrusor hyperreflexia: a dual center study with long term follow up. J Urol 1997; 158:2087–2093.
76. Chancellor MB, DeGroat WC. Intravesical capsaicin and resiniferatoxin therapy: spicing up the ways to treat the overactive bladder. J Urol 1999; 162:3–11.
77. Diokno A, Taub M. Ephedrine in treatment of urinary incontinence. Urology 1975; 5:624–627.
78. Awad S, Downie J, Kirutula J. Alpha adrenergic agents in urinary disorders of the proximal urethra: I. Stress incontinence. Brit J Urol 1978; 50:332–336.
79. Stewart B, Borowsky L, Montague D. Stress incontinence: conservative therapy with sympathomimetic drugs. J Urol 1976; 115:558–562.
80. Neergaard L. An FDA warning on cold and diet drugs. Philadelphia Inquirer Nov. 7, 2000.
81. Kernan WN, Viscoli CM, Brass LM. Phenylpropanolamine and the risk of hemorrhagic stroke. N Engl J Med 2000; 343:1932.
82. Abramowicz M, Zuccotti G. Phenylpropanolamine and other OTC alpha-adrenergic agonists. Med Lett Drugs Ther 2000; 42:113.
83. Gilja I, Radej M, Kovacic M. Conservative treatment of female stress incontinence with imipramine. J Urol 1984; 132:909–914.
84. Lin H-H, Sheu BC, Lo M-Cea. Comparison of treatment outcomes of imipramine for female genuine stress incontinence. Brit J Obstet Gynaecol 1999; 106:1089–1092.
85. Thor KB, Katofiasc MA. Effects of duloxetine, a combined serotonin and norepinephrine reuptake inhibitor, on central neural control of lower urinary tract function in the choralose anesthetized female cat. J Pharmacol Exptl Therap 1995; 274:1024.
86. Hextall A. Oestrogens and lower urinary tract functions. Maturitas 2000; 36:83–87.

14

Behavioral Treatments

Diane K. Newman
University of Pennsylvania Medical Center, Philadelphia, U.S.A

I. INTRODUCTION

Behavior modification is an accepted treatment option for persons with urinary lower urinary tract symptoms (LUTS) which include urinary incontinence (UI) and overactive bladder (OAB), which include urgency, frequency, with or without urge UI and nocturia. These interventions improve symptoms through identification of lifestyle habits and changing a person's behavior, environment or activity that are contributing factors or triggers (1). Interventions such as bladder retraining and pelvic floor muscle rehabilitation attempt to decrease incontinence and OAB symptoms through increasing awareness of the function and coordination of the bladder and pelvic floor muscle so as to gain muscle identification, control, and strength and to decrease bladder overactivity. These interventions are often referred to as behavioral treatments, and involve learning new skills through extensive one-on-one patient instruction on techniques for preventing urine loss, urgency, and other symptoms.

These treatments have a growing body of clinical research. The Agency for Health Care Policy and Research (AHCPR) clinical practice guideline on urinary incontinence in adults recommended these treatments as first line interventions (2,3). AHCPR is now known as the Agency for Healthcare Research and Quality (AHRQ). These guidelines defined behavioral interventions as a group of therapies used to modify stress, urge, or mixed urinary incontinence by changing the person's bladder habits or by teaching new skills. They have been defined to include lifestyle changes (e.g., cessation of smoking, weight reduction, elimination of dietary bladder irritants, adequate fluid intake, bowel regulation, moderation of physical activities, and exercises), toileting programs (e.g., habit training and prompted voiding), bladder training, pelvic floor muscle training or rehabilitation utilizing methods such as biofeedback, vaginal weights, and pelvic muscle electrical stimulation. This chapter outlines the current research as well as clinical practice on the use of behavioral treatment, specifically lifestyle or self-care practices, scheduled toileting programs, bladder training and pelvic muscle rehabilitation. Despite the high level of evidence supporting the effectiveness of behavioral therapy, there are few demonstrations of outcomes obtained when this research is translated into clinical practice. A common complaint of behavioral treatments is that the outcome reflects the combination of these treatments as opposed to a single intervention. More research on clinical effectiveness is needed to encourage health care clinicians, specifically doctors and nurses, to incorporate behavioral therapy instruction into standard treatment care protocols.

II. LIFESTLE CHANGES/BEHAVIOR MODIFICATION

In many instances, lifestyle practices can be the contributing cause of LUTS, especially in women. The following is the current summary of these practices.

A. Smoking

Conditions exist in which increased intra-abdominal pressure may promote the development of UI and urinary urgency, particularly in women. These conditions include pulmonary diseases such as asthma, emphysema, and chronic coughing such as seen in persons who smoke. Smoking increases the risk of developing all forms of UI, and stress UI in particular, depending on the number of cigarettes smoked. There may be several causes of the increased risk of stress UI in smokers. Smokers have stronger, more frequent, and more violent coughing, which may lead to earlier development of anatomic and pressure damage of the urethral sphincteric mechanism and of vaginal supports (4). Violent and frequent, prolonged coughing can increase downward pressure on the pelvic floor, causing repeated stretch injury to the pudendal and pelvic nerves. Smoking is also the most important etiological factor in bladder cancer. There is felt to be antiestrogenic hormonal effects of products found in tobacco products. These effects are felt to affect the production of collagen synthesis. Nicotine has been shown to contribute to large phasic bladder contractions in animal studies through the activation of purinergic receptors and has been postulated to similarly affect the human bladder (5,6). There may also be an association between nicotine and increased detrusor contractions.

Bump and McClish (7) demonstrated that women who previously smoked had a 2.2-fold increase and those who currently smoked have a 2.5-fold increase in stress UI. One case control study of 80 incontinent and 80 continent women established a strong statistical relationship between cigarette smoking and urinary incontinence (8). Nuotio et al. (9) showed a correlation between smoking and urinary urgency in a population based survey of 1059 women and men aged 60–89 years. A large cross-sectional study evaluated multiple risk factors for incontinence, including smoking in women attending antenatal care (10). Smokers were more likely to report incontinence than nonsmokers. The previous research was concentrated in women, but Koskimaki et al. (11) showed an increased risk of LUTS in a survey of 2128 middle-aged and elderly men who smoked currently or formerly. LUTS symptoms included incomplete bladder empting and hesitancy, daily frequency, nocturia, urgency, and urge incontinence. The effects of smoking on LUTS are probably mediated through the development of BPH. In men, tobacco products may increase accumulation of androgens in the prostate gland. The study also found that in men, the risk of LUTS decreased, disappearing 40 years after cessation of smoking. No data have been reported examining whether smoking cessation in women resolves incontinence. However, in clinical practice, women who smoke are educated on the relationship between smoking and UI, and strategies designed to discourage women from smoking are often suggested; however, no evidence supports their effectiveness (12).

B. Obesity

Obesity has been identified as an independent risk factor for the development of stress and mixed UI in women (13–16). Research looking at the relationship between obesity and incontinence used body mass index (BMI). A BMI of ≤ 29 is considered normal or low weight, and a BMI of ≥ 30 a high weight or obese. The stress UI seen in obesity may be secondary to increases in intra-abdominal pressure on the bladder and greater urethral mobility. Also, obesity may impair blood flow or nerve innervation to the bladder. Elia et al. (13) reported on 540 women who responded to a questionnaire of which BMI status was attained. The association between BMI and UI was statistically significant. Mommsen and Foldspang (16) reported on 2589 women in Denmark who responded to a mailed questionnaire. BMI was found to correlate with urge UI in women who reported having one or more episodes of cystitis. It was hypothesized that poor personal hygiene in obese women may lead to an infectious process. Mommsen also found a relationship between stress UI and an increased BMI. Dwyer et al. (17) found women with genuine stress UI or with detrusor instability to have a higher mean BMI than the general population of the same age. Roe and Doll (18) reported on 6139 (53% response rate) respondents to a British postal survey on incontinence status. Significantly more obese respondents have UI than continent respondents. This association was more prevalent in obese women than men. Brown et al. (19) studied 2763 women who completed questionnaires on prevalence and type of incontinence as part of a randomized trial of estrogen hormone therapy. A higher BMI and higher waist-to-hip ratio were found to be predictors of stress UI and also of mixed UI when the major component was stress. This study found that the prevalence of at least weekly stress UI increased by 10% per 5 units BMI. Højberg et al. (10) found that BMI > 30 and smoking were possible risk factors for women attending antenatal care who were 16 at weeks' gestation.

Weight loss is an acceptable treatment option for morbidly obese women. Research has shown that stress UI symptoms decrease in morbidly obese women who undergo extreme weight loss after gastric bypass surgery (20). At this time, there is little information on whether weight loss resolves incontinence in women who are moderately obese. Subak et al. (21,22) showed that improvement in UI was seen when participants lost as little as 5% from baseline weight so weight loss is recommended in clinical practice to all women who have a BMI > 30. Clinicians might suggest self-weight programs such as Weight Watchers or depending on the BMI refer the women to a physician-monitored weight loss program or possibly weight reduction surgery.

C. Dietary Habits

There are components of everyday diet and bodily functions that can "trigger" LUTS which if eliminated through modification can also decrease their effects. These components include amount of fluid intake; the ingestion of certain beverages, foods, and medications; and maintaining normal bowel regulation (23).

1. Fluid Management

Individuals may subscribe to either a restrictive or excessive fluid intake behavior. Adequate fluid intake is needed to eliminate irritants from the bladder. Underhydration may play a role in the development of urinary tract infections (UTIs) and decreases the functional capacity of the bladder (24). Surveys of community-residing elders report self-care practices to include the self-imposed restrictions of fluids, as they fear UI, urinary urgency, and frequency (25,26). Adequate fluid intake is very important for older adults, who already have a decrease in their total body weight and are at increased risk for dehydration.

However, the research showing the relationship of quantity of fluid intake to urinary symptoms is inconclusive. In a geriatric population, there appears to be a strong relationship between evening fluid intake, nocturia, and nocturnal voided volume (27). Nygaard and Linder (28) surveyed teachers and questioned their voiding habits at work, allotted breaks, bladder complaints including UTIs, and incontinence. Teachers who drank less while working to decrease their voiding frequency had a twofold higher risk of UTI than those who did not report self-imposed fluid restriction. There was no association between UTI and either voiding infrequently at work or the mean number of voids at work. Fitzgerald et al. (29) surveyed women who worked for a large academic center. Of the 1113 women surveyed, 21% (n = 232) reported UI at least monthly. Incontinent women were significantly older and had a higher BMI than continent women. One of the strategies women in this study used to avoid urinary symptoms was limiting fluids and avoiding caffeinated beverages.

Wyman et al. (30) reported a positive relationship between fluid intake and severity of UI in women with stress UI over age 55 years. However, in this same study there was no correlation in women with detrusor instability. In a randomized trial, Dowd (31) assigned 32 women to one of three groups: group 1 increased fluid intake by 500 cc over baseline; group 2 decreased by same amount; and group 3 maintained baseline level. The authors reported that 20 women who had fewer incontinent episodes at the end of the trial attributed this to drinking more fluids. Women in this study noted that it was easier to limit daily intake than to increase it. The recommended daily fluid intake is 1500 mL, but many feel that a more appropriate intake is 1800–2400 mL/d. To be adequately hydrated, it is felt that older patients must consume at least 1500–2000 mL/d of liquids (32). Many patients, especially women who are dieting or who actively exercise, may drink excessive fluids that may total more than 4000 mL/d. If they are experiencing UI, they should be encouraged to decrease the amount.

The timing of fluid may be important in persons who have problems with nocturia. Aging causes an increase in nocturia, defined as the number of voids recorded from the time the individual goes to bed with the intention of going to sleep, to the time the individual wakes with the intention of rising. Nocturia is an average of greater than 2 nocturnal voids per night. Nocturia can be diagnosed as nocturnal polyuria (NP), which causes the largest amount of urine production to occur at rest while the person is supine. Chronic medical conditions such as congestive heart failure, venous stasis with peripheral edema, hypoglycemia, excess urine output, obstructive sleep apnea, and diuretics as well as evening/nighttime fluid consumption are causes of NP. During the night, there is a lower level of physical activity, and body fluid moves more quickly from one part of the body to another, causing an increase in the amount of urine in the bladder. To decrease nocturia precipitated by drinking fluids primarily in the evening or with dinner, the person should be instructed to reduce fluid intake after 7 PM and shift intake toward the morning and afternoon.

2. Influence of Bladder Irritants

The type of fluid or food is felt to be important (33). Caffeine is an ingredient found in certain beverages, foods, and medications and is felt to impact LUTS by causing a significant rise in detrusor pressure (34). Caffeine has been shown to have an excitatory effect on detrusor muscle contraction (35).

The consumption of caffeinated beverages, foods, and medications should not be underestimated. In the United States, >80% of the adult population consumes caffeine in the form of coffee, tea, or soft drinks on a daily basis. It is estimated to average ~200 mg d, which is equivalent to two 7.5-oz cups of brewed coffee (36). Additionally, the U.S. Food and Drug Administration (FDA) has listed >300 drugs that are bought off over the counter (OTC) in pharmacies and retail drug stores that contain caffeine. Caffeine is usually listed on the label of the products.

In addition to caffeine, alcohol is also felt to have a diuretic effect that can lead to increased frequency. Alcohol causes a release of antidiuretic hormone (ADH) from the posterior pituitary (34). Alcohol with dinner may be a contributing factor for nocturia. Anecdotal evidence suggests that eliminating dietary factors such as artificial sweeteners (aspartame) and certain foods (e.g., highly spiced foods, citrus juices, and tomato-based products) may play a role in continence (37).

Research has shown that urine leakage decreased (63%) when caffeine consumption was reduced from 23 to 14 g (38). Arya et al. (39) found that women (N = 20) with higher caffeine intake (484 ± 123 mg/d) had a 2.4-fold increased risk for detrusor instability than women (N = 10) with a low caffeine intake (194 ± 84 mg/d). There was also a correlation between current smoking and caffeine intake. Bryant et al. (40) conducted a prospective randomized controlled trial of persons with symptoms of urgency, frequency, and urge UI who routinely ingested 100 mg or more of caffeine per day. Both groups were taught bladder training, but the intervention group was also instructed to reduce caffeine intake. Significant improvement in urine loss was seen in the intervention group. Results in this study appeared to affect the OAB symptom of urgency. A 37% reduction was found among low users (100–200 mg of caffeine), a 5% reduction was found among medium users (201–300 mg) and a 4% increase was found among the high users (>301 mg). Tomlinson et al. (38) showed in 34 women with symptoms of UI (mostly mixed) who decreased caffeine intake (from 900 mL/d to 480 mL/d), episodes of daily urine loss also decreased (from 2.33 to 1.0 mg/d).

Even though current research is not conclusive, clinicians should assess all patients with LUTS for amount of daily caffeine intake. Patients should be advised about the possible adverse effects caffeine may have on the detrusor muscle and the possible benefits of reduction of caffeine intake (41). The patient should be instructed to switch to caffeine-free beverages and foods or eliminate them and see if symptoms decrease or resolve. Patient Guide #1 lists the caffeine intake of common products. Patients need to read product labels. Herbal teas that are felt to be more "natural" usually contain caffeine unless stated otherwise. Patients seem to think that iced tea has less caffeine than hot tea. In many patients who ingest large quantities, total elimination may be unrealistic. It is recommended that patients with incontinence and OAB avoid excessive caffeine intake (e.g., no more than 200 mg/d; 2 cups).

D. Bowel Regularity

Chronic constipation and straining during defecation can contribute to LUTS and pelvic organ prolapse. The close proximity of the bladder and urethra to the rectum and their similar nerve innervations make it likely that there are reciprocal effects between them (42). Constipation is defined as having fewer than three stools per week. Usually a patient's definition of constipation is considerably broader, however, and includes straining during defecation, painful defecation, dry hard stools, small stools, and incomplete or infrequent stool evacuation. Studies of severely constipated women who have strained during defecation over a prolonged period have demonstrated changes in pelvic floor neurological function (43).

Lubowski et al. (44) reported that denervation of the external anal sphincter and pelvic floor muscles may occur in association with a history of excessive straining on defecation. Many believe that if these are lifetime habits, they may have a cumulative effect on pelvic floor and bladder function. Spence-Jones et al. (45) found that straining excessively at stool was significantly more common in women with stress UI and in women with prolapse. Moller et al. (46) reported an almost uniform positive association between straining at stool and constipation and LUTS in women (N = 487) 40 years of age. Moller postulated that chronic constipation and repeated straining efforts induced progressive neuropathy in the pelvic floor. Charach et al. (47) examined the effect of alleviating constipation on LUTS in 52 patients aged 65–89. After constipation treatment with laxatives (e.g., Senokot, lactulose) subjects reported fewer episodes of urgency and frequency.

As there are data to suggest that chronic constipation and straining may be risk factors for the development of LUTS, self-care practices that promote bowel regularity should be an integral part of any treatment care plan. Suggestions to reduce constipation include the addition of fiber to the diet, increased fluid intake, regular exercise, digital stimulation, and establishment of a routine defecation schedule (see Patient Guide #2). Improved bowel function can also be achieved by determining a timetable for bowel evacuation so that the patient can take advantage of the urge to defecate. The schedule should be determined by the patient's bowel elimination pattern and previous time pattern for defecation. The patient should be taught never to ignore the "call to stool," the feeling that the bowel needs to be emptied.

Combining fluid management, elimination of bladder irritants, and regulation of bowels may be the yield the maximum benefit. Dougherty et al. (48) conducted a randomized, controlled trial in women (N = 218) aged 55 years and older that incorporated reduction of caffeine consumption, adjusting the amount and timing of intake, and making dietary changes to promote bowel regularity, which were termed "self-monitoring activities." Women in the intervention group also received bladder training and biofeedback-assisted pelvic muscle exercises. Two hundred eighteen women with stress, urge, or mixed UI were randomized, and 178 completed one or more follow-ups. At 2 years the intervention group UI severity decreased by 61%. Self-monitoring activities and bladder training accounted for most of the improvement.

III. TOILETING PROGRAMS

The Cochrane Collaboration has published systematic reviews for toileting programs which include prompted voiding, habit training, and timed or schedule voiding (49–51). Each of these toileting programs are caregiver dependent, which is defined as the need of a professional or family caregiver to assist with toileting. These programs can be utilized to improve continence, and the choice of which program is needed is determined by the cognitive status of the individual, the variability of the voiding pattern, and the need for psychological reinforcement for adherence to the regimen (52).

A. Dependent Scheduled Toileting Programs

A caregiver-dependent program that provides toileting on a scheduled time basis may be the simplest initial approach. If residents in institutions like nursing homes or patients living at home have an available and willing caregiver, a timed toileting program should be established, as at least 60% of care-dependent patients can benefit. The premise of these programs is that if the person is toileted on a preplanned schedule, the bladder will be emptied before incontinence occurs. These patients may have mobility or cognitive impairment and may need assistance (e.g., one-person assist), but may be able to cooperate with toileting. Studies suggest that while fewer than 20% of frail elders become completely dry, 30–50% of incontinent elders improve with reduction in the number and amount of incontinence episodes.

B. Habit Training

Habit training, first described in England as "bladder drill," is toileting a person on a rigid, fixed schedule. Toileting takes place whether or not a sensation to void is present but is usually only followed during waking hours. The goal is to keep the person dry, and no effort is made to motivate the person to resist urgency and to delay urination. Prefixed times such as every 2 h have been adopted for toileting programs in institutions such as nursing homes. However, a more realistic schedule may be related to certain daily routines such as upon awakening, mid-morning before or after meals, and at bedtime.

C. Prompted Voiding

Prompted voiding (PV) is a type of scheduled toileting program that employs behavior modification to reinforce both appropriate toileting behaviors and the individuals' desire to stay dry. PV is used for patients who are able to recognize urine leakage and are able to respond (will void) when prompted. PV stresses active communication and interaction between a caregiver and patient allowing the patient to take an active part in their incontinence and toileting behavior. Characteristics of "high responders" (53,54) or those who were more likely to make the greatest improvement in their incontinence include:

Has a bladder capacity of at least 200 cc and < 600 cc
Maximum voided volume > 150 cc
Postvoid residual < 200 cc
Has a small number (<4 times/12 h) of incontinent episodes per day
Responds to caregivers if prompted (asked and taken to the toilet) to void
Ability to ambulate independently or with assistance of one person

There are five major steps of a prompted voiding program that includes scheduled checking to allow the patient to request toileting, discussing with the patient the incontinence problem, prompting the patient to void, providing positive reinforcement to the patient for making an effort to use the toilet, and if incontinent, indicate to the patient that the expectation is that they stay dry.

Like habit training, this program is for frailer, older patients who require assistance from family members and/or professional caregivers. At least 25–40% of patients respond well to PV while approximately 38% cannot successfully toilet even when provided assistance by caregivers (53,55).

Another caregiver-dependent PV program involves toileting residents and other care-dependent patients at times when they are most likely need to void, which are determined by tracking voiding and UI and determining patterns using computerized recordings of wetness (56,57).

Despite documented research and positive outcomes, PV interventions have not been adopted by the staff in institutionalized settings such as nursing homes. There is a wide gap between what is known and what is actually used. Research has documented the success of a program called Behavioral Supervision Model, which defines responsibilities of staff members for the prompted voiding intervention, staff feedback regarding performance, and consequences based on staff performance evaluation (58). A novel staffing model that employed a "designated" versus an "integrated" role in nursing homes of the certified nursing assistant (CNA) in the delivery of a restorative care (walking program, exercise therapy) may have application to delivery of continence care (59).

D. Independent Bladder Training

Bladder training is also commonly referred to as bladder *retraining*, as well as bladder discipline, bladder drill, and bladder reeducation and is an education program that involves learning and independent micturition behavior by the patient.

E. Bladder Training

Bladder training (BT) requires patients to resist the sensation of urgency, to postpone voiding, and to urinate by the clock rather than in response to an urge. Mechanisms of action are not well understood, but it is felt that bladder retraining improves cortical inhibition over detrusor contractions, facilitates cortical ability over urethral closure during bladder filling, strengthens pelvic striated muscles, and alters behaviors that affect continence (e.g., frequent response to urgency). The goals of a BT program are to:

Improve bladder overactivity by controlling urgency and decreasing frequency
Increase bladder capacity
Reduce urge incontinence episodes

Jeffcoate and Francis (60) originally introduced bladder training that was called "bladder drill" by implementing the program in hospitalized patients with bladder dysfunction secondary to psychological disorders. At that time, it was prescribed for functional disorders of the bladder for which surgical intervention was not expected to be successful. The management regimen included education followed by a strict schedule of voluntary voiding with specific instructions to avoid responding prematurely to urinary urgency. This type of bladder training was the basis of a randomized controlled clinical trial of 123 women with detrusor instability, stress, and mixed UI. Results on the group taught BT reduced number of incontinent episodes by 57% and quantity of urine loss was reduced by 54% (61). In addition, BT significantly improved the quality of life, specifically in the ability to carry out activities and relationships, to tolerate and control symptoms and in improved ability to cope (62).

In the behavioral intervention research that focuses on persons with urge or mixed incontinence, BT is an integral component. The Cochrane database includes a systematic review of bladder training (63). BT is most appropriate for patients who have:

Stress, urge, or mixed incontinence
Cognition; are mentally intact
Ability to sense the urinary urge sensation
Comprehension; can read and follow instructions
Motivation; willing to comply with a structured education program

Prior to beginning a BT program, the patient should be educated about the lower urinary tract, causes of urinary incontinence, and concepts of bladder urgency using easy-to-understand visual aids such as "the urinary urge" (see Patient Guide #3). Education should include the fact that "continence" is a learned behavior and the importance of the brain's control over lower urinary tract function. The clinician initiates the program by assigning a voluntary voiding schedule, which includes voiding every 30–60 min (64). The voiding intervals are based on the baseline micturition frequency as determined by the bladder diary. The initiation of BT with very short voiding intervals is particularly important for patients who are experiencing urgency, as the shorter intervals will decrease or eliminate these symptoms (61,65). The goal is for the patient to void "before" the urge sensation of bladder fullness. Depending on the patient's ability to keep the schedule and/or evidence of reduction of incontinence episodes and/or urinary urgency and frequency, the scheduled intervals between voiding is increased by 30 min until the patient can achieve a goal of voiding every 3–4 hr. In many cases, patients find this schedule difficult. Therefore the patient should be told to adhere to this schedule at least 75% of the day, and it is not realistic to expect patients to maintain this voiding schedule during the night. The use of reminders such as a kitchen timer or stop watch can be beneficial to helping the patient keep on a schedule (66). Self-monitoring through the use of bladder diaries is used to evaluate adherence and to determine the next weekly voiding interval.

Another essential part of BT patient education focuses on the cortical ability to delay voiding and strategies for distraction. Concentration on an attentional task is useful in distracting the individual from the sensation of urgency (65). The patient is taught methods to resist or inhibit the urge sensation so that an expanded voiding interval can be adopted. Improving the ability to suppress the urge sensation and eventually diminish urgency will enable the patient to adopt a more normal voiding pattern. There are several bladder control strategies or techniques used to inhibit the urge sensation (67). They include:

Slow, deep breathing to consciously relax the bladder to combat a stressful rush to the toilet

Performing five or six rapid, deliberate, and intense pelvic muscle contractions, or "quick flicks" which are 2–3 sec in duration

As with most behavioral interventions, the relationship between the clinician and patient is very important to the success of the retraining. The clinician must monitor the patient's progress and provide praise and encouragement where appropriate. The use of a signed patient agreement or "contract" with the patient stating personal outcome goals can be helpful in motivating the patient to adhere to the program and outlines expectations. It has been shown that women with incontinence have diverse goals for incontinence treatment, which in some cases may be improvement in urine leakage and not continence (68).

It is felt by most experts that combining behavioral interventions with treatments such as drug therapy would increase symptom reduction. Mattiasson et al. (69) reported on a multicenter, single-blind Scandinavian study of 505 subjects, predominantly women (mean age 63) with symptoms of OAB with and without urge incontinence that were either treated with tolterodine 2 mg BID or tolterodine 2 mg BID and bladder retraining (BT). Subjects in the BT group were provided with a written information sheet that outlined the principles of BT and explained simple techniques that could be used to help improve bladder control. Both groups received bladder diaries to track outcomes. Seventy-eight percent of subjects completed 24 weeks of treatment. The median percent reduction of voiding frequency for those receiving drug therapy plus BT was 33% compared with 25% reduction in those subjects on drug therapy alone. There was no significant difference between the groups in relation to reduction in incontinence episodes or urgency. The authors term this approach as a "minimalist" approach, as there was no physician or other professional. They feel this negates the need for an extensive personal interaction between the patient and clinician; however, this is the only study that has shown this technique. Other such programs have not been successful (70).

IV. PELVIC MUSCLE REHABILITATION

A. Pelvic Muscle Exercises

Dr. Arnold Kegel, an obstetrician-gynecologist, introduced pelvic muscle exercises in the late 1940s by implementing a comprehensive program of progressive contractions of the levator ani muscle that incorporated biofeedback technology and was under direct supervision of a trained nurse. Dr. Kegel demonstrated in several clinical trials that practicing these exercises decreased stress urinary incontinence in childbearing women (71,72). These Kegel exercises, or as they have become know as pelvic muscle exercises (PMEs) or pelvic floor muscle training (PFMT), have been shown to decrease LUTS of incontinence, urgency, and frequency (3).

The actual effects of PMEs on lower urinary tract function is not completely understood; some studies show a relationship between changes in various measures of pelvic floor strength, such as anal sphincter strength or increased urethral closure pressure and resistance, all of which will prevent urine leakage (73–77). The proposed mechanisms of action for PMEs are that:

1. A strong and fast pelvic muscle contraction closes the urethra and increases urethral pressure to prevent leakage during sudden increase in intra-abdominal pressure (e.g., during a cough) (78,79). Urethral compression can be maximized by timing the muscle contraction at the exact moment of intra-abdominal force (called the "knack") (80–83).

2. Rising intra-abdominal pressure (e.g., during coughing, laughing, sneezing) exerts a downward (caudal) pressure or force on the bladder and urethra (84). Contraction of the levator ani exerts a counterbalancing upward (cephalic) force by lifting the endopelvic fascia upon which the urethra rests and pressing it upward toward the pubic symphysis, creating a mechanical pressure rise (85,86).

3. Muscle contraction causes a pelvic muscle "reflex" contraction that precedes increased bladder pressure and may inhibit bladder overactivity. The aim is to acquire learned reflex activity.

As part of a rehabilitation program, PMEs increases support to the urethral sphincter and detrusor muscle, thus preventing stress, urge, and mixed UI and is most appropriate in patients:

Who do not have cognitive impairments
Have the motivation to comply with the program
Have a pelvic floor that is neurologically intact

The goal of PFMT is to isolate the pelvic floor muscle, specifically the levator ani (80,87–89). The PFMs are a striated, skeletal muscle group under voluntary control. PMEs consist of repeated, high-intensity pelvic floor muscle contractions of two types of muscle fibers: type I, slow-twitch muscle fibers, and type II, fast-twitch muscle fibers. At least 80% of the levator ani muscle is type 1 muscle fibers. These fibers produce less force on contraction and assist in improving muscle endurance by generating a slower, more sustained, but less intense, contraction. Over time the continuous, though lower-intensity contraction of these muscle fibers maintains a general level of support and urethral closure pressure. Type I muscle fibers are also fatigue resistant. The second group is type II, or fast-twitch, fibers, which aid in strong and forceful contractions. These fibers come into play during sudden increases in intra-abdominal pressure by contributing to urethral closure. By exercising these fibers, pelvic muscle strength will increase. Muscle inactivity, aging, and innervation damage can contribute to a decrease in the proportion of type II fibers. As type II fibers fatigue easily, patients are taught to perform rapid, repeated contractions in exercising them (75,76).

The functional demands on the fibers of PFM include sustaining force over time, especially during increases in intra-abdominal pressure, developing force quickly and contracting and relaxing voluntarily (90). During voiding, the person must relax the PFM to open the external urethral sphincter to allow voiding. When these muscles do not function properly, women in particular may develop stress UI, fecal incontinence, and pelvic organ prolapse.

Dr. Kegel described four phases in the performance of PMEs (91):

1. Awareness of the function and coordination of the PFM muscle. For older adults and persons whose pelvic muscle is severely relaxed, this may take several weeks.

2. Gains over muscle identification, control, and strength. Muscle strength is the maximal force that can be generated by the PFM. Although the PFM is not flexible, the muscle must adapt to different or changing requirements so the PFM must have contractibility and build force quickly when contracting.

3. Firmness, thickening, broadening, and bulking of the muscles to increase muscle endurance. Muscle endurance is a performance characteristic of the ability of the PFM to

execute repeated contractions to and initial level of strength often called a "submaximum" contraction.

4. Improvements of the symptoms indicate that the muscles are strengthening. At this point some patients feel that their LUTS are so improved that regular exercising is no longer needed.

For muscle contractility to improve, the initial muscle strength, power, endurance, repetitions, and fatigue must be considered together with the principles of muscle training (92). The following are the definitions for determining pelvic muscle contractility:

> Strength—the maximum force or contraction that a muscle can generate.
> Power—the ability for the muscle to "contract-relax" as quickly and strongly as possible, until the muscle fatigues. These are often called "quick flicks."
> Endurance—this is the time, up to 10 sec, that the maximum muscle contraction can be maintained or repeated, before a reduction in power of 50% or more is detected. In other words, the muscle contraction is timed until the muscle fatigues.
> Repetitions—the number of repetitions (up to 10) of the muscle contraction of equal force that can be repeated. Use at least a 5-sec muscle relaxation between each two contraction; easily fatigable muscles need a chance to recover, without permitting excessive rest periods for strong muscles.
> Fatigue—failure to maintain the required or expected force of the pelvic muscle contraction for more than one or two times in succession.

The following definitions can be applied to pelvic floor muscle dysfunction:

1. Low-tone is the clinical finding of an impaired ability to isolate and contract the pelvic floor muscles in the presence of a weak and atrophic PFM. Ideally, the patient will gain the ability to recognize the difference between relaxation and contraction.

2. High-tone refers to the clinical condition of hypertonic, spastic PFM with resultant impairment of muscle isolation, contraction and relaxation. A high resting baseline with high variability and occasional spasms may be seen in patients with chronic pelvic pain syndromes. In some cases, this excessive, elevated resting tone may be created unconsciously. Therapeutic exercise is important in the management of pelvic pain as the patient often has a reduced level of activity related to the prolonged nature of their pain. Rehabilitating the pelvic muscle can be central in resolving pain when muscle spasm is present. Using PMEs on patients with high-tone to enhance muscle relaxation is referred to as "downtraining." Teaching a muscle to relax is often more difficult than teaching it how to contract (uptraining), as the feeling of relaxation is small.

The patient should be cautioned not to:

1. Perform these exercises during voiding and not to stop and start urine flow as a form of exercising. This exercise has good face validity for effectiveness because many patients initially report an inability to stop the urine flow when it begins. However, there is some controversy over this practice because it is nonphysiological and can be harmful (93).

2. Over-exercise the pelvic muscle. Women can develop levator ani myalgia by performing excessive PFM exercises to reduce incontinence (94). Start slowly, building gradually.

Patients should be instructed on the correct technique of pelvic muscle exercises. Patients have a difficult time identifying and isolating this muscle. Without sufficient information, women may mistakenly bear down or exercise ineffectively. Specifically, women are told to "draw in" and "lift up" of the perivaginal and anal sphincter muscles. Once patients are able to identify the muscle, they are instructed to perform a series of "quick flicks," or 2-sec contractions, followed by sustained (endurance contractions) contractions of 5 sec and longer as part of a daily exercise regimen (see Patient Guide #4). At least 10 sec of relaxation is recommended between contractions. Encourage the patient to aim for a high level of concentrated effort with each pelvic muscle contraction, as greater contraction intensity is associated with improvement in pelvic muscle strength (74,76).

Patients are given verbal and written instructions for a daily exercise program based on the baseline assessment of the patient's PFMs strength, contraction, and endurance during the initial assessment session. Visual aids are helpful (see Figs. 1, 2). Patients should be encouraged to aim for a high level of concentrated effort with each pelvic muscle contraction, as greater contraction intensity is associated with improvement in pelvic muscle strength (74,76). Patients are instructed to exercise at least twice daily and to perform the exercises in three positions—lying, sitting, and standing. A minimum of 30–45 PMEs per day is recommended (95). A gradual increase in number of contractions over a period of PME practice has been shown to increase muscle strength significantly and decrease urine loss. The patient should be instructed to contract the muscle at the time of the UI episode (81,95). Contracting it before sneezing, coughing, lifting, standing or swinging a golf club can prevent stress UI from occurring (see Patient Guide #4). The muscle also can be contracted when a strong urge to void occurs. Results may not occur until after 6–8 weeks of exercise, and optimal results usually take longer. Self-monitoring practice through the use of a calendar record, audio, and video taped material that review the exercises can improve protocol compliance (37,96).

Most clinicians in this field have relied on the use of verbal and written instructions for patients to use for home practice of PMEs, not the use of a home biofeedback device. There is a paucity of research on the use of a home biofeedback device to aid in performing these exercises at home while providing information to the clinician and patient about the success of the muscle contraction (97,98).

Teaching women to strengthen the pelvic floor muscle as part of a comprehensive behavioral program has been demonstrated to be effective in 50–60% of women with SUI. However, even after they have learned to do that, there is the additional problem that many find too burdensome—the daily exercises necessary to increase muscle strength and control. As a result, the noncompliance rate for this therapy can be high, varying from 10% to 40%. This can

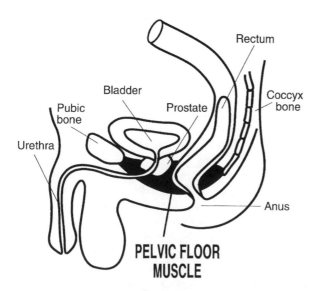

Figure 1   Pelvic floor muscle in men. © 1995 Diane K Newman

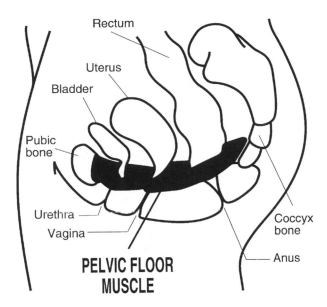

Rectum

Uterus

Bladder

Pubic
bone

Urethra

Vagina

Coccyx
bone

Anus

**PELVIC FLOOR
MUSCLE**

Figure 2   Pelvic floor muscle in women. © 1995 Diane K Newman

be frustrating to clinicians who provide these treatments, as poor outcome may be secondary to noncompliance and out of their control.

Research in the area of PMEs is extensive but long-term results have been reported only rarely (99). Cammu et al. (100) found that in women who had been successful with PMEs initially, two-thirds maintained their success 10 years later. Practice of PMEs in primiparas results in fewer UI symptoms during late pregnancy and postpartum (101).

Subak and colleagues (22,23) conducted a randomized trial for community dwelling women who at least reported one UI episode per week. Women were randomly assigned to the behavioral therapy (n = 77) and control (n = 75) group. Women in the behavioral therapy were asked to keep urinary diaries and attend six weekly 20-min group instructional sessions with three to five participants on bladder retraining and written and verbal instructions on PMEs, which was termed a "low-intensity" behavioral therapy. Women in the control group did not receive any instructions but were asked to keep urinary diaries for 6 weeks. At 6 weeks, the treatment group had a 50% reduction in mean number of incontinence episodes compared with a 15% reduction or the control group. They also experienced improved diurnal and total incontinence frequencies.

The Association of Women's Health Obstetric and Neonatal Nurses (AWHONN) tested the efficacy of a bladder and pelvic floor muscle training program in real-world ambulatory care settings (88,102,103). Twenty-one clinical sites participated yielding a sample of 132 women with a mean age of 51 years that originally screened positive for incontinence, received instruction in bladder and pelvic floor muscle training, and persisted to a point of follow-up 4 months posttreatment. Significant reductions were noted between pre- and posttreatment in the frequency of incontinent episodes, the volume of leakage per episode, the cost of self-management, and the frequency of nocturia. Simultaneously, significant improvements were reported in indices reflecting quality of life. Specifically, women indicated that the incontinence was less bothersome and that they were avoiding fewer activities because of their incontinence. These results demonstrate the effectiveness of an evidence-based protocol in actual clinical settings and warrant the implementation of the protocol by nurses in general ambulatory women's health care settings across the United States (104).

B. Use of EMG or Manometric Measurement

Pelvic floor muscle strength is either measured by electromyography (EMG) or manometric pressure. Most clinicians who specialize in this field prefer EMG measurements. EMG is the graph of the electrical activity of a muscle and as a practical indicator of muscle activity has been defined as:

> The study of electrical potentials generated by the depolarization of muscle
> A monitor of bioelectrical activity correlating to motor unit activity; it does not measure the muscle contractility itself but the electrical correlate of the muscle contraction
> An indicator of the physiological activity

The advantage of EMG over manometric pressure is that, provided the machinery is of sufficient sophistication with adequate filtering, EMG apparatus can engage the use of the newer types of electrodes that are lightweight and designed to stay in place, hence allowing more functional positions during assessment and treatment (92). An added benefit is that EMG can be multichannel, which allows the simultaneous reinforcement of contractions of the pelvic floor muscles and inhibition of accessory muscles (e.g., abdominal muscle contractions). A common error in contracting the PFM is to simultaneously contract the abdominal, gluteal, or adductor muscles. This may mask the strength of the PFM contraction. Abdominal contraction increases intra-abdominal pressure, which mechanically elevates bladder pressure, so it is important to measure concurrent use of abdominal contraction (105). For the PMR treatment to be successful, it is essential that the patient be able to isolate the pelvic floor muscles. When an additional muscle group is contracting at the same time of the pelvic floor, it is called "recruitment." Monitoring for accessory muscle recruitment during initial EMG and subsequent visits are necessary until recruitment stops and should be considered on all patients.

The use of multichannel EMG can be especially helpful in patients who are having difficulty identifying and isolating the correct muscle. Four methods of EMG measurements have been used in the investigation of lower urinary tract dysfunction (106):

> Vaginal sensor
> Anal sensor or plug electrode (anorectal)
> Surface skin electrodes
> Needle electrodes

Vaginal and anal sensors are designed to provide accurate detection of EMG muscle activity. The accuracy of longitudinal sensing electrodes has been shown to be virtually identical to the gold standard, inserted needle electrodes. The use of vaginal or rectal sensors is contraindicated in the following:

> Active vaginal infection or genital disease
> Severe pelvic pain where insertion of the sensor causes vaginal or rectal discomfort
> Pregnancy
> Recent (within last 6 months) pelvic or rectal surgery
> Untreated atrophic vaginitis
> Dyspareunia
> Menstrual period

In these cases consider the use of skin surface electrodes. Surface skin electrodes are relatively non-invasive and well tolerated. They give quantitative information about muscle activity rather than data for qualitative analysis. The first choice of electrode placement is at the 10 and 4 o'clock or 9 and 3 o'clock position on either side of the anus (see Fig. 3). Electrodes should be

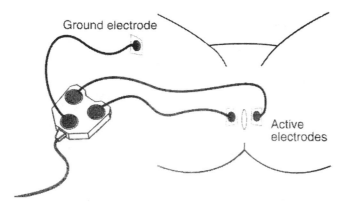

Figure 3 Surface skin electrode placement

placed close to the anus without touching the other sensor or without sensors overlapping. Needle electrodes are primarily used during urodynamic testing. The EMG data are measured in microvolts. The actual threshold of pelvic muscle strength required for maintaining continence is unknown at this time as is unknown the normal values for pelvic muscle strength. The baseline and all follow-up EMG recordings should include two set of measurements of:

First Set:

Maximum or "short/quick" muscle contractions of 2-sec duration
Resting muscle activity of 2-sec duration

Second set:

Sustained or "long" muscle contractions (5, 10, or 30 sec); the clinician should not go directly from 3- to 10-sec muscle contractions but increase in increments of 5 sec as patient's ability warrants
Resting muscle activity of 5-sec duration or for the same length of time as muscle contraction

The ability to relax one's pelvic muscle following a contraction is of most importance if one is to gain control and coordination of these muscles.

Manometry is the use of an instrument to detect, assess, and record pressure. A pressure perineometer consists of a vaginal or rectal probe with a connector tube to a manometer. Dr. Arnold Kegel first used the term "perineometer" for a vaginal pressure gauge specific to the PFM. He developed this instrument for both diagnosis and nonsurgical treatment for women with stress UI and pelvic muscle relaxation. Perineometers aim to show changes in pressure caused by the contraction of the perivaginal musculature, to be observed on a manometer gauge. The pressure changes can be measured in centimeters of water (cmH_2O) or millimeters of mercury (mm Hg). Depending on the sophistication of the equipment, the pressure changes may be shown on a dial, a digital readout, a bar chart, or a graphical representation. Different types of probes—air-filled, water-filled, individually made, and mass produced—have been reported and can be performed by inserting sensors into the vagina or rectum. Although manometry and pressure sensors are available with certain clinical systems and have been used in several clinical trials, they are primarily used for treatment of rectal dysfunction (e.g. constipation, fecal incontinence), not for treatment with LUTS. Theofrastous, Wyman et al. (107) used two water-filled balloon manometric devices to measure vaginal and abdominal pressures. The group who received a pelvic floor muscle training regimen demonstrated a 15–23% improvement in pelvic muscle strength.

C. Application of Biofeedback Therapy

The use of biofeedback therapy is a method of assessment and treatment of pelvic floor dysfunction. Biofeedback relayed using EMG, when used as part of a pelvic muscle rehabilitation program, is a method by which the patient is immediately made aware of the physiologic state of the PFM. Feedback to the patient is in the form of tactile, verbal, visual, or auditory methods. Biofeedback treatment may assist muscles that have increased tension even when the patient or clinician cannot detect it. This is particularly true of the pelvic floor muscles, as denervation damage may lead to impaired sensation. High levels of resting activity and fleeting muscle spasms may be only visualized using EMG biofeedback instruments. Muscle training that utilizes EMG biofeedback may improve the effectiveness of the muscle relaxation efforts while strengthening weak pelvic muscles. A biofeedback-assisted exercise program that stabilizes the pelvic floor muscles can reduce and eliminate symptoms of pelvic floor dysfunction as seen in chronic pelvic pain syndromes.

Generally, visual, auditory, or verbal feedback techniques are used for neuromuscular conditioning. These methods help to reinforce a particular task being performed. For example, the display on a monitor screen of the pressure, or the EMG changes of the anal sphincter, provide instant visual feedback to the patient regarding their performance. Similarly, during muscle contraction the intensity (pitch of the electrical activity) of the sphincter muscle provides corresponding auditory feedback to the patient regarding their performance. To determine PFM strength, two indices recommended as outcome of muscle strength tests that can be recorded on the EMG are the peak muscle contraction value and the average score. EMG or manometry can record the following variables of the PFM:

> Strength—recorded as the peak or maximum contraction that has the highest waveforms indicating ability to sustain the muscle contraction
> Endurance—average muscle contraction measured across the waveform
> Contractibility—the rate of the original rise of the muscle contraction

Throughout the treatment session, the clinician reinforces the patient's behavior and provides compliments and other appropriate advice. This constitutes verbal feedback to the patient and is an essential part of a behavioral treatment program. All three maneuvers are complimentary.

Motivation and active participation play a big part in the success of biofeedback therapy. For incontinence and other LUTS, biofeedback therapy uses computer graphs or lights as a teaching tool to help the patient identify and learn to control the correct muscles. Biofeedback helps the patient locate the pelvic muscles by changing the graph or light when the patient contracts or tightens the correct muscle.

Different biofeedback methods can be used in pelvic floor muscle (PFM) reeducation, including proprioception and verbal encouragement during:

1. Digital (e.g., vaginal or rectal) PFM assessment of the levator ani muscle is a form of biofeedback and is an important component of teaching correct pelvic muscle contraction and muscle awareness (108). Verbal feedback of a voluntary contraction can also encourage and assist in enhancing patient effort. A digital measure of pelvic muscle strength can be performed based on pressure, duration of contraction, and displacement of the examiner's finger. Palpation of muscular attachments along the pubic arch and the insertion of the levator ani and coccygeus muscles are part of the assessment. The levator ani can be palpated just superior to the hymeneal ring. Palpate the levators at the 4 and 8 o'clock positions to determine if that reproduces any discomfort or

tenderness. There are several different grading systems (examples are found in Tables 1 and 2) that can be used to assess and document pelvic muscle strength in women. Using the scale described in Table 1, a scale, assess *pressure*, which is defined as the strength of contraction on the finger. Scores range from 0 for no pressure felt to 5 for strong compression, where the examiner's finger(s) are gripped. Ask the patient to squeeze hard and count in seconds to determine the *duration* of the contraction, which is recorded in seconds. Note the *displacement in plane* by the amount of movement of your finger(s) when the patient contracts her muscle. The rating scale starts with 1, which is no displacement, to 5 when the examiners finger are moved upward and drawn in by the contraction of the pelvic muscle. It may be helpful to perform a digital PMA pre- and posttreatment to determine the increase in muscle strength, strength, and ability to isolate the levators.

2. Manometric and EMG biofeedback helps in PFM awareness, but also provides interest, challenge, and reward for effort, a greater feeling of control, and progress in monitoring (109).

Research is extensive detailing the efficacy of the use of biofeedback-assisted behavioral therapy for PFMT (110–116). The 1996 guideline on Urinary Incontinence in Adults (3) outlined the research that demonstrated that PMEs are indicated for patients with stress incontinence and can reduce urgency and prevent urge UI. Pelvic floor reeducation has proven to be effective in women with sphincter deficiency and detrusor instability. More recent research has supported this claim (101,117,118). Behavioral modifications, pelvic muscle rehabilitation, and bladder retraining programs have successfully decreased UI in homebound elders (119,120). A study of men with urinary incontinence following radical prostate surgery showed that 88% of the treatment group achieved continence in 3 months compared to 56% of the control group (121).

Wyman and colleagues (122) randomized 204 women into three groups. Group 1 was encouraged to use bladder training with the voiding interval set at 30 or 60 min and increased by 30 min each week. Group 2 received pelvic muscle instruction that included four office biofeedback sessions; women were instructed to perform five fast and 10 sustained contractions twice a day and work up to a total of 50 contractions by the third week. Participants were also instructed to use pelvic muscle contractions for urge inhibition and preventive contractions with exertional events. Group 3 received a combination of the two therapies. There were no significant differences found pretreatment in any of the outcome variables. At the short-term follow-up 2 weeks after treatment, the combination therapy group had significantly fewer incontinent episodes, better quality of life, and greater satisfaction with treatment. However, by 3 months posttreatment, all three treatment groups had improved relative to baseline status. The absence of differences among the three groups led the investigators to conclude that the type of therapy (bladder or pelvic floor muscle training) may be less important than participation in a structured intervention program.

Dougherty and colleagues (48) randomized 218 women, aged 55 and older who were provided treatment in their home by a trained nurse practitioner. Group 1 was a control group. Group 2 received a behavioral management for continence (BMC) program that consisted of sequenced phases: (a) self-monitoring, (b) bladder training, and (c) biofeedback-assisted pelvic muscle exercises. The BMC treatment was not found to have a significant impact on either urinary frequency or voiding intervals. Amount of urine loss decreased in 61% of the BMC over the 2 years of follow-up, whereas the control group's urine loss worsened by 184%. However, both the BMC and control groups' episodes of urine loss decreased (70% and 16%, respectively).

Burgio and associates (123) compared the effectiveness of anorectal biofeedback-assisted behavioral therapy for PFMT with drug therapy and placebo control and showed that the behavioral intervention was more effective with 80% of those receiving behavioral experienced a reduction in incontinence episodes compares with 68.5% if those receiving drug therapy and only 39.4% of those receiving placebo.

Table 1 Pelvic Muscle Rating Scale

				Grade		
	0	1	2	3	4	5
Pressure	None	Flick, more than one point, but not a full circumference (instant, mild pressure)	Felt at more than one point but not a full circumference (instant, mild pressure)	Loose hold (full circumference)	Snug (full circumference)	Strong compression of fingers
Displacement	None	Base lifting	Base to midfinger	Base to fingertip; lifting, gentle lift at tip	Base to fingertip; lifting, strong lift at tip	Vigorous drawing up and in
Duration		Seconds maintained				

Source: Brink et al. (124).

Table 2 Modified Oxford Scale for Pelvic Muscle Assessment

	Grade	Description
Nil	0	No discernible PFM contraction
Flicker	1	Feels like a flicker or a pulsation and represents a very weak contraction
Weak	2	Weak contraction, is detected as an increase in muscle tension, without any discernible lift or tightening
Moderate	3	A moderate contraction characterized by a degree of lifting of the posterior vaginal wall, tightening of the examiner's finger (pubovisceralis) and drawing in of the perineum. A grade 3 as well as a grade 4 and 5 contraction is generally discernible on visual perineal inspection.
Good	4	Produces elevation of the posterior vaginal wall against resistance (applied as pressure to the posterior vaginal wall) and drawing in of the perineum. If two fingers (index and middle) are placed laterally in the vagina and separated, a grade 4 contraction can squeeze them together against resistance.
Strong	5	Strong resistance can be given against elevation of the posterior vaginal wall and approximation of the index and middle fingers.

Clinician-supervised PME with biofeedback is felt to provide the most favorable long-term results and many multidisciplinary pelvic floor dysfunction or "continence" centers provide these services (37). Berghmans et al. (125,126) reviewed the literature regarding biofeedback-assisted PMEs in women with stress and urge UI and felt there was a need for more research to support these more intensive therapy regimens.

The most recent study was conducted by Burgio and colleagues (127) in women (n = 222) who had urge UI. Women were randomized to three treatment groups:

Group 1 received behavioral training that consisted of bladder retraining and PMEs with anorectal biofeedback. They had four clinic visits with nurse practitioners at 2-week intervals with a home program of PMEs.

Group 2 received behavioral training without biofeedback but digital pelvic muscle assessment with information on muscle isolation and correct identification and was given a home program of PMEs.

Group 3 were given a 20-page self-administered booklet that included an 8-week step-by-step, self-help instructions on bladder retraining, and PMEs.

Results indicated that the outcomes of the three groups were not significantly different. Group 1 had 63.1% reduction in frequency of UI episodes, group 2 had 69.4% reduction in frequency of

UI episodes, and group 3 58.6% reduction in frequency of UI episodes. However, patients' perceptions of treatment were significantly better for groups 1 and 2.

D. Combining Behavioral Treatments with Drug Therapy

In addition, a more recent study (128) examined the effects of combining behavioral treatment and drug treatment for urge UI in ambulatory women. Subject's reduction of incontinence went from a mean 57.5% with behavioral therapy to a mean 88.5% overall reduction with combined behavioral and drug (anticholinergic) treatment. The majority of the PME research used biofeedback therapy to teach and train the PFM.

E. Use of Vaginal Weights

Vaginal weights are another example of a biofeedback technique, which educates women on contraction of the PFMs. They have been most successful in woman with stress incontinence, and can be used by the patient as part of a structured resistive pelvic muscle exercise program. The weights are made of plastic and shaped like cones and are of increasing weights. The user is instructed to insert the lightest weight into the vagina, in the position of a tampon. It should be inserted so that it cannot be felt protruding from the opening of the vagina. The user then walks around for up to 15 min. If the weight is retained during this time, the next-heaviest weight is introduced and the procedure is repeated until a weight of a certain weight slips out. The woman uses that weight to practice holding it in, by contracting the pelvic muscles, for up to 15 min BID. When the woman can successfully hold one weight, she is told to switch to a heavier one. To increase the exercise value of these weights, the woman is instructed to practice retaining the weight during coughing, jumping, or any stress-provoking act that causes incontinence. Theoretically, when the weight is placed in the vagina, it provides sensory feedback and prompts a pelvic floor muscle contraction to keep it from slipping out. The perceived advantages of vaginal weight training are that it involves less teaching time, can be self-taught, may be motivational, and can be used with minimal supervision. There is strong evidence that indicates it is an effective treatment for stress UI in pre- and postmenopausal women (12), However, the evidence is inconclusive regarding the superiority of vaginal weight training over PMEs alone or electrical stimulation; further there appears to be no added benefit to use of vaginal weight training with PMEs (129,130). Although vaginal weight training may take less instructional time in terms of office practice, it may be less acceptable to some women than PFME alone as noted by higher attrition rates in some clinical trials (131). Reasons given for their nonuse were aesthetic dislike, unpleasantness, discomfort, difficulty of insertion, or bleeding (132).

F. Pelvic Floor Electrical Stimulation

Pelvic floor electrical stimulation (PFES) is the application of a low grade of electrical stimulation to the pelvic floor muscles (PFMs) to stimulate the muscle to contract. PFES has a twofold action: contraction of pelvic floor muscles, and inhibition of unwanted detrusor contractions. PFES for stress UI is the result of stimulation of afferent fibers of the pudendal nerve activating both the pelvic floor and periurethral muscles. For urge UI bladder inhibition occurs through pudendal (afferent) to pelvic (efferent) nerve reflex and a pudendal to hypogastric reflex. The application of electric current to the pelvic floor muscles produces a reflex muscle contraction without any effort on the part of the patient. Pelvic muscle electrical stimulation combined with biofeedback may prove useful in that the electrical stimulation provides a passive contraction with increased awareness of pelvic muscle contractions.

The parameters of most stimulation units include the waveform, the current intensity, the pulse frequency, the ramping of impulses, and the on/off timing. The muscle contraction, called neuromuscular stimulation, is a useful addition to pelvic floor exercises in the rehabilitation of weakened pelvic muscles and is very beneficial for both men and women who are unable to contract these muscles on command, as it leads to an improved comprehension of the activity of the muscles and subsequently better active contraction. Also, PFES is used with patients as an adjunct treatment to:

Assist with identification and isolation of pelvic muscle
Increase pelvic muscle strength
Decrease unwanted or uninhibited detrusor (bladder) muscle contraction
Assist with normalizing pelvic muscle relaxation

There are no documented side effects to electrical stimulation of the pelvic floor, but PFES is contraindicated in the following:

Complete denervation of the pelvic floor (will not respond)
Dementia
Demand cardiac pacemaker
Unstable or serious cardiac arrhythmia
Pregnancy or planning/attempting pregnancy
Rectal bleeding
Active infection (UTI/vaginal)
Unstable seizure disorder
Swollen, painful hemorrhoids
Presence of vaginal vault prolapse
Pelvic surgery in past 6 months

Electrical stimulation is usually performed initially in the clinician's office than prescribed as a home program using a battery-operated home unit. The delivery of the electrical current to the tissues is via a sensor, which may be on the surface of the skin (skin electrodes around the anus) or by vaginal or rectal sensors and is used in conjunction with biofeedback. The home program consists of using the stimulator for 15 min BID for several weeks to months, although the length of time and number of treatments is highly variable. However, with the wide variations in stimulation parameters including time, intensity, and frequency of sessions, it is difficult to make comparisons across studies. Given the equivocal results, the benefit of electrical stimulation in stress, urge, and mixed UI in women remains controversial (12).

There does not appear to be any consistency to PFES protocols used in clinical practice to treat patients with stress, urge and mixed incontinence. The research in this area is confusing because information is lacking on detail of stimulation parameters (intensity, pulse duration), time PFES is used by the patient, devices used and methods of delivery (133–138). The Cochrane Database did not find any significant differences between the addition of PFES to a PME program for self-reported cure (139).

Goode et al. (140) conducted a RCT of the effect of PFES to a behavioral intervention program in women with stress only or mixed UI. This study was similar to their previous research (127) except that PFES was added. Women (N = 200) underwent an 8-week treatment program and were asked to complete a daily bladder diary. Women were randomized to three groups:

- Group 1 received behavioral training that consisted of anorectal biofeedback-assisted PMEs, home exercises, and bladder control strategies.
- Group 2 received same program as Group 1 with PFES (performing both office and home stimulation) using a vaginal sensor.
- Group 3 or control condition consisting of a self-administered self-help book on behavioral treatments.

Results indicated that the addition of PFES did not seem to enhance the results of behavioral training alone however, behavioral training with or without PFES were significantly more effective than the self-help book. Actual results showed that behavioral training resulted in a mean 68.6% reduction in frequency of UI episodes, behavioral training with PFES resulted in a 71.9% mean reduction and treatment with the self-help book a 52.5% reduction. The authors felt that the two treatments of PMEs and PFES may overlap. This reinforces other research noted in this chapter on behavioral interventions that suggest that this treatment is optimally implemented in a clinical practice setting with trained professionals (doctors, nurse practitioners or nurses) to ensure that patients are exercising the correct muscle. Also, a stepped approach in which biofeedback and PFES are added to a less invasive program such as PMEs and lifestyle changes is the preferred clinical approach and is supported by current reimbursement (141).

REFERENCES

1. Nygaard I, Bryant C, Dowell C, Wilson PD. Lifestyle interventions for the treatment of urinary incontinence in adults. Cochrane Incontinence Group, Cochrane Database of Systematic Reviews. Issue 2, 2002.
2. Diokno AC et al. (1992).
3. Fantl J, Newman D, Colling J. Urinary incontinence in adults: acute and chronic management. Clinical practice guideline No. 2, 1996 update (ACHCPR publication No. 96-0692. Rockville, MD: U.S. Department of Health and Human Services. Public Health Services, Agency for Health Care and Policy Research).
4. Bump RC, McClish DM. Cigarette smoking and pure genuine stress incontinence of urine. A comparison of risk factors and determinants between smokers and nonsmokers. Am J Obstet Gynecol 1994; 170(2):579–582.
5. Koley B, Koley J, Saha JK. The effects of nicotine on spontaneous contractions of cat urinary bladder in situ. Br J Pharmacol 1984; 83:347–355.
6. Ruggieri MR, Whitmore KE, Levine RM. Bladder purinergic receptors. J Urol 1990; 144:176–181.
7. Bump RC, McClish DM. Cigarette smoking and urinary incontinence. Am J Obstet Gynecol 1992; 167(5):1214–1218.
8. Tampakoudis P, Tantanassis T, Grimbizis G, Papeletsos M, Mantalenakis S. Cigarette smoking and urinary incontinence in women—a new calculative method of estimating the exposure to smoke. Eur J Obstet Gynecol Reprod Biol 1995; 63:17–30.
9. Nuotio M, Jylha M, Koivisto AM, Tammela TLJ. Association of smoking with urgency in older people. Eur Urol 2001; 40:206–212.
10. Højberg KE, Salvig JD, Winslow NA, Lose G, Secher NJ. Urinary incontinence: prevalence and risk factors at 16 weeks of gestation. Br J Obstet Gynaecol 1999; 106:842–850.
11. Koskimaki J, Hakama M, Huhtala H, Tammela TLJ. Association of smoking with lower urinary tract symptoms. J Urol 1998; 159:1580–1582.

12. Wilson D, Bo K, Hay-Smith J, Nygaard I, Staskin D, Wyman J. Conservative management in women. In: Abrams P, Cardozo L, Khoury S, Wein A, eds. Incontinence. Plymouth: Health Publications Ltd, 2002:571–624.

13. Elia G, Dye TD, Scariati PD. Body mass index and urinary symptoms in women. Int Urogyncol J 2001; 12:366–369.

14. Brown NJ et al. (1996).

15. Burgio KL, Matthews KA, Engel BT. Prevalence, incidence and correlates of urinary incontinence in healthy, middle-aged women. J Urol 1991; 46:1255–1259.

16. Mommsen S, Foldspang A. Body mass index and adult female urinary incontinence. World J Urol 1994; 19:319–322.

17. Dwyer PL, Lee ETC, Hay DM. Obesity and urinary incontinence in women. Br J Obstet Gynaecol 1998; 95:91–96.

18. Roe B, Doll H. Lifestyle factors and continence status: comparison of self-report data from a postal survey in England. JWOCN 1999; 26(6):312–319.

19. Brown JS, Grady D, Ouslander JG, Herzog AR, Varner RE, Posner SF. Prevalence of urinary incontinence and associated risk factors in postmenopausal women. Obstet Gynecol 1999; 94(1):66–70.

20. Bump RC, Sugerman H, Fantl JA, McClish DM. Obesity and lower urinary tract function in women: effect of surgically induced weight loss. Am J Obstet Gynecol 1992; 166:392–399.

21. Subak LL, Quesenberry CP, Posner SF, Cattolica E, Soghikian K. The effect of behavioral therapy on urinary incontinence. Obstet Gynecol 2002; 100(1):72–78.

22. Subak LL, Johnson C, Whitcomb E, Boban D, Saxton J, Brown JS. Does weight loss improve incontinence in moderately obese women? Int Urogynecol J 2002; 13:40–43.

23. Newman DK, Giovanni D. Overactive bladder: a nursing perspective. Am J Nurs 2002; 102(6):36–46.

24. Dowd TT, Campbell JM, Jones JA. Fluid intake and urinary incontinence in older community-dwelling women. J Community Health Nurs 1996; 13(3):179–186.

25. Engberg SJ, McDowell BJ, Burgio KL, Watson JE, Belle S. Self-care behaviors of older women with urinary incontinence. J Gerontol Nurs 1995; 21(8):7–14.

26. Johnson TM, Kincade JE, Bernard SL, Busby-Whitehead J, DeFriese GH. Self-care practices used by older men and women to manage urinary incontinence: results from the national follow-up survey on self-care and aging. J Am Geriatr Soc 2000; 48(8):894–902.

27. Griffiths DJ, McCracken PN, Harrison GM, Gormley EA. Relationship of fluid intake to voluntary micturition and urinary incontinence in geriatric patients. Neurourol Urodyn 1993; 12:1–7.

28. Nygaard IE, Linder M. Thirst at work—an occupational hazard? Int Urogyn Pelvic Floor Dysfunc 1997; 8(6):340–343.

29. Fitzgerald S, Palmer MH, Berry SJ, Hart K. (2000) Urinary incontinence: impact on working women. AAOHN J 48(3):112–118.

30. Wyman JF, Elswick RK, Wilsom MS, Fantl JA. Relationship of fluid intake to voluntary micturitions and urinary incontinence in women. Neurourol Urodyn 1991; 11(3): 463–473.

31. Dowd (1991).

32. Kayser-Jones J, Schell ES, Porter C, Barbaccia JC, Shaw H. Factors contributing to dehydration in nursing homes: inadequate staffing and lack of professional supervision. J Am Geriatr Soc 1999; 47:1187–1194.

33. Dallosso HM, McGrother CW, Matthews RJ, Donaldson MMK, Leicestershire MRC Incontinence Study Group. The association of diet and other lifestyle factors with overactive bladder and stress incontinence: a longitudinal study in women. BJU International 2003; 92:69–77.

34. Creighton SM, Stanton SL. Caffeine: does it affect your bladder? Br J Urol 1990; 66:613–614.

35. Lee JG, Wein AJ, Levin RM. The effect of caffeine on the contractile response of the rabbit urinary bladder to field stimulation. Gen Pharmacol 1993; 24(4):1007–1011.

36. Lamarine RJ. Selected health and behavioral effects related to the use of caffeine. J Community Health 1994; 19(6):449–466.

37. Newman DK. Managing and treating urinary incontinence. Baltimore: Health Professions Press, 2002.

38. Tomlinson B, Dougherty M, Pendergast J, Boyington A, Coffman M, Pickens S. Dietary caffeine, fluid intake and urinary incontinence in older rural women. Int Urogynecol J 1999; 10:22–28.

39. Arya LA, Myers DL, Jackson ND. Dietary caffeine intake and the risk for detrusor instability: a case-control study. Obstet Gynecol 2000; 96(1): 85–89.

40. Bryant CM, Dowell CJ, Fairbrother G. Caffeine reduction education to improve urinary symptoms. Br J Nursing 2002; 11(8):560–565.

41. Gray M. Caffeine and urinary continence. JWOCN 2001; 28:66–69.

42. Dohil R, Roberts E, Jones K, Jenkins HR. Constipation and reversible urinary tract abnormalities. Arch Dis Child 1994; 70:56–57.

43. Snooks SJ, Barnes PRH, Setchell M, Henry MM. Damage to the innervation of pelvic floor musculature in chronic constipation. Gastroenterology 1985; 89:977–981.

44. Lubowski DZ, Swash M, Nicholls RJ, Henry MM. Increase in pudendal nerve terminal motor latency with defaecation straining. Br J Surg 1988; 75:1095–1097.

45. Spence-Jones C, Kamm MA, Henry MM, Hudson CN. Bowel dysfunction: a pathogenic factor in ureterovaginal prolapse and urinary stress incontinence. Br J Obstet Gynaecol 1994; 101:147–152.

46. Moller LA, Lose G, Jorgensen T. Risk factors for lower urinary tract symptoms in women 40 to 60 years of age. Obstet. Gynecol 2000; 96(3):446–451.

47. Charach G, Greenstein A, Rabinovich P, Groskopf I, Weintraub M. Alleviating constipation in the elderly improves lower urinary tract symptoms. Gerontology 2001; 47:72–76.

48. Dougherty MC, Dwyer JW, Pendergast JF, Boyington AR, Tomlinson BU, Coward RT, Duncan RP, Vogel B, Rooks LG. A randomized trial of behavioral management for continence with older rural women. Res Nurs Health 2002; 25:3–13.

49. Eustice S, Roe B, Paterson J. Prompted voiding for the management of urinary incontinence in adults. Cochrane Incontinence Group, Cochrane Database of Systematic Reviews, Issue 2, 2002.

50. Ostaszkiewicz J, Johnston L, Roe B. Habit retraining for the management of urinary incontinence in adults. Cochrane Incontinence Group, Cochrane Database of Systematic Reviews, Issue 2, 2002.

51. Ostaszkiewicz J, Johnston L, Roe B. Timed voiding for the management of urinary incontinence in adults. Cochrane Incontinence Group, Cochrane Database of Systematic Reviews, Issue 2, 2002.

52. Lekan-Rutledge D, Colling J. Urinary incontinence in the frail elderly. Am J Nurs 2003; March(suppl).

53. Ouslander JG, Schnelle JF, Uman G, Fingold S, Nigam JG, Tuico E, Bates-Jensen B. Predictors of successful prompted voiding among incontinent nursing home residents. JAMA 1995; 273(17):1366–1370.

54. Lekan-Rutledge D. Diffusion of innovation: a model for implementation of prompted voiding in long term care settings. J Gerontol Nurs 2000; 26(4):25–33.

55. Engberg SJ, Sereika SM, McDowell BJ, Weber E, Brodak I. Effectiveness of prompted voiding in treating urinary incontinence in cognitively impaired homebound older adults. JWOCN 2002; 29(5):252–265.

56. Colling J, Ouslander J, Hadley BJ, Eisch J, Campbell E. The effects of patterned urge response toileting (PURT) on urinary incontinence among nursing home residents. J Am Geriatr Soc 1992; 40:135–141.

57. Colling J, Owen TR, McCreedy M, Newman DK. The effects of a continence program on frail community-dwelling elderly persons. Urol Nurs 2003; April 23(2):117–122; 127–131.

58. Burgio LD, Burgio K. Institutional staff training and management: a review of the literature and a model for geriatric long-term care facilities. Int J Aging Hum Dev 1990; 30:287–302.

59. Remsburg R, Armacost K, Radu C, Bennett R. Two models of restorative nursing care in the nursing home: designated versus integrated restorative nursing assistants. Geriatr Nurs 1999; 20(6):321–326.

60. Jeffcoate TNA, Francis WJA. Urinary incontinence in the female. Am J Obstet Gynecol 1966; 94:604–618.
61. Fantl JA, Wyman JF, McClish DK, Harkins SW, Elswick RK, Taylor JR. Efficacy of bladder training in older women with urinary incontinence. JAMA 1991; 265(5):609–613.
62. Wyman J, Fantl J, McClish D, Harkins S, Uebersax J, Ory M. Quality of life following bladder training in older women with urinary incontinence. Int Urogyn Pelvic Floor Dysfunc J 1997; 8(4):223–229.
63. Roe B, Williams K, Palmer M. Bladder training for urinary incontinence in adults. Cochrane Incontinence Group, Cochrane Database of Systematic Reviews. Issue 2, 2002.
64. Tobani L, Fantl JA. Urinary incontinence in women and the use of bladder training for its management. Mature Med 1999; March/April:90–93.
65. Wyman JF, Fantl JA. Bladder training in ambulatory care management of urinary incontinence. Urol Nurs 1991; 11(3):11–17.
66. Newman DK. The Urinary Incontinence Sourcebook. 2nd ed. California: Lowell House, 1999.
67. Sampselle CM. Behavioral intervention for urinary incontinence for women: evidence for practice. J Midwifery Women's Health 2000; 45(2):94–103.
68. Sale PG, Wyman JF. Achievement of goals associated with bladder training by older incontinent women. Res Briefs 1994; 93–96.
69. Mattiasson A, Blaakaer J, Hoye K, Wein AJ, Tolterodine Scandinavian Study Group. Simplified bladder training augments the effectiveness of tolterodine in patients with an overactive bladder. BJU Int 2003; 91:54–60.
70. Visco AG, Weidner AC, Cundiff GW, Bump RC. Observed patient compliance with a structured bladder retraining program. Obstet Gynecol 1999; 181(6):1392–1394.
71. Kegel AH. Progressive resistance exercise in the functional restoration of the perineal muscles. Am J Obstet Gynecol 1948; 56(2):238–248.
72. Kegel AH. Physiologic therapy for urinary incontinence JAMA 1951; 146:915–917.
73. Benvenuti F, Caputo GM, Bandinelli S, Mayer F, Biagini C, Sommavilla A. Re-educative treatment of female genuine stress incontinence. Am J Phys Ther 1987; 66:155–168.
74. Bo K et al. (1990).
75. Ferguson K, McKey PL, Bishop KR, Kloen P, Verheul JB, Dougherty MC. Stress urinary incontinence: effect of pelvic muscle exercise. Obstet Gynecol 1990; 73:671–675.
76. Dougherty M, Bishop K, Mooney R, Gimotty P, Williams B. Graded pelvic muscle exercise. Effect on stress urinary incontinence. J Reprod Med 1993; 39(9):684–691.
77. Boyington A, Dougherty M. Pelvic muscle exercise effect on pelvic muscle performance in women. Int Urogynecol J 2000; 11:212–218.
78. Theofrastous JP, Wyman JF, Bump RC. The relationship between urethral and vaginal pressures during pelvic floor muscle contraction. Neurourol Urodyn 1997; 16:553–558.
79. Bo K, Talseth T. Change in urethral pressure during voluntary pelvic floor muscle contraction and vaginal electrical stimulation. Int Urogynecol J 1997; 8:3–7.
80. Miller JM. Criteria for therapeutic use of pelvic floor muscle training in women. JWOCN 2002; 29(6):301–311.
81. Miller J, Aston-Miller J, DeLancey J. The knack: use of precisely-timed pelvic muscle contraction can reduce leakage in SUI. Neurourol Urodyn 1996; 15:302–393.
82. Miller JM, Ashton-Miller JA, DeLancey JOL. A pelvic muscle precontraction can reduce cough-related urine loss in selected women with mild SUI. J Am Geriatr Soc 1998; 46:870–874.
83. Miller JM, Perucchini D, Carchidi L, DeLancey JOL, Ashton-Miller JA. Pelvic floor muscle contraction during a cough and decreased vesical neck mobility. Obstet Gynecol 2001; 97(2):255–260.
84. Viktrup L, Bump R. Simplified neurophysiology of the lower urinary tract. Prim Care Update Ob/Gyns 2003; 10(5):261–264.
85. DeLancey JO. Stress urinary incontinence: where are we now, where should do we go? Am J Obstet Gynecol 1996; 175:311–319.

86. Brubaker et al. (1993).

87. Miller J, Kasper C, Sampselle C. Review of muscle physiology with application to pelvic muscle exercise. Urol Nurs 1994; 14(3):92–97.

88. Newman DK. Continence for Women: Research-Based Practice. Association of Women's Health, Obstetric and Neonatal Nurses: Washington, DC, 2000.

89. Dougherty M. Current status of research on pelvic muscle strengthening techniques. JWOCN 1998; 25(2):75–83.

90. Ashton-Miller J, Howard D, DeLancey J. The functional anatomy of the female pelvic floor and stress continence control system. Scand J Urol Nephrol Suppl 2001; 207:1–7.

91. Newman DK, Smith DA. Pelvic muscle reeducation as a nursing treatment for incontinence. Urol Nurs 1992; 12(l):9–15.

92. Newman DK. Clinical Manual—Pelvic Muscle Rehabilitation. Prometheus: Dover, NH, 2003:89–98.

93. Sampselle C, DeLancey J. The urine stream interruption test and pelvic muscle function. Nurs Res 1992; 41(2):73–77.

94. DeLancey JO, Sampselle CM, Punch MR. Kegel dyspareunia: levator ani myalgia caused by overexertion. Obstet Gynecol 1993; 82(40):658–659.

95. Newman DK. Stress urinary incontinence in women. Am J Nurs 2003; 103(8):46–55.

96. Gallo M, Staskin D. Cues to action: pelvic floor muscle exercise compliance in women with stress urinary incontinence. Neurourol Urodyn 1997; 16:167–177.

97. Hirsch A, Weirauch G, Steimer B, Bihler K, Peschers U, Bergauer F, Leib B, Dimpfl T. Treatment of female urinary incontinence with EMG-controlled biofeedback home training. Int Urogynecol J 1999; 10:7–10

98. Aukee P, Immonen P, Penttinen J, Laippala P, Airaksinen O. Increase in pelvic floor muscle activity after 12 weeks' training: a randomized prospective pilot study. Urology. 2002; 60(6):1020–1024.

99. Bo K, Talseth, T. Long-term effect of pelvic floor muscle exercise 5 years after cessation of organized training. Obstet Gyncol 1996; 87:261–265.

100. Cammu H, Van Nylen M, Amy JJ. A 10-year follow-up after Kegel pelvic floor muscle exercises for genuine stress incontinence. BJU Int 2000; 85:655–658.

101. Sampselle CM, Miller JM, Mims BL, DeLancey JOL, Ashton-Miller JA, Antonakos CL. Effect of pelvic muscle exercise and transient incontinence during pregnancy and after birth. Obstet Gynecol 1998; 91(3):406–412.

102. Sampselle CM, Wyman JF, Thomas KK, Newman DK, Gray M. Continence for women: evaluation of AWHONN's third research utilization project. J Obstet Gynecol Neonat Nurs 2000a; 29(1):9–17.

103. Sampselle CM, Wyman JF, Thomas KK, Newman DK, Gray M. Continence for women: a test of AWHONN's evidence-based protocol in clinical practice. J Obstet Gynecol Neonat Nurs 2000b; 29(1):18–26.

104. Newman DK, Palmer MH, Mason D. The state of the science on urinary incontinence. Am J Nurs 2003; March(suppl):1–72.

105. Sapsford R, Hodges P. Contraction of the pelvic floor muscles during abdominal maneuvers. Arch Phys Med Rehabil 2001; 82:1081–1088.

106. Workman D, Cassis J, Dougherty M. Validation of surface EMG as a measure of intravaginal and intraabdominal activity: implications for biofeedback-assisted Kegel exercises. Psychophysiology 1993; 30:120.

107. Wyman JF et al. (2002).

108. Bo K, Finckenhagen B. Vaginal palpation of pelvic floor muscle strength: inter-test reproducibility and comparison between palpation and vaginal squeeze pressure. Acta Obstet Gynaecol Scand 2001; 80:883–887.

109. Morkved S, Bo K, Fjortoft T. Effect of adding biofeedback to pelvic muscle exercise training to treat urodynamic stress incontinence. Obstet Gynecol 2002; 100(4):730–739.

110. Baigis-Smith J, Smith D, Rose M, Newman D. Managing urinary incontinence in community-residing elderly persons. Gerontologists 1989; 29(2): 229–233.

111. Burns PA, Pranioff K, Nochajski TH, Hadley EC, Levy KJ, Ory MG. A comparison of effectiveness of biofeedback and pelvic muscle exercise treatment of stress-incontinence in older community-dwelling women. J Gerontol 1993; 48(4):167–174.

112. Burgio K, Whitehead WE, Engel BT. Urinary incontinence in the elderly: bladder-sphincter biofeedback and toileting skills training. Ann Intern Med 1985; 104:507–515.

113. Burgio K, Robinson J, Engel B. The role of biofeedback in Kegel exercise training for stress urinary incontinence. Am J Obstet Gynecol 1986; 154(1): 58–64.

114. Burgio KL, Stutzman RE, Engel BT. Behavioral training for post-prostatectomy urinary incontinence. J Urol 1989; 141:303–306.

115. Burton et al. (1988).

116. McDowell BJ, Burgio KL, Dombrowski M, Locher JL, Rodriguez E. An interdisciplinary approach to the assessment and behavioral treatment of urinary incontinence in geriatric outpatients. J Am Geriatr Soc 1992; 40:370–374.

117. Holtedahl K, Verelst M, Schiefloe A. A population based randomized, controlled trial of conservative treatment for urinary incontinence in women. Acta Obstet Gynaecol Scand 1998; 77:671–677.

118. Sampselle et al. (2000).

119. McDowell BJ, Engberg S, Sereika S, Donovan N, Jubeck ME, Weber E, Engberg R. Effectiveness of behavioral therapy to treat incontinence in homebound older adults. J Am Geriatr Soc 1999; 47(3):309–318.

120. Flynn L, Cell P, Luisi E. Effectiveness of pelvic muscle exercises in reducing urge incontinence among community residing elders. J Gerontol Nurs 1994; May 20(5):23–27.

121. Van Kampen M, De Weerdt W, Van Poppel H, DeRidder, Feys M, Baert, L. Effect of pelvic-floor re-education on duration and degree of incontinence after radical prostatectomy: a randomized controlled trial. Lancet 2000; 355:98–102.

122. Wyman JF, Fantl JA, McClish DK, Bump RC. Continence Program for Women Research Group. Comparative efficacy of behavioral interventions in the management of female urinary incontinence. Am J Obstet Gynecol 1998; 179(4):999–1007.

123. Burgio K, Locher J, Goode P, Hardin M, McDowell B, Dombrowski M, Candib D. Behavioral vs. drug treatment for urge urinary incontinence in older women. JAMA 1998; 280(23):1995–1999.

124. Brink CA, Sampselle CM, Well TJ, Diokno AC, Gillis GL. A digital test for pelvic muscle strength in older women with urinary incontinence. Nurs Res 1989; 38:196–197.

125. Berghmans LCM, Hendricks HJM, Bo K. Conservative treatment of stress urinary incontinence in women: a systematic review of randomize clinical trails. Br J Urol 1998; 82:181–191.

126. Berghmans LCM, Hendricks HJM, De Bie RA, Van Waalwijk ESC, Van Doorn, Bo K, Van Kerrebroeck PEV. Conservative treatment of urge urinary incontinence in women: a systematic review of randomized clinical trials. BJU Int 2000; 85:254–263.

127. Burgio K, Goode PS, Locher JL, Umlauf MG, Roth DL, Richter HE. Behavioral training with and without biofeedback in the treatment of urge incontinence in older women. JAMA 2002; 288(18):2293–2299.

128. Burgio K, Locher J, Goode P. Combined behavioral and drug therapy for urge incontinence in older women. J Am Geriatr Soc 2000; 48:370–374.

129. Herbison P, Plevnik S, Mantle J. Weighted vaginal cones for urinary incontinence (Cochrane Review). In: The Cochrane Library, Issue 1, 2002. Oxford: Update Software.

130. Glazener CM, Herbison GP, Wilson PD, MacArthur C, Lang GD, Gee H. Conservative management of persistent postnatal urinary and faecal incontinence: randomised controlled trial. Br Med J 2001; 323(7313):593–596.

131. Cammu H, Van Nylen M. Pelvic floor exercises versus vaginal weight cones in genuine stress incontinence. Eur J Obstet Gynecol Reprod Biol 1998; 77:89–93.

132. Wyman JF. Treatment of urinary incontinence men and older women. Am J Nurs 2003; March(suppl).

133. Bent AF, Sand PK, Ostergard DR, Brubaker L. Transvaginal electrical stimulation in the treatment of genuine stress incontinence and detrusor instability. Int Urogynecol J 1993; 14:9–13.

134. Brubaker L, Benson JT, Bent A, et al. Transvaginal electrical stimulation for female urinary incontinence. Am J Obstet Gynecol 1997; 177:536–540.

135. Luber KM, Wolde-Tsadik G. Efficacy of functional electrical stimulation in treating genuine stress incontinence: a randomized clinical trial. Neurourol Urodyn 1997; 16:543–551.

136. Richardson DA, Miller KL, Siegel SW, Karram MM, Blackwood NB, Staskin DR. Pelvic floor electrical stimulation: a comparison of daily and every-other-day therapy for genuine stress incontinence. Urology 1996; 48:110–118.

137. Sand PK, Richardson DA, Staskin DK, Swift SE, et al. Pelvic floor electrical stimulation in the treatment of genuine stress incontinence: a multicenter, placebo-controlled trial. Am J Obstet Gynecol 1995; 173:72–79.

138. Yamanishi T, Yasuda K, Sakakibara R, Hattori T, Suda S. Randomized, double-blind study of electrical stimulation for urinary incontinence due to detrusor overactivity. Urology 2000; 55:353–357.

139. Hay-Smith EJC, Bo K, Berghmans LCM, Hendriks HJM, de Bie RA, van Wallwijk, van Doorne ESC. Pelvic floor muscle training for urinary incontinence in women (Cochrane Review). In: The Cochrane Library, 2002, Issue 2. Oxford: Update Software Ltd.

140. Goode PS, Burgio KL, Locher JL, Roth DL, Umlauf MG, Richter HE, Varner RE, Lloyd LK. Effect of behavioral training with or without pelvic floor electrical stimulation on stress incontinence in women: a randomized controlled trial. JAMA 16 Jul 2003; 290(3):395–397.

141. Medicare Coverage Issues Manual. Rockville, MD: Center for Medicare and Medicaid Services, Dept of Health and Human Services; 2000.

142. Agency for Health Care Policy & Research, Public Health Service. Urinary Incontinence in Adults: Clinical Practice Guideline (AHCPR Pub. No. 92-0038). Rockville, MD: U.S. Dept of Health and Human Services, 1992.

143. Brubaker L, Benson JT, Bent A, Clark A, Shott S. Transvaginal electrical stimulation for female urinary incontinence. Am J Obstet Gynecol 1997; 177(3):536–540.

144. Burgio K, Engel T. Biofeedback-assisted behavioral training for elderly men and women. J Am Geriatr Soc 1990; 38:338–340.

145. Burns P, Pranikoss K, Nochajski T, Desotelle P, Harwood M. Treatment of stress incontinence with pelvic floor exercises and biofeedback. J Am Geriatr Soc 1990; 38:341–344.

146. Cammu H, Van Nylen M, Derde M-P, DeBruyne R, Amy JJ. Pelvic physiotherapy in genuine stress incontinence. Urology 1991; 38(4):332–337.

147. Dietz H, Wilson P, Clarke B. The use of perineal ultrasound to quantify levator activity and teach pelvic floor muscle exercises. Int Urogynecol J 2001; 12:166–169.

148. Engberg SJ, McDowell BJ, Weber E, Brodak I, Donovan N, Engberg R. Assessment and management of urinary incontinence among homebound older adults: a clinical trial protocol. Adv Prac Nurs Q 1997; 3(2):48–56.

149. Ferrie BG, Smith JS, Logan D, Lyle R, Paterson PJ. Experience with bladder training in 65 patients. Br J Urol 1984; 56:482–484.

150. Fischer W, Linde A. Pelvic floor findings in urinary incontinence—results of conditioning using vaginal cones. Acta Obstet Gynaecol Scand 1997; 76: 455–460.

151. Laycock J, Brown J, Cusack C, Green S, Jerwood D, Mann K, McLachlan Z, Schofield A. Pelvic floor reeducation for stress incontinence: comparing three methods. Br J Community Nurs 2001; 6(5):230–237.

152. Lekan-Rutledge D, McConnell ES, Anderson RA, Corazzini-Gomez K. Evidence-based practice in long term care: promoting sustainability of prompted voiding. Unpublished manuscript, 2002.

153. Luber KM, Wolde-Tsadik G. Efficacy of functional electrical stimulation in treating genuine stress incontinence: a multicenter, clinical trial. Physiotherapy 1997; 79:553–540.

154. Nygaard I, Kreder K, Lepic M, Fountain K, Rhomberg A. Efficacy of pelvic floor muscle exercises in women with stress, urge, and mixed urinary incontinence. Am J Obstet Gynecol 1995; 174(1): 120–125.

155. Palmer MH, Fitzgerald S, Berry SJ, Hart K. Urinary incontinence in working women: an exploratory study. Women Health. 1999; 29(3):67–80.
156. Theofrastous JP, Wyman JF, Bump RC, et al. Effects of pelvic floor muscle training on strength and predictors of response in the treatment of urinary incontinence in women. Neurourol Urodyn 2002; 21:486–490.

Patient Guide #1: Caffeine Chart

Source of caffeine		Serving Size	Caffeine (mg)
Coffee:	Brewed, drip	8 oz.	100–164
	Brewed, percolated	8 oz.	80–135
	Instant	8 oz.	50–75
	Decaffeinated	5 oz.	2–4
Tea (black or green)	1-min brew	5 oz.	20–34
	3-min brew	5 oz.	35–46
	5-min brew	5 oz.	39–50
Instant tea		5 oz	30
Iced tea		12 oz.	67–76
Hot chocolate		5 oz.	2–15
Soft drinks	Jolt Cola	12 oz.	71
	Mountain Dew	12 oz.	54
	Coca-Cola	12 oz.	60
	Diet Coke	12 oz.	46
	Tab	12 oz.	49
	Pepsi-Cola	12 oz.	43
	Diet Pepsi	12 oz.	36
	Dr. Pepper	12 oz.	60
	Red Bull	12 oz.	106
Chocolate desserts	Brownie (with nut)	1.25 oz.	8
	Cake	1/16 of 9″	14
	Ice cream	2/3 cup	5
	Pudding	2 cup	6
Chocolate candy	Milk chocolate	1 oz.	1–15
	Sweet, dark chocolate	1 oz.	20
	Baking chocolate	1 oz.	25–35
Painkillers	Anacin	2 tablets	64
	Excedrin	2 tablets	130
	Vanquish	2 tablets	66
	Midol	2 tablets	64
	Darvon compound	2 tablets	65
	Fiorinal	2 tablets	80
	Norgesic	2 tablets	30
Cold/allergy	Dristan	2 tablets	32
	Sinarest	1 tablet	30
Stimulants	No-Doz	2 tablets	200
	Vivarin	1 tablet	200

Patient Guide #2: Maintaining Bowel Regularity

Sometimes urinary incontinence, urgency, and frequency may be aggravated by increased pressure on the bladder from the pressure related to *constipation* or *stool (hard) impaction*. Eating foods that have a lot of fiber helps overcome this problem. Fiber-rich foods include whole-grain breads, brown or wild rice, cereals, nuts, and raw fruits and vegetables. Apricot juice has more fiber content than prune juice. Another way to increase your fiber is by using a special bran recipe.

How to make "Special Bran Recipe"
Mix together:

1 cup applesauce	You can buy unprocessed wheat bran in the
1 cup coarse unprocessed wheat bran	grocery or health food stores. This type of bran
$\frac{3}{4}$ cup prune juice	is different from bran cereal.

Refrigerate mixture and take 2 tablespoons of the mixture every day. Take the mixture in the evening for a morning bowel movement. Increase the bran mixture by one tablespoon until your bowel movements become regular. If the amount exceeds 4 tablespoons, take the mixture in divided doses in the morning and evening. Always drink one large glass of water with the mixture.

What if I don't like the "Special Bran Recipe"?
Add unprocessed wheat bran to your diet. Start by using 1–2 tablespoons every day. If necessary for regulation, increase bran slowly over several weeks to approximately 6 tablespoons every day. Mix bran in foods like applesauce, cereals, or sauces, or use it as a spice in gravies or puddings. Sprinkle bran on ice cream, vegetable and fruit salads, or cottage cheese. Add to muffins, breads, and cookies when baking.

When will I notice a change?
You may notice effects on bowel function 3–5 days after starting bran or other natural remedies. You should continue to use these remedies.

Will bran and other natural remedies harm me?
No! The normal reaction to bran is stomach bloating and increased gas. These symptoms usually last for only the 1st week. If symptoms last longer, contact your nurse or doctor.

© 2001 Diane K. Newman

Patient Guide #3: Bladder Retraining—Controlling Urgency and Frequency

---

Frequency is voiding often, usually eight times or more in a 24-h period. Frequency can worsen if you get into the habit of voiding "just in case," which means that the bladder never fills completely and holds only a small amount of urine. It is better to wait until the bladder is full.

Urgency is a sudden need to void immediately that can cause urine leakage on the way to the bathroom. Urgency follows a wave pattern; it starts, grows, peaks and then subsides until it stops.

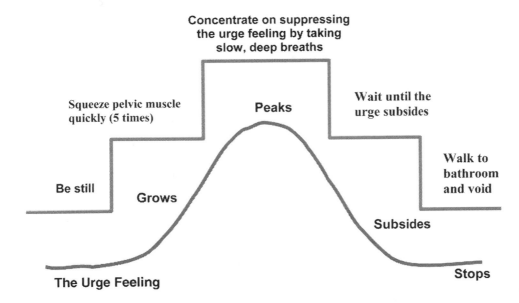

The key to controlling the urinary urge is *not* to respond by rushing to the bathroom. Rushing causes movement, which jiggles your bladder, which in turn increases the feeling of urge.

Controlling the urge
The goal is for you to be voiding no more than every ____ hours. If you get the *urge* to void and it is not yet your scheduled voiding time, stop all activity and sit down if possible. Then try one or more of the following techniques that may help the urge to subside allowing the bladder to relax and give you more time to get to the bathroom:

Take some slow, deep breaths through your mouth, concentrating on your breathing, or
Tighten your pelvic muscle *quickly and hard* several times in a row.
Use mental distraction strategies such as concentrating on an activity, such as counting backward from 100 by sevens, or reciting the words of a favorite song or nursery rhyme.

© 2001 Diane K. Newman

Patient Guide #4: Pelvic Muscle Exercises & the "KNACK"

WHAT IS THE PELVIC MUSCLE? – Your pelvic muscle provides support to your bladder, and rectum and, in women, the vagina and the uterus. If it weakens or is damaged, it cannot support these organs and their position can change. This can cause problems with the organs normal function. Keeping the muscle strong can help prevent bladder control problems and unwanted urine leakage.

FINDING THE PELVIC MUSCLE – Without tensing the muscles of your leg, buttocks or abdomen, imagine that you are trying to control the passing of gas or pinching off a stool. Or imagine you are in an elevator full of people and you feel the urge to pass gas. What do you do? You tighten or pull in the ring of muscle around your rectum – your pelvic muscle. You should feel a lifting sensation in the area around the vagina or a pulling in of your rectum.

EXERCISE REGIMEN – There are two types of muscle contractions you will need to practice – **Short** (2 second) or **Quick** contractions and **Slow** (3 or 5 or 10 second) or **long** contractions. To do the short or quick muscle contractions, contract or tighten your pelvic muscle quickly and hard and immediately relax it. For the slow or long (sustained) contractions, contract or tighten your pelvic muscle and hold for a count of (3 or 5 or 10 as prescribed) seconds, then relax the muscle completely for the same amount of time. It is equally important to control when your muscle tightens and relaxes. Be sure to relax completely between each muscle tightening.

WHERE TO PRACTICE – You should do the exercises in these positions:
> *Lying Down* – Lie on your back with your head on a pillow, knees bent and feet slightly apart.
> *Sitting* – Sit upright in a firm seat and straight-back chair, knees slightly apart, feet flat on the floor or legs stretched out in front and crossed at the ankles.
> *Standing* – Stand and lean on a back of a chair, knees slightly bent with feet shoulder width apart and toes slightly pointed outward. You can also lean on the kitchen counter with your hips flexed.

PERFORMING THE "KNACK" – In addition to doing your prescribed set of pelvic muscle exercises, you should start contracting your pelvic muscle at the time your incontinence occurs. Timing your pelvic muscle contraction to when your incontinence is most likely to occur is called the "KNACK." This is the skill of consciously timing an intentional contraction of the pelvic muscles just before and throughout the activity that causes an increase in your urine leakage (incontinence) or bladder control problem such as urgency.

HOW TO DO THE "KNACK" – The "KNACK" is an acquired motor skill that requires you to anticipate your urine leakage. Any activity, which increases pressure in your abdomen, may cause you to lose urine. Examples of such activities are: coughing, sneezing, laughing, bending/lifting, carrying objects, sitting down, standing up, and going up/down stairs. During these activities, pressure is placed on the bladder, forcing urine to leak out. You should practice the "KNACK" by contracting the pelvic floor muscles:

- Immediately before initiating a hard cough and maintaining the contraction throughout the cough
- Do *5 quick pelvic muscle contractions when you get a strong urge* that you cannot control.
- Tighten your muscle on the way to the bathroom. Remember, the more exercising you do:
  - The stronger your pelvic muscles will get.
  - The faster they will get stronger.
  - The easier it will be to maintain muscle strength.

REMEMBER – It may take some time to translate the "KNACK" successfully into daily life.

MAKING THE EXERCISES PART OF YOUR DAILY ACTIVITY – Once your muscles are stronger and you incontinence and urgency are better, you should do these exercises as part of your daily routine (activities you do on a daily basis). This means you do both types of exercises, short and long muscle contractions. You do not have to keep a formal count of the number of times you do each exercise. Just do them several times in a row and often enough to make them a habit. Do your exercises when you are:

- Standing at the sink and brushing your teeth
- Sitting in the car at a stop light.
- Reading a book in bed.
- Going for a walk.
- Talking on the phone.

YOU MUST PRACTICE SO THAT EXERCISING BECOMES A HABIT.
ALMOST LIKE A REFLEX ACTION!!

15

Pessaries and Vaginal Devices for Stress Incontinence

G. Willy Davila and Minda Neimark
Cleveland Clinic Florida, Weston, Florida, U.S.A.

I. INTRODUCTION

Pessaries and other intravaginal devices have long been used for the treatment of pelvic floor dysfunction in women. Initial descriptions of vaginal device use entailed intravaginal placement of objects to support genital prolapse and/or administer therapeutic chemicals. Specific applications of pessaries for women with stress urinary incontinence (SUI) are rather recent. Owing to the high coexistence of genital prolapse and urinary incontinence, it is likely that many women who were fit with a pessary for genital prolapse noted an improvement in their urinary incontinence. Alternatively, women with exteriorized prolapse may have occult stress incontinence which is uncovered upon being fit with a vaginal pessary for reduction of the prolapse.

The concept of intravaginal device use as an option for SUI treatment is very useful for the practicing clinician. As our population ages, with an increased incidence of pelvic floor dysfunction, alternatives to surgery become more desirable. There are many urogynecologic indications for pessary usage (Table 1). In addition, technological developments have led to innovative designs of intravaginal devices with specific purposes such as elevation of the urethrovesical junction (UVJ) (Fig. 1). To achieve continence, a device should provide elevation

Table 1 Indications for Pessary Use

Vaginal and uterine prolapse
Stress incontinence
Patient unable to safely undergo pelvic reconstructive surgery
Desire to delay surgery
Evaluation of continence mechanism in moderate to severe vaginal prolapse
Preoperatively demonstrate effectiveness of urethropexy for SUI
Pregnant patient with incompetent cervix/premature delivery/multiple gestation
Genital prolapse in the neonate
Low back/pelvic pain secondary to genital prolapse
Postoperative usage following pelvic reconstructive surgery to prevent recurrence

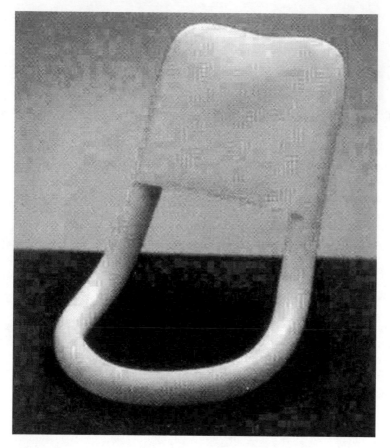

Figure 1 Intravaginal devices specifically useful for enhancing bladder neck support: (a) Smith-Hodge pessary; (*continued*)

and support of the urethrovesical junction and/or extrinsically enhance urethral sphincteric function by compression. While doing this, outflow obstruction should be avoided to prevent significant urinary retention and its consequences.

II. PESSARIES AND STRESS INCONTINENCE

Voiding difficulty, bladder outlet obstruction, and occult stress incontinence may coexist in a patient with severe prolapse. The initial descriptions of vaginal pessary use for stress urinary incontinence were not in its therapy, but rather in the uncovering of occult stress incontinence in women with advanced degrees of prolapse (1). It was suggested that the mechanism of continence in women with severe prolapse is urethral obstruction, which increases maximum urethral closure pressure and pressure transmission ratio. It has been demonstrated that up to 70% of women with moderate to severe pelvic organ prolapse will demonstrate stress incontinence once the prolapse has been reduced (2–5). Subsequently, Bhatia and colleagues described the impact of a Smith-Hodge pessary on urodynamic parameters in women with stress urinary incontinence (6). A pessary's effect on urethral mobility and urodynamic parameters were described and noted to be similar to those of a successful bladder neck

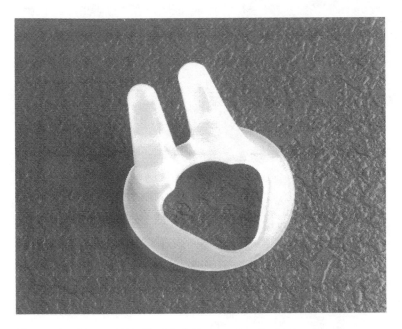

Figure 1   (b) Introl Bladder Neck Support Prosthesis; (*continued*)

suspension (Table 2). No evidence of urinary outflow obstruction was found. The use of Smith-Hodge pessaries for stress incontinence was popularized as a result of these data.

A "pessary test" was suggested for identification of occult stress incontinence in women with advanced degrees of genital prolapse, and as a prognostic test for success of anti-incontinence surgery—similar to a Bonney or Marshall test (7,8). Similarity in changes in continence mechanism with improvements in functional urethral length, urethral pressure profiles, and cough profiles was demonstrated in those who became asymptomatic with a pessary and those who underwent a Burch urethropexy. Smith-Hodge, Ring, and Gellhorn pessaries are most frequently used for this evaluation (2–4,9). When using this test, care must be taken to avoid compressing the urethra and causing outflow obstruction. Smith-Hodge pessaries are especially useful for this purpose owing to the notched nature of the retropubic square end (Fig. 1a). Another practical feature of the Hodge pessary is the ability to modify its shape by folding it into a better-fitting device for an individual patient. The curvature of the pessary frequently requires shape adjustment in order to achieve a snug retropubic fit.

Other intravaginal devices have also been studied for the nonsurgical treatment of SUI. Contraceptive diaphragms, owing to their retropubic placement, may result in improved bladder neck support. In one study, complete resolution of SUI was reported in 91% of women fit with a diaphragm (10). Discomfort with the device in place led to discontinuation by 16% of the women. In addition, contraceptive diaphragms have been associated with the occurrence of urinary tract infections due to their effect on urethral outflow (11). Diaphragm fitting rings can also be effective in treating SUI in some women (12). Diaphragms and fitting rings may be useful in the patient with mild SUI and minimal prolapse. However, if significant prolapse is present or urine loss occurs with minimal exertion, diaphragms may not be strong enough to provide sufficient urethrovesical junction (UVJ) support.

Vaginal tampons have also been used for SUI. Many women have reported that SUI is improved during menses when a tampon is in place. Tampons have been listed as effective

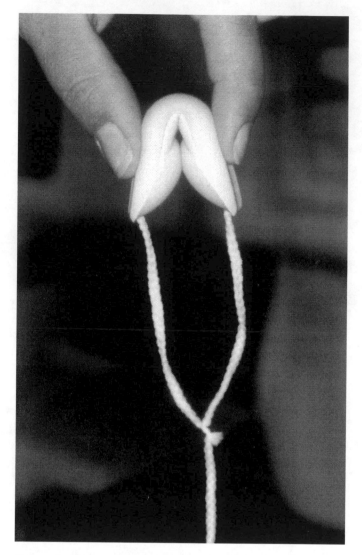

Figure 1   (c) Continence Guard; (*continued*)

conservative options for the management of SUI (13). When compared to a Hodge pessary, a super tampon was found to be equally effective in reducing urine loss during an exercise session (14). In this study, the devices were used only during exercise sessions, and urodynamics was not performed. Thus, the author's conclusions may not be applicable to many women with SUI. However, the wide availability and low cost of tampons make them an attractive first-line intravaginal therapy for SUI. Importantly, extra-absorbent tampons should not be left in place for more than 6 h at a time in order to avoid the risk of toxic shock syndrome.

Innovative devices specifically designed to elevate the bladder neck in a manner similar to a bladder neck suspension have recently been studied. The Introl Bladder Neck Support Prosthesis (BNSP) (Uromed Corp., Needham, MA) is available in the Far East but not widely used in the United States, despite approval by the FDA (Fig. 1b). It is a silicone ring-shaped device with two prongs at one end. Upon insertion, the prongs fit retropubically to provide

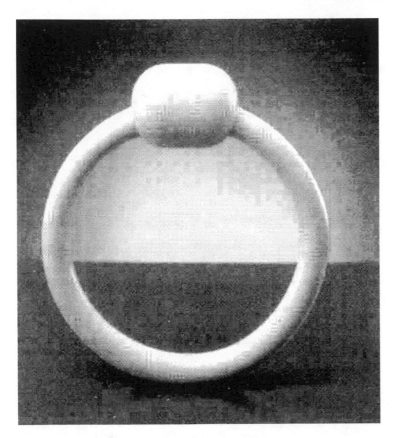

Figure 1   (d) Continence Ring.

bladder neck support (Fig. 2). It was shown to reduce urine loss by 80% in most users with stress incontinence, with urodynamic effects similar to a bladder neck suspension (15). A multicenter study evaluating women with stress and mixed incontinence confirmed these findings (16). Fluoroscopic evaluation of a woman with a BNSP in place helps us understand the effect of a vaginal device in enhancing bladder neck and proximal urethral support (Fig. 3). Its widespread use was limited by its cost and by the difficulties encountered in individualized fitting. Women who used the BNSP only during specific physical activities (i.e., jogging, tennis, etc.) were noted to be the most successful subgroup of users.

A disposable intravaginal device specifically designed to provide urethral support during exertion has been available in Europe. The Continence Guard is a single-use polyurethane foldable device (Fig. 1c). Thyssen and Lose showed that 95% of their study population were either dry or improved with the Continence Guard in place (17). Significant reduction in urine loss on a 24-h pad test, without alteration in uroflowmetry parameters, was noted (18). A multicenter study of this device revealed objective improvement in 75% of the study population, with 46% being dry on a pad test (19).

Most recently, in the United Kingdom, a cylindrical vaginal device designed to provide bladder neck support in women with stress incontinence has been marketed (Contiform, Bard Limited Forest House, West Sussex, U.K.). Its cylindrical design prevents its collapse during

Table 2   Urodynamic Effects of Pessaries

1. Enhance bladder neck support—normalize Q-tip angle
2. Lengthen urethra—increase functional urethral length
3. Enhance urethral sphincteric mechanism—increase urethral closure pressure
4. Enhance urethral dynamic function—increase pressure transmission ratio
5. Allow normal voiding—no effect on uroflow parameters

strenuous activities. It is reported to not cause outflow obstruction and results in continence in 85% of users (Bard Limited Forest House, data on file).

Multiple other devices are being marketed for intravaginal treatment of SUI. However, most have not undergone scientific study. Many commonly available pessaries have been modified by adding a "cushion" at one end to enhance urethral compression (Fig. 1d). Care must be taken to avoid urethral obstruction during usage.

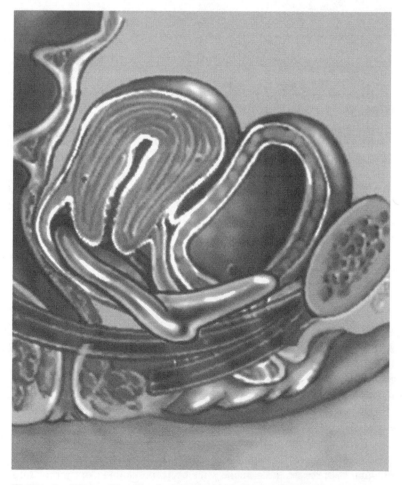

Figure 2   Effect of intravaginal device in bladder neck support—lateral view.

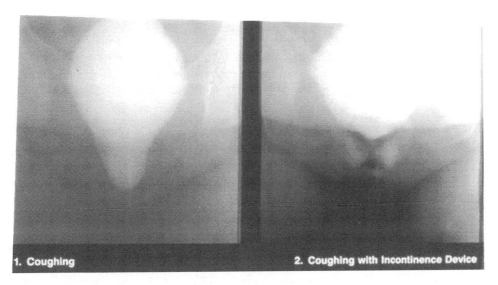

1. Coughing   2. Coughing with Incontinence Device

Figure 3 Fluoroscopic appearance of intravaginal device enhancing proximal urethral support.

III. HISTORICAL PESSARY APPLICATIONS

In the 1800s, Hugh Lenox Hodge designed the lever pessary to treat uterine retroversion thought to be a cause of pelvic pain (20). As modifications of the lever pessary were made, other indications were proposed for its use. In 1961, Vitsky suggested that cervical incompetence was due to a lack of central uterine support. Uterine retroversion has also been associated with infertility and pelvic pain. Placing a lever pessary would displace the cervix posteriorly, thus lifting the weight of the uterus off of the incompetent cervix (21). Women diagnosed with an incompetent cervix were treated during pregnancy with a Hodge pessary from 14 to 38 weeks' gestation, with an 83% successful pregnancy rate (22). Currently, cervical cerclage is the treatment of choice for women with cervical incompetence. There is great controversy regarding the possible causative role of uterine retroversion in many gynecologic conditions including pelvic pain, infertility, and sexual dysfunction.

IV. PESSARIES FOR GENITAL PROLAPSE

Use of vaginal devices for prolapse reduction and administration of chemicals is documented as far back as during the early Egyptian civilization. Written documentation of efforts to reduce genital prolapse with vaginal objects dates back as far back as the fifth century. Modernization of the pessary came with the discovery of vulcanization of rubber and a better understanding of female anatomy. Since then, multiple modifications in pessary design and material selection for manufacture have been made (23).

Advances in gynecologic surgery and anesthesia over the last several decades have reduced the need for pessary usage in the treatment of prolapse and incontinence. However, the recent increase in the elderly population requiring conservative treatment of prolapse and incontinence has led to a resurgence of pessary use (24). In addition, there remains a very acceptable role for therapeutic use of a vaginal pessary in the premenopausal patient. In a recent survey administered to members of the American Urogynecologic Society, 77% of the respondents used pessaries as a first-line therapy for prolapse, and only 12% reserved pessaries for women who were not surgical candidates. In addition, 92% of the physicians surveyed believed that pessaries relieved symptoms associated with pelvic organ prolapse, and 48% felt they had a therapeutic benefit in addition to relieving the symptoms (25).

In a simple prospective protocol for pessary management, patients with symptomatic pelvic prolapse were given the option of pessary use versus surgery or expectant management. If the vaginal pessary was chosen as the method of treatment, the patient was fitted with a ring pessary or a pessary that could be retained without difficulty. The patient then followed up at scheduled intervals to evaluate pessary effectiveness. Sixty-six percent of those who used a pessary for >1 month remained users after 12 months. Fifty-three percent of the patients continued to wear the pessary after 36 months (26). A retrospective series of 107 patients who were fit with a Gellhorn, cube, or ring pessary for symptomatic vaginal prolapse for various indications including medically unfit for surgery, awaiting surgery, or desired conservative management, confirmed that at least 50% of the women continued use of their pessary without complications at follow-up (27). Of those who continued pessary use, 20% were patients who initially desired surgery but later declined because of their satisfaction with the vaginal pessary.

At our center, pessaries are frequently used as first-line therapy for prolapse and incontinence. Review of our usage trends reveals rather equivalent use of the Smith-Hodge and Continence Ring pessaries for SUI. For advanced degrees of prolapse, our most commonly used pessary is the Gelhorn. Cube pessaries should only be used with extreme caution in women who will be compliant with follow-up, as the suctioned adherence to the vaginal sidewalls may lead to significant mucosal erosions and ulcerations. A significant number of women who wear pessaries for SUI or prolapse eventually become frustrated with the efforts required for safe pessary use, and opt for surgical management.

V. PESSARY TYPES

Many different types of pessaries are available, most made of medical-grade silicone or rubber. Although the majority were designed for specific types of prolapse, clinical use is typically based on a "best fit" choice (Table 3). Whichever pessary is chosen, it must fit snugly without causing discomfort to the patient, allowing her to void easily. The health care provider must be prepared to try several different types and sizes until the correct pessary is found for each individual patient.

VI. PERCEIVED DRAWBACKS TO PESSARY USE

Clinicians may be hesitant to recommend pessary use by women with SUI. Various factors account for this reluctance. Owing to variations in pelvic anatomy, optimal fitting of a pessary may be challenging. In addition, the large number of pessary types, each with various sizes, further complicates the process. Because pessary fitting is a trial- and error-process, a clinician must have a large inventory of pessaries of varying sizes in order to accomplish appropriate fitting of patients. An appropriately fit pessary is comfortable, remains in place with ambulation, and allows for normal voiding.

Pessary care recommendations should be followed closely for safe long-term use (Table 4). The patient who cannot self-care for the pessary must be seen by the clinician on a regular basis. We recommend scheduled office visits for pessary care every 6 weeks. Patients must be encouraged to use intravaginal estrogen cream regularly. Some patients may be able to perform pessary self-care if removal is facilitated by attaching a string (dental floss or suture) to the pessary.

Table 3 Pessary Types and Indications

Pessary	Sizes	Cystocele		Enterocele	Rectocele	Vault prolapse	Stress incontinence
		Small	Large				
Smith-Hodge	0–9	X		X			X
Risser	0–9	X		X			X
Marland	2–8	X					X
Incontinence Dish (mm)	55–85	X					X
Incontinence Ring	0–10	X					X
Ring (with or without support)	0–9	X	X	X	X		X
Gerhrung (with or without knob)	0–9	X			X		X
Gellhorn (inches)	$1\frac{1}{2}$–$3\frac{1}{2}$	X	X	X	X	X	
Schaatz (inches)	$1\frac{1}{2}$–$3\frac{1}{2}$	X		X	X	X	
Doughnut (inches)	2–$3\frac{3}{4}$	X	X	X	X	X	
Inflatable (inches)	2–$3\frac{1}{4}$	X	X	X	X	X	
Cube	0–7	X	X	X	X	X	

Source: Ref. 23.

Table 4   Pessary Care Recommendations

Remove at least two nights per week
Leave out overnight
Insert 1–2 g estrogen cream during night while pessary is out
Wash pessary with soap and water
Reinsert using water-soluble lubricant
Report any unusual discharge, bleeding, or discomfort
Report any changes in bladder or bowel function
Have pelvic examination every 6–12 months

Source: Ref. 23.

Cost issues must also be considered. In many cases, reimbursement by insurance companies does not cover the entire cost of a pessary. Additionally, no optimal distribution systems through pharmacies or durable medical supply houses exist. The physician is thus typically at financial risk when fitting pessaries.

Patients themselves may be hesitant to accept pessaries for SUI treatment. The common notion that pessaries are used solely by elderly women with prolapse and contraindications to surgical intervention frequently dissuades younger women from considering their use. Nevertheless, young women of reproductive age are often ideal candidates for pessary treatment of SUI (Table 5).

VII.   THE PATIENT WHO CANNOT BE FIT WITH A PESSARY

Not all female candidates can be successfully fit with a pessary. Typical reasons for inability to be fit include vaginal scarring with loss of vaginal caliber or length from previous surgery, severe urogenital atrophy, vaginal pain, and markedly restricted or enlarged vaginal introitus. In women with restricted caliber, use of a vaginal tampon may reduce stress incontinence. In those with significantly increased vaginal caliber, performing a perineoplasty and subsequent refitting with a pessary should be considered. For elderly women with severe genital prolapse who are not, and will not become, sexually active, and cannot be fit with a pessary, consideration should be given to a colpocleisis performed under regional or local anesthesia.

VIII.   CONTRAINDICATIONS TO PESSARY USE

Although the pessary can be a valuable tool in the treatment of stress incontinence and genital prolapse, there are certain patients for whom pessary use may be considered contraindicated (Table 6).

Table 5   Ideal Candidate for Pessary Usage for SUI

Reproductive age
Comfortable with genital contact (i.e., tampon user)
Adequate manual dexterity
Usage primarily for specific activities (i.e., running)
Compliant with safe usage recommendations
Urethral hypermobility
Well-estrogenized vagina
Unscarred vagina

Table 6 Contraindications to Pessary Use

Severe atrophic tissues
Erosive or ulcerative changes in the vaginal mucosa
Inability to remove pessary on a regular basis
Undiagnosed vaginal bleeding
Undiagnosed vaginal discharge
Vaginal or cervical cancer
Noncompliance in follow-up
Impaired mental capacity

IX. SUMMARY

The concept of using an intravaginal device for treatment of stress incontinence is attractive to many women suffering from stress urinary incontinence. Various devices specifically designed to provide bladder neck support during exertional activities have been developed and proven to be effective. Motivated patients who wish to avoid surgical therapy are the optimal candidates for vaginal pessary use. Although several limiting factors may arise, including difficulty with insertion and removal, interference with sexual activity, pelvic discomfort, and associated vaginal discharge, vaginal devices are a valuable conservative option for the treatment of stress incontinence.

REFERENCES

1. Richardson DA, Bent AE, Ostergard DR. The effect of uterovaginal prolapse on urethrovesical pressure dynamics. Am J Obstet Gynecol 1983; 146:901–905.
2. Bergman A, Koonings PP, Ballard CA. Predicting postoperative urinary incontinence development in women undergoing operation for genitourinary prolapse. Am J Obstet Gynecol 1988; 158:1171–1175.
3. Veronikis DK, Nichols DH, Wakamatsu MM. The incidence of low-pressure urethra as a function of prolapse-reducing technique in patients with massive pelvic organ prolapse (maximum descent at all vaginal sites). Am J Obstet Gynecol 1997; 177:1305–1314.
4. Rosenzweig BA, Pushkin S, Blumenfeld D, Bhatia NN. Prevalence of abnormal urodynamic test results in continent women with severe genitourinary prolapse. Obstet Gynecol 1992; 79:539–542.
5. Chaikin DC, Groutz A, Blaivas JG. Predicting the need for anti-incontinence surgery in continent women undergoing repair of severe urogenital prolapse. J Urol 2000; 163:531–534.
6. Bhatia NN, Bergman A, Gunning JE. Urodynamic effects of a vaginal pessary in women with stress urinary incontinence. Am J Obstet Gynecol 1983; 147:876–884.
7. Bhatia NN, Bergman A. Pessary test in women with urinary incontinence. Obstet Gynecol 1985; 65:220–226.
8. Bergman A, Bhatia NN. Pessary test: simple prognostic test in women with stress urinary incontinence. Urology 1984; 24:109–110.
9. Romanzi LJ, Chaikin DC, Blaivas JG. The effect of genital prolapse on voiding. Urology 1999; 161:581–586.
10. Suarez GM, Baum NH, Jacobs J. Use of standard contraceptive diaphragm in the management of stress urinary incontinence. Urology 1991; 37:119–122.
11. Fihn SD, Johnson C, Pinkstaff C, Stamm WE. Diaphragm use and urinary tract infections: analysis of urodynamic and microbiological factors. J Urol 1986; 136:853–856.
12. Realini JP, Walters MD. Vaginal diaphragm rings in the treatment of stress urinary incontinence. J Am Board Fam Pract 1990; 3:99–103.

13. Marshall S. Conservative management of stress urinary incontinence [letter]. Urology 1991; 38:294.

14. Nygaard I. Prevention of exercise incontinence with mechanical devices. J Reprod Med 1995; 40:89–94.

15. Davila GW, Ostermann KV. The bladder neck support prosthesis: a nonsurgical approach to stress incontinence in adult women. Am J Obstet Gynecol 1994; 171:206–211.

16. Davila GW, Neal D, Horbach N, Preacher J, Doughtie JD, Karram M. A bladder neck support prosthesis for women with stress and mixed incontinence. Obstet Gynecol 1999; 93:938–942.

17. Thyssen HH, Lose G. Long term efficacy and safety of a disposable vaginal device (Continence Guard) in the treatment of female stress incontinence. Int Urogyn J Pelvic Floor Dysfunct 1997; 8:130–133.

18. Thyssen H, Lose G. New disposable vaginal device (Continence Guard) in the treatment of female stress incontinence. Design, efficacy and short-term safety. Acta Obstet Gynaecol Scand 1996; 75:170–173.

19. Hahn I, Milsom I. Treatment of female stress urinary incontinence with a new anatomically shaped vaginal device (Conveen Continence Guard). Br J Urol 1996; 77:711–715.

20. Miller DS. Contemporary use of the pessary. In: Sciarra JJ, ed. Gynecology and Obstetrics. Vol 1. Philadelphia: Lippencott-Raven, 1992:1–12.

21. Vitsky M. Simple treatment of the incompetent cervical os. Am J Obstet Gynecol 1961; 81:1194–1197.

22. Oster S, Javert CT. Treatment of the incompetent cervix with the Hodge pessary. Obstet Gynecol 1966; 28:206–208.

23. Davila GW. Vaginal prolapse: management with nonsurgical techniques. Postgrad Med 1996; 99:171–176, 181, 184–185.

24. Poma PA. Nonsurgical management of genital prolapse: a review and recommendations for clinical practice. J Reprod Med 2000; 45:789–797.

25. Cundiff GW, Weidner AC, Visco AG, Bump RC, Addison WA. A survey of pessary use by members of the American Urogynecologic Society. Obstet Gynecol 2000; 95:931–935.

26. Wu V, Farrell SA, Baskett TF, Flowerdew G. A simplified protocol for pessary management. Obstet Gynecol 1997; 90:990–994.

27. Sulak PJ, Kuehl TJ, Shull BL. Vaginal pessaries and their use in pelvic relaxation. J Reprod Med 1993; 38:919–923.

16
Current Role of Transvaginal Needle Suspensions

Firouz Daneshgari
The Cleveland Clinic Foundation, Cleveland, Ohio, U.S.A.

I. INTRODUCTION

The modern era of surgical treatment of stress urinary incontinence (SUI) began in 1892 when Poussan (1) proposed the concept of urethral meatus advancement, and it followed an amazing and sometimes convoluted path through the 20th century. Transvaginal needle suspension (TVNS) was introduced in the 1950s as a simpler and less invasive treatment for SUI in women.

II. DEVELOPMENT AND EVOLUTION OF TRANSVAGINAL NEEDLE SUSPENSIONS

In 1959, Armand Pereyra (2) introduced a novel approach to surgical treatment of the patient with genuine SUI. His decision on switching from the traditional Marshall-Marchetti-Krants procedure was based on the failure of cases he observed, which he attributed to "strands of fibrous material between the relaxed tissues and the posterior aspects of the symphysis." Therefore, he postulated that if the tissues could be suspended from the rectus fascia, traction from coughing and Valsalva maneuver would not encourage disruption of the repair. Pereyra devised the principle of the needle suspension with the design of a ligature carrier. His first published results reported 28 successful procedures and two failures.

In 1973, Thomas Stamey (3) from California described several modifications of the needle suspension. The main revision was the use of cystoscopy to determine the position of the bladder neck with accuracy and hence to place the sutures in close proximity to this point.

In 1979, Shlomo Raz (4), from the University of California at Los Angeles, reported a modification of the Pereyra procedure using a curvilinear incision and including the paravaginal tissues within the helical suture. Cobb and Radge (5), in 1978, suggested the use of a double-pronged needle passer in order to reduce the number of passages of a needle through the tissue. In 1989, Raz et al. (6) also described the "four-corner suspension"—a TVNS operation that repairs anterior vaginal wall prolapse in addition to producing an anti-incontinence effect due to its ability to place the bladder neck in the high retropubic position.

279

III. SURGICAL TECHNIQUES

Regardless of the specific modifications, the general principles of the needle suspension remain the same. These include suspension/elevation of the bladder neck and of the proximal urethra (by vaginal wall or synthetic material) by use of a nonabsorbable suture. The details of surgical techniques of various TVNS are discussed in another chapter.

IV. LEVEL OF EVIDENCE

No discussion on the assessment of a treatment option for UI could be complete without a discussion on the issue of level of evidence. The evidence required in the medical literature is limited to data reported in clinical trials, specifically excluding expert opinion. This is similar to that required to determine the final judgment of a jury in a legal proceeding, which must be based on the material evidence presented during the trial. The judgment (opinion) of the jury is not evidence. Evidence is factual information presented.

Attempts to find such evidence have led several national and international organizations to conduct exhaustive searches of the literature with the aim of providing some guidelines to clinicians for UI management. In this regard, four documents have been released over the past decade:

1. AHCPR's Clinical Practice Guideline reports on UI in adults in 1992 and 1996 (7).
2. The report of the AUA Clinical Guidelines Panel on surgical management of female SUI (8).
3. The report of the World Health Organization First and Second International Consultations on Incontinence (ICI) (9,10).

All these documents were based on a review of the *existing* literature by panels of experts who subsequently formulated the recommendations.

The AHCPR Report and ICI addressed the issue of data quality by dividing the level of evidence into High (or A) Best: where the recommendation is supported by scientific evidence from properly designed and implemented controlled trials providing statistical results that consistently support the panel's recommendation; Intermediate (or B) Acceptable: where the recommendations are supported by scientific evidence from properly designed and implemented clinical series that support the guideline statement; and Low (or C) Marginal: the recommendation is supported by expert opinion.

V. REPORTED OUTCOMES

In 1997, the AUA Female Stress Urinary Incontinence Clinical Guidelines Panel published guidelines for the surgical treatment of stress incontinence (8). The AUA report on surgical management of female SUI was based on a final review of 282 articles by a selected panel of experts that included treatment outcome reports in clinical trials including nonrandomized controlled trials. Four major surgical techniques were studied: retropubic suspensions, transvaginal suspensions, anterior repairs, and sling procedures. The following criteria were reviewed in these trials: cure/dry, cure/dry/improved postoperative urgency, retention, hospital days, resumption of normal activities, transfusion, general conservative complications, intraoperative complications, preoperative complications, subjective complications, and complications requiring surgery. Based on this review, the panel concluded that (a) retropubic suspensions and slings are the most efficacious procedures for long-term success on the basis of cure/dry rates, but (b) retropubic suspensions and sling procedures are associated with slightly higher complication rates (including postvoiding dysfunction) and with a longer convalescence, and (c) anterior repairs are the least likely to be efficacious over time.

The level of evidence for the AUA guidelines recommendation was "Low (or C) Marginal" by ICI's and AHCPR's guidelines. Despite that, however, these recommendations have encouraged many urologists in the United States to use the sling as the primary procedure for stress incontinence. This trend is illustrated clearly by comparing the results of two surveys in which American urologists were asked what procedure they used for stress incontinence related to urethral hypermobility. In the 1996 report, 71% of urologists used needle suspensions and 25% used retropubic suspensions (11). In the 2001 report, 38% of urologists used needle suspensions, 16% used retropubic suspensions, and 44% used slings for type I stress incontinence; for type II stress incontinence, the corresponding numbers were 14%, 17%, and 68%, respectively (12).

VI. COMPLICATIONS

The reported incidence of de novo detrusor instability following needle suspensions has varied between zero and 20%, with a mean incidence in the region of 5.8%. Voiding disorders may also follow this procedure, with a mean of 5.8% and a range of 1–24% (13).

VII. CURRENT STATUS

One of the historical attractions of the TVNS was the minimally invasive advantage they had over the alternatives of retropubic suspensions and pubovaginal slings. In addition, urologists and gynecologists were originally taught to use retropubic or needle suspensions if the patient had urethral hypermobility or anatomical incontinence. Sling operations were reserved for cases of intrinsic urethral sphincter deficiency because they had higher morbidity. However, with the improved understanding of the pathophysiology of SUI, we now believe that it is the hammock support of the bladder neck or the urethra and not the intrapelvic position of the urethra that helps the SUI. The surgical consequence of this enhanced understanding is that the surgeons no longer pull the slings with tension. Moreover, with improved techniques, suture material, and availability of allograft fascia, the morbidity of sling procedures has decreased significantly (14,15). The combination of a low rate of long-term cure by TVNS, decreased morbidity, and the ease of performing pubovaginal sling procedures has increasingly created a situation where the use of TVNS as a primary treatment option for even simple SUI is rapidly decreasing.

REFERENCES

1. Poussan. Arch Clin Bord 1892; 1.
2. Pereyra AJ. A simplified surgical procedure for the correction of stress urinary incontinence in women. West J Obstet Gynecol 1959; 67:223–226.
3. Stamey TA. Cystoscopic suspension of the vesical neck for urinary incontinence. Surg Gynecol Obstet 1973; 136:547–554.
4. Raz S. Modified bladder neck suspension for female stress incontinence. Urology 1981; 17:82–85.

5. Cobb OE, Radge H. Simplified correction of female stress incontinence. J Urol 1978; 141:38–42.
6. Raz S, Klutke CG, Golomb J. Four-corner bladder and urethral suspension for moderate cystocele. J Urol 1989; 142(3):712–715.
7. Clinical Practice Guideline: Urinary Incontinence in Adults: Acute and Chronic Management. U.S. Department of Health and Human Services. Public Health Service, Rockville, MD. Agency for Health Care Policy and Research, 1996; AHCPR publication No. 96-0682.
8. Leach GE, Dmochowski RR, Appell RA, Blaivas JG, Hadley HR, Luber KM, Mostwin JL, O'Donnell PD, Roehrborn CG. Female Stress Urinary Incontinence Clinical Guidelines Panel. Summary report on surgical management of female stress urinary incontinence. J Urol 1997; 158(3 Pt 1):875–880.
9. Abrams P, Khoury S, Wein A, eds. Incontinence. First International Consultation on Incontinence, Monaco, July 28–July 1, 1988.
10. Abrams P, Carduzo L, Khoury S, Wein A, eds. Incontinence. 2nd International Consultation on Incontinence, Paris, July 1–3, 2001.
11. Gee WF, Holtgrewe HL, Albertsen PC. Practice trends of American urologists in the treatment of impotence, incontinence and infertility. J Urol 1996; 156:1778–1782.
12. Kim HL, Gerber GS, Patel RV. Practice patterns in the treatment of female urinary incontinence: a postal and Internet survey. Urology 2001; 57:45–48.
13. Jarvis FJ. Surgery for genuine stress incontinence. Br J Obstet Gynaecol 1994; 101:371–373.
14. Chaikin DC, Rosenthal J, Blaivas JG. Pubovaginal fascial sling for all types of stress urinary incontinence: long-term analysis. J Urol 1998; 160:1312–1316.
15. Barnes NM, Dmochowski RR, Park R, Nitti VW. Pubovaginal sling and pelvic prolapse repair in women with occult stress urinary incontinence: effect on postoperative emptying and voiding symptoms. Urology 2002; 59(6):856–860.

17

Anterior Vaginal Wall Suspension

Tracey Small Wilson and Philippe E. Zimmern
University of Texas Southwestern Medical Center, Dallas, Texas, U.S.A.

I. EVOLUTION

Raz described the first four-corner bladder and urethral suspension procedure in 1989 (1). He recognized that many anti-incontinence procedures failed because they addressed anterior vaginal wall prolapse or urethral hypermobility rather than addressing the two together. For example, the Kelly-type plication corrected the cystocele by reapproximation of the pubocervical fascia, but it was associated with a high failure rate for stress urinary incontinence (SUI) (50–80%) (2) partly because it did not support the proximal urethra and bladder neck. Conversely, the Marshall-Marchetti-Krantz (MMK) bladder neck suspension corrected urethral hypermobility but not the cystocele. Raz believed that bladder base descent and urethral hypermobility must be corrected at the time of cystocele repair regardless of whether incontinence existed. At that time, the only procedure accomplishing this combined goal was the retropubic Burch cystourethropexy. Raz therefore drew from his experience with the modified Peyrera needle suspension procedure to develop a vaginal technique that would simultaneously address urethral hypermobility and anterior vaginal wall prolapse.

Raz's original modification of the Pereyra suspension procedure incorporated the urethropelvic ligament, pubocervical fascia, and vaginal wall (without its epithelium) into helical suspensory sutures (3). He further modified this procedure to develop the four-corner bladder neck suspension (1). By combining this initial set of helical sutures (placed at the bladder neck) with a second set (placed at the level of the cystocele base), Raz created four sites, or "corners," from which the proximal urethra and bladder base were suspended. Via an inverted U-shaped incision, these nonabsorbable sutures were placed very lateral (as with the Burch suspension) to minimize the risk of outflow obstruction. They were then transferred suprapubically by a ligature carrier and secured to the anterior rectus fascia. This procedure essentially resuspended the anterior vaginal wall without repairing the fascial defect.

In his initial series of 120 patients with grade 2 or 3 cystocele Raz reported a 94% and 98% subjective correction of incontinence and cystocele, respectively. Obstruction was relieved in 84% of patients, preoperative detrusor instability improved in 54%, and de novo urge occurred in 5% (1). Despite these successes, patients continued to experience a significant amount of suprapubic discomfort and cystocele recurrence.

Bruskewitz et al. compared several different anchoring materials and their rate of tissue pull through and local tissue reaction in the rabbit abdominal wall (4). He concluded that loops of suture material had a lower incidence of tissue pull-through and tension loss over time. He believed this was due to a lower initial tension and a greater cross-sectional area of the anchor material.

Using Bruskewitz's findings, Leach and Zimmern modified the Raz four-corner suspension to obtain a broader anterior vaginal wall anchor (5). They believed that broader support of the upper vagina would protect the bladder neck repair and distribute pressure more evenly during stress maneuvers. Their distal sutures were placed in the vaginal wall at the bladder neck level and did not incorporate the urethropelvic ligaments. Proximal sutures were placed in a helical fashion at the cystocele base to provide broader and stronger support of the upper anterior vaginal wall. If the uterus was present, these helical sutures incorporated the cardinal ligaments; if absent, they incorporated the scar of the vaginal cuff.

Long-term results of the four-corner procedure were reported in 1997 (6). Using both subjective and objective outcomes, Dmochowski et al. (6) evaluated 47 patients after a mean of 37 months (range 15–80 months) and found an 87% subjective cure or improvement rate. Standing voiding cystourethrogram revealed recurrent cystocele, grade I or II (Baden-Walker classification) (7), in 57%. This moderate recurrence rate was attributed to possible suture pull-through from the cardinal ligament complex or apical cuff. Upon more careful evaluation of those patients with recurrent cystoceles, the recurrent fascial defect was found to be centrally located. Further modifications were therefore imposed. The current procedure, described below, is referred to as an anterior vaginal wall suspension (AVWS).

II. INDICATIONS

The AVWS is indicated in patients diagnosed with SUI due to urethral hypermobility and a small to moderate cystocele (grade I or II) with no midline fascial defect, as seen on voiding cystogram (VCUG). Upper vaginal suspension sutures support and elevate the cystocele base, while the distal sutures support the bladder neck, thereby correcting urethral hypermobility. Patients with large cystoceles (grade III or IV) due to a central defect are best served with an anterior colporrhaphy or an abdominal sacrocolpopexy along with support of the bladder neck (8).

The AVWS is not indicated in patients with SUI due to intrinsic sphincteric deficiency (ISD) alone, and no urethral hypermobility. This procedure does not provide sufficient urethral coaptation to ensure dryness in this population. If the patient has a cystocele in association with ISD (as diagnosed by physical examination and urodynamics), a pubovaginal sling along with support of the upper anterior vagina or an anterior colporrhaphy is indicated depending, on the extent of the cystocele. Simultaneous correction of the cystocele is indicated to avoid excessive angulation at the urethrovesical junction, which could produce outflow obstruction.

III. OPERATIVE TECHNIQUE

After induction of general anesthesia, the patient is placed in the high dorsal lithotomy position using candy-cane stirrups. The lower abdomen, perineum, and vagina are properly prepped and draped, and a ring retractor is positioned to aid visualization. A urethral catheter is inserted, and the balloon is palpated to identify and mark the bladder neck. Marking sutures are now placed at the vaginal apex—one in the midline and one 1.5 cm lateral to the midline on each side. Beginning ∼1.5 cm lateral to the bladder neck, an incision is made in the anterior vaginal wall and extended proximally to the level of the marking sutures—lateral to the cervix or to the vaginal apex. The same procedure is repeated on the opposite side (Fig. 1). The area of anterior vaginal wall between the incision lines will serve as the elevating vaginal wall plate and is

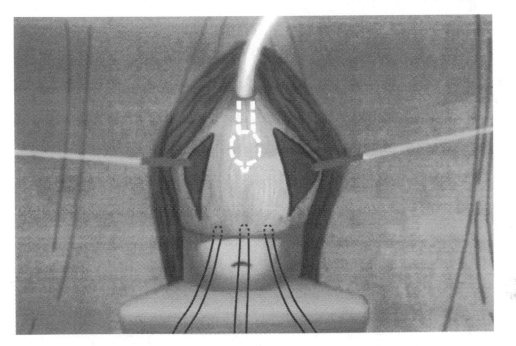

Figure 1   Initial setup of AVWS. Three marking sutures are placed at vaginal apex. Bilateral anterior vaginal incisions are made extending from the level of the bladder neck to the vaginal cervix or cuff.

usually 3 cm in width and 4–8 cm in length depending upon the length of the anterior vaginal wall (average 6 cm). In the presence of a moderate cystocele, the redundant vaginal wall lateral to these incisions should be excised lengthwise, preserving 0.5–1 cm of tissue laterally in order to recreate the lateral sulcuses upon closure of the vaginal wall.

The 3 × 4–8 cm in situ anterior vaginal wall plate is now divided into equal quadrants using a marking pen. The first of four No. 1 polypropylene sutures is placed into the scar of the vaginal cuff or cardinal ligament and run distally in a helical fashion to the level of the midvagina (half the length of the vaginal plate). The helical bites should traverse medially to the middle of the vaginal plate and should incorporate the vaginal wall, excluding the epithelium. The second suture is then placed at the level of the midvagina and run distally by two to three helical passes to the bladder neck area (Fig. 2). The third and fourth sutures are placed similarly on the opposite side.

A 3–4 cm transverse suprapubic incision is then made two fingerbreadths above the level of the pubic symphysis and carried down to the level of the rectus fascia. This incision should be as close to midline as possible to avoid genitofemoral nerve involvement. Owing to the risk of bleeding, placement of the four suspension sutures and suprapubic incision are done before entering the retropubic space. Blunt or sharp dissection at the level of the bladder neck is now performed to develop the plane laterally between the endopelvic fascia and the pubic bone. Once this space is cleared of all adherent tissue, the deep endopelvic fascia is perforated, which allows entrance into the retropubic space. The retropubic space is then developed anteriorly using a sweeping motion of the finger along the inside surface of the pubic bone. It is critical to keep the catheter on gravity drainage to ensure bladder emptiness during this maneuver.

In a virgin case, there is little to no resistance entering the retropubic space at the site of the lateral defect. However, after a Burch or MMK procedure, there may be a significant amount of

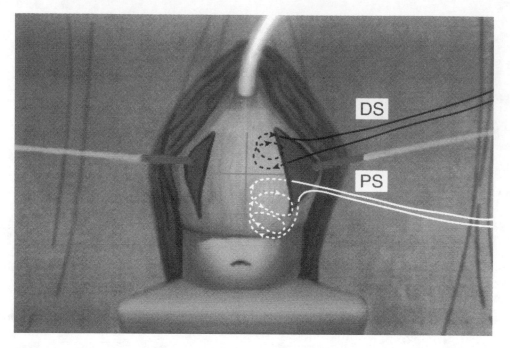

Figure 2   Placement of suspension sutures. Note division of vaginal plate into quadrants. PS, proximal sutures; DS, distal sutures.

retropubic scarring, which increases the risk of bladder injury during finger dissection or needle passage. Once it is felt that only rectus fascia and muscle remain between a finger in the suprapubic incision and one in the retropubic space, each of the four suspension sutures is transferred to the suprapubic position using a ligature carrier. We use a double-pronged ligature carrier; however, a single pronged instrument may be necessary in obese patients or in those with significant abdominal wall and/or retropubic scarring. When possible, the proximal suspension sutures (adjacent to cervix) are placed more lateral and cephalad than the distal suspension sutures (Fig. 3).

    After intravenous indigo carmine is given, cystoscopy with a 70° lens is performed to exclude intravesical suture placement and/or bladder perforation and to confirm ureteral integrity. If sutures are present in the bladder, they should be removed via the vaginal side and repositioned. A large bladder perforation should be closed in multiple layers immediately with possible interposition of a fat graft (9) (in this instance, the anti-incontinence procedure may need to be aborted). The vaginal wall incisions are now closed with running 2-0 absorbable suture. Using a rubber-shod right-angle clamp, each suture is grasped ~1.5–2 cm above the rectus fascia and tied above the clamp as an assistant supports the vaginal plate in a position parallel to the floor. This maneuver provides adequate support without over correction. An antibiotic-soaked vaginal pack is inserted, and the suprapubic incision is closed.

IV. OUTCOMES

Both subjective and objective outcome measures have been used to assess effectiveness of the AVWS. Lemack and Zimmern reported midterm results of the AVWS in 61 of 102 women who

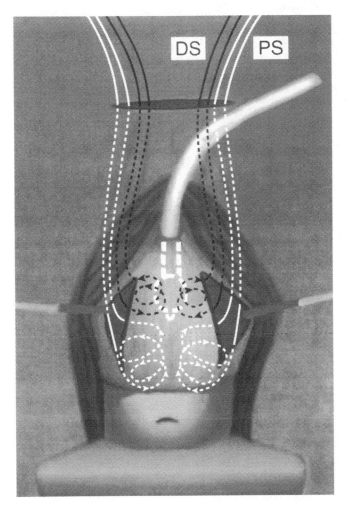

Figure 3   Final appearance of suspension sutures. Note that sutures cover the entire vaginal plate. Proximal sutures (PS) are placed more lateral and cephalad than distal sutures (DS).

had responded to questionnaires at a mean of 25 months following AVWS (10). Seventy-seven percent of patients were subjectively cured or improved of their stress incontinence. Using a visual analog scale and the quality-of-life question—"If you were to spend the rest of your life with your urinary condition just the way it is now, how would you feel about that?"—the median preoperative score was 6.7 (0, pleased; 10, terrible), and declined postoperatively to a median response of 2. Eight percent experienced de novo urge incontinence, and diuretic use was the only poor prognostic indicator. The standing voiding cystourethrogram (VCUG) has been used as an objective outcome tool for anti-incontinence procedures (11). Showalter et al. (12) compared the VCUG of 76 continent control patients to two surgical groups: group 1, 52 patients who underwent an AVWS for urethral hypermobility and grade I or II cystocele; group 2, 36 patients with grade III or greater cystocele who underwent formal anterior colporrhaphy. After 3–6 months, there was no difference in the urethral angle in patients who had undergone the AVWS compared to controls. There was also a significant reduction in the lateral height of the cystocele following AVWS and anterior colporrhaphy (Figs. 4, 5).

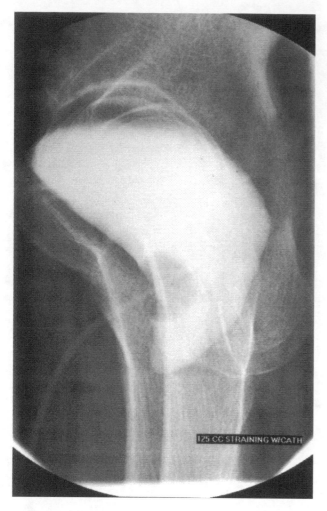

Figure 4   Preoperative lateral VCUG demonstrating urethral hypermobility (urethral angle of 60–70°) associated with a mild cystocele.

Sexual function following AVWS has also been assessed. Lemack and Zimmern subjectively evaluated 93 women at least 1 year following an AVWS alone or in combination with a posterior colporrhaphy (13). Sixty percent of patients responded to a mailed questionnaire. The same percentage of patients was sexually active postoperatively as preoperatively; however, only 20% noted dyspareunia postoperatively, compared to 29% preoperatively. Eighteen percent of patients reported intercourse to be worse postoperatively, but these were not the same patients who reported dyspareunia. Thus, the etiology of this finding remains unclear. Only one of 29 patients who had undergone an AVWS alone reported sexual inactivity due to loss of libido or inability to have intercourse. The AVWS did not seem to adversely affect the majority of women who were sexually active, and the incidence of symptomatic vaginal narrowing was rare.

Other investigators have also utilized the anterior vaginal wall in anti-incontinence procedures. Appell described the in situ vaginal wall sling, which utilizes the anterior vaginal wall for support of the proximal urethra and bladder neck (14). This vaginal wall support is

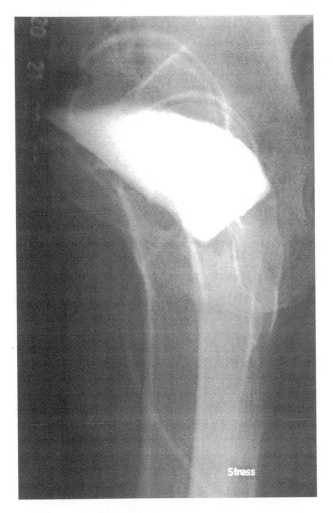

Figure 5 Postoperative lateral VCUG demonstrating a normal urethral angle and a well-supported bladder base.

anchored to the pubic bone, thereby limiting the amount of retropubic dissection. Kaplan also described his long-term results with the vaginal wall sling (15). The AVWS is not a sling procedure but does utilize the vaginal wall as a supporting structure.

There are many advantages to using the anterior vaginal wall in anti-incontinence procedures. Namely, it does not require a separate harvesting incision (as is necessary for autologous fascia); one avoids the risk of tissue contamination and disease transmission that is a small but potential risk with allograft and xenograft materials; and there is less risk of infection and erosion than is seen with synthetic materials.

The AVWS most resembles the Burch bladder neck suspension, which has recognized durability and effectiveness in correcting stress urinary incontinence due to urethral hypermobility. A recent meta-analysis found the Burch procedure to be 85% successful after 4 years (16). Like the Burch procedure, support of the AVWS is based on a broad vaginal anchor. The retropubic dissection common to both procedures promotes scarring in this region, which further enhances the vaginal support. The vaginal support in the Burch procedure is anchored to

Cooper's ligament, whereas the anchoring point for the AVWS is the rectus muscle tendon as it inserts into the back of the pubic symphysis. The transvaginal approach for the AVWS allows repair of concomitant pelvic prolapses through the same incision. In addition, lack of a Pfannenstiel incision reduces postoperative incisional pain and allows for a shorter convalescence following the AVWS.

V. CONCLUSION

The AVWS procedure is a reliable surgical option for the patient with stress urinary incontinence due to urethral hypermobility in the presence of a small to moderate cystocele. It is favorable to the patient due to its shortened convalescence and reduced postoperative morbidity. From a surgeon's perspective, it is easy to teach and reproducible. Midterm results of the AVWS are respectable, and its long-term results are forthcoming.

REFERENCES

1. Raz S, Klutke C, Golomb J. Four-corner bladder and urethral suspension for moderate cystocele. J Urol 1989; 142:712–715.
2. Stanton SL, Hilton P, Norton C, Cardozo L. Clinical and urodynamic effects of anterior colporrhaphy and vaginal hysterectomy for prolapse with and without incontinence. Br J Obstet Gynaecol 1982; 89:459–463.
3. Raz S. Modified bladder neck suspension for female stress incontinence. Urology 1981; 17:82–85.
4. Bruskewitz RC, Nielsen KT, Graversen PH, Saville WD, Gasser TC. Bladder neck suspension material investigated in a rabbit model. J Urol 1989; 142:1361–1363.
5. Zimmern PE, Leach GE, Sirls L. Four-corner bladder neck suspension. In: Leach GE, ed. Atlas of the Urologic Clinics of North America. Philadelphia: W.B. Saunders, 1994:29–36.
6. Dmochowski RR, Zimmern PE, Ganabathi K, Sirls GL, Leach GE. Role of the four-corner bladder neck suspension to correct stress incontinence with a mild to moderate cystocele. Urology 1997; 49:35–40.
7. Baden WF, Walker TA. Surgical Repair of Vaginal Defects. Philadelphia: J.B. Lippincott, 1992.
8. Miyazaki FS, Miyazaki DW. Raz four corner suspension for severe cystocele: poor results. Int Urogynecol J Pelvic Floor Dysfunc 1994; 5:94–97.
9. Hernandez RD, Himsl K, Zimmern PE. Transvaginal repair of bladder injury during vaginal hysterectomy. J Urol 1994; 152:2061–2062.
10. Lemack GE, Zimmern PE. Questionnaire-based outcome after anterior vaginal wall suspension for stress urinary incontinence (abstract). J Urol 2000; 163(4):73.
11. Zimmern PE. The role of voiding cystourethrography in the evaluation of the female lower urinary tract. Prob Urol 1991; 5:23–41.
12. Showalter PR, Zimmern PE, Roehrborn CG, Lemack GE. Standing cystourethrogram: an outcome measure after anti-incontinence procedures and cystocele repair in women. Urology 2001; 58:33–37.
13. Lemack GE, Zimmern PE. Sexual function after vaginal surgery for stress incontinence: results of a mailed questionnaire. Urology 2000; 56:223–227.
14. Appell RA. In situ vaginal wall sling. Urology 2000; 56:499–503.
15. Kaplan SA, Te AE, Young GP, Andrade A, Cabelin MA, Ikeguchi EF. Prospective analysis of 373 consecutive women with stress urinary incontinence treated with a vaginal wall sling: the Columbia–Cornell University experience. J Urol 2000; 164:1623–1627.
16. Leach GE, Dmochowski RR, Appell RA, Blaivas JG, Hadley HR, Luber KM, Mostwin JL, O'Donnell PD. Report on the Surgical Management of Female Stress Urinary Incontinence Clinical Practice Guidelines. Baltimore: American Urological Association, 1997.

18
Retropubic Urethropexy

Jeffrey L. Cornella
Mayo Clinic Scottsdale, Scottsdale, Arizona, U.S.A.

I. INTRODUCTION

The suprapubic approach to anterior segment or urethrovaginal stabilization is known as retropubic urethropexy. Retropubic urethropexy (RPU) procedures have a long and important history in pelvic surgery. They remain an essential contribution to the surgical armamentarium for the management of female urinary incontinence. This chapter will review the history, techniques, and pertinent literature of the retropubic urethropexies—open and laparoscopic.

II. RETROPUBIC URETHROPEXY VERSUS PUBOVAGINAL SLING

The past several years have seen an increasing trend for selection of the pubovaginal sling as a primary incontinence procedure in the United States. There were two phenomena that accelerated this trend. The first was accumulating data on the poor outcomes of needle-suspension procedures. The second was the development of a less invasive pubovaginal sling, in the form of the transvaginal tape procedure (TVT) (1). Additionally, the misconception of intrinsic sphincteric deficiency as an entity with a possible laboratory diagnosis further resulted in increased numbers of patients receiving slings. Practice trends may reach the point where the majority of patients are simply relegated to a TVT procedure, with little clinical evaluation or attention to paravaginal anatomy.

Caution should be exhibited prior to relegating all patients to TVT-like procedures. First of all, the strong objective data on TVT procedures only extends 5–7 years (2). The Burch urethropexy has 10- to 20-year objective data in several studies showing a high cure rate for stress urinary incontinence (3–5). It is unclear how the TVT will perform at 10 years plus compared to other procedures, especially if stretching of the sling material occurs.

Additionally, the TVT only supports the urethra, and if the patient has a paravaginal defect, which is often the case, the patient would be best served with a site-specific repair of the paravaginal area and retropubic urethropexy. If this is not done, the patient may continue to show anterior wall descent and additional symptoms.

The majority of patients with low urethral pressures or low Valsalva leak-point pressures are candidates for urethropexy, as the subsequent section on patient selection in this chapter will emphasize.

III. HISTORY OF RETROPUBIC URETHROPEXY

In many respects the retropubic urethropexy was introduced in the United States by the work of George Reaves White (6). White studied anatomy under Josef Halban in Vienna, just after the turn of the 20th century. The 1909 and 1912 articles regarding a radical cure for cystocele by White documented both a vaginal and an abdominal approach to the anterior segment (6,7). The anterior approach was a retropubic vaginopexy in the form of a paravaginal defect repair (PVDR). The anterior sulcus of the vaginal was reattached to the appropriate anatomic site, the arcus tendineus fascia pelvis (ATFP). This technique was lost for decades until its resurrection by the work of A. Cullen Richardson in the late 1970s.

In the interim, 30 years before the articles of Richardson, a different procedure for fixation of the urethra was described. This procedure was not a site-specific repair, but rather fixed the urethra to the posterior symphysis and disregarded the anterior lateral sulcus. Marshall et al. reported their female incontinence procedure in 1949 (8). Thousands of women have since received the Marshall-Marchetti-Krantz (MMK) procedure and its modifications for the control of urinary stress incontinence. It consists of fixation of the urethra and bladder by a bilateral series of three chromic sutures to the periosteum of the symphysis.

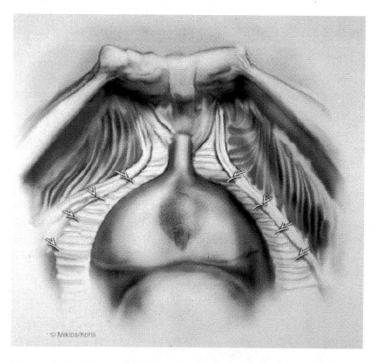

Figure 1   Tied paravaginal sutures attaching anterior lateral sulcus of vagina to obturator internis muscle along the white line (ATFP). (Used with permission of John Miklos.)

A patient who did not receive this intended procedure because of a weak periosteum was responsible for precipitating a new point of attachment and thus a different retropubic urethropexy. The operating surgeon was John Christopher Burch, and he chose as a new site of attachment, the iliopectineal ligament of Cooper (9). This procedure, performed in 1958, eventually became known as the Burch procedure. It would become the gold standard of the retropubic urethropexies. It has the largest literature and greatest long-term follow-up of any operation for female urinary incontinence. It is often the Burch procedure that other techniques for urinary incontinence are compared to in randomized studies. It will be the main procedure emphasized in this chapter, given the strong foundation of underlying literature.

IV. TECHNIQUES AND EFFICACY OF OPEN PROCEDURES

A. Paravaginal Defect Repair

The anterior lateral sulcus of the vagina is normally attached to the arcus tendineus fascia pelvis and portions of the levator musculature. The majority of anterior compartment defects, which are often referred to as cystoceles, are related to detachment and separation of this anatomic site (10). Restoration of the anatomy via the abdomen offers a symmetrical and complete repair without potentially inducing neuropathy by penetration of the urogenital diaphragm. It is a site-specific repair that often results in the cure of female urinary stress incontinence. A series of sutures attach the anterior lateral sulcus to the ATFP or white line of the obturator internis muscle.

It is not considered a standalone incontinence operation used by the majority of surgeons who treat female urinary stress incontinence, owing to a lack of prospective studies documenting its efficacy. The single prospective study that compared the PVDR to the Burch procedure for the treatment of female urinary incontinence showed a significantly higher failure rate in those patients receiving the paravaginal defect repair (11). Enrollment in this study by Mario Colombo was discontinued after 36 patients owing to the high failure rate of the PVDR for incontinence. Colombo reported the cure as 61% ($P < .004$) in the PVDR group and 100% ($P < .02$) 18 of 18 in the Burch group.

This failure may be secondary to persistent or recurrent urethrovesical junction descent from relaxation of the anterior vaginal wall in the midline, despite the restoration of paravaginal anatomy. The may be evidenced by the fact that in Colombo's study all of the postoperative Burch patients had a negative urethral angle on cotton swab testing, but only 33% of the PVDR patients. Patients who continued to have midline urethral descent despite paravaginal support demonstrated high rates of failure. Thus, patient selection in the office by documenting lack of urethral descent during instrumental support of the anterior lateral sulci may be beneficial in increasing the cure rate in PVDR patients.

Concomitant PVDR at the time of urethrolysis for the management of voiding dysfunction secondary to urethropexy is a consideration. Webster et al. reported 15 women with voiding dysfunction following cystourethropexy who underwent takedown and substitution with a PVDR (12). All 13 women who had symptoms of bladder instability experienced resolution of their symptoms, and of seven patients who required intermittent self-catheterization preoperatively, only one required catheterization postoperatively. A successful outcome was achieved in 14 of 15 patients. The article underscores the anatomic correction of the PVDR technique, which does not result in elevation of the urethrovesical junction beyond its normal anatomic position.

To treat patients receiving a Burch or MMK procedure adequately who have a concomitant paravaginal defect, a PVDR may be accomplished simultaneously. This is often referred to as a paravaginal-plus or MMK-plus procedure. In this setting the Burch procedure would be seen as the primary incontinence operation, and the PVDR corrects a defect and further supports the anterior vaginal wall.

1.   Technique of Outpatient Mini-Incision Paravaginal Defect Repair

Long-acting local anesthetic is infiltrated into the fascia prior to closing the fascia and skin. A 4-cm transverse suprapubic incision is made followed by a 4-cm fascial incision. The fascia is mobilized off the underlying rectus muscle followed by lateral dissection into the space of Retzius. A mini-Bookwalter retractor is placed followed by entry into the bladder dome. The surgeon's left hand is placed within the vagina and fiberoptic light facilitates visualization. The surgeon begins on the left side with identification and delineation of the full length of the anterior lateral sulcus. A gauze stick facilitates additional retraction of the bladder, and the anterior lateral sulcus is elevated with the vaginal hand. Vessels will be noted coursing in a longitudinal course along the sulcus. The obturator foramen is palpated, and care is taken to avoid the nerve and vessels including the aberrant branch of the obturator vein. Sutures are placed initially into the obturator internis when operating on the patient's left side and in the anterior lateral sulcus when operating on the patient's right side. A single bite is taken into the obturator internis at the level of the ATFP, and double bites are taken into the vaginal sulcus. Two to five sutures are placed along the sulcus from an area just inferior to the ischial spine to the symphysis pubis. In elderly patients, the arcuate line may not be visible and the attachment of the vagina is along a course 1–1.5 to 2 cm below the obturator foramen. Bites into the obturator internis as $\sim$3–4 mm deep and 1 cm long, avoiding vital structures that are 7.5 mm deep. The ureter courses 2.5–3 cm medial to the superior aspect of the anterior lateral sulcus. Delineation of the ureter is possible by use of the vaginal finger palpating the structure against the abdominal finger. The sutures are tied on the left side of the patient prior to placing sutures on the right. If a concomitant Burch urethropexy is done, the paravaginal sutures are tied first to establish the proper length of the Burch sutures as they course up to Cooper's ligament.

B.   Marshall-Marchetti-Krantz

The MMK procedure was first accomplished in a female on June 8, 1944 (13). Modifications of the MMK must involve suturing of the periurethral tissues to the midline cartilage or periosteum of the symphysis pubis in order to maintain this designation. Mainprize and Drutz in a review of 56 articles through the year 1988 stated that the overall success rate was 86.1% in 2712 cases (13). They noted that even in repeat procedures, the cure rate was high at 84.5%. Lee et al. noted in a series of 549 patients followed 2–16 years a 91% subjective cure rate in 227 primary patients and a 90% subjective cure rate in 322 repeat procedures (14).

Colombo et al. reported a randomized comparison between the MMK and the Burch procedure (15). A full urodynamic investigation was done 6 months after surgery. The cure rate for the MMK was noted be 65% on urodynamic testing and a subjective cure rate of 85% at mean 3.5 years. The Burch procedure was found to have an objective cure rate of 80%.

The MMK is effective in patients with low urethral pressures if they have hypermobility of the urethra. Quadri et al. did a prospective, randomized comparison of the MMK and the Burch urethropexy in patients with low urethral pressures who demonstrated urethral descent (16). Only 15 patients were studied in each group. At 1 year, stress tests were negative in 93% of women who underwent the MMK procedure and 53% of those who underwent the Burch procedure.

In their review, Mainprize and Drutz (13) reported the overall complication rate was 21.1% with 5% wound complication rate, a 3.8% urinary tract infection rate, and a 2.5%

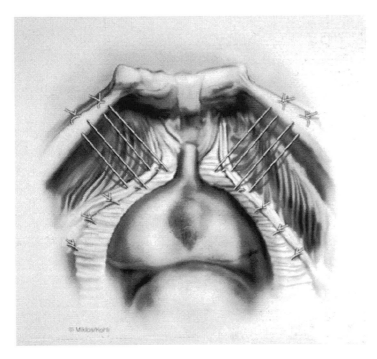

Figure 2 Completed paravaginal defect repair and Burch urethropexy. The paravaginal sutures are tied first and determine length of the Burch sutures. The latter are tied without additional tension. This stabilizes, but does not elevate the anterior vagina. (Used with permission of John Miklos.)

incidence of osteitis pubis. Kammerer reported 15 cases of osteitis pubis diagnosed after 2030 MMK procedures at the Mayo Clinic (17).

1. Technique of the Outpatient Mini-Incision MMK Procedure

Long-acting local anesthetic is infiltrated into the fascia prior to closing the fascia and skin. A 4-cm transverse suprapubic incision is made followed by a 4-cm fascial incision. The fascia is mobilized off the underlying rectus muscle followed by lateral dissection into the space of Retzius. A mini-Bookwalter retractor is placed followed by entry into the bladder dome. The surgeon's left hand is placed within the vagina, and fiberoptic light facilitates visualization. The bladder dome is opened to facilitate precise suture placement. The urethrovesical junction is palpated with one finger in the bladder and two fingers of the vaginal hand separated by the catheter. The vaginal hand is positioned with each finger on the urethrovesical junction, and the abdomen hand retracts fat medially, allowing visualization of the white periurethral tissue. Permanent sutures are placed with the needle initially entering closest to the urethra and then coursing lateral in a perpendicular direction for a distance of 1 cm. The sutures are check after placement by palpating with a finger in the bladder to determine distance lateral to the urethra and position relative to the urethrovesical junction. A total of four sutures are placed, two on each side of the urethra with the secondary sutures just distal to the initial urethrovesical junction sutures. All sutures are passed through the midline cartilage of the symphysis taking care to ensure that they are in the inferior aspect of the cartilage, thus avoiding overelevation. The cartilage of the symphysis has less blood supply than surrounding tissues and an aseptic technique is essential. Needles passing through the vagina should be cut and replaced with a

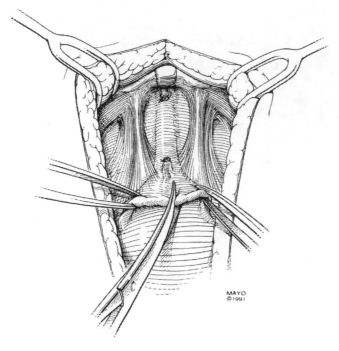

Figure 3 A small cystotomy allows precise suture placement, ability to check the bladder for suture material and ureteral efflux, and placement of a suprapubic catheter. (Used with permission of the Mayo Foundation.)

clean free-Mayo needle prior to passing through cartilage. The sutures are tied and the bladder is examined to ensure that it is free of suture material and the ureters are examined for efflux. The bladder is then closed in a double layer closure with 2-0 Chromic with incorporation of a 16-gauge catheter into the apex of the incision. The catheter is placed through a right lower quadrant stab incision.

C. Burch

In 1961 Burch reported a series 53 retropubic urethropexies (9). In seven of these patients the ATFP served as the area of attachment for the periurethral sutures. In 46 cases the iliopectineal ligament was used. In 1968 Burch reported a 9-year experience with the operation resulting in a 93% cure rate with only 12.5% of the 143 patients having a 5-year follow-up (18). Only 12 patients in the series had undergone a previous incontinence operation. The operative technique was described in detail and included three sutures of 2-0 Chromic attaching the periurethral tissues directly to Cooper's ligament. Postoperative enterocele occurred in 7.6% of patients despite cul-de-sac reinforcement being added to the procedure early in the series.

The majority of Burch procedures performed today are similar to the modification reported by Emil A. Tanagho (19). The article, which did not describe Tanagho's results, was presented at the Western section meeting of the American Urologic Association in Coronado in 1976. Tanagho placed his sutures in a far-lateral position, used two sutures bilaterally (No. 1 Dexon), and emphasized avoidance of undue tension on the anterior vaginal wall. He commented that two fingers could be placed between the symphysis and urethra, stressing that the vagina did not have to be contiguous with Cooper's ligament.

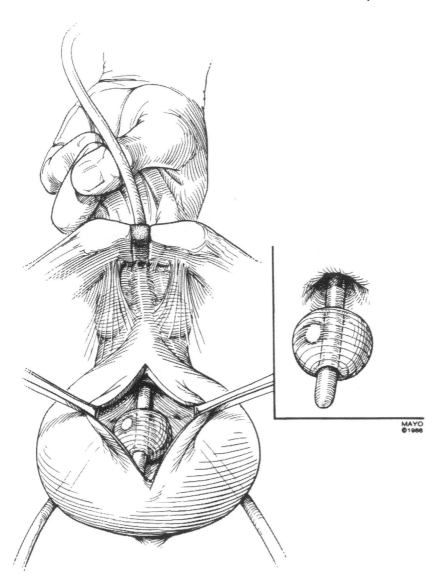

Figure 4   The surgeon's vaginal hand supports the urethrovesical junction, with one finger on each side of the catheter. Combined intravesical palpation and vaginal palpation allows precise delineation of the bladder neck and lateral distance of sutures from the urethra. (Used with permission of the Mayo Foundation.)

The concept of not overelevating the vaginal wall at the time of retropubic urethropexy was an important one and it presaged the hammock hypothesis of John O.L. DeLancey (20). Patients could experience cure with less risk of urinary retention and bladder overactivity secondary to obstruction. It is consistent with the concepts of the hammock hypothesis that Burch procedures should stabilize and not elevate the anterior vaginal wall. Tanagho's modification by its lateral placement of sutures, reduced compression, and overelevation of the urethra. It is important when reviewing articles describing Burch results to note the technique utilized and to what degree the anterior vaginal wall was elevated. Articles that

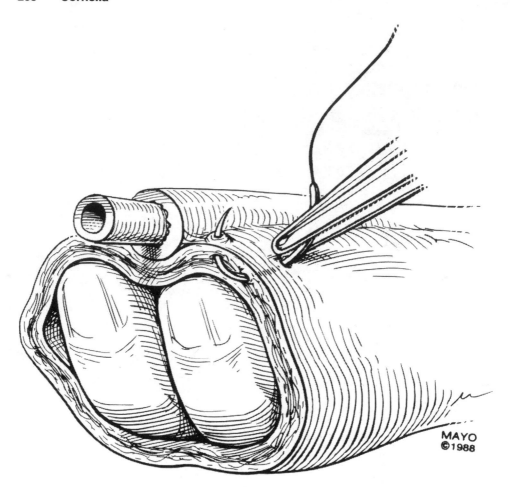

Figure 5 Sutures are placed 3–4 mm lateral to the urethra. A 22-guage catheter is in the urethra. The surgeon's two fingers straddle the urethra. (Used with permission of the Mayo Foundation.)

describe apposition of the wall to Cooper's ligament or significant elevation will have a higher incidence of prolonged voiding dysfunction and enterocele formation.

There are several studies that document long-term results of the Burch urethropexy. Herbertsson and Iosif studied 72 women who underwent Burch colposuspension with pre-operative and postoperative urodynamics (21). Objective follow-up occurred a mean of 9.4 years later. The objective surgical cure rate was 90.3% (a negative stress test with at least 300 cc within the bladder. The enterocele formation rate in this study was 4%.

Feyereisl et al. reported urodynamic outcome in 87 patients, 5–10 years after Burch urethropexy (3). Patients with greater than grade I prolapse or cystocele were excluded. Inclusion criteria included objective stress leakage in the absence of detrusor instability and documented hypermobility of the urethra. Stress incontinence was objectively cured in 81.6% of patients. Cure was defined as a dry, symptom-free patient, without objective loss during coughing in the standing position with 400 cc of bladder volume.

Alcalay et al. reported a 10- to 20-year follow-up of the Burch colposuspension (4). This was a longitudinal retrospective study with a long-term follow-up including symptom review, uroflowmetry, and an extended pad test. Objective cure was defined as inability to demonstrate stress incontinence during clinical examination and provocative urodynamics. The authors stated that cure on incontinence is time dependent, with a decline for 10–12 years when a plateau of 69% is reached.

Langer et al. reported a long-term (10–15 years) follow-up after Burch colposuspension in 127 patients (5). An additional postoperative urodynamic examination was accomplished at least 10 years after surgery in 109 patients. The cure rate was 93.7%, with cure defined as subjective and objective dryness. Following surgery there was an improvement in symptoms of frequency ($P < .001$), urgency ($P < .01$), and urge incontinence ($P < .001$).

1. Prospective, Randomized Studies Comparing Burch Urethropexy and Anterior Colporrhaphy

Anterior colporrhaphy or the Kelly procedure was utilized in the management of female urinary incontinence for decades. It became popular after the concepts of the paravaginal defect were lost to common awareness and before creation of other retropubic urethropexies. There remain proponents of the procedure for incontinence correction to date, despite a preponderance of objective evidence supporting retropubic urethropexy for this indication. There are now several prospective, randomized studies comparing Burch urethropexy to anterior colporrhaphy.

In 1995 Bergman and Elia reported a 5-year objective follow-up of a surgical comparison between three procedures for the treatment of urinary incontinence (22). The series consisted of 127 patients without a history of previous incontinence surgery. Multichannel urodynamics were performed preoperatively and at 3 months, 12 months, and 5 years postoperatively. Patients were randomized to the anterior colporrhaphy with Kelly plication, Pereyra procedure, and the Burch urethropexy. Ninety-three subjects were available for the 5-year objective follow-up. The success rates were 37% for the anterior colporrhaphy, 43% for the Pereyra procedure, and 82% for the Burch urethropexy. Seventy percent of the colporrhaphy patients had a urethrovesical junction descent at 5 years, compared with 7% of the Burch patients. Many patients who had cure at 1 year but demonstrated a positive cotton swab test, were noted to be failures at 5 years.

Kammerer-Doak performed a randomized trial comparing the Burch urethropexy to the modified anterior colporrhaphy (23). Thirty-five patients were randomized with preoperative and postoperative urodynamic testing as a component of the study. Objective cures 1 year after surgery showed 16 of 18 (89%) of Burch patients were cured compared to five of 16 (31%) of colporrhaphy patients. Subjective and objective ratings of incontinence severity by questionnaires and pad testing were significantly lower for the Burch patients than for the colporrhaphy patients. Mobility of the urethrovesical junction was lower for the Burch patients.

Liapis et al. reported a randomized study of three operations for stress incontinence, the MMK, Burch, and anterior colporrhaphy (24). The patients were examined clinically and urodynamically preoperatively and 60 months after surgery. There was a significant difference in results between the procedures at 5 years. The cure rate was 89% for the Burch procedure and 56% and 67% for the AC and MMK, respectively ($P < .001$).

2. Technique of Mini-Incision Outpatient Modification of the Burch Urethropexy

Long-acting local anesthetic is infiltrated into the fascia prior to closing the fascia and skin. A 4-cm transverse suprapubic incision is made followed by a 4-cm fascial incision. The fascia is mobilized off the underlying rectus muscle in the usual fashion followed by lateral dissection into the space of Retzius. A mini-Bookwalter retractor is placed followed by entry into the bladder dome. A suture tag is placed at the superior aspect of the bladder incision. The surgeon's left hand is placed within the vagina, and fiberoptic light facilitates visualization. Two sutures of No. 1 Ethibond are placed on each side of the urethra, taking double bites with each suture through almost full-thickness vagina. The initial suture is at the urethrovesical junction, and the second suture is 1 cm inferiorly. All sutures are at least 4 mm lateral to the urethra. Precise placement of each suture is confirmed by subsequent palpation via the cystotomy. The lateral distance from the urethra, the position relative to the urethrovesical junction, the affect on the urethra with suture elevation, and the distance of the lower suture from the urethral meatus are noted. The retractor is removed from each side during placement of sutures through Cooper's ligament. The rectus muscle on the side of placement is retracted with Greene retractors. Each strand of the suture pairs is placed through the ligament, with the second strand of each pair taking a second bite into the ligament. Needles, which have passed through the vagina, are removed and replaced with free-Mayo needles prior to passage through Cooper's ligament. The interior of the bladder is then examined for absence of suture material and bilateral efflux of urine via the ureters. The Foley catheter is removed and a cotton swab test is performed with the table and patient's back parallel to the floor. A zero to $-10°$ angle to the horizontal is established by elevating or loosening the sutures. The goal of the procedure is stabilization rather then elevation. The sutures are then tied with precise square knots, maintaining equal and opposite tension on the strands while tying. The bladder is then closed in a double layer closure with 2-0 Chromic with incorporation of a 16-gauge catheter into the apex of the incision. The catheter is placed through a right lower quadrant stab incision.

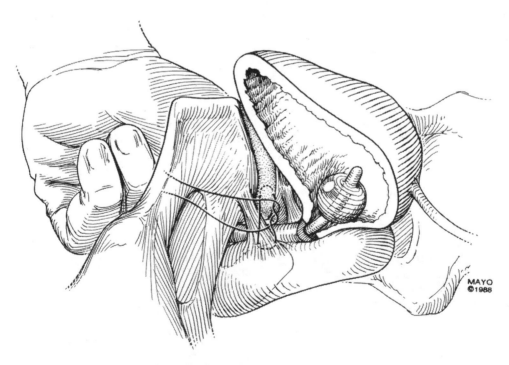

Figure 6 The Marshall-Marchetti-Krantz sutures are placed into the vagina and cartilage of the symphysis. After placing a double bite into the vagina, the needle is removed and replaced with a new free-Mayo needle prior to placement into the cartilage. This decreases risk of infection. A total of four sutures are placed. (Used with permission of the Mayo Foundation.)

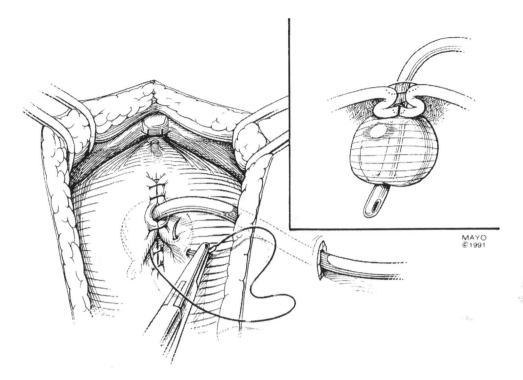

Figure 7 The bladder is closed in a double-layer closure incorporating the catheter into the incision. (Used with permission of the Mayo Foundation.)

V. PATIENT SELECTION FOR SURGERY

Patients with genuine stress urinary incontinence and hypermobility of the urethra in the absence of severe bladder overactivity are candidates for Burch urethropexy. This includes patients with low urethral closure pressures or low Valsalva leak-point pressures if they also demonstrate urethral hypermobility.

The best definition of intrinsic sphincteric deficiency is functional: stress urinary incontinence despite complete support of the urethra in the absence of uninhibited bladder contractions. These patients are not candidates for urethropexy because they lack urethral mobility.

Bergman et al. performed a study showing that patients who have $<30°$ of urethral descent with urinary stress incontinence have a 55% failure rate associated with Burch urethropexy (25). Data on the transvaginal tape (TVT) procedure show that individuals with a nonmobile urethra and stress incontinence are also at increased risk of failure with TVT surgery (2).

Patients with low urethral pressures who have urethral junction rotation are not at increased risk of failure following Burch urethropexy. Sand et al. performed a prospective randomized comparison of the pubovaginal sling procedure and the Burch urethropexy in patients with low urethral pressures (26). The cure rate was comparable in the two procedures.

Hsieh et al. confirmed this in a separate study (27). The aim of their study was to determine whether an isolated low Valsalva leak-point pressure could be an independent risk factor for Burch failure in patients with a normal maximum urethral closure pressure. Twenty-four women with objectively proven stress incontinence, Valsalva leak-point pressures $<60\,cmH_2O$ and

MUCP values $>20 \, cmH_2O$ were evaluated preoperatively and postoperatively. At >1-year follow-up, 22 of the 24 (91.7%) patients were objectively continent.

Patients with preoperative hypermobility of the urethra who demonstrate stress incontinence postoperatively, despite restoration of urethral support, have intrinsic sphincteric deficiency. This may occur after any operation for stress incontinence, including on occasion the pubovaginal sling procedure. This failure must be secondary to occult deficiency in nerve, muscle, and connective tissue that could not be diagnosed preoperatively. This occult deficiency results in deficient urethral resistance despite restored urethral support after surgery. We have no urodynamic parameters that predict which preoperative patients will fall into this group. The future may hold promise in diagnosing this tendency through laboratory assessment of deficient muscle, nerve, and connective tissue.

As an example of such assessment, Kenton et al. reported on the role of urethral electromyography in predicting patients who have preoperative urethral hypermobility, but fail to have their stress leakage repaired with Burch urethropexy (28). Eighty-nine women who underwent preoperative testing with urethral EMG and cystometrograms were also assessed postoperatively. Fifty-nine of 74 women (80%) were objectively cured, and 15 women had persistent urinary stress incontinence at 3 months. Women who were cured did not differ from those who failed in age, parity, menopausal status, maximum urethral closure pressure, Valsalva leak-point pressure, maximum cystometric capacity, and detrusor instability or prolapse stage. Electrical activity of the urethra was calculated in these patients during rest, voluntary urethral squeezing, repetitive coughing, and bladder filling. There was no difference in any EMG parameters between the two groups when measured at rest, with urethral squeezing, or during bladder filling. Women who were cured did demonstrate better motor unit action potential activation with repetitive coughing than those with persistent leakage.

VI. LAPAROSCOPIC BURCH PROCEDURES

Vancaille and Schuessler reported the first laparoscopic colposuspension (MMK) case series in 1991 (29). The literature reflects a lack of standardization and precise outcome measurements. Prospective, randomized comparisons of laparoscopic to open technique include the studies by Summitt et al. and Fatthy et al. (30,31). Comparable rates of stress incontinence cure were noted between the two groups in each of the studies. Prospective, randomized studies that show increased cure by open technique include Burton et al. (32) and Su et al. (33). Su examined success at 1 year and showed an 84% cure with the laparoscopic approach and a 95.6% cure with the open technique. The randomized study by Burton included a 3-year follow-up with a 40% failure rate in the laparoscopic group compared with a 15% failure rate in the open group.

Several authors have reported an increased complication rate with the laparoscopic approach. Speights et al. reported on frequency of lower urinary tract injury at laparoscopic Burch and PVDR (34). There were no ureteral injuries, and four patients of 171 had cystotomies.

Walter et al. compared morbidity and costs of laparoscopic versus open Burch when performed with concomitant vaginal prolapse repairs (35). A retrospective review of 76 laparoscopic and 143 open Burch procedures with at least one concomitant vaginal repair for symptomatic prolapse was accomplished. The group with open urethropexy had an older age, greater degree of prolapse, fewer concurrent hysterectomies, and a greater number of vaginal procedures than the group with the laparoscopic Burch procedures. There were minimal differences in complications. There were no differences in estimated blood loss, operative time, hemoglobin change, hospitalization, or hospital charges between the two groups. Considering that a significant percentage of incontinent patients require some type of concomitant prolapse repair, the benefits of laparoscopy in this setting is less evident. Kholi et al. showed that despite shorter hospital stay, the direct costs of laparoscopic Burch were higher than those of the open technique (36).

Persson et al. showed the benefit of two sutures on each side of the urethra in comparison to one (37). Objective cure rate was 83% in the women with two sutures, compared to the 58% of patients with one suture.

The current literature would indicate additional large prospective, randomized studies with adequate power are needed.

VII. LONG-TERM BLADDER COMPLICATIONS OF RETROPUBIC URETHROPEXY

Symptoms of voiding dysfunction and de novo detrusor instability are most likely increased by excessive elevation of the vagina and secondarily the bladder trigone at urethropexy. Greater elevation may result in obstruction and secondary effects on bladder muscle. The benefit of stabilization and not elevation may be an important factor to consider in decreasing postoperative complications of voiding dysfunction.

Alcalay et al. noted that the most frequent complication in their series was de novo detrusor instability (DI) (14.7%) (4). The rate of de novo DI was commensurate between those having primary or secondary operations. The authors noted that the development of de novo DI is a bad prognostic factor for long-term objective cure. Women who developed postoperative DI continued to have symptoms of urgency and urgency incontinence for >10 years. In addition, Alcalay et al. noted that 22% of patients still complained of voiding dysfunction 10 years or more after surgery, and four of these patients underwent urethrotomy. The authors found that preoperative factors had poor predictive value for postoperative voiding dysfunction.

In an earlier study, Stanton's group had followed 92 patients with no evidence of preoperative DI on urodynamics who had undergone Burch urethropexy. Postoperative urodynamics showed that 75 (81.5%) had stable bladders and 17 (18.5%) had unstable bladders (38).

In Langer et al.'s 10-year follow-up objective study, the incidence of de novo DI was 16.6% and 18.7% of postoperative patients developed anatomical defects (5). De novo DI appeared in 12 of 17 patients during the first year of follow-up. It took longer for the majority of anatomical defects to become manifest.

In the study by Feyereisl et al., the prevalence of postoperative DI was noted to be 14.9% and the prevalence of late voiding difficulties was 4.6% (3). In the study by Kammerer et al., the complication rate was no different in the Burch group compared to the anterior colporrhaphy group (23).

De novo DI complicated the postoperative course in two of 40 (5%) patients in the prospective study of Colombo et al. (this was half the amount noted in the MMK group) (11).

Vierhout et al. reviewed six studies totaling 396 patients who had undergone urethropexy. Sixty-eight (17%) developed de novo DI (39). The prevalence varied from 5% to 27% in the different studies.

Current knowledge indicates that patients with mixed incontinence who demonstrate DI at low bladder volumes are at higher risk of failure from retropubic urethropexy. This does not mean that patients with detrusor instability demonstrated at higher volumes are not candidates for urethropexy. The majority of female incontinent patients over the age of 60 probably have mixed incontinence. Colombo, in a retrospective study, showed that in a group of mixed-incontinence patients, the objective stress incontinence cure rate 2 years after urethropexy was 75% (40). To be considered cured, patients had to be subjectively free of any incontinence symptoms.

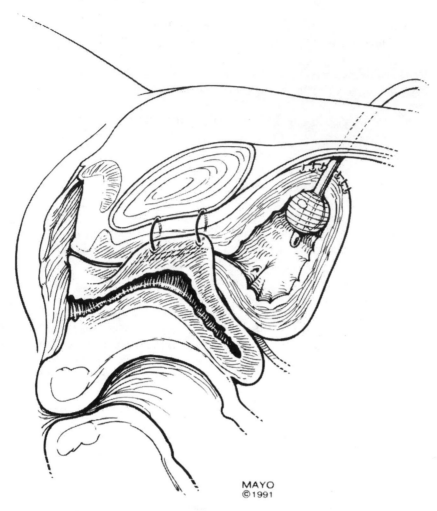

MAYO
©1991

Figure 8   The completed Marshall-Marchetti-Krantz procedure. The sutures are in the lower one-half of the symphysis avoiding excessive elevation. (Used with permission of the Mayo Foundation.)

The incidence of long-term urinary retention and its adverse sequelae after urethropexy is more difficult to estimate. The studies have not reported specific residual urine amounts at 5–10 years of follow-up. It is unclear in Alcalay et al.'s study how many patients had persistently high residual urine values in the group of voiding dysfunction patients (4). Four of 366 patients had subsequent urethrotomy. Residual urine values were not reported in the 10- to 20-year follow-up category. Feyereisl et al. in their 5- to 10-year follow-up of Burch urethropexy patients noted a residual urine value >60 mL in 16% of patients (3). The number of patients demonstrating long-term residual urine determinations >150 mL or 200 mL is not reported.

The risk of enterocele or rectocele formation after colposuspension may also be decreased by avoidance of excessive elevation of the vagina. Some series show up to a 26.7% risk of prolapse following colposuspension (41).

Demirci and Petri have documented a review of perioperative complications in the Burch literature (42). Wiskind et al. reported a need for blood transfusion in 0.7–2.3% of cases (41).

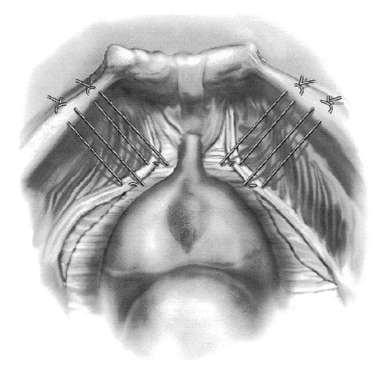

Figure 9   The Burch sutures are placed with each strand of the suture pair going through Cooper's ligament. Stabilization and not elevation of the anterior wall is achieved in order to decrease the risks of voiding dysfunction and bladder overactivity. (Used with permission of John Miklos. Copyright John Miklos.)

VIII.   CONCOMITANT GYNECOLOGIC SURGERY AND RETROPUBIC URETHROPEXY

Objective studies of hysterectomy at the time of urethropexy show no effect on incontinence cure or longevity of cure. Meltomaa et al. in a recent prospective study looked at morbidity and long-term subjective outcome between Burch colposuspension alone and Burch with concomitant abdominal hysterectomy (43). There was no difference in subjective short- and long-term (5 years) outcome. Complications related to operation occurred in 29.2% of the Burch group and 46.2% of the Burch/hysterectomy group. Complications were mainly related to infection and postoperative anemia. The reoperation rate was 1.5% for the Burch group and 2.6% for the Burch/hysterectomy group.

Sze et al. compared the surgical morbidity, postoperative course, and hospital charges of Burch colposuspension performed in conjunction with abdominal versus vaginal hysterectomy (44). The abdominal route had significantly longer hospital stays and higher hospital charges than the vaginal group.

IX.   CONCLUSION

The retropubic urethropexy remains an important procedure in the surgical management of female urinary incontinence. Burch urethropexy has a replete literature with some of the longest objective follow-up series of any incontinence procedure. It is effective in patients with low urethral pressure who have hypermobility of the urethra. It can be accomplished with a mini-incision allowing precise placement of sutures, and allows performance of a concomitant PVDR with site-specific correction of paravaginal defects.

REFERENCES

1. Ulmsten U, Henriksson L, Johnson P, Varhos G. An ambulatory surgical procedure under local anesthesia for treatment of female urinary incontinence. Int Urogynecol J 1996; 7:81–86.
2. Nilsson CG, Kuuva N, Falconer C, Rezapour M, Ulmsten U. Long-term results of the tension-free vaginal tape (TVT) procedure for surgical treatment of female stress urinary incontinence. Int Urogynecol J 2001; Suppl. 2:S5–S14.
3. Feyereisl J, Dreher E, Haenggi W, Zikmund J, Schneider H. Long-term results after Burch colposuspension. Am J Obstet Gynecol 1994; 171:647–652.
4. Alcalay M, Monga A, Stanton SL. Burch colposuspension: a 10–20 year follow up. Br J Obstet Gynaecol 1995; 102:740–745.
5. Langer R, Lipshitz Y, Halperin R, Pansky M, Bukovsky I, Sherman D. Long-term (10–15 years) follow-up after Burch colpsuspension for urinary stress incontinence. Int Urogynecol J 2001; 12:323–327.
6. White GR. A radical cure by suturing lateral sulci of vagina to white line of pelvic fascia. JAMA 1909; 21:1707–1708.
7. White GR. An anatomical operation for the cure of cystocele. Am J Dis Wom Child 1912; 65:286–290.
8. Marshall VF, Marchetti AA, Krantz KE. The correction of stress incontinence by simple urethrovesical suspension. Surg Gynecol Obstet 1949; 88:509.
9. Burch JC. Urethrovesical fixation to Cooper's ligament for correction of stress incontinence, cystocele, and prolapse. Am J Obstet Gynecol 1961; 81:281.
10. Richardson CA, Lyon JB, Williams NL. A new look at pelvic relaxation. Am J Obstet Gynecol 1976; 126:568–571.
11. Colombo M, Milani R, Vitobello D, Maggioni A. A randomized comparison of Burch colposuspension and abdominal paravaginal defect repair for female stress urinary incontinence. Am J Obstet Gynecol 1996; 175:78–84.
12. Webster GD, Kreder KJ. Voiding dysfunction following cystourethropexy. J Urol 1990; 144:670–673.
13. Mainprize TC, Drutz HP. The Marshall-Marchetti-Krantz procedure: a critical review. Obstet Gynecol Surv 1988; 43:724–729.
14. Lee RA, Symmonds RE, Goldstein RA. Surgical complications and results of modified Marshall-Marchetti-Krantz procedure for urinary incontinence. Am J Obstet Gynecol 1979; 53:447–450.
15. Colombo Colombo M, Scalambrino S, Maggioni A, Miliani R. Burch colposuspension versus modified Marshall-Marchetti-Krantz urethropexy for primary genuine stress urinary incontinence: a prospective, randomized trial. Am J Obstet Gynecol 1994; 171:1573–1579.
16. Quadri G, Magatti F, Belloni C, Barisani D, Nicola N. Marshall-Marchetti-Krantz urethropexy and Burch colposuspension for stress urinary incontinence in women with low pressure and hypermobility of the urethra: early results of a prospective randomized clinical trial. Am J Obstet Gynecol 1999; 181:12–18.
17. Kammerer-Doak DN, Cornella JL, Magrina JF, Stanhope CR, Smilack J. Osteitis pubis after Marshall-Marchetti-Krantz urethropexy: a pubic osteomyelitis. Am J Obstet Gynecol 1998; 179:586–590.
18. Burch JC. Cooper's ligament urethrovesical suspension for stress urinary incontinence. Am J Obstet Gynaecol 1968; 6:764–774.
19. Tanagho EA. Colpocystourethropexy: the way we do it. J Urol 1976; 116:751–753.
20. DeLancey JOL. Structural support of the urethra as it relates to stress urinary incontinence: the hammock hypothesis. Am J Obstet Gynecol 1994; 170:1713–1720.

21. Herbertsson G, Iosif GS. Surgical results and urodynamic studies ten years after retropubic urethropexy. Acta Obstet Gynaecol Scand 1993; 72:299–301.
22. Bergman A, Elia G. Three surgical procedures for genuine stress incontinence: five-year follow-up of a prospective randomized study. Am J Obstet Gynecol 1995; 173:66–71.
23. Kammerer-Doak DN, Dorin MH, Rogers RG, Cousin MO. A randomized trial of Burch urethropexy and anterior colporrhaphy for stress urinary incontinence. Obstet Gynecol 1999; 93:75–78.
24. Liapis AE, Asimiadis V, Loghis CD, Pyrogiotis E, Zourlas PA. A randomized prospective study of three operative methods for genuine stress incontinence. J Gynecol Surg 1996; 12:7–13.
25. Bergman A, Koonings PP, Ballard CA. Negative Q-tip test as a risk factor for failed incontinence surgery in women. J Reprod Med 1989; 34:193–197.
26. Sand PK, Winkler H, Blackhurst DW, Culligan PK. A prospective randomized study comparing modified Burch retropubic urethropexy and suburethral sling for treatment of genuine stress incontinence with low-pressure urethra. Am J Obstet Gynecol 2000; 182:30–34.
27. Hsieh GC, Klutke JJ, Kobak WH. Low Valsalva-leak point pressure and success of retropubic urethropexy. Int Urogynecol J 2001; 12:46–50.
28. Kenton K, Fitzgerald MP, Shott S, Brubaker L. Role of urethral electromyography in predicting outcome of Burch retropubic urethropexy. Am J Obstet Gynecol 2001; 185:51–55.
29. Vancaille TG, Schuessler W. Laparoscopic bladderneck suspension. J Laparoendosc Surg 1991; 1:169–173.
30. Summitt RL, Lucente V, Karram MM. Randomized comparison of laparoscopic and transabdominal Burch urethropexy for the treatment of genuine stress incontinence. Obstet Gynecol 2000; 95(Suppl):2.
31. Fatthy H, El Hoa M, Samaha I, Abdallah K. Modified Burch colposuspension: laparoscopy versus laparotomy. J Am Assoc Gynecol Laparosc 2001; 8:99–106.
32. Burton G. A three year randomized urodynamic study comparing open and laparoscopic colposuspension. Neurourol Urodyn 1993; 16:353–354.
33. Su TH, Wang KG, Hsu CY. Prospective comparison of laparoscopic and traditional colposuspension in the treatment of genuine stress incontinence. Acta Obstet Gynecol 1997; 76:576–582.
34. Speight SE, Moore RD, Miklos JR. Frequency of lower urinary tract injury at laparoscopic Burch and paravaginal repair. J Am Assoc Gynecol Laparosc 2000; 7:515–518.
35. Walter AJ, Morse AN, Hammer RH, Hentz JG, Magrina JF, Cornella JL, Magtibay PM. Laparoscopic versus open Burch retropubic urethropexy: comparison of morbidity and costs when performed with concurrent vaginal prolapse repairs. Am J Obstet Gynecol 2002; 186:723–728.
36. Kholi N, Jacobs PA, Sze EHM, Roat TW, Karram MM. Open compared with laparoscopic approach to Burch colposuspension: a cost analysis. Obstet Gynecol 1997; 90:411–415.
37. Persson J, Wolner-Hanssen, P. Laparoscopic Burch colposuspension for stress urinary incontinence: a randomized comparison of one to two sutures on each side of the urethra. Obstet Gynecol 2000; 95:151–155.
38. Cardozo LD, Stanton SL, Williams JE. Detrusor instability following surgery for genuine stress urinary incontinence. Br J Urol 1979; 51:204–207.
39. Vierhout ME, Mulder AFP. De novo detrusor instability after Burch colposuspension. Acta Obstet Gynaecol Scand 1992; 71:414–416.
40. Colombo M, Zanetta G, Vitobello D, Milani R. The Burch colposuspension for women with and without detrusor overactivity. Br J Obstet Gynaecol 1996; 103:255–260.
41. Wiskind AK, Creighton SM, Stanton SL. The incidence of genital prolapse after the Burch colposuspension. Am J Obstet Gynecol 1992; 167:399–405.
42. Demirci F, Pertri E. Perioperative complications of Burch colposuspension. Int Urogynecol J 2000; 11:170–175.
43. Meltomaa SS, Haarala MA, Taalikka MO, Kiiholma PJA, Alanen A, Makinen JI. Outcome of Burch retropubic urethropexy and the effect of concomitant abdominal hysterectomy: a prospective long-term follow-up study. Int Urogynecol J 2001; 12:3–8.
44. Sze EHM, Kohli N, Miklos JR, Roat TW, Karram MM. Comparative morbidity and charges associated with route of hysterectomy and concomitant Burch colposuspension. Obstet Gynecol 1997; 90:42–45.

19

Laparoscopic Treatment of Urinary Stress Incontinence

Thomas L. Lyons
Center for Women's Care and Reproductive Surgery, Atlanta, Georgia, U.S.A.

I. INTRODUCTION

The treatment of urinary incontinence is a costly endeavor in the United States with over billion dollars spent each year when all forms of management are considered, including the sale of adult diapers and the cost of medical and surgical care. Incontinence remains the most common cause for tertiary admission for long-term custodial care in the older patient.

Since urinary stress incontinence (USI) is the most common type of incontinence and the numbers of this diagnosis are increasing owing to the active postreproductive years population, the incidence of this already common disorder is becoming more frequent. Stress incontinence occurs almost exclusively in women and is stated to occur, at least to some degree, in 85% of women over the age of 18. The majority of women with USI are multiparous, and pregnancy or parturition, with its accompanying hormonal effects, pelvic floor, and pelvic neurological damage, is at the basis for the problem. In a majority of cases, patients are able to manage their symptoms using one or a combination of medical therapies, behavior modification, and pelvic floor conditioning. These therapies include Kegel exercises, behavior modification, electrical or ultrasonic stimulation of pelvic musculature, and a number of pharmacologic agents that act in a neuroleptic manner to improve urethral sphincter tone. However, if these alternatives have been exhausted, then surgery is the appropriate solution. The goal of surgery in this and every instance is to provide an effective solution with minimal medical and economic morbidity.

Because of the pandemic nature of USI and the difficulty of reliably correcting the problem with existing surgical techniques, over 300 surgical procedures have been developed over the years to deal with the problem (1–11). Similarly, as minimally invasive techniques have been applied in this area, a multitude of variations and new procedures have been proposed, many of which have "borrowed" names from traditional procedures whether the laparoscopic procedure resembled the old procedure or not. This means that some "laparoscopic Burch" procedures are not Burch procedures in the real sense of the word. The purpose of this chapter is to present some of the variations which have been proposed and what available data are present on these modifications. In addition, we will attempt to carefully describe the procedure that we currently perform and present the data and rationale that supports this approach.

Most gynecologists will agree that the gold standard surgically speaking in the treatment of USI is retropubic culposuspension (Burch procedure) (2,3). The Marshall, Marchetti, Krantz

309

(MMK) procedure is also included in this discussion (1). We also include the paravaginal repair, which was described by Richardson in the mid-1970s, as a component of this type of repair that is referred to as "site-specific defect repair of the pelvic floor" (4). The other type of surgical treatment recommended for USI is the suburethral sling procedure (11). This is the preferred method by most urologists, and although we have performed these procedures with laparoscopic assistance, we do not suggest that this should be the norm. It is important to apply a global approach to pelvic floor reconstruction, as rarely do the defects described here exist in absence of corresponding defects of the posterior compartment. Therefore, when the treatment of USI is considered, all defects are approached and treated at the same time. This invariably improves outcomes not only in the short term, but also extended follow-up is improved.

II. HISTORICAL CONTEXT

Originally, vaginal approaches to this USI problem were considered the only alternative to pessaries and nonsurgical methods of improving continence. In fact, the problem was rarely discussed and the initial descriptions of anterior colporrhaphy with the Kelley Kennedy plication in 1913 were rapidly accepted over the existing techniques, which had greater morbidity with uniformly poor outcomes (5). The subsequent development of vaginal approaches progressed under the auspices of proficient surgeons such as Nichols and Richardson into the latter half of the 20th century (4,6). Still, however, there were treatment failures particularly, over long-term follow-up.

Midcentury, a retropubic approach to the problem was suggested by Marshall, Marchetti, and Krantz (MMK) (1). This retropubic urethropexy seemed to improve outcomes but also brought new morbidity of osteitis pubis and urinary retention. A decade later the Burch modification was proposed and later modified by Tanangho and others into the procedure that is currently being used by most gynecologists and urologists (12). The clinical success rates quoted short term are in the high 80% range for this procedure.

Despite the excellent clinical outcomes, there was concern regarding the morbidity associated with the need for laparotomy to perform these procedures which gave rise to a number of new procedures. One group of these procedures were called the "needle procedures." Most notable among these proposed procedures were those described by Raz (7), Pereyra (8), Stamey (9), and Gittes (10). In further investigations these procedures have yielded relatively disappointing success rates of 50–70% (13).

The sling procedures which were first applied in the 1970s have produced good clinical outcomes, particularly in those patients with intrinsic sphincter deficiency (ISD) and mixed incontinence (11). These procedures also have morbidities that include the need for laparotomy in some cases and the potential for rejection/infection of the sling material itself. Although many of these problems have been obviated, very few gynecologists perform sling procedures routinely, and most urologists who use them do not approach the posterior and/or concomitant anterior compartment defects.

The late 1980s and the 1990s brought the replacement of a number of laparotomy-based gynecologic procedures with laparoscopic alternatives. In most instances, the laparoscopic approaches have produced similar clinical results with significant reductions in overall costs and morbidity. Logically, applications of minimally invasive techniques to USI and defects of the anterior compartment were the next step in this area. A Medline search of information on this application in 2002 reveals a wealth of papers on the laparoscopic applications to USI. However, standardization of these papers is difficult to assess but will be presented in the next segment of this discussion.

The first report of laparoscopic retropubic treatment of USI was by Vancaille and Shuessler, a gynecologist and an urologist, respectively, in 1991 (14). Vancaille has subsequently developed his techniques after Zacharin, the well-known Australian surgeon (15), while other gynecologists in the United States, including Lui, Lyons, and others, have pursued a site-specific approach to retropubic repairs (16–19). Table 1 summarizes the results of a Medline search on laparoscopic applications to USI.

III. TECHNIQUE

The technique that will be described here is the favored technique in our institution and this technique is similar to that of Lui, Miklos, and Wattiez. There are differences, but those

Table 1 Laparoscopic Urinary Stress Incontinence Procedures—Clinical Outcomes[a]

Reference	Patients (n)	Follow-up (months)	Cure rate (%)
Vancaillie et al. (14)	9	3	100
Liu et al. (18)	107	3–27	97.2
Liu (19)	58	24	94.8
Burton (20)	30	12	73
Gunn et al. (21)	15	4–9	100
Liu (22)	132	24	96.2
Nezhat (23)	62	8–30	91.9
Lam et al. (24)	15	9	98
Langebrekke et al. (25)	8	3	88
Lyons et al. (26)	20	12	92
Lyons (27)	38	18	90
Polascik et al. (28)	12	21–36	83
Von Theobald et al. (29)	37	42	86
Cooper et al. (30)	113	1–28	87
Kung et al. (31)	31	14–30	97
Nieves (32)	35	4–30	90
Radomski (33)	34	12–26	85
Shwayder (34)	20	12–54	100
Burton (35)	30	36	60
Lobel et al. (36)	35	1–51	68.6
Papasakelariou et al. (37)	32	24	90.6
Su et al. (38)	46	12	80.4
Das (39)	10	36	90
Lee et al. (40)	48	26	93.8
Miannay et al. (41)	36	17	79
Ross (42)	48	30–41	89
Saidi et al. (43)	70	5–27	91.4
Fatthy et al. (44)	34	18	87.9
Lee et al. (45)	150	36	90.7
Zullo et al. (46)	30	12	89

[a]Patient reports no loss of urine with Valsalva.

differences are predominately typical surgeon-specific idiosyncrasies. After an accurate diagnosis is made, the patient is prepped for surgery with a magnesium citrate bowel prep and is consented for pelvic floor reconstruction. If there are indications for hysterectomy, then hysterectomy is performed with laparoscopic supracervical hysterectomy (LSH), the preferred procedure. This allows excellent ability to reconstruct the pericervical ring of fascia and also facilitates the repair of the posterior compartment and vault support.

The patient is positioned as shown in Figure 1. Dual monitors placed at the patient's feet are at or above eye levels for surgeon comfort. The trocar placement is as shown in Figure 2. The midline trocars are 10/12 mm in diameter and allow for passage of the laparoscope in the subumbilical site and the introduction and extraction of curved needles of adequate size through the suprapubic site. The lateral trocars are 5 mm in diameter and are placed well lateral to the rectus muscles and as high as the suprapubic midline trocar at least four fingerbreadths above the symphysis. This allows an adequate angle to access both the space of Retzius and the posterior cul-de-sac. A 20-cc bulb Foley catheter is placed in the bladder.

After completion of the hysterectomy, posterior compartment repair is accomplished which usually includes a high McCall's culdoplasty and vault suspension. This is performed with #0 Ethibond (Ethicon Inc., New Brunswick, NJ) suture in an ipsilateral fashion. A relaxing incision is made medial to the ureter on each side to identify and avoid kinking of the ureter with this suspension procedure.

The space of Retzius is entered by making an incision in the anterior wall peritoneum ~1 inch above the symphysis pubis. This incision is extended bilaterally to the obliterated umbilical ligaments. Blunt and sharp dissection is used to identify first the symphysis and Cooper's ligaments and then the lateral pelvic sidewall, obturator neurovascular canal, neurovascular bundle, the ischial spine, the arcus tendinius (White's line of the pelvis), the arcus of the levator ani, and the paravaginal fascia (Fig. 3). The entire area is cleared or fat and areolar

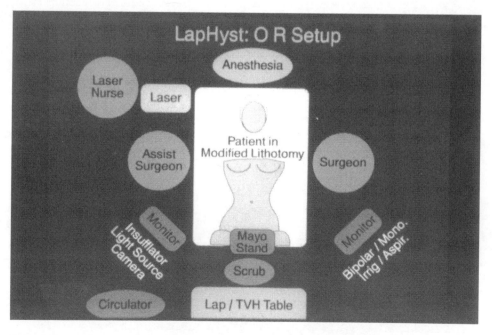

Figure 1

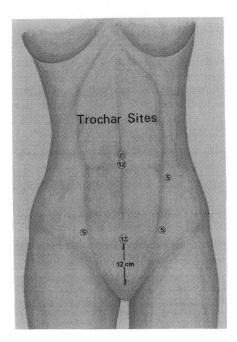

Figure 2

tissue (Tanangho modification) (12). Then the endopelvic fascia of the vagina is then sutured using #2-0 Ethibond (Ethicon Inc., New Brunswick, NJ) to the corresponding arcus tendinius fascia pelvis, thus correcting the lateral cystocele defect. This suture can be placed as an interrupted suture or in a running fashion. After both paravaginal defects have been repaired in

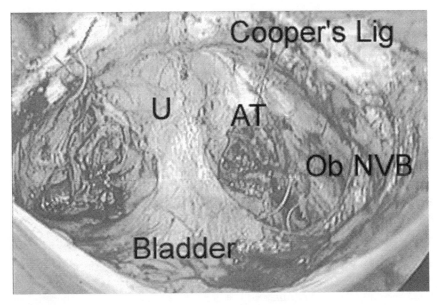

Figure 3

Table 2 Follow-up Laparoscopic Burch Urethropexy[a]

Suture	Success % (N)	Failure % (N)
Vicryl	50% (14)	50% (14)
Ethibond	76% (60)	24% (19)

[a]Based on 80.7% response rate.

this fashion then the Burch sutures are placed. Ethibond #0 suture is placed in an interrupted figure of eight fashion through the endopelvic fascia 1–2 cm lateral to the urethra with one suture at the midurethral level and one at the urethrovesical junction. These sutures are then taken through Cooper's ligament and tied, stabilizing the urethra and the U/V junction. This repair corresponds to the paravaginal-plus repair described by Shull in the late 1980s and constitutes completion of the repair of the anterior compartment. The anterior peritoneal defect is closed using #2-0 Vicryl (Ethicon Inc., New Brunswick, NJ) in a running purse-string manner.

Cystoscopy is performed 5 min after 5 cc of indigo carmine is injected intravenously documenting ureteral patency and the absence of suture material in the bladder. A 17 or 19 Fr cystoscope with 70° lens is helpful in this portion of the procedure. Absence of ureteral effluent requires investigation of ureteral patency. The catheter is removed as soon as the patient is ambulatory and the patient is allowed to void. Voiding abnormalities are common in the first few days but resolve rapidly. In the patient who is unable to void 5 h after the catheter is removed, the catheter is replaced and left overnight. Virtually all patients are able to void by morning. However, all patients are counseled about voiding difficulties postprocedure and are taught self-catheterization for this instance. Patients are discharged from the facility when discharge criteria are met and they wish to leave. This means that all patients are discharged within 23 h, and the average discharge is accomplished in 11 h. Patients are encouraged to resume most normal activity as soon as they feel comfortable but are restricted from intercourse and repetitive straining or heavy lifting for 4–6 weeks.

It is important to note at this time in the technical segment of this chapter that the use of permanent suture material is significant when treating support type defects. The present author's experience confirms this need. Table 2 summarizes the early experience in laparoscopic Burch procedures when first absorbable, and then permanent materials were used. Success rates have been maintained since that time when using permanent suture material.

Other described techniques involve the use of Prolene or other mesh materials and stapling or tacking devices to attach the mesh to Cooper's ligament and the paravaginal fascia, respectively (47), the use of the laparoscope to facilitate the performance of a "needle" or a sling procedure (36), and the placement of sclerotic materials into the space of Retzius under laparoscopic guidance all being described as a laparoscopic Burch procedure. Representative data from these techniques are included in Table 1. Conclusions regarding the efficacy of these procedures are left to the reader.

IV. DISCUSSION

Ultimately, there are a number of factors that will eventually contribute to the adoption of laparoscopically directed pelvic floor reconstruction. These are the same factors that should govern the adoption of any surgical or medical procedure. First and foremost, the procedure must accomplish the task that it is proposed to do. There seems to be ample evidence that this goal can be achieved with laparoscopic retropubic culposuspension. In the data generated to date, although little level I evidence is available, it appears that in competent hands results should be equivalent at worst.

Secondly, morbidity should be improved or no worse than existing techniques. Again, the evidence appears convincing that laparoscopic procedures definitely reduce short-term morbidity and mortality when compared to laparotomy procedures. There are some who argue that laparoscopy has a morbidity in and of itself, but the arguments for this position thus far have remained unconvincing. Medicolegally speaking, entry into the abdomen has a definable morbidity whether that entry is made laparoscopically or via laparotomy.

Thirdly, there is the question of cost. There certainly is no question that cost is and should be an issue in the performance of surgery. We must look, therefore, at cost and not at "charges," which some would have us believe are the actual costs of surgery. Charges are what the hospital or facility charges the patient or the patient's insurer for the procedure and almost always bear only a vague resemblance to the actual cost of the procedure. Operating-room time is an issue, and, early in the learning curve, any new procedure will take more time, but it is our observation that this is no longer an issue once proficiency is gained. No special materials or devices are needed for this procedure, although some have been suggested. Intangible costs of more rapid return to work have not been addressed in the literature to date but based on information derived from work done with laparoscopic cholecystectomy and laparoscopic hysterectomy the cost savings from these procedures could be substantial (48,49).

Finally, there is the question of technical training and credentialing. The procedures described are not new procedures as such but only different modes of access to perform "tried-and-true" procedures. Certainly, suturing laparoscopically is one of the more difficult skills to learn by the novice laparoscopist, but it does not represent a barrier that is in any way unreachable by a surgeon who is willing to practice this technique and apply it in his or her practice. The potential reduction in morbidity for that surgeon's patients is well worth the extra efforts involved. There have also been concerns that somehow adoption of these procedures would signal an end to vaginal surgery and its attendant discipline. It is this author's belief that the further anatomic knowledge that is attainable with laparoscopic surgery can serve to improve the vaginal skills of the operator and potentially open more vaginal opportunities for possible success in correcting these defects.

Pelvic floor reconstruction is a discipline that, in reality, has only one century of history. In that period of time, great strides have been made and many solutions have been found to these problems that affect women in their day-to-day lives. At the same time, advances have been made in surgery that have made surgical procedures safer and more effective for our patients. At the end of the 20th century, operative laparoscopy entered the scene and has made an impact on numerous gynecologic and general surgical procedures (50). Owing to the technical difficulty of some of these procedures, assimilation into the mainstream of therapeutic options has been less rapid (51). Lack of level I evidence has been suggested as the reason for this slow uptake, but since there is a dearth of such evidence for existing procedures, it is doubtful that this is the case. How best to perform pelvic floor reconstruction, and what are the anatomic and what are the physiologic explanations for these disorders and their attendant symptomologies are questions for which answers remain lacking. This is truly a surgical field that is a "work in progress." It is felt that if laparoscopically directed approaches can further any of this knowledge, anatomically or surgically, then the effort was well spent.

REFERENCES

1. Marshall VF, Marchetti AA, Krantz KE. The correction of stress incontinence by simple vesicourethral suspension. Surg Gynecol Obstet 1949; 88:590.
2. Burch JC. Urethrovaginal fixation to Cooper's ligament for correction of stress incontinence, cystocele, and prolapse. Am J Obstet Gynecol 1961; 81:281–286.
3. Burch JC. Cooper's ligament urethrovesical suspension for stress urinary incontinence. Am J Obstet Gynecol 1968; 100:764–771.
4. Richardson AC, Edmonds PB, Williams N. Treatment of stress urinary incontinence due to paravaginal fascial defect. Obstet Gynecol 1982; 57:357–360.
5. Kelly HA. Incontinence of urine in women. Uro Certan Rev 1913; 17:291–299.
6. Nichols DH, Ponchak SF. Treating incontinence transvaginally. Cont Obstet Gynecol Suppl 1986; 109–121.
7. Raz S, Sussman FM, Erickson DB, Bugg KS, Nitti VW. The Raz bladder neck suspension results in 206 patients. J Urol 1992; 148:845–850.
8. Pereyra AS. A simplified procedure for correction of stress incontinence. J Surg Gynecol Obstet 1959; 67:223–226.
9. Stamey TA. Endoscopic suspension of the vesicle neck for urinary incontinence in females: a report on 203 consecutive patients. Am Surg 1980; 192:465–471.
10. Gittes RF. No incision pubovaginal suspension for stress incontinence. J Urol 1987; 138:568–574.
11. Ridley JH. Appraisal of the Goebell-Frangenheim-Stoeckel sling procedure. Am J Obstet Gynecol 1966; 95:714–721.
12. Tanagho EA. Culpocystourethropexy: The way we do it. J Urol 1976; 116:751–753.
13. Bergman A, Ballard CA, Konings PP. Comparison of three different surgical procedures for genuine stress incontinence: prospective randomized study. Am J Obstet Gynecol 1989; 160:1102–1107.
14. Vancaillie TG, Schuessler W. Laparoscopic bladder neck suspension. J Laparosc Endosc Surg 1991; 1:169–173.
15. Zacharin RF. The anatomic supports of the female urethra. Obstet Gynecol 1968; 32:754–759.
16. Miklos JR, Kohli N. Laparoscopic paravaginal repair plus Burch urethropexy: review and descriptive technique. Urology 2000; 56:64–69.
17. Wattiez A, Boughizane S, Alexandre F, Canis M, Mage G, Pouly JL. Laparoscopic procedures for stress incontinence and prolapse. Curr Opin Obstet Gynecol 1995; 7:317–321.
18. Liu CY, Paek W. Laparoscopic retropubic colposuspension (Burch procedure). J Am Assoc Gynecol Laparosc 1993; 1:31–35.
19. Liu CY. Laparoscopic retropubic colposuspension (Burch procedure). A review of 58 cases. J Reprod Med 1993; 38:526–530.
20. Burton GA. A randomized comparison of laparoscopic and open colposuspension. Neurourol Urodyn 1994; 13:487–498.
21. Gunn GC, Cooper RP, Gordon NS, Gagnon L. Use of a new device for endoscopic suturing in the laparoscopic Burch procedure. J Am Assoc Gynecol Laparosc 1994; 2:65–70.
22. Liu CY. Laparoscopic treatment of genuine urinary stress incontinence. Baillieres Clin Obstet Gynaecol 1994; 8:789–798.
23. Nezhat CH, Nezhat F, Nezhat CR, Rottenberg H. Laparoscopic retropubic cystourethropexy. J Am Assoc Gynecol Laparosc 1994; 1:339–349.
24. Lam AM, Jenkins GJ, Hyslop RS. Laparoscopic Burch colposuspension for stress incontinence: preliminary results. Med J Aust 1995; 162:18–21.
25. Langebrekke A, Dahlstrom B, Eraker R, Urnes A. The laparoscopic Burch procedure. A preliminary report. Acta Obstet Gynaecol Scand 1995; 74:153–155.
26. Lyons TL, Winer WK. Clinical outcomes with laparoscopic approaches and open Burch procedures for urinary stress incontinence. J Am Assoc Gynaecol Laparosc 1995; 2:193–198.
27. Lyons TL. Minimally invasive retropubic colposuspension. Gynaecol Endosc 1995; 4:189–194.

28. Polascik TJ, Moore RG, Rosenberg MT, Kavoussi LR. Comparison of laparoscopic and open retropubic urethropexy for treatment of stress urinary incontinence. Urology 1995; 45:647–652.

29. Von Theobald P, Guillaumin D, Levy G. Laparoscopic preperitoneal colposuspension for stress incontinence in women. Technique and results of 37 procedures. Surg Endosc 1995; 9:1189–1192.

30. Cooper MJW, Cario G, Lam A, Carlton M. A review of results in a series of 113 laparoscopic colposuspensions. Aust NZ J Obstet Gynaecol 1996; 36:44–48.

31. Kung RC, Lie K, Lee P, Drutz HP. The cost effectiveness of laparoscopic versus abdominal Burch in women with urinary stress incontinence. J Am Assoc Gynecol Laparosc 1996; 3:537–544.

32. Nieves A. Long-term results of laparoscopic Burch. J Am Assoc Gynecol Laparosc 1996; 3:S35.

33. Radomski SB, Herschorn S. Laparoscopic Burch bladder neck suspension: early results. J Urol 1996; 155:515–518.

34. Shwayder JM. Laparoscopic Burch cystourethropexy compared with the transperitoneal and extraperitoneal approaches. J Am Assoc Gynecol Laparosc 1996; 3:S46–S47.

35. Burton GA. A three-year randomized urodynamic study comparing open and laparoscopic colposuspension. Neurourol Urodynam 1997; 16:353–354.

36. Lobel RW, Davis GD. Long-term results of laparoscopic Burch urethropexy. J Am Assoc Gynecol Laparosc 1997; 4:341–345.

37. Papasakelariou C, Papasakelariou B. Laparoscopic bladder neck suspension. J Am Assoc Gynecol Laparosc 1997; 4:185–189.

38. Su TH, Wang KG, Hsu CY, Wei HJ, Hong BK. Prospective comparison of laparoscopic and traditional colposuspensions in the treatment of genuine stress incontinence. Acta Obstet Gynecol Scand 1997; 76:576–582.

39. Das S. Comparative outcome analysis of laparoscopic colposuspension, abdominal colposuspension and vaginal needle suspension for female urinary incontinence. J Urol 1998; 160:368–371.

40. Lee CL, Yen CF, Wang CJ, Huang KG, Soong YK. Extraperitoneal colposuspension using CO_2 distension method. Int Surg 1998; 83:262–264.

41. Miannay E, Cosson M, Lanvin D, Querleu D, Crepin G. Comparison of open retropubic and laparoscopic colposuspension for treatment of stress urinary incontinence. Eur J Obstet Gynecol Reprod Biol 1998; 79:159–166.

42. Ross JW. Multichannel urodynamic evaluation of laparoscopic Burch colposuspension for genuine stress incontinence. Obstet Gynecol 1998; 91:55–59.

43. Saidi MH, Sadler RK, Saidi JA. Extraperitoneal laparoscopic colposuspension for genuine urinary stress incontinence. J Am Assoc Gynecol Laparosc 1998; 5:247–252.

44. Fatthy H, El Hao M, Samaha I, Abdallah K. Modified Burch colposuspension: laparoscopy versus laparotomy. J Am Assoc Gynecol Laparosc 2001; 8:99–106.

45. Lee CL, Yen CF, Wang CJ, Jain S, Soong YK. Extraperitoneal approach to laparoscopic Burch colposuspension. J Am Assoc Gynecol Laparosc 2001; 8:374–377.

46. Zullo F, Palomba S, Piccione F, Morelli M, Arduino B, Mastrantonio P. Laparoscopic Burch colposuspension: a randomized controlled trial comparing two transperitoneal surgical techniques. Obstet Gynecol 2001; 98:783–788.

47. Ou CS, Presthus J, Beadle E. Laparoscopic bladder neck suspension using hernia mesh and surgical staples. J Laparoendosc Surg 1993; 3:563–566.

48. Demco L. Hysterectomy panel discussion. J Am Assoc Gynecol Laparosc 1994; 13:287–295.

49. Bass EB, Pitt HA, Lillemoe KD. Cost-effectiveness of laparoscopic cholecystectomy versus open cholecystectomy. Am J Surg 1993; 165:466–471.

50. Soper, NJ, Brunt LM, Kerbl K. Laparoscopic general surgery. N Engl J Med 1994; 330:409–419.

51. Levy BS, Hulka JS, Peterson HB. Operative laparoscopy: AAGL membership survey. J Am Assoc Gynecol Laparosc 1994; 14:301–314.

20

Insertion of Artificial Urinary Sphincter in Women

H. Roger Hadley
Loma Linda University, Loma Linda, California, U.S.A.

I. INTRODUCTION

The artificial urinary sphincter (AUS) is an effective alternative to the urethral sling or periurethral injection therapy for the treatment of urinary incontinence in women as a result of intrinsic sphincteric deficiency (ISD) or type III stress urinary incontinence (1,2). In women with anatomic (type II) urinary incontinence associated with poor bladder neck support (hypermobility), the AUS is rarely inserted in deference to the more commonly used urethral sling or standard bladder neck suspension.

Intrinsic sphincter deficiency in women may be associated with or due to scarring following multiple prior anti-incontinence operations, neurologic disorders (myelomeningocele, sacral cord tumor, or peripheral neuropathy), radical pelvic operations (abdominoperineal resection or radical hysterectomy), pelvic radiation therapy, and estrogen deficiency, or senile changes of the urethra and vagina. Because intrinsic sphincter deficiency leads to inadequate urethral closure, a standard bladder neck suspension is unlikely to alleviate the patient's stress urinary incontinence. Operative management, therefore, is directed toward improving urethral closure with a suburethral sling, periurethral bulking agents, or insertion of the AUS.

The AUS is a manufactured device that includes a pump, a reservoir to store and regulate the pressure of the hydraulic fluid, and a cuff designed to provide a uniform circumferential compression on the urethra and bladder neck (Fig. 1). To empty her bladder the patient cycles the pump component of the AUS which is placed in the subcutaneous tissue of the labia majora. The American Medical System AS-800 is the only artificial sphincter currently commercially available and can be implanted using either a transvaginal or transabdominal approach.

This chapter describes the technique of transvaginal implantation of the artificial urinary sphincter in the treatment of incontinence due to intrinsic sphincter deficiency (type III stress urinary incontinence).

II. URINARY INCONTINENCE DUE TO SUSPECTED INTRINSIC SPHINCTER DEFICIENCY

Evaluation of the incontinent female patient should include a history, physical examination, radiographic evaluation, and urodynamic studies. The patient with genuine stress urinary

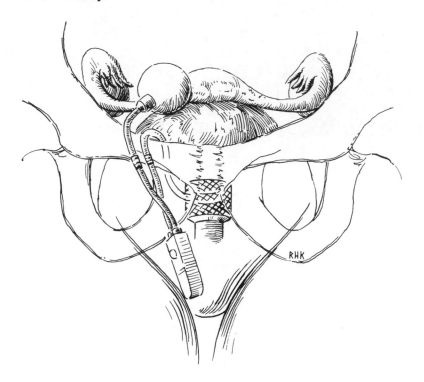

Figure 1   The AS-800 AUS in a woman. The cuff is placed around the bladder neck, the pressure-regulating balloon in the prevesical space, and the pump in the labia majora. (From Ref. 14.)

incontinence due to intrinsic sphincter deficiency will report loss of urine with abdominal straining that may or may not be associated with urgency. Previous anti-incontinence procedures, radical pelvic operations, history of orthopedic or neurologic disorders, and currently used medications (including replacement hormones) constitute important historical information.

Physical examination includes measurement of postvoid residual volume and an assessment of vaginal wall integrity and pelvic floor support. With the bladder filled to near capacity, the patient is assessed for stress urinary incontinence in the supine and/or upright position. Not only is it imperative to witness the loss of urine simultaneous to abdominal straining, but it is also important to make note of the severity of incontinence—i.e., losses of large volumes of fluid with minimal provocation. The Q-tip deflection test is used to assess urethral mobility. Neurologic examination of the lower extremities and perineum is performed to evaluate the lower lumbar and sacral cord segments. Cystourethroscopy is done to assess urethral coaptation, bladder trabeculation, and the unlikely presence of a fistula.

Radiographic evaluations may include a standing voiding cystourethrogram with resting and straining views. A well-supported urethra with an open bladder neck not associated with a bladder contraction is consistent with primary urethral insufficiency.

Urodynamic studies include a filling cystometrogram and measurement of urethral leak point pressure. Leakage of urine associated with a leak point pressure of $<80-100 \, cmH_2O$ in the absence of a detrusor contraction supports the diagnosis of intrinsic sphincter deficiency. Women with severe leakage (e.g., $<40-50 \, cmH_2O$) may need to be identified in a separate category, since these patients do not respond as well to traditional treatments as compared to their counterparts with higher pre-treatment leak point pressures.

Video urodynamics, if available, provides a concurrent fluoroscopic and urodynamic assessment that allows a simultaneous and perhaps a more accurate evaluation of the cause and type of urinary incontinence.

A. Patient Selection

Implantation of an AUS is reserved for those who have genuine stress urinary incontinence despite a well-supported bladder neck and no significant bladder instability. If the incontinent patient has concomitant vesical instability, simultaneous pharmacologic or operative management may be required to achieve urinary continence.

In the patient with urinary incontinence due to primary urethral insufficiency, conservative measures should be tried before operative intervention. These nonoperative measures include timed voiding, fluid restriction, pelvic floor exercises, systemic or topical estrogens, α-receptor agonists, and anticholinergic medications. If the patient continues to be incontinent despite conservative treatment, placement of the artificial urinary sphincter may be considered.

Because the more commonly used modes of therapy—urethral sling and periurethral bulking agents—have not been as successful in patients with severe incontinence and low leak point pressures, the AUS should be seriously considered and, indeed, may be best suited in these patients since it is designed to provide a uniform circumferential compression on the incompetent bladder neck.

B. Technique

The artificial urinary sphincter is composed of three parts: the inflatable cuff, the pressure-regulating balloon, and the pump (Fig. 1). The cuff is placed circumferentially around the bladder neck, the pressure-regulating balloon is positioned in the prevesical space, and the pump is put in the labia majora. When the pump is squeezed, fluid moves from the cuff to the balloon reservoir. This decompression of the cuff opens the bladder neck and allows the patient to void. After 1–2 min the pressure-regulating balloon automatically reinflates the cuff, which then reestablishes urethral coaptation and continence.

Three different techniques have been described for the transvaginal placement of the artificial urinary sphincter (1,3,4). The inherent advantage of the transvaginal approach is the possibility of dissection of the urethrovaginal plane, which is often obliterated after previous anti-incontinence procedures. The transvaginal technique allows dissection of the urethrovaginal plane under direct vision.

A vertical incision is made in the anterior vaginal wall (Fig. 2). The incision extends from a point midway between the bladder neck and the external meatus to the proximal bladder neck. A plane under the vaginal wall is created on each side of the incision with sharp dissection. The dissecting scissors are first pointed laterally to the pubis ramus and then upward toward the ipsilateral shoulder of the patient (Fig. 3). Sufficiently thick vaginal flaps are created in anticipation of closure of the vagina over the soon-to-be-placed cuff of the artificial urinary sphincter. If the patient has not had a previous bladder neck operation, blunt finger dissection may be performed to separate the endopelvic fascia from its lateral attachments to the pubic rim. The finger should sweep from lateral to medial, creating a window into the retropubic space. In the patient with dense scar tissue, sharp dissection will be required to enter the retropubic space. The urethra and bladder neck can then be separated posteriorly and laterally from the vagina and the pelvic side wall with sharp and blunt dissection. A similar procedure is followed on the opposite side.

The posterior aspect of the bladder neck is dissected free from the underlying anterior vaginal wall. It is important to mobilize the bladder from the vaginal wall without extending the

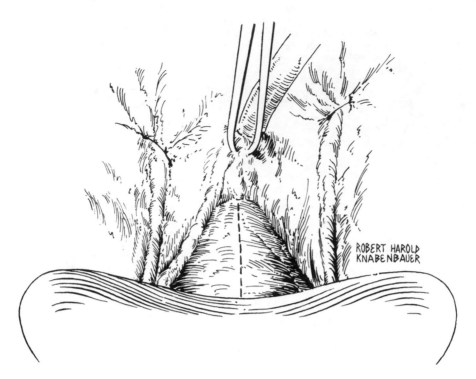

Figure 2   With the patient in the modified dorsolithotomy position, a vertical incision is made in the anterior vaginal wall. (From Ref. 14.)

vaginal incision toward the apex of the vagina. Leaving an intact thick vaginal wall underneath the bladder neck will lessen the likelihood of cuff erosion into the vagina.

Attention is next directed to the anterior aspect of the proximal urethra or bladder neck to free its attachments from the overlying symphysis pubis. If possible, blunt finger dissection should be used to perform this part of the procedure. However, in the patient who has had a previous retropubic operation, dense scarring may be encountered in the anterior portion of the urethra. Overly aggressive dissection may lead to unintentional bladder opening or urethral tear. The dissection on the anterior side of the urethra may be particularly difficult because of its relative inaccessibility through the transvaginal approach. To facilitate exposure of the top side of the urethra a separate suprameatal incision may be used. The previously placed Foley catheter is retracted downward, and a small (1–2 cm), crescent-shaped incision is made above the external meatus (Fig. 4A). Sharp dissection is then done in the midline below the symphysis pubis (Fig. 4B). After the bladder is allowed to drop away from its attachments to the symphysis, lateral blunt dissection can be easily performed to complete the dissection to the retropubic space previously opened through the vaginal incision. Thus, a circumferential dissection is completed around the bladder neck. However, if one is readily able to free the urethra from its anterior attachments through the vaginal incision alone, this suprameatal dissection is not necessary.

After the proximal urethra has been freed circumferentially, a broken-back small vascular clamp (Dale femoral-popliteal anastomosis clamp, Pilling 35-3543) is passed around the urethra from the left to right. The cuff-measuring tape is grasped and passed around the urethra (Fig. 5), and the circumference of the urethra is measured. If the circumference is equivocal, it is best to err in favor of a slightly larger cuff size. Using a curved clamp, the appropriate-size cuff of the

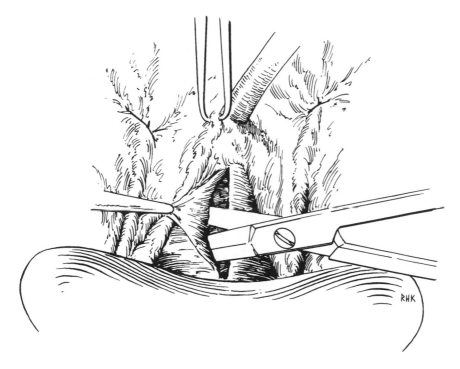

Figure 3   Using a combination of sharp and blunt dissection, the retropubic space is entered lateral to the bladder neck. (From Ref. 14.)

artificial urinary sphincter is placed around the proximal urethra (Fig. 6). If the pump of the artificial urinary sphincter is to be inserted into the right labium majus, the cuff is withdrawn from right to left. If, however, the pump is to be placed in the left labia majora, the cuff should be withdrawn from left to right. The cuff is then locked in place (see Fig. 6) and rotated 180° so that the hard-locking button lies on the anterior aspect of the urethra, away from the anterior vaginal wall (Fig. 7).

A 4-cm transverse suprapubic incision is made on the side that the pressure-regulating balloon and pump mechanism will be implanted. The tubing passer is passed antegrade under fingertip guidance from the suprapubic incision lateral to the midline and down to the vaginal incision on the ipsilateral side of the bladder neck. (This operative step is similar to passing a needle carrier under fingertip guidance during a Pereyra-type bladder neck suspension.) The cuff tubing is attached to the tubing passer and then withdrawn up to the suprapubic incision. The anterior rectus sheath is incised transversely, and the prevesical space is developed adjacent to the bladder. The pressure-regulating balloon is then inserted in the prevesical space. In women, the 51–60 cmH$_2$O pressure balloon reservoir is routinely used.

From the suprapubic incision a subcutaneous tunnel is created through which the pump will be inserted into the labia majora. The pump is passed into the labia majora to the level of the urethra with the deactivation button facing anteriorly.

Filling of the cuff and reservoir is performed according to the instructions specified by the manufacturer. The tubings are trimmed to the appropriate lengths and then irrigated to remove any air or debris from the system.

The suprapubic and vaginal wounds are irrigated with copious amount of antibiotic solution. The wounds are then closed in multiple layers with absorbable sutures to ensure good

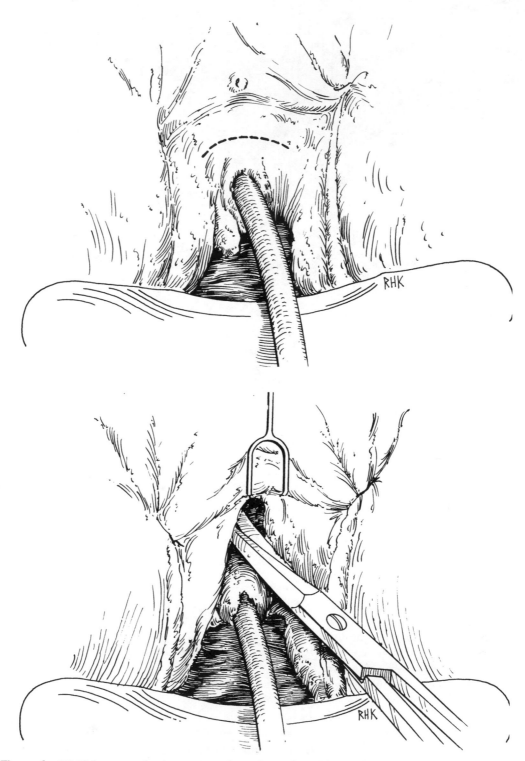

Figure 4 (A) If dense scarring is encountered anterior to the urethra, a separate incision is made above the urethral meatus. (B) The suprameatal dissection is done in the midline just below the symphysis pubis. (From Ref. 14.)

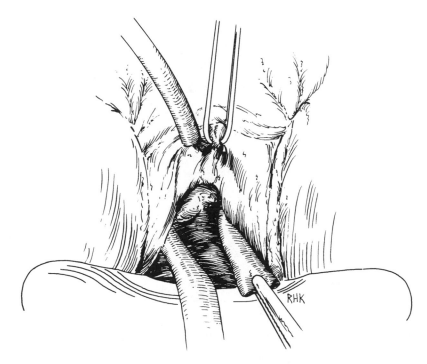

Figure 5 A Penrose drain is placed around the bladder neck to demonstrate the completed circumferential dissection. (From Ref. 14.)

coverage of the prosthesis with healthy overlying tissue. If the integrity of the vaginal wall appears to be compromised, an interposition of a vascularized flap (e.g., Martius flap) should be considered. The pump is left in the deactivated mode for 6 weeks.

A vaginal gauze pack is placed and removed on the first postoperative day. The Foley catheter is removed on the third postoperative day.

III. DISCUSSION

Favorable outcomes of transvaginal placement of the AUS have been published. Appell reported a series of 34 patients in whom the artificial urinary sphincter was placed through simultaneous vaginal and abdominal incisions (1). Nineteen patients underwent follow-up of 3 years. The overall continence rate was 100%. Three patients, however, required revisionary operations for inadequate cuff compression and connector leak. Abbassian described the implantation of the artificial urinary sphincter in four patients utilizing the vaginal incision alone (4). At mean follow-up of 14 months, all patients were dry.

The potential advantage of the artificial urinary sphincter over the urethral sling is the capability to place a known circumferential compressive force around the entire urethra rather than a single force on the posterior surface of the urethra. Women with severe leakage (e.g., <40–$50\,cmH_2O$) do not respond as well to traditional treatments as compared to their counterparts with higher pretreatment leak point pressures. The AUS may therefore be the preferred treatment in those patients with severe symptoms of stress incontinence associated with very low leak-point pressures.

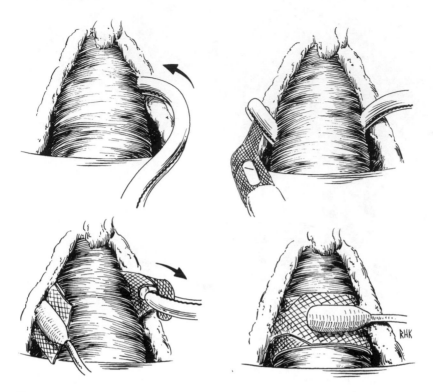

Figure 6 The cuff of the artificial urinary sphincter is passed around the bladder neck and then locked in place. (From Ref. 14.)

In addition, a decreased likelihood of urinary retention and bladder instability may be associated with the artificial urinary sphincter. The incidence of prolonged postoperative urinary retention after the urethral sling operation has been reported to be up to 10%, especially in patients with a preoperative hypotonic bladder (5). Persistent postoperative frequency and urgency due to bladder instability has been demonstrated in 6–18% of patients after placement of the pubovaginal sling in the treatment of type III stress urinary incontinence (6,7). In our experience of 25 patients who underwent transvaginal placement of the AS-800 artificial urinary sphincter for primary urethral insufficiency, seven patients had preoperative hypotonic bladder documented on urodynamic studies. Follow-up lasted from 3 to 16 months (mean, 7.3 months). None of the patients developed clinically significant postoperative frequency or urgency. All seven patients were dry and able to void spontaneously with or without abdominal straining. Prolonged (i.e., >1 month) urinary retention requiring intermittent catheterization was not demonstrated by any of the patients who had hypocontractile bladders preoperatively (8).

The continence rate of the AUS successfully implanted either by the transvaginal or transabdominal approach in women who have not had an erosion in either the bladder or vagina has been very good. A recent series of more than 200 women undergoing a transabdominal placement of the AUS reported a continence rate of >90% with a mean follow-up of 3.9 years. In this same series the explantation rate was 6% (12).

Long-term reliability of the artificial sphincter, regardless of the technique of implantation, is reported sparingly in the urological literature. Our experience from the artificial sphincter in both men and women indicates that the revision rate from all causes is ~50% at 5 years and >90% at 10 years. Similar 10-year revision rates have been reported from Fulford et al. (13).

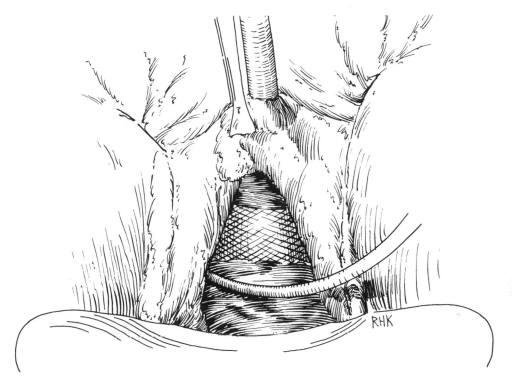

Figure 7   The cuff is rotated 180° clockwise so that the hard-locking button lies anterior to the urethra, away from the anterior vaginal wall. (From Ref. 14.)

Erosion of the AUS, like all nonhuman implantable devices, is a risk that cannot be completely avoided. Extrusion may occur if the pump erodes through the skin of the labium or the cuff erodes into the urethra or the vagina. Device erosion has been attributed to poor circulation, low-grade infection, technical difficulties, and shifting of the cuff (4). Cuff erosion commonly occurs in patients who have undergone prior pelvic irradiation (9). Our earlier experience included two patients who had been previously irradiated for cervical carcinoma. Both patients developed repeated cuff erosion into the vagina despite multiple revisionary operations. With the use of a low-pressure-regulating balloon (51–60 cmH$_2$O pressure), delayed primary activation of the cuff, and exclusion of the patient with prior pelvic radiotherapy, the incidence of device erosion may be much reduced (1,9). In the past, mechanical malfunction of the artificial urinary sphincter has been common, revision occurring in 31–43% of women with the device (10,11). However, since the introduction of the newly improved cuff design and the in situ activation-deactivation control assembly of the AS-800 model in 1983, the incidence of mechanical malfunction has dramatically decreased (2).

IV.   SUMMARY

Intrinsic urethral deficiency in women with stress urinary incontinence associated with a nonmobile, well-supported urethra and bladder neck is certainly a challenge in management to the urinary incontinence specialist. Many of these patients have undergone previous unsuccessful anti-incontinence operations. The artificial urinary sphincter is a viable alternative treatment modality to the urethral sling or periurethral injection therapy for these difficult patients. It may be the most appropriate mode of treatment for those patients with severe stress incontinence since these patients have not responded well to the customary urethral slings and periurethral bulking agents.

The advantage of the transvaginal approach in the placement of the artificial urinary sphincter is that it offers the surgeon the ability to dissect through the difficult urethrovaginal plane under direct vision. In the patient with abundant scar tissue, the addition of a suprameatal incision reduces the likelihood of an inadvertent cystotomy or urethral injury during the anterior dissection of the urethra.

With familiarization of the implantation technique, the use of a low-pressure-regulating balloon reservoir ($51-60$ cmH$_2$O pressure), delayed primary activation of the cuff, and selective patient criteria (e.g., exclusion of patients with prior pelvic irradiation), the artificial urinary sphincter can result in reasonable long-term social continence in patients with urinary incontinence due to intrinsic urethral insufficiency. In the subgroup of patients with a combination of hypotonic bladder and intrinsic sphincteric incompetence, the artificial urinary sphincter may be the initial treatment of choice over the urethral sling because of its lower incidence of prolonged postoperative urinary retention and vesical instability.

REFERENCES

1. Appell RA. Techniques and results in the implantation of the artificial urinary sphincter in women with type III stress urinary incontinence by a vaginal approach. Neurourol Urodyn 1988; 7:613–619.
2. Webster GD, Perez LM, Khoury JM. Management of type III stress urinary incontinence using artificial urinary sphincter. Urology 1992; 39(6):499–503.
3. Hadley R. Transvaginal placement of the artificial urinary sphincter in women. Neurourol Urodyn 1988; 7:292–293.
4. Abbassian A. A new operation for insertion of the artificial urinary sphincter. J Urol 1988; 140:512–513.
5. Blaivas JG, Jacobs BZ. Pubovaginal fascial sling for the treatment of complicated stress urinary incontinence. J Urol 1991; 145:1214–1218.
6. Blaivas JG, Olsson CA. Stress incontinence: classification and surgical approach. J Urol 1988; 139:727.
7. McGuire EJ, Bennett CJ, Konnak JA. Experience with pubovaginal slings for urinary incontinence at the University of Michigan. J Urol 1987; 138:525.
8. Wang Y, Hadley HR. Artificial urinary sphincter in the female: is it procedure of choice for the patient with type III urinary incontinence associated with an acontractile bladder?. J Urol 1992; 147(4):377A.
9. Duncan HJ, Nurse DE, Mundy AR. Role of the artificial urinary sphincter in the treatment of stress incontinence in women. Br J Urol 1992; 69:141.
10. Donovan MG, Barrett DM, Furlow WL. Use of the artificial urinary sphincter in the management of severe incontinence in females. Surg Gynecol Obstet 1985; 161:17.
11. Light JK, Scott FB. Management of urinary incontinence in women with the artificial urinary sphincter. J Urol 1985; 134:476–478.
12. Costa P. The use of an artificial urinary sphincter in women with type III incontinence and a negative Marshall test. J Urol 2001; 165(4):1172–1176.
13. Fulford SCV, Sutton C, Bales G. The fate of the "modern" artificial urinary sphincter with a follow-up more than 10 years. Br J Urol 1997; 79:713–716.
14. Wang Y, Hadley R. Artificial sphincter: transvaginal approach. In: Raz, S, ed. Female Urology. 2nd ed. Philadelphia: W.B. Saunders, 1996.

21
Urethral Injectables in the Management of SUI and Hypermobility

Sender Herschorn and Adonis Hijaz
University of Toronto and Sunnybrook and Women's Health Sciences Centre, Toronto, Ontario, Canada

I. INTRODUCTION

Murless, in 1938, first reported on injection of sodium morrhuate around the urethra by (1), and since then various materials have been injected for urinary incontinence as an alternative to surgery. Quackels (2) reported paraffin wax in 1955, and Sachse (3) used sclerosing agents in 1963. The initial results were poor, and significant complications such as pulmonary emboli and urethral sloughing were seen. Polytetrafluoroethylene (Teflon) paste, was first introduced by Berg (4) and then popularized by Politano (5) in the 1970s. Shortliffe et al. (6) published the first report on glutaraldehyde cross-linked collagen, and more recently autologous fat injection (7) has been described. Newer agents, such as silicone microparticles (8) and injectable microballoons, have also been reported (9).

Despite a tremendous growth in interest recently in injectable agents, there have been few published prospective randomized trials comparing different agents or injectables to other treatments for SUI. Outcome measures have not been standardized. This article will summarize the properties, published results, and complications of the various agents as well as examine some of the controversies.

II. MECHANISM OF ACTION OF INJECTABLES

It is generally agreed that these agents improve intrinsic sphincter function. Collagen injections have been reported (10,11) to augment urethral mucosa and to improve coaptation and intrinsic sphincter function as evidenced by an increase in posttreatment abdominal leak pressure (12–14). Initial investigators with collagen (15,16) postulated obstruction as a mechanism of action, but Monga et al. (11) showed that successfully treated patients have an increased area and pressure transmission ratio in the first quarter of the urethra. They suggested that placement of the injectable at the bladder neck or proximal urethra prevents bladder neck opening under stress. Proper placement of the injectable, possibly just below the bladder neck, rather than actual quantity (17) of the agent improves intrinsic sphincter deficiency (ISD).

The ideal injectable agent (18) should be easily injectable and conserve its volume over time. If unsuccessful, it should not interfere with subsequent surgical intervention. It should also be biocompatible, nonantigenic, noncarcinogenic, and nonmigratory. To date, no substance has met all of these requirements.

III. PATIENT SELECTION

Patients with ISD and normal detrusor function are candidates for injectable agents (19). McGuire et al. (20) identified these patients with the use of abdominal leak pressures to measure the strength of the intrinsic sphincter. Low leak pressures (<65 cmH$_2$O) correlate well with type 3 videourodynamic findings, i.e., a poorly functioning bladder neck and proximal urethra (ISD), and higher leak pressures correlated with types 1 or 2 hypermobility.

The presence of ISD is the primary indication for the use of injectable agents in patients with stress incontinence (10). Since ISD can coexist with hypermobility (21), injectables have been administered to patients with hypermobility to improve the ISD component of their incontinence. Furthermore, elderly women with hypermobility, who are poor operative risks, have also been injected (22).

IV. INJECTION TECHNIQUES

The materials can be administered under local anaesthesia with cystoscopic control as an outpatient procedure. Both the *periurethral* and *transurethral* methods are done to implant the agent within the urethral wall, preferably into the submucosa or lamina propria. It is thought that the implant should be positioned at the bladder neck or proximal urethra. Different sites can be chosen such as 3 and 9 o'clock or 4 and 8 o'clock positions. The needle size depends on the viscosity of the injectable. Pre- and postoperative antibiotics are usually administered. The technique of injection is seen in Figures 1 and 2.

With the periurethral approach, perimeatal blebs are raised with 1% or 2% lidocaine at the 3 and 9 o'clock or 4 and 8 o'clock positions ~3–4 mm lateral to the urethral meatus. A 20F urethroscope with a 30° telescope is inserted into the urethra after instillation of topical urethral lidocaine. The periurethral needle is introduced and advanced parallel to endoscope sheath until its position can be seen cystoscopically just below the bladder neck within the mucosa. Care must be taken to prevent the needle from getting to close to or entering the urethral lumen as rupture of the mucosa and extravasation will occur. Rocking the needle will confirm the position of the tip. If penetration of the mucosa occurs, the needle should removed and repositioned. The substance is injected either unilaterally or bilaterally to create the appearance of "prostatic" lobes. The patient is asked to cough or strain in the supine and then upright position. If leakage still occurs, more agent may be given. If no leakage is seen, the procedure may be terminated. The patient then voids and can be discharged. Acute retention can be treated by insertion of a fine 8F catheter.

The implant can also be injected transurethrally through the cystoscope with specially designed needles. Teflon, silicone microparticles, and fat, owing to their high viscosity, may require the use of injection guns.

A. Collagen

Glutaraldehyde cross-linked collagen or Gax-collagen is a highly purified suspension of bovine collagen in normal saline containing at least 95% type I collagen and 1–5% type III

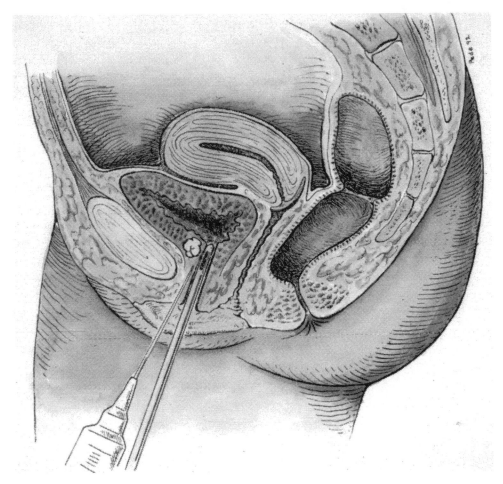

Figure 1   Periurethral collagen injection. The 20F cystoscope with a 30° lens is positioned in the urethra while the substance is injected into the bladder neck region.

collagen (23). This cross-linking makes the Gax-collagen resistant to the fibroblast-secreted collagenase. As a result of this, the Gax-collagen is only very slightly resorbed. The implant causes no inflammatory reaction or granuloma formation and is colonized by host fibroblasts and blood vessels. It is not known to migrate. However, it does degrade over time and is replaced by host collagen, to explain its persistence (23).

Since 2–5% of patients (24) are sensitized to collagen through dietary exposure, all patients must undergo a skin test into the volar aspect of the forearm 30 days prior to treatment. Positive responders should be excluded.

1.   Collagen Results

Numerous reports of its efficacy, safety, ease of administration, and relative lack of morbidity have appeared since the first description of collagen injections for urinary incontinence. Our original report, with short-term follow-up of 6 months (12), showed a cured and improved rate of 90.3%. With longer follow-up the success rate decreased, but there were still long-term cures. Table 1 lists various reported series.

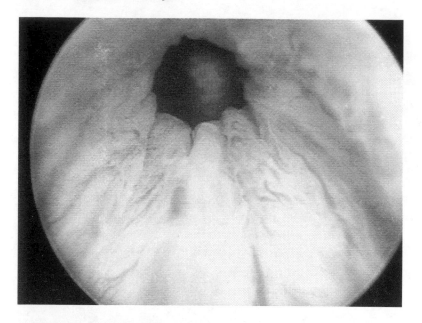

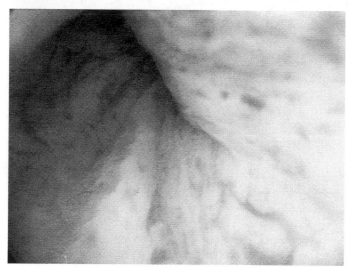

Figure 2   (a) Cystoscopic view of the open bladder neck region prior to injection. (b) Collagen has been injected via the periurethral route on the patient's left side. Note the intraluminal bulking effect of the agent.

Persistence of the implant itself has been demonstrated with magnetic resonance imaging of the urethra at intervals of up to 22 months after injection although the measured volume was less than that injected (25). Early results are generally good with success rates of 72–100% (Table 1). Maintenance of good results in the long term may be from durability of the initial procedure itself or from reinjections with additional collagen. It is important for authors to differentiate the durability of the original procedure(s) from reinjections or top-ups by reporting the follow-up period starting from after the last injection.

Table 1 Comparison of Collagen Parameters and Results

Study	No. pts.	Type of incontinence	Follow-up (mo.)	No. pts. dry (%)	No. pts. improved (%)	No. pts. failed (%)
Stricker and Haylen (26)	50	ISD	Mean: 11 Range: 1–21	21 (42)	20 (40)	7 (14)
Kieswetter et al. (27)	16	Not specified	9	7 (44)	7 (44)	2 (12)
Eckford and Abrams (15)	25	Not specified	3	16 (64)	4 (16)	5 (20)
O'Connell et al. (28)	44	42 with ISD 2 hypermobile	1–2(longest 7)	20 (45)	8 (18)	16 (37)
Moore et al. (29)	11	Types 1 and 3	2	1 (9)	7 (63)	2 (18)
Winters and Appell (13)	50	ISD	>12	48 (96) dry or socially continent		2 (4)
McGuire and Appell (10)	17	Mobile	>12	8 (47)	3 (17)	6 (35)
	137	ISD	>12	63 (46)	47 (34)	29 (19)
Faerber (22)	12	Type 1	10.3 (Range 3–24)	10 (83)	2 (17)	0
Monga et al. (11)	60	Some hypermobile	3 (N = 59)	27 (46)	24 (40)	
			12 (N = 54)	22 (40)	20 (37)	
			24 (N = 29)	14 (48)	6 (20)	
Richardson et al. (14)	42	ISD	46 (10–66 after 1st injection)	17 (40)	18 (43)	7 (17)

(continued)

Table 1 *Continued*

Study	No. pts.	Type of incontinence	Follow-up (mo.)	No. pts. dry (%)	No. pts. improved (%)	No. pts. failed (%)
Herschorn et al. (30)	181	Type 1: 54	Mean: 22 (Range 4–69)	42 (23)	94 (52)	45 (25)
		Type 2: 67	>=24 (N = 62)	27 (43.5)	29 (46.8)	6 (9.7)
		Type 3: 60	>=36 (N = 25)	13 (52)	8 (32)	4 (16)
Smith et al. (31)	94	Type 3	Median: 14	36 (38.3)	27 (28.7)	31 (33)
Khullar et al. (17)	21	Not specified	24 (minimum)	10 (48)	2 (9)	9 (43)
Swami et al. (32)	107	Some hypermobile	24 (minimum)	27 (25)	43 (40)	37 (35)
Cross et al. (33)	103	Type 3	Median: 18 (Range 6–36)	Substantially improved 103 (74)	29 (20)	7 (6)
Groutz et al. (34)	63	Type 3	Mean 6.4 + 4.9	13%	10% good 17% fair 42% poor	18%
Bent et al. (35)	90	Type 1 & 2	12	19 (21%)	19 (21%)	62 (58%)
Corcos and Fournier (36)	40	Type 1 (8) Type 2 (20) Type 3 (12)	Av 52; 47–55	12 (30%)	16 (40%)	12 (30%)

Longer-term results of more than 1–2 years vary from 57%, cure and improved (17), to 94% (36). Most patients need one or two treatment sessions with means of 5.6–15 cc collagen. Since patients are treated at different times and durations of follow-up vary, the Kaplan-Meier curve can be useful to display the persistence of a good result. In our series (30), the probability of remaining dry was 72% at 1 year, 57% at 2 years, and 45% at 3 years (Fig. 3). Winters and Appell (13) also reported a similar 50% rate of complete continence in the multicentre trial after 2 years. Corcos and Fournier reported a 4-year follow-up with 40% improvement and 30% cure rates (36). Additional administration of collagen usually resulted in restoration of continence, and this has to be factored into the reporting.

Berman and Kreder (37) analyzed the cost effectiveness of collagen versus sling cystourethropexy for type 3 incontinence. They concluded that surgery was more cost effective than collagen.

2. Collagen and Hypermobility

The use of collagen for patients with hypermobility has been reported. Moore et al. (29) included patients with both type 1 and type 3 abnormalities. Faerber (22) treated elderly patients with type 1 abnormality. In the report by McGuire and Appell (10), the results at >1 year in women with ISD were similar to those in women with hypermobility, although there were far more women with ISD. However, Appell (19) subsequently reported that these patients with hypermobility all required bladder neck surgery within 2 years. Monga et al. (11) included patients with hypermobility and found that cure rates were not reduced for women with up to 2.5 cm of movement. In our series of 181 patients there was no significant difference in outcome in patients with or without hypermobility (30). Steele et al. (38) found that urethral mobility did not significantly affect the success rate. As a matter of fact, four of six patients with urethral hypermobility were dry at the 6-month follow-up examinations; however, among the 19 women

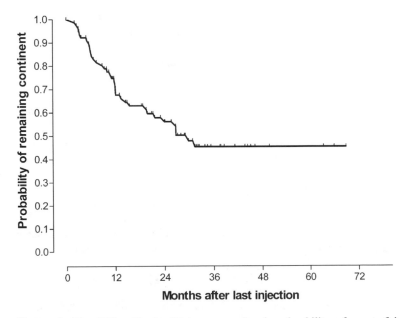

Figure 3   Durability: Kaplan-Meier curve showing durability of cure of incontinence after the last collagen injection in 78 patients. (From Ref. 30.)

without hypermobility, only a 32% remained dry. Corcos and Fournier found no difference between patients with and without bladder neck hypermobility in their 4-year follow-up on 40 patients (36).

3. Collagen Complications

Treatment-related morbidity has been minimal. Urinary retention ranges from 1% to 21% (12,13,19) and can be managed with intermittent catheterization or short-term foley. Urinary tract infection occurs in 1−25% (12,13,19). Extravasation resolves quickly with flushing away of the dilute collagen suspension and sealing over of the small needle site. Hematuria can occur in 2% of patients (19). Another rare complication is periurethral abscess formation (39).

Other complications include de novo instability, seen in 11 of 28 elderly women (39%) treated by Khullar et al. (17). Stothers et al. reported de novo urgency with urgency incontinence in 43 of 337 patients (12.9%), 21% of whom did not respond to anticholinergics (40).

Another rare complication is a reaction in the previously negative skin test site following a urethral collagen injection (24). This occurred in three patients (1.9%) and was associated with arthralgias in two. This reaction has been reported before in the dermatologic literature (41), and two negative pretreatment skin tests have been suggested to prevent it. The potential for hypersentivity reactions is present since antibody production is stimulated by collagen injection (42).

B. Polytetrafluoroetylene Paste (PTFE, Teflon, Urethrin)

Polytetrafluoroetylene Paste (Teflon) is composed of equal parts Teflon paste and glycerine with polysorbate 20 (43). Teflon is a resin polymer with a very high molecular weight and high viscosity, and is composed of small particles (40 μm in diameter). It is inert and stable, and does not induce an allergic response. However, it does cause a local inflammatory response with histiocytes phagocytizing the particles and coalescing to form foreign body giant cells and a granuloma. There is also fibrous tissue ingrowth that adds to the bulk formed by the Teflon. Owing to the small particle size, Malizia et al. (44) also showed distant migration of teflon particles to pelvic nodes, lung, brain, and kidneys of experimental animals.

Teflon paste has been used to treat urinary incontinence since 1964, but it was not reported until 1975, by Berg (4). Since that time, numerous reports relating to its use in treating incontinence have appeared in the literature. Although not approved in the United States, Teflon has been approved in Canada and in other countries.

It may be injected via the periurethral route and volumes of up to 10−20 cc are reported. The procedure is done under local or spinal anesthesia, and repeats may be done after 6 months. We have modified the procedure by injecting small amounts (2.5 cc) via the periurethral approach under local anesthetic (45). Heating the Teflon reduces its viscosity and allows injection without a gun.

1. Teflon Results

Table 2 lists various series. There are wide-ranging outcomes with longer-term series showing poorer results (33−76% cure and improved) than those of short-term series (57−86%) (46−54).

2. Teflon Complications

Since relatively large volumes of Teflon have been injected with the patient under general anesthesia, the incidence of urinary retention at 25% (46) is higher than that of collagen. Irritative voiding symptoms have also been seen transiently in 20% (48). Urinary infection is

Table 2 Teflon Results for Female Stress Incontinence

Study	No. pts.	Follow-up (mo.)	Pts. dry (%)	Pts. improved (%)	Pts. failed (%)
Politano et al. (46)	51	6	26 (51)	10 (20)	15 (29)
Lim et al. (47)	28	—	6 (21)	9 (33)	13 (46)
Schulman et al. (48)	56	3	39 (70)	9 (16)	8 (4)
Deane et al. (49)	28	3–24	9 (32)	8 (28)	11 (40)
Beckingham et al. (50)	26	36	2 (7)	7 (27)	17 (66)
Harrison et al. (51)	36	61	4 (11)	8 (22)	24 (67)
Lotenfoe et al. (52)	21	11	8 (38)	4 (19)	9 (43)
Lopez et al. (53)	74	31	41 (56)	15 (20)	18 (24)
Vesey et al. (54)	36	9 (3–36)	20 (56)	4 (11)	12 (33)
Herschorn and Glazer (45)	46	12	14 (31)	19 (41)	13 (28)

rare at 2% (47). Perineal discomfort may occur in 5% (46), and transient fever in 10–15% of patients. Perforation and extravasation can occur and, if recognized at the time of injection, the Teflon should be removed.

Although Teflon particles can migrate (44), only one case of clinical significance has been reported in the literature in humans. Claes et al. (55) described a woman previously treated with large volumes of periurethral Teflon for urinary incontinence who later presented with lymphocytic alveolitis and fever. Light microscopy showed Teflon particles in the lungs. She was treated successfully with steroids. Mittleman and Marraccini (56) reported an incidental finding of postmortem interstitial pulmonary granulomas in a previously asymptomatic man who had received Teflon. Kiilhoma et al. (57) reported three complications out of 22 women—a sterile periurethral abscess, a urethral diverticulum, and a urethral granuloma—that all required surgical intervention. In another case, the material migrated into the bulbar corpus spongiosum causing perineal pain for 3 months necessitating medication for pain relief (58).

Although neoplastic transformation was hypothesized (44), there has never been a clinical occurrence reported. Furthermore, in a long-term rat study, Dewan et al. (59) demonstrated no increase in tumor risk and no tumors found at the injection site.

Despite the potential for complications with Teflon the actual rate of reported problems is low. However, Teflon is rarely used as an injectable now.

C. Autologous Fat

Autologous fat has been used for aesthetic and defect reconstruction since the 1980s (60). Although fat is biocompatible and readily available, 50–90% of the transferred adipose tissue graft may not survive (61). Graft survival depends on minimal handling, low suction pressure during liposuction, and the use of large-bore needles. Smaller grafts survive better than larger ones (62).

The procedure involves harvesting abdominal wall fat by liposuction either under local (63) or general anesthesia (64). The injection is usually carried out via the periurethral route with a 16- or 18-gauge needle. Postprocedure care may involve intermittent catheterization or even a suprapubic tube (64).

1. Autologous Fat Results

A number of reports of urethral fat injections have been published and appear in Table 3. Most of the series report short-term results with success apparently lower than that of other injectables,

Table 3   Results of Autologous Fat Injection

Study	No. pts.	Follow-up (mo.)	No. pts. dry (%)	No. pts. improved (%)	No. pts. failed (%)
Cervigni and Panei (7)	14	9.7	8 (57)	4 (29)	2 (14)
Santarosa and Blaivas (65)	12	11	7 (58)		5 (42)
Trockman and Leach (63)	32	6	4 (12)	14 (44)	14 (44)
Haab et al. (66)	45	7	6 (13)	13 (29)	26 (58)
Su et al. (64)	26	Mean 17.4; range 12–30	13 (50)	4 (15)	9 (35)
Palma et al. (67)	30	12	1 injection: 4/13 (34) 2 injections:11/17 (67)		

apart from the study of Su et al. (64) with a follow-up of more than 12 months. Palma et al. (67) showed that repeat injections improved the cure rate from 31% to 64%. Haab et al. (66) reported a comparative study with collagen. After a mean of 7 months, 13% of the women with fat injection were cured versus 24% of the women with collagen injections. The subjective improvement rate was also higher with the collagen. Lee and colleagues reported a randomized double-blind study of autologous fat versus saline injection (68). At 3 months, six of 27 (22.2%) and six of 29 (20.7%) women were cured or improved in the fat and saline groups, respectively. In this study periurethral fat injection did not appear to be more efficacious than placebo in treating stress urinary incontinence.

2.   Autologous Fat Complications

Reported complications are similar to other injectables with urinary infection, retention, hematuria, and extravasation. Additional problems, such as pain, with donor site, the abdominal wall, hematomas, and infection may also be seen. Other noteworthy complications are urethral pseudolipoma (69) and fat embolism (39), one of which was fatal (70).

D.   Silicone Microimplants

Silicone microimplants (8) are solid polydimethylsiloxane (silicone rubber) particles suspended in a nonsilicone carrier gel that is absorbed by the reticuloendothelial system and excreted unchanged in the urine. Since 99% of the particles are between 100 and 450 μm in diameter, the likelihood of migration is low. Henly et al. (71) demonstrated distant migration of small particles, <70 μm, but no migration of particles >100 μm in diameter. Although there was a typical histiocytic and giant cell reaction within the injection site, there was no granuloma formation in response to the larger particles. Since the substance is quite viscous, it must be injected with an injection gun and a 16-gauge tip transurethral needle.

1.   Silicone Microimplant Results

Hariss et al. (8) reported on 40 patients followed for a minimum of 3 years at which time 16 (40%) were dry, 7 (18%) were improved, and 17 (42%) failed. Twelve of the 16 required one injection, and four needed two injections to become dry. Sheriff et al. (72) reported an overall success of 48% in 34 patients after unsuccessful stress incontinence surgery, and Koelbl et al. (73)

reported a 60% success rate in 32 women after 12 months but noted a time-dependent decrease in success. Radley et al. (74) reported a success rate of 61% (19.6% cured and 41.1% improved) in 60 women after a mean of 19 months. Barranger et al. (75), in a group of 21 patients, reported a dry rate of 19%, improved rate of 38%, and failure rate of 52% at a median follow-up of 31 months. Interestingly, they did not observe a time-dependent decrease in results.

2.   Silicone Microimplant Complications

Self-limited side effects of hematuria, dysuria, frequency, and retention have been reported in a minority of patients. The lack of a granulomatous reaction and migration of the large silicone particles may provide some benefit over Teflon, although no long-term data are available. Despite the laboratory and clinical evidence of safety with the large particles concerns still exist about the small silicone particle migration and long-term tissue response to the injection (71).

E.   Other New Injectables

Calcium hydroxylapatite, which is a normal constituent of bone, can be manufactured into particles of a spherical mean diameter of 100 μm. There is one report of its use in 10 women with ISD and limited hypermobility (76). After 1 year, seven reported substantial improvement, two improved, and one had no change. No significant complications were reported.

Another new synthetic agent, Durasphere, is composed of nonabsorbable pyrolytic zirconium oxide beads suspended in a carrier gel. The nonreactive beads range in size from 251 to 300 μm. Lightner et al. (77) reported results of a randomized trial compared to bovine collagen. At 1 year after the last treatment, 49 (80.3%) of 61 women in the Durasphere group had an improvement in Stamey continence grade of 1 or more, compared with 47 (69.1%) of 68 women in the collagen group. The difference was not statistically significant. There was also no difference in number of injections or pad weight test. However, the injected initial and repeat injection volume of Durasphere was significantly less than those of collagen. Adverse events were similar, but more women had posttreatment urgency and acute retention with Durasphere. Pelvic x-rays taken at 1 and 2 years after injection showed stability of the bulking agents at the injection site. This suggests potential durability. In another, small series of 13 women, Pannek and colleagues (78) reported a decline in success from 76.9% at 6 months to 33% at 12 months. In contrast to the previous study, they demonstrated particle migration locally and to distant sites on follow-up plain x-rays.

V.   IMPLANTABLE MICROBALLOONS

To obviate the degradation and movement of injectable materials, Atala and coworkers (79) developed a self-detachable implantable balloon system. The balloon is a silicone elastomer with a check valve that prevents escape of the solution that is injected at the time of implant. The filling solution is a biocompatible cross-linked hydrogel that maintains its volume within the silicone shell. The balloons are inserted into the submucosal area, usually periurethrally, with cystoscopic control.

Pycha et al. (9) reported that eight (42%) of 19 women were dry and seven (36.8%) were improved after a mean of 14.4 months. The patients with hypermobility had a poor outcome. Rare complications included bladder instability and balloon extrusion.

VI. CONCLUSIONS

Considerable progress has been made since the introduction of collagen injections. Injectable agents are used for buttressing the ISD component of the incontinence, but patients with concomitant hypermobility may benefit as well. They have also been administered to elderly patients who were not surgical candidates. However, there are still a number of areas in which further study is needed.

Durability is a concern. Although long-term successes have been reported with collagen and Teflon, the results of both deteriorate over time. Similarly autologous fat and silicone microimplants yield poorer long-term than short-term results. Comparisons of injectables and injectables to surgery have been done to a limited degree and prospective studies have yet to be reported. Despite the ease of the technique and the attractiveness to patients of an outpatient procedure that can be repeated if necessary, the cost-effectiveness of injectable agents relative to other treatments, such as newer, minimally invasive surgical procedures, still has to be addressed.

Safety of the material is also a concern. All of the injectables have excellent safety profiles, although the risk of migration and granuloma formation with Teflon has prevented its widespread use. Rare but serious complications have also been reported with collagen and autologous fat. The long-term risks of silicone microparticles, carbon beads, and balloons are unknown. Longer-term and comparative studies may settle these issues.

An exciting experimental model of using injected muscle derived cells into the bladder and urethra has been reported (80). There was persistence of the injected muscle cells compared to injected collagen. This may ultimately lead to additional treatments for stress incontinence.

Despite the shortcomings of the technology, the lack of long-term data, and the continuing need for an ideal agent, injectables are a viable minimally invasive alternative. Furthermore, since they do work in patients with hypermobility, this has lead to an increase our knowledge of the pathophysiology of stress incontinence. The two major components in stress incontinence, ISD, and hypermobility can be considered as interdependent and not separate entities. The relative importance of each component in any patient is variable, so the result of bulking in one patient with hypermobility may not the same as that in another. Other than the challenges mentioned above, it would be beneficial to identify factors in patients with hypermobility that would predict for success with injectables. More work also needs to be done to find out whether results can be improved by injecting the agent at sites other than the bladder neck.

REFERENCES

1. Murless BC. The injection treatment of stress incontinence. J Obstet Gynaecol Br Emp 1938; 45:67–73.
2. Quackels R. Deux incontinences après adénectomie guéries par injection de paraffine dans la périnée. Acta Urol Belg 1955; 23:259–262.
3. Sachse H. Treatment of urinary incontinence with sclerosing solutions. Indications, results, complications. Urol Int 1963; 15:225–244.
4. Berg S. Polytef augmentation urethroplasty. Correction of surgically incurable urinary incontinence by injection technique. Arch Surg 1973; 107:379–381.
5. Politano VA, Small MP, Harper JM, Lynne CM. Periurethral Teflon injection for urinary incontinence. J Urol 1974; 111:180–183.
6. Shortliffe LMD, Freiha FS, Kessler R, Stamey TA, Constantinou CE. Treatment of urinary incontinence by the periurethral implantation of glutaraldehyde cross-linked collagen. J Urol 1989; 141:538–541.

7. Cervigni M, Panei M. Periurethral autologous fat injection for type III stress urinary incontinence. J Urol 1993; 149(Part 2):403A.

8. Harriss DR, Iacovou JW, Lemberger RJ. Peri-urethral silicone microimplants (Macroplastique) for the treatment of genuine stress incontinence. Br J Urol 1996; 78:722–728.

9. Pycha A, Klingler CH, Haitel A, Heinz-Peer G, Marberger M. Implantable microballoons: an attractive alternative in the management of intrinsic sphincter deficiency. Eur Urol 1998; 33:469–475.

10. McGuire EJ, Appell R. Transurethral collagen injection for urinary incontinence. Urology 1994; 43:413–415.

11. Monga AK, Robinson D, Stanton SL. Periurethral collagen injections for genuine stress incontinence. Br J Urol 1995; 76:156–160.

12. Herschorn S, Radomski SB, Steele DJ. Early experience with intraurethral collagen injections for urinary incontinence. J Urol 1992; 148:1797–1800.

13. Winters JC, Appell R. Periurethral injection of collagen in the treatment of intrinsic sphincter deficiency in the female patient. Urol Clin North Am 1995; 22:673–678.

14. Richardson TD, Kennelly MJ, Faerber GJ. Endoscopic injection of glutaraldehyde cross-linked collagen for the treatment of intrinsic deficiency in women. Urology 1995; 46:378–381.

15. Eckford SD, Abrams P. Para-urethral collagen implantation for female stress incontinence. Br J Urol 1991; 68:586–589.

16. Appell RA. New developments: injectables for urethral incompetence in women. Int Urogynecol J 1990; 1:117–119.

17. Khullar V, Cardozo LD, Abbott D, Anders K. GAX collagen in the treatment of urinary incontinence in elderly women: a two year follow up. Br J Obstet Gynaecol 1997; 104:96–99.

18. Kershen RT, Atala A. New advances in injectable therapies for the treatment of incontinence and vesicoureteral reflux. Urol Clin North Am 1999; 26:81–94.

19. Appell RA. Periurethral injection therapy. In: Walsh PC, Retik AB, Vaughan ED Jr, Wein AJ, eds. Campbell's Urology. 7th ed. Philadelphia: W.B. Saunders, 1998:1109–1120.

20. McGuire EJ, Fitzpatrick CC, Wan J, Bloom D, Sanvordenker J, Ritchey M, Gormley EA. Clinical assessment of urethral sphincter function. J Urol 1993; 150:1452–1454.

21. Raz S, Little N, Juma S. Female urology. In: Walsh PC, Retik AB, Stamey TA, Vaughan ED, eds. Campbell's Urology. 6th ed. Philadelphia: W.B. Saunders, 1992:2782–2828.

22. Faerber GJ. Endoscopic collagen injection therapy in elderly women with type I stress urinary incontinence. J Urol 1996; 155:512–514.

23. Remacle M, Bertrand B, Eloy P, Marbaix E. The use of injectable collagen to correct velopharyngeal insufficiency. Laryngoscope 1990; 100:269.

24. Stothers L, Goldenberg SL. Delayed hypersensitivity and systemic arthralgia following transurethral collagen injection for stress urinary incontinence. J Urol 1998; 159:1507–1509.

25. Carr LK, Herschorn S, Leonhardt C. Magnetic resonance imaging of intraurethral collagen injected for stress urinary incontinence. J Urol 1996; 155:1253–1255.

26. Stricker P, Haylen B. Injectable collagen for type III female stress incontinence: the first 50 Australian patients. Med J Aust 1993; 158:89–91.

27. Kieswetter H, Fischer M, Wöber L, Flamm J. Endoscopic implantation of collagen (GAX) for the treatment of urinary incontinence. Br J Urol 1992; 69:22–25.

28. O'Connell HE, McGuire EJ, Aboseif S, Usui A. Transurethral collagen therapy in women. J Urol 1995; 154:1463–1465.

29. Moore KN, Chetner MP, Metcalfe JB, Griffiths DJ. Periurethral implantation of glutaraldehyde cross-linked collagen (contigen?) in women with type I or type III stress incontinence: quantitative outcome measures. Br J Urol 1995; 75:359–363.

30. Herschorn S, Radomski SB. Collagen injections for genuine stress urinary incontinence: patient selection and durability. Int Urogynecol J 1997; 8:18–24.

31. Smith DN, Appell RA, Winters JC, Rackley RR. Collagen injection therapy for female intrinsic sphincteric deficiency. J Urol 1997; 157:1275–1278.

32. Swami S, Batista JE, Abrams P. Collagen for female genuine stress incontinence after a minimum 2-year follow-up. Br J Urol 1997; 80:757–761.

33. Cross CA, English SF, Cespedes RD, McGuire, EJ. A followup on transurethral collagen injection therapy for urinary incontinence. J Urol 1998; 159:106–108.
34. Groutz A, Blaivas JG, Kessler SS, Jeffrey P, Chaikin D. Outcome results of transurethral Collagen injection for female stress incontinence: assessment by urinary incontinence score. J Urol 2000; 164:2006–2009.
35. Bent AE, Foote J, Siegel S, Faerber G, Chao R, Gormley EA. Collagen implant for treating stress urinary incontinence in women with urethral hypermobility. J Urol 2001; 166:1354–1357.
36. Corcos J, Fournier C. Periurethral collagen injection for the treatment of female stress urinary incontinence: 4-year follow-up results. Urology 1999; 54(5):815–818.
37. Berman CJ, Kreder KJ. Comparative cost analysis of collagen injection and fascia lata sling cystourethropexy for the treatment of type III incontinence in women. J Urol 1997; 157:122–124.
38. Steele AC, Kohli N, Karram MM. Periurethral collagen injection for stress incontinence with and without urethral hypermobility. Obstet Gynecol 2000; 95:327–331.
39. Sweat SW, Lightner DJ. Complications of sterile abscess formation and pulmonary embolism following periurethral bulking agents. J Urol 1999; 161:93–96.
40. Stothers L, Goldenberg SL, Leone EF. Complications of periurethral collagen injection for stress urinary incontinence. J Urol 1998; 159:806–807.
41. Elson ML. The role of skin testing in the use of collagen injectable materials. J Derm Surg Oncol 1986; 15:301.
42. McClelland M, DeLustro F. Evaluation of antibody class in response to bovine collagen treatment in patients with urinary incontinence. J Urol 1996; 155:2068–2073.
43. Diagnostic and Therapeutic Technology Assessment (DATTA). Use of Teflon preparations for urinary incontinence and vesicoureteral reflux. JAMA 1993; 269:2975–2980.
44. Malizia AA, Reiman HM, Myers RP, Sande JR, Barham SS, Benson RC, Dewanjee MK, Utz WJ. Migration and granulomatous reaction after periurethral injection of Polytef (Teflon). JAMA 1983; 251:3277–3281.
45. Herschorn S, Glazer AA. Early experience with small volume periurethral teflon for female stress urinary incontinence. J Urol 2000; 163:1838–1842.
46. Politano VA. Periurethral polytetrafluoroethylene injection for urinary incontinence. J Urol 1982; 127:439–442.
47. Lim KB, Ball AJ, Feneley RCL. Periurethral teflon injection: a simple treatment for urinary incontinence. Br J Urol 1983; 55:208–210.
48. Schulman CC, Simon J, Wespes E. Endoscopic injections of Teflon to treat urinary incontinence in women. Br Med J 1984; 288:192.
49. Deane AM, English P, Hehir M, Williams JP, Worth PHL. Teflon injection in stress incontinence. Br J Urol 1985; 57:78–80.
50. Beckingham IJ, Wemyss-Holden G, Lawrence WT. Long-term follow-up of women treated with perurethral Teflon injections for stress incontinence. Br J Urol 1992; 69:580–583.
51. Harrison SC, Brown C, O'Boyle PJ. Periurethral Teflon for stress urinary incontinence: medium-term results. Br J Urol 1993; 71:25–27.
52. Lotenfoe R, O'Kelly JK, Helal M, Lockhart JL. Periurethral polytetrafluoroethylene paste injection in incontinent female subjects: surgical indications and improved surgical technique. J Urol 1993; 149:279–282.
53. Lopez AE, Padron OF, Patsias G, Politano VA. Transurethral polytetrafluoroethylene injection in female patients with urinary incontinence. J Urol 1993; 150:856–858.
54. Vesey SG, Rivett A, O'Boyle PJ. Teflon injection in female stress incontinence. Effect on urethral pressue profile and flow rate. Br J Urol 1988; 62:39–41.
55. Claes H, Stroobants D, Van Meerbeek J. Pulmonary migration following periurethral polytetrafluoroethylene injection for urinary incontinence. J Urol 1989; 142:821–822.
56. Mittleman RE, Marraccini JV. Pulmonary Teflon granulomas following periurethral Teflon injection for urinary incontinence. Arch Pathol Lab Med 1983; 107:611–612.
57. Kiilhoma PJ, Chancellor MB, Makinen J, Hirsch IH, Klemi PJ. Complications of teflon injection for stress urinary incontinence. Neurourol Urodyn 1993; 12:131–137.

58. Stanisic TH, Jennings CE, Miller JI. Polytetrafluoroethylene injection for post-prostatectomy incontinence: experience with 20 patients during 3 years. J Urol 1991; 146:1575–1577.

59. Dewan PA, Owen AJ, Byard RW. Long-term histologic response to subcutaneously injected polytef and bioplastique in a rat model. Br J Urol 1995; 76:161–164.

60. Billings E, May JW. Historical review and present status of free fat graft autotransplantation in plastic and reconstructive surgery. Plast Reconst Surg 1989; 83:368–381.

61. Horl HW, Feller AM, Bieuner E. Technique for liposuction fat re-implantation and long-term evaluation by magnetic resonance imaging. Ann Plast Surg 1991; 26:248–258.

62. Bircoll M, Novack BH. Autologous fat transplantation employing liposuction techniques. Ann Plast Surg 1987; 18:327–329.

63. Trockman BA, Leach GE. Surgical treatment of intrinsic urethral dysfunction: injectables (fat). Urol Clin North Am 1995; 22:665–671.

64. Su T-H, Wang K-G, Hsu C-Y. Periurethral fat injection in the treatment of recurrent genuine stress incontinence. J Urol 1998; 159:411–414.

65. Santarosa RP, Blaivas JG. Periurethral injection of autologous fat for the treatment of sphincteric incontinence. J Urol 1994; 151:607–611.

66. Haab F, Zimmern PE, Leach GE. Urinary stress incontinence due to intrinsic sphincteric deficiency: experience with fat and collagen periurethral injections. J Urol 1997; 157:1283–1286.

67. Palma PC, Riccetto CL, Herrmann V, Netto NR Jr. Repeat lipoinjections for stress urinary incontinence. J Endourol 1997; 11:67–70.

68. Lee P, Kung R, Drutz HP. Periurethral autologous fat injection as treatment for female stress urinary incontinence: a randomized double-blind control trial. J Urol 2001; 165(1):153–158.

69. Palma PC, Riccetto CL, Netto NR Jr. Urethral pseudolipoma: a complication of periurethral lipo-injection for stress urinary incontinence in a woman. J Urol 1996; 155:646.

70. Currie I, Drutz HP, Beck J, Oxorn D. Fat embolism following periurethral injection of autologous fat — case report and review of the literature. Int Urogynecol J 1997; 8:377.

71. Henly DR, Barrett DM, Weiland TL, O'Connor MK, Malizia AA, Wein AJ. Particulate silicone for use in periurethral injections: local tissue effects and search for migration. J Urol 1995; 153:2039–2043.

72. Sherriff MKM, Foley S, McFarlane J, Nauth-Misir R, Shah PJR. Endoscopic correction of intractable stress incontinence with silicone misro-implants. Eur Urol 1997; 32:284–288.

73. Koelbl H, Saz V, Doerfler D, Haeusler G, Sam C, Hanzal E. Transurethral injection of silicone microimplants for intrinsic sphincter deficiency. Obstet Gynecol 1998; 92:332–336.

74. Radley SC, Chapple CR, Mitsogiannis IC, Glass KS. Transurethral imlantation of Macroplastique for the treatment of female stress urinary incontinence secondary to urethral sphincter deficiency. Eur Urol 2001; 39:383–389.

75. Barranger E, Fritel X, Kadoch O, Liou Y, Pigné A. Results of transurethral injection of silicone micro-implants for females with intrinsic sphincter deficiency. J Urol 2000; 164(50):1619–1622.

76. Mayer R, Lightfoot M, Jung I. Preliminary evaluation of calcium hydroxylapatite as a transurethral bulking agent for stress urinary incontinence. Urology 2001; 57:434–438.

77. Lightner D, Calvosa C, Andersen R. A new injectable agent for treatment of stress urinary incontinence: results of a multicenter, randomized, double-blind study of Durasphere. Urology 2001; 58:12–15.

78. Pannek J, Brands FH, Senge T. Particle migration after transurethral injection of carbon coated beads for stress urinary incontinence. J Urol 2001; 166:1350–1353.

79. Yoo JJ, Magliochetti M, Atala A. Detachable seld-sealing membrane system for the endoscopic treatment of incontinence. J Urol 1997; 158:1045–1048.

80. Yokoyama T, Yoshimura N, Dhir R, Qu Z, Fraser MO, Kumon H, De Groat WC, Huard J, Chancellor MB. Persistence and survival of autologous muscle derived cells versus bovine collagen as potential treatment of stress urinary incontinence. J Urol 2001; 165:271–276.

22

Vaginal Sling Surgery: Overview, History, and Sling Material

Keith J. O'Reilly*
Tripler Army Medical Center, Honolulu, Hawaii, U.S.A.

Kathleen C. Kobashi
Virginia Mason Medical Center, Seattle, Washington, U.S.A.

I. INTRODUCTION

The pubovaginal sling (PVS) is considered the gold standard for the treatment of female stress urinary incontinence (SUI). Originally described for the treatment of intrinsic sphincter deficiency (ISD), PVSs have been utilized to treat other types of SUI. There have been many modifications to the technique over the years, but the principles behind the PVS still hold today. The sling is placed beneath the proximal urethra and bladder neck to provide support and compression and to prevent proximal urethral descent during increased intra-abdominal pressure. Numerous materials have been utilized over the years to construct slings, and newer materials continue to be introduced in an attempt to decrease morbidity and improve durability of the procedure and patient satisfaction. This chapter will discuss the history of the PVS and examine the various materials used to construct slings as well as the different fixation techniques available.

II. HISTORY

The PVS was first described in 1907 by Van Giordano (1). The sling was constructed using gracilis muscle. Goebell, in 1910, described a sling constructed from the pyramidalis muscle (2). This was later modified by Frangenheim in 1914, who incorporated the overlying rectus fascia in a flap (3). Stoeckel then added a plication of muscular structures around the bladder neck via a vaginal approach (4). Common to all these operations was the belief that muscle placed around the bladder neck would acquire a sphincterlike function. Later, in 1933, Price described the first sling constructed from fascia lata (5). In this procedure, the fascia lata was passed beneath the urethra from a suprapubic approach, and the ends of the fascia were secured to the rectus muscle. In 1942, Aldridge described the use of a fascial sling that compressed the urethra during times of increased intra-abdominal pressure (6). Rectus fascia without muscle was passed through the retropubic space, and the ends were sutured beneath the urethra. This became a classic technique

---

Current affiliation: Madigan Army Hospital, Tacoma, Washington, U.S.A.

and was used for many years. In 1962, Narik and Palmrich modified the Aldridge technique by leaving the external oblique aponeurosis attached to the pubic tubercle and then suturing the ends beneath the proximal urethra (7). Complications associated with these procedures included urethrovaginal fistulas, urethral slough, outlet obstruction, and retropubic abscess. Given the high complication rates, slings fell out of favor for several years.

McGuire and Lytton revived the pubovaginal sling procedure for type III SUI in 1978 using autologous rectus fascia (8). They described a combined abdominal and vaginal approach and reported an 80% success rate for ISD. Blaivas and Jacobs then modified the procedure by penetrating the endopelvic fascia and by completely detaching the rectus fascia from the abdominal wall (9). Subsequent studies have confirmed that there is no difference in efficacy between free and pedicled fascial flaps for sling surgery (10). The results obtained by McGuire and Lytton have been further corroborated by other reports and therefore confirm the success and durability of the autologous fascia pubovaginal sling procedure for stress urinary incontinence (11–15). In 1996, the American Urological Association Clinical Guidelines Panel performed a meta-analysis of the literature regarding anti-incontinence procedures (16). The panel reported an overall success rate with slings of 82–84% at 48 months, regardless of sling material or anchoring technique employed.

III. CHOICE OF SLING MATERIALS

A. Autologous Fascia/Tissue

Numerous materials such as autologous fascia, cadaveric fascia, and synthetics have been used for pubovaginal slings with varying results. The choice of sling material ultimately depends on the preferences of the patient and the surgeon. Each material has its own advantages, disadvantages, and inherent complications.

Autologous fascia has been the gold standard material for the pubovaginal sling. Table 1 summarizes several authors' results with autologous fascia. Complications related to the sling material are extremely rare, primarily consisting of de novo detrusor instability or urinary retention.

Rectus fascia has been the most commonly used fascia and has proven long-term results. The fascia is harvested via a Pfannenstiel incision. In most cases, an adequate piece of fascia can be harvested despite prior lower abdominal surgery. One advantage of using rectus fascia is that following the harvesting of the fascia, no repositioning of the patient is necessary. Disadvantages include a limitation in the maximum length of fascia attainable, increased patient morbidity secondary to pain at the incision site, potential for abdominal wall hernia, and a theoretical

Table 1 Contemporary Results of the Pubovaginal Sling Using Autologous Fascia

Author	n	Type of fascia	Success (%)	Follow-up (mos.)	Postop retention	De novo urgency	Sling erosion
Morgan (17)	247	Rectus	88	52	2.4	7	0
Chaikin (18)	251	Rectus	92	36	2	3	0
Govier (14)	32	Fascia lata	87	14	3	9	0
Beck (19)	170	Fascia lata	92	NR	"High"	<1	0
Haab (20)	40	13 Rectus; 27 fascia lata	86	48	2.7	10	0

concern of poorer tissue quality if there has been prior lower abdominal surgery or radiation therapy to the area. The tensile strength of rectus fascia has been found to be approximately four times less than that of fascia lata (21).

Conversely, autologous fascia lata has been favored over rectus fascia by some authors because of improved tensile strength and better length, which can make adjustment of the sling tension easier. Fascia lata is also thought to provide long segments of unscarred fascia, which translates into more equal distribution of pressure on the urethra and more uniform urethral closure. There are also fewer postoperative activity restrictions than with the use of rectus fascia. Disadvantages include the time to harvest and reposition the patient, pain at the harvest site, muscle herniation at the harvest site, and cosmetic issues (22). In one study, 38% of patients were unhappy with the appearance of the leg scars (23).

Another source of autologous tissue that has been utilized as a sling material is an in situ vascularized island of anterior vaginal wall. In 1996, Kaplan et al. compared the safety and efficacy of an autologous rectus fascial sling versus a modified vaginal wall sling for ISD (24). Both procedures were effective in treating incontinence, but the authors were able to demonstrate that the vaginal wall sling was associated with a significantly shorter hospital stay, decreased catheter time, decreased pain, and fewer days lost from work. In a follow-up report, Kaplan et al. demonstrated durable results of the vaginal wall sling at a mean of 39 months (25). Subjectively, 93% of women were either satisfied or very satisfied. Recurrent stress incontinence occurred in 4%, and there was an 8% incidence of de novo instability and/or urge incontinence. Concerns with regard to the use of vaginal wall slings include the development of suburethral inclusion cysts reported by Su and Woodman (26,27). Additionally, the harvesting of vaginal mucosa from the anterior wall may affect pelvic support as demonstrated by the 7% incidence of new pelvic prolapse associated with this procedure. Lastly, vaginal tissue quality may vary depending on the estrogen status of the patient, exposure to radiation, and prior surgeries.

B. Allograft Fascia

Allografts are tissue harvested from human donors, usually cadavers, and transplanted into a human recipient. Soft tissue allografts have been used in clinical practice for more than 20 years. Orthopedic surgeons have used fascia lata allografts in the reconstruction of the anterior cruciate ligament, and ophthalmologists have used it in orbital floor repair. However, cadaveric fascia was not widely used in incontinence surgery until 1996 (28).

An important issue concerning the use of cadaveric fascia lata is the potential of transmitting infectious disease, such as HIV and other viruses. The risk of HIV transmission from soft tissue allografts is one in 1.7 million to one in 8 million, which is lower than the risk of HIV infection from a blood transfusion (29,30). Simmonds et al. documented the only case of HIV transmission due to tissue transplantation, which developed in a woman who received a bone allograft in 1985 from a seronegative donor (31). Since 1985, not only have all donors have been screened for HIV and other viruses, but more than 60,000 organ transplants and 1 million tissue plants have been performed without an increase in disease transmission (30).

Another potential risk of transplantation of cadaveric fascia is the transmission of prions. Prions are proteinacious particles that are the causative agents of spongiform encephalopathy, of which the most common is Creutzfeldt-Jakob disease. Prions are very resistant to treatments that target nucleic acids such as radiation (32). However, prions may be destroyed by denaturing agents. One manufacturer (Mentor Corporation, Santa Barbara, CA) has designed a treatment process that addresses the risk of prion disease without affecting the tensile strength of the graft (33). The patented processing technique involves gamma irradiation followed by solvent dehydration. Despite the theoretical risk and heightened worldwide awareness of prion-transmitted diseases, there are no cases of a transmissible spongiform encephalopathy associated with cadaveric fascia lata (32).

The Food and Drug Administration (FDA) regulates licensed tissue banks that process cadaveric fascia. Tissue banks are required to perform an extensive process of donor selection, donor testing, and a multistep tissue processing in order to remove tissue antigenicity and the risk of disease transmission. Prior to harvesting, donors are screened for a history of carrying hepatitis and other viruses. Serologic tests for HIV, hepatitis B, hepatitis C, HTLV-1, and syphilis are then performed.

The tissue is processed by one of several techniques: freeze-drying alone, gamma irradiation with freeze-drying, or solvent dehydration. There is some concern that different processing techniques may alter the tensile strength of the allograft. Lemer et al. demonstrated that the tensile strength and tissue consistency was decreased in freeze-dried fascia as compared to solvent-dehydrated fascia, acellular dermal grafts, and autologous fascia (35). Conversely, Sutaria and Staskin found no statistical difference in the tensile strengths of freeze-dried, gamma-irradiated and freeze-dried, or solvent-dehydrated gamma-irradiated fascia (36).

Allograft fascia lata is an attractive alternative to autologous fascia lata because it avoids foreign body reactions associated with synthetic grafts. Early reports have demonstrated that operative time, hospital stay, and postoperative time may be decreased with the use of allograft fascia (37,38). With respect to effectiveness, early results with cadaveric fascia lata have been promising. Amundsen et al. reported on the results of 104 patients who underwent a pubovaginal sling using a 2 × 15 cm strip of freeze-dried, nonirradiated cadaveric fascia lata. With a follow-up of 19.5 months, 87% were significantly improved (37). They also reported no adverse events related to the fascia. Brown and Govier compared 121 consecutive women who underwent a pubovaginal sling using cadaveric fascia with a group of 46 women who underwent a pubovaginal sling using autologous fascia (34). With a mean follow-up of 12 months in the cadaveric fascia lata group, 85% were cured of their SUI. These results were very similar to those achieved with autologous fascia. Cadaveric fascia lata has also been used to address not only SUI, but also pelvic organ prolapse. Kobashi and Leach reported on a new technique using solvent dehydrated cadaveric fascia lata to perform simultaneous transvaginal sling and cystocele repair. The authors reported that no recurrent cystoceles occurred and that 72% of patients were completely dry at a follow-up of 6 months (39).

The results attained with cadaveric fascia have been promising, and there have been minimal complications secondary to the cadaveric fascia. However, the follow-up has been short, and there is question regarding the durability of fascia lata. Chaikin and Blaivas described a case of an early failure of a cadaveric fascial sling in which the holding sutures had pulled through (40). Fitzgerald and Brubaker reported on 35 patients who underwent a pubovaginal sling with freeze-dried and irradiated cadaveric fascia (41). They reported a 69% cure rate, but eight patients (23%) were considered to be failures. Of these, seven (20%) were initially cured of their stress incontinence but went on to develop subjective and objective failure by 6 months. At reoperation, there were either remnants of the fascia or no evidence of fascia at all. Carbone et al. recently reported on their series of cadaveric fascial slings, which demonstrated a 40% failure rate along with a reoperative rate of 16.9% (42). At the time of reoperation, the fascial sling was noted to be attenuated or fragmented. The fascia used in this series was obtained from several tissue banks and processed by irradiation. It is becoming apparent that processing techniques, in addition to surgical technique employed, play a role in the short- and, presumably, long-term success of a procedure.

The fate of fascial allografts is well documented in the orthopedic literature, but there is little data in the urological literature, and there has been no good animal model studied. The process of incorporation is multifactorial and is heavily dependent on tissue, donor, and recipient factors. The process of incorporating fascial allografts involves initial donor fibrocyte death followed by neovascularization, fibroblast migration, remodeling, and maturation (41). Variations in harvesting site and processing techniques affect the quality of the tissue. It has been shown that solvent-dehydrated cadaveric fascia lata and cadaveric dermal allografts have significantly higher tensile strength and less tissue variability than does freeze-dried cadaveric fascia lata (35).

Though cadaveric fascia lata is FDA approved, there are no regulations regarding the quality or thickness of the fascia that is harvested, a fact that may be reflected in the variable results from one center to another (34,37,38,41,42). This concern can be addressed by using a commercially available solvent dehydrated product in which the tissue consistency and strength may be more similar to that of autologous fascia. Also, the characteristics of the donor, including age and comorbidities, must be considered. Little is known about what role the recipient plays in graft incorporation and the healing process. Will surgical outcome vary with the recipient's ability to incorporate the allograft? What role do recipient comorbidities and immune reaction play? Does the existence of scarring from prior surgery inhibit neovascularization of the graft and fibroblast proliferation? Although graft antigenicity is lessened after processing, an immune reaction still occurs. What patient characteristics will facilitate or hinder the fibroblast proliferation and remodeling along the graft? Still another unresolved issue is the ideal length of fascial strip to be used and the method of fixation. The lengths of fascia used by Amundsen et al. (37) and Govier et al. (34) (2×15 cm and 2×24 cm, respectively) were longer than those used by Fitzgerald (41) and Carbone (42) (2×10 cm and 2×7 cm, respectively), and different methods of fixation were used by each group. So it may be that the technique, not the fascia, is the cause for varying success. More than likely, it is both.

In summary, the use of cadaveric fascia lata as sling material for a PVS is safe and effective. It is associated with a shorter operative time and decreased postoperative pain. However, controversy does exist with regard to its durability. Studies with longer follow-up will be needed to further clarify its role as a sling material.

C. Synthetic Materials

In recent years there has been interest in using synthetic materials as an alternative to autologous fascia in the pubovaginal sling procedure in order to decrease operative time, postoperative pain, and need for hospitalization, and, in theory, to improve the durability of the results. There is no question that autologous slings have good long-term cure rates, and failures are usually apparent within the first 3 months. However, autologous fascia is subject to the same cellular degeneration and fascial tears experienced by host tissues that contributed to the original problem of SUI. In theory, the ideal sling material should last the lifetime of a patient and should not be at risk for degradation. It is believed that the biomechanical properties of synthetic material are superior to those of autologous tissue. The question is whether this will translate into improved long-term durability with synthetic slings. The first synthetic sling, which utilized nylon, was described in 1965 (43). Since that time a number of different synthetic materials, such as polytetrafluoroethylene (Gore-Tex), polypropylene (Marlex), polyethylene (Mersilene, Silastic), and nonabsorbable polyester impregnated with bovine collagen matrix (ProteGen), have been used as sling material. SUI cure rates using synthetic slings have been reported to be 77–90% at a mean follow-up of 4–8 years (44–47). Despite apparent long-term durability, synthetic slings are more prone to infection and erosion. In their review of the literature, the AUA Clinical Guidelines Panel found reports of only 12 of 1715 patients (.007%) with vaginal or urethral erosion of autologous fascial slings. In contrast, 41 of 1515 patients (.027%) with synthetic slings had erosion of the material into the vagina or urethra (16). The incidence of erosion and infection has varied with the type of material utilized. Polymeric silicone, polytetrafluoro-ethylene, and polyester have the highest incidence of erosion ranging from 11% to 55% (48,49). Owing to the problems with erosions and infections, the woven polyester slings were withdrawn from the U.S. market.

Kobashi et al. reported a multicenter review of 34 patients who required removal of the woven polyester sling secondary to erosion, infection, or pain (48). The most common presenting complaints were delayed vaginal discharge (62%), vaginal pain (62%), suprapubic pain (32%), and recurrent urinary tract infection (15%). Other symptoms included recurrent stress incontinence, vaginal bleeding, and irritative voiding symptoms. The mean time interval from sling insertion to removal was 7.95 months (range 1–22 months). Vaginal erosions alone occurred in 50%, urethral erosions occurred in 20%, and urethrovaginal fistulas occurred in 17%. Treatment was surgical removal of all the foreign material, following which only 20% of patients were dry.

The mechanism behind the erosion of the synthetic slings through the vagina and urethra appears to be multifactorial. Possible mechanisms of erosion may be considered according to the site of erosion and the material used. Vaginal erosions may occur as a result of delayed infection of the synthetic sling which leads to separation of the vaginal incision, vaginal erosion of the sling material, and subsequent onset of vaginal discharge (48). Urethral erosion may occur secondary to excessive tension of the sling on the urethra or unrecognized urethral injury at the time of insertion. The weave properties of different sling materials and tissue reaction to the synthetic material are also important factors. It is important that the material be able to be incorporated by the host tissue. Smooth-surfaced materials are poorly incorporated and may be prone to complications (49). Tissue reaction to the material may create inflammation and subsequent wound breakdown and erosion. Efforts to decrease inflammation have included extensive irrigation with antibiotic solutions, impregnating the mesh with antibiotics, and covering the mesh in a plastic sheath at the time of implantation to prevent contamination.

One of the new and promising synthetic slings used today is composed if a polypropylene (Prolene) mesh. The mesh tape is placed around the midurethra without tension. The mesh can be placed via either the tension-free vaginal tape (TVT) technique (Gynecare, Falls Church, VA), first described in 1996 by Ulmsten et al. (50), or the new SPARC procedure, recently introduced by American Medical Systems (Minnetonka, MN). Regardless of the approach used, this procedure can be carried out under local anesthesia in ~30 min in an outpatient setting. A small vaginal incision is made along the anterior wall of the vagina, and the dissection carried laterally on either side of the midurethra. With the TVT technique, trocars with the tape attached are passed through the urethropelvic ligament, behind the symphysis, and out through the lower abdomen. Conversely, the SPARC procedure involves passage of thin trocars under finger guidance from two small suprapubic incisions to the vaginal incision, similar to the technique of needle passage in the traditional bladder neck suspensions. Theoretically, SPARC allows a more controlled passage of the trocars between the suprapubic and vaginal incisions.

Minuscule "spikes" along the edges of the polypropylene mesh anchor the sling to the patient's tissue, securing it in place in a tension-free fashion. Regardless of which of the two techniques is used to place and position the tape, the theories behind the mechanism of anti-incontinence are similar. One theory is that the narrow ribbon at the midurethra attempts to re-create the normal urethral support mechanisms and kink the urethra with increased abdominal pressure. This mechanism requires hypermobility and is therefore not suitable for the fixed urethra. A second theory is that, as increased intra-abdominal pressure causes urethral mobility, the tape also migrates distally and anteriorly, resulting in compression of the urethra between the tape and pubic bone (51).

Early results with the TVT revealed a cure rate of 80%, and local tolerance of the tape has been high. Haab et al. reported on 62 patients with a minimum of 1-year follow-up. They reported a cure rate of 87%, with another 9.6% who were improved and 3.3% in whom the procedure failed. De novo detrusor instability was noted in 6.4%; 59 of 63 patients (93.7%) were able to void immediately; and all patients voided spontaneously within 4 days. There was no evidence of outlet obstruction, infections, or erosions; however, there were six bladder perforations (52). Ulmsten et al. recently reported on the 3-year results of the TVT in 50 consecutive patients followed prospectively. They reported a cure rate of 86% with an additional 11% who were significantly improved. There were no cases of retention or major intra- or postoperative complications. There were no signs of deterioration of the results over the 3 years, nor were there any erosions or rejection of the tape (53).

The concept of using a synthetic sling material is appealing because it does not have the morbidity of harvesting the graft. The material is permanent, and the results of the procedure should therefore be durable. There is also no risk of transmissible disease. In the past, synthetics have been associated with higher complication rates mainly due to erosions and infections. However, it appears that the composition of the synthetic material used is of utmost importance. This is exemplified by a report from Ulmsten and Petros, who performed a procedure using polytetrafluoroethylene versus polyethylene terephthalate as the sling material. They reported a 10% rate of erosion at one year (54). This is in contrast to the polypropylene mesh now used. The polypropylene mesh has large interstices that allow in-growth of fibroblasts and hence, incorporation by the host tissue. TVT is gaining popularity in the United States, and there have been over 100,000 cases performed worldwide. Erosions have been rare. Both the TVT and SPARC using the polypropylene mesh are promising techniques, but, as with all procedures, further studies with adequate follow-up are imperative to properly establish their role in the armamentarium of treatment of female SUI.

D. Sling Fixation Techniques

With the evolution of the pubovaginal sling, there has been a shift in the fixation techniques employed. Originally, the rectus fascia was left attached to the pubic tubercle. Further modifications involved detaching the fascia from the bone and fixing it to or over the rectus fascia. These forms of fixation necessitate a suprapubic incision that may be prone to infection and hernia. Injury to the urethra and bladder may occur with passing the fascial strip from the vaginal incision to the abdominal incision. Also, persistent pain secondary to nerve entrapment may occur when suprapubic fixation is used. Nevertheless, the suprapubic fixation of a pubovaginal sling is fast and inexpensive, and has proven durable and effective over the long term.

Since the goal of the pubovaginal sling is to recreate a hammocklike support beneath the urethra, the type of material used as well as the point of fixation for this material is important to the success of the procedure. The previous transvaginal needle suspensions that were fixed to the rectus fascia were prone to failure over time. One theory for the cause of failure was that the sutures pulled through the periurethral tissue. As the rectus muscles move with Valsalva maneuver, so may the sutures supporting the sling. This change in tension may predispose sutures to pull through the periurethral tissue or the sling material. In the animal model, this has been found to be dependent on the amount of tension and the characteristics of the tissue being fixed (55). The Burch bladder neck suspension involves secure fixation to Cooper's ligament and has demonstrated durable results (16). This procedure requires an abdominal incision and hence has the potential of increased patient morbidity.

Newer techniques of fixation have moved toward a completely transvaginal approach. Bone anchors placed transvaginally to the underside of the pubic bone have recently gained tremendous popularity. Bone anchor suture fixation in a cadaveric model has been found to be more stable than fixation to the rectus fascia but no better than fixation to Cooper's ligament (56,57). Several bone anchor systems are now commercially available. Several early reports utilizing bone anchors to perform a transvaginal sling have been promising (58). The pubovaginal sling procedure using allograft fascia and bone anchors can be performed with minimal morbidity and on an ambulatory basis. There are increased costs associated with the anchoring systems, but this cost must be weighed against decreased operative time, decreased hospital stay, and decreased patient convalescence. Long-term data on the efficacy of these procedures are necessary, and follow-up is ongoing.

One of the major concerns associated with the use of bone anchors is the potential for the development of osseous complications in the form of osteomyelitis or osteitis pubis. Osteitis pubis is a noninfectious inflammatory condition that causes pain in the pubic bone. Osteomyelitis is a pyogenic infection of the bone and marrow. Both conditions present with similar symptoms but vary with regard to treatment. Osteitis pubis represents an inflammation of the pubic bone secondary to periosteal trauma. It may also present with suprapubic pain, leukocytosis and radiographic changes such as irregular bone margins and widening of the symphysis. This condition is generally not progressive and responds to conservative measures such as non steroidal anti-inflammatory medications and physical therapy.

Osteomyelitis may present with suprapubic pain, difficult ambulation, and/or a wide-based gate. A key point in the history is that the pain is progressive. Patients may also describe fevers, chills, or erythema of the suprapubic skin. There may be an associated leukocytosis and an elevation in the erythrocyte sedimentation rate (ESR). Radiographic evaluation can be performed with plain anteroposterior radiography, CT scan, MRI, or bone scan. The findings may vary from irregular bony margins, widening of the pubic symphysis, and superficial bone destruction early in the disease to localized bone destruction and sequestration later in the process. While a bone scan may be positive in both osteomyelitis and osteitis pubis, a negative bone scan generally indicates that there is no osteomyelitis. Cultures are obtained via needle aspiration prior to instituting treatment. Osteomyelitis is treated with a 4- to 6-week course of antibiotics. However, if there is evidence of necrosis, surgical debridement is needed in addition to antibiotics.

Historically, the risk of infectious osseous complications associated with all forms of pelvic surgery is 1–3% (59). More specific to anti-incontinence procedures is a 0.76% risk of osseous infection associated with the Marshall-Marchetti-Krantz retropubic urethropexy (60). Leach reported five cases of infected bone anchors requiring removal following implantation of 7000 anchors (61). In an extensive Medline review, Rackley et al. found six reported cases of osteomyelitis involving bone anchors in 1018 procedures (0.6%) (59). Interestingly, all of the infections reported occurred in cases in which the bone anchors were placed from a suprapubic approach. There have been no formally reported cases of infectious complications associated with the transvaginal placement of the bone anchors. The reason for this is unclear and may represent a reporting bias given that there have been twice as many reported cases of suprapubic versus transvaginal anchor placement (62). Also, the technique, type of anchor used, and the amount of dissection required are different between the two types of bone anchors.

The organisms isolated from the reported cases of osteomyelitis included *Pseudomonas*, *Staphylococcus aureus*, *Entercoccus*, and *Citrobacter*. Coincidentally, these are the same organisms that have been isolated from infections complicating pelvic surgery that does not require bone anchors (59). Prophylaxis is of the utmost importance in preventing this dreaded complication. First, the urinary tract should be sterile prior to the procedure. Second, prophylactic antibiotics with a broad range of coverage against gram-positive, gram-negative, and anaerobic organisms should be given prior to the procedure. At the authors' institution, intravenous cefazolin and gentamycin are administered preoperatively followed by an oral fluoroquinolone postoperatively for 1 week. In patients who are allergic to penicillin, vancomycin is substituted perioperatively. With this regimen there have been no infectious complications in over 250 cases involving transvaginal bone anchor placement (58).

In summary, bone anchor technology offers a secure form of fixation for the pubovaginal sling. It is technically easier to perform and is associated with decreased operative time and postoperative pain. It allows the procedure to be performed transvaginally, which may be of benefit to patients who are morbidly obese or who have had prior lower abdominal surgery. Also, the incidence of voiding dysfunction and de novo urgency after these procedures is minimal (62). The infectious risks as reported in the literature are no greater than what is historically reported for other pelvic procedures not using bone anchors. Patients must be counseled carefully on the potential risks of this technology. In addition, as with any new technique, long-term follow-up is necessary to further define its role in the treatment of SUI.

In an attempt to offer the same secure fixation as bone anchors but avoid the osseous complications, there are new reports of performing transvaginal fixation to Cooper's ligament using commercially available needle devices (63). The new techniques are promising; however, they may be difficult in patients who have undergone prior anti-incontinence procedures secondary to scarring, but appropriate follow-up of new procedures will continue to advance the techniques available.

IV. CONCLUSION

The field of female urology is expanding and undergoing rapid advances. New techniques and materials are being introduced into the market every year. This makes it difficult for the clinician to decide which material and technique is safe and effective. Currently, the pubovaginal sling procedure using autologous fascia is the gold standard for the treatment of female SUI. Autologous fascia has the longest follow-up, most durable results, and a favorable risk-benefit ratio with regard to potential complications. The results obtained with cadaveric fascia, polypropylene mesh, and bone anchors are promising, but the follow-up is still immature. Ultimately it is the decision of the patient and the surgeon as to what material is to be used for the transvaginal or pubovaginal sling, and both parties must be aware of the risks and benefits of the material and anchoring technique chosen.

REFERENCES

1.   Ridley JH. The Goebel-Stoeckel sling operation. In: Mattingly RF, Thompson JD, eds. TeLinde's Operative Gynecology. Philadelphia: Lippincott Williams and Wilkins, 1985.
2.   Goebel R. Zur operitaven beseitigung der angebornen incontinentia vesicae. Zeitscher Gynakol 1910; 2:187–191.
3.   Frangenheim P. Zu operativen behandlung der inkontinenz der mannlichen harnohre. Ver Dtsch Ges Chir 1914; 43:149–154.
4.   Stoeckel W. Uber die verwendung der museuli pyramidalis bei der operitaven behandlung der incontinentia urinae. Zentralbl Gynakol 1917; 41:11–19.
5.   Price PB. Plastic operations for incontinence of urine and feces. Arch Surg 1933; 26:1043–1048.
6.   Aldridge AH. Transplantation of fascia for relief of urinary stress incontinence. Am J Obstet Gynecol 1942; 44:398–411.
7.   Narik G, Palmrich AH. A simplified sling operation suitable for routine use. Am J Obstet Gynecol 1962; 84:400–403.

8. McGuire EJ, Lytton B. Pubovaginal sling procedure for stress incontinence. J Urol 1978; 119:82–84.
9. Blaivas JG, Jacobs BZ. Pubovaginal sling in the treatment of complicated stress incontinence. J Urol 1991; 145:1214–1218.
10. Fokaefes ED, Lampel P, Hohenfellner M, Lazica M, Thuroff JW. Experimental evaluation of the free versus pedicled fascial flaps for sling surgery of stress urinary incontinence. J Urol 1997; 157:1039–1043.
11. McGuire EJ, Bennett CJ, Konnak JA, Sonda P, Savastano JA. Experience with pubovaginal slings for urinary incontinence at the University of Michigan. J Urol 1987; 138:525–526.
12. Blaivas JG, Salinas J. Type III stress urinary incontinence: importance of proper diagnosis and treatment. Surg Forum 1984; 35:473–478.
13. Mason RC, Roach M. Modified pubovaginal sling for treatment of intrinsic sphincter deficiency. J Urol 1996; 156:1991–1994.
14. Govier FE, Gibbons RP, Correa RJ, Weissman RM, Pritchett TR, Hefty TR. Pubovaginal slings using fascia lata for the treatment of intrinsic sphincter deficiency. J Urol 1997; 157:117–121.
15. Carr LK, Walsh PJ, Abraham VE, Webster GD. Favorable outcome of pubovaginal slings for geriatric women with stress incontinence. J Urol 1997; 157:125–128.
16. Leach GE, Dmochowski RR, Appell RA, Blaivas JG, Hadley HR, Luber KM, Mostwin JL, O'Donnell PD, Roehrborn CG. Female stress urinary incontinence clinical guidelines panel summary report on the surgical management of female stress urinary incontinence. J Urol 1997; 158:875–880.
17. Morgan TO, Westney OL, McGuire EJ. Pubovaginal sling: 4-year outcome analysis and quality of life assessment. J Urol 2000; 163:1845–1848.
18. Chaikin DC, Rosenthal J, Blaivas JG. Pubovaginal fascial sling for all types of stress urinary incontinence: long term analysis. J Urol 1998; 160:1312–1316.
19. Beck RP, McCormick S, Nordstrom L. The fascia lata sling procedure for treating genuine stress incontinence of urine. Obstet Gynecol 1988; 72:699–703.
20. Haab F, Trockman BA, Zimmern PE, Leach GE. Results of pubovaginal sling for the treatment of intrinsic sphincter deficiency determined by questionnaire analysis. J Urol 1997; 158:1738–1741.
21. Crawford JS. Nature of fascia lata and its fate after implantation. Am J Ophthalmol 1969; 67:900–904.
22. Wheatcroft SM, Vardy SJ, Tyers AG. Complications of fascia lata harvesting for ptosis surgery. Br J Ophthalmol 1997; 82(3):333–334.
23. Naugle TC Jr, Fry CL, Sabtier RE, Elliott LF. High leg incision fascia lata harvesting. Ophthalmology 1997; 104(9):1480–1488.
24. Kaplan AA, Santarosa RP, Te AE. Comparison of fascial and vaginal wall slings in the management of intrinsic sphincter deficiency. Urology 1996; 47:885–889.
25. Kaplan SA, Te AE, Young GPH, Andrade A, Cabelin MA, Ikeguchi EF. Prospective analysis of 373 consecutive women with stress urinary incontinence treated with vaginal wall sling: the Columbia-Cornell university experience. J Urol 2000; 164:1623–1627.
26. Su TH, Huang JP, Wang YL, Yang JM, Wei HJ, Huang CL. Is modified in situ vaginal wall sling operation the treatment of choice for recurrent genuine stress incontinence? J Urol 1999; 162:2073–2077.
27. Woodman PJ, Davis GD. The relationship of the in-situ advancing vaginal wall sling to vaginal epithelial inclusion cyst. Int Urogynecol 2000; 11:124–126.
28. Handa VL, Jensen JK, Germain MM. Banked human fascia lata for the suburethral sling procedure: a preliminary report. Am J Obstet Gynecol 1996;88:104-106.
29. Buck BE, Malinin TI. Human bone and tissue allografts. Preparation and safety. Clin Orthop 1994; 8:303–306.
30. Tomford WW. Transmission of disease through transplantation of musculoskeletal allografts. J Bone Joint Surg 1995; 77:1742–1745.
31. Simonds RJ, Holmberg SD, Hurwitz RL. Transmission of human immunodeficiency virus type 1 from a seronegative organ and tissue donor. N Engl J Med 1992; 326:726.
32. Cashman NR. A prion primer. Can Med Assoc J 1997; 1997:1381.
33. Tutoplast® processed fascia lata package inset, Biodynamics International, Inc.

34. Brown SL, Govier FE. Cadaveric versus autologous fascia lata for the pubovaginal sling: surgical outcomes and patient satisfaction. J Urol 2000; 164:1633–1637.

35. Lemer ML, Chaikin DC, Blaivas JG. Tissue strength analysis of autologous and cadaveric allografts for the pubovaginal sling. Neurourol Urodynam 1999; 18:497–503.

36. Sutaria PM, Staskin DR. Tensile strength of cadaveric fascia lata allograft is not affected by current methods of tissue preparation. J Urol 1998; 161(4):Abstract 1194.

37. Amundsen CL, Visco AG, Ruiz HE, Webster GD. Outcome in 104 pubovaginal slings using freeze dried allograft fascia lata from a single tissue bank.

38. Wright EJ, Iselin CE, Carr LK, Webster GD. Pubovaginal sling using cadaveric fascia allograft fascia for the treatment of intrinsic sphincter deficiency. J Urol 1998; 160:759–761.

39. Kobashi KC, Mee SL, Leach GE. A new technique for cystocele repair and transvaginal sling: the cadaveric prolapse repair and sling (CaPS). Urology 2000; 56:9–14.

40. Chaikin DC, Blaivas JG. Weakened cadaveric fascial sling: unexpected cause of failure. J Urol 1998; 160:2151.

41. Fitzgerald MP, Mollenhauer, Brubaker L. Failure of allograft suburethral slings. Br J Urol Int 1999; 64:785–788.

42. Carbone JM, Kavaler E, Raz S. Disappointing early results with bone anchored cadaveric fascia pubovaginal sling (abstract 736). J Urol 2000; 163:166.

43. Zoedler D, Boeminghaus H. On indication and technique of suspension plastic surgery. Z Urol Nephrol 1965; 58:459–461.

44. Staskin DR, Choe JM, Breslin DS. The Goretex sling procedure for female sphincteric incontinence: indications, technique, and results. World J Urol 1997; 15:295–298.

45. Yamada T, Arai G, Masuda H. The correction of type 2 stress incontinence with polytetra-fluoroethylene patch sling: 5 year mean follow-up. J Urol 1998; 160:746–750.

46. Morgan TE, Farrow GA, Stewart FE. Marlex sling operation for the treatment of recurrent stress urinary incontinence: a 16-year review. Am J Obstet Gynecol 1985; 151:224–229.

47. Bryans Fe. Marlex gauze hammock sling operation with coopers ligament attachment in the management of recurrent urinary stress incontinence. Am J Obstet Gynecol 1979; 133:292–295.

48. Kobashi KC, Dmochowski R, Mee SL, Mostwin J, Nitti VW, Zimmern PE, Leach GE. Erosion of woven polyester pubovaginal sling. J Urol 1999; 162:2070–2072.

49. Duckett JRA, Constantine G. Complications of silicone sling insertion fro stress urinary incontinence. J Urol 2000; 163:1835–1837.

50. Ulmsten U, Henriksson L, Johnson P, Varhos G. An ambulatory surgical procedure under local anesthesia for treatment of female urinary incontinence. Int Urogynecol J 1996; 7:81–86.

51. Klutke JJ, Carlin BI, Klutke CG. The tension-free vaginal tape procedure: correction of stress incontinence with minimal alteration in proximal urethral mobility. Urology 2000; 55:512–514.

52. Haab F, Sananes S, Amaranco G, Ciofu C, Uzan S, Gattegno B, Thibault P. Results of the tension-free vaginal tape procedure for the treatment of type ii stress urinary incontinence at a minimum follow-up of 1 year. J Urol 2001; 165:159–162.

53. Ulmsten U, Johnson P, Rezapour M. A three-year follow-up of tension free vaginal tape procedure for surgical treatment of female stress urinary incontinence. Br J Obstet Gynaecol 1999; 106:345–350.

54. Ulmsten U, Petros P. Intravaginal slingplasty (IVS): an ambulatory surgical procedure for treatment of female urinary incontinence. Scand J Urol Nephrol 1995; 29:75–82.

55. Bruskewitz R, Nielsen K, Graversen P. Bladder neck suspension material investigation in a rabbit model. J Urol 1989; 142:1361–1363.

56. Klutke J, Bullock A, Klutke C. Comparison of anchors used in anti-incontinence surgery. Urology 1998; 52:979–981.

57. Winters J, Fonetnot C, Glowacki C. A comparison of the biochemechanical properties of periosteal suture fixation and bone anchor fixation to the pubic bone. Urology 2000; 55:866–869.

58. Begley SJ, Kobashi KC. Cystocele repair with concomitant sling: current techniques (in press).

59. Rackley RA, Abdelmalak JB, Madjar S, Yanilmaz A, Appell RA, Tchetgen MB. Bone anchor infections in female reconstructive procedures: a literature review of series and case reports. J Urol 2001; 165:1975–1978.

60. Kammerer-Doak DN, Cornella JL, Magrina JF. Osteitis pubis after Marshall-Marchetti-Krantz urethropexy: a pubic osteomyelitis. Am J Obstet Gynecol 1998; 179:586–589.

61. Leach GE. Local anesthesia for urologic procedures. Urology 1996; 48:284–288.

62. Winters JC, Scarpero HM, Appell RA. Use of bone anchors in female urology. Urology 2000; 56(suppl 6A):15–22.

63. Koduri S, Goldberg RP, Sand PK. Transvaginal therapy of genuine stress incontinence. Urology 2000; 56:23–27.

23

Use of Cadaveric Fascia Lata Allograft for Pubovaginal Slings

Matthew B. Gretzer and E. James Wright
The Johns Hopkins Medical Institutions, Baltimore, Maryland, U.S.A.

I. INTRODUCTION

The pubovaginal sling has become a favored treatment option for stress urinary incontinence (SUI). While initially indicated for treating SUI secondary to intrinsic sphincter deficiency, it has proven versatile for the management of urethral hypermobility (type 2 incontinence) (1). Originally introduced by Giordano (2) in 1907, the concept of suburethral support was reintroduced in 1978 by McGuire and Lytton (3). This work described successful results using autologous rectus fascia for sling construction and set the stage for ongoing exploration into sling materials and techniques to minimize morbidity, operative time, and time of recovery. Many options are available, and the quest for a gold standard continues.

Autologous fascia has endured the test of time as a safe and effective material; however, the added morbidity and time associated with procurement propel the search for alternative sling materials. Current options for pubovaginal sling materials include allografts (cadaveric fascia lata and dermis), xenografts (porcine dermis and small intestinal submucosa, bioengineered collagen matrices, and a host of synthetic materials including Marlex, Gore-Tex, and polypropylene. While synthetic materials have exhibited durable results without the time and morbidity of harvest, concern over the potential for urethral erosion and other complications has often overshadowed their successful application (4–6). Cadaveric fascia lata allografts (CFLA) have been available for more than 20 years and are well described in the orthopedic (7,8) and ophthalmologic (9) literature. This experience of safety and stability over time has extended to new applications in urologic and urogynecologic reconstructive surgery. This chapter describes the technical and material aspects of CFLA sling and justifies its role in effective incontinence therapy.

II. PREOPERATIVE EVALUATION

Selection of patients for pubovaginal sling is well described elsewhere in this volume. All patients should have an accurate urogynecologic history and physical exam. The presence and symptoms of pelvic organ prolapse should be evaluated for consideration of concomitant repair. A voiding diary, pad test, and urodynamic evaluation are helpful in the overall assessment of symptoms and outcome from intervention. After urine studies have excluded infectious processes, those with a history of prior pelvic surgery may undergo cystoscopy to evaluate for the presence of foreign body or other intravesical pathology.

III. SURGICAL TECHINIQUE

Numerous techniques are described for pubovaginal sling placement. Among these are variations in the choice of incision, extent of urethropelvic ligament perforation, degree of urethrolysis, sling dimensions, and choice of fixation. While refinements continue, an evidenced-based, universally accepted approach remains to be established. Ultimately, the chosen method should allow easy reproducibility and achieve an outcome that approximates published standards. The technique described below satisfies these requirements and offers the surgeon a method for sling placement associated with minimal morbidity, surgical efficiency, and favorable outcome.

Two factors associated with successful pubovaginal sling surgery are accurate placement at the urethrovesical junction and correct tension. Inappropriate sling placement or excessive tension risks postoperative voiding dysfunction or urinary retention. Undue laxity may result in continued incontinence.

A. Anesthesia/Position

Regional or general anesthesia may be used without particular advantage to either technique for sling surgery. Preoperative antibiotics should be administered. The patient is placed in the modified lithotomy position with the knee and hip at 90° flexion so as to minimize neural stretch. Following suprapubic, vaginal and perineal preparation, a 16Fr Foley catheter is placed into the bladder and the balloon filled with 10 cc of fluid.

B. Allograft Preparation

As there are different sources for allograft material, specific tissue bank recommendations for preparation prior to the start of the operation should be followed. A 2 × 13 cm strip of fascia is created, and the ends are bound through and through with O-PGA suture to prevent dissection along the fiber planes (Fig. 1A). While debate continues as to optimal sling dimensions, we believe the technique descried provides a sling long enough for fixation in the retropubic space without reliance on suspension sutures or bone fixation, yet not so long as to require passage through the rectus fascia for proper tensioning. Two delayed absorbable or monofilament sutures of equal length are placed through the bound ends of the sling in a helical fashion to provide temporary suspension. The ends of these sutures are made even to allow symmetric sling placement (Fig. 1B).

C. Vaginal Dissection

The urethrovesical junction is identified by palpation of the Foley balloon through the anterior vaginal wall and labeled with a skin marker (Fig. 2). The anterior vaginal wall has no reliable landmarks to identify this position. Estimation of the bladder neck "by eye" is discouraged, as this may result in placement of the sling too distal from the bladder neck. Two longitudinal incisions are made on either side of the vesicle neck mark, forming an H configuration (Fig. 2). A subepithelial tunnel is made at the vesical neck. Potts scissors angled "on the flat" at a 45°

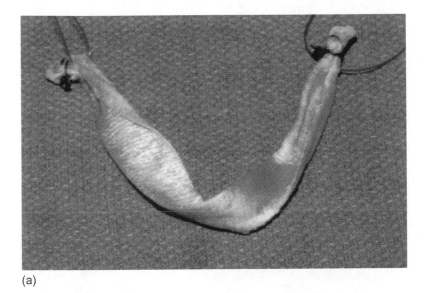

(a)

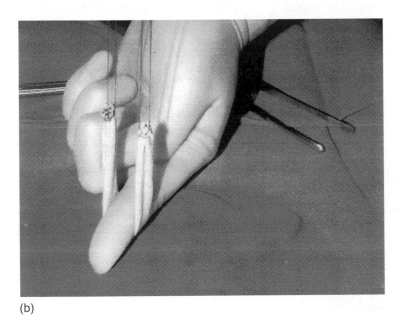

(b)

Figure 1   (A) A 2 × 13 cm strip of fascia is created with the ends bound through and through with O-PGA suture. (B) Two delayed absorbable or monofilament sutures of equal length are placed through the bound ends of the sling in a helical fashion to provide temporary suspension.

angle can aid this dissection (Fig. 3). This tunnel ensures accurate placement of the sling preventing cephalad or caudad displacement, and eliminating the need for additional fixation.

Flaps are raised laterally from the vaginal wall incisions. Dissection of the vaginal epithelium from the underlying urethropelvic ligament laterally on each side is extended to the urethropelvic ligament. With the bladder empty, the urethropelvic ligament is perforated using scissors pointed somewhat superiorly and laterally. This allows entry into the retropubic space.

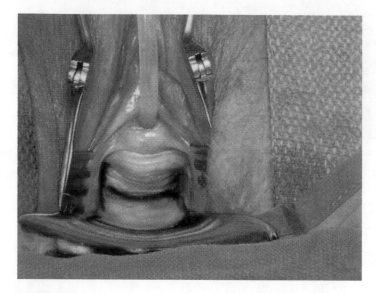

Figure 2   Location of the urethrovesical junction is marked, and two longitudinal incisions are made on either side of the vesical neck mark, forming an H configuration.

The space is dissected digitally, freeing the bladder from the symphysis pubis to create a space for the sling to traverse the retropubic space through the endopelvic fascia.

A 1- to 2-cm midline suprapubic incision is made and a ligature carrier passed through the rectus fascia and guided through the retropubic space to emerge in the vaginal introitus. Lateral

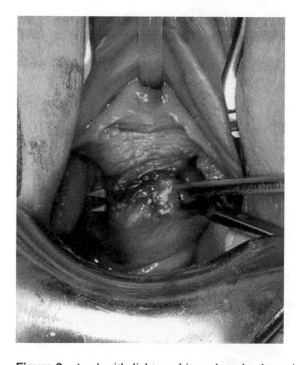

Figure 3   A subepithelial tunnel is made under the vesical neck using Potts scissors.

extension of this incision is avoided in order to reduce damage to cutaneous nerves and the possible risk of postoperative pain. One should also avoid placing the abdominal incision directly over the pubis, as this may cause discomfort during intercourse after the suspending sutures are tied.

D. Sling Placement

The suspension suture is passed on the ligature carrier and transferred to the suprapubic incision. The opposite end of the sling is passed through the subepithelial tunnel (Fig. 4) and process repeated. Following sling placement, Indigo Carmine is administered intravenously, and cystoscopy is performed to inspect bladder or ureteral injury. A $70°$ lens simplifies evaluation of the anterior wall and superior bladder neck, where most injuries occur as the ligature carrier is passed. The position of the sling at the bladder neck can be examined on exiting the bladder by gently pulling on the suspension sutures. Following bladder inspection, the suspending sutures are tied.

As stated above, proper sling tension is imperative to successful outcome. One method to ensure a tension-free position of the sling is to place the arms of a forceps on either side of the sling as it exits the subepithelial tunnel (Fig. 5A). Tying the sutures over the rectus fascia in this manner limits both sling redundancy and excessive tension (Fig. 5B). A cystoscope with downward traction on the urethra can accomplish the same goal. Repeat cystoscopy can be done to check the urethra for undue cephalad angulation and confirm proper laxity. The course of the urethra should be unimpeded, and suprapubic pressure should allow for crede voiding.

The suprapubic and vaginal incisions are closed with absorbable suture. The vagina can be packed with gauze soaked with either povidine iodine (Betadine) or estrogen cream according to preference. The vaginal pack is removed the morning following surgery. A cystotomy or Foley catheter can be used for 24 h or longer, after which time a voiding trial can be initiated.

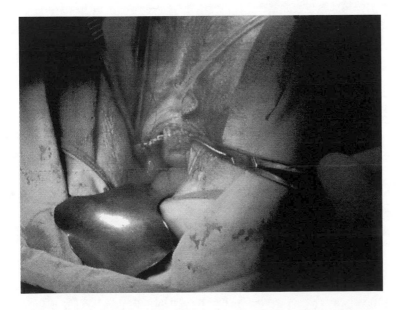

Figure 4 The opposite end of the sling is passed through the subepithelial tunnel.

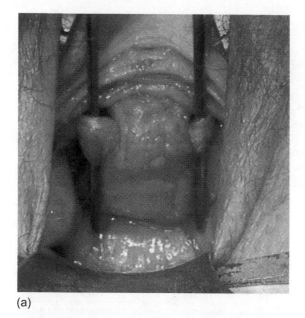

(a)

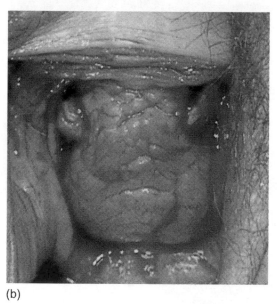

(b)

Figure 5   (A) Placing arms of forceps on either side of the sling as it exits the tunnel to ensure a tension-free position of the sling. (B) Tension-free sling position after tying sutures over rectus muscle.

IV. OUTCOMES

Enthusiasm for cadaveric fascial slings has increased with increasing availability of allograft tissue, awareness of savings in time and morbidity, and published efficacy. Since 1996, reports continue to emerge supporting favorable outcomes using fascial allografts (10–15). These results, described in Table 1, appear comparable to studies examining fascial autografts using

Table 1 Results of Pubovaginal Sling Using Fascial Allografts

Author	Processing method	#Pts.	F/u(mean)	% Improved (0–2 pads/d)	% "Cure" (0 pads/d)
Elliot (14)	Solvent-dried, +IR[a]	26	15 mo.	92	77
Amundsen (13)	Freeze-dried, −IR	104	19 mo.	84	63
Wright (10)	Freeze-dried, −IR	59	12 mo.	98	N.A.
Handa (12)	Freeze-dried, −IR	16	12 mo.	85	79
Brown (11)	Freeze-dried, ?IR	121	12 mo.	83	74
Fitzgerald (15)	Freeze-dried, +IR	35	6 mo.	83	69

[a]IR, gamma irradiation.

rectus fascia and fascia lata (11,16–20). The latter are shown in Table 2. The most notable difference in assessing these outcomes is a shorter follow-up available for the allograft cohorts. These comparisons are perhaps hindered by variability in methods used to evaluate outcomes, which include validated postal survey questionnaires, third-party telephone interviews, and clinical examination. In most of these critiques, patients using less than one pad per day without significant urge symptoms or retention were designated as having a favorable outcome. Better standardization of outcome measures is necessary to improve direct comparison, and future studies should strive to adhere to ICS recommendations for outcome evaluation. Nevertheless, outcomes measured in a variety of ways appear to be fairly consistent between allograft and autograft fascial slings.

Given a shorter evaluation horizon for cadaveric allograft slings, questions remain about their long-term effectiveness, durability, and potential for autolysis (21–23). Allograft and autograft fascia exhibit significant histologic variability in vivo, ranging from minimal change to neovascularization to complete replacement (24). While yielding an overall success rate of 83%, Fitzgerald et al. (15,21) observed a 17% failure rate of cadaveric fascial slings within 5 months after surgery. At reoperation in seven of 35 patients, no consistent histologic pattern emerged in the grafts to explain a lack of efficacy. Similarly, Blander et al. described histologic findings in five "failed" slings (22). The adverse outcomes in this series included de novo retention as well as recurrent SUI. No distinct histologic pattern emerged for either outcome. Curiously, absence of allograft and presumed autolysis did not preclude persistent urinary retention.

Table 2 Results of Pubovaginal Sling Using Fascial Autografts

Author	Processing method	#Pts.	F/U (mean)	% Improved (0–2 pads/d)	% "Cure" (0 pads/d)
Haab (16)	RFA[a]	40	4 yr.	86	46
Iglesia (17)	RFA	50	3 mo.	94	73
Chaikin (18)	RFA	251	3 yr.	92	73
Morgan (19)	RFA	247	4 yr.	88	82
Brown (11)	FLA[b]	46	3.5 yr.	85	73
Breen (20)	FLA	72	2 yr.	90	N.A.

[a]RFA, rectus fascia lata.
[b]FLA, fascia lata.

It appears that both autograft and allograft fascial slings have a high success rate as well as a demonstrable failure rate (25,26). Most overt failures occur early, within the first 6–12 months, irrespective of the material used (11,15,19). With lengthening follow-up, fewer failures due to recurrent SUI are seen after 1 year, with most studies reporting a "cure" rate approaching 15% lower than the rate of improvement and overall patient satisfaction. The source of these differences is not well studied. Whether due to unrecognized host vs. graft reactions or other specific patient characteristics remains a focus for further investigation.

Another area of continuing concern in the use of allograft fascia is a potential for disease transmission. In an attempt to minimize risk from tissue transplantation, the FDA established standards for donor screening (27) which currently include HIV, hepatitis, and history of cancer, neurodegenerative conditions, syphilis, and rabies. Following the introduction of PCR and DNA probing techniques, identification of these diseases has nearly eliminated any risk of donor transmission. In more than 60,000 organ transplants and 1 million of tissue transplants, only one case has been reported of HIV transmission. This case was identified from a bone graft. Since the introduction of strict guidelines in 1985, no cases of HIV transmission have been reported (28) in organ or soft tissue transplants. Further review of the literature does not identify a single case of disease originating from transplanted allograft fascia (29).

Beyond concern for identifiable pathogens is concern regarding potential risk of prion transmission. In proteinacious substances implicated in various forms of spongiform encephalopathy including Creutzfeld-Jacob disease, scrapie, and mad and cow disease (30–32), prions defy culture and characterization. While prions are resistant to methods aimed at destroying nucleic acids, they may be inactivated by denaturing detergents or chemotropic ions (31,32). These processes must be weighed against damage to the tissue rendering it unsuitable for transplant. To date, no case of prion infection has been described in a patient who had not received tissue with origin in or proximity to brain, dura mater, cornea, pituitary extracts, or brain stimulation electrodes. More than 200,000 soft tissue transplants are done annually, while fewer than 200 cases of prion related encephalopathy have been documented since their classification. It is unlikely that cadaveric fascia lata represents a prion reservoir.

In addition to donor screening, tissue preparation methods strive to eliminate disease transmission risk. Allograft processing involves combinations of bactericidal and antiviral solutions, flash freezing, freeze-drying, solvent dehydration, and gamma irradiation. These methods render the material sterile and virtually free of cellular elements to the extent that it will not impair its suitability for transplantation. Beyond specific requirements, processing methods are proprietary. Lack of standardization may account for variability in allograft tissue, although studies suggest ex vivo durability is independent of processing technique (33,34). Cellular elements and nucleic acid can persist in allograft fascia (35,36), but the degree to which this contributes to outcome or risk is uncertain.

In comparing the performance of allograft fascia to autografts and synthetics, questions about strength arise. This is especially true in the face of variations in tissue processing. That such processing may affect the strength and durability of allograft tissue is speculative. While studies (33,34,36) from both orthopedic and urologic literature reveal maximum load to failure values of 315 Newtons and 250 Newtons for solvent-dried and freeze-dried cadaveric tissue, respectively, these forces (500–700 lb) likely exceed those generated physiologically at the bladder neck and proximal urethra. Consequently, it is not clear that the ex vivo strength of fascial allografts is related to in vivo success of pubovaginal sling. Data are not available reporting the tensile strength necessary for success of the pubovaginal sling in vivo. A single study by Kim et al. evaluated an in vivo model of cadaveric allograft application in an animal model (37). Using the "trouser tear test," these authors found similar decreases in durability of both autologous and allograft fascia over time. The clinical implications of their findings are unclear.

V. CONCLUSION

Cadaveric fascia allografts offer decreases in operative time and morbidity relative to autografts (39). Current evidence supports this material as a safe and viable option among the vast array of available options (40). There is a measurable failure rate of allograft fascia which seems to manifest in the first 6–12 months of application. This rate does not appear to be significantly different from the failure rate of autograft fascia. Therefore, the search for a conclusive gold standard continues. Consistent "cure" rates of 80–86% can be obtained with most sling procedures, while patient "satisfaction" rates remain between 92% and 96%.

REFERENCES

1. McGuire EJ, O'Connell, HE. Surgical treatment of intrinsic urethral dysfunction. Slings Urol Clin North Am 1995; 22:657.
2. Giordano D. In Twentieth Congress. Franc de Chir. 1907.
3. McGuire EJ, Lytton B. Pubovaginal sling procedure for stress incontinence. J Urol 1978; 119(1):82–84.
4. Morgan JE, Farrow GA, Stewart FE. The Marlex sling operation for the treatment of recurrent stress urinary incontinence: a 16-year review. Am J Obstet Gynecol 1985; 151(2):224–226.
5. Weinberger MW, Ostergard DR. Long-term clinical and urodynamic evaluation of the polytetrafluoroethylene suburethral sling for treatment of genuine stress incontinence. Obstet Gynecol 1995; 86(1):92–96.
6. Bent AE, Ostergard DR, Zwick-Zaffuto M. Tissue reaction to expanded polytetrafluoroethylene suburethral sling for urinary incontinence: clinical and histologic study. Am J Obstet Gynecol 1993; 169(5):1198–1204.
7. Noyes FR, Barber-Westin, SD. Reconstruction of the anterior cruciate ligament with human allograft. Comparison of early and later results. J Bone Joint Surg Am 1996; 78(4):524–537.
8. Cooper JAB. History of soft tissue allografts in orthopedics. Sports Med Arthrosc Rev 1993; 1:2–16.
9. Bedrossian EH Jr. Banked fascia lata as an orbital floor implant. Ophthal Plast Reconstr Surg 1993; 9(1):66–70.
10. Wright EJ. Pubovaginal sling using cadaveric allograft fascia for the treatment of intrinsic sphincter deficiency. J Urol 1998; 160(3 Pt 1):759–762.
11. Brown SL, Govier FE. Cadaveric versus autologous fascia lata for the pubovaginal sling: surgical outcome and patient satisfaction. J Urol 2000; 164(5):1633–1637.
12. Handa VL. Banked human fascia lata for the suburethral sling procedure: a preliminary report. Obstet Gynecol 1996; 88(6):1045–1049.
13. Amundsen CL. Outcome in 104 pubovaginal slings using freeze-dried allograft fascia lata from a single tissue bank. Urology 2000; 56(6 suppl 1):2–8.
14. Elliott DS, Boone TB. Is fascia lata allograft material trustworthy for pubovaginal sling repair? Urology 2000; 56(5):772–776.
15. Fitzgerald MP, Mollenhauer J, Brubaker L. Failure of allograft suburethral slings. BJU Int 1999; 84(7):785–788.
16. Haab F. Results of pubovaginal sling for the treatment of intrinsic sphincteric deficiency determined by questionnaire analysis. J Urol 1997; 158(5):1738–1741.
17. Iglesia CB. Effect of preoperative voiding mechanism on success rate of autologous rectus fascia suburethral sling procedure. Obstet Gynecol 1998; 91(4):577–581.
18. Chaikin DC, Rosenthal J, Blaivas JG. Pubovaginal fascial sling for all types of stress urinary incontinence: long-term analysis. J Urol 1998; 160(4):1312–1316.
19. Morgan TO Jr, Westney OL, McGuire EJ. Pubovaginal sling: 4-year outcome analysis and quality of life assessment. J Urol 2000; 163(6):1845–1848.
20. Breen JM, Geer BE, May GE. The fascia lata suburethral sling for treating recurrent urinary stress incontinence. Am J Obstet Gynecol 1997; 177(6):1363–1365; discussion 1365–1366.

21. FitzGerald MP. Functional failure of fascia lata allografts. Am J Obstet Gynecol 1999; 181(6):1339–1344; discussion 1344–1346.
22. Blander DS, Zimmern PE. Cadaveric fascia lata sling: analysis of five recent adverse outcomes. Urology 2000; 56(4):596–599.
23. Huang YH, Lin AT, Chen KK. High failure rate using allograft fascia lata in pubovaginal sling surgery for female stress urinary incontinence. Urology 2001; 58:943.
24. FitzGerald MP, Mollenhauer J, Brubaker L. The fate of rectus fascia suburethral slings. Am J Obstet Gynecol 2000; 183(4):964–966.
25. Decter RM. Use of the fascial sling for neurogenic incontinence: lessons learned. J Urol 1993; 150(2 Pt 2):683–686.
26. Chaikin DC, Blaivas JG. Weakened cadaveric fascial sling: an unexpected cause of failure. J Urol 1998; 160(6 Pt 1):2151.
27. Administration, FDA. The FDA Iteragency Guidelines for Human Tissue Intended for Transplantation. Washington: FDA, 1993.
28. Simonds RJ, Hulmder SD, Hurwitz RL. Transmission of human immunodeficiency virus from seronegative organ tissue donors. N Engl J Med 1992; 326:726.
29. Parizek J, Mericka P, Husek P. Detailed evaluation of 2959 allogenic and zenogenic dense connective tissue grafts (fascia lata, pericardium, and dura mater) used in the course of 20 years for duraplasty in neurosurgery. Acta Neurochir 1997; 139:827–838.
30. Prusiner SB. Novel proteinaceous infectious particles cause scrapie. Science 1982; 216(4542):136–144.
31. Prusiner SB. Prions. Proc Natl Acad Sci USA 1998; 95(23):13363–13383.
32. Cashman NR. A prion primer. Can Med Assoc J 1997; 157(10):1381–1385.
33. Hinton R. A biomechanical analysis of solvent-dehydrated and freeze-dried human fascia lata allografts. A preliminary report. Am J Sports Med 1992; 20(5):607–612.
34. Sutaria PM, Staskin DR. Tensile strength of cadaveric fascia lata allograft is not affected by current methods of tissue preparation (abstract). J Urol 1999; 161:1194.
35. Sadhukhan P, Rackley RR, Bandyopadhyay S. Extraction of celluar genetic material from human fascia lata allografts. In: AUA Annual Meeting, Dallas, 1999.
36. Fitzgerald MP, Mollenhauer J, Brubaker L. The antigenicity of fascia lata allografts. BJU Int 2000; 86(7):826–828.
37. Lemer ML, Chaikin DC, Blaivas JG. Tissue strength analysis of autologous and cadaveric allografts for the pubovaginal sling. Neurourol Urodyn 1999; 18(5):497–503.
38. Kim HL, LaBarbera MC, Patel RV. Comparison of cadaveric and autologous fascia using an in vivo model. Urology 2001; 58:800.
39. Labasky RF, Soper T. Reduction of patient morbidity and cost using frayed cadaveric fascia lata for pubovaginal sling. J Urol 1997; 154(Abstract 1794):459.
40. Wright EJ. Current status of fascia lata allograft slings treating urinary incontinence: effective or ephemeral? Tech Urol 2001; 7(2):81–86.

24

Autologous Fascia Lata Sling Cystourethropexy

Karl J. Kreder
University of Iowa, Iowa City, Iowa, U.S.A.

I. INTRODUCTION

Pubovaginal sling cystourethropexy has recently become one of the primary surgical treatment options for women with urinary incontinence. The procedure has evolved over time with regard to clinical indications, patient selection criteria, surgical techniques, and sling materials. This chapter reviews the historical development of pubovaginal sling cystourethropexy using fascia lata. The selection of graft materials is considered and the utility of fascia lata emphasized.

II. HISTORY

The idea of using autologous graft material as a sling behind or around the urethra for treatment of urinary incontinence is not actually a new concept. In 1907 Giordano (1) described mobilizing the distal end of the gracilis muscle and wrapping it around the urethra. In 1910 Goebell (2) introduced the use of a sling of pyramidalis muscle sutured behind the urethra. This technique was subsequently modified by Frangenheim (3) and Stoeckel (4). Squire (5) described the use of the levator ani muscles, and Martius (6) advocated use of the bulbocavernosus muscles as pedicled flap grafts to support the urethra. In 1942, Aldridge (7) described the use of bilateral strips of rectus fascia, passed through the rectus abdominis muscles and sutured together posterior to the urethra. Narik and Palmrich (8) described the creation of a sling from the fascia of the inguinal aponeurosis of the external oblique muscles. They advocated preserving the attachment of the fascia at the level of the pubic tubercle. These techniques eventually fell out of favor because of a significant complication rate, including prolonged urinary retention, sling erosion, iatrogenic bladder and urethral injuries, and recurrent incontinence.

Price first reported using a fascia lata sling in a female with sacral agenesis (9). Beck and colleagues described the use of fascia lata for the creation of a suburethral sling for the treatment of recurrent urinary incontinence (10–12). Originally, the procedure was considered a secondary procedure to be used in cases of failed prior surgical repair, or in patients who lacked substantial pubovaginal tissues. Beck's group reported a 92% overall cure rate in 170 women treated with fascia lata pubovaginal sling cystourethropexy for recurrent stress urinary incontinence (SUI) (12). Others have demonstrated similar results using this technique (Table 1).

Table 1 Fascia Lata Sling Results

Authors	No. of patients	Dry (%)	Improved (%)	Failed (%)
Griebling et al. (35)	30	26 (87)	4 (13)	0 (0)
Govier et al. (36)	30	21 (70)	6 (20)	3 (10)
Handa et al. (59)	14	11 (79)	1 (7)	2 (14)
Ogundipe et al. (57)	8	7 (88)	0 (0)	1 (11)
Karram et al. (58)	10	9 (90)	1 (10)	0 (0)
Beck et al. (12)[b]	170	157 (92)	4 (2)	9 (5)
Addison et al. (56)	97	84 (87)	8 (8)	5 (5)
Low et al. (55)	43	37 (86)	4 (9)	2 (5)
Ridley (50)	36	30 (86)	4 (11)	2 (6)
Total	438	382 (87)	32 (7)	24 (5)

[a]UDS: urodynamic studies.
[b]Cumulative data include patients previously reported in Ref. 10 and 11.
Source: Ref. 64.

III. INDICATIONS

A. Intrinsic Sphincter Deficiency

For many years, the primary indication for fascia lata sling cystourethropexy has been the management of women with SUI who demonstrate a significant component of intrinsic sphincter deficiency (ISD). ISD has multiple etiologies, including neurologic, anatomic, and primary causes (13–15). Neurologic factors include disruption of the sacral nerve roots S2–S4 during major pelvic surgery, loss of autonomic neural control associated with myelodysplasisa, radiation therapy, lumbosacral spinal cord injuries, or anterior spinal artery syndrome. Anatomic causes of ISD include congenital defects such as spinal dysraphism, periurethral scarring from prior anti-incontinence surgery, or urethral atrophy due to estrogen deficiency in postmenopausal women. Although idiopathic ISD has been described, the etiology of ISD can usually be identified (16).

Several diagnostic modalities have been used to identify ISD, including cystourethroscopy, cystography, multichannel urodynamics with measurement of abdominal leak-point pressure, urethral pressure profilometry, and videourodynamics. ISD is classically diagnosed by an open bladder neck at rest on erect cystography and a low Valsalva leak-point pressure (VLPP) (15). The VLPP is a reasonably simple test that generally correlates with the degree of urethral dysfunction (17,18).

B. Urethral Hypermobility (Type II Incontinence)

SUI caused by urethral hypermobility has traditionally been treated surgically with vaginal or abdominal-urethral suspension procedures. Recently, however, it has been recognized that pubovaginal sling cystourethropexy may be used for the management of patients with isolated type II or combined ISD and type II stress urinary incontinence (19–23). Specifically, the overall success rates for slings appear to be greater than those for needle suspension procedures and comparable to the Burch procedure. As shown in Table 1, a review of the published literature on pubovaginal slings reveals that 87% of patients overall are dry postoperatively, with an additional 7% significantly improved. In comparison, several recent studies of the long-term results for needle suspension procedures revealed that 20–47% of patients were dry, with

29–71% categorized as improved (24–26). Although more long-term data are necessary, it also appears that the results of pubovaginal sling cystourethropexy are durable. Finally, the procedure could potentially prevent some of the treatment failures associated with traditional urethral suspension procedures. The incidence of ISD appears to be higher in older women, and, as patients age, many may develop ISD. This anatomic change is not addressed by standard cystourethropexy procedures, which may explain why some patients develop recurrent incontinence over time. Theoretically, a sling cystourethropexy performed initially for stress incontinence caused by urethral hypermobility may prevent recurrent incontinence caused by the subsequent development of ISD.

In the author's early experience with pubovaginal sling cystourethropexy for the treatment of patients with combined urethral hypermobility and ISD (20), 11 patients with isolated ISD and 16 with combined ISD and urethral hypermobility who underwent pubovaginal sling cystourethropexy were evaluated. The preoperative diagnoses were confirmed in all patients with multichannel urodynamics; mean follow-up in this study was 22 months. Of the 11 patients with isolated ISD, six (55%) were dry, two (18%) had continued urge with incontinence, two (18%) developed de novo urge with incontinence, and one (9%) had continued stress incontinence. In comparison, 13 of the 16 patients (81%) with combined ISD and urethral hypermobility were dry, three (19%) had continued urge with incontinence, and none had de novo urge or continued stress incontinence.

Others have also shown pubovaginal sling cystourethropexy to have promising results in women with urethral hypermobility, both with and without concomitant ISD. O'Donnell reported the utility of creation of a pubovaginal sling and simultaneous retropubic bladder neck suspension in patients with combined type II and type III incontinence (21). Cross et al. reported the results of pubovaginal sling cystourethropexy in 124 patients treated for SUI (22): 50% of the patients in this series had ISD, 35.4% had type II incontinence, and 14% had both diagnoses. The overall cure rate for SUI was 90% at a mean follow-up of 19 months. Zaragoza (23) reported complete continence after a mean follow-up of 25 months in 95% of 38 women with type II incontinence and 96% of 22 women with type III incontinence.

These early data support the use of pubovaginal sling procedures as a primary surgical treatment in women with SUI due to either type II, type III, or combined incontinence.

C. Other Indications

Pubovaginal sling cystourethropexy has been utilized to treat incontinence in a variety of complex patient populations. Woodside reported that two women with incontinence after pelvic trauma and urethral injury were continent at 6 and 15 months, respectively, after pubovaginal sling cystourethropexy (27). Chancellor et al. described the use of pubovaginal sling cysto-urethropexy in the management of women with urethral dysfunction secondary to long-term indwelling catheter drainage (28). Ghoniem and Monga reported the combined use of a pubovaginal sling and a Martius flap graft for patients with vesicovaginal fistula involving the internal sphincter (29). Swierzewski and McGuire reported the simultaneous performance of urethral diverticulectomy and pubovaginal sling cystourethropexy (30).

Gormley et al. (31) reported an overall continence rate of 92% in 15 adolescent females after pubovaginal sling cystourethropexy. Mean follow-up was 54 months. Ten of the patients in this series had spinal dysraphism, three were incontinent after pelvic trauma, and two underwent concomitant augmentation cystoplasty for poor bladder compliance. Secondary procedures were required in three patients, including repeat sling in two, and repeat bladder augmentation in one. Pérez et al. reported a continence rate of 58.3% in 24 girls who underwent rectus fascia sling cystourethropexy (32). The majority of these patients had neurogenic bladder secondary to spinal dysraphism, and the highest success rates were identified in those who underwent combined pubovaginal sling and augmentation cystoplasty. Walker et al. (33) successfully used a modification of the rectus fascia sling for both male and female patients with incontinence associated with neurogenic bladder. In this case the fascia was wrapped around the urethra to cause luminal apposition.

Pubovaginal sling cystourethropexy has also been used successfully in elderly women. Carr et al. (34) reported resolution of stress incontinence symptoms in all 19 geriatric women (median age 72 years) treated with rectus fascia sling cystourethropexy. Mean follow-up was 22 months. Similar results were reported by Griebling et al. in a cohort analysis of our older and younger pubovaginal sling patients (35). At a mean follow-up of 10.5 months, 65% of 26 older women (mean age 67.6 years) were dry, and 27% significantly improved. Of the 28 younger women (mean age 48.9 years), 82% were dry and 18% were significantly improved.

IV. SURGICAL TECHNIQUE

A. Fascia Lata Graft Harvest

Fascia lata grafts can be harvested by a variety of methods. In one technique, the skin and subcutaneous tissues overlying the fascia lata of the lateral thigh and upper leg are incised along the entire length of the planned graft. However, several modifications have been described to obviate the need for such a long incision. Govier (36) described making three small incisions perpendicular to the planned graft. Dissection is then carried down to the fascia lata along the entire length of the graft beneath the skin and subcutaneous tissues. A strip of fascia lata $\sim$24 × 2.5 cm is harvested, cleared of fat, and tailored to a 2-cm width.

Beck et al. (10) described the use of a fascial stripper to obtain the fascia lata graft. A modification of Beck's technique is described below (37). A line is drawn from the anterior superior iliac spine to the lateral epicondyle of the knee. A 3-cm-long longitudinal incision is then created just proximal to the distal mark (Fig. 1A), and dissection is carried down to the level of the fascia lata. Two small parallel incisions are made longitudinally in the distal fascia lata. The tissue is then raised off the underlying muscle, and a suture of 0-Prolene is secured in the distal end of the fascia. A Crawford fascial stripper (Fig. 1B; Karl Stortz Medical Instruments, St Louis, MO) is then used to harvest a strip of fascia lata which is $\sim$20 × 2 cm in dimension (Fig. 1C). A second 0-Prolene suture is secured in the proximal end of the graft, which is placed in saline for future use. The subcutaneous tissues and skin are closed with absorbable sutures. A compressive elastic bandage is wrapped around the thigh and proximal leg to provide hemostasis. The bandage is usually removed 8 h postoperatively, and early ambulation is encouraged.

B. Sling Placement

The sling placement procedure we utilize is a modification of the techniques described by Beck et al. (10–12) and McGuire and Lytton (38). The patient is placed in the dorsal lithotomy position, and the lower abdomen and vagina are prepared and draped. A small transverse lower abdominal incision is made, and dissection is carried down to the rectus abdominis fascia just superior to the symphysis pubis. A Foley catheter and a weighted vaginal speculum are placed. The vaginal mucosa is incised longitudinally on either side of the urethra at the level of the bladder neck. A tunnel is then created in the retropubic space on either side of the urethra, using sharp and blunt dissection. This tunnel is dissected to the level of the posterior rectus abdominis fascia (Fig. 2). A space is created between the urethra and the vaginal mucosa, and the fascia lata graft is placed in

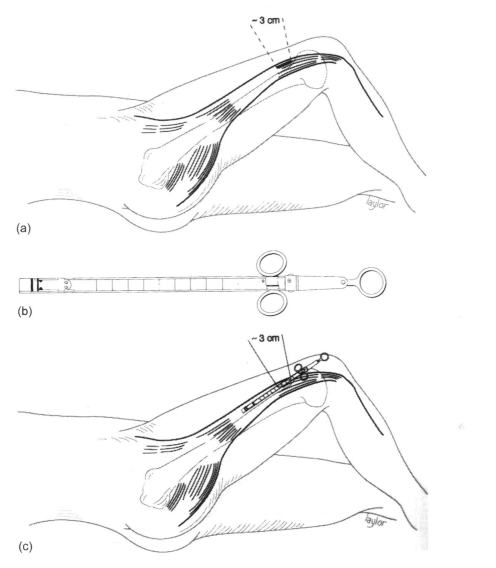

Figure 1 (A) Location of the 3-cm incision over the underlying fascia lata. (B) The Crawford fascial stripper (Karl Stortz Medical Instruments, St Louis, MO). (C) Harvest of the 20 × 2 cm section of fascia lata using the Crawford fascial stripper.

position posterior to the urethra. A tonsil clamp is then used to pierce the rectus abdominis fascia just lateral to the midline. The clamp is passed by fingertip guidance through the previously created retropubic tunnel to the vagina. The ends of the 0-Prolene sutures at one end of the sling are then grasped with the clamp and brought out through the abdominal incision. The procedure is repeated on the contralateral side (Fig. 3). The sling is tied without any tension on the graft. Cystoscopy is performed to ensure that no iatrogenic bladder or ureteral injuries have occurred. The abdominal and vaginal incisions are closed and a vaginal pack is placed. A new Foley catheter is placed to provide postoperative bladder drainage. The vaginal pack is removed on postoperative day 1, and the catheter is removed on day 7. The patient is instructed to perform postvoid self-catheterization until residual urine volumes are consistently below 100 mL.

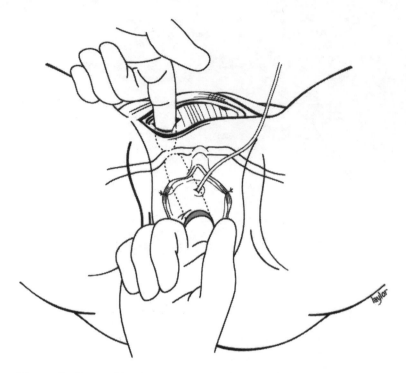

Figure 2 Retropubic dissection prior to placement of the fascia lata sling.

C. Suture Techniques

A number of different techniques have been described to secure the sling. Initially, the fascial sling was secured directly to the rectus fascia on each side. Subsequently, the technique was modified to that described by Govier et al. (36), whereby the two ends of the sling are tied over the rectus fascia without anchoring the sling directly to the rectus fascia. Pérez et al. (32) described securing the ends of the fascial graft to Cooper's ligament with or without crossing the ends of the graft across the midline to improve urethral coaptation. Ghoniem (38) described wrapping the sling around the urethra at the level of the bladder neck.

Various techniques have been advocated to secure the sling at the level of the bladder neck. Gormley et al. (31) described suturing the midportion of the sling to the periurethral fascia. Govier et al. (36) used three interrupted absorbable sutures to tack the sling to the bladder and urethra. It is likely not necessary to secure the sling at the urethra, provided a submucosal tunnel is created for placement of the sling.

D. Sling Tension

Most authors now agree that proper sling placement using a tension-free technique is critical for a satisfactory surgical outcome. Excessive sling tension has been identified as a significant risk factor for persistent postoperative urinary retention. We prefer a technique in which the ends of the graft are brought up to the rectus abdominis fascia, allowed to settle into position by gentle traction on the Foley catheter, and secured to the rectus abdominis fascia as previously described. The urethra is carefully inspected after this procedure to ensure that it is in an anatomic position without evidence of overcorrection.

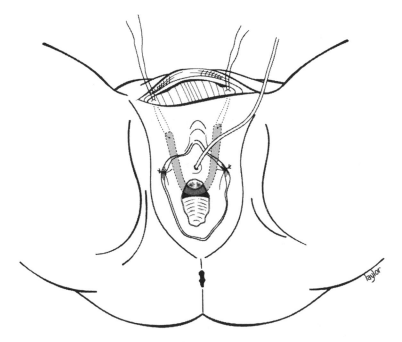

Figure 3   Fascia lata sling in place, just prior to tying the sutures.

Other authors have utilized different techniques for adjusting sling tension intraoperatively. Beck et al. (12) used intraoperative urethral manometry to create an intraurethral pressure of 50–90 cmH$_2$O at the sling site. MeGuire et al. (39) described adjusting sling tension by endoscopic observation with direct visualization of mucosal "soft" coaptation. Govier (36) described adjusting the sling tension until one finger could be placed between the suture and the anterior abdominal wall. Rovner et al. (40) have described using a cystoscope sheath placed transurethrally to stabilize the urethral angulation when the sling is secured to the rectus abdominis fascia.

E. Selection of Graft Material

A wide variety of materials have been used as grafts for pubovaginal sling cystourethropexy. Currently, the most common include autologous rectus fascia or fascia lata, or allogenic fascia. Permanent and absorbable synthetic materials have also been used (41–44), but these do present a higher risk of infection and erosion. The reported rates of urethral erosion and need for graft explantation with synthetic materials have ranged from 14% to 23% (43–48).

Autologous materials have the advantage of low erosion rates and no potential for transmission of viral disease or infection. Theoretically, fascia lata offers several advantages over rectus fascia. It generally has greater tensile strength than rectus fascia and is less affected by the patient's nutritional status or prior abdominal surgery (14). The use of fascia lata also minimizes the risk of developing an abdominal wall hernia, which may occur after rectus fascia harvest. The disadvantage of using autologous fascia is the time required for harvest and additional morbidity associated with the harvest site (i.e., pain, hematoma).

Synthetic graft materials do offer the advantage of decreased overall surgical time because the graft harvesting step is eliminated. Cadaveric allogrant fascia lata has been used by a number of authors (49–54). However, there is some concern about possible transmission of viral or infectious disease, as well as the possibility of graft autolysis.

V.   CLINICAL RESULTS

A review of the literature regarding fascia lata pubovaginal sling cystourethropexy revealed an overall success rate of 87% in 438 reported patients. An additional 7% of patients had improvement of incontinence symptoms, and only 5% experienced no improvement over base-line. These data are summarized in Table 1. It should be noted that these studies represent a compilation of several variations in surgical technique and patient selection.

Early reports by both Ridley (50) and Low (55) suggested that pubovaginal sling procedures with fascia lata were effective for the management of SUI. More recent studies have confirmed these findings. At a mean follow-up of 10 months, Griebling et al. (35) reported that 26 of 30 patients (87%) who had undergone a pubovaginal sling cystourethropexy with a fascia lata graft for treatment of SUI were dry, and four (13%) were improved. In comparison, 11 of 21 patients (52%) who had undergone pubovaginal sling with a rectus fascia graft were dry, eight (38%) were improved, and two (10%) were unchanged from preoperative baseline. Govier et al. treated 32 females for ISD with fascia lata sling cystourethropexy (36). At a median follow-up of 14 months, 87% required no pads (chart review), and 70% required no pads (independent patient survey). Eighty percent of the patients claimed they would choose to undergo the procedure again.

In 1988, Beck et al. (12) reported their 22-year experience of 170 patients treated for SUI with fascia lata pubovaginal sling cystourethropexy. The overall symptomatic cure rate was 92.4%. At that time they recommended the procedure be reserved for patients with recurrent SUI or those not amenable to other therapy. Similarly, Addison et al. (56) reported the results of pubovaginal sling procedures performed for recurrent SUI over a 25-year period. The overall cure rate for these 97 patients was 87%, with an additional 8% improved after surgery. They recommended that the procedure be used primarily for recurrent incontinence. Only three patients in this series underwent pubovaginal sling placement as the initial surgical treatment for incontinence. The authors also recommended that the procedure should usually be performed in conjunction with anterior colporrhaphy.

Ogundipe et al. (57) compared the use of fascia lata and synthetic graft material in a small prospective study. The found 100% cure in the eight patients treated with a synthetic graft, and 87.5% in the eight patients treated with a fascia lata graft at 6 months follow-up. Postoperative urodynamic evaluation revealed no significant differences between the two groups. Although not statistically significant, there was a slightly higher complication rate in the group treated with the synthetic slings.

Karram and Bhatia (58) described the use of a patch of fascia lata as a suburethral support. The 5×7 cm patch was secured under the urethra with nonabsorbable helical sutures placed laterally and brought up to the rectus abdominis fascia.

Handa et al. (59) recently reported the use of banked fascia lata grafts taken from cadaveric donors. They reported an overall subjective cure rate of 86% and an objective cure rate of 79%. One patient in this series experienced persistent urinary retention, which has required continued clean intermittent self-catheterization.

VI.   COMPLICATIONS

Prolonged urinary retention, urgency, and urge incontinence are the most commonly reported complications after pubovaginal sling cystourethropexy. Anatomic or functional obstruction may occur if the sling is tied with excessive tension. Significant postoperative bladder outlet obstruction usually occurs in <5% of patients (14). Beck reported a mean interval of 59.6 days between surgery and the return of consistent voiding function (12). In this author's experience, however, most patients are able to void spontaneously within 2 weeks of surgery.

Several different surgical techniques have been described to release the sling tension in cases of prolonged obstruction (60–62). In a recent series of 54 women treated at our institution with pubovaginal sling cystourethropexy (30 fascia lata sling, 21 rectus fascia sling, three vaginal wall sling), the overall complication rate was 37% (32). However, the majority of these complications were minor and self-limited. Only two women experience prolonged urinary retention, which has required intermittent self-catheterization.

De novo detrusor instability is a troubling complication of pubovaginal sling cystourethropexy, reported to occur in up to 15–20% of patients. These symptoms may severely affect a patient's overall quality of life, and often require treatment with anticholinergic medication.

Other complications are less common. Brodak et al. (63) reported the development of a levator hernia through the pelvic floor 18 months after sling cystourethropexy performed in combination with transvaginal vesicovaginal fistula repair. Govier et al. (36) reported that one patient needed physical therapy for prolonged leg pain after the fascia lata graft harvest. Addison et al. (56) reported eight bladder lacerations in a series of 97 patients who underwent

Table 2 Complications of Fascia Lata Sling Cystourethropexy

Authors	No. of patients	Complications
Griebling et al. (35)[a]	30 (54 total)	10, urinary tract infection 2, wound infection 1, vaginal hemorrhage, incisional hernia, thigh hematoma, thrombophlebitis, allergic reaction, hypotension, death
Govier et al. (36)	30	1, leg pain, sling revision
Handa et al. (59)	14	2, wound infection 1, persistent retention
Ogundipe et al. (57)	8	none reported
Karram et al. (58)	10	none reported
Beck et al. (12)[b]	170	26, pyrexia 14, pyuria 9, pulmonary atelectasis 8, wound infection 6, wound seroma 5, sling revision
Addison et al. (56)	97	8, bladder perforation 6, persistent retention 5, enterocele 2, wound infection 1, pulmonary embolus, thrombophlebitis
Low et al. (55)	43	3, genitourinary fistula (deemed not from sling), wound infections (number not cited)
Ridley (50)	36	8, pyruria

[a]Includes complications from 24 additional patients (21 rectus fascia sling, 3 vaginal wall sling).
[b]Cumulative data include patients previously reported in Refs. 10 and 11.

pubovaginal sling over a 25-year period. In all cases the injury was identified intraoperatively and repaired immediately. No long-term sequelae were reported in these cases. In addition, five patients in their series developed enteroceles, of which three required subsequent surgical repair. The complications listed in the published reports on fascia lata sling cystourethropexy are summarized in Table 2.

Pubovaginal sling cystourethropexy using autologous fascia lata as the graft material is an appealing surgical option for the treatment of urinary incontinence in women. It has shown its usefulness as both a primary operation and a secondary procedure in cases of prior failed surgical repair. A review of the reported literature on fascia lata pubovaginal slings reveals an overall cure rate of 87%, with an additional 7% reporting symptomatic improvement over baseline. The selection of fascia lata as the graft material offers several advantages: it is durable and readily available in most patients, it can be harvested in a minimally invasive fashion, and the risks of postoperative complications such as abdominal hernia are minimized. The technique has shown promise in the management of complex patient populations, including adolescents, the elderly, and patients with neurologic causes of incontinence, particularly when combined with augmentation cystoplasty. In addition, the procedure has been used successfully to treat incontinence caused by pure ISD, urethral hypermobility, or combined etiologies.

REFERENCES

1. Giordano D. Vingtieme Congres Français de Chirurgie. Paris, 1907:506.
2. Goebell R. Zur operativen beseitigung der angeborenen incontinentia vesicae. Ztschr Gyniikol Urol 1910; 2:187–191.
3. Frangenheim P. Zur operativen behandlung der inkontinenz der mannlichen hamrohre. Verhandl Deutsch Gesellsch Chir 1914; 43:149–152.
4. Stoeckel W. Aber die Verwendung der Musculi pyramidales bie der operativen behandlung der incontinentia urinae. Zentralbl Gyniiko 1917; 41:11–19.
5. Squire JB. Postoperative urinary incontinence: urethroplastic operation. Med Rec 1911; 79:868.
6. Martius H. Sphincter- und hamrohrenplastik aus clem musculus bulbocavernosus. Chirurgie 1929; 1:769–773.
7. Aldridge AH. Transplantation of fascia for relief of urinary stress incontinence. Am J Obstet Gynecol 1942; 44:398–411.
8. Narik G, Palmrich AH. A simplified sling operation suitable for routine use. Am J Obstet Gynecol 1962; 84:400–405.
9. Price PB. Plastic operation for incontinence of urine and of feces. Arch Surg 1933; 26:1043.
10. Beck RP, Grove D, Arnusch D, Harvey J. Recurrent urinary stress incontinence treated by the fascia lata sling procedure. Am J Obstet Gynecol 1974; 120:613–621.
11. Beck RP, Lai AR. Results in treating 88 cases of recurrent urinary stress incontinence with the Oxford fascia alata sling procedure. Am J Obstet Gynecol 1982; 142:649–651.
12. Beck RP, McCormick S, Nordstrom L. The fascia lata sling procedure for treating recurrent genuine stress incontinence of urine. Obstet Gynecol 1988; 72:699–703.
13. Haab F, Zimmern PE, Leach GE. Female stress urinary incontinence due to intrinsic sphincteric deficiency: recognition and management. J Urol 1996; 156:3–17.
14. Haab F, Zimmern PE, Leach GE. Diagnosis and treatment of intrinsic sphincter dysfunction in females. AUA Update Series. Lesson 35, Vol. XV. American Urological Association: Baltimore, MD, 1996:282–287.
15. Blaivas JG. Intrinsic shpincter deficiency. In: Walsh PC, Retik AB, Stamey TA, Vaughan ED, Wein AJ, eds. Campbell's Urology, Update 17. Philadelphia: W.B. Saunders, 1996:1–11.
16. Horbach NS, Ostergard DR. Predicting intrinsic urethral sphincter dysfunction in women with stress urinary incontinence. Obstet Gynecol 1994; 84:188–192.

17. McGuire EJ, Fitzpatrick CC, Wan J, Bloom D, Sanvordenker J, Ritchey M, Gormley EA. Clinical assessment of urethral sphincter function. J Urol 1993; 150:1452–1457.
18. McGuire EJ, Cespedes RD, O'Connoll HE. Leak-point pressures. Urol Clin North Am 1996; 23:253–262.
19. Leach GE, Dmochowski RR, Appell RA, Blaivas JG, Hadley HR, Luber KM, Mostwin JL, O'Donnell PD, Roehborn CG. Female stress urinary incontinence clinical guidelines panel summary report on surgical management of female stress urinary incontinence. J Urol 1997; 158:875–880.
20. Kreder KJ, Austin CJ. Treatment of stress urinary incontinence in women with urethral hypermobility and intrinsic sphincter deficiency. J Urol 1996; 156:1995–1998.
21. O'Donnell PD. Combined Raz urethral suspension and McGuire pubovaginal sling for treatment of complicated stress urinary incontinence. J Ark Med Soc 1992; 88:389–392.
22. Cross CA, McGuire EJ, Cespedes RD. Our experience with pubovaginal slings in patients with stress urinary incontinence. J Urol 1997; 157:460A, abstract 1797.
23. Zarazoga MR. Expanded indications for the pubovaginal sling: treatment of type 2 or 3 stress incontinence. J Urol 1996; 156:1620–1622.
24. Christensen H, Laybourne C, Eickhoff JH, Fromdt-Moller C. Long-term results of the Stamey bladder-neck suspension procedure and of the Burch colposuspension. Scand J Urol Nephrol 1997; 31:349–353.
25. Trockman BA, Leach GE, Hamilton J, Sakamoto M, Santiago L, Zimmern PE. Modified Pereyra bladder neck suspension: 10-year mean followup using outcomes analysis in 125 patients. J Urol 1995; 154:1841–1847.
26. Korman HJ, Sirls LT, Kirkemo AK. Success rate of modified Pereyra bladder neck suspension determined by outcomes analysis. J Urol 1994; 152:1453–1457.
27. Woodside JR. Pubovaginal sling procedure for the management of urinary incontinence after urethral trauma in women. J Urol 1987; 138:527–528.
28. Chancellor MB, Erhard MJ, Kilholma PJ, Karasick S, Rivas DA. Functional urethral closure with pubovaginal sling for destroyed female urethral after long-term urethral catheterization. Urology 1994; 43:499–505.
29. Ghoniem GM, Monga M. Modified pubovaginal sling and Martius graft for repair of the recurrent vesicovaginal fistula involving the internal urinary sphincter. Eur Urol 1995; 27:241–245.
30. Swierzeski SJ III, McGuire EJ. Pubovaginal sling for treatment of female stress urinary incontinence complicated by urethral diverticulum. J Urol 1993; 149:1012–1014.
31. Gormley EA, Bloom DA, McGuire EJ, Ritchey ML. Pubovaginal slings for the treatment of urinary incontinence in female adolescents. J Urol 1994; 152:822–825.
32. Pérez LM, Smith EA, Broecker BH, Massad CA, Parrott TS, Woodward JR. Outcome of sling cystourethropexy in the pediatric population: a critical review. J Urol 1996; 156:642–646.
33. Walker RD III, Flack CE, Hawkins-Lee B, Kim DJ, Parramore H, Hackett RL. Rectus fascial wrap: early results of a modification of the rectus fascial sling. J Urol 1995; 154:771–774.
34. Carr LK, Walsh PJ, Abraham VE, Webster GD. Favourable outcome of pubovaginal slings for geriatric women with stress incontinence. J Urol 1997; 157:125–128.
35. Griebling TL, Schrepferman CG, Nygaard IE, Kreder KJ. Sling cystourethropexy for treatment of women with stress urinary incontinence: comparison of older and younger patients. J Am Geriatr Soc 1997; 45:S42, abstract P125.
36. Govier FE, Gibbons RP, Correa RJ, Weismann RM, Pritchett TR, Hefty TR. Pubovaginal slings using fascia lata for the treatment of intrinsic sphincter deficiency. J Urol 1997; 157:117–121.
37. Kreder KJ, Nygaard IE. Fascia lata sling cystourethropexy. J Urol 1995; 153:205A, abstract V-7.
38. Ghoniem GM. Bladder neck wrap: a modified fascial sling in treatment of incontinence in myelomeningocele patients. Eur Urol 1994; 25:340–342.
39. McGuire EJ, Bennett CJ, Konnak JA, Sonda LP, Savastano JA. Experience with pubovaginal slings for urinary incontinence at the University of Michigan. J Urol 1987; 138:525–526.
40. Rovner ES, Ginsberg DA, Raz S. A method for intrtoperative adjustment of sling tension: prevention of outlet obstruction during vaginal wall sling. Urology 1997; 50:273–276.
41. Fianu S, Söderberg G. Absorbable polyglactin mesh for retropubic sling operations in female urinary stress incontinence. Gynecol Obstet Invest 1983; 16:45–50.

42. Morgan JE, Heritz DM, Stewart FE, Connolly JC, Farow GA. The polypropylene pubovaginal sling for the treatment of recurrent stress urinary incontinence. J Urol 1995; 154:1013–1014.
43. Errando C, Batista JE, Artano P. Polytetrafluorethylene sling for failure in female stress incontinence surgery. Worl J Urol 1996; 14(suppl 1):S48–S50.
44. Norris JP, Breslin DS, Staskin DR. Use of synthetic material in sling surgery: a minimally invasive approach. J Endourol 1996; 10:227–230.
45. Ghoniem GM, Shaaban A. Suburethral slings for treatment of stress urinary incontinence. Int Urogynecol J 1994; 5:228–239.
46. Bent AE, Ostergard DR, Zwick-Zafutto M. Tissue reaction to expanded polytetrafluorethylene suburethral sling for urinary incontinence: clinical and histologic study. Am J Obstet Gynecol 1993; 169:1189–1204.
47. Weinberger MW, Ostergard DR. Long-term clinical and urodynamic evaluation of the polytetrafluorethylene suburethral sling for treatment of genuine stress incontinence. Obstet Gynecol 1995; 86:92–96.
48. Weinberger MW, Ostergard DR. Postoperative catheterization, urinary retention, and permanent voiding dysfunction after polytetrafluorethylene suburethral sling placement. Obstet Gynecol 1996; 87:50–54.
49. Labasky RF, Soper T. Reduction of patient morbidity and cost using frozen cadaveric fascia lata for the pubovaginal sling. J Urol 1997; 157:459, abstract 1794.
50. Ridley JH. Appraisal of the Goebell-Frangenheim-Stoeckel sling procedure. Am J Obstet Gynecol 1966; 95:714–721.
51. Carbone JM. Pubovaginal sling using cadaveric fascia and bone anchors: disappointing early results. J Urol 2001; 165:1605–1611.
52. Amundsen CL. Outcome in 104 pubovaginal slings using freeze-dried allograft fascia lata from a single tissue bank. Urology 2000; 56(suppl 6A):2–8.
53. Fitzgerald MP, Mollenhauer J, Bitterman P, Brubaker L. Functional failure of fascia lata allografts. Am J Obstet Gynecol 1999; 181:1339–1346.
54. Singla AK. The use of cadaveric fascia in the treatment of stress urinary incontinence in women. BJU Int 2000; 85:264–269.
55. Low JA. Management of severe anatomic deficiencies of urethral sphincter function by a combined procedure with a fascia lata sling. Am J Obstet Gynecol 1969; 105:149–155.
56. Addison WA, Haygood V, Parker RT. Recurrent stress urinary incontinence. Obstet Gynecol Annu 1985; 14:254–265.
57. Ogundipe A, Rosenzweig BA, Karram MM, Blumenfeld D, Bhatia NN. Modified suburethral sling procedure for treatment of recurrent or severe stress urinary incontinence. Surg Gynecol Obstet 1992; 175:173–176.
58. Karram MM, Bhatia NN. Patch procedure: modified transvaginal fascia lata sling for recurrent or severe stress urinary incontinence. Obstet Gynecol 1990; 75:461–463.
59. Handa VL, Jensen JK, Germain MM, Ostergard DR. Banked human fascia lata for the suburethral sling procedure: a preliminary report. Obstet Gynecol 1996; 88:1045–1049.
60. Carr LK, Webster GD. Voiding dysfunction following incontinence surgery: diagnosis and treatment with retropubic or vaginal urethrolysis. J Urol 1997; 157:821–823.
61. Ghoneim GM, Elgamasy A-N. Simplified surgical approach to bladder outlet obstruction following pubovaginal sling. J Urol 1995; 154:181–183.
62. Raz S. Atlas of Transvaginal Surgery. Philadelphia: W.B. Saunders, 1992.
63. Brodak PP, Juma S, Raz S. Levator hernia. J Urol 1992; 148:872–873.
64. Griebling TL, Berman CJ, Krader KJ. Fascia lata sling cyfousethropexy for the management of female urinary incontinence. Int Urogynecol 1998; 9:165–173.

25

The In Situ Anterior Vaginal Wall Sling

Howard B. Goldman
University Hospitals of Cleveland, CASE School of Medicine, Cleveland, Ohio, U.S.A.

I. INTRODUCTION

Over the past decade the surgical treatment of woman with stress urinary incontinence has undergone tremendous evolution. A number of studies evaluating urologists' practice patterns have demonstrated a clear shift from bladder neck suspensions, either retropubic or transvaginal, to slings (1,2). While much of this may be due to a better understanding of the mechanisms of stress urinary incontinence (SUI), in all likelihood the development of "minimally invasive" sling procedures with less patient morbidity and which are easier for surgeons to perform has significantly contributed to this shift in preferences as well.

Initially, autologous fascia, either rectus fascia or fascia lata, was the most common material used for pubovaginal slings. It remains the gold standard. In an effort to reduce the morbidity and discomfort associated with fascial harvest, other materials have been used for sling formation. Synthetic materials offer ease of availability, but they may have a higher rate of infection and erosion, and they can be costly. Cadaveric and other biologic tissues are easily obtainable, but they too can be costly, have at least a theoretic risk of transmission of infection, and may not offer comparable uniform strength and durability. On the other hand, the in situ anterior vaginal wall sling (AVWS) avoids the morbidity of autologous fascial harvest, does not have an increased rate of infection or erosion, is available at no cost, and avoids any risk of infectious disease transmission.

Raz first introduced the AVWS in 1989 (3). This technique uses in situ vaginal wall over the bladder neck and proximal urethra as the sling material, thus making fascial harvest unnecessary. Various modification of Raz's original technique have been introduced, but the concept of an in situ patch of tissue functioning as a backboard beneath the bladder neck and proximal urethra remains the same.

II. PATIENT SELECTION

Most women with documented SUI are candidates for an AVWS. However, patients with a history of prior vaginal surgery who have significant scarring of the anterior vaginal wall may not be suitable. In addition, postmenopausal women with very thin or significantly irritated vaginal skin may not be ideal candidates for an AVWS. In these cases a 6- to 8-week course of hormone replacement via vaginal cream may restore some of the suppleness of the vaginal wall. Other women with severe vaginal stenosis either secondary to previous surgery or postmenopausal changes may not be best served with an AVWS.

Furthermore, women with significant intrinsic sphincteric deficiency may not be ideal candidate for an AVWS. A number of studies that reviewed outcomes in women after an AVWS showed a trend toward higher failure rates in those patients with lower Valsalva leak-point pressures (VLPP). Studies by Raz, Litwiller, Su, and Goldman note this and based on these findings women with a VLPP <50 cm H_2O may do better with a fascial or other type of sling (3–6).

III. SURGICAL TECHNIQUE

After appropriate anesthesia has been achieved, the patient is placed in a modified dorsolithotomy position, the hair over the pubic bone is shaved, and the vagina and lower abdomen are prepped and draped in the usual fashion. A single dose of a broad-spectrum intravenous antibiotic is administered. Labial retraction sutures, a weighted vaginal speculum, and a Foley catheter are placed.

The bladder neck is identified by placing gentle traction on the Foley catheter and palpating the Foley balloon through the vaginal wall. A "Block A" is marked on the anterior vaginal wall (AVW), with the top of the "A" at a point halfway between the bladder neck and the urethral meatus and the proximal transverse marking of the "A" just proximal to the bladder neck. The legs of the "A" connect both transverse markings laterally and continue proximally along the anterior vaginal wall for a distance just greater than the distance between the two transverse markings.

Using a No. 15 blade on a long-handled scalpel, incisions are made along the markings. (Some find that infiltration of saline or lidocaine with epinephrine into the AVW facilitates dissection.) It is easiest to start at the proximal AVW along one leg of the "A" and incise to the midpoint of the top of the "A" and then repeat that incision on the other side. Then the transverse incision near the bladder neck can be made. The box between the transverse incisions will become the sling, while the area between the legs of the "A" will become a flap of AVW that will cover the sling. Of note, some surgeons incise only around the sling (not forming a flap) or just make the lateral sling incisions and do not cover the sling with a flap of AVW.

At this point, the vaginal skin between the legs of the "A" is dissected from the underlying pubocervical fascia but left attached proximally (Fig. 1). The rectangle of skin that will be used as the sling is freed distally and laterally from any attachments but left completely in situ. Using first sharp and then blunt dissection, the lateral spaces are opened along the periurethral fascia until the underside of the pubis is easily palpated. (Some prefer to continue the dissection further and perforate the endopelvic fascia.)

A 3-cm transverse incision is made one fingerbreadth above the pubis. A Stamey needle is passed from each lateral edge of the incision through the rectus fascia and under finger guidance into the vagina. Cystoscopy is performed to ensure no bladder perforation. If perforation is noted, the needle is removed and replaced. A No. 1 polypropylene suture is passed in a horizontal mattress configuration incorporating the pubocervical fascia and vaginal wall through each lateral edge of the sling. (Helical or other types of suture attachment through the sling edges can be done instead.) Both ends of each suture are passed through the corresponding Stamey eye and brought up to a prepubic position (Fig. 2). The previously formed flap is advanced over the sling and the vaginal wall is closed with a running, locking 2-0 polyglactin suture (Fig. 3). The weighted vaginal speculum is removed. (Some prefer to place transvaginal bone anchors

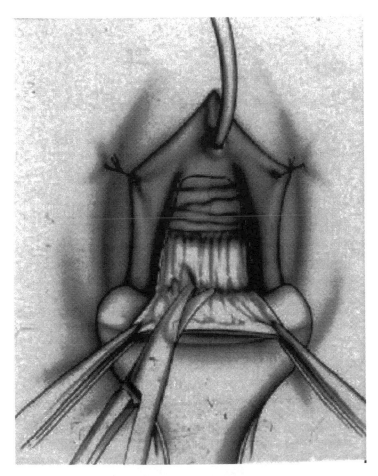

Figure 1   Incisions of "Block A" and preparations of flap. (Courtesy of R.A. Appell.)

and sutures transvaginally, thus avoiding the prepubic incision. Long-term success rates of this modification are unknown.)

At this point, the prepubic sutures can be stabilized or tied according to the surgeon's preference. One technique is to pass one end of each set of sutures through periosteum or rectus fascia with a Mayo needle and then loosely tie the two ends of the suture together on each side. Others prefer to tie both sets of suture ends across the midline in one large knot. Still others use bone anchors or have another system for tying the sutures down with the appropriate minimal tension.

Scarpa's fascia is approximated with a 3-0 chromic suture, and the skin is closed with a running 4-0 polyglactin subcuticular suture. Steri-Strips and a dressing are applied to the prepubic wound and a vaginal packing impregnated with either hormonal cream or antibiotic ointment is placed. The labial retraction sutures are removed and the procedure is completed. (For bladder drainage, a urethral or suprapubic catheter can be left in place for a few days or the patient can be given an opportunity to void postoperatively. If she cannot, intermittent catheterization can be instituted.)

Patients are discharged on oral analgesics and instructed to avoid heavy lifting or strenuous activity for 4–6 weeks.

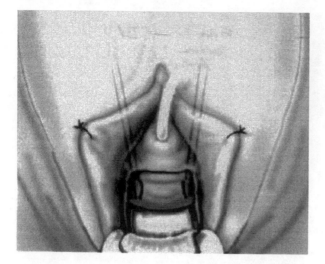

Figure 2   Placement of sutures through the anterior vaginal wall sling. (Courtesy of R.A. Appell.)

IV.   RESULTS

The reported success rates for the AVWS range from a high of 100% to a low of 61% (subjective cure) (7,5). The majority of authors report success in 70–95% of patients (Table 1). Some of the differences in the reported outcomes may be due to variations in the definition of success.

There are three studies of note that have a documented average follow-up longer than 2 years. Litwiller et al. reported on a series of 42 evaluable patients followed for an average of 31 months. They noted resolution of SUI in 71% (4). Lobel and Sand reported an 80% success rate in a series of 90 patients followed for an average of 26 months (8). The largest series, which

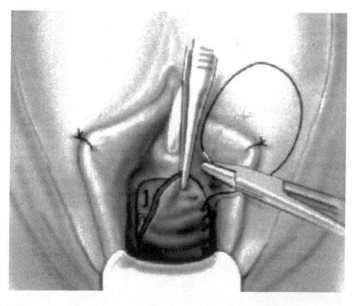

Figure 3   Closure of the anterior vaginal wall flap over the sling. (Courtesy of R.A. Appell.)

Table 1 Reports of Efficacy of AVWS

Author	No. of patients with follow-up	Percent with prior procedure	Length of follow-up (months)	Successful outcome
Raz (3)	26	100	10–28	85% (excellent 77%, very good 8%)
Juma (11)	54	89	23.9	94.4% (excellent 90.7, very good 3.7%)
Couillard (7)	18	100	18	100% (all dry)
Pidutti (12)	12	100	17.3	92% (excellent 67%, improved 25%)
Lessans (13)	29	25	7	82% (dry 41%, improved 41%)
Raz (10)	160	54	1	93% (SUI resolved)
Kaplan (9)	36	100	? (likely 16)	97% (SUI resolved)
Liwiller (4)	42	72	31	71% (SUI resolved) (92% in those with LPP > 60)
Lobel (8)	90	33	26	80% (70% complete or almost complete cure; 10% somewhat improved)
Masoudi (14)	23	17	13	85% (SUI cured or improved)
Cummings (15)	16	?	8.1	88% (75% dry; 13% improved but using pads)
Su (5)	23	100	15	60.9% (subjective cure) 34.8% (objective cure)
Kaplan (9)	335	?	39.8	96% (SUI resolved)
Goldman (6)	39	51	19	79.5% (SUI resolved) (93% in those with VLPP > 50)

consisted of a combination of patients treated at three different centers, was reported by Kaplan et al. (9), who noted a 96% success rate in a group of 373 patients followed for an average of 40 months. Importantly, the success rate for patients with follow-up exceeding 5 years was 94%. It should be noted that Raz et al. (10), in another large study of 160 patients followed for an average of only 17 months, reported a 93% success rate, which is similar to the result of Kaplan et al.

Various authors evaluated possible patient factors that may predict a successful outcome. Goldman et al. noted an overall 80% success rate (6). However, they noted that the majority of their failures were in those with lower Valsalva leak-point pressures (VLPP). After using receiver operator characteristic curves to identify a VLPP that predicted a successful outcome, they found that those with a VLPP of 50 cmH$_2$O or higher had a success rate of 93%, whereas those with a VLPP less than 50 cmH$_2$O had a success rate of 40% (4). Similarly, Litwiller et al. noted a success rate of 92% in their patients with isolated hypermobility, whereas those with pure ISD and a mixed problem had success rates of 72% and 62%, respectively. In addition, Su et al.(5) found that patients with an objective cure had higher maximal urethral closure pressures than those who failed. Finally, Raz et al. noted a trend toward late recurrence of stress incontinence in their group of patients with intrinsic sphincter deficiency (ISD) (10). Thus, a number of reports support the concept that patients with a lower VLPP (VLPP <50 cmH$_2$O per Goldman et al.) and more significant ISD have a worse outcome than those with a higher VLPP. In contrast, Kaplan et al. found no difference in outcome between patients with ISD (VLPP <60 cmH$_2$O) and those with anatomic incontinence (VLPP > 60 cmH$_2$O) (9). Their findings are clearly different from those of the aforementioned groups, and this difference is difficult to explain.

V. COMPLICATIONS

Significant intraoperative hemorrhage is rare, and its rate of occurrence is similar to that seen in other sling procedures. Infection, usually a urinary tract infection or a prepubic or suprapubic wound infection, occurs in $<5\%$ of patients. Rare cases of inclusion cyst formation in the buried piece of AVW have been reported (16). Delayed spontaneous voiding or chronic retention occurs in $<5\%$, whereas de novo detrusor instability and/or obstructive voiding complaints may occur in as many as 15% of cases. Urethrolysis may be necessary on occasion. Significant failure—persistent SUI—occurs in 5–25% of patients.

VI. CONCLUSIONS

The in situ AVWS is a technically straightforward, minimally invasive procedure for treatment of female SUI. It minimizes patient morbidity and avoids some of the potential problems associated with use of synthetic or biologic materials. Reported success rates range from 70% to 95%, with the largest series reporting successful outcomes in $>90\%$ of patients. Some authors report that success rates are lower in patients with lower VLPP values, but not all studies support that concept.

REFERENCES

1. Kim HL, Gerber GS, Patel RV, Hollowell CM, Bales GT. Practice patterns in the treatment of female urinary incontinence. A postal and internet survey. Urology 2001; 57:45.
2. Leach GE, Dmochowski RR, Appell RA, Blaivas JG, Hadley HR, Luber KM, Mostwin JL, O'Donnell PD, Roehrborn CG. Female stress urinary incontinence clinical guidelines panel summary report on surgical management of female stress urinary incontinence. J Urol 1997; 158:875.
3. Raz S, Siegel AL, Short JL, Synder JA. Vaginal wall sling. J Urol 1989; 141:43.
4. Litwiller SE, Nelson RS, Fone PD, Kim KB, Stone AR. Vaginal wall sling: long-term outcome analysis of factors contributing to patient satisfaction and surgical success. J Urol 1977; 157:1279.
5. Su T, Huang J, Wang Y, Yang J, Wei H, Huang C. Is modified in-situ vaginal wall sling operation the treatment of choice for recurrent genuine stress incontinence? J Urol 1999; 162:2073.
6. Goldman HB, Rackley RR, Appell RA. The in situ anterior vaginal wall sling: predictors of success. J Urol 2001; 166:2559.
7. Couillard DR, Deckard-Janatpour KA, Stone AR. The vaginal wall sling: a compressive suspension procedure for recurrent incontinence in elderly patients. Urology 1994; 43:203.
8. Lobel RW, Sand PK. Long-term results of vaginal wall suburethral sling. J Urol 1997; 157:459A.
9. Kaplan SA, Te AE, Young GPH Andrade A, Cabelin MA, Ikeguchi EF. Prospective analysis of 373 consecutive women with stress urinary incontinence treated with a vaginal wall sling: The Columbia–Cornell University experience. J Urol 2000; 164:1623.

10. Raz S, Stothers L, Young GPH, Short J, Marks B, Chopra A, Wahle GR. Vaginal wall sling for anatomical incontinence and intrinsic sphincter dysfunction: efficacy and outcome analysis. J Urol 1996; 156:166.

11. Juma S, Little NA, Raz S. Vaginal wall sling: four years later. Urology 1992; 39:424.

12. Piduitti RW, George SW, Morales A. Correction of recurrent stress urinary incontinence by needle urethropexy with a vaginal wall sling. Br J Urol 1994; 73:418.

13. Lessans KD, Gordon DA, Despradel V, Witmore KE. Modified vaginal wall sling with pubic bone anchors for the treatment of stress urinary incontinence. J Urol 1996; 155:699A.

14. Masoudi JF, Whitmore KE, Gordon DA, Lessans KD, Campion MJ. Modified vaginal wall sling with bone anchors for the treatment of urinary incontinence and cystocele. J Urol 1997; 157:460A.

15. Cummings JM, Parra RO, Boulher JA. Comparison of vaginal wall sling with pubovaginal sling for stress incontinence from intrinsic sphincteric deficiency. J Urol 1997; 157:461A.

16. Woodham PJ, Davis GD. The relationship of the in situ anterior vaginal wall sling to a vaginal epithelial cyst. Int Urogynecol J Pelvic Floor Dysfunct 2000; 11:124.

26
CATS: Cadaveric Transvaginal Sling

Dawn M. Bodell
Tower Urology Institute for Continence, Los Angeles, California, U.S.A.

Gary E. Leach
Tower Urology Institute for Continence, Los Angeles, California, U.S.A.

I. INTRODUCTION

Pubovaginal/transvaginal slings have become the gold standard for the treatment of all types of female stress urinary incontinence, whether the stress urinary incontinence (SUI) is secondary to intrinsic sphincter deficiency (ISD) or hypermobility of the urethra (1). The author's sling procedure of choice is the cadaveric transvaginal sling procedure (CATS).

II. INDICATIONS AND PATIENT SELECTION

A successful sling procedure requires an appropriate preoperative evaluation, starting with the history and physical exam. The key components of the history should include the impact the incontinence has on the patient's quality of life. The SEAPI incontinence score facilitates a subjective assessment of the patient's symptoms (Appendix A). The physical examination should document urethral hypermobility or a fixed urethra and provide documentation of pelvic relaxation. Patients with pelvic prolapse should have the prolapse repaired simultaneously with the sling procedure (2). Patients with stress urinary incontinence and a fixed or extremely elevated urethra should also have urethrolysis performed in order to release the urethra from the surrounding scar tissue and fixation, and thus allow the sling to apply adequate urethral compression (3). Prior to performing a sling procedure, a urodynamic evaluation should be completed to confirm stress urinary incontinence, exclude detrusor instability at low bladder volumes, and evaluate the patient's ability to empty the bladder.

III. FASCIA

The choices of fascia for the sling can be autologous or allograft fascia. Cadaveric fascia has become a more popular choice of material than autologous material for a multitude of reason, including shortening of operative time and hospital stay, while decreasing postoperative pain and shortening the recuperation period.

Tutoplast, produced by Mentor Corporation, is a solvent-dehydrated, gamma-irradiated fascia, which is our fascia of choice. The Tutoplast processing includes a five-step process:

1. *Screening*:   The U.S. Food and Drug Administration serologically screens donor candidates and the fascia. The fascia is inspected for cleanliness, quality, structure, and size. Donor tissue will be rejected if there is an adverse medical or social history that might be suspicious for any infectious disease or malignancy.
2. *Processing*:   The fascia is cleaned in a saline solution and then osmotically treated. This treatment destroys any bacteria or viruses.
3. *Denaturization*:   NaOH and H_2O_2 treatment inactivates any prions, destroys any remaining viruses, and removes all antigens. Exposure time to NaOH is limited in this step to avoid any significant weakening of the collagen.
4. *Preservation*:   Water is extracted from the tissues via organic solvents, to preserve the dense collagenous fiber structure.
5. *Gamma irradiation*:   The fascia is cut to the appropriate size and treated with gamma irradiation to sterilize the tissue. The amount of radiation is limited to <2.5 Mrad, to limit weakening of the fascia.

Testing of the solvent-dehydrated fascia revealed significantly higher stiffness, higher maximum load to failure, and higher maximum load per unit width of graft with the solvent-dehydrated fascia (4). Boone reviewed 26 stress urinary incontinent patients who underwent a pubovaginal sling with cadaveric fascia lata (Tutoplast), with a minimum follow-up of 12 months (5). The outcome results reported 25 of 26 (96%) patients to be "significantly" improved postoperatively. Twenty-four of 26 (92%) of the patients wore no more than one pad daily, and 77% of the patients were completely dry. Only two patients required more than one pad: one of the patients went from four pads to two pads. Two patients experienced de novo urgency, which was controlled with anticholinergics. No patient underwent a second operation. This study supports the longer-term sling results obtained with solvent dehydrated cadaveric fascia lata.

Conversely, Raz et al. performed 154 consecutive bone-anchored cadaveric fascia pubovaginal slings with a follow-up of 10.6 months (6). The type of fascia used in theses cases was freez-dried fascia from a California tissue bank. Of the 154 patients, 58 (37.6%) had recurrent incontinence (grades 2–3), with 26 (16.9%) patients having undergone a second pubovaginal sling procedure. Average time to reoperation was 9 months. Attenuated, fragmented, or absent fascia was noted at the time of reoperation. This study demonstrated that all cadaveric fascia is not "created equally." Lemer et al. (7) compared autologous rectus fascia, dermal graft, solvent-dehydrated cadaveric fascia lata, and freeze-dried cadaveric fascia lata. The cadaveric freeze-dried fascia lata had the weakest tensile strength of all the tissues studied. Also, the freeze-dried cadaveric fascia had the most inconsistencies in the tissues among the other fascias compared. Solvent-dehydrated cadaveric fascia and dermal grafts were identical to native autologous rectus fascia with regard to tensile strength and tissue stiffness. Thus, the use of the tissue bank "frozen" fascia was a significant factor accounting for the poor sling results obtained by Raz. Also, the authors avoid the use of synthetic sling materials because allograft fascia has a significantly lower infection and erosion rate, when compared to synthetic materials (8–11).

In conclusion, the choice of the appropriate sling material is extremely important. For the transvaginal sling procedure, the authors use the 2×7 cm strip of cadaveric solvent dehydrated allograft fascia lata.

IV. BONE ANCHORS

In 1949, the Marshall-Marchetti-Krantz vesicourethropexy was one of the first procedures to use bone fixation as part of a suspension procedure for the correction of female stress urinary incontinence (12). In 1988, Leach described a suprapubic bone fixation technique for needle suspension procedures (13). This technique fixed the suspension sutures directly into the pubic tubercle, utilizing a strong Mayo needle, as opposed to securing the suspension suture to the rectus fascia. This bone fixation technique alleviated the complication of ilioinguinal nerve entrapment caused by the sutures being placed laterally in the rectus fascia, thereby decreasing postoperative pain from nerve entrapment. Benderev developed his modification of needle suspension using bone anchors with the Vesica procedure (14). Nativ further modified the placement of bone anchors by using an entirely transvaginal approach to complete the cystourethropexy which was further developed into a sling procedure (15). The technique employed a drill and transvaginal bone anchor system. This entirely transvaginal technique revolutionized the sling procedure.

Advantages of this transvaginal bone anchor fixation include minimal postoperative pain and bleeding. Since no needles or sutures are passed through the retropubic space, the risk of bladder perforation is significantly decreased. Also, utilizing the author's transvaginal sling technique outlined below, the endopelvic fascia is not routinely perforated during the procedure. Thus, it is possible that the risk for postoperative vaginal prolapse and recurrent stress incontinence may be reduced when the endopelvic fascia remains intact (16).

There is also a decreased rate of bone infection with the transvaginal bone anchors when compared to suprapubic anchor placement. Rackley et al. (17) found no pubic bone infections in 314 patients who had undergone a transvaginal sling with bone anchor placement compared to a .86% osseous complication rate associated with suprapubic bone anchors. The reported rate of osseous infections from a Marshall-Marchetti-Krantz retropubic urethropexy was .76%, with an overall incidence of an infectious bone bone anchor complications in female pelvic reconstructive procedures was found to be .6% (18).

V. SURGICAL TECHNIQUE

A. Preoperative Preparation

Prior to performing a sling procedure, the urine is confirmed to be sterile. Patients are taught how to do self-catheterization preoperatively, or a suprapubic catheter may be placed at the time of the procedure for those patients with documented incomplete bladder emptying and inability to perform self-catheterization. A providone iodine vaginal douche is performed the night before surgery. Perioperative antibiotics are given, preferably a first-generation cephalosporin, ampicillin, or vancomycin (if a penicillin allergic), combined with an aminoglycoside. When timing allows, patients with vaginal wall atrophy are instructed to use an estrogen vaginal cream three times a week for 4–6 weeks preoperatively.

B. Operative Procedure

Patients are placed in the dorsal lithotomy position. A Foley catheter is inserted, and a Scott retractor (Lonestar, Houston, TX) is secured to the medial buttocks with towel clamps. Palpation of the foley balloon identifies the bladder neck. The anterior vaginal epithelium is injected with plain saline and an inverted "U" shaped incision is made from the mid-urethra to the bladder neck. (Fig. 1). The inverted "U" flap is mobilized to the bladder neck. Stopping the vaginal wall flap dissection at the level of the bladder neck prevents the sling from migrating above the

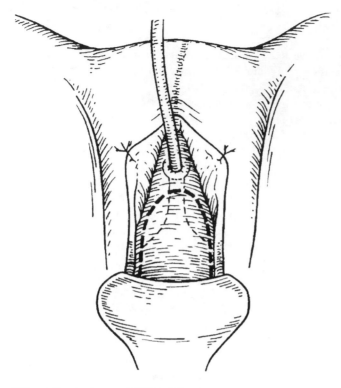

Figure 1   An inverted "U" incision is made in the anterior vaginal wall.

bladder neck. Sharp lateral dissection at the level of the bladder neck cleans off the undersurface of the pubic bone for accurate placement of the bone anchors. As previously mentioned, the endopelvic fascia is not routinely perforated, to minimize the chance of significant bleeding in the space of Retzius and to maintain the integrity of the endopelvic fascia.

Prior to placing the bone anchors, suspension sutures and anchors need to be chosen. Two types of bone anchors are available: an anchor with polypropolene (prolene) suture attached to the bone screw, and a "loop"-type anchor through which a suture of the surgeon's choice can be placed (Fig. 2). The choice of suture depends on the patient. A suture is threaded through the loop screw.

Once the pubic bone is cleared of tissue posteriorly, the transvaginal bone anchor is placed. Before placing the anchor, the bladder is drained to minimize the risk of bladder perforation. To avoid injury to the bladder or bladder neck during the bone anchor placement, the backside of a forceps is used to retract the bladder medially away from the anchor placement site. The drill is positioned on the underside of the pubic bone so that the anchor is flush with the bone (Fig. 3). Once the drill is activated, a change in tone of the drill motor confirms that the anchor is firmly placed into the bone. Once the anchor is seated, the drill is removed and the attached suture is vigorously pulled upon to confirm secure anchor placement. This same bone anchor insertion process is completed on the contralateral side.

A 2 × 7 cm piece of Tutoplast fascia is soaked in antibiotic solution. The edge of the fascia is folded over to minimize the risk of suture "pull-through" by cross-hatching the fascial fibers (Fig. 4). An 18-gauge needle facilitates atraumatic passage of the suture through the overlapping end of the sling (Fig. 5). The bladder neck suture is placed more medially through fascia than the distal suture, to keep the fascial strip tight against the bladder neck. Once both

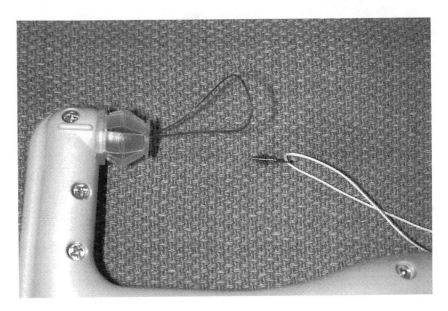

Figure 2   Drill and loop screw with suture attached to the screw.

ends of the suture attached to the bone anchor are brought through the end of the sling, the suture is tied flush to the bone anchor. A 2-0 Vicryl suture secures the distal edge of the sling to the periurethral tissues to prevent "rolling" of the sling toward the bladder neck. The correct suture tension, while tying the sling in place, is determined by folding over the fascial strip and placing an Allis clamp on the folded portion of the fascia and then stretching the fascia to the contralateral bone anchor site (Fig. 6). Once the proper tension is determined, the suspension

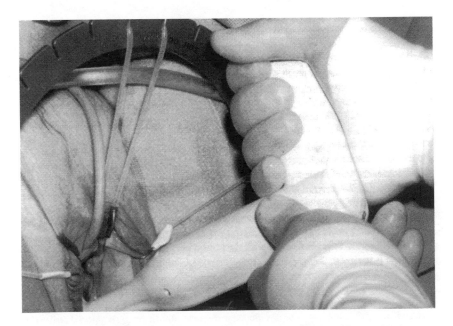

Figure 3   The bone anchor drill is positioned on the underside of the pubic bone.

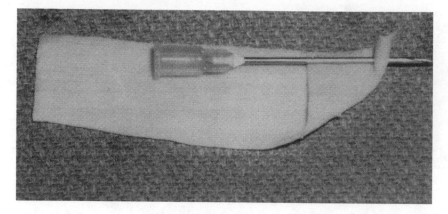

Figure 4   The edge of the fascial sling is folded over to minimize the risk of suture "pull through."

sutures are passed through the free end of the sling in the same fashion as the other side. The sutures are tied snugly (without any clamp between the urethra and the sling), to create a well supportive "backstop" for the urethra. To eliminate the stress incontinence, it is critical that the sling not be tied too loosely.

A 2-0 Vicryl suture secures the distal edge of the sling to the periurethral tissue. Cystoscopy with a 30° lens confirms the absence of bladder or urethral injury from the bone anchor placement. Antibiotic solution is used to irrigate the vaginal incision throughout the procedure. The Foley catheter is placed to drainage and the vaginal incision is closed with a running 2-0 Vicryl suture. An antibiotic-soaked vaginal packing is placed.

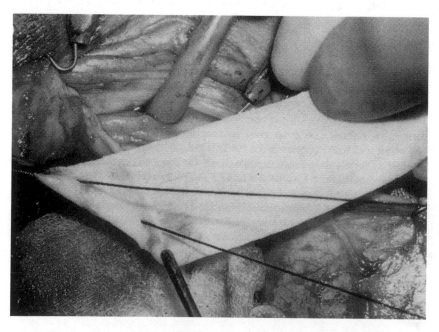

Figure 5   The sutures attached to the bone anchor are placed atraumatically through the fascial strip with the more proximal suture placed more medially.

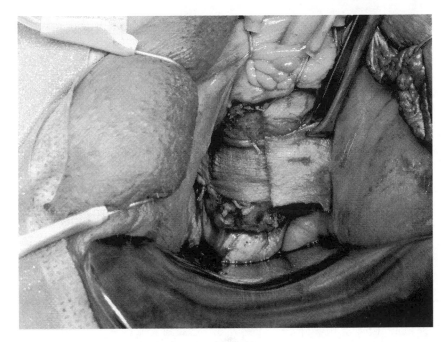

Figure 6   Folding over an adequate amount of the sling ensures proper sling tension.

C. Postoperative Care

The vaginal packing and Foley catheter are removed on the first postoperative day. Patients are given a voiding trial and the postvoid residual urine volume is checked. When postvoid residuals are >100 mL, patients are reinstructed in self-catheterization. When patients have a suprapubic catheter (SPT), postvoid residuals can be checked via the SPT. Intravenous antibiotics are discontinued on the first postoperative day, and patients are started on an oral antibiotic (cephalosporin or a fluoroquinolone). Oral antibiotics are continued for 1 week to minimize the risk of osteitis pubis or wound infection. Most patients have minimal postoperative pain that is controlled with acetominophen. For 6 weeks, patients are instructed to comply with complete pelvic rest (i.e., nothing in the vagina: no tampons or intercourse) and to avoid heavy lifting.

VI. RESULTS

A. The AUA Guidelines Panel

The American Urological Association Guidelines Panel did an in depth data analysis, reviewing over 5000 articles, related to the surgical treatment of female stress urinary incontinence. Practice recommendations were formulated based on reported surgical outcomes obtained with the different types of anti-incontinence procedures. The panel compared four general groupings of procedures: transvaginal suspensions, anterior repairs, retropubic suspensions, and slings. "Cure/dry" rate and "cure/improved" rates were tabulated with this meta-analysis with 3 follow-up periods: 12–23 months, 24–47 months, and 48 months or longer. There was no statistical difference in outcomes within each group of procedures at any time interval. Among the different anti-incontinence procedures, there was a statistical difference in outcomes only at a follow-up period of >48 months.

Slings and retropubic suspensions had the best long-term success rate of 83% and 84%, respectively. The panel concluded that the most effective surgical procedures (at >48-month follow up) were obtained with slings and retropubic suspensions (Fig. 7).

The panel also examined complication rates for synthetic slings. Based on the literature reviewed, synthetic slings had a higher erosion and infection rate than the "nonsynthetic" slings. The risk of vaginal erosion for synthetic slings was .7%, compared to .01% for autologous slings. The risk of urethral erosion with synthetic slings was 2%, compared to only .3% with autologous slings (Table 1).

A more global assessment of the "success rates" should also include patient satisfaction and a patient generated confidential questionnaire. Sirls et al. did an outcome analysis of 151 patients, with a 25-month follow up, who had undergone a modified Pereyra bladder neck suspension (19). The study consisted of a retrospective chart review and a simultaneous, confidential patient questionnaire, which was reviewed by a second party. The confidential questionnaire results revealed a cure in 47% of the patients and improvement of SUI in 65% of the patients. In contrast, the results with the simultaneous retrospective chart review revealed a cure in 72% of the patients and 89% of the patients were improved. Sirls concluded that the way postoperative data was obtained greatly impacted outcome results. Although the surgical results are significantly less "optimistic" with subjective questionnaires than with chart review, clearly, subjective questionnaires most accurately assess patient satisfaction and surgical outcomes. Thus, the authors have evaluated their transvaginal sling results utilizing a confidential questionnaire completed by the patients and reviewed by an independent party at 6-month intervals following the sling procedure.

Since there are no standardized definitions for surgical outcomes following anti-incontinence surgery, Groutz et al. (20) conducted a study to develop an outcome instrument incorporating multiple noninvasive outcome measures including a 24-h voiding diary, a 24-h pad test, uroflowmetry, postvoid residual urine, and a postoperative patient questionnaire (20). Ninety-four pubovaginal sling patients were studied, with a minimum follow-up of 1 year (mean 3.4 years). The outcome data were formulated into an incontinence score, which is the sum of

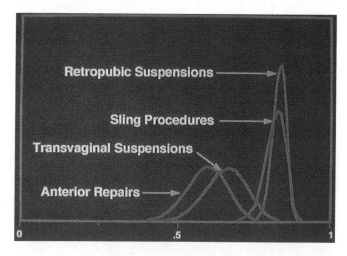

Figure 7 AUA outcomes data of 4 categories surgical procedures at >48 months follow-up. (© 1994, 1995, 1996, 1997 American Urological Association, Inc. All rights reserved.)

Table 1 Comparative Complication Rates for Sling Materials

Complications	Autologous materials (1715 pts)	Homologous materials (414 pts)	Synthetic materials (1515 pts)
Vaginal erosion	1 pt (0.0001)	0	10 pts (0.0007)
Urethral erosion	5 pts (0.003)	0	27 pts (0.02)
Fistula	6 pts (0.0003)	0	4 pts (0.002)
Wound sinus	3 pts (0.0002)	0	11 pts (0.007)
Wound infection	11 pts (0.006)	9 pts (0.02)	15 pts (0.009)
Seroma	6 pts (0.003)	0	1 pt (0.0007)

three categories: a 24-h voiding diary, 24-h pad test, and a patient questionnaire (Appendix B). Cure is classified as a score of 0 and failure as a score of 6. With this new response score, only 47% were defined as totally cured (zero score following the sling). These results more accurately represent realistic outcomes following the sling procedure.

B. Cadaveric Transvaginal Sling (CATS) Results

The CATS procedure has been performed on 229 patients with 186 patients followed for more than 1 year. The age range was from 23 to 90 years (mean 63 years). Patients are followed closely with follow-up visits and confidential questionnaires competed every 6 months after the sling to obtain accurate long-term outcome data. The longest follow-up has been 43 months with a mean follow up of 21.2 months. On the confidential questionnaire, 50/186 (27%) of the patients reported 100% improvement, 105/186 (54%) were >80% improved, and 118 (69%) were >50% improved. Persistent urgency was noted in 32 (17%), and de novo urgency in 20 (11%). Mean SEAPI scores were 6.2 preoperatively and 2.4 postoperatively, representing a significant decrease ($P < .0001$). Overall, 109/186 (56%) of patients were >80% satisfied with the procedure on a visual analog scale (with a mean satisfaction score of 67%), and 69% would recommend the surgery to a friend.

Fifty-eight (31%) reported <50% improvement. Of these, 18 (9.7%) had stress urinary incontinence, 23 (12.3%) had mixed incontinence, five (2.7%) had urge incontinence, and four (2.1%) patients were not clear regarding the cause of their dissatisfaction. Eight of 58 (35%) patients had no incontinence but based their dissatisfaction on urinary urgency. Few late failures at >1 year were reported (6/58; 10.3%). The majority of failures (40/58; 65%) experienced recurrent incontinence within 3 months following surgery. No unexpected postoperative urinary retention occurred. Complications included osteitis pubis (without osteomyelitis), managed in two patients with nonsteroidal medication, and wound separation in three patients, which healed secondarily.

VII. CONCLUSIONS

The AUA guidelines panel recommendations support the use of the sling as a first-line treatment for female stress urinary incontinence. Patient selection and appropriate preoperative evaluation are critical to the success of the sling procedure. Utilizing nonfrozen cadaveric fascia lata (Tutoplast) obviates the need for tissue harvesting and decreases postoperative pain. Also, the complications associated with the use of synthetic sling materials are avoided. Results with the transvaginal sling, incorporating the use of transvaginal bone anchors and Tutoplast cadaveric fascia, are encouraging.

REFERENCES

1. Leach GE, Dmochowski RR, Appell RA. Female stress urinary incontinence clinical guidelines panel summary report on surgical management of female stress urinary incontinence. J Urol 1997; 158:875–880.
2. Kobashi KC, Mee SL, Leach GE. A new technique for cystocele repair and transvaginal sling: the cadaveric prolapse repair and sling (CaPs). Urology 2000; 56:9–14.
3. Leach GE. Urethrolysis. Urole Clin North Am 1994; 2:23–27.
4. Jinnah RH, Johnson C, Warden K, Clarke HJ. A biomechanical analysis of solvent-dehydrated and freeze-dried human fascia lata allografts. A preliminary report. Am J Sports Med 1992; 20(5): 607–612.
5. Elliot DS, Boone TB. Is fascia lata allograft material trustworthy for pubovaginal sling repair? Urology 2000; 56:772–776.
6. Carbone JM, Kavaler E, Raz S. Pubovaginal sling using cadaveric fascia and bone anchors: disappointing early results. J Urol 2001; 165:1605–1611.
7. Lemer ML, Chaikin DC, Blaivas JG. Tissue strength analysis of autologous and cadaveric allografts for the pubovaginal sling. Neurourol Urodyn 1999; 18:497–503.
8. Bent AE, Ostergard DR, Zwick-Zaffuto M. Tissue reaction to expanded polytetrafluoroethylene suburethral sling for urinary incontinence: clinical and histology study. Am J Obstet Gynecol 1993; 169:1198–1207.
9. Choe JM, Kothandapani R, James L. Autologous, cadaveric, and synthetic materials used in sling surgery: comparative biomechanical analysis. Urology 2001; 58:482–486.
10. Leach GE, Kobashi KC, Mee SL. Erosion of woven polyester synthetic (ProteGen) pubovaginal sling. J Urol 1999; 161:106.
11. Duckett JR, Constantine G. Complications of silicone sling insertion for stress urinary incontinence. J Urol 2000; 163:1835–1837.
12. Marshall VF, Marchetti AA, Krantz DE. The correction of stress incontinence by simple vesico-urethral suspension. Surg Gynecol Obstet 1949; 88:509.
13. Leach GE. Bone fixation technique for transvaginal needle suspension. Urology 1988; 31:388–390.
14. Benderev T. Anchor fixation and other modifications of endoscopic bladder neck suspension. Urology 1992; 40:409–418.
15. Nativ O, Levine S, Madjar S. Incisionless per vaginal bone anchor cystourethropexy for the treatment of female stress incontinence: experience with the first 50 patients. J Urol 1997; 158:1742–1744.
16. Kohle N, Sze EHM, Roat TW. Incidence of recurrent cystocele after transvaginal needle suspension procedures with and without concomitant anterior colporrhaphy. Am J Obstet Gynecol 1996; 175:1476–1480.
17. Rackley RR, Abdelmalak JB, Madjar S. Bone anchor infections in female pelvic reconstructive procedures: a literature review of series and case reports. J Urol 2001; 165:1975–1978.
18. Kammerer-Doak DN, Cornella JL, Magrina JF. Osteitis pubis after Marshll-Marchetti-Krantz urethropexy: a pubic osteomyelitis. Am J Obstet Gynecol 1998; 179:586.
19. Sirls LT, Keoleian CM, Korman HJ, Kirkemo AK. The effect of study methodology on reported success rates of the modified Pereyra bladder neck suspension. J Urol 1995; 154:1732–1735.
20. Groutz A, Blaivas JG, Rosenthal VE. A simplified urinary incontinence score for the evaluation of treatment outcomes. Neurourol Urodyn 2000; 19:127–135.

Appendix A   SEAPI Incontinence Score (Subjective)

S	Stress related	0 = no urine loss
		1 = loss with strenuous activity
		2 = loss with moderate activity
		3 = loss with minimal activity, or gravitational incontinence
E	Empting ability	0 = no obstructive symptoms
		1 = minimal symptoms
		2 = significant symptoms
		3 = voiding only in dribbles, or urinary retention
A	Anatomy	0 = no descent during strain
		1 = descent, not to introitus
		2 = descent though introitus with strain
		3 = Through introitus without strain
P	Protection	0 = never used
		1 = used only for certain occasions
		2 = used daily for occasional accidents
		3 = used continually for frequent accidents or constant leaking
I	Inhibition	0 = no urgency incontinence
		1 = rare urgency incontinence
		2 = urgency incontinence once a week
		3 = urgency incontinence at least once a day

Source: Ref. 1.

Appendix B   Groutz and Blaivas Response Score for Assessment of Surgical Outcomes of Anti-Incontinence Procedures

1. 24-h voiding diary
    a. No urinary incontinence (urge or stress) episodes: 0 points
    b. 1–2 incontinence episodes: 1 point
    c. ≥3 incontinence episodes: 2 points
2. 24-h pad test
    a. Total weight gain of the pads ≤8 g: 0 points
    b. Total weight gain of the pads 9–20 g: 1 point
    c. Total weight gain of the pads >20 g: 2 points
3. Patient questionnaire
    a. Patient considers herself as cured: 0 points
    b. Patient considers herself as improved: 1 point
    c. Patient considers the operation to have failed: 2 points
The response scores the sum of the above subscores and is classified as:
    Cure: total score 0
    Good response: total score 1–2
    Fair response: total score 3–4
    Poor response: total score 5
    Failure: total score 6

Source: Ref. 20.

27

Tension-Free Vaginal Tape: An Innovative, Minimally Invasive Pubovaginal Sling for Female Stress Urinary Incontinence

Vincent R. Lucente*
Pennsylvania State University, College of Medicine, Hersey, Pennsylvania, U.S.A.

Marisa A. Mastropietro[†]
Lehigh Valley Hospital, Allentown, Pennsylvania, U.S.A.

I. INTRODUCTION

The first surgical approach for the treatment of female stress urinary incontinence (SUI) was published in 1914 by Howard Kelly, describing his technique of urethral plication (1). Since then, over 100 surgical procedures and various modifications have been described in the literature. The fact that our knowledge of the functional anatomy of the urethra and the physiology of the normal continence mechanism continues to evolve is no doubt interrelated to why such a plethora of surgical procedures has been reported.

Despite the growing body of comparative studies, a systematic review of the literature in 1996 by Black and Downs could not determine the "best procedure" for surgical treatment of female SUI based on scientific evidence (2). More recently, however, an expert clinical panel of the American Urological Association concluded that retropubic suspensions and slings provide the most effective long-term cure rate. The sling operation, however, was associated with significant complications (3). The higher incidence of postoperative voiding dysfunction and the potential for sling erosion is often cited as the rationale against sling procedures as the primary surgery of choice for correcting female SUI (4). Improved techniques and new sling materials have contributed to a gradual lowering of these complication rates (5,6). Another advantage of sling procedures is that they are more effective in women with intrinsic sphincter deficiency (ISD), which has been identified as a significant risk factor in reducing long-term surgical success.

As with all other surgeries, the traditional sling procedure, despite its success to date, is faced with today's challenge, if not the defined trend of modern surgery, that is to be performed less invasively with consistent results and fewer complications. In 1995 Ulmsten and Petros

---

Current affiliation: Institute for Female Pelvic Medicine and Reconstructive Surgery, Allentown, Pennsylvania, U.S.A.
[†]*Current affiliation*: Lincoln Hospital, Bronx, New York, U.S.A.

responded to this challenge by introducing an innovative minimally invasive pubovaginal sling procedure—the tension-free vaginal tape (TVT) (7).

II. HISTORICAL BACKGROUND

The TVT procedure was developed based on a theory regarding the urethral continence mechanism postulated by Ulmsten. His hypothesis was a significant shift from widely held previous views: Enhorning's theory of abdominal pressure transmission, which required proper elevation of the bladder neck into the abdominal pressure zone (8), and DeLancey's theory of a vaginal hammock providing active (muscular) and passive (connective tissue) support to the urethra (9). Ulmsten's theory is based on the concept that the urethral continence mechanism is controlled by the interplay of three anatomical structures and their associated function: the tension of the pubourethral ligaments, the muscular activity of the pubococcygeus and levator ani, and the condition of the suburethral vaginal hammock (10,11). These three structures are thought by Ulmsten to be connected to each other via the vagina and surrounding connective tissue "glue." Ulmsten considers these structures to be closely integrated in a complicated coordination to close, as well as open the bladder neck and urethra. Although defects in any one of these structures or in their interplay may result in urinary incontinence and/or voiding dysfunction, it is the tension in the pubourethral ligaments that is most essential for the correct interplay between the muscular component and the vaginal hammock (Fig. 1). If tension within the pubourethral ligaments is inadequate, forward contraction of the pubococcygeus muscle and backward-downward contraction of the remaining levator muscles will be ineffective in "kinking" the urethra during stress. Ulmsten refers to this kink in the urethra as the urethral "knee," demonstrated on lateral urethrocystography and located just distal to the maximum urethral closing pressure zone, which corresponds to the location of the insertion of pubourethral ligaments (Fig. 2).

Based on his integral theory, Ulmsten introduced the first TVT procedure as a simple ambulatory surgical procedure referred to as the intravaginal slingplasty (IVS) (7). This initial TVT procedure varied slightly from the current technique. The IVS procedure involved a single 2-cm vertical suprapubic incision and a concomitant "double-breast" vaginal plasty in cases where there was excessive vaginal tissue noted. In addition, the sling material itself was not made of the current unique TVT prolene, but rather a variety of materials including Mersilene, Gortex, Teflon, and Lyodura. In 1996, Ulmsten reported on an improved surgical technique and instrumentation for the IVS procedure, establishing the TVT procedure as it is known today (12). This modification also included the sling material being solely of a prolene mesh, 40-cm-long and 10-mm-wide covered by a plastic sheath swedged on two stainless steel needles. A recent study examining the initial stiffness and peak breaking load of commonly used sling materials demonstrated that the TVT prolene has by far the lowest initial stiffness (Fig. 3). The TVT elastic limit is only reached at an elongation of almost 50% of its initial length although at relatively low forces. Its fracture point is reached at very high elongation and on exertion of a relatively high force. It may be that the unique biomechanical properties of the TVT prolene have contributed to the fact that the material seems unusually biocompatible in its current use as a suburethral sling (13). Additional instrumentation consists of a reusable stainless steel introducer handle along with a reusable rigid Mandarin (catheter guide) (Fig. 4).

III. SURGICAL TECHNIQUE

The TVT procedure is most often performed under local anesthesia with intravenous sedation. This approach allows the patient to participate in the "cough test," an important step for correctly

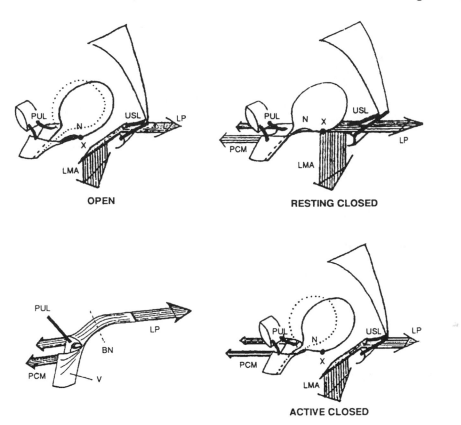

Figure 1   Opening and closure of inner urethra and bladder neck is mainly controlled by three anatomical structures; the tension of the pubourethral ligaments (PUL), the activity of the pubococcygeus muscles (PCM) and levator muscles (LP = levator plate; LMA = longitudinal muscle of the anus), and the condition of the suburethral vaginal hammock, i.e., the vaginal wall on which urethra and bladder neck are lying. All structures are connected to each other via the vagina and connective tissue "glue." The tension in the pubourethral ligaments is essential for correct interplay between the muscles and the vaginal hammock. Opening of the urethra and bladder neck occurs when PCM stop their forward contraction, when PUL has an adequate tension securing bladder neck in correct anatomical position and when there is backward-downward contraction of the levator muscles. Hereby the suburethral vaginal hammock is loosened allowing the inner urethra and bladder neck to funnel. Forward contraction of PCM and backward contraction via levator muscles actively closes (kinks) the inner urethra and bladder neck provided there is adequate tension in PUL. In the lower panel the forces acting on the inner part of the urethra and bladder neck (BN) are simplified. The importance of the interplay among PUL, PCM, vaginal hammock, and levator plate on closing and opening of inner urethra and bladder neck is obvious. USL, uterosacral ligaments; N, free nerve terminals or stretch receptors in the bladder base and inner part of urethra; X, the site where vagina is fixed to the bladder base. (From Ref. 7.)

placing the Prolene tape. For patients undergoing concomitant pelvic reconstructive or obliterative vaginal surgery, regional anesthesia may be required. For this clinical scenario at least one study has suggested that epidural regional anesthesia is preferable to a spinal block (14). If general anesthesia is indeed necessary, reproducing the cough test by simulating the abdominal forces of a cough via a brisk and vigorous credé maneuver is recommended. The credé maneuver, however, is not analogous to a cough in the awake patient. Therefore, caution should be exercised when using this maneuver to adjust the TVT under general anesthesia, as it has been suggested in at least one study to be associated with a potential for increased postoperative voiding dysfunction and/or retention as well as de novo detrusor instability (15).

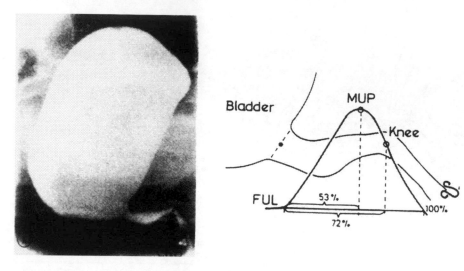

Figure 2 Urethral pressure profile measurement and lateral urethrocystography in a continent female. As seen the "urethral knee" indicating the main position/fixation of the pubourethral ligament is located just distal to the high pressure zone of the urethra. It is important that the sling is positioned at the urethral knee. FUL, functional urethral length; MUP, maximum urethral pressure. (From Ref. 7.)

    The procedure is performed with the patient in the dorsal lithotomy position with the lower extremities supported in adjustable Allen-type stirrups. The degree of Trendelenburg is important, as this will affect the angle or tilt of the pubic symphysis, which can affect the technical aspects of navigating the TVT needles safely through the retropubic space with constant and direct contact with the posterior aspect of the pubic symphysis. An 18 Fr Foley catheter is inserted into the urethra, and the bladder is emptied. A local anesthetic is applied suprapubically at two points, 1–2 cm above the pubic symphysis and 2–3 cm lateral to midline.

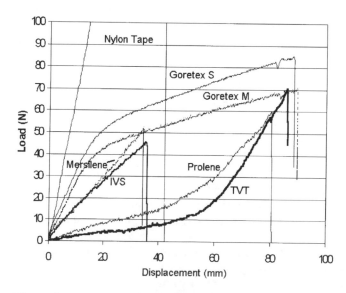

Figure 3 Typical load-deformation curves for the seven tested permanent materials. (From Ref. 13.)

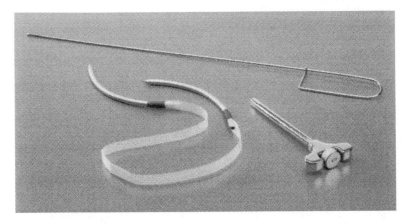

Figure 4 Tension-free vaginal tape system (Gynecare, Somerville, NJ) consists of (clockwise from top) rigid catheter guide, stainless-steel needle introducer, and TVT device with polypropylene mesh attached to stainless-steel needles. (From Ref. 61.)

The abdominal skin, underlying rectus muscle and fascia, and the posterior aspect of the pubic bone are infiltrated bilaterally. Two small abdominal skin incisions (0.5–1.0 cm) are then made at these points. No further abdominal dissection is necessary. A Sims speculum is then inserted into the vagina to allow visualization of the anterior vaginal wall. The external urethral meatus is easily visualized, and the indwelling Foley bulb is utilized to identify the location of the internal urethral egress. Using these two anatomical landmarks, the region of the midurethra is easily identified. The same local anesthetic solution is then injected into the vaginal submucosa at the level of the midurethra along the midline and slightly lateral to each side of the urethra. Allis clamps are then placed on the vaginal wall at the level of midurethra bilaterally for counter-traction as a small sagittal incision (1.5 cm) is made in the midline. The incision should begin ∼0.5–1 cm proximal to the external urethral meatus.

Following the midline scalpel incision, Allis clamps are replaced on the cut edges of the vaginal wall, and Metzenbaum scissors are utilized to minimally dissect the vaginal wall bilaterally, freeing it from the underlying periurethral tissue and developing a small tunnel bilaterally. This dissection should be limited to a depth of only 1–1.5 cm. The surgeon should take great care to avoid puncturing through the pubocervical fascia or injuring the urethra. After the vaginal incision and periurethral dissection are completed, additional local anesthetic solution should be administered bilaterally. Using a long spinal needle and an examination finger within the vaginal canal for guidance, the needle is placed through the vaginal incision periurethrally until the bevel of the needle reaches the inferior and posterior aspect of the pubic symphysis. Approximately 15–20 cc additional local anesthetic solution is placed at this location bilaterally.

The bladder is then drained via the Foley catheter, and a rigid catheter guide (Mandarin) is inserted into the catheter. The handle of the rigid catheter guide is then deviated to the ipsilateral side of the anticipated passage of the forthcoming TVT device. Gentle pressure inward or cephalad will further encourage retraction of the ventral aspect of the bladder dome away from the posterior aspect of the pubic symphysis. (Figs. 5,6) With the aid of introducer handle, the surgeon places the tip of the needle into the previously developed periurethral tunnel, utilizing both hands to correctly and safely pass the needle. The needle is directed only slightly lateral, most often in direct alignment with the patient's ipsilateral axilla. An additional reference point is the previously made ipsilateral suprapubic incision. The TVT needle is steadily and gradually

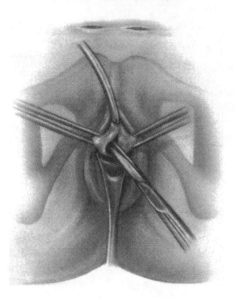

Figure 5 Paraurethral dissection is performed after an initial midline incision on the anterior vaginal mucosa at the level of the midurethra. Note the small suprapubic abdominal stab incisions bilaterally. (From Ref. 61.)

advanced by applying gentle pressure with the palm of the vaginal hand and continued with vaginal finger guidance and slight pressure from the second hand placed on the introducer handle. As the needle tip passes through the pubocervical fascia, a distinct drop in resistance can be appreciated.

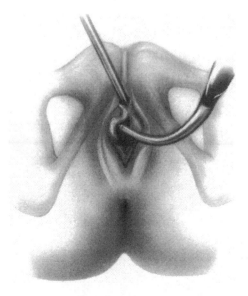

Figure 6 After bilateral dissection of the paraurethral space, the rigid catheter guide is inserted into the urinary catheter. The handle of the guide is deflected to the ipsilateral side and the needle is inserted into the paraurethral space. (From Ref. 61.)

At this point, with downward deflection of the introducer handle the surgeon guides the needle superiorly through the space of Retzius with the needle being immediately opposed to the backside of the pubic symphysis. (Figs. 7,8) As the needle opposes the underside of the rectus muscle and fascial sheath, significant resistance is again appreciated. The introducer handle is then utilized to apply pressure directly anterior, advancing the needle up through the previously made abdominal incision. The surgeon's nondominant hand is placed suprapubically to further guide the needle tip up through the abdominal incision (Fig. 9).

The rigid catheter guide and Foley catheter are removed, and diagnostic urethrocystoscopy is performed to evaluate for any unintentional injury of the urethra or bladder. Once correct needle placement is confirmed, the needle is passed completely up through the abdominal incision. The steps of the procedure are then repeated on the opposite side. Care should be taken to ensure the tape is not twisted under the urethra (Fig. 10).

After correct placement of the TVT device and before removal of the protective sheath, a cough test is performed to identify the correct positioning of the tape. The cough test is conducted with a full bladder (250–300 mL saline) (Fig. 11). Once the proper positioning of the tape is obtained, the plastic sheath is removed and the prolene mesh is left in place without tension under the midurethra. The abdominal ends of the tape are cut just below the skin's surface. The procedure is completed with closure of the abdominal and vaginal incisions (Fig. 12).

IV. MECHANISM OF ACTION

Since its inception the TVT procedure has generated much debate as to its mechanism of action. With that in mind, researchers have examined a wide range of outcomes from its effect on voiding and urodynamic parameters to radiologic and connective tissue changes.

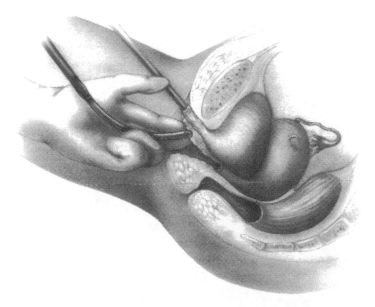

Figure 7   The tip of the needle is angulated laterally and the endopelvic fascia is perforated just behind the inferior surface of the pubic symphysis. (From Ref. 61.)

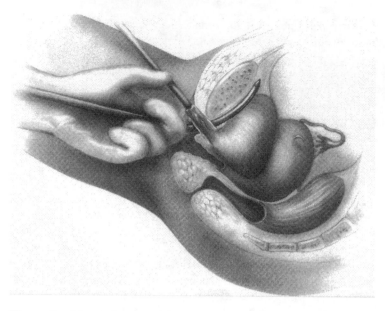

Figure 8   After perforation of the endopelvic fascia, the tip of the needle is guided through the retropubic space along the backside of the pubic symphysis. (From Ref. 61.)

Historically, GSI patients have been examined for urethral hypermobility as a contributing factor to their symptoms, and anti-incontinence procedures have long been directed toward the resolution of hypermobility as a way to restore the urethra back to its abdominal position, thereby improving the pressure transmission ratio. Recent studies have demonstrated that despite

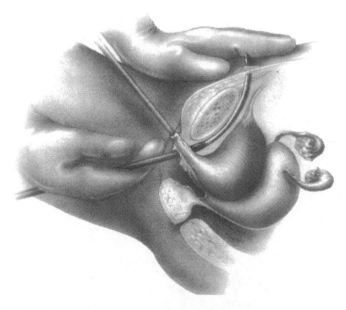

Figure 9   After perforation of the rectus fascia, a hand is used to palpate the needle tip suprapubically and guide the needle to the abdominal incision. (From Ref. 61.)

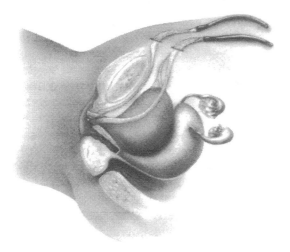

Figure 10   After the technique is repeated on the other side, the TVT sling is in place with the tape lying flat against the posterior surface of the midurethra. (From Ref. 61.)

postoperative persistence of urethral hypermobility, cure rates for the TVT procedure have been maintained and equal to the Burch colposuspension (16–18).

In one recent study, further evaluation of urodynamic indices revealed a decrease in resting maximum urethral closing pressure along with an increase in dynamic maximum urethral closing pressure and in resting and dynamic functional urethral length, although statistical significance was not reached (19). Another study, however, demonstrated no change in

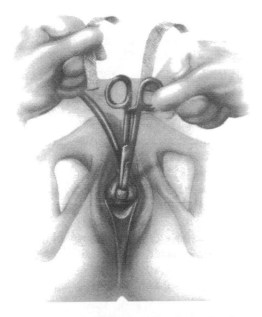

Figure 11   The needles are detached and an instrument is placed between the tape and the urethra. Gentle traction on each end brings the tape in contact with the urethra and correct tension is adjusted with an intraoperative cough stress test. (From Ref. 61.)

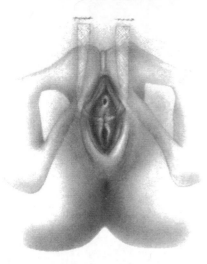

Figure 12 The incisions are closed. The completed procedure allows fixation of the tape below the midurethra with the ends just below the skin level. (From Ref. 61.)

maximum urethral closing pressure while revealing an increase in the pressure transmission ratio, which has been demonstrated with other anti-incontinence procedures, such as the Burch colposuspension and needle suspension procedure (18).

Other researchers have questioned whether the TVT's success is contingent upon an outflow obstruction at the urethral "knee." A few early reports have suggested this as a possible mechanism based on an increased urethral resistance and elevated postvoid residual volumes along with decreased maximum flow rates as seen on pressure flow studies during follow-up at less than 1 year (20,21).

In an attempt to explain the TVT mechanism on an anatomic basis, both radiologic and histologic studies have been initiated. Initial studies utilizing ultrasound and magnetic resonance imaging revealed that the tape remained in either the middle or distal urethra and demonstrated convexity toward the urethra. The tape maintained its position at the abdominal wall in all patients evaluated (22). Biochemical analyses from paraurethral connective tissue biopsies up to 2 years postoperatively demonstrated no change in the amount of collagen present, although registering increased collagen metabolism (23).

V. PROCEDURAL OUTCOMES

A. Clinical Results

With the initial introduction of the intravaginal slingplasty (IVS), 50 patients were surgically treated for pure genuine stress incontinence (GSI) or mixed incontinence with predominant stress incontinence symptoms. Seventy-eight percent of patients were cured of stress incontinence symptoms while 12% demonstrated significant improvement (7). Expanding on this initial report, a case series using only a Prolene sling in patients with primary SUI demonstrated 84% cure with 8% improvement at 2 years follow-up (12). In 1999, Ulmsten and colleagues reported on the surgical outcome of TVT at 3 years including an 86% cure rate with 12% significantly improved (24). Other authors reported similar success rates (19,25–30). With time, additional clinical research continued to demonstrate the high success rates associated with the TVT procedure. Nilsson and colleagues reported a sustained objective cure rate of 84.7% along with 10.6% significantly improved after ~5 years. All patients in this multicenter trial demonstrated preoperative SUI. Complications were few in number: 3.3% retropubic hematoma, 1.1% bladder perforation, and 3.3% intraoperative bleeding of >200 mL. No surgical intervention was required. Transient voiding dysfunction (<4 days postoperatively) was present in 4.4%. Interestingly, of the patients with preoperative urgency symptoms, 56% were relieved of their symptoms. Six percent of patients reported de novo urge symptoms postoperatively, but no urodynamic proven detrusor instability was demonstrated (31).

B. Subpopulation Studies

In addition to the sustained high cure rates of the TVT in the patient with primary GSI, similar success rates have been reported in subgroups of GSI patients. Azam and colleagues reported on a cohort of patients with recurrent SUI without ISD after multiple procedures including needle suspension procedures, Burch and MMK colposuspensions, urethral bulking agents, anterior colporrhaphy, with Kelly plications and vaginal sling procedures. At the 1-year follow-up after TVT, a cure rate of 81% along with a success rate of 87% was demonstrated in a patient population of 67 women with a median of two prior surgical procedures (32). This was reproduced at a mean follow-up of 4 years with 82% cured and 9% significantly improved (33).

Early reports of the TVT procedure in patients with ISD as defined by a low urethral closure pressure (MUCP < 20 cmH$_2$O) demonstrated a high patient satisfaction rate of 85%, equal to that of patients with normal urethral closure pressure, despite a significantly lower objective cure rate of only 37% at a follow-up of only 1 year (34,35).

One study has specifically examined TVT outcomes in ISD patients refractory to periurethral collagen injection. No significant difference with regard to success or complication rates was demonstrated (36). A long-term study of patients with ISD demonstrated a sustained cure rate after TVT of 74% with an additional 12% significantly improved after 4 years (37). Furthermore, in patients experiencing mixed urinary incontinence, the TVT procedure resulted in a cure rate of 85% and 4% improvement for both stress and urge symptoms at a mean follow-up of 4 years (38).

There have been a few recent reports specifically examining the safety and efficacy of performing the TVT procedure in obese patients. These studies have shown no difference in success or complication rates when compared to normal-weight patients (39,40).

The low procedural morbidity and the opportunity to use local anesthesia would seem to make the TVT procedure well suited for the elderly patient population. We performed a retrospective review of 83 women age ≥ 70 years (advanced elderly), who underwent a TVT procedure for GSI, comparing the outcomes to 179 patients with age < 70 years (41). Several differences were noted between the groups. The advanced elderly patients presented with a higher rate of overactive bladder symptoms; a greater percentage (19%) had also undergone prior periurethral collagen injections, and they experienced an increase in combined prolapse surgery with the anticipated findings of increased operative time and increased estimated blood loss. The success rate, defined as subjective cure, was similar with a 95.2% for the advanced elderly patients and a 98.9% cure rate for the control group. Two smaller studies reporting on 45 women and 18 women, respectively, have also demonstrated the safety and efficacy of TVT when performed in the advanced elderly (42,43). It appears from these preliminary studies that age alone does not appear to decrease the success rate of the TVT procedure as a treatment for female GSI.

VI. POTENTIAL COMPLICATIONS

In general, the complications associated with a TVT procedure occur far less frequently than similar pubovaginal sling-type procedures. Table 1 demonstrates the reported incidence of such minor and major complications according to data gathered and reported by Gynecare in over 200,000 worldwide cases. The more minor complications include transient voiding dysfunction, urinary retention, retropubic bleeding and/or hematoma formation, perforation of the bladder, and localized infection. Complications more typically associated with the use of synthetic materials with sling procedures, such as complete graft erosion, rejection, sinus tract formation, or development of a fistula, have not been reported. There have been cases of localized erosion or vaginal extrusion, as well as obturator nerve irritation, retained plastic sheath, and vaginal wall laceration, however, these appear to be extremely rare occurrences.

Most concerning to surgeons performing the TVT procedure are the rare but nonetheless significant vascular injuries that have been reported during tape placement. These injuries have involved the obturator, external iliac, femoral, and inferior epigastric vessels. Additionally, significant hemorrhage has been reported from venous bleeding in the retropubic space, possibly from the inferior vesical veins or, alternatively, disruption of the venous supply along the posterior aspect of the pubic symphysis (44,45). To avoid vascular injury it is imperative that the operating surgeon maintain the curved TVT tunneler (trocar) in direct contact with the posterior aspect of the pubic bone medial to the pubic tubercle. Any inadvertent lateral or cephalad migration of the tunneler could potentially result in vascular injury. One recent study described the proximity of the major vessels in the retropubic space and anterior abdominal wall to the TVT needle (46). The study was performed on 10 fresh frozen cadavers, during which measurements from the lateral aspect of the needle to the medial aspects of the vessels were obtained and recorded. All vessels measured were lateral to the TVT needle. The vessels studied included a superficial epigastric, inferior epigastric, external iliac, and obturator (Table 2). Based on this study, the authors concluded that the TVT needle, if laterally directed or externally rotated during the course of insertion, could result in major vascular injury. Venous bleeding that is not readily controlled by direct pressure or vaginal packing can be managed with the placement of a 30-cc Foley balloon inflated to a 50-cc volume, upon which significant traction is placed, taping the Foley to the medial aspect of the thigh. This will effectively tamponade most venous bleeding in the retropubic space, which will encourage effective coagulation and clot formation (47). Hematomas usually present within the first 12 h of surgery. The presentation is that of significant pressurelike discomfort in the suprapubic or vaginal area. The diagnosis can be obtained by a careful bimanual exam and confirmed by ultrasound investigation. Most hematomas will resolve spontaneously without intervention; however, ultrasound-guided

Table 1 Gynecare TVT Tension-free Support for Incontinence: Statement Regarding Complications

Complication	U.S.	Non-U.S.	Total	%
Vascular injury	3	25	28	0.01
Vaginal mesh exposure	13	2	15	0.008
Urethral erosion	8	0	8	0.004
Bowel perforation	4	6	10	0.005

Source: Gynecare, Somerville, NJ.

Table 2   Vessel Distance from TVT Needle

Vessel	TVT needle Mean cm	(range)	Midpubic bone Mean cm	(range)
Superficial epigastric	3.9	(0.9–6.7)	7.2	(4.4–9.3)
Inferior epigastric	3.9	(1.9–6.6)	7.4	(4.8–10.0)
External iliac	4.9	(2.9–6.2)	8.3	(6.5–10.9)
Obturator	3.2	(1.6–4.3)	6.9	(5.2–8.4)

Source: Ref. 46.

drainage should be considered for larger hematomas (>8 cm), as the likelihood of potential infection is increased.

The most common procedure associated infection is that of an acute bacterial cystitis. One must remember this is a nosocomial infection when prescribing antibiotic therapy. True wound infections following a TVT procedure are rare. This may be a result of the protective nature of the plastic tape, which minimizes the likelihood of bacterial inoculation or contamination during placement, passage, and subsequent tape adjustment. Additionally, Prolene as a graft material has been associated with less risk of infection than other synthetic materials (48). The liberal use of preoperative topical estrogen, in either cream or suppository form, may help reduce the incidence of vaginal atrophy or mucosal irritation, which may contribute to wound infection. Treatment of wound infection includes broad-spectrum antibiotics and pelvic rest. Surgical debridement or intervention is most often not required.

Bladder perforation during the TVT procedure has been reported in most all clinical studies. It is the most frequently reported complication occurring on average ~6% of the time. It is more commonly seen in patients who have undergone a previous retropubic suspension. The perforation rate tends to vary, depending on surgeon experience and patient population from as low as 0% to as high as 23.1%. The surgeon should avoid the tendency to place the TVT needle more laterally after encountering a bladder perforation. Ideally, one should assess the location of the inadvertent puncture and readjust placement accordingly. In general, perforations occur at the 10 and 2 o'clock positions, safely away from the trigone and ureteral orifices. If such perforation occurs, the TVT tunneler is withdrawn and redirected with closer adherence to the posterior aspect of the pubic symphysis in conjunction with perhaps improved deviation of the bladder with gentle inward pressure (cephalad) of the indwelling rigid catheter, helping to elongate the bladder to a more elliptical shape rather than a bulbous contour, thus increasing the distance between the bladder and the posterior aspect of the pubic symphysis. For more midline perforations, some lateral correction may be warranted—however, never beyond the pubic tubercle. These patients should have continuous bladder drainage via an indwelling Foley catheter for 24–48 h.

A variable incidence of voiding dysfunction including urinary retention has been reported after the TVT procedure. Contributing factors include preoperative detrusor hypocontractility, patient age, anesthesia type, and failure to adhere to the standardized technique of tape adjustment including utilization of an intraoperative cough test. For patients who are unable to initiate a void postoperatively, conservative management can be employed with an indwelling catheter for 24–48 h. The possibility of a hematoma should also be entertained and an appropriate evaluation performed. If the patient continues to be unable to void beyond 72 h, surgical intervention can be employed via a simple opening of the vaginal incision under local anesthesia with bilateral downward pulling of the mesh lateral to the urethra on both sides for a limited distance (5–6 mm). After 10 days, this "loosening" of the mesh is often not possible. These patients should be instructed on intermittent self-catheterization and scheduled for a potential surgical release in 4–6 weeks. This time frame will allow the tissue to heal and the mesh to become fixed laterally at the level of the pubocervical fascia. Persistent retention or refractory voiding dysfunction is relatively uncommon—however, one that can be successfully managed with a fairly simple surgical midline release of the Prolene tape. Rardin and colleagues recently described a collective series of 848 women over a 2-year period who underwent a TVT procedure. Among these patients, 19 (2.2%) had severe voiding dysfunction, described as either urinary retention, significant incomplete bladder emptying, or severe urgency or urge-related incontinence, refractory to conservative management. These patients underwent a vaginal TVT surgical release: 15 by midline tape transection, and four by midline tape excision of a 2- to 11-mm segment. All patients had at least partial resolution of voiding dysfunction immediately following the takedown procedure. Ten of the 19 women had complete resolution of symptoms. Twelve of the 19 patients (63%) remained completely continent after the release, three (60%) had only mild incontinence described as still being significantly improved or baseline, and only four patients (21%) had recurrence of their stress urinary incontinence (49).

VII. TVT WITH CONCOMITANT SURGERY

It has been well recognized that proper identification and correction of pelvic support defects in addition to performing surgery for incontinence improves patient outcomes (50–52). The incidence of pelvic organ prolapse requiring concomitant reconstructive pelvic surgery at the time of surgery for SUI has been reported to be as high as 42% (53). Several reports on the clinical outcomes of patients undergoing the TVT procedure have included patients receiving concomitant surgery for pelvic organ prolapse (30,54). Only a few studies have specifically examined the safety and efficacy of the TVT in combination with reconstructive pelvic surgery.

Jomaa was the first to report on combining the TVT procedure with an anterior and/or posterior colporrhaphy in 32 patients under local anesthesia. Ninety-three patients were cured with a mean hospital stay of 2 days (55). We performed a retrospective review comparing 47 patients who underwent TVT with concomitant vaginal surgery (TVT +) to 133 patients who underwent TVT alone (TVT) (56). Concomitant vaginal surgery consisted of one or more of the following procedures: sacrospinous ligament fixation (one), vaginal hysterectomy (one), enterocele repair (4), anterior colporrhaphy (eight), posterior colporrhaphy (13), LeFort colpocleisis (14), or perineorrhaphy (15). The mean operative time and estimated blood loss was appropriately increased as anticipated in the TVT + group. The hospital stay was also marginally increased; however, most often remained <24 h. The only operative complication was that of bladder perforation, which was similar in the two groups, occurring in 6.4% of the TVT + patients and 6.8% of the TVT patients; no patients developed any wound infection or tape rejection. Twenty-four-hour spontaneous micturition rates were also similar in the two groups. One hundred thirty-one patients (98.5%) of the TVT group reported a subjective cure versus 47 (100%) of the TVT + group. Lastly, 41% of the TVT + had local anesthesia with sedation, 58% had regional anesthesia, and only 2% (one patient) received general anesthesia, whereas 96% of the TVT group had local anesthesia, 4% had regional, and 0.8% (one patient) underwent general. In conclusion, we have found that the TVT pubovaginal sling can be safely and effectively performed with concomitant vaginal surgery without significant increase in morbidity.

VIII. COMPARATIVE STUDIES

Although there are several ongoing studies comparing the clinical outcome of the TVT procedure to that of the Burch colposuspension, only a few have reported on preliminary findings or conclusions. One of the earlier studies involves comparing the open Burch colposuspension to the TVT. In this study the Burch procedure was found to have a significantly greater blood loss and increased hospital stay, yet a similar success rate at 6 months (57). Vassallo and colleagues reported on a retrospective analysis among women who underwent either a TVT or laparoscopic Burch procedure for treatment of SUI. Seventy-four women were identified and followed for at least 1 year. The overall objective cure rates were comparable with 88% for the laparoscopic Burch and 92% for the TVT procedure. There were no significant differences in time to resumption of normal voiding or related irritative bladder symptoms such as urgency, frequency, and/or urge incontinence. There was a trend toward increasing intraoperative complications among the TVT group; however, this did not reach statistical significance. The TVT patients were noted to have a shorter operative time as well as a shorter hospital stay (58). In terms of cure and improvement rates, Fotte reported the opposite finding, with a higher rate among patients undergoing laparoscopic colposuspension (59). The laparoscopic colposuspension group had a cure or improved rate of 94%, versus 82% for the TVT group. The laparoscopic group did require a significantly longer operative time, but had less intraoperative and post-operative complications. Voiding difficulty was significantly less in the laparoscopic group, 0% versus 18%.

A. TVT-OBTURATOR

The worldwide adaptation of retropubic TVT has been associated with a number of intraoperative complications including bladder perforations, urethral injuries, retropubic hematoma formation, and rarely, complications with significant consequences such as injury to bowel, major blood vessels and nerves. Consistent with the spirit of improving procedural safety, recent modifications in the method of placement of the tension free mid urethral sling have taken place. To avoid blind passage of introducers into the retropubic space, a unique approach using the obturator foramina has been developed.

The transobturator approach was first described by Dr. Emmanuel DeLorme in France in September of 2001 (62). DeLorme used an Emmet needle the path of which carried it through a skin incision in the thigh fold, through the inferior-medial aspect of the obturator foramen, the anterior recess of the ishiorectal fossa under the levator muscles, and through the pubocervical fibromuscular tissue to exit a suburethral incision. The tape was then withdrawn through the same path. The same procedure was performed on the opposite side to form the midurethral sling. Initial data have demonstrated similar cure rates when compared to traditional retropublic placement with a lower incidence of bladder injury (63). As the obturator approach was adopted by others however, lower urinary tract injuries were experienced. Vaginal tears and groin hematomas have also since been reported (64–66).

In an attempt to further improve upon the intraoperative safety profile of a obturator approach, Dr. Jean de Leval more recently described a transobtuator technique of tape placement with a helical passer that begins at the vaginal incision, follows the same path and exists the skin 2 cm lateral to the thigh fold thus earning it the "inside-out" designation. Initial reports are encouraging suggesting a similar efficacy with no reported adverse events thus far reported (67). Long term data demonstrating sustained efficacy of the TVT-Obturator approach are eagerly awaited.

IX. CONCLUSION

The TVT procedure has been proven to be an effective minimally invasive approach to the surgical management of female stress urinary incontinence. The TVT-obturator system will most likely result in additional patient safety. With TVT's widespread use, both clinical success and patient safety will only be achieved through continued close adherence to the technical aspects of the procedure as originally described. It has been referred to as perhaps the most exciting and most innovative procedure for stress incontinence in the last 40 years (60).

REFERENCES

1. Kelly H, Dunn Wm. Urinary incontinence in women without manifest injury to the bladder: a report of cases. Surg Gynecol Obstet 1914; 18:444.
2. Black NA, Down SH. The effectiveness of surgery for stress incontinence in women: a systematic review. Br J Urol 1996; 78:497.
3. Leach GE, Dmochowski RR, Appell RA. Female stress urinary incontinence clinical guidelines panel summary report on surgical management of female stress urinary incontinence. American urological association. J Urol 1997; 158:875.
4. Ostergard DR. Primary slings for everyone with genuine stress incontinence? The argument against. Int Urogynecol J 1997; 8:321.
5. Chan PT, Fournier C, Corcos J. Short-term complications of pubovaginal sling procedure for genuine stress incontinence in women. Urology 2000; 55:207.
6. Chaikin DC, Rosenthal J, Blavis JG. Pubovaginal fascial sling for all types of stress urinary incontinence: long-term analysis. J Urol 1998; 160:1312.
7. Ulmsten U, Petros P. Intravaginal slingplasty (IVS): an ambulatory surgical procedure for treatment of female urinary incontinence. Scand J Urol Nephrol 1995; 29:75–82.
8. Enhorning G. Simultaneous recording of the intravesical and intraurethral pressure. Acta Obstet Gynecol Scand 1961; 276(suppl):1–89.
9. DeLancey JOL. Structural support of the urethra as it relates to stress urinary incontinence: the hammock hypothesis. Am J Obstet Gynecol 1994; 170:1713–1723.
10. Petros P, Ulmsten U. An integral theory of female urinary incontinence: experimental and clinical considerations. Acta Obstet Gynecol Scand. 1990; 69(suppl 153).
11. Petros P, Ulmsten U. An integral theory and its method for the diagnosis and management of female incontinence. Scand J Urol Nephrol 1993; (suppl 153).
12. Ulmsten U, Henrixsson L, Johnson P, Morrows V, Arhos G. An ambulatory surgical procedure under local anesthesia for treatment of female urinary incontinence. Int Urogynecol J 1996; 7:81–86.
13. Dietz HP, Vancaillie P, Suehla M. Mechanical properties of implant materials used in incontinence surgery. 31st Annual Meeting of the International Continence Society, Seoul, South Korea, Sept 18–21, 2001.
14. Wang AC, Chen M. Randomized comparison of local versus epidural anesthesia for tension free vaginal tape operation. J Urol 2001; 165:1177–1180.
15. Hammer R, Magtibay P. Efficacy of tension free vaginal tape under general anesthesia. 22nd Annual Scientific Meeting of the American Urogynecologic Society, Chicago, Oct 25–27, 2001.
16. Klutke JJ, Carlin Bl, Klutke CG. The tension-free vaginal tape procedure: correction of stress incontinence with minimal alteration in proximal urethral mobility. Urology 2000; 55:512–514.
17. Atherton MJ, Stanton SL. A comparison of bladder neck movement and elevation after tension-free vaginal tape and colposuspension. Br J Obstet Gynecol 2000; 107:1366–1370.
18. Mutone M, Mastropietro M, Brizendine E, Hale D. Effect of tension-free vaginal tape procedure on urodynamic continence indices. Obstet Gynecol 2001; 98(4):638–645.
19. Wang AC. An assessment of early surgical outcome and urodynamic effects of TVT. Int Urogynecol J 2000; 11:282–284.
20. Bower WF, Morris A, O'Sullivan R, Moore KH. Voiding parameters after simple TVT. 31st Annual Meeting of the International Continence Society, Seoul, South Korea, Sept 18–21, 2001.

21. Hardart A, Klutke JJ, Klutke CG, Carlin B. Altered voiding after the tension-free vaginal tape procedure: is increased resistance the mechanism of therapy? Obstet Gynecol 2000; 94(4, Part 2):55S.

22. Tunn R, Schuettoff S, Beyersdorff D. Visualization of the prolene tape and its topography (following TVT plasty) by introital ultrasound and MR imaging. 31st Annual Meeting of the International Continence Society, Seoul, South Korea, Sept 18–21, 2001.

23. Falconer C, Ekman-Ordeberg G, Malmstrom A, Ulmsten U. Clinical outcome and changes in connective tissue metabolism after intravaginal slingplasty in stress incontinent women. Int Urogynecol J 1996; 7:133–137.

24. Ulmsten U, Johnson P, Rezapour M. A three year follow-up of tension free vaginal tape for surgical treatment of female stress urinary incontinence. Br J Obstet Gynaecol 1999; 106:345–350.

25. Ulmsten U, Falconer C, Johnson P. Multicenter study of TVT for surgical treatment of SUI. Int Urogynecol J 1998; 9:210–213.

26. Olsson I, Kroon UB. A 3 year post op evaluation of TVT. Gynecol Obstet Invest 1999; 48:267–269.

27. Nilsson CG, Kuuva N. The TVT procedure is successful in the majority of women with indications for surgical treatment of urinary stress incontinence. Br J Obstet Gynaecol 2001; 108:414–419.

28. Soulie M, Cuvillier X, Benaissa A. The TVT procedure in the treatment of female urinary stress incontinence: a French prospective multicentre study. Eur Urol 2001; 39:709–715.

29. Haab F, Sananes S, Amarenco G. Results of the TVT procedure for the treatment of type II SUI at a minimum follow-up of 1 yr. J Urol 2001; 165(1):159–162.

30. Meschia M, Pifarotti P, Bernasconi F, Guercio E. TVT: analysis of outcomes of complications in 404 stress incontinent women. Int Urogynecol J 2001; 12(suppl 2):S24–S27.

31. Nilsson CG, Kuuva N, Falconer C. Long-term results of the tension-free vaginal tape (TVT) procedure for surgical treatment of female stress urinary incontinence. Int Urogynecol J 2001; 12(suppl 2):S5–S8.

32. Azam U, Frazer MI, Kozman EL. The tension-free vaginal tape procedure in women with previous failed stress incontinence surgery. J Urol 2001; 166(2):554–556.

33. Rezapour M, Ulmsten U. Tension-free vaginal tape (TVT) in women with recurrent stress urinary incontinence—a long-term follow-up. Int Urogynecol J 2001; 12(suppl 2):S9–S11.

34. Kulseng-Hanssen S. Success of TVT operation in patients with low urethral pressure. 31st Annual Meeting of the International Continence Society, Seoul, South Korea, Sept 18–21, 2001.

35. Ohkawa A, Kondo A, Baba S. TVT operation is it effective for those patients suffered from type III incontinence? 31st Annual Meeting of the International Continence Society, Seoul, South Korea, Sept 18–21, 2001.

36. Murphy M, Horton TR, Druckenmiller J, Lucente V. Tension free vaginal tape for the treatment of ISD refractory to periurethral collagen injection. 22nd Annual Scientific Meeting of the American Urogynecologic Society, Chicago, Oct 25–27, 2001.

37. Rezapour M, Falconer C, Ulmsten U. Tension-free vaginal tape (TVT) in stress incontinent women with intrinsic sphincter deficiency (ISD)—a long-term follow-up. Int Urogynecol J 2001; 12(suppl 2):S12–S14.

38. Rezapour M, Ulmsten U. Tension-free vaginal tape (TVT) in women with mixed urinary incontinence—a long-term follow-up. Int Urogynecol J 2001; 12(suppl 2):S15–S18.

39. Chung MK, Bradley AF, Chung RP. TVT for treatment of urinary incontinence in obese women. 21st Annual Scientific Meeting of the American Urogynecologic Society, Hilton Head, SC, Oct 25–28, 2000.

40. Rufford I J, Toozs-Hobson P, Cardozo LD. Where surgeons dare; the effect of body weight on TVT success rates. 31st Annual Meeting of the International Continence Society, Seoul, South Korea, Sept 18–21, 2001.

41. Horton TR, Druckenmiller J, Lucente V. Pubovaginal sling use and tension-free vaginal tape in advanced elderly women. 22nd Annual Scientific Meeting of the American Urogynecologic Society, Chicago, Oct 25–27, 2001.

42. Nilsson C. The effect of age and time on the outcome of TVT surgery. 31st Annual Meeting of the International Continence Society, Seoul, South Korea, Sept 18–21, 2001.

43. Fischer M. Tension-free vaginal tape (TVT) in the elderly. 31st Annual Meeting of the International Continence Society, Seoul, South Korea, Sept 18–21, 2001.

44. Walters MD, Tulikangas PK, Lasala C, Muir T. Vascular injury during tension-free vaginal tape procedure for stress urinary incontinence. Obstet Gynecol 2001; 98(5)Part 2:957–959.

45. Tim K, Kim H, Lee S. Vascular injury following tension-free vaginal tape (TVT and stress incontinence). 31st Annual Meeting of the International Continence Society, Seoul, South Korea, Sept 18–21, 2001.

46. Muir T, Tulikangas PK, Paraiso MF, Walters MD. The relationship of tension-free vaginal tape insertion to the vascular anatomy of the retropubic space and the anterior abdominal wall. 22nd Annual Scientific Meeting of the American Urogynecologic Society, Chicago, Oct 25–27, 2001.

47. Katske FA, Raz S. Use of a Foley catheter to obtain transvaginal tamponade. Urol 1983; 21:627.

48. Iglesia CB, Fenner DE, Brubaker L. The use of mesh in gynecological surgery. Int Urogynecol J Pelvic Floor Dysfunct 1997; 8:105–115.

49. Rardin C, Lucente V, Miklos J. Takedown of tension-free vaginal tape for the treatment of refractory postoperative voiding dysfunction. 22nd Annual Scientific Meeting of the American Urogynecologic Society, Chicago, Oct 25–27, 2001.

50. Drutz HP, Alnaif B. Surgical management of pelvic organ prolapse and stress urinary incontinence. Clin Obstet Gynecol 1998; 41:786–793.

51. Bruce RG, El-galley RE, Galloway NT. Paravaginal defect repair in the treatment of female urinary incontinence and cystocele. Urology 1999; 54:647–651.

52. Serels SR, Rackley RR, Appell RA. In situ slings with concurrent cystocele repair. Tech Urol 1999; 5:129–132.

53. Ng CS, Rackley RR, Appell RA. Incidence of concomitant procedures for pelvic organ prolapse and reconstruction in women who undergo surgery for stress urinary incontinence. Urology 2001; 57(5):911–914.

54. Tamussino K, Hanzal E, Kolle D. The Austrian tension-free vaginal tape registry. Int Urogynecol J 2001; 12(suppl 2):S28–S29.

55. Jomaa M. Combined tension-free vaginal tape and prolapse repair under local anesthesia in patients with symptoms of both urinary incontinence and prolapse. Gynecol Obstet Invest 2001; 51:184–186.

56. Horton TR, Druckenmiller J, Lucente V. Concomitant vaginal surgery with tension-free vaginal tape pubovaginal sling for treatment of female stress urinary incontinence and pelvic support defects. 27th Scientific Meeting of the Society of Gynecologic Surgeons, Lake Buena Vista, FL, March 5–7, 2001.

57. Ward KL, Hilton P, Browning J. A randomised trial of colposuspension and tension-free vaginal tape (TVT) for primary genuine stress incontinence. 30th Annual Meeting of the International Continence Society, Tampere, Finland, Aug 28–31, 2000.

58. Vassallo B, Murphy M, Lucente V, Karram M. TVT versus laparoscopic burch: a retrospective review at 1–4 years. 27th Scientific Meeting of the Society of Gynecologic Surgeons, Lake Buena Vista, FL, March 5–7, 2001.

59. Fotte A. Which is the best minimally invasive procedure? TVT versus laparoscopic colposuspension. 31st Annual Meeting of the International Continence Society, Seoul, South Korea, Sept 18–21, 2001.

60. Stanton SL. Some reflections on tension-free vaginal tape—a new surgical procedure for treatment of female urinary incontinence. Int Urogynecol J 2001; 12 (suppl 2):S1–S2.

61. Kohli N, Miklos JR, Lucente V. Tension-free Vaginal Tape: a minimally invasive technique for treating female SUI. Contemp Ob/Gyn May 1999.

62. De Lorme E. *Prog. Urol.* 2001; 11:1306–1313 La bandelette trans-obturatrice: un procede mini-invasif pour traiter l'incontinence urinair d'effort de la femme.

63. Droupy et al. Abstract #779 EUA March 2003 Trans-obturator urethral support for female stress urinary incontinence: 1 year outcome of a new surgical procedure.

64. Dargent D, Bretones S, George P, Mellier G. *Gynécol Obstét Fertil* 2002; 30:576–82 Insertion of a suburethral sling through the obturator membrane in the treatment of female urinary incontinence.

65. Costa et al. Abstract #334 ICS October 2003 Trans-obturator tape (TOT) for female stress urinary incontinence: Preliminary results of a prospective multicenter register.

66. Hermieu JF, et al. *Progres en Urologie* 2003; 13:115–117 Plaie vesicale apres bandelette trans-obturatrice.

67. Leval J de, European Urology. 2003; 44:724–730 Novel surgical technique for the treatment of female stress urinary incontinence: Transobturator vaginal Tape inside-out.

28
Distal Urethral Polypropylene Sling

Larissa V. Rodríguez
University of California Los Angeles, Los Angeles, California, U.S.A.

I. INTRODUCTION

The etiology of stress urinary incontinence is not completely understood. In the past, bladder neck suspensions were performed in order to correct anatomic abnormalities, and bladder neck and urethral hypermobility. These procedures were attractive because of their simplicity, low morbidity, and excellent early success. With time, the successes seen with these procedures have not proven to be durable, and alternative surgical procedures have been developed.

Sling procedures for the treatment of female stress urinary incontinence have been used for almost 100 years. The first sling, described in 1907 by Von Giordano, used gracilis muscle wrapped around the urethra (1). The procedure was reintroduced in 1978 by McGuire and Lytton, who suspended a piece of rectus fascia under the bladder neck for the treatment of intrinsic sphincter deficiency (2). Because of the initial relatively high incidence of complications associated with pubovaginal slings, such as sling erosion and urinary retention, these procedures did not achieve popularity until the last decade. Since then, multiple variations in surgical technique have been reported using new sling materials and anchoring techniques to increase both durability and ease of placement, and decrease surgical morbidity.

Until recently, the indications for bladder neck suspensions were type I and II stress incontinence, and slings were reserved for only type III incontinence. With the poor long-term durability of needle suspension procedures, interest has been renewed in sling procedures (3–6). A meta-analysis of various surgical techniques for the treatment of stress incontinence showed pubovaginal slings to have superior durability to needle suspension procedures, and similar durability to retropubic suspension (4). Slings have been shown to be as effective as and more durable than bladder neck suspensions for the treatment of all types of stress incontinence, and their popularity has therefore spread. Many new procedures and materials have emerged. Recent studies have focused on new materials, innovative ways to anchor the sling, changes in location of the sling, and broadening the application of slings for multiple types of incontinence. This plethora of procedures has led to an increased need for well-controlled, objective outcome studies in order to understand the impact of these surgeries on our patients.

The success of new techniques for the treatment of stress urinary incontinence has broadened our understanding of the pathophysiology of the disease and has led to new theories to explain the anatomic and physiologic processes that lead to incontinence in the female.

For example, the success of distal urethral slings suggests that, contrary to previous thinking, the correction of anatomic hypermobility is not necessary to correct stress incontinence (7).

Most sling procedures can be categorized by location of the sling: (1) the proximal urethra and bladder neck; (2) mid to distal urethra (Table 1), and the choice of sling material (Table 2). This chapter will discuss the technique and mechanism of cure of distal urethral slings and describe our current technique and results.

II. PATHOPHYSIOLOGY

Female stress incontinence has been categorized as occurring with or without urethral hypermobility (8,9). Classically, sling procedures have been reserved for the treatment of individuals with stress incontinence without urethral hypermobility (2). The AUA guidelines for the treatment of stress urinary incontinence (SUI) demonstrated excellent long-term durability of these procedures, and subsequent authors have demonstrated excellent cure rates for pubovaginal slings performed on patients with urethral hypermobility as well (4,10,11).

Several recent investigations have called into question the mechanism by which sling procedures correct stress incontinence. Theories ranging from a backboard that improves coaptation to frank urethral kinking leading to mild obstruction have been reported. Fulford and coworkers demonstrated significant increases in both postvoid residual and voiding pressures, with a concomitant decrease in peak flow rates in individuals treated with pubovaginal slings (12). Similarly, Klutke and coworkers demonstrated a tendency toward obstructed voiding patterns in patients who had undergone successful anti-incontinence procedures (13). These results have not been supported by several other studies, which have shown no evidence of obstruction on postoperative urodynamics in patients treated with slings (14). Ongoing efforts to define outflow obstruction in women may be helpful in studying the mechanism of success of sling procedure (7,15). At this time it is impossible to tell how these procedures correct urinary incontinence.

The use of distal urethral slings has broadened our understanding of urethral support and the mechanism of continence. Using the tension-free vaginal tape procedure Klutke and coworkers have demonstrated high rates of cure of stress incontinence without correcting urethral hypermobility (16). Thus, it seems that the anatomic correction of bladder neck hypermobility is not as important as previously thought in the prevention of stress urinary incontinence.

The proximal urethra and bladder neck are supported by the urethropelvic ligament. This is the primary mechanism of continence in women, responsible for passive continence. A defect in this support leads to bladder neck hypermobility and opening of the bladder neck. Since up to

Table 1   Variables Between Sling Procedures

Location	Anchoring method	Sling length
Bladder neck/proximal urethra Mid and distal urethra	None (TVT) Absorbable sutures Nonabsorbable sutures Bone anchors	Anterior vaginal wall only Vaginal wall + retropubic space Vaginal wall + retropubic space + suprapubic

Table 2   Currently Utilized Sling Materials

Material			
Autologous	Cadaveric	Synthetic	Other
Vaginal wall	Fascia lata	PTFE/Gore-Tex	Cadaveric fascia
Rectus fascia		Polypropylene (Prolene)	Pelvicol
Fascia lata		Polypropylene (Marlex)	DuraDerm
		Polyester (Prote-Gen)	Repliform
		Polyethylene (Mersilene)	DermMatrix
			AlloDerm
			Stratasis
			SABRE

50% of women with hypermobility do not suffer from urinary incontinence, we know that a defect to this area alone is not sufficient to cause urinary incontinence.

Unlike bladder neck suspensions and the pubovaginal sling, distal urethral slings do not cure SUI by correcting hypermobility. The distal urethral complex is composed of the pubourethral ligaments, the intrinsic sphincteric mechanism of the urethra, the extrinsic sphincter, and the levator muscle located immediately distal to the pubourethral ligament. All these elements interact and have a role in providing resting tonicity to the middistal urethra, induce urethral coaptation, and respond protectively at the time of increased intra-abdominal pressures by increasing urethral resistance. They not only provide anatomic support but also contribute to the normal function of the urethra. For simplicity, we refer to everything proximal to the pubourethral ligaments as proximal urethra and everything distal as distal urethra. Past surgical procedures have targeted the proximal urethra and bladder neck by elevating the bladder neck to an intra-abdominal position, fixing the proximal urethra to the pubic bone, or increasing the resistance of the proximal urethra. Newer procedures supporting the distal urethra work by a different mechanism. Anatomically, the distal suburethral slings both bring the urethra closer to the pubic bone and provide support posteriorly. The distal slings leave the bladder neck and urethra intact and hypermobile. The distal urethral function is altered, allowing for increased segmental distal urethral resistance and better urethral coaptation. The proximity of the urethra to the symphysis pubis allows for a more efficient impact of the levator musculature on the urethra at the time of increased intra-abdominal pressures. In addition, the sling itself may also provide support posteriorly to provide a "distal backboard," which also contributes to better urethral coaptation.

Thus continence can be achieved by correcting the proximal urethral sphincter (proximal urethra and bladder neck) in procedures such as bladder neck and retropubic suspensions or proximal urethral slings, correcting the distal urethral sphincter as with the transvaginal tape procedure (TVT; Ethicon) and other distal suburethral slings, or addressing the intrinsic mechanism of the urethra with the use of injectables.

III. MID TO DISTAL SUBURETHRAL SLINGS

The TVT procedure was introduced by Ulmsten et al. in 1996 (17). It has been shown to be an effective therapy for the treatment of stress incontinence (7,13,17–29). Based on similar anatomic location and mechanisms of cure as the TVT, other procedures have been described. Such procedures include SPARC (American Medical Systems), Safyre (Promedon, Argentina), and SABRE (Mentor) among others. Since some of these procedures will be discussed in other sections of this book, we will not focus on them in this chapter. Although a significant body of literature exists regarding outcomes of surgery and complications from the TVT, very few data are available on these newer procedures. All these techniques involve placement of a synthetic sling at the level of the mid to distal urethra, and all are commercial product that include placement needles or passers and prefabricated slings. As such, they can be costly. They differ primarily in the approach to placement (from suprapubic area to vagina or vice versa, from vagina to the suprapubic area) and in the particular hardware necessary for their placement.

Although simple to perform, these procedures require special instrumentation, and their price is prohibitive in many parts of the world. In addition, for some of these procedures, the technique for placement is blind without finger guidance, and this has lead to high rates of bladder perforations, rare cases of injuries to the bowel or major vessels, and even death (30–32).

We have described the placement of a mid to distal urethral polypropylene sling (DUPS) for the treatment of SU (33,34). Unlike other distal urethral slings, our procedure is inexpensive with an approximate cost of $15 for the mesh, does not require special instrumentation, and is placed only within the retropubic space. The procedure is simple and quick, with an average operating room time of 28 min. The rest of this chapter will focus on the surgical technique and outcomes of the DUPS.

IV. DUPS: AN INEXPENSIVE ALTERNATIVE TO COMMERCIALLY AVAILABLE PRODUCTS

A. Surgical Technique

A 1 × 10 cm thinly woven polypropylene (Ethicon, Inc.) mesh is prepared and 0 polyglactin (Vicryl) suture is placed at each end. The patient is placed in high dorsal lithotomy position. The lower abdomen and genitalia are prepped and draped in a sterile fashion. The labia are retracted laterally with stay sutures. A Lowsley retractor is used to place a suprapubic tube. A 16F Foley catheter is inserted per urethra, and the bladder is emptied. A weighted vaginal speculum is used for exposure. An Allis clamp is used to grasp the anterior vaginal wall just proximal to the meatus. Two oblique lateral incisions are made in the anterior vaginal wall (Fig. 1). One additional Allis clamp is placed at the distal portion of each of the oblique incisions to aid in the exposure. The dissection is carried out laterally over the glistening periurethral fascia toward the ipsilateral shoulder. A small window into the retropubic space is made at the level of the mid to distal urethra (Fig. 2).

A suburethral tunnel is created in the anterior vaginal wall 1.5 cm from the urethral meatus, using a fine, right-angle clamp (Fig. 3). The sling is transferred underneath the suburethral tunnel (Fig. 4). A suprapubic puncture is made just above the symphysis. A double-pronged needle (Cook Urological, Inc., Spencer, IN) is passed under finger control through the fascia and retropubic space to the level of the oblique vaginal incision, and the previously placed polyglactin sutures from the polypropylene mesh are transferred to the suprapubic incision. A similar maneuver is done on the other side. Cystoscopy is performed to rule out bladder or urethral perforation.

To guarantee tying of the sling under no tension, one Allis clamp is placed through each vaginal incision to firmly hold the sling in the horizontal position while the assistant ties the polyglactin sutures suprapubically (Fig. 5). The suture knots are located 3 mm bellow the skin and are not immediately above the fascia. The retropubic space is irrigated with betadine solution. The vaginal incisions are closed with 3.0 polyglactin. A subcuticular stitch with 4.0 polyglactin is used to close the suprapubic incision. A vaginal pack and dressing are applied.

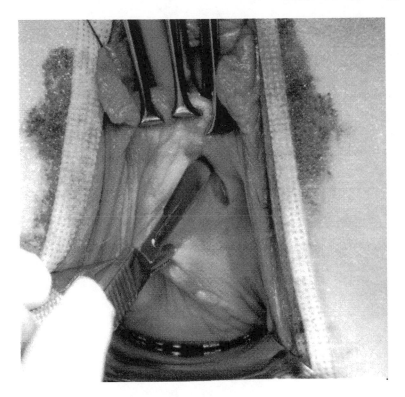

Figure 1 Vaginal exposure and lateral incisions.

Postoperatively, the vaginal pack is removed in the recovery room, 2 h after the procedure. The suprapubic tube is capped and the patient is instructed to void every 3 h and record her postvoid residual. The patient is discharged home. The suprapubic tube is removed once postvoid residuals are <50 cc.

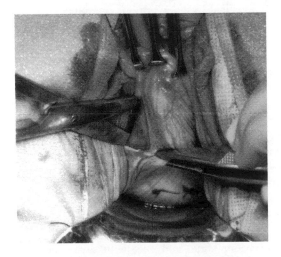

Figure 2 Entering the retropubic space.

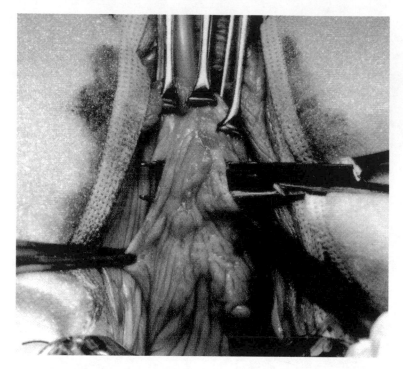

Figure 3 Suburethral vaginal tunnel.

B. Surgical Outcomes

From November 1999 to February 2002, 301 patients underwent the polypropylene sling for the treatment of SUI. The average age was 59.3 years (41–83). Our series consists of a complex SUI population. Of the 301 patients, 62% suffered from mixed incontinence and 139 (46%) of the patients had failed an average of 1.6 (1–5) prior anti-incontinence procedures. In addition, 55% of the patients had concomitant prolapse surgery with 33% of patients undergoing a concomitant rectocele repair, 7% a cystocele repair, and 10% a vaginal hysterectomy among others.

When reporting perioperative complications we evaluated all patients who underwent the polypropylene sling procedure. In this group, there were 301 patients with an average follow up of 10.3 months (1–23 months). Complications occurred in $<0.3\%$ of patients except development of cystocele, which occurred in 2% of patients. Of these seven patients, none had cystocele repair at the time of the sling surgery. Four of these patients had symptomatic cystoceles that required surgical repair. No patients developed urethral erosion or permanent retention. Three patients had prolonged voiding dysfunction requiring intermittent catheterization for a maximum of 3 months. This resolved, and they are voiding spontaneously without residual. One patient developed a vaginal erosion of the polypropylene mesh. This patient originally had urethral erosion from a cadaveric fascial sling with abscess formation. At the time of her procedure, the cadaveric fascial sling was removed, the urethra was reconstructed, and the polypropylene sling was placed. To date, no other patients have required removal of the sling because of pain, infection, or erosion.

The surgical failure rate for this procedure is 2.3%, with seven patients in our series requiring further intervention. Of these patients, four were treated successfully with durasphere injections, two were treated with repeat polypropylene sling, and one, with severe urethral incompetence, was treated with a spiral sling. The de novo urge incontinence rate was 6.8%.

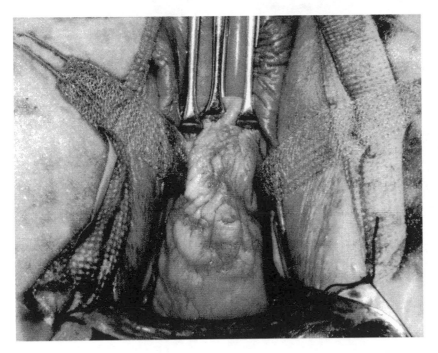

Figure 4   The sling is placed under the vaginal tunnel.

It is always difficult to report success and failure rates in anti-incontinence surgery since how these terms are defined can change these rates by up to 50%. Although the Urodynamic Society and the American Urologic Association have made genuine attempts to standardize the evaluation of treatment outcomes in urinary incontinence, most of these recommendations are not being followed, and there are no specific recommendations as to how to assess patient quality of life (QOL) or how to gather this information (35,36). Although a number of validated questionnaires are available to assess QOL issues in the incontinent population, the means for conducting this assessment is still nonstandardized (37). One thing is known; numerous studies have demonstrated lower cure rates when patients subjective outcomes are compared to physician assessment and objective cure rates on physical exam, pad tests, or UDS (3,38,39). In addition, clinical outcomes do not always translate into patient satisfaction (40). Examples of this phenomenon include diverging success rates reported for particular procedures. One such procedure is the pubovaginal sling where physicians report success rates of 70–100% compared to subjective cure rates of 46–55% (10,41–44). These discrepancies are seen across the board with abdominal urethropexy having objective cure rates of 93% versus subjective cure rates of 54% (45). Sirls et al. compared retrospective chart reviews following modified Pereyra bladder neck suspension and found disparate success rates of 72% cure rates using chart reviews versus 47% using patient questionnaires (39). In a recent randomized study comparing the TVT to colposuspension, the objective cure rated defined as a negative pad test and a negative cystometry was 66% in the TVT group versus 57% in the colposuspension group (46). More interesting, when patients filled out validated question-naires, only 59% and 53% of patients reported cure of SUI, respectively. In addition, only 36% and 28% reported no leakage of urine under any circumstance.

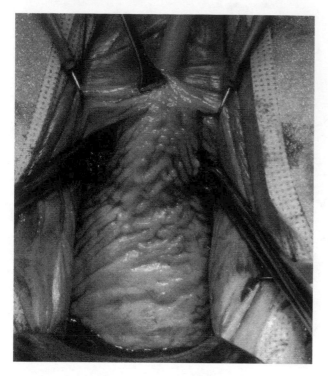

Figure 5   Adjusting sling tension using two Allis clamps.

In light of the biases present when members of the medical staff are involved in gathering outcome data, we chose to evaluate our patients with patient self-assessment. Of the 301 patients there were 92 patients with a minimum follow-up of 12 months (mean 16; range 12–23). Patients were evaluated by self-reported questionnaires looking at the presence, absence, and frequency of symptoms, bother from symptoms (short form of the urogenital distress inventory, UDI-6), and global quality of life question related to urinary symptoms. Self-assessment questionnaires were available on 76 (83%) of the 92 patients with a minimum 1-year follow-up. Eighty-four percent of patients reported symptoms of SUT never or less than once a week, with 69% never experiencing SUI. On the UDI-6, 86% of the patients reported either never or rarely being bothered by symptoms of SUI. The postoperative mean QOL related to urinary symptoms was 1.5 (scale of 0–6), between pleased and mostly satisfied.

Patients were asked to list the number of pads used per day regardless of the indication (SUI, UI, protection, hygiene, etc.). The mean number of pads used before surgery was 2.5 and postoperatively 0.8 ($P < .05$). Postoperatively, 61% of patients reported never wearing pads. There was no statistically significant difference between maximum flow rates and postvoid residuals obtained before and after surgery. In addition, patients were asked to rate their percent improvement in a scale of 0–100%. The patients reported an average improvement of 86% after surgery.

Combining all the available data, we defined failures as patients who reported being <50% improved, had a positive Marshall's test on physical exam, or reported severe symptoms of or bother from SUI on questionnaires. With this definition, the failure rate was 11%, and the cure or improved rate 89%. Objective cure rate, defined as a negative stress test on physical exam with the patient in the standing and lithotomy positions, was 92%.

V. CONCLUSIONS

The etiology of female SUI appears to be more complex than previously understood. Although the proximal urethra is the primary continence mechanism, the distal urethra appears to play an essential role as a compensatory mechanism. Repairs directed at either the bladder neck or the distal urethra appear to be effective. The middistal suburethral polypropylene sling offers an inexpensive, safe, and simple alternative treatment for patients with SUI. The procedure offers high objective but lower patient-determined, subjective cure rates.

Although numerous sling procedures have been described, their efficacies are highly variable. It is clear that variations in how authors measure success, and the lack of objective outcome analysis, have made it very difficult to evaluate all these procedures. There is a need for well-controlled, randomized outcome studies before definite determinations regarding the efficacy and durability of these procedures can be made.

REFERENCES

1. Von Giordano D. Twentieth congress. Fr Chir 1907; 506.
2. McGuire EJ, Lytto B. Pubovaginal sling procedure or stress incontinence. J Urol 1978; 119:82.
3. Korman HJ, Sirls LT, Kiekemo AK. Success rate of modified Pereyra bladder neck suspension determined by outcomes analysis. J Urol 1994; 152:1453.
4. Leach GE, Dmochowski RR, Appell RA, Blaivas JG, Hadley HR, Luber KM. Female stress urinary incontinence clinical guidelines panel summary report on surgical management of female stress urinary incontinence. The American urological association. J Urol 1997; 158:875.
5. Elkabir JJ, Mee AD. Long-term evaluation of the Gittes procedure for urinary stress incontinence. J Urol 1998; 159:1203.
6. Walker GT, Texter JH Jr. Success and patient satisfaction following the Stamey procedure for stress urinary incontinence. J Urol 1992; 147:1521.
7. Klutke JJ, Carlin BI, Klutke CG. The tension-free vaginal tape procedure: correction of stress incontinence with minimal alteration in proximal urethral mobility. Urology 2000; 55:512.
8. Blaivas JG, Olsson CA. Stress incontinence: classification and surgical approach. J Urol 1988; 139:727.
9. Blaivas JG, Appell RA, Fantl JA, Leach G, McGuire EJ, Resnick NM. Definition and classification of urinary incontinence: recommendations of the urodynamic society. Neurourol Urodyn 1997; 16:149.
10. Cross CA, Cespedes RD, McGuire EJ. Our experience with pubovaginal slings in patients with stress urinary incontinence. J Urol 1998; 159:1195.
11. Chaikin DC, Rosenthal J, Blaivas JG. Pubovaginal fascial sling for all types of stress urinary incontinence: long-term analysis. J Urol 1998; 160:1312.
12. Fulford SC, Flynn R, Barrington J, Appanna T, Stephenson TP. An assessment of the surgical outcome and urodynamic effects of the pubovaginal sling for stress incontinence and the associated urge syndrome. J Urol 1999; 162:135.
13. Klutke JJ, Klutke CG, Bergman J, Elia G. Urodynamics changes in voiding after anti-incontinence surgery: an insight into the mechanism of cure. Urology 1999; 54:1003.
14. Kuo HC. Videourodynamic results after pubovaginal sling procedure for stress urinary incontinence. Urology 1999; 54:802.
15. Lemack GE, Zimmern PE. Pressure flow analysis may aid in identifying women with outflow obstruction. J Urol 2000; 163:1823.
16. Blaivas JG, Groutz A. Bladder outlet obstruction nomogram for women with lower urinary tract symptomatology. Neurourol Urodyn 2000; 19:553.
17. Ulmsten U, Henriksson L, Johnson P, Varhos G. An ambulatory surgical procedure under local anesthesia for treatment of female urinary incontinence. Int Urogynecol J Pelvic Floor Dysfunct 1996; 7:81.

18. Lebret T, Lugagne PM, Herve JM, Barre P, Orsoni JL, Yonneau L. Evaluation of tension-free vaginal tape procedure. Its safety and efficacy in the treatment of female stress urinary incontinence during the learning phase. Eur Urol 2001; 40:543.

19. Jeffry L, Deval B, Birsan A, Soriano D, Darai E. Objective and subjective cure rates after tension-free vaginal tape for treatment of urinary incontinence. Urology 2001; 58:702.

20. Haab F, Sananes S, Amarenco G, Ciofu C, Uzan S, Gattegno B. Results of the tension-free vaginal tape procedure for the treatment of type II stress urinary incontinence at a minimum followup of 1 year. J Urol 2001; 165:159.

21. Brophy MM, Klutke JJ, Klutke CG. A review of the tension-free vaginal tape procedure: outcomes, complications, and theories. Curr Urol Rep 2001; 2:364.

22. Carlin BI, Klutke JJ, Klutke CG. The tension-free vaginal tape procedure for the treatment of stress incontinence in the female patient. Urology 2000; 56:28.

23. Azam U, Frazer MI, Kozman EL, Ward K, Hilton P, Rane A. The tension-free vaginal tape procedure in women with previous failed stress incontinence surgery. J Urol 2001; 166:554.

24. Rezapour M, Falconer C, Ulmsten U. Tension-free vaginal tape (TVT) in stress incontinent women with intrinsic sphincter deficiency (ISD)—a long term follow-up. Int Urogynecol J Pelvic Floor Dysfunct 2001; 12(suppl 2):S12.

25. Rezapour M, Ulmsten U. Tension-free vaginal tape (TVT) in women with recurrent stress urinary incontinence—a long-term follow up. Int Urogynecol J Pelvic Floor Dysfunct 2001; 12(suppl 2):S9.

26. Nilsson CG, Kuuva N, Falconer C, Rezapour M, Ulmsten U. Long-term results of the tension-free vaginal tape (TVT) procedure for surgical treatment of female stress urinary incontinence. Int Urogynecol J Pelvic Floor Dysfunct 2001; 12(suppl 2):S5.

27. Nilsson CG, Kuuva N. The tension-free vaginal tape procedure is successful in the majority of women with indications for surgical treatment of urinary stress incontinence. Br J Obstet Gynaecol 2001; 108:414.

28. Niemczyk P, Klutke JJ, Carlin BI, Klutke CG. United States experience with tension-free vaginal tape procedure for urinary stress incontinence: assessment of safety and tolerability. Tech Urol 2001; 7:261.

29. Moran PA, Ward KL, Johnson D, Smirni WE, Hilton P, Bibby J. Tension-free vaginal tape for primary genuine stress incontinence: a two-centre follow-up study. BJU Int 2000; 86:39.

30. Kuuva N, Nilsson CG. A nationwide analysis of complications associated with the tension-free vaginal tape (TVT) procedure. Acta Obstet Gynecol Scand 2002; 81:72.

31. Madjar S, Tchetgen MB, Van Antwerp A, Abdelmalak J, Rackley RR. Urethral erosion of tension-free vaginal tape. Urology 2002; 59:601.

32. Klutke C, Siegel S, Carlin B, Paszkiewicz E, Kirkemo A, Klutke J. Urinary retention after tension-free vaginal tape procedure: incidence and treatment. Urology 2001; 58:697.

33. Rodriguez LV, Raz S. Polypropylene sling for the treatment of stress urinary incontinence. Urology 2001; 58:783.

34. Rodriguez LV, Berman J, Raz S. Polypropylene sling for treatment of stress urinary incontinence: an alternative to tension-free vaginal tape. Tech Urol 2001; 7:87.

35. Lee RS, DeAntoni E, Daneshgari F. Compliance with recommendations of the urodynamic society for standards of efficacy for evaluation of treatment outcomes in urinary incontinence. Neurourol Urodyn 2002; 21:482.

36. Blaivas JG, Appell RA, Fantl JA, Leach G, McGuire EJ, Resnick NM. Standards of efficacy for evaluation of treatment outcomes m urinary incontinence: recommendations of the urodynamic society. Neurourol Urodyn 1997; 16:145.

37. Corcos J, Beaulieu S, Donovan J, Naughton M, Gotoh M. Quality of life assessment in men and women with urinary incontinence. J Urol 2002; 168:896.

38. Deval B, Jeffry L, Al Najjar F, Soriano D, Darai E. Determinants of patient dissatisfaction after a tension-free vaginal tape procedure for urinary incontinence. J Urol 2002; 167:2093.

39. Sirls LT, Keoleian CM, Korman HJ, Kirkemo AK. The effect of study methodology on reported success rates of the modified Pereyra bladder neck suspension. J Urol 1995; 154:1732.

40. Eisen SV. Assessment of subjective distress by patients' self-report versus structured interview. Psychol Rep 1995; 76:35.

41. Chaikin DC, Blaivas JG. Weakened cadaveric fascial sling: an unexpected cause of failure. J Urol 1998; 160:2151.

42. Morgan TO Jr, Westney OL, McGuire EJ. Pubovaginal sling: 4-year outcome analysis and quality of life assessment. J Urol 2000; 163:1845.

43. Haab F, Trockman BA, Zimmern PE, Leach GE. Results of pubovaginal sling for the treatment of intrinsic sphincteric deficiency determined by questionnaire analysis. J Urol 1997; 158:1738.

44. Hassouna ME, Ghoniem GM. Long-term outcome and quality of life after modified pubovaginal sling for intrinsic sphincteric deficiency. Urology 1999; 53:287.

45. Tegerstedt G, Sjoberg B, Hammarstrom M. Clinical outcome or abdominal urethropexy-colposuspension: a long-term follow-up. Int Urogynecol J Pelvic Floor Dysfunct 2001; 12:161.

46. Ward K, Hilton P. Prospective multicentre randomised trial of tension-free vaginal tape and colposuspension as primary treatment for stress incontinence. BMJ 2002; 325:67.

29

Transvaginal Cooper's Ligament Sling for the Treatment of Stress Urinary Incontinence and Low-Pressure Urethra

Sanjay Gandhi and Peter K. Sand
Evanston Continence Center, Northwestern University, Evanston, Illinois, U.S.A.

I. INTRODUCTION

Many consider retropubic urethropexies and bladder neck slings to be the standard of care surgeries for the surgical treatment of stress urinary incontinence (SUI). Although the increased enthusiasm for midurethral tape procedures has shifted some focus from these traditional operations, they still enjoy the best long-term results.

In women with intrinsic sphincteric deficiency and urethral hypermobility, surgical treatment focuses on increasing urethral resistance. Standard colposuspensions, such as the Burch or Marshall-Marchetti-Krantz retropubic urethropexies, improve the support of the sphincteric unit without obstruction. Most reports suggest that these procedures are less successful in patients with intrinsic sphincteric deficiency (1–4). McGuire first suggested that failure of multiple incontinence procedures was associated with the presence of low resting urethral pressure (<20 cmH$_2$O) with or without urethral hypermobility (1). Hilton and Stanton reported that patients whose surgery failed had relatively lower proximal or maximal urethral closure pressures postoperatively than those with a successful surgery (2). Sand and colleagues reported a 54% failure rate for Burch colposuspension in patients with a maximum urethral closure pressure ≤ 20 cmH$_2$O, compared with 18% in women with "normal" urethral pressures (4). Other studies (3,5) have confirmed these findings and have been used to justify the use of sling procedures for the treatment of intrinsic sphincteric deficiency.

Since the introduction of the laparoscopic retropubic urethropexy (6), there has been significant enthusiasm for minimal-access techniques. Minimally invasive vaginal sling procedures along with the availability of allografts and xenografts enable the surgeon to recreate the bladder neck support offered by slings, but without the morbidity of an abdominal incision and a graft harvest. In response to this trend, we developed an entirely transvaginal sling procedure with the graft tied to Cooper's ligament with no intervening suture bridges (7).

II. PROCEDURE

Cooper's ligament—as opposed to rectus fascia-is utilized as the anchoring structure for this sling to allow for an immobile suspension point to remove anterior mobility as a variable while tensioning

429

the sling. Cooper's ligament has been proven a strong structure for supporting the bladder neck abdominally and has been used for abdominal-vaginal slings. The Capio CL device (Boston Scientific, Natick, MA) is used to place sutures into Cooper's ligament (Fig. 1). The sling material is tied such that it directly apposes the ligament without intervening suture bridges. In theory, this technique creates a sling that is independent of abdominal-wall activity and changes in rectus muscle tone.

A Foley catheter is inserted to drain the bladder and identify the urethrovesical junction. Dilute vasopressin solution is injected beneath the epithelium of the anterior vaginal wall. An inverted midline T-incision is made on the anterior wall of the vagina extending from the base of the bladder to approximately 2 cm proximal to the external urethral meatus. The vaginal epithelium is sharply dissected from the underlying endopelvic connective tissue bilaterally to the level of the descending pubic rami. Metzenbaum scissors are used to perforate right against the rami at the level of the bladder neck to avoid bladder injury and to assure proper entrance into the retropubic space (Fig. 2). On entry into the retropubic space, Cooper's ligament is palpated and cleared of any fatty tissue. This may be challenging in women with prior retropubic operations, but it does not prevent us from placing sutures in Cooper's ligament. Especially in patients with prior incontinence operations, lysis of any urethral attachments to the pubis allows mobility of the urethrovesical segment and facilitates proper positioning of the sling at the bladder neck.

The Capio CL device is used to deliver permanent monofilament sutures bilaterally into Cooper's ligament (Figs. 3, 4). A laminated tape measure is backloaded onto one suture and used to measure the distance from the suture insertion in the ligament to the bladder neck. Doubling of

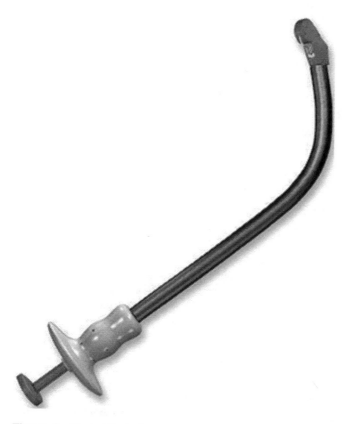

Figure 1   Capio CL device.

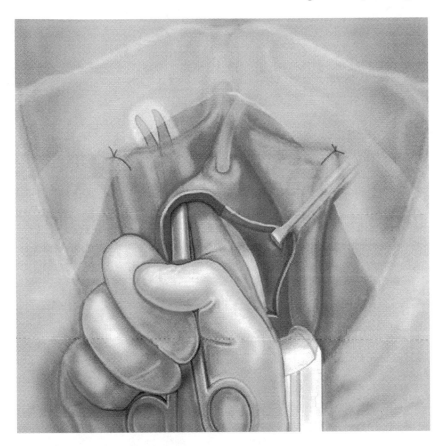

Figure 2   Entry into retropubic space.

this length defines the sling length required. Anterior colporrhaphy, if needed, is performed prior to measuring the length of the sling. If cadaveric fascia is to be used, the ends are airplane-folded to prevent suture pull through as previously described (8). Both suture ends are passed through the ends of the sling graft previously pierced with 16-gauge angiocaths. The sling is then tied in place bilaterally to Cooper's ligament with no suture bridges between the sling and the ligament. Other surgeons have used a similar technique to place a suture suspended sling (Fig. 5). Although some authors have suggested avoiding straightening a folded sling (9), we prefer anchoring the anterior and posterior edges of the sling periurethrally to prevent the sling from rolling up when fascia is used. The vagina is then closed.

III. MATERIAL

The choice of sling material has generated much controversy in the literature. Although many case series have described success rates for sling procedures, only a handful have described the in vivo tissue changes that occur and might affect operative success. Because of significant local complications associated with synthetic materials, many surgeons have used autologous fascia, but it is associated with increased operative time, convalescence, and pain. Cadaveric allograft fascia might offer decreased operating-room time and patient morbidity, but there has been controversy as to their durability (10–12). Different tissue processing techniques may affect the

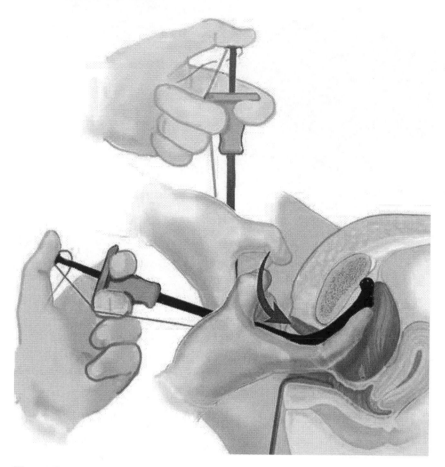

Figure 3   Inserting device behind pubic bone.

durability of allografts; solvent dehydration may provide an advantage over freeze-dried tissues as it preserves the tensile strengths of collagen in in vitro studies (13,14).

We initially used freeze-dried cadaveric fascia in 68% of our cohort. We are currently using porcine dermis for our slings: it is easier to manipulate, remains intact in vivo for at least 2 years, and does not require airplane-folding the ends to prevent suture pullout as described with fascial allografts (14,15). In the absence of a randomized trial comparing sling materials, we cannot be sure which is best (16).

IV.   OUTCOMES

In our initial case series, we operated on 105 women with SUI, low urethral closure pressure, and urethral hypermobility. These women all had a transvaginal Cooper's ligament anchored sling. Subjective stress and urge incontinence symptoms were assessed, and patients underwent urodynamic testing preoperatively and at 14 weeks postoperatively. Objective assessment at 1 year included a standing stress test at 250 mL and structured pelvic examination.

Women in the cohort had an average age of 70 years and an average mean body mass index of 26.8 kg/m (2). On preoperative questionnaires 71% of women had symptoms of stress

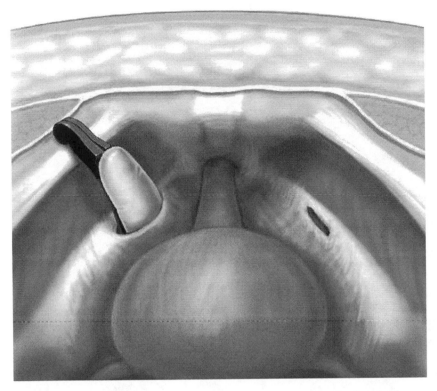

Figure 4 Retropubic view of device in proper position over Cooper's ligament.

incontinence while 77% had urge incontinence. On preoperative urodynamic testing, the mean preoperative closure pressure was 12.3 cm H_2O, and 78% of our cohort had concomitant detrusor overactivity on urethrocystometry. All women had SUI and a low-pressure urethra on urodynamic testing with and without support of concomitant prolapse.

At 14 weeks follow-up, 64 of 91 women (70%) had objective cure of their stress incontinence, while 20 women (22%) developed type III stress incontinence with operative correction of their urethral hypermobility. Seven women (8%) had recurrent stress incontinence with urethral hypermobility. Sixty-seven percent of women with objective failures at 14 weeks were asymptomatic of stress incontinence. Overall, 16 of 91 women were symptomatic of stress incontinence postoperatively. Of those women with preoperative detrusor overactivity, 90% had persistent detrusor overactivity on urodynamic testing, and 48% of women without preoperative detrusor overactivity developed de novo detrusor overactivity.

At 1-year follow-up, 84% of women had subjective cure of their stress incontinence while 42% had a subjective cure of their urge incontinence. Eighty-eight percent of those tested had a negative stress test and an objective cure of their preoperative stress incontinence. Voiding dysfunction was similar to other sling procedures that have been documented in previous studies (17–19). The median time to normal voiding for the cohort was 10 days. The majority of patients used clean intermittent self-catheterization. Ninety percent of women were voiding with normal residuals (<50 mL) by 6 weeks. Frequently, patients who underwent the sling procedure described a delay in initiation of voiding and a less forceful stream. We had two women who underwent urethrolysis for prolonged retention and who are currently voiding well.

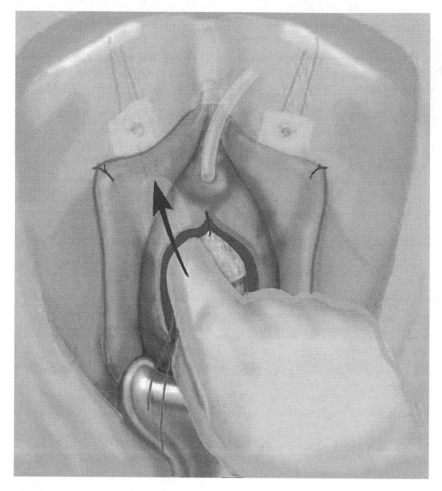

Figure 5 Tying sling into place from Cooper's ligament to Cooper's ligament.

V. COMPLICATIONS

There were no intraoperative complications directly related to the sling procedure. One woman had a stroke in the evening after surgery; one woman developed a retropubic hematoma that was drained percutaneously; and there were two fascial erosions into the vagina that were managed in the office. Fewer than 5% of women had significant long-term voiding dysfunction requiring self-catheterization beyond 12 months. Two women underwent urethrolysis to address postoperative retention and did well.

VI. CONCLUSION

Women in this cohort, who on average were older, were mildly overweight, had detrusor overactivity, and had low closure pressures, have had good resolution of their stress incontinence with the transvaginal Cooper's ligament sling. The procedure is minimally invasive and provides the additional supportive benefits of a sling in preventing recurrent anterior vaginal wall prolapse. Because of anterior anchoring to Cooper's ligament which is immobile, retention and pareuresis are less common than we have seen with pubovaginal slings. These Capio CL transvaginal slings are also associated with far less pain and offer the cosmetic advantage of no abdominal incision. This also makes them ideal outpatient procedures. This operation has become our standard for women with intrinsic sphincter insufficiency, replacing the need for pubovaginal or transvaginal bone-anchored slings.

REFERENCES

1. McGuire EJ. Urodynamic findings in patients after failure of stress incontinence operations. Prog Clin Biol Res 1981; 78:351.
2. Hilton P, Stanton SL. Urethral pressure measurement by microtransducer: the results in symptom-free women and in those with genuine stress incontinence. Br J Obstet Gynaecol 1983; 90:919–933.
3. Bowen LW, Sand PK, Ostergard DR, Franti CE. Unsuccessful Burch retropubic urethropexy: a case-controlled urodynamic study. Am J Obstet Gynecol 1989; 160:452–458.
4. Sand PK, Bowen LW, Panganiban R, Ostergard DR. The low pressure urethra as a factor in failed retropubic urethropexy. Obstet Gynecol 1987; 69:399–402.
5. Koonings PP, Bergman A, Ballard CA. Low urethral pressure and stress urinary incontinence in women: risk factor for failed retropubic surgical procedure. Urology 1990; 36:245–248.
6. Vancaillie TG, Schuessler W. Laparoscopic bladderneck suspension. J Laparoendosc Surg 1991; 1:169–173.
7. Koduri S, Goldberg RP, Sand PK. Transvaginal therapy of genuine stress incontinence. Urology 2000; 56:23–27.
8. Sutaria PM, Staskin DR. Cadaveric allograft strength: an assessment of the effects of preservation techniques and the methods of suture fixation using two separate experimental models. Neurourol Urodyn 1999; 18:324–325.
9. Wright EJ. Current status of fascia lata allograft slings treating urinary incontinence: effective or ephemeral? Tech Urol 2001; 7:81–86.
10. Carbone JM, Kavaler E, Hu JC, Raz S. Pubovaginal sling using cadaveric fascia and bone anchors: disappointing early results. J Urol 2001; 165:1605–1611.
11. Fitzgerald MP, Mollenhauer J, Brubaker L. Failure of allograft suburethral slings. BJU Int 1999; 84:785–788.
12. Elliott DS, Boone TB. Is fascia lata allograft material trustworthy for pubovaginal sling repair? Urology 2000; 56:772–776.
13. Kobayashi T, Takei T, Yagi R. Reconstruction of the four major ligaments in an unstable knee joint after dislocation by solvent-preserved human fascia lata transplantation. Arch Orthop Trauma Surg 1989; 108:246–249.
14. Lemer ML, Chaikin DC, Blaivas JG. Tissue strength analysis of autologous and cadaveric allografts for the pubovaginal sling. Neurourol Urodyn 1999; 18:497–503.
15. Chaikin DC, Blaivas JG. Weakened cadaveric fascial sling: an unexpected cause of failure. J Urol 1998; 160:2151.
16. Choe JM, Kothandapani R, James L, Bowling D. Autologous, cadaveric, and synthetic materials used in sling surgery: comparative biomechanical analysis. Urology 2001; 58:482–486.
17. McLennan MT, Melick CF, Bent AE. Clinical and urodynamic predictors of delayed voiding after fascia lata suburethral sling. Obstet Gynecol 1998; 92:608–612.
18. Richter HE, Varner RE, Sanders E, Holley RL, Northen A, Cliver SP. Effects of pubovaginal sling procedure on patients with urethral hypermobility and intrinsic sphincteric deficiency: would they do it again? Am J Obstet Gynecol 2001; 184:14–19.
19. Beck RP, McCormick S, Nordstrom L. The fascia lata sling procedure for treating recurrent genuine stress incontinence of urine. Obstet Gynecol 1988; 72:699–703.

30

Management of Postoperative Detrusor Instability and Voiding Dysfunction

Peter O. Kwong and O. Lenaine Westney
University of Texas Health Science Center, Houston, Texas, U.S.A.

I. INTRODUCTION

Stress urinary incontinence (SUI) is frequently encountered in urology and urogynecology. Today there are multiple surgical procedures, each with several variations for correcting SUI. The selected surgery depends on the etiology (urethral hypermobility vs. intrinsic sphincter deficiency) of the incontinence, and surgeon preference.

Anti-incontinence procedures have reported very good outcomes, with success rates ranging from 80% to 95% initially (1). The Female Stress Urinary Incontinence Clinical Guidelines Panel summary reported 48-month cure rates of 84% and 83% for retropubic suspensions and suburethral slings, respectively (2).

Although the surgical procedures to correct SUI have been reasonably successful, there are potential complications including persistent stress urinary incontinence, urethral erosion, de novo detrusor instability, and urethral obstruction (3). Iatrogenic urethral obstruction occurs in 5–20% following anti-incontinence procedures (4,5). With the Marshall-Marchetti-Krantz retropubic suspension, urethral obstruction rates range from 5% to 20% (6,7). Holschneider et al. reported a 5–7% obstruction rate with transvaginal needle suspensions (8). With respect to pubovaginal slings, there is a 2–12% prolonged urinary retention rate (beyond 4 weeks) and a 3–24% de novo urgency rate (9). The Female Stress Urinary Incontinence Clinical Guidelines Panel noted a prolonged retention rate and de novo urgency rate of 6–11% and 3–11% in sling procedures, 3–7% and 8–16% in retropubic suspensions, and 4–8% and 3–10% in transvaginal needle suspensions (2).

Tension-free vaginal tape (TVT), which is supposed not to cause obstruction because it ideally is placed tension free, is not immune from inducing iatrogenic urethral obstruction requiring tape division (10,11). Carlin et al.'s TVT series of more than 100 patients had 3% de novo urgency and <1% prolonged urinary retention (12). Even the minimally invasive transurethral injection of collagen has a 13% incidence of de novo detrusor instability and a 2% incidence of urinary retention (13).

Postoperative urgency and urge incontinence may be due to urethral obstruction or due to detrusor instability, which may be de novo or preexisting. Detrusor instability has been defined urodynamically as an involuntary detrusor contraction of any magnitude with an urge or increased detrusor pressure of $15\,cmH_2O$ or greater without urge (14). Forty percent to 55% of patients with SUI also have coexisting urge incontinence and urgency that are not demonstrated urodynamically. Hence, the distinction between motor urgency (with involuntary detrusor contractions) and sensory urgency (without involuntary detrusor contractions) has been identified to describe symptomatology that fails to correlate with urodynamic findings. In patients with urge incontinence, urodynamic evidence of detrusor instability is present in 50–90% (15). Preexisting urge incontinence resolves in 50–80% after correction of the SUI (9,15). While many series have failed to reveal any preoperative parameter to predict whose urge incontinence will resolve postoperatively, a recent study by Schrepferman et al. showed that patients with SUI and preoperative low-pressure (detrusor contractions $<15\,cmH_2O$) motor urgency were much more likely (92% cure) to have resolution of urgency symptoms postoperatively, in contrast to those with high-pressure motor urgency (27.8% cure) or with sensory urgency (39.3% cure) (15).

In lieu of detrusor instability (persistent or de novo), the post-operative development of voiding dysfunction may be due to iatrogenic urethral obstruction. The cause of the obstruction is usually secondary to over-correction of the urethrovesical angle (urethral hypersuspension) by excess tension of the suspension sutures (retropubic or sling), urethral distortion by a suture placed to close to the urethra or by buckling of the sling material (3,16). The obstruction then leads to obstructive and/or irritative voiding symptoms or urge incontinence. These symptoms can be very distressing to the patient, as she has now traded stress urinary incontinence for what many consider more problematic and unpredictable-urge incontinence. Thus, the patient should be informed preoperatively about the possible post-operative complications and the plan to treat them if the complications arise (3).

II. PRESENTATION OF POSTOPERATIVE VOIDING DYSFUNCTION

Urethral obstruction following anti-incontinence surgery often presents as urinary retention or obstructive voiding symptoms (hesitancy, incomplete bladder emptying, weak urinary stream, urinary straining), but many patients present primarily with irritative voiding symptoms (urgency, frequency, nocturia) and urge incontinence. Recurrent urinary tract infections may also point to occult outlet obstruction. Upon further evaluation, these patients usually demonstrate elevated postvoid residuals (3). In studies of patients who developed urethral obstruction after anti-incontinence surgery, 60–84% presented with obstructive symptoms, and 55–75% presented with irritative symptoms (1,3,16). Therefore, one must suspect iatrogenic urethral obstruction in any patient who presents with obstructive and/or irritative voiding symptoms or recurrent urinary tract infections (UTIs) following an anti-incontinence procedure.

It is not unusual to see a brief period of voiding dysfunction and poor bladder emptying during the immediate postoperative period. This may be explained by a local inflammatory reaction in the area of the surgical dissection. These symptoms are usually transient and normal voiding returns when the response resolves (usually within 2–4 weeks). During this period, the patient is instructed to perform self-catheterization after voiding until postvoid residuals are $<60\,mL$, which indicates return of efficient bladder emptying (9). If voiding dysfunction persists beyond 6–12 weeks or if urinary retention persists beyond 4 weeks, then one should begin to be concerned about urethral obstruction and initiate a formal workup for the voiding dysfunction.

III. EVALUATION OF VOIDING DYSFUNCTION

The evaluation of prolonged voiding dysfunction following anti-incontinence surgery includes a complete history and physical, a postvoid residual, and full urodynamic study (filling and voiding phases). The history includes a voiding diary, current voiding pattern (daily number of episodes of frequency/urgency/nocturia, amount of incontinence, obstructive symptoms), type and date of the anti-incontinence surgery, and prior surgeries or treatments that may affect urination and voiding pattern prior to the anti-incontinence procedure. The physical examination should be thorough—abdominal, pelvic, and neurological. One should note the position of the urethra and whether it is mobile or fixed against the retropubis with Valsalva, urine leakage with Valsalva or cough, and presence of any pelvic organ prolapse. With frank urethral hypersuspension, the urethra is fixed in a high retropubic position, at times creating a relative anterior vaginal wall prolapse (4).

A post-void residual urine volume should also be obtained in all patients regardless of specific symptomatology. A large postvoid residual in the patient with frequency suggests that an underlying obstruction may be the cause of the irritative voiding symptoms (3).

Cystoscopy may also be performed, looking for urethral distortions or suture/sling erosion. Careful examination may document severe anterior deviation due to excessive suture or sling tension. Additionally, irritative symptoms and/or UTIs may herald exposure of synthetic material to the urinary stream.

The urodynamic evaluation includes a free-flow measurement, a multichannel fluoroscopic urodynamic study with provocative maneuvers to evaluate bladder compliance, instability, and persistent SUI. A pressure-flow voiding study is performed to evaluate maximum detrusor pressure during voiding, looking for evidence of obstruction. Fluoroscopic cysto-urethrography is helpful in identifying the specific site of obstruction. However, in females, definitive evidence of voiding dysfunction (especially obstruction) on urodynamic studies has proven to be very difficult, with no consistent findings.

The diagnosis of bladder outlet obstruction (BOO) in females has gradually evolved as it has become apparent that the criteria classically used to diagnose obstruction in males do not apply in females. Women normally have significantly lower voiding detrusor pressures than males. Many women void by relaxing the pelvic floor muscles or by abdominal straining with very low or no detrusor pressure. This has led several investigators to redefine the criteria for diagnosing BOO obstruction in females (17).

Farrar et al. diagnosed obstruction primarily by flow rates, using $Q_{max} < 15$ mL/sec with a voided volume of at least 200 mL as criteria for obstruction. They believed that relative BOO with low Q_{max} may exist even with normal or low detrusor pressure (18). Massey and Abrams defined female BOO if two or more of four parameters were present, including $Q_{max} < 12$ mL/sec, detrusor pressure at $Q_{max} > 50$ cmH$_2$O, urethral resistance ($P_{det}Q_{max}/Q_{max}^2$) > 0.2, or significant postvoid residual (PVR) with high pressure or resistance (19). Axelrod and Blaivas proposed the BOO criteria of $P_{det} Q_{max} > 20$ cmH$_2$O and $Q_{max} < 12$ mL/sec (20). Later, Nitti et al. recommended video fluorourodynamics during voiding to diagnose BOO by radiographic evidence of obstruction (closed or narrow bladder neck or discrete area of urethral narrowing with proximal dilatation), not using any strict pressure-flow criteria. However, they did note that patients with radiographic evidence of BOO had lower mean Q_{max}, higher mean $P_{det} Q_{max}$, and higher mean PVR than patients with no obstruction. As with all of the other studies, there was wide variability in the urodynamic parameters (17).

Chassagne et al. analyzed clinically obstructed women to define a set of cutoff urodynamic parameters to diagnose BOO in women. The parameters of $Q_{max} < 15$ mL/sec and $P_{det} Q_{max} > 20$ cmH$_2$O were used (21). However, Q_{max} was obtained with a transurethral catheter in place during the pressure-flow study. The transurethral catheter can lead to test-induced BOO due to urethral irritation and/or relative mechanical obstruction of the urethra. Therefore, Groutz et al. compared the "free" Q_{max} from the uroflow study and the Q_{max} from the pressure-flow study, finding that "free" Q_{max} was significantly higher than Q_{max}, while the voided volume was the same (22). However, Lemack and Zimmern's study did not reveal any significant difference (23).

Most recently, Blaivas and Groutz compared 50 unobstructed female controls with 50 women with obstruction as defined by the presence of one or more of three parameters, including (a) free Q_{max} ≤ or 12 mL/sec in repeated flow studies with a sustained detrusor contraction and with P_{det} Q_{max} ≥ 20 cmH$_2$O; (b) radiographic evidence of BOO during a sustained detrusor contraction of at least 20 cmH$_2$O and low Q_{max}; and (c) sustained detrusor contraction of at least 20 cmH$_2$O but unable to void. From their study, they constructed a nomogram that used the two parameters of free Q_{max} and P_{det} max to diagnose BOO in females. The nomogram was able to separate obstructed from unobstructed women and also distinguished three zones of BOO severity (mild, moderate, and severe). The three zones also correlated with symptom scores from the AUA symptom index scale. They further emphasized that the nomogram should be used only to help in the diagnosis of BOO in female, not to direct treatment (24).

There are no standardized criteria for obstruction in this patient population. Normally, obstruction is characterized on pressure-flow study by elevated detrusor pressure (>30–50 cmH$_2$O) with low flow rate (<12–15 mL/sec). However, in the female with obstruction, this finding is often absent. Nitti and Raz demonstrated urodynamic evidence of obstruction in only 56% of their patients who underwent and responded well to urethrolysis, while Carr and Webster reported urodynamic evidence of obstruction in only 22% (16,25). One subset of patients who responded well to urethrolysis despite documented low detrusor pressure and low flow rate or urinary retention may be explained by the fact that some women void by urethral relaxation without obvious detrusor activity. These patients likely had a relative urethral obstruction (16).

Evidence of uninhibited bladder contractions (motor urgency) may also be absent despite subjective symptoms of urgency and urge incontinence (sensory urgency). In Cross et al.'s study, only 30% with urge incontinence demonstrated urodynamic evidence of detrusor instability. Other authors note that there are no preoperative factors, including urodynamic parameters and type of and time from anti-incontinence surgery, that predicted success of the urethrolysis (3,4,16,26). Even those with no detrusor contraction by urodynamic study responded well to urethrolysis. However, there is a trend toward a lower success rate in patients with preexisting low bladder contractility, large postvoid residual, or detrusor instability (1,25,27).

Owing to the variability of urodynamic findings in females with voiding dysfunction after anti-incontinence surgery and no consistent urodynamic parameter that predicts outcome of urethrolysis, many physicians do not base their decision to perform urethrolysis on the urodynamic study alone. According to Carr and Webster, the best indicators of obstruction after anti-incontinence surgery are new irritative or obstructive voiding symptoms or urge incontinence in addition to a physical exam that reveals urethral hypersuspension. The absolute criterion for urethrolysis is the correlation between the time of onset voiding dysfunction and the anti-incontinence surgery (16,28). Goldman et al. further report that the urodynamic study is not required in a patient who had documented normal voiding pattern prior to the anti-incontinence surgery, a clear temporal relationship between the anti-incontinence surgery and the onset of voiding dysfunction, and a large postvoid residual (3). They had seven patients who fit these criteria, five (75%) of whom responded well to urethrolysis.

IV. TREATMENT

A. Conservative Management

Conservative measures can be tried initially with the hope that the voiding dysfunction will improve or resolve spontaneously. Intermittent self-catheterization can be employed if urinary retention or inefficient bladder emptying is the main problem. The decision to pursue a non-operative course should also be based on knowledge regarding the material of the suspension sutures and sling material. For example, synthetic sling and suture materials are less likely to change with respect to urethral compression than an absorbable suture and organic sling combination.

For irritative voiding symptoms and detrusor instability, anticholinergic agents may be used to give relief, but using anticholinergics in the face of obstruction may exacerbate poor bladder emptying. The exact time course of the irritative symptom resolution is not well documented in most incontinence procedure series. However, Cross et al. reported that 22 of 26 (85%) of patients with de novo urge incontinence/urgency treated with anticholinergics and timed voiding were symptom free within 3 months (29). In addition to pharmaceutical treatment, other conservative therapeutic options including behavioral therapy, pelvic floor exercises, biofeedback, and electrical stimulation, all of which are covered in other chapters, should be utilized.

The likelihood of spontaneous resolution or improvement of voiding dysfunction due to obstruction is small if it has not occurred after 6–12 weeks postoperatively because the periurethral scarring has fixed the proximal urethra and bladder neck to the retropubis. Thus, surgical mobilization via urethrolysis is often required to correct the iatrogenic urethral obstruction produced by hypersuspension of the urethra and bladder neck.

B. Surgical Management

1. Urethrolysis

The primary surgical approach to urethral obstruction is urethrolysis—transvaginal, retropubic, or infrapubic (30–32). As previously stated, the timing of intervention is generally related to the

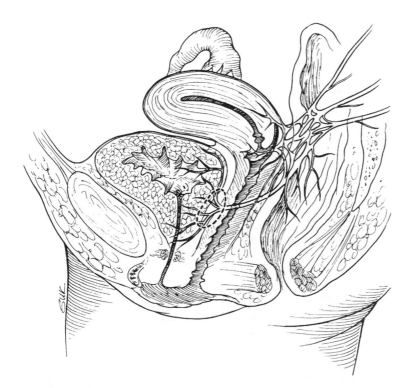

Figure 1   Inferior hypogastric innervation to the bladder.

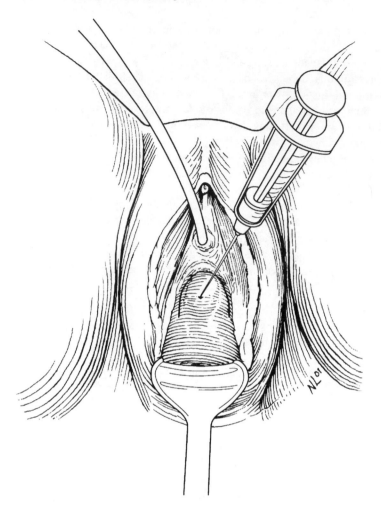

Figure 2   Injection of subtrigonal local anesthetic.

severity of the obstruction and the material used for the procedure. The selection of urethrolysis technique is based on the number of prior attempt at urethrolysis, the type of anti-incontinece procedure, and surgical experience. The individual techniques will be discussed in the following chapter.

2.   Other Surgical Procedures

If the symptoms are primarily those of detrusor instability and if urethrolysis fails to improve the problem, other surgical options may be entertained, assuming that mechanical obstruction has been eliminated. These procedures include partial bladder denervation (the Ingelman-Sundberg procedure), detrusor myectomy, sacral nerve stimulation, and augmentation cystoplasty. Detrusor myectomy, sacral nerve stimulation, and augmentation cystoplasty are covered in other sections of this text.

In the 1950s, Ingelman-Sundberg originally described the bladder denervation procedure, which relieved detrusor instability by disrupting the inferior hypogastric innervation to the

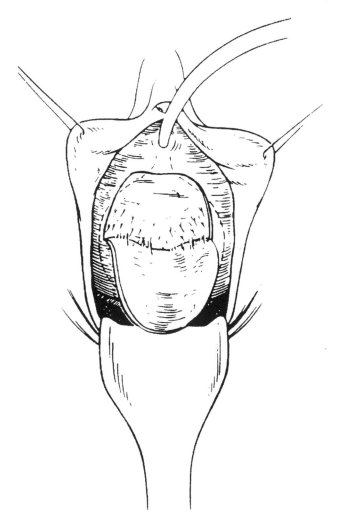

Figure 3   Inverted-U incision for subtrigonal dissection.

bladder (33) (Fig. 1). It was believed that the sensory input from the trigone was decreased while normal voiding and bladder sensation continued. Later modifications led to less extensive dissection in the transvaginal approach to the partial bladder denervation procedure for the treatment of refractory detrusor instability.

To determine who will most likely benefit from the partial bladder denervation procedure, patients are initially screened by transvaginally injecting approximately 10 mL of 0.25% bupivacaine into the subtrigonal area using a 22-gauge spinal needle to temporarily block the nerves that would be transected by the denervation procedure (Fig. 2) Patients who experienced significant relief of symptoms during the following 24 h would then be offered the partial bladder denervation procedure (34).

The patient is placed in a dorsal lithotomy position, and a 16F Foley catheter is placed into the bladder. A weighted vaginal speculum is placed for retraction. An inverted-U incision centered over the trigone is made on the anterior vaginal wall. With plane of dissection super-ficial the bladder serosa, the vaginal epithelium and perivesical fascia are sharply dissected off of the trigone, thus disrupting the innervation to this area (Fig. 3). The limits of the dissection are extended laterally and posteriorly to the terminal branches of the pelvic nerves. The vaginal mucosa incision is closed with locked running or interrupted 2-0 chromic suture; a betadine-soaked or estrogen cream–impregnated vaginal pack is placed. The procedure takes ~15–20 min. The vaginal pack and Foley catheter are removed the next day, checking the postvoid residual to confirm adequate bladder emptying.

Response rates have been demonstrated to be durable with a long-term positive response (median follow-up of 44.1 months) of 68%, with complete response in 54% and partial response in 14% (35). Thus, the Ingelman-Sundberg partial-bladder denervation procedure offers a minimally invasive option in those determined to be responders by pretest injection.

V. CONCLUSION

The surgical correction of SUI is commonly performed with very high rates of cure of the SUI. However, postoperative voiding dysfunction can decrease the patient's satisfaction with the procedure. The signs of obstruction may be UTIs, irritative symptoms, or obstructive symptoms. While the irritative symptoms may resolve spontaneously or respond to conservative measures, patients having persistent symptoms require further workup including a urodynamic evaluation. Often the only indication for additional surgery (i.e., urethrolysis) may be a temporal relationship of onset of symptoms to the anti-incontinence surgery. For those who fail to improve after urethrolysis and continue to have primarily severe irritative voiding symptoms without evidence of obstruction, the Ingelman-Sundberg partial bladder denervation, detrusor myectomy, sacral nerve stimulator, or augmentation cystoplasty are options.

REFERENCES

1. Foster HE, McGuire EJ. Management of urethral obstruction with transvaginal urethrolysis. J Urol 1993; 150:1448–1451.
2. Leach, GE, Dmochowski RR, Appell RA, Blaivas JG, Hadley HR, Luber KM, Mostwin JL, O'Donnell PD, Roehrborn CG. Female stress urinary incontinence clinical guidelines panel summary report on surgical management of female stress urinary incontinence. J Urol 1997; 158:875–880.
3. Goldman HB, Rackley RR, Appell RA. The efficacy of urethrolysis without resuspension for iatrogenic outlet obstruction. J Urol 1999; 161:196–198.
4. Cross CA, Cespedes RD, English SF, McGuire EJ. Transvaginal urethrolysis for urethral obstruction after anti-incontinence surgery. J Urol 1998; 159(4):1199–1201.
5. Appell RA. Editorial: urinary incontinence. J Urol 1994; 152:103–104.
6. Zimmern PE, Hadley HR, Leach GE, Raz S. Female urethral obstruction after Marshall–Marchetti–Krantz operation. J Urol 1987; 138:517–520.
7. McDuffie RW Jr, Litin RB, Blundin, KE. Urethrovesical suspension (Marshall–Marchetti–Krantz): experience with 204 cases. Am J Surg 1981; 141:297–298.
8. Holschneider CH, Solh S, Lebhertz TB, Montz FJ. The modified Pereyra procedure in recurrent stress urinary incontinence: a 15-Year review. Obst Gynecol 1994; 83:573–578.
9. Westney OL, McGuire EJ. Pubovaginal sling. Atlas Urol Clin North Am 2000; 8(1):23–39.
10. Romanzi LJ, Blaivas JG. Protracted urinary retention necessitating urethrolysis following tension-free vaginal tape surgery. J Urol 2000; 164:2022–2023.
11. Choe JM. Tension-free vaginal tape: is it truly tension-free? J Urol 2001; 166:1003.
12. Carlin BI, Klutke JJ, Klutke CG. The tension-free vaginal tape procedure for the treatment of stress incontinence in the female patient. Urol 2000; 56(6)(suppl 1):28–31.

13. Dmochowski RR, Appell RA. Injectable agents in the treatment of stress urinary incontinence in women: where are we now? Urol 2000; 56(6)(suppl 1): 32–40.
14. Carlson KV, Rome S, Nitti VW. Dysfunctional voiding in women. J Urol 2001; 165:143–148.
15. Schrepferman CG, Griebling TL, Nygaard IE, Kreder KJ. Resolution of urge symptoms following sling cystourethropexy. J Urol 2000; 164:1628–1631.
16. Carr LK, Webster GD. Voiding dysfunction following incontinence surgery: diagnosis and treatment with retropubic or vaginal urethrolysis. J Urol 1997; 157:821–823.
17. Nitti VW, Tu LM, Gitlin J. Diagnosing bladder outlet obstruction in women. J Urol 1999; 161:1535–1540.
18. Farrar DJ, Osborne JL, Stephenson TP, Whiteside CG, Weir J, Berry J, Milroy EJG, Turner Warwick R. A urodynamic view of bladder outflow obstruction in the female: factors influencing the results of treatment. Br J Urol 1975; 47:815–822.
19. Massey, JA, Abrams PA. Obstructed voiding in the female. Br J Urol 1988; 61:36–39.
20. Axelrod SL, Blaivas JG. Bladder neck obstruction in women. J Urol 1987; 137:497–499.
21. Chassagne S, Bernier PA, Haab F, Roehrborn CG, Reisch JS, Zimmern PE. Proposed cutoff values to define bladder outlet obstruction in women. Urology 1998; 51:408–411.
22. Groutz A, Blaivas JG, Chaiken DC. Bladder outlet obstruction in women: definition and characteristics. Neurourol Urodyn 2000; 19:213–220.
23. Lemack GE, Zimmern PE. Pressure flow analysis may aid in identifying women with outflow obstruction. J Urol 2000; 163: 1823–1828.
24. Blaivas JG, Groutz A. Bladder outlet obstruction nomogram for women with lower urinary tract symptomatology. Neurourol Urodynam 2000; 19:553–564.
25. Nitti VW, Raz S. Obstruction following anti-incontinence procedures: diagnosis and treatment with transvaginal urethrolysis. J Urol 1994; 152:93–98.
26. Dmochowski RR, Leach GE, Zimmern PE, Roskamp DA, Ganabathi K. Urethrolysis to relieve outlet obstruction after prior incontinence surgery. J Urol 1997; 151:420. Abstract.
27. Austin P, Spyropoulos E, Lotenfoe R, Helal M, Hoffman M, Lockhart JL. Urethral obstruction after anti-incontinence surgery in women: evaluation, methodology, and surgical results. Urology 1996; 47(6):890–894.
28. Carr LK, Webster GD. Bladder outlet obstruction in women (Urodynamics II). Urol Clin North Am 1996; 23(3):385–392.
29. Cross CA, Cespedes RD, McGuire EJ. Our experience with pubovaginal slings in patients with stress urinary incontinence. J Urol 1998; 159:1195–1198.
30. McGuire EJ, Letson W, Wang S. Transvaginal urethrolysis after obstructive urethral suspension procedures. J Urol 1989; 142:1037–1039.
31. Webster GD, Kreder KJ. Voiding dysfunction following cystourethropexy: its evaluation and management. J Urol 1990; 144:670–673.
32. Petrou SP, Brown JA, Blaivas JG. Suprameatal transvaginal urethrolysis. J Urol 1999; 161:1268–1271.
33. Westney OL, McGuire EJ. Surgical procedures for the treatment of urge incontinence. Tech Urol 2001; 7(2):126–132.
34. Cespedes RD, Cross CA, McGuire EJ. Modified Ingelman–Sundberg bladder denervation procedure for intractable urge incontinence. J Urol 1996; 156:1744–1747.
35. Westney OL, Lee JT, McGuire EJ, Palmer JL, Cespedes DA, Amundsen CL. Long-term results of Ingelman–Sundberg denervation procedure for urge incontinence refractory to medical therapy. J Urol 1999; 161:77. Abstract.

31

Postoperative Complications of Sling Surgery

Elizabeth A. Miller and George D. Webster
Duke University Medical Center, Durham, North Carolina, U.S.A.

I. INTRODUCTION

The sling procedure for the treatment of urinary incontinence in women was described by Goebell in 1910 using gracilis muscle (1) and was later modified by Aldrigde in 1942 (2), who first described using abdominus rectus fascia for urethral compression. Since its inception in the early part of the 20th century, the sling procedure had been modified and ultimately replaced by other forms of anti-incontinence surgery, such as the retropubic and transvaginal bladder neck suspensions. The concept of using a fascial strip to provide compression of the urethra was revitalized in 1978, when McGuire et al. (3) described its use in the treatment of type III stress urinary incontinence (SUI), or incontinence secondary to intrinsic sphincter deficiency (ISD). Until very recently, the sling procedure was thought to only be effective in the treatment of ISD, and anatomic descent was best treated with bladder neck suspension procedures. However, it is now widely accepted as an effective treatment for type II SUI, or incontinence resulting from urethral hypermobility/anatomic descent. The sling procedure has now gained widespread use by both urologists and gynecologists. Cure rates for both types II and III incontinence range from 75% to 93%, with 95–98% of women reporting significant improvement in symptoms (4,5). However, along with its success and expanded utility has come a greater knowledge of the complication profile. We are now aware of several well-described complications of the sling procedure: urethral obstruction, de novo urgency, urethral/vaginal erosion, and infection. This chapter will review the diagnosis and management of the most commonly described complications of the sling procedure.

II. URETHRAL OBSTRUCTION

A. Clinical Presentation

Urethral obstruction is an uncommon but very disturbing complication of sling surgery. The incidence of unintended urethral obstruction following the sling procedure varies and is reported to be between 1% and 4% (4,5). Common presenting symptoms of urethral obstruction other than urinary retention include new-onset urgency or urge incontinence and incomplete bladder emptying. Fifty-five percent to 93% of women complain of irritative symptoms immediately following surgery (7,8). A similarly high percentage (64–81%) either are performing intermittent catheterization for incomplete emptying or are in urinary retention (68). Not all women display obstructive symptoms, yet have urethral obstruction. In a series of women with urethral obstruction resulting from bladder neck suspension and sling procedures, one-third complained exclusively of irritative symptoms without other signs of obstruction such as retention or high postvoid residual urine volumes (9). Identification of women with urethral obstruction resulting in obstructive or irritative symptoms can be problematic, since detrusor hypocontractility and de novo urge, respectively, share this symptomatology. Urodynamic assessment, cystoscopy, and vaginal examination can help identify urethral obstruction.

B. Diagnosis: Urodynamics

Urodynamic evaluation can aid in the identification of functional obstruction following a sling procedure. The urodynamic definition of urethral obstruction in women has not been agreed upon; however, several definitions have been offered (Table 1). Nitti et al. (10) suggest that the use of video fluoroscopy may be the most sensitive tool for the detection of obstruction. Using video to identify obstruction, they found that obstructed women had higher detrusor pressures at peak flow (42.8 vs. 22.1 cmH$_2$O) and lower peak flow rates (9 vs. 20 cmH$_2$O) than unobstructed women.

Using the criteria of PDET >30–40 cmH$_2$O and PFR <15 cc/sec, Amundsen (7), Carr (11), and Nitti and Raz (12) show that only 33%, 22%, and 56%, respectively, showed no signs of obstruction, but were likely obstructed based on the temporal relationship between onset of symptoms and anti-incontinence surgery. In all three series, urethrolysis was at least 75% successful. Additionally, urodynamic evidence of obstruction does not predict favorable surgical outcomes following urethrolysis. Cross et al. (9) showed that in a comparison of those with and without urodynamics signs of obstruction, the two groups did equally well after urethrolysis. Amundsen et al. (7), in a study of 32 women, showed that of the 93.5% who had good outcomes, 41% showed no evidence of obstruction on urodynamics. In Goldman's study of 31 women, seven did not have preoperative urodynamics, and five of these (75%) had good results following takedown, a success rate similar to that of those who had had urodynamics.

Based on this information, it has been concluded that urodynamic evaluation may not be necessary in the evaluation of urethral obstruction following sling procedures. These authors feel that sufficient valuable information is obtained from the study despite these reports to justify its continued use, but certainly that equivocal studies should not be used to exclude women from a sling takedown. The most important information in making the diagnosis of urethral obstruction is the temporal relationship of the onset of symptoms to the sling procedure.

Table 1 Urodynamic Criteria for Urethral Obstruction

Author	PDET[a] (cmH$_2$O)	PFR[b] (cc/sec)
Axelrod et al. (34)	>20	<15
Massey et al. (35)	>50	<12
Petrou et al. (15)	>20	<12
Amundsen et al. (7)	<15	<12
Nitti et al. (10)	Flouroscopically	

[a]PDET: detrusor pressure at peak flow rate.
[b]PFR: peak flow rate.

C. Diagnosis: Cystoscopy and Vaginal Examination

Cystoscopy has also proven to be of benefit in diagnosing urethral obstruction in women after a sling procedure. Cystoscopy provides information on the urethral axis, the presence of urethral erosion, and loss of urethral mobility as identified by loss of the ability to sagitally rotate the urethra, all of which are important elements in diagnosing urethral obstruction. Additionally, the site of sling obstruction can often be seen as a posterior "knucle" in the urethra while viewing the lumen with a $0°$ or $30°$ lens. An estimate of the urethrovesical angle is obtained by measuring the angle of the cystoscope from horizontal that is required to maintain the urethral lumen in the center of the cystoscopic field during urethroscopy. A normal urethrovesical angle with the patient in the dorsal lithotomy position ranges from $0°$ to $30°$, where the horizontal axis is zero. An obstructed urethra following a sling procedure often demonstrates negative (the eyepiece of the cystoscope deflecting toward the floor) angulations, up to $60°$ or more. This negative angulation is the result of excessive elevation of the mid to proximal urethra by a sling which is too tight. Obstruction may also be suspected if rotation of the cystoscope in the sagittal plain is restricted. Finally, sling erosion at the mid to proximal urethral is usually easily identified with urethroscopy. Complete inspection of the bladder ensures that there is no suture or sling material inside the bladder, causing irritative symptoms.

   Vaginal examination in obstructed women following a pubovaginal sling procedure often demonstrates retropubic angulation of the anterior vaginal wall at the level of the mid to proximal urethra. The vaginal examination is also important in identifying other vaginal pathology that may or may not be related to sling obstruction, such as vaginal erosions and prolapse. Concurrent pathologies should be treated at the time of incision of the obstructing sling.

D. Treatment

Obstruction following a pubovaginal sling procedure can be treated by incising the sling or by performing urethrolysis. Several approaches to sling incision or takedown have been described (7,8). Our preferred technique is to incise the sling in the midline direcely beneath the urethra. The sling is approached through a midline anterior vaginal wall incision, the incision being carefully deepened until the often pristine and usually easily identifiable transversely oriented fibers of the sling are encountered. The sling is often deeply located and the bladder may fold over the sling, making the dissection quite intimidating. Repeated palpation of the sling over the shaft of the cystoscope will help direct the dissection (6). The sling is circumferentially isolated (Fig. 1) and incised in the midline and generally the urethra immediately sags between the separated sling ends, confirming the release. Occasionally, more urethral mobility is needed and the sling ends may be further dissected off of the urethra laterally (Fig. 2). Intraoperatively, the success of the procedure may be determined by creding the full bladder and observing the resulting urinary stream and by confirming restoration of adequate sagittal mobility using the cystoscope. Amundsen et al. reported that 93.5% achieved efficient voiding within 1 week of the procedure. Sixty-seven percent with urge incontinence had resolution of their symptoms. Only three of 32 women in this study reported SUI symptoms following sling takedown; one of these went on to receive periurethral collagen injection therapy.

   Others have reported that urethrolysis can be performed for sling obstruction with equally effective results. Vaginal urethrolysis for obstruction following abdominal and transvaginal bladder neck suspension procedures was described by Zimmern (13) and Kreder (14) and applied by several others in the treatment of sling and bladder neck suspension obstruction. Its use in the treatment of sling obstruction has never been evaluated exclusively, since most reported series include both sling and bladder neck suspensions without stratifying by procedure. However, according to recent reports (8,9), the technique has been found to be effective for both,

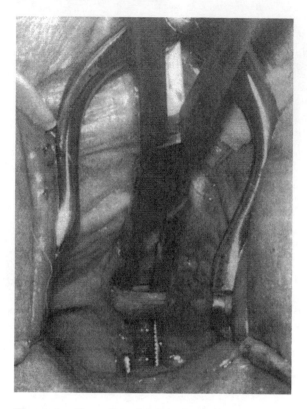

Figure 1 Circumferential dissection of the sling in preparation for incision.

but it requires considerably more dissection than simple midline sling incision. We feel the formal urethrolysis should be reserved for those in whom sling incision fails.

A variety of vaginal incisions can be employed for urethrolysis, including inverted U-shaped, midline, paramedian, or suprameatal (15). The vaginal epithelium is elevated on either side of the urethra, at the level of the obstruction (usually mid to proximal urethra). The vesicopelvic and endopelvic fascial layers are incised sharply, and the retropubic attachments of the urethra to symphysis are released. The endpoint of dissection is marked by achieving sufficient urethral mobility as demonstrated by posterior rotation of the urethra while applying pressure on the Foley catheter or a transurethral instrument (9) or complete circumferential mobilization of the urethra from the undersurface of the symphysis (8). Although outcome measures vary by study, 84–87% of women have significant improvement in voiding efficiency (8,9), with a similar improvement in irritative symptoms (85%) and an overall cure rate of 72% for both irritative and obstructive symptoms (9). Application of a Martius labial fat pad flap is often necessary to prevent recurrence of urethral-symphyseal attachment with recurrent obstruction in cases of secondary urethrolysis.

Recurrent incontinence following surgery to relieve sling obstruction ranges from 0% to 23%. The variation likely depends on the degree to which the urethra is mobilized. The suprameatal approach is a unique approach to urethrolysis that limits lateral dissection and is said to prevent recurrent incontinence (15). This technique uses an inverted U-shaped incision from 9 to 3 o'clock 1 cm anterior to the urethral meatus. The plane between the urethra and undersurface of the symphysis is developed, allowing direct visualization of the sling. This technique differs from the previously described transvaginal urethrolysis in that the tethering

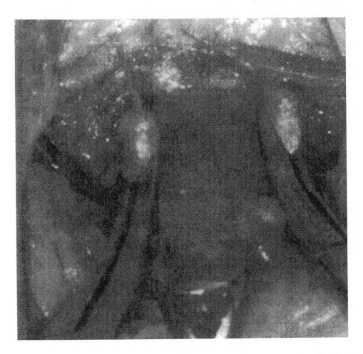

Figure 2 Clamped incised ends of the sling in preparation for further mobilization.

attachments can be released under direct vision, while the lateral vesicopelvic ligament is left intact. Petrou et al. believe that by maintaining continuity of the vesicopelvic ligament, recurrent incontinence can be prevented. There were no patients in their series of 12 women who complained of posturethrolysis incontinence, compared with 2.5–19% in other transvaginal urethrolysis series (8,9). However, resolution of retention was not as good in this series compared to others (Table 2).

Outcomes of urethrolysis or sling takedown may be dependent on the degree to which the urethra is mobilized, or the presling anatomy is restored. Most women find the symptoms of obstructions to be more bothersome than those of recurrent incontinence, and therefore are more willing to trade the latter for resolution of irritative and obstructive symptoms. Therefore, the goal of sling takedown or urethrolysis should be restoration of normal and efficient voiding.

E. Prevention of Urethral Obstruction

To our knowledge, there have been no practically useful and proven techniques to prevent urethral obstruction during sling placement. However, most agree that there should be no tension

Table 2 Outcomes of Urethrolysis or Sling Incision for Treatment of Sling Obstruction

Author	Resolution of retention (%)	Resolution of urgency (%)	Recurrent incontinent (%)
Amundsen et al. (5)	93.5	67	9
Cross et al. (13)	87	85	2.5
Goldman et al. (8)	84	NA	19
Petrou et al. (15)	65	67	0

on the sling and therefore no visible compression of the urethra once the sling is secured in place with the patient in the dorsal lithotomy position. Urethral compression by the sling is activated during rises in intraabdominal pressure, as shown flouroscopically by Ghoneim et al. (16) They showed flouroscopically that during straining the sling moves upward and cephalad, while the bladder base moves downward and caudad. Appropriate tension, therefore, allows for urethral compression during rises in intra-abdominal pressure only.

Several ideas have been proposed to identify the appropriate tension intraoperatively. Measuring urethral pressure during the sling placement has been proposed but has not been proven technically practical (3). Yamada et al. proposed ultrasounding the urethra-vesical angle to identify inappropriate angulation of the urethra during sling placement. Finally, Blaivas and Jacobs recommend placing downward tension on a cystoscope placed in the urethra while securing the sling. The authors prefer to hold the sling several millimeters from the urethra, while the assistant ties the suspending prolene sutures suprapubically. In this way, the sling is positioned loosely beneath the urethra.

It is certainly true to say that sling tension probably needs to vary from patient to patient depending on the degree of urethral hypermobility, the rigidity of the urethra, and perhaps even the magnitude of the intrinsic sphincter deficiency. This is an evolving science, and at present we have no objective way by which to determine the individual patient's needs. Indeed, it is also evident to all who perform pubovaginal sling surgery that sling tension seen at surgery may be very different from what is seen several weeks later. We believe that it may be possible that the sling, in some cases, shrinks during the remodeling process, or that the tension in the surgical position may not translate into that which exists in the upright, ambulatory position, so that despite appropriate tension placed at the time of surgery, urethral obstruction develops.

III. DE NOVO URGE

The etiology of new urge symptoms (de novo urge) after pubovaginal sling procedure is not known. The incidence is reported to range from 7% to 17.5% (5,17,19). This incidence is somewhat lower (0–15.6%) in recent outcome studies of the polypropylene mesh midurethral sling (TVT or SPARC systems) (22,23). Often a thorough evaluation including vaginal examination, cystoscopy, and urodynamics in a patient with new-onset urgency after a sling procedure will reveal obstruction. Irritative symptoms will resolve in up to 67–85% following incision of the obstruction sling, or urethrolysis without additional treatments, as was discussed in the previous section. When obstruction has been definitively ruled out, de novo urge is present by exclusion.

De novo urge may resolve within several months of the sling procedure. Kaplan et al. (19) report one of the largest prospective analysis of the pubovaginal sling procedure. In this series, 30 of 373 women developed de novo urge, and eight of these (26%) had resolution of their symptoms by the average 40-month follow-up interval. In a similar series of women undergoing fascial sling, Juma et al. (24) found that 50% of those who reported initial de novo urge had persistent urge several months after the sling procedure. Although most long-term studies have not identified rates of de novo urge resolution, from our experience, most urge incontinence that is seen in the early postoperative period, without coexistence of obstruction, will resolve. In the interim, symptoms can be managed with a combination of behavioral therapy, pelvic floor reeducation and strengthening, and anticholinergic medication such as tolterodine (Detrol) or oxybutynin (Ditropan) with excellent results. If conservative management is not effective in controlling irritative symptoms, the diagnosis of urethral obstruction should be readdressed.

IV. URETHRAL EROSION OR VAGINAL EXTRUSION

A. Clinical Presentation

Erosion of sling material either into the urethra or through the vaginal epithelium is rare and is seen most commonly when synthetic sling material is used. The incidence of synthetic sling erosion ranges widely, from 0% to 23% (25,26,28). However, more contemporary series have reported lower erosion rates. The Female Stress Urinary Incontinence Clinical Guidelines Panel of 1997 performed a rigorously selected meta-analysis of the incontinence literature dating from 1994 to 1997, and found the incidence of vaginal and urethral erosions with synthetic material was 0.007% and 0.02%, respectively (29). In one of the largest and most recently reported synthetic sling experiences to date, Choe and Staskin (25) report that five of 141 (4%) consecutive Gortex patch slings developed vaginal erosions, and there were no urethral erosions. Vaginal erosion rates with polypropylene mesh slings using the TVT system are similarly low, 0.4%, with no reported urethral erosions (22). Kobashi et al. (30) found the prevalence of vaginal erosions to be more common than urethral extrusion. Their study reviewed 34 women who presented with woven polyester sling erosion: 50% vaginal, 20% urethral, and 17% concurrent urethrovaginal. Erosion using autologous or allogenic fascial slings is reported to be 0.007% according to the Female Stress Urinary Incontinence Clinical Guidelines Panel, and reported only in case series (31,32). Autologous and allogenic fascial erosions more commonly involve the urethra as the result of excessive sling tension during initial placement. Amundsen and Webster (33) recently reported a series of nine patients who developed urethral erosion and sling obstruction. The nine slings involved included: allograft fascia lata (5), autologous rectus (1), woven polyester treated with bovine collagen (2), and Prolene mesh (1).

We feel that it is important to differentiate between urethral and vaginal erosion of sling material. In the former, the sling material is surgically removed from the urethral lumen, and the urethra is closed, while vaginal expulsion of sling material can be treated more conservatively (see Sec. IV.C below).

B. Diagnosis

Chronic vaginal discharge and vaginal pain or pressure are the most common presenting symptoms of vaginal erosion. Vaginal examination may reveal granulation tissue, without overt evidence of erosion. However, careful examination will uncover sling material beneath the granulation tissue in most cases. Symptoms of urethral erosion include dysuria and urethral pain, irritative voiding symptoms, recurrent incontinence or urinary retention, and macro- or microscopic hematuria. In Amundsen's recent report of sling urethral erosions (33), 50% presented with retention, while the remaining had urge incontinence requiring at least three pads per day. Urethral erosion should also be suspected when a patient complains of persistent dysuria, without evidence of urinary tract infection. The diagnosis is made by urethroscopy, which reveals the sling as a glistening white material within the urethral lumen or at the 6 o'clock position. Erosions of either type have been reported to occur up to 4 years from the time of the initial surgery. Golomb et al. (32) report a case of an autologous fascial sling in which the patient developed an acute UTI and urinary retention. The catheterization was traumatic, and shortly thereafter the patient developed severe irritative symptoms. Barbalias and Barbalias (28) similarly report two patients in which their Gortex sling erosion presented 3.5 years after initial placement. Therefore, the index of suspicion for a vaginal or urethral erosion should remain high when women present with classic symptoms of erosion, despite the time interval between placement and presentation.

C. Treatment

Treatment of urethral or vaginal erosion requires sling removal. Synthetic sling material must be removed completely. Autologous and allogenic material should be removed at the site of erosion, but residual material located lateral to the urethra and within the retropubic space may be left in situ (32,33). Suspending sutures for both synthetic and autologous/allogenic may also remain in place. Synthetic slings are associated with a variable degree of scar. Some are encased in a pseudosheath and are easily removed (30). Others are heavily embedded in dense fibrosis. Autologous and allogenic slings are usually found with very little reactive tissue and well preserved (7). After removing sling material, the urethra may be primarily closed with absorbable suture, or left open to heal with catheter stenting. We prefer primary closure of the urethra. Martius labial fat flaps may be used to cover the urethra in the event that urethral damage is significant, or vaginal and urethral erosions have occurred concurrently and where fistula development is feared. Extensive vaginal erosion may be covered with a Martius skin island pedicle flap. When treating urethral erosions, a urethral catheter is usually left in place for 7 days, or alternatively, the urine may be diverted with a suprapubic catheter for a similar amount of time. Some recommend a voiding cystourethrogram prior to suprapubic tube removal to ensure urethral integrity.

Vaginal erosions of autologous or allogenic sling material very often epithelialize over and do not need surgical revision. This process can be aided with the use of topical estrogen cream. When synthetic material has eroded through the vaginal epithelium, it can be locally excised with good success.

V. CONCLUSION

In summary, the sling procedure for stress urinary incontinence is a safe and effective procedure. The most common complications, urethral obstruction, de novo urge, and sling erosion, are uncommon and can usually be managed effectively.

REFERENCES

1. Goebell R. Zur operativen beseitigung der angebornen inctoninentia vesicae. Ztschr Gynak 1910; 2:187–190.
2. Aldridge A. Transplantation of fascia for relief of urinary stress incontinence. Am J Obstet Gynecol 1942; 44:398–342.
3. McGuire E, Lytton B. Pubovaginal sling procedure for stress incontinence. J Urol 1978; 1191:82–84.
4. Wright JE, Carr LK, Webster GD. Pubovaginal sling using cadaveric allograft fascia for the treatment of intrinsic sphincter deficiency. J Urol 1998; 160:759–762.
5. Cross CA, McGuire EJ. Our experience with pubovaginal slings in patients with stress urinary incontinence. J Urol 1998; 159:1195–1198.
6. Webster GD. Cadaveric fascia slings. Atlas of the Urol Clinics of North America 2000; 81:41–49.
7. Amundsen CL, Webster GD. Variations in strategy for the treatment of urethral obstruction after a pubovaginal sling procedure. J Urol 2000; 164:434–437.
8. Goldman HB, Rackley RR, Appell RA. The efficacy of urethrolysis without re-suspension for iatrogenic urethral obstruction. J Urol 1999; 1611:196–198; discussion 198–199.
9. Cross CA, Cespedes RD, English SF, McGuire EJ. Transvaginal urethrolysis for urethral obstruction after anti-incontinence surgery. J Urol 1998; 1594:199–1201.
10. Nitti VW, Gitlin J. Diagnosing bladder outlet obstruction in women. J Urol 1999; 161:535–1540.

11. Carr LK, Webster GD. Voiding dysfunction following incontinence surgery: diagnosis and treatment with retropubic or vaginal urethrolysis. J Urol 1997; 1573:821–823.
12. Nitti VW, Raz S. Obstruction following anti-incontinence procedures: diagnosis and treatment with transvaginal urethrolysis. J Urol 1994; 1521:93–98.
13. Zimmern PE, Hadley HR, Leach, GE, Raz S. Female urethral obstruction after Marshall-Marchetti-Krantz operation. J Urol 1987; 138:517.
14. Webster GD, Kreber KJ. Voiding dysfunction following cystourethropexy: its evaluation and management. J Urol 1990; 144:670–673.
15. Petrou SP, Brown JA, Blaivas JG. Suprameatal transvaginal urethrolysis. J Urol 1999; 1614:1268–1271.
16. Ghoniem GM, Kapoor DS. Nonautologous sling material. J Urol 2001; 2(5):357–363.
17. Kuo H. Anatomical and functional results of pubovaginal sling procedure using polyproplyene mesh for the treatment of stress urinary incontinence. J Urol 2001; 166:152–157.
18. McGuire EJ, O. C. H. Surgical treatment of intrinsic urethral dysfunction. Urologic Clinics of North America 1995; 223:657–664.
19. Kaplan SA, Te AE, Young GP, Andrade A, Cabelin MA, Ikeguchi EF. Prospective analysis of 373 consecutive women with stress urinary incontinence treated with a vaginal wall sling: the Columbia–Cornell University experience. J Urol 2000; 1645:1623–1627.
20. Morgan T, O Jr, Westney OL, McGuire EJ. Pubovaginal sling: 4-Year outcome analysis and quality of life assessment. J Urol 2000; 1636:1845–1848.
21. Chaikin DC, Rosenthal J, Blaivas JG. Pubovaginal fascial sling for all types of stress urinary incontinence: long-term analysis. J Urol 1998; 1604:1312–1316.
22. Abouassaly R, Corcos J. Complications of tension-free vaginal tape surgery: a multi-institutional review of 242 cases. AUA Annual Meeting 2002.
23. White M, Katz D, Stone AR. Tension free vaginal tape versus pubovaginal sling: is there a difference in quality of life? AUA Annual Meeting 2002.
24. Juma S, Little NA, Raz S. Vaginal wall sling: four years later. Urology 1992; 395:424–428.
25. Choe JM, Staskin DR. Gore-Tex patch sling: 7 years later. Urology 1999; 544:641–646.
26. Hom D, Desautel MG, Lumerman JH, Feraren RE, Badlani GH. Pubovaginal sling using polypropylene mesh and vesica bone anchors. Urology 1998; 515:708–713.
27. Bent AE, Ostergard DR, Zwick-Zaffuto M. Tissue reaction to expanded polytetrafluoroethylene suburethral sling for urinary incontinence: clinical and histologic study. Am J Obstet Gynecol 1993; 1695:1198–1204.
28. Barbalias G, Barbalias D. Use of slings made of indigenous and allogenic material (Gortex) in type III urinary incontinence and comparison between them. Eur Urol 1997; 31:394–396.
29. Leach GE, Appell RA. Female Stress Urinary Incontinence Clinical Guidelines Panel summary report on surgical management of female stress urinary incontinence. J Urol 1997; 157:875.
30. Kobashi KC, Dmochowski R, Mee SL, Mostwin J, Nitti VW, Zimmern PE, Leach GE. Erosion of woven polyester pubovaginal sling. J Urol 1999; 1626:2070–2072.
31. Handa VL, Stone A. Erosion of a fascial sling into the urethra. Urology 1999; 545:923.
32. Golomb J, Groutz A, Mor Y, Leibovitch I, Ramon J. Leibovitch J. Management of urethral erosion caused by pubovaginal fascial sling. Urology 2001; 571:159–160.
33. Amundsen CL, Webster GD. Continence outcome and management following urethral erosion of the pubovaginal sling. AUA Annual Meeting 2002.
34. Axelrod SL. Bladder neck obstruction in women. J Urol 1987; 137:497.
35. Massey JA. Obstructed voiding in the female. B J Urol 1988; 61:36.

32

Detrusor Myomectomy

Patrick J. Shenot
Thomas Jefferson University, Philadelphia, Pennsylvania, U.S.A.

I. INTRODUCTION

The efficacy of enterocystoplasty has been demonstrated in numerous studies. Clinical success, measured by improved patient quality of life and decreased upper urinary tract complications, has been clearly established. The requirement of bowel segment isolation and reanastomosis, however, has a significant risk of early complications, such anastomotic leakage or intestinal obstruction.

Potential long-term sequelae of enterocystoplasty include bowel dysfunction, metabolic derangements, and spontaneous perforation of the intestinal segment. Urinary retention requiring intermittent catheterization may be required for at least 15% of patients following enterocystoplasty (1). Enterocystoplasty may also predispose to the subsequent development of malignancy. A growing number of malignancies have been reported in the world literature in patients who have undergone enterocystoplasty (2–4).

Detrusor myomectomy, also termed bladder autoaugmentation, is a technique that increases bladder capacity and lowers intravesical storage pressures without the use of intestinal segments. By utilizing only autologous bladder tissue, it is hoped that low-pressure bladder storage will be assured while also minimizing the risk of complications by eliminating involvement of the gastrointestinal system in this urologic reconstruction procedure.

Autoaugmentation of the urinary bladder is accomplished by disruption of the detrusor musculature to an extent significant to permit the eventual formation of a large bladder diverticulum, which can effectively reduce abnormal contractility and improve the functional capacity of the bladder. The disruption of the detrusor can be accomplished using a simple incision, referred to as a myomyotomy, although greater success has been achieved with myomectomy, where a patch of detrusor muscle is actually removed from the anterior surface of the bladder.

II. HISTORY OF ENTEROCYSTOPLASTY AND DETRUSOR MYOMECTOMY

Anticholinergic and other pharmacological agents are often effective in decreasing uninhibited detrusor contractions. These medications also represent the first line of treatment for the high-pressure, noncompliant, small-capacity bladder, although patients usually require an intermittent catheterization program once satisfactory storage pressure is achieved. When medical therapy fails to improve continence and bladder storage parameters, surgical bladder augmentation is often employed.

Tizzoni and Foggi reported the first use of small intestine as a tissue graft for bladder augmentation, enterocystoplasty, in dogs in 1888 (5). Ten years later, the first human ileocystoplasty was performed by Mikulicz (6). Currently, enterocystoplasty remains the standard treatment for the surgical correction of the small-capacity, poorly compliant bladder that is unresponsive to medical therapy. This technique is also useful in patients with intractable urge incontinence who have failed less invasive therapies.

Although generally effective, potential problems may be associated with the use of gastrointestinal segments for bladder augmentation. In the case of intestinal segments, these structures tend to retain at least some of their absorptive function. The reabsorption of urinary solutes may result in the development of electrolyte abnormalities, especially during periods of dehydration or in patients with renal insufficiency (7). In the creation of intestino-intestinal and intestino-vesical anastomoses, one must be aware of the potential for anastomotic leakage, fistula formation, and possibly intestinal obstruction to occur postoperatively.

Several other concerns have arisen with the development of bladder augmentation techniques. Mucus, produced by the intestinal segment, has proved bothersome and may partially occlude drainage catheters, requiring intermittent irrigation of the bladder. In some patients, bowel peristalsis has contributed to episodic urinary leakage after intestinal bladder augmentation. Deficiency of vitamin B_{12} may result in pernicious anemia in those with isolation of the terminal ileum from the fecal stream, while adenocarcinoma has developed in some patients in the bowel segments used for bladder augmentation. These problems, as well as the direct complications of a bowel segment isolation, have encouraged the development of alternative methods to improve urinary storage without involvement of the gastrointestinal system.

During the past 30 years, various nonintestinal materials have been studied for potential application during bladder augmentation. Many investigators have tried a variety of natural or synthetic tissues including free fascial grafts, lyophilized dura, pericardium, and placental membranes. In addition, the use of synthetic materials such as polytetrafluoroethylene (Teflon), felt, and a gelatin sponge material has been attempted (8–12). None of these materials have proven to be suitable for bladder augmentation because of the development of infections, rejection, scarring and graft contracture, metaplastic bone and/or calculus stone formation, or urinary fistula formation.

Cartwright and Snow in 1989 reported a technique which they named bladder autoaugmentation (13,14). The principle of this surgical technique is that the detrusor muscle over the dome of the bladder is excised leaving the underlying bladder urothelium intact. A large bladder diverticulum results in augmented bladder capacity and permits the low-pressure storage of urine. Since no other tissue is used, the term autoaugmentation was coined. Both myomyotomy and myomectomy have been advocated for bladder autoaugmentation. Most experienced investigators recommend the more extensive myomectomy rather than a simply myomyotomy because of improved success rates. There is little evidence to support the routine use of detrusor myomyotomy.

Detrusor myomectomy in adults may offer many advantages over enterocystoplasty. Because intestinal manipulation is avoided, anastomotic complications and electrolyte problems should not occur. The entire procedure may be performed extraperitoneally, which also will minimize effects on the intestine. It is possible that autoaugmentation is ideal for the patient who has undergone previous abdominal surgery and is left with significant intraperitoneal scarring, or who could be at risk for the short bowel syndrome if an intestinal segment was isolated for use in enterocystoplasty.

III. TECHNIQUES OF DETRUSOR MYOMECTOMY

A. Preoperative Preparation

Preoperatively, all patients should undergo a thorough medical evaluation including videourodynamics to determine the functional status of the bladder and sphincter. Surgical intervention is appropriate if alternative therapies have failed to improve symptoms of frequency, urgency, and incontinence. Although intermittent catheterization is not required in all patients, the ability and willingness of patients to perform this postoperatively should be confirmed before contemplating this procedure. Clean intermittent catheterization technique should ideally be taught before the procedure as part of routine preoperative teaching. We routinely utilize both mechanical and antibiotic bowel preparation prior to surgery. If detrusorectomy is found to be technically impossible intraoperatively, conventional enterocystoplasty can be accomplished if the bowel preparation has been performed. Intravenous antibiotics are administered pre-operatively.

B. Operative Technique

The urethral meatus is prepped into the operative field to allow placement of an indwelling urethral catheter with self-retaining balloon. The retropubic space may be exposed using either a Pfannensteil or low midline abdominal incision. The bladder is exposed and filled with saline. The catheter may be connected with a Y connector to both a normal saline reservoir for irrigation and a drainage bag to facilitate distension and emptying of the bladder during dissection. The anterior wall of the bladder is identified, with gentle blunt and sharp dissection used to free the peritoneum from the bladder surface (Fig. 1). Detrusor myomectomy may be performed using either the intraperitoneal or extraperitoneal approach. At the present time, most surgeons experienced in this technique strongly recommend an extraperitoneal approach so that the peritoneum can act to reinforce to bladder diverticulum created by the myomectomy, preventing

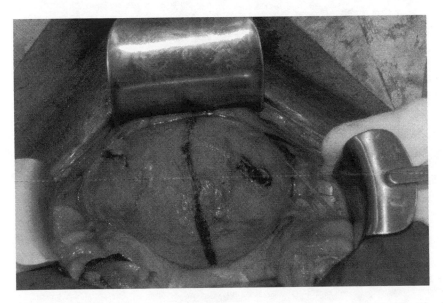

Figure 1 Extraperitoneal exposure of the anterior wall and dome of the bladder. The detrusor is scored with electrocautery in the midline.

intraperitoneal leak and decreasing the risk of rupture. Once adequate exposure is achieved, the detrusor muscle is scored in the midline using needle-tip electrocautery.

The incision is extended from anterior to posterior over the entire dome of the bladder. After the detrusor has been divided through three-fourths of its thickness, the muscle is separated from the urothelium using a fine hemostat or a Kitner dissector. The remaining detrusor fibers overlying the epithelium are gently spread apart with a hemostat until they are disrupted. Thus, the bladder epithelium becomes exposed along the entire length of detrusor incision (Fig. 2). Although not technically demanding, this dissection can be tedious, especially in highly trabeculated bladders. It is imperative to minimize inadvertant tears of the bladder epithilium as these can prevent adequate bladder distension and make the subsequent dissection much more difficult.

The detrusor margin on one side of the incision is then grasped with Allis clamps while the bladder is fully distended. A plane is developed using blunt dissection between the detrusor muscle and the intact bladder epithelium, proceeding laterally. This plane of dissection is maintained while keeping the epithelium intact. The dissection progresses laterally in each direction up to the entire dome until at least one-half to two-thirds of the detrusor muscle of the entire bladder is stripped away from the epithelium.

During the myomectomy, the bladder is repeatedly emptied and filled with saline through the urethral catheter to facilitate the dissection. Small openings in the epithelium are repaired with the application of a right-angle clamp to the opening which is then secured with a 4-0 chromic ligature. After the detrusor is freed from the mucosal epithelium, the redundant detrusor

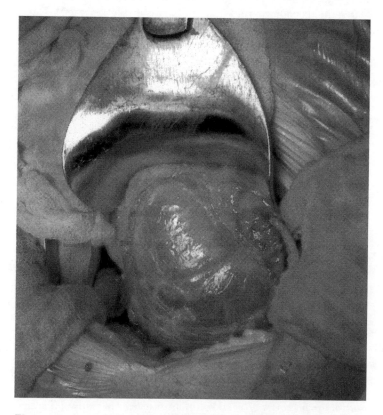

Figure 2   Epithelium bulging through detrusor myomotomy.

flaps are excised. We attempt to remove the detrusor from the entire anterior and lateral surfaces of the bladder (Fig. 3). To achieve this extensive myomectomy, the superior vascular bladder pedicles must be sacrificed, with the dissection extending laterally and inferiorly to the level of the inferior bladder pedicle. Bilateral psoas hitches may be performed using absorbable suture to prevent reannealment of the cut detrusor edges, although this is usually unnecessary. At the completion of the procedure, the prevesical space should be drained.

C. Postoperative Care

The surgical result of myomectomy is that of a thin, quite large diverticular patch of bladder epithelium, bulging from the bladder as it is filled. An exposed segment of very thin mucosa may be at increased risk of rupture because of increased wall tension at large capacity. The mucosal diverticulum, however, may become protected by a layer of peritoneum and omentum of adequate thickness to reduce the risk of rupture. Postoperatively, a urethral catheter is left indwelling. Cyclic distension and drainage of the bladder with saline irrigant may help avoid scarring of the autoaugmentation in the contracted position. Alternatively, the catheter may be put to 20 cm of back pressure by draping it over the bedrail. Cystography is performed 3–5 days postoperatively. If no extravasation is evident, the indwelling catheter is removed, and, if necessary, the patient may begin an intermittent catheterization program. Initially, intermittent catheterization is performed every 3–4 h. As the diverticulum created by the autoaugmentation matures, the interval between catheterizations can be lengthened. Patients are maintained on a prophylactic regimen of antimicrobial therapy at least until the indwelling catheter is removed. Postoperatively, patients are evaluated with a videourodynamic evaluation 3 months following surgery (Fig. 4). Urodynamic follow-up is most important in patients with poor compliance who are at risk for upper urinary tract compromise. Anticholinergic agents may be administered to

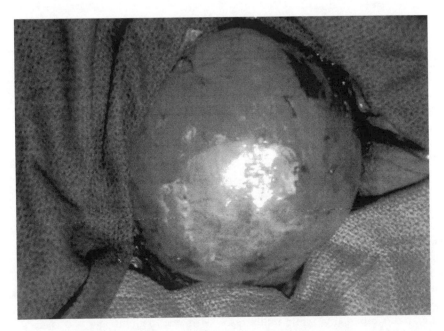

Figure 3   Completed detrusor myomectomy. Note the Foley catheter balloon visible through the thin translucent bladder epithelium.

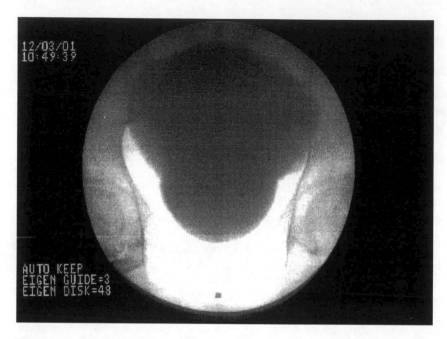

Figure 4   Cystogram obtained from videourodynamic study 3 months following detrusor myomectomy. The large augmented segment is clearly seen arising from the bladder dome.

assure low-pressure urinary storage. The anticholinegic regimen can eventually be tapered and ultimately discontinued.

IV. CLINICAL RESULTS OF DETRUSOR MYOMECTOMY

Following initial success with an animal model, Cartwright and Snow (13,14) utilized this technique in seven pediatric patients with both neurogenic and nonneurogenic voiding dysfunction. This procedure resulted in marked clinical improvement in five patients, although one showed only modest improvement and one eventually required enterocystoplasty. Bladder capacity improved in three of the five patients studied urodynamically, while compliance improved in four.

After performing this procedure on 19 patients, Cartwright and Snow have noted that although bladder capacity did not consistently increase after autoaugmentation, most patients developed improvement in their urinary storage pressure. Thus, urinary storage occurs under lower pressure postoperatively, accompanied not only by improved continence but also by improvement in upper urinary tract dilatation.

Stohrer and associates in Germany performed the first autoaugmentation on an adult bladder in 1989. Since then, Stohrer et al. have reported their experience in 29 patients with neurogenic and nonneurogenic voiding dysfunction (15). In this report, the majority of patients were able to void spontaneously postoperatively. Preoperatively, three patients required intermittent catheterization for urinary drainage, while postoperatively, an intermittent catheterization program was used by 12 patients. Preoperatively, five patients demonstrated vesicoureteral reflux radiographically, while reflux resolved in two patients and was reduced from bilateral to unilateral in two additional patients. No complications occurred as a result of autoaugmentation. Subjective success was reported as excellent in 16 patients and as good in eight cases. A later study by the same investigators confirmed the efficacy of this procedure in 50 patients treated with this technique. (16).

In 1994, Kennelly and associates reported on the treatment of a small capacity, poorly compliant bladder with autoaugmentation in five patients, 18–73 years old (17). Operative time averaged only 106 min, and the hospital stay was only 6 days for this patient group. No postoperative complications occurred. In follow-up ranging from 12 to 82 weeks, bladder capacity increased from 75 mL to 310 mL, or from 40% to 310%. Compliance improved in all patients. While three patients demonstrated reflux preoperatively, this resolved in one patient and improved in two patients. Of four patients who were incontinent preoperatively, three became continent and extended the interval between catheterizations. Upper tract function remained stable, and no patient required enterocystoplasty to control elevated intravesical pressure.

Leng and colleagues reported on a heterogeneous group of 61 patients who had undergone 37 primary detrusor myomectomies and compared their outcomes to 32 enterocystoplasties (18). Eight patients with detrusor instability underwent detrusor myomectomy. All eight demonstrated urodynamic improvement, with all but one patient spontaneously voiding postoperatively. One patient reported persistent urge incontinence and subsequently underwent enterocystoplasty. Leng et al. also noted clinical and urodynamic improvement in three of six patients with radiation cystitis who underwent this procedure. They report an overall 73% success rate in this diverse group of patients treated with primary detrusor myomectomy. Of note, the rate of serious complications was 22% in patients undergoing enterocystoplasty but only 3% in those treated with primary detrusor myomectomy.

Given that autoaugmentation is successful in improving urinary storage, refinement of the technique could reduce operative time, hospital stay, and the rate of complications. The recent trend in minimally invasive surgery has spurred several investigators to employ laparoscopy to achieve bladder autoaugmentation (19–21). This alternative surgical approach has been reported in very small numbers of patients with limited follow-up. To date, this approach has not been widely utilized.

V. APPLICATION OF DETRUSOR MYOMECTOMY

Although detrusor myomectomy offers definite advantages when compared to traditional techniques, it is clear that the results of this procedure with regard to increases in bladder capacity and reduced detrusor overactivity indicate that this technique is inferior to conventional enterocystoplasty. With any novel technique, enthusiastic preliminary reports are often made before the potential complications have been realized. The number of cases reported is small with relatively short follow-up. Currently, detrusor myomectomy should be offered only to highly selected patients who would otherwise be candidates for conventional enterocystoplasty. The ability to improve urinary storage capacity in patients with intractable urge incontinence without disturbance of the gastrointestinal system may greatly reduce the rate of serious complications. Since this is an extraperitoneal procedure, it may be ideal for patients with previous intraperitoneal surgery. Lastly, the laparoscopic approach to detrusor myomectomy may evolve into viable minimally invasive procedure for the treatment of refractory detrusor overactivity.

REFERENCES

1. Mundy AR, Stephenson TP. "Clam" ileocystoplasty for the treatment of refractory urge incontinence. Br J Urol 1988; 140:641–646.

2. Filmer RB, Spencer JR. Malignancies in bladder augmentation and intestinal conduits. J Urol 1990; 143:671–678.
3. Hasegawa S, Ohshima S, Kinukawa T, Matsuura O, Takeuchi Y, Hattori R, Murakami S. Adenocarcinoma of the bladder 29 years after ileocystoplasty. Br J Urol 1988; 61:162.
4. Ali-El-Dein B, El-Tabey N, Abdel-Latif M, Abdel-Rahim M, El-Bahnasawy MS. Late uro-ileal cancer after incorporation of ileum into the urinary tract. J Urol 2002; 167:84–88.
5. Tizzoni G, Foggi A. Die Wiederhestellung der Harnbalase. Centralbl Chir 1888; 15:921.
6. Miculicz J. Zur Operation der angeborenen Blasenspalte. Zentralb Chir 1898; 26:641.
7. Nurse DE, Mundy AR. Metabolic complications of cystoplasty. Br J Urol 1989; 63:165–170.
8. Kelami A, Dustmann HO, Ludtke-Handjery A, Carcamo V, Herold G. Experimental investigations of bladder regeneration using Teflon felt as a bladder wall substitute. J Urol 1970; 104:693–698.
9. Kelsmi A. Lyophilized human dura as a bladder wall substitute: experimental and clinical results. J Urol 1971; 105:518–522.
10. Fishman LJ, Flores FN, Scott FB, Spjut HJ, Morrow B. Use of fresh placental membranes for bladder reconstruction. J Urol 1987; 138:1291–1294.
11. Telly O. Segmental cystectomy with peritoneoplasty. Urol Int 1970; 25:236.
12. Taguchi H, Ishizuka E, Saito K. Cystoplasty by regeneration of the bladder. J Urol 1977; 118: 752–756.
13. Cartwright PC, Snow BW. Bladder autoaugmentation: early clinical experience. J Urol 1989; 142: 520–521.
14. Cartwright PC, Snow BW. Bladder autoaugmentation: partial detrusor excision to augment the bladder without use of bowel. J Urol 1989; 142:1050–1053.
15. Stohrer M, Kramer A, Goepel M, Lochner-Ernst D, Kruse D, Rubben H. Bladder autoaugmentation— an alternative for enterocystoplasty. Neurourol Urodyn 1995; 14:11–23.
16. Stohrer M, Kramer G, Goepel M, Lochner-Ernst D, Kruse D, Rubben H. Bladder autoaugmentation in adult patients with neurogenic voiding dysfunction. Spinal Cord 1997; 35:456–462.
17. Kennelly MJ, Gormley EA, McGuire EJ. Early clinical experience with adult bladder autoaugmentation. J Urol 1994; 152:303–306.
18. Leng WW, Blalock J, Fredrikkson WH, English SH, McGuire EJ. Enterocystoplasty or detrusor myomectomy? Comparison of indications and outcomes for bladder augmentation. J Urol 1999; 16:758–763.
19. Ehrlich RM, Gershman A. Laparoscopic seromyotomy (autoaugmentation) for nonneurogenic bladder in a child: initial case report. Urology 1993; 42:175–178.
20. McDougal EM, Clayman RV, Figenshau RS, Pearle MS. Laparoscopic retropubic autoaugmentation of the bladder. J Urol 1995; 153:123–126.
21. Braren V, Bishop MR. Laparoscopic bladder autoaugmentation in children. Urol Clin North Am 1998; 25:533–540.

33

Management of Refractory Detrusor Instability: Anterior Flap Extraperitoneal Cystoplasty

Eric S. Rovner
University of Pennsylvania School of Medicine, Philadelphia, Pennsylvania, U.S.A.

David A. Ginsberg
University of Southern California School of Medicine, Los Angeles, California, U.S.A.

Shlomo Raz
David Geffen School of Medicine at UCLA, Los Angeles, California, U.S.A.

I. INTRODUCTION

Enlargement or augmentation cystoplasty may be useful in a number of clinical situations, including the treatment of decreased functional or organic bladder capacity. In general, conservative therapy including behavioral modification, intermittent catheterization, anti-cholinergic medication, and/or electrical stimulation is successful in treating the majority of these patients. However, a number of patients will be refractory to these conservative measures and will continue to have unacceptable symptoms of frequency, urgency, urge incontinence, and perhaps even upper urinary tract deterioration due to high-pressure storage of urine. It is this group of patients in whom augmentation cystoplasty may have a therapeutic role. Neuromodulation is a promising new alternative therapy in a subset of this patient population, but long-term data are still lacking.

Many methods and approaches exist for bladder augmentation using varying segments of bowel (ileum, colon, etc.) (1–3), or urothelium (4) including autoaugmentation (5). All of these procedures have the common goals of providing drainage of the upper urinary tract into a low-pressure, high-capacity urinary reservoir. The use of bowel for enlargement cystoplasty has many well-documented disadvantages and has historically been associated with morbidity (6). Among the problems associated with enterocystoplasty are a large abdominal incision and intraperitoneal exploration with subsequent disruption of the gastrointestinal tract in order to harvest the bowel segment. This often results in a prolonged postoperative ileus requiring nasogastric tube decompression, especially in the neurogenic population who have neurogenic bowel in addition to their neurogenic bladder. Devastating complications associated with standard enterocystoplasty include intraperitoneal abscess, fistula, bowel obstruction, and prolonged ileus. The anterior flap extraperitoneal cystoplasty (AFEC) is a modification of the standard enterocystoplasty intended to minimize the preoperative, intraoperative, and postoperative complications historically associated with this procedure.

The AFEC is a variation of the standard cup-patch technique popularized by Goodwin and associates at UCLA (7). AFEC is performed through an extraperitoneal approach to the bladder with retrieval and then harvest of an ileal segment through a small peritoneal window. Care is taken to avoid significant manipulation of the intraperitoneal contents by working through a small peritoneotomy. Reconstitution of the GI tract (ileoileostomy) is performed extraperitoneally and then the anastomosed bowel is returned into the peritoneal cavity through the small peritoneal window. The peritoneal window is closed against the base of the mesentery of the harvested bowel segment, sealing the vesicointestinal anastomosis from the peritoneal cavity and placing the harvested segment in an extraperitoneal location adjacent to the bladder. A broad-based anterior bladder flap is fashioned and reflected cephalad where a wide vesicointestinal anastomosis is performed extraperitoneally. We feel this modified technique of augmentation cystoplasty may be associated with a faster return to bowel function and a shorter hospital stay.

We do not perform AFEC in the presence of multiple previous abdominal and pelvic surgeries where scar or adhesions may limit the ability to remain extraperitoneal or may limit the mobility of the bowel segment. We also do not perform AFEC if concomitant intra-abdominal or ureteric surgery is to be performed. Patients with renal insufficiency may not be candidates for AFEC, as the interposition of bowel in the urinary tract may lead to the provocation or aggravation of metabolic complications due to the reabsorption of certain urinary constituents. Patients with significant urethral disease (stricture, etc.), which may limit the ability to perform clean intermittent catheterization (CIC), or those who are unable or unwilling to perform CIC are likewise not good candidates for AFEC. Finally, patients with Crohn's disease, short gut syndrome, or other bowel conditions potentially affecting GI function and viability are not offered AFEC.

II. TECHNIQUE

Preoperative evaluation includes a thorough medical history with special attention toward previous abdominal surgery and the presence of GI disease which would limit use of the ileum (Crohn's disease, etc.), physical examination, upper urinary tract imaging, determination of renal function (serum creatinine), and videourodynamics—including an assessment of sphincteric function. Finally, an assessment is made of the patient's willingness and ability to perform clean intermittent catheterization, as this is critical to both long-term success and patient satisfaction.

Bowel preparation begins at home 2 days preoperatively and consists of a clear liquid diet and mild laxatives. The patient is brought into the hospital on the day of surgery, and intravenous antibiotics are administered preoperatively. The patient is placed in the supine position maintaining access to the urethra. A nasogastric tube is not routinely placed. A Foley catheter is placed per urethra.

Through a Pfannenstiel or lower midline incision the retropubic space is entered. The dome of the bladder is visualized and the unopened peritoneum is swept off the posterior bladder (Fig. 1). A small peritoneotomy (Fig. 2) is performed and a segment of ileum is grasped and brought into the extraperitoneal space through the peritoneal window. The operative field is isolated to prevent gross contamination and a 15- to 20-cm segment of ileum is selected based on an adequate vascular supply. This segment is isolated on its mesentery, using hemostats and the GIA stapling device. The gastrointestinal (GI) tract is then reconstituted with a side-to-side, functional end-to-end stapled anastomosis reinforced with nonabsorbable suture. The GI

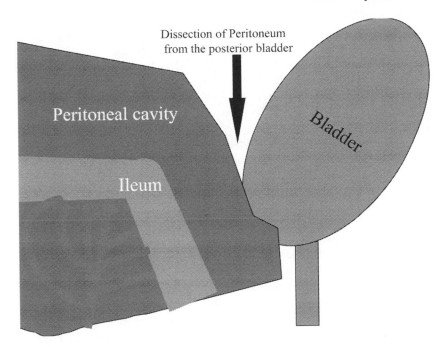

Figure 1 The retropubic space is entered and the peritoneum is swept off the posterior bladder. (Drawing courtesy of Shlomo Raz.)

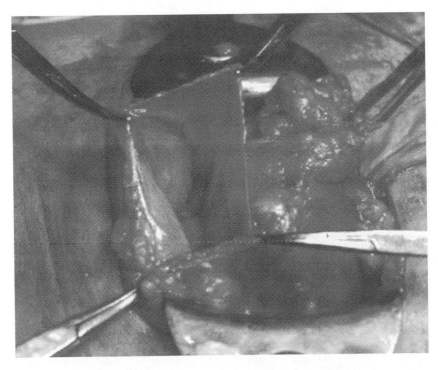

Figure 2 A small peritoneal window is made to gain access to the intraperitoneal contents. (Photograph courtesy of Shlomo Raz.)

anastomosis is placed back into the peritoneal cavity, and the peritoneum is circumferentially closed about the base of the mesentery of the isolated ileal segment leaving this portion extraperitoneal (Fig. 3). It is important that the peritoneotomy not be closed too tightly, resulting in compression of the mesenteric blood supply to the augment segment. If this occurs, the bowel segment may appear ischemic or have an appearance of vascular congestion secondary to poor venous return, and the peritoneal closure should be loosened.

The isolated ileal segment is opened, irrigated with an antibiotic solution, folded into a "U" configuration (Fig. 4) and detubularized eccentrically using the electrocautery (Fig. 5). The medial aspects of the detubularized bowel are now anastomosed, forming a patch (Fig. 6).

An anterior bladder flap is now created by incising on the posterior bladder wall in the shape of an inverted "U" (Fig. 7). This flap is raised as caudally as possible in order to create maximum mobility of the anterior flap. The anterior bladder flap has four advantages: (a) a wide based flap avoids an hourglass configuration of the augmented bladder; (b) the posterior placement of the flap puts the mesentery in a position where internal herniation is unlikely; (c) the bladder can be additionally incised in the anterior midline to obtain more bladder edge for the anastomosis if necessary; and (d) the anterior bladder flap may be advanced cephalad towards the ileal segment, which may be helpful in patients with a short or relatively immobile mesentery (8).

The ileal segment is anastomosed to the bladder and bladder flap using two layers of absorbable suture (Fig. 8). Prior to closure of the augmented bladder a suprapubic tube is placed to allow dual drainage of the augmented bladder. A Penrose drain is left in the retropubic space.

Beginning postoperative day 1, the augmented bladder is irrigated twice daily with saline to prevent the formation of inspissated mucous plugs. The Foley catheter is removed 2–3 weeks postoperatively after a radiograph confirms a well-healed augment without extravasation, and the patient is instructed to void and check postvoid residuals through the suprapubic tube.

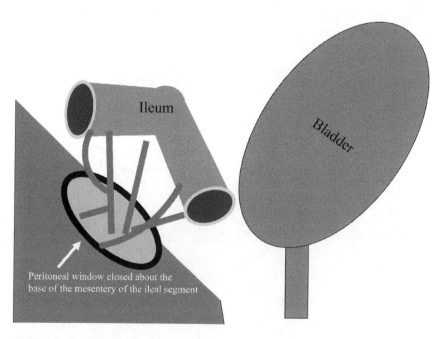

Figure 3   The peritoneal window is closed around the base of the mesentery of the ileal segment. (Drawing courtesy of Shlomo Raz.)

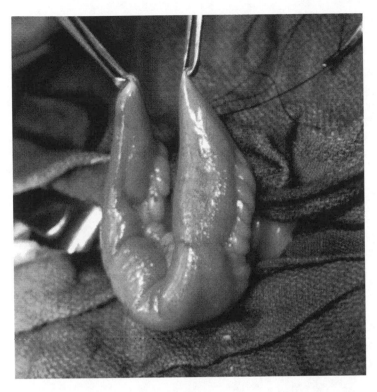

Figure 4 The ileal segment is placed into a "U" configuration. (Photograph courtesy of Shlomo Raz.)

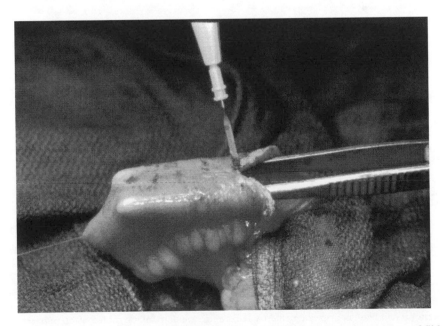

Figure 5 The ileal segment is debularized eccentrically. (Photograph courtesy of Shlomo Raz.)

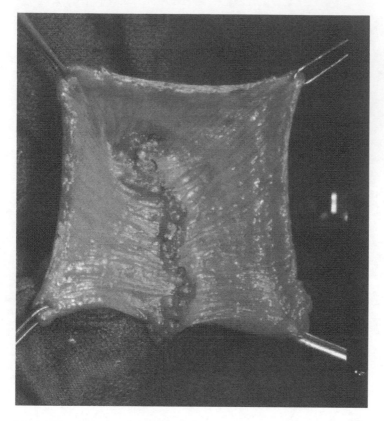

Figure 6   After detubularization the medial walls of the ileal patch are anastomosed, forming a patch. (Photograph courtesy of Shlomo Raz.)

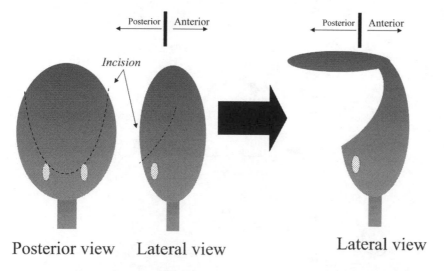

Figure 7   An anterior based bladder flap is created by incising as caudally as possible on the posterior bladder wall in the shape of an inverted "U."

(a)

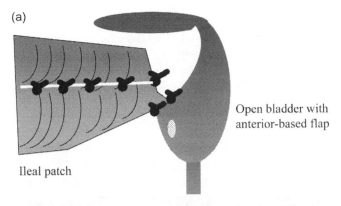

Open bladder with
anterior-based flap

Ileal patch

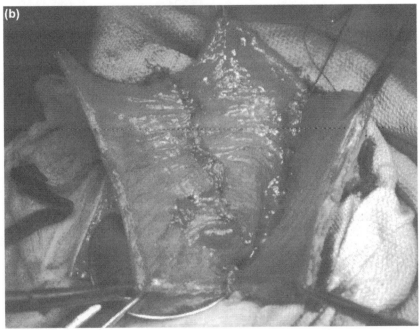

Figure 8   (a) Diagram of anastomosis of the ileal patch to the bladder. (b) Intraoperative photograph of
the anastomosis of the ileal patch to the bladder. (Courtesy of Shlomo Raz.)

If the residuals remain high, the patient is reinstructed on the technique of clean intermittent
catheterization, and the suprapubic tube is removed.

III. RESULTS

In 1997, Albo and coworkers reported their initial experience with AFEC (9). There were 23 women
and four men. Fourteen patients were noted to have a defined neurologic condition and detrusor
hyperreflexia, and 13 were considered to have nonneurogenic voiding dysfunction. All patients had
failed conservative therapy. Of the 27 patients, 25 had an "uneventful" postoperative convalescence
from AFEC without requiring nasogastric decompression. In these 25 patients the mean time to oral

(enteral) nutrition was 3.5 days and mean hospitalization was 5.5 days. Complications included one patient with a prolonged ileus and one patient with clostridium difficile enterocolitis. An additional patient required emergent laparotomy 3 months postoperatively for a bladder perforation after failing to catheterize as instructed. Overall, at a mean follow-up of 9 months, 92% of patients were cured or experienced marked improvement in voiding symptoms. Forty-four percent of patients still required anticholinergic therapy postoperatively, and 60% of patients were on CIC. There was no difference in success between neurogenic and nonneurogenic groups.

Subsequently, Rovner and colleagues reported on an update of this series (10). Forty-two patients (24 nonneurogenic and 18 neurogenic) were followed for a mean of >15 months following AFEC. Overall, 90% of patients were tolerating a regular diet by postoperative day 5. Range of inpatient hospital stay was 3–22 days, with >80% discharged by postoperative day 6. At a mean follow-up of over 15 months >80% of patients were cured or significantly improved from symptoms of urinary urgency and frequency, and almost 90% were cured or significantly improved with regard to preoperative symptoms of urge incontinence. There have been no cases of fistula or small bowel obstruction. Other than the complications noted above, two additional patients had a postoperative GI hemorrhage requiring transfusion.

IV. CONCLUSIONS

We have found AFEC to be a simple and effective method of augmentation cystoplasty in select patients. Theoretically, extraperitoneal performance of the procedure and minimal handling of the bowel and peritoneal contents should reduce perioperative morbidity and complications. Isolation of the vesicointestinal anastomosis from the peritoneum minimizes risks of urinary fistula formation, uncontrolled urinary extravasation, and intraperitoneal abscess formation and infection. In addition, the risk of postoperative intraperitoneal adhesions and subsequent bowel obstruction is potentially reduced owing to the minimal disruption of the peritoneum. Principles of AFEC include minimal intraperitoneal bowel manipulation, an extraperitoneal bowel resection, and vesicointestinal anastomosis performed and isolated outside the peritoneal cavity. Limited bowel manipulation and isolation of the peritoneal contents from the vesicointestinal anastomosis may allow an earlier return of bowel function, shorter hospital stay, and reduced perioperative morbidity.

REFERENCES

1. Gil-Vernet JM Jr. The ileocolic segment in urologic surgery. J Urol 1965; 94:418.
2. Smith RB. Use of ileocystoplasty in the hypertonic neurogenic bladder. J Urol 1975; 113:125.
3. Luangkhot R, Peng BCH, Blaivas JG. Ileocystoplasty for the management of refractory neurogenic bladder: surgical technique and urodynamic findings. J Urol 1991; 146:1340.
4. Churchill BM, Aliabadi H, Landau EH. Ureteral bladder augmentation. J Urol 1993; 150:716–720.
5. Cartwright PC, Snow BW. Bladder autoaugmentation: early clinical experience. J Urol 1989; 142(2 Pt 2):505–508.
6. Khoury JM, Timmons SL, Corbel L, Webster GD. Complications of enterocystoplasty. Urology 1992; 40:9.
7. Goodwin WE, Winter CC, Barker UF. Cup-patch technique of ileocystoplasty for bladder enlargement or partial substitution. Surg Gynecol Obstet 1959; 108:240.
8. Chopra A, Stothers L, Raz S. Bladder augmentation. Urol Clin North Am 1995; 3(2):81–93.
9. Albo M, Raz S, Dupont MC. Anterior flap extraperitoneal cystoplasty. J Urol 1997; 57(6):2095–2098.
10. Rovner ES, Ginsberg DA, Albo ME, Raz S. Anterior flap extraperitoneal cystoplasty (AFEC): a simplified method of ileal augmentation cystoplasty. J Urol 1997; 157(4):397A.

34

Laparoscopic Enterocystoplasty

Raymond R. Rackley and Joseph B. Abdelmalak
Cleveland Clinic Foundation, Cleveland, Ohio, U.S.A

I. INTRODUCTION

When a patient with bladder dysfunction due to noncompliance or reduced functional capacity does not benefit from conventional therapies, one choice for treatment is augmentation cystoplasty. This procedure involves anastomosing a segment of bowel to the urinary bladder in order to create a large, fully functional storage container that can be emptied at the patient's will. The procedure is typically performed using an open laparotomy incision and can utilize several different portions of bowel, as long as the segments have good blood supplies and are of adequate size (1). Each segment of bowel has its own advantages and disadvantages, and the decision as to which portion to use is based on the history and current and future needs of the patient, and the preference of the surgeon. This highly effective reconstructive technique protects the upper urinary tract while allowing the patient to regain continence (2–5). First performed in a dog in 1888, enterocystoplasty was later shown to be successful in human subjects (6), and is currently the most widely accepted method of treating refractory bladder dysfunction.

Although this procedure has a high success rate, many patients opt not to seek treatment owing to the stigmas of open surgery namely complications, pain, and morbidity. Additional consequences of open surgery include delayed postoperative recoveries, increased metabolic needs for wound healing, and prolonged hospital stays. These consequences are most prolific in the elderly and in patients with previously diagnosed neurologic and other comorbid conditions, and can be potentially avoided by the use of a laparoscopic approach. Patients who have undergone enterocystoplasty using this technique report less postoperative pain and morbidity, improved comesis, and shorter hospital stays and recuperation times than those who have received the surgery through conventional open methods. In addition, it has been shown that laparoscopy notably reduces the number and severity of intra-abdominal adhesions associated with open surgery (7).

Laparoscopic bladder augmentation is a technically complex procedure in which the main goal is to achieve the benefits of open surgery while avoiding its detriments. However, the mechanical difficulties associated with laparoscopic bladder augmentation have greatly limited its use, despite the prevalence of similar techniques in other routine urological surgeries. In this article, the authors illustrate their method of reconstructive laparoscopic enterocystoplasty as it has developed through their experience with 17 patients.

II. INDICATIONS AND PATIENT SELECTION

Laparoscopic augmentation cystoplasty provides a surgical solution for those patients with noncompliant small bladders that have not responded to more traditional therapies. Using a minimally invasive approach, the procedure involves making an incision of the bladder wall for anastomosis of a segment of bowel. Patients with ventriculoperitoneal shunts (such as those with a myelomingocele) are likely to have intra-abdominal adhesions that may interfere with laparoscopic techniques. For patients with neurogenic bladder dysfunction, they will need to perform clean intermittent catheterization for extended periods of time following the operation in order to effectively empty their bladders. Lastly, a continent catheterizable abdominal stoma (in addition to bladder augmentation) may be necessary for patients who are not able to catheterize themselves via the urethra.

Before the operation, upper and lower urinary tract studies are valuable for establishing a baseline evaluation. Urodynamics and cystoscopy are also helpful; they provide information regarding the competence of the urinary sphincter. Additionally, one may obtain routine laboratory studies, including: renal function and serum electrolytes, a whole blood cell count, urinalysis, and a urine culture (when appropriate).

III. PATIENT PREPARATION

Two days prior to surgery, the patient should be placed on a clear liquid diet; on the day preceding the operation, a bowel preparation must be performed. Preoperative antibiotics are recommended for bowel and urinary tract surgical prophylaxis, as are antifungal medications when appropriate. Owing to chronic constipation, patients with neurological diseases may require more time for an adequate bowel preparation.

The procedure begins with the patient fitted in pneumatic compression stockings and situated in the supine position. Padded shoulder braces are used to prevent patient sliding during extreme excursions in the head-down or Trendelenberg position. Next, he/she is anesthetized and intubated, followed by the insertion of an oral gastric tube. The patient is then moved to the low-lithotomy position where he/she remains for the rest of the operation. The patient's arms are tucked and protected along the sides so as to facilitate the surgical team's ability to direct their operative movements deep into the pelvis.

During the first few procedures, cystoscopy was used to aid in the insertion of internal-external ureteral stents (7F, 90 cm; Circon Surgitek, Santa Barbara, CA) into the renal pelvis, which provided both intraoperative and postoperative drainage. Maximal intraoperative drainage of urine was obtained by leaving the straight ends of the stents outside the external urethral meatus and securing them to a 20–24F urethral catheter. However, the use of these internal-external ureteral stents prevented effective bladder irrigation by interfering with the formation of an adequate seal of the urethra around the urethral catheter. It was later found that ureteral stents were unnecessary, as it is possible to provide effective intraoperative urine and pelvic fluid drainage by intermittently opening the 20–24F urethral catheter without losing the pneumoperitoneum during the procedure.

IV. SURGICAL TECHNIQUE (9)

There are many features essential to a successful bladder augmentation. First, a segment of bowel must be chosen based on a broad, well-vascularized mesenteric pedicle. This portion must then be excised, and the remaining segments of bowel joined together. Next, the bowel segment must be detubularized and reconfigured while avoiding peritoneal soiling of bowel contents. After this has been accomplished, the bladder should be mobilized, and an adequate-size cystotomy performed. Lastly, the bowel segment should be anastomosed to the bladder, creating a tension-free, watertight, full-thickness seal, and the surgeon should confirm adequate postoperative urinary drainage.

Several ports are useful for the manipulation of laparoscopic tools. The first, a disposable 10- to 12-mm port with occluding balloon and cuff, is introduced through an incision made at the umbilical crease and is guided into the peritoneal cavity under direct vision. A 10-mm 10° laparoscope can later be inserted through this port. Next, two ports are introduced paraumbilically in order to facilitate suturing. These ports are 10 and 5 mm and are located bilaterally at the lateral borders of the rectus muscle at the level of the umbilicus (Fig. 1). One last 5-mm port should be placed medially to the left anterior superior iliac spine. The introduction of additional ports may be beneficial; their location will depend on the segment of bowel being used and the surgeon's preference.

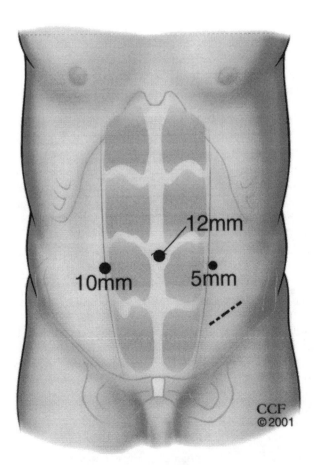

Figure 1 Options for selection of port sizes and location in laparoscopic enterocystoplasty procedures. (Courtesy Cleveland Clinic Foundation.)

V. BOWEL SELECTION AND MOBILIZATION

While many segments of bowel may be used for laparoscopic enterocystoplasty, a chosen section must meet the following requirements: (a) a length of 15–20 cm ensures that an adequate augmented bladder capacity will be obtained; (b) the bowel segment should reach the area of the bladder neck without tension; and (c) the bowel mesentery must contain an adequate blood supply. These criteria are the same as for open enterocystoplasty, and the selection of a portion of bowel is based on the clinical requirements of the patient.

When ileum is to be used for augmentation, *ileocystoplasty*, the surgeon must first identify the ileocaecal junction. The section of bowel to be used for augmentation must be located at least 15 cm proximal to the ileocaecal junction in order to preserve absorptive bowel functions after the segment is removed. The portion selected is then clamped off using small, 5-mm laparoscopic bowel clamps. Inserting a 5-mm laparoscope into the lower left port and illuminating the area will help to identify the vascular mesenteric pedicle associated with this segment of bowel. Portions of the mesentery adjacent to the proximal and distal ends of the selected section of bowel are then scored with laparoscopic electrosurgical scissors, which facilitates subsequent extracorporeal identification.

The use of sigmoid colon, *sigmoidocystoplasty*, is suggested for patients who meet the following criteria: (a) neurogenic bladder dysfunction accompanied by defecating dysfunction with a resultant redundant sigmoid colon; (b) ability to perform intermittent catheterization via the urethra; and (c) do not require a continent catheterizable stoma. Removing this segment of bowel can be done in a similar manner as above, with the additional insertion of a 10-mm port medial to the level of the right anterior iliac spine. This aids in mobilization of the bowel segment so that it may be manipulated via the extension of the lower left abdominal port (Fig. 2).

For patients who *do* require a continent catheterizable stoma, the right colon and terminal ileum should be used. The peritoneum lateral to the cecum and ascending colon, and the peritoneum of the terminal aspect of the Z line are incised, and the entire right colon and terminal ileum are mobilized for extracorporeal manipulation via the extended incision of the umbilical port. This is facilitated by making certain that the patient's thighs are kept in a low position with low lithotomy. Once incised, the cecum and ascending colon are anastomosed to the bladder, while the 10–12 cm of terminal ileum is used to create a catheterizable channel and stoma at the umbilicus.

VI. EXCLUSION AND REANASTOMOSIS OF THE BOWEL

The umbilical port is removed after exsufflation of the pneumoperitoneum. Next, the umbilical incision is enlarged circumumbilically (it may also need to be extended an extra 2 cm in obese cases) in order to allow for delivery of the preselected bowel segment. Care must be taken to ensure proper proximal-distal orientation of the loop and to avoid twisting of the mesenteric pedicle. Using traditional open surgical techniques, the selected portion of bowel and its mesenteric pedicle is then divided between clamps and isolated as described above in ileocystoplasty (Fig. 3). Bowel anastomosis is performed cephaled to the excluded segment of bowel using traditional open surgical techniques, and the mesenteric defect is repaired. The bowel is then immediately returned to the abdomen via the umbilical port, which ensures that the umbilical incision will not need to be enlarged should the reanastomosed bowel or the reconfigured bowel segment for augmentation become edematous.

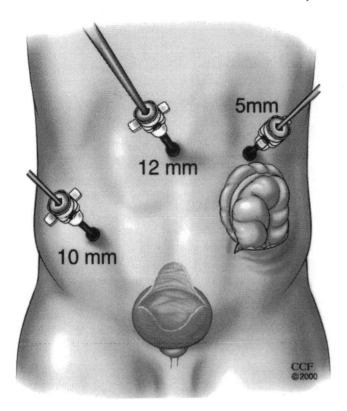

Figure 2   Selection of port sizes and location for laparoscopic sigmoidocystoplasty. (Courtesy Cleveland Clinic Foundation.)

VII. REFASHIONING OF THE ISOLATED BOWEL SEGMENT

The isolated bowel segment should be draped in moist warm sponges and irrigated with normal saline until the returning irrigation is clear. Next, an incision is made along the border of the bowel, opposite the side of the mesentery. A U-shaped plate is created by a side-to-side anastomosis with 2-0 Vicryl sutures (Fig. 4) when using the small bowel or sigmoid colon. The refashioned bowel segment is then reintroduced to the peritoneal cavity. Ports are replaced in order to reestablish the pneumoperitoneum. In ileocystoplasty, this involves inserting a disposable 10- to 12-mm blunt-tip port with a fascial retention balloon and foam cuff to minimize gas leakage. In sigmoidocystoplasty, it involves reducing the lower left incision to accommodate a 10-mm port. A laparoscope can then be inserted, and the isolated bowel segment can be oriented and inspected to exclude torsion of the pedicle.

When the right colon and terminal ileum are to be used, as in patients who require a catheterizable stoma, the cecum and proximal colon must be detubularized, and the appendix removed. The terminal ileum is then plicated over a 16F red rubber catheter using a gastrointestinal anastomosis stapling device (GIA stapler), and the ileocecal junction is imbricated and intussuscepted to augment the continence mechanism of the ileocecal valve using 2-0 silk sutures (Fig. 5). To facilitate intracorporeal laparoscopic identification and manipulation, orientation sutures are placed at the cephalic end (undyed, 2-0 Vicryl on a CT-1 needle) and the caudal end (dyed, 2-0 Vicryl on a CT-1 needle) of the bowel patch. The 16F red rubber catheter is then secured to the terminal end of the catheterizable segment of the ileum with

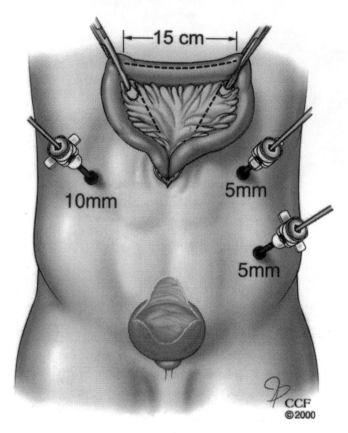

Figure 3 Extracorporeal isolation and manipulation of the small bowel via the umbilical port site. (Courtesy Cleveland Clinic Foundation.)

a 2-0 silk suture for atraumatic intracorporeal manipulation and for delivering this terminal segment to the umbilicus for stoma maturation at the end of the procedure. The isolated bowel patch is then returned to the abdominal cavity and the infraumbilical incision is closed over a 10- to 12-mm blunt-tip port with a fascial retention balloon and foam cuff, which minimizes gas leakage for the remainder of the operation. As in ileo- and sigmoidocystoplasty, once the pneumoperitoneum has been reestablished, the laparoscope is inserted and the bowel segment is oriented and inspected to rule out torsion of the pedicle.

While both isolation of the bowel section for augmentation and reestablishing bowel continuity can be done laparoscopically, we prefer to perform them extracorporeally by delivering the bowel outside the abdomen through the umbilical or lower port sites. This offers many advantages: (a) it makes it easier to obtain a precise measurement of the bowel segment; (b) the vascularity of the mesentery can be ensured before an incision is made; (c) if the mesentery is long enough to be delivered outside the body without evidence of ischemia, then it should be an adequate length to reach the bladder neck without tension; (d) the reanastomosis of the bowel can be performed with increased confidence using open surgical techniques; (e) likewise, the detubularization and modification of the bowel segment can be performed quickly by open suturing techniques; (f) irrigation of the excluded loop can be performed without peritoneal spillage, which minimizes the chance of pelvic abscess formation; and (g) this approach yields significant savings in overall operative time and cost.

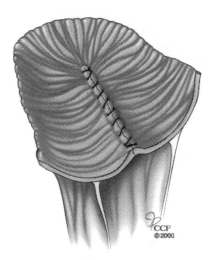

Figure 4   Detubularization and reconfiguration of the isolated bowel segment. (Courtesy Cleveland Clinic Foundation.)

VIII. BLADDER MOBILIZATION AND CYSTOTOMY

For the remainder of the operation, the patient should be placed in the Trendelenberg position. This ensures that the bowel loops do not encroach upon the pelvic cavity, and aids in the subsequent steps of the procedure. The next step in mobilization of the bladder is distension of the bladder with saline via the urethral catheter. Finally, an incision is made through the peritoneum surrounding the bladder. It originates at the medial border of the left medial umbilical ligament and continues linearly to the right medial umbilical ligament. The median umbilical ligament is taken down during the procedure using electrosurgical scissors,

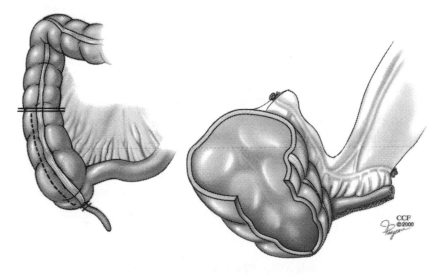

Figure 5   Detubularization and reconfiguration of the right colon and ileum for cecocolocystoplasty in preparation for formation of a catheterizable stoma. (Courtesy Cleveland Clinic Foundation.)

and when needed, the lateral peritoneum incisions can be extended along the medial umbilical ligaments to increase exposure. Another means for increasing exposure is dissection of the loose areolar tissue surrounding the bladder; this allows for greater access to the bladder neck and perivesical spaces.

The cystostomy begins with a curvilinear incision through the bladder wall. The apex of the incision is at the bladder neck, and the base extends posteriorly past the midcoronal plane of the bladder dome (Figs. 2, 3). This type of incision greatly disrupts the musculature of the bladder, facilitates the anastomosis of bowel, and is particularly useful in patients in whom the presence of a uterus may prevent an adequate cystostomy incision.

IX. ENTEROVESICAL ANASTOMOSIS

There are many possible methods of securing the bowel to the bladder. However, to ensure a watertight anastomosis, we prefer to begin by attaching the "posterior" wall of the reconfigured bowel patch to the apical portion of the bladder flap and continue suturing in a medial (point A) to lateral (points B and C) direction on each side (Fig. 6). Beginning the anastomosis at the "anterior" wall of the bowel segment may impede the closing of the posterior segment, as this portion will be difficult to visualize owing to the constraints of the pelvic anatomy.

Using laparoscopic suturing (5-mm needle holder and a 5-mm grasper) and intracorporeal knot-tying techniques, we finish the anastomosis by securing the anterior portion of the bowel segment to the bladder. The bladder is then distended with saline to confirm a watertight anastomosis (Fig. 7), and a Jackson-Pratt drain is inserted into the pelvic cavity through the lower lateral five port sites. In female patients, bladder drainage is maintained with a 20–24F

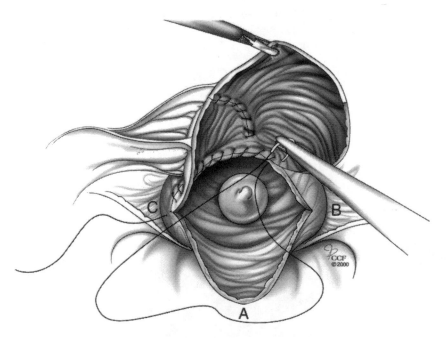

Figure 6 Intracorporeal suturing of the isolated bowel segment to the bladder. Point A is at the apical aspect of the newly formed bladder flap that was derived from the anterior aspect of the bladder wall near the bladder neck when the cystotomy incision was made. (Courtesy Cleveland Clinic Foundation.)

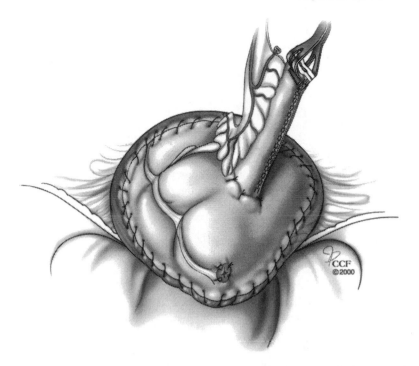

Figure 7   Completed view of the bowel to bladder anastomosis in preparation for maturation of the catheterizable stoma to the umbilicus. (Courtesy Cleveland Clinic Foundation.)

urethral catheter. A smaller urethral catheter is preferred for males; therefore, a suprapubic tube is placed through the bladder wall and extends to the outside of the body through the lower port site. Any 10-mm port sites, as well as the umbilical incision, are closed in layers.

When patients require a catheterizable stoma, the isolated ileal segment is positioned with the attached red rubber catheter is secured with an endoclamp via the umbilical port. Once the pneumoperitoneum has been decompressed, the terminal end of the ileal segment is delivered to the umbilicus and secured to the anterior rectus fascia and skin; 4-0 chromic sutures are used to perform a Y-V flap maturation of the stoma to the skin of the umbilicus. In obese patients, the use of the umbilicus as the site of stoma formation decreases the amount of ileum needed to mature the stoma to the skin. Finally, to optimize bladder drainage and healing of the newly created channel, a 16F catheter is isolated through the stoma and into the bladder.

X.   POSTOPERATIVE MANAGEMENT

The oral-gastric decompression tube is removed, the patient is extubated, and the Jackson-Pratt drain is taken out once drainage is <25 mL or fluid chemistries indicate peritoneal fluid. The patient is allowed to leave the hospital if afebrile and has completed three consecutive meals, the first tending to be consumed the first postoperative day. Patients are discharged with the indwelling urethral catheter for drainage and are instructed to perform daily bladder irrigation using 100 mL sterile saline via the uretheral catheter, they are also given daily low-dose antibiotics for prophylaxis. At 3 weeks postoperative, the urinary catheter is removed and intermittent catheterization is begun. While the catheter at the umbilical stoma is usually capped at the time of hospital discharge, it may be used to flush out the bladder during daily irrigation practices in the weeks following surgery.

XI. RESULTS (TABLE 1)

Seventeen laparoscopic enterocystoplasties were performed in patients with neurogenic bladder dysfunction between June 1999 and November 2001, including five ileocystoplasties, three sigmoidocystoplasties, one colocystoplasty, and eight cecocolocystoplasties with a continent catheterizable ileal stoma. Blood loss for all procedures was minimal, averaging 175 mL and not exceeding 250 mL. The entire operation lasted an average of 7.0 h (range 5.3–8 h), with laparoscopic suturing taking a mean 2.4 h (range 1.7–3.1 h). Sixteen of 17 patients were able to resume eating 24 h postsurgery, and patients were ready to be discharged from the hospital an average of 5.7 days (range 3–7 days) after the procedure. This, along with the fact that patients did not need long-term care, was remarkable considering that most of the patients suffered from underlying neurological conditions. The only complications that accompanied these procedures were a trocar-induced rectus sheath hematoma during a sigmoidocystoplasty and a self-limited paralytic ileus. The former was controlled laparoscopically, and the latter through conservative treatment.

Each patient consented to participate in our follow-up study that consisted of filling out validated surveys about their bladder control (BLCS) and bowel control (BWCS) before and after the surgery. Two male (14.4%) and 12 female (85.6%) patients with an average age of 40 years (range 18–62) were able to complete at least the 6th month postoperative questionnaires

Table 1 Laparoscopic Enterocystoplasty Cases

ID	Age (yr)	Sex	Primary disease	Op. T (h)	Bl. L (mL)	H. S (d)	Bowel used
1	27	M	Sensory urgency	6.15	300	10	Ileum
2	49	F	MS	7	350	9	Sigmoid colon
3	30	F	SCI	7	200	5	Cecum and rt colon and ileum
4	48	F	TM	3.15	60	6	Ileum
5	36	F	MS	8	150	6	Cecum and rt colon and ileum
6	62	M	MS	5	300	4	Ileum
7	18	F	SCI	8	110	6	Cecum and rt colon and ileum
8	46	F	MS	8	125	6	Cecum and rt colon and ileum
9	52	F	MS	5.15	200	5	Sigmoid colon
10	23	F	Spina bifida	8	200	6	Rt colon
11	38	F	MS	7	350	7	Cecum and rt colon and ileum
12	45	F	SCI	9.15	550	5	Cecum and rt colon and ileum
13	31	F	SCI	9	300	4	Cecum and rt colon and ileum
14	58	F	MS	4	150	4	Ileum
15	27	F	SCI	7	200	3	Sigmoid colon
16	39	M	MS	8	200	4	Cecum and rt colon and ileum
17	49	F	DI	8	200	3	Ileum

Op. T (h), operative time (h); H. S (d), hospital stay; Bl. L (mL), blood loss (mL); MS, multiple sclerosis; SCI, spinal cord injury; TM, transversmyelitis; DI, detrusor instability.

based on a mean follow-up of 17 months (range 7–27). Significant improvement in bladder control was seen with a decline in average score on the BLCS from 14.9 ± 5.0 to 1.6 ± 1.8, $P = .0002$. However, there was no significant change in bowel function, with an average preoperative BWCS score of 6.4 ± 6.5 and a mean postoperative score of 5.3 ± 6.0, $P = .30$. It is important to emphasize that bowel function control score did not decrease despite the removal of a segment of bowel for bladder augmentation.

XII. SUMMARY

As in open enterocystoplasty, laparoscopic bladder augmentation uses various segments of bowel to enlarge the bladder and to restore compliance. While benefits of laparoscopic surgery include decreased pain, morbidity, and recovery time (an attractive option to those with complex comorbid illnesses), a major drawback of this type of surgery is cost. However, as surgeons become more familiar with laparoscopic techniques, reusable equipment is implemented, cost-saving strategies are employed, and surgical time and length of hospital stay decrease, a decline in overall cost become apparent (4).

For those who undergo laparoscopic augmentation cystoplasty owing to neurogenic bladder dysfunction, a significant improvement in bladder control without impairment of bowel control has been documented. Our experience demonstrates that laparoscopic augmentation cystoplasty technique may be a practical alternative to traditional open enterocystoplasty in improving the quality of life of our patients.

REFERENCES

1. Novick AC. Augmentation cystoplasty. In: Operative Urology. Baltimore: Williams and Wilkins, 1982:98.
2. Hasan ST, Marshall C, Robson WA, Neal DE. Clinical outcome and quality of life following enterocystoplasty for idiopathic detrusor instability and neurogenic bladder dysfunction. Br J Urol 1995; 76:551–557.
3. Mundy AR, Stephenson TP. Clam: ileocystoplasty for the treatment of refractory urge incontinence. Br J Urol 1985; 57:641–646.
4. Rink RC, Adams MC. Augmentation cystoplasty. In: Marshal F, ed. Textbook of Operative Urology. Philadephia: W.B. Saunders, 1990:914–926.
5. Smith JJ, Swierzewewski SJ. Augmentation cystoplasty. Urol Clin North Am 1997; 24:745–754.
6. Mikulicz J. Zur Operation der angeborenen Blasenspalte. Zentralbl Chir 1899; 26:641.
7. Garrard CL, Clements RH, Nanney L, Davidson JM, Richards WO. Adhesion formation after laparoscopic surgery. Surg Endosc 1999; 13:10–13.
8. Hobart MG, Gill IS, Schweizer D, Schweizer D, Bravo EL. Financial analysis of needlescopic versus open adrenalectomy. J Urol 1999; 162(4):1264–1267.
9. Rackley RR, Abdelmalak BJ. Laparoscopic augmentation cystoplasty: surgical technique. Urol Clin North Am 2001; 28:663–670.

35

Management of Refractory Detrusor Instability: Sacral Nerve Root Stimulation

Patrick J. Shenot
Thomas Jefferson University, Philadelphia, Pennsylvania, U.S.A.

I. INTRODUCTION

Clinical manifestations of urinary voiding dysfunction include urge incontinence, urgency-frequency, and urinary retention. Patients with nonobstructive urinary retention have few treatment options except intermittent catheterization. The treatment of refractory detrusor overactivity represents one of the most challenging problems in urology. Conservative treatment rarely results in a durable cure of patients with urge incontinence and bladder overactivity. Pharmacologic and behavioral techniques result in total cure in <50% of patients (1). Once behavioral and pharmaceutical options have failed, these patients have been traditionally been offered more invasive treatments such as bladder augmentation. While effective, this technique is highly invasive and irreversible, and it carries significant complication rates. Other minimally invasive surgical treatments for refractory detrusor overactivity, such as transvaginal detrusor denervation, produce unreliable results. Detrusor myomectomy represents a potential treatment option, but this technique has not been widely studied. Sacral neuromodulation offers an alternative, reversible minimally invasive treatment for patients with urge incontinence, urinary urgency-frequency syndrome, and nonobstructive, nonneurogenic urinary retention refractory to conservative therapy.

II. HISTORY

Although neurostimulation techniques for urinary incontinence were first applied in the 1960s, the foundation for sacral neuromodulation arose out the neurostimulation program at the University of California, San Francisco. Following extensive animal studies, a clinical program at this institution was initiated that laid the foundation for the clinical application of this therapy. Tanagho and Schmidt reported on a diverse group of patients who benefited from neuromodulation of sacral the nerve roots (1,2). It was demonstrated that electrical stimulation of the sacral nerve root could reduce inappropriate neural activity to inhibit the overactive detrusor. Promising results at this and other centers led to the commercial development of the InterStim device (Medtronic Inc, Minneapolis, MN), large-scale clinical trials, and FDA approval for the treatment of refractory urge incontinence in 1997. Further testing and clinical trials resulted in subsequent approval of the device (April 1999) for significant symptoms of urgency-frequency and nonobstructive urinary retention. This implantable sacral neurostimulation system comprises a neurostimulator, an extension cable, and a quadripolar stimulating electrode that is implanted in one of the sacral foramen, most commonly S3. Although other stimulation systems have been studied, this is the only device that has gained widespread acceptance.

Despite recent advances in the clinical application of sacral nerve stimulation, the exact mechanism by which it works is not understood. The finding that sacral neuromodulation can be used to treat both detrusor overactivity and urinary retention suggests that in patients with voiding dysfunctions it has a conditioning effect on neural excitability and can restore neural equilibrium between facilatory and inhibitory influences although the exact mechanism of action in each of these conditions may be different (4). The basic principles of neuromodulation are that electrical stimulation is intrinsically inhibitory and that activity in one neural pathway can influence activity in other pathways. It is generally assumed that sacral nerve stimulation results in afferent inhibition of sensory processing in the spinal cord. Evidence suggests that this occurs via a polysynaptic reflex mechanism, but it is unclear whether such a reflex is at a segmental level within the sacral cord or involves spinobulbospinal pathways (5). Proposed mechanisms of afferent stimulation include direct activation of afferents fibers in the sacral nerve root or perhaps activation of the pelvic floor with subsequent amplification of afferent impulses (6).

III. PATIENT SELECTION

Sacral neuromodulation may be considered for patients with urge incontinence, urinary urgency-frequency syndrome, and nonobstructive urinary retention who have failed more conservative forms of management. These patients should have undergone a comprehensive evaluation, including a thorough medical history; general, neurologic, and pelvic examinations; urinalysis; culture; voiding diary; and postvoid residual (PVR) urine determination. Diagnostic testing, such as cystoscopy, urine cytology, and urodynamics, should be considered to rule out any treatable conditions. An accurate, complete voiding diary is critical to document baseline voiding behaviors and judge the patient's response to therapy. Patients being evaluated for this therapy should be willing and competent to completely and accurately fill out voiding diaries at various time points during evaluation.

Attempts at conservative management should be made using some combination of altered fluid intake, medication, pelvic floor exercises (with or without biofeedback), and bladder interval training. Only after a patient fails a diligent attempt at conservative therapy should SNS be considered. Patients with neurologic disorders, such as multiple sclerosis, are potential beneficiaries of this therapy, but experience is limited and it is unknown how the progressive nature of these conditions will impact on long-term results of this treatment (7). In addition, the foreseeable need for magnetic resonance imaging (MRI) studies represents a relative contraindication to this procedure.

IV. TEST PROCEDURE

A. Acute Nerve Stimulation Testing

Acute nerve stimulation testing is done with the patient in the prone position. Pillows may be placed under the lower abdomen to achieve slight flexion of the hips to position the sacrum horizontally. The sacral area is prepared with povidone-iodine and sterile drapes are placed to allow visual observation of the motor responses of the pelvic floor, calves, and feet. Using palpation of bony landmarks or fluoroscopy, the approximate location of the S3 foramina are located at the level of the greater sciatic notch about one finger width from the midline (Fig. 1) Local anesthesia is then achieved by infiltrating the subcutaneous tissue and periostium taking care not to infiltrate the foramen itself. An insulated foramen needle is placed in the appropriate foramen at an angle of approximately 60° relative to the skin (Fig. 2). The needle is stimulated using an external stimulator at a set frequency and pulse width while the voltage is gradually increased. The sensory and motor responses to stimulation are recorded (Table 1). Sensory responses to S3 stimulation typically include a pulling sensation in the rectum which extends forward to the scrotum or labia. Motor responses to S3 stimulation include contraction of the

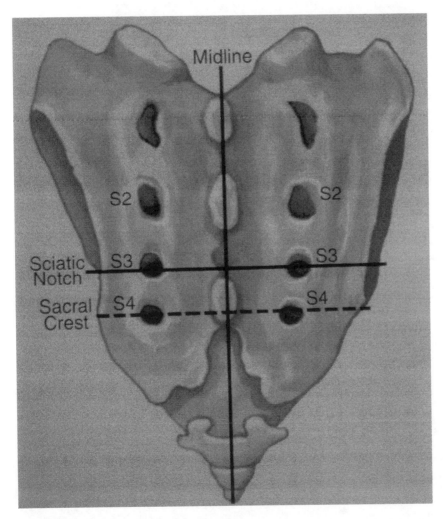

Figure 1   Sacral anatomy. The S3 foramen lies at the level of the sciatic notch one finger breadth from the midline. This is a valuable radio graphic landmark that aides the in locating the S3 foramen. The S4 foramen lies at the sacral crest, where the sacrum flattens out and serves as a useful topographic landmark. (Courtesy of Medtronic, Inc.)

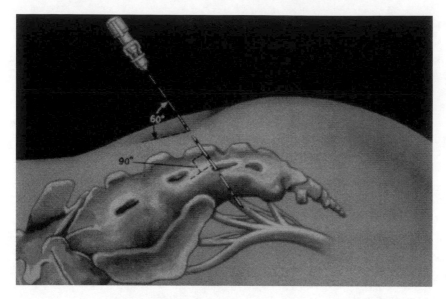

Figure 2   The insulated foramen needle is advanced at an angle of 60° to the skin and perpendicular to the bony surface of the sacrum. (Courtesy of Medtronic, Inc.)

levators ("bellows" response of the perineum) and plantar flexion of the great toe. S2 stimulation leads to "clamp" response of the anal sphincter and lateral leg rotation. S4 stimulation results in a perineal bellows response but no lower extremity motor response. Occasionally, stimulation at S4 will produce a better response owing to variations in neural anatomy. In difficult cases, it is sometimes helpful to map the sacral responses during acute nerve stimulation testing to determine the appropriate foramen in which the temporary or permanent lead should be placed (Fig. 3). Fluoroscopy may be invaluable in locating and placing the foramen needle, but radiographic information should only serve to confirm the impressions derived from stimulation responses.

Table 1   Important Responses to Acute Sacral Nerve Root Stimulation

| Nerve root | Response to acute stimulation | | |
	Pelvic floor	Ipsilateral lower extremity	Sensation
S2. Primary somatic contributor of pudendal nerve for external sphincter, leg, foot	Contraction ("clamp") of anal sphincter	Lateral leg/hip rotation, plantar flexion of entire foot, contraction of calf	Contraction of base of penis or vagina
S3. Virtually all pelvic autonomic functions and striated muscle (levator ani)	Pelvic floor bellows	Plantar flexion of great toe; other toes show variable response	Pulling in rectum, extending to scrotum or labia
S4. Pelvic autonomic and somatic; no leg or foot	Pelvic floor bellows	No lower-extremity motor stimulation	Pulling in rectum only

Figure 3 Intraoperative fluoroscopic "map" showing foramen needles in S2, S3, and S4 in a patient under general anesthesia during permanent implantation. The characteristic leg rotation noted upon stimulation of S2 indicates that the S3 foramen is located one segment lower.

B. Subchronic Phase: Peripheral Nerve Evaluation (PNE)

Once the desired responses are obtained, the test stimulation lead is inserted through the needle, and the needle is removed. The lead is securely taped to the skin and attached to the external stimulator. The patient is able to adjust the voltage amplitude so that he/she maintains the maximum comfortable level of stimulation. Sacral radiographs are obtained to document lead placement. These may aid in placing the permanent lead in the same position in those patients who proceed to permanent implantation. Voiding diaries are kept for 3–7 days before the leads are removed. PNE is considered successful if there is significant (>50%) objective improvement in the particular parameter being evaluated. A voiding diary is then repeated when the patient's symptoms return to baseline to exclude the rare patient who derives long-term benefit from subchronic stimulation. Repeat testing may be considered in patients who had a suboptimal response to PNE. In one series, 65% of patients with a positive test stimulation were identified during the first test stimulation, 21.5% during a second stimulation, and 13.5% during additional testing (unpublished data from Medtronic to the FDA). Patients with a positive response are offered permanent neurostimulator implantation.

V. PERMANENT NEUROSTIMULATOR IMPLANTATION

Permanent implantation may be performed either under general anesthesia with nonparalytic agents or using a combination of local anesthetics and intravenous sedation. Broad-spectrum antibiotics are administered perioperatively, and the patient is positioned as previously described. Acute nerve stimulation testing is performed to locate the desired motor response, which should correspond to that noted during earlier testing. Once the desired foramen and responses are noted, a paramedian incision is made directly over the needle. The incision is carried down to the level where the foramen needle enters the lumbodorsal fascia. The fascia is clean of overlying fat using a Kitner dissector, the hub of the foramen needle is cut off, and a 14-gauge angiocatheter sheath is placed over the needle and through the foramen. A quadripolar lead is placed through the angiocatheter, and the catheter is removed. The lead tested to assure desired motor responses in at least three of the four levels, and the locking collar is placed at the location where the lead perforates the lumbodorsal fascia. The collar is secured to the fascia using nonabsorbable sutures to prevent lead migration. A second incision is made over the upper buttock 3–5 cm below the iliac crest, and a subcutaneous pocket is created for the neurostimulator. A tunneling device is utilized to transfer the free end of the lead to the buttock incision. A connecting lead is secured between the quadripolar stimulating lead and the neurostimulator. The neurostimulator is placed in the subcutaneous pocket, and both incisions are closed in layers with absorbable suture. A radiograph is obtained to document placement (Fig. 4). Alternatively, the neurostimulator may be placed subcutaneously in the anterior abdominal wall using a longer connecting lead, but this technique has fallen out of favor owing to the need to reposition the patient and excellent patient tolerance for buttock placement (8). The patient is discharged within 23 h and returns 1 week later for initial activation of the neurostimulator.

A. Two-Stage Implantation

Two-stage sacral neurostimulator implantation is an alternative method that may increase the number of patients who may benefit from this therapy (9). The technique involves acute stimulation testing as previously described. Instead of placing a temporary lead, the permanent

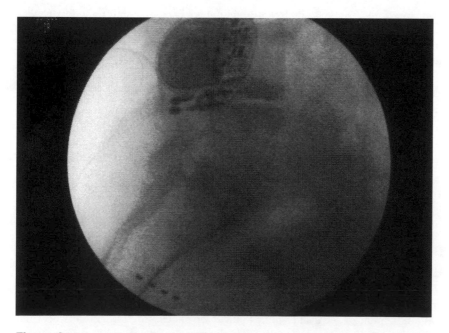

Figure 4   Intra-operative fluoroscopic view following placement of quadripolar electrode and permanent neurostimulator. AP and lateral pelvic radiographs are taken immediately following implantation to document lead placement.

quadripolar electrode lead is placed in the desired foramen and tunneled to the proposed site for permanent neurostimulator placement in the upper buttock. A small incision is made and the permanent lead is connected to a percutaneous extension wire, which is then tunneled to the contralateral side and brought through a small skin puncture. The extension wire is connected to an external neurostimulator. In the next 5–7 days voiding diaries are obtained. If the desired objective and subjective improvement is noted, the percutaneous extension is removed and the permanent neurostimulator is placed as the second stage procedure. If the trial is unsuccessful, the leads are removed using local anesthesia. Future developments may include the development of a permanent electrode that can be placed percutaneously without fear of lead migration.

The two-stage technique offers several advantages. Because the lead is fixed to the lumbodorsal fascia with sutures, the problems encountered with early lead displacement inherent to PNE are obviated. The use of a quadripolar lead for test stimulation allows greater flexibility in the setting of stimulation parameters that should increase the percentage of responders who will then qualify for permanent neurostimulator implantation.

Although there are some concerns about infection, the long subcutaneous tunnel through which the percutaneous extension is placed minimizes this risk. This technique, which received FDA approval in 2001, is commonly utilized in patients who have failed a percutaneous trial. It is rapidly gaining favor as the initial technique (in lieu of PNE) for the initial testing of this form of therapy. Bilateral sacral nerve root stimulation has been utilized in select cases, but to date there is no convincing evidence that this will significantly improve clinical efficacy (10). An alternative approach involves the bilateral implantation of cuff electrodes following sacral laminectomy. This technique may improve the efficacy of chronic sacral neuromodulation by preventing lead migration, but the procedure is much more invasive and the necessity for sacral laminectomy may limit patient acceptance.

B. Postimplantation Activation and Programming

Within 1 week of implantation, the neurostimulator is activated. A console programmer allows transcutaneous adjustment of stimulation parameters including amplitude, rate of stimulation, pulse width, and either continuous or cycling mode. After basic parameters are set, the patient can easily adjust the amplitude of stimulation within limits set by the treating physician by using a small handheld programmer. The patient is instructed to turn the stimulator up to the maximum comfortable level. Patients with urinary retention are instructed to turn the device off to void. The neurostimulator battery has an estimated lifespan of 7–10 years.

VI. EFFICACY OF SACRAL NERVE STIMULATION

During the 1980s and 1990s, a number of centers in Europe and the United States reported on their experience with SNS for various urinary voiding dysfunctions (11–15). These were case series that lacked control groups and simply compared the clinical symptoms of patients before and after neurostimulator implantation. The most convincing evidence for the efficacy of sacral neuromodulation was derived from a prospective, randomized study (MDT-103) conducted at 16 centers in North America and Europe. This study included patients with urge incontinence, urinary urgency-frequency, and urinary retention who had failed standard medical therapy and who demonstrated at least a 50% improvement from baseline during test stimulation. These patients were randomized to either the treatment (immediate implantation) group or control (delayed implantation) group (Fig. 5).

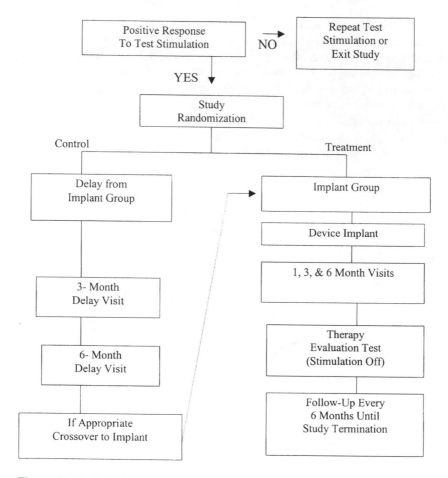

Figure 5   Design of MDT-103, a multicenter, prospective randomized controlled trial of 581 patients with urge incontinence, significant urgency-frequency, or urinary retention who failed standard treatment or standard treatment was deemed medically inappropriate. (From Refs. 16–19.)

A.   Results of the Multicenter Randomized Controlled Trial (MDT-103)

1.   Urge Incontinence

It is clear that sacral neuromodulation decreases both the frequency and the severity of leakage in patients with refractory urge incontinence (16). After 6 months, 77% of patients who were randomized to neurostimulator implantation experienced no heavy leaking episodes compared to 8% in the control (no implant) group. Forty-seven percent of those treated achieved complete continence at 6 months compared to none in the control arm. Clinical efficacy was sustained for 18 months with 52% of patients being completely dry and 24% showing >50% improvement. The same group later reported that sacral nerve stimulation is a durable and effective treatment for refractory urge incontinence with sustained long-term benefit through an average of 30.8 months.

2.   Urinary Frequency

Hassouna and associates studied 51 patients with refractory urgency-frequency who successfully completed test stimulation in a randomized controlled study (18). Compared to the control group, the treatment group demonstrated significantly improvements in the number of voids daily, volume voided per void, and degree of urgency before void. Symptoms returned to baseline when the neurostimulators were turned off 6 months following implantation. Approximately half of the patients (48%) reported either a 50% or greater decrease in urinary frequency or complete resolution of urinary frequency (fewer than eight voids per day). Improvement in urinary urgency was reported by 83%. These responses remained essentially unchanged through the 18-month follow-up period. Favorable urodynamic responses were seen in those patients with detrusor instability noted during initial evaluation.

3. Urinary Retention

Sacral neuromodulation has proven effective in selected patients with nonobstructive retention (19). Compared to the control group, the treatment group had statistically and clinically significant reductions in the catheter volume per catheterization. Of the patients treated with implants, 69% eliminated catheterization at 6 months and an additional 14% had a 50% or greater reduction in catheter volume per catheterization. Successful results were achieved in 83% of the implant group with retention compared to 9% of the control group at 6 months. Temporary inactivation of sacral nerve stimulation therapy resulted in a significant increase in residual volumes. The efficacy of sacral nerve stimulation was sustained through 18 months after implantation.

B. Complications

Percutaneous test stimulation has been proven to be exceedingly safe. The most common adverse event in 914 test stimulations in MDT-103 was lead migration which occurred in 11.8% of procedures (Medtronic Inc., unpublished data to FDA). Technical problems and pain were the two next most common events, occurring in <3% of patients. The rate of complications requiring surgical intervention associated with test stimulation was noted in one patient (0.1% of procedures). This involved a test stimulation electrode that became dislodged during routine removal requiring surgical removal.

There is a relatively high incidence of adverse events associated with sacral nerve stimulator implants. Evaluation of the safety of sacral nerve stimulation was established by pooling safety data in a population of 219 patients with implants for urge incontinence, urgency-frequency, and retention. Pooling of safety data from these three indications was justified based on the identical study protocol, devices, efficacy results, and safety profile (18). The probability of postimplant adverse events that exceeded 5% at 12 months included pain at neurostimulator site (15.3%), new pain (9.0%), suspected lead migration (8.4%), infection (6.1%), transient sensation of electrical shock (5.5%), and pain at the lead site (5.4%). Surgical revision of the implanted neurostimulator or lead system was performed in 33.3% of cases patients to resolve an adverse event. There were no reports of serious adverse device effects or of permanent injury associated with the devices or use of sacral nerve stimulation. It is expected that as implanting physicians gain experience in this technique and technical improvements in this device are introduced, the moderately high complication rates should fall.

VII. CONCLUSION

The management of voiding dysfunction remains one of the most challenging problems faced by the practicing urologist. Although the mode of action of sacral neuromodulation is poorly understood, controlled studies have clearly shown the superiority of this treatment to conservative therapy. Implantation and testing techniques are easily learned by surgeons with particular interest in voiding dysfunction. The use of sacral nerve modulation via an implantable system is an effective, minimally invasive, potentially reversible tool for the management of refractory voiding dysfunction. Improvements in the technical design of the neurostimulation system promise to simplify the techniques of testing and implantation and reduce the significant complication rate of this therapy.

The field of neurostimulation is rapidly evolving. Since the completion of earlier studies on sacral nerve stimulation, procedural advances including new, less invasive technology and surgical techniques have led to greater acceptance among the patient and physicians. A tined quadripolar stimulation lead and introducer system, approved by the FDA in 2002, has significantly decreased the invasiveness of sacral nerve stimulation using the Interstim system. Tined leads offer sacral nerve stimulation through a sutureless anchoring procedure. This procedure can be conducted under local anesthesia. This allows for the evaluation of patient sensory response during the implant procedure ensuring optimal lead placement. This improved technique results in faster patient recovery times as a result of a minimized surgical incision.

Electrical stimulation of the pudendal nerve has been demonstrated to inhibit detrusor activity. Chronic neurostimulation of pudendal afferents may provide effective treatment for disorders of detrusor overactivity. There are significant technical challenges inherent to placing and maintaining an electrode near the pudendal nerve in humans. The development of new implantable microstimulators has made chronic implantation or pudendal neurostimulators feasible. The bion® (Advanced Bionics, Sylmar, California) is a new generation generic implantable microstimulator implanted using minimally invasive techniques. The bion® microstimulator contains a rechargeable battery, sophisticated electronics, and stimulating electrodes in a 3 mm × 28 mm cylinder and weighing only 0.75 grams. It is implanted through the use of a needle-like instrument. The bion® has received CE Mark approval for use in urinary urge incontinence in the European Union and is currently in a U.S. Phase II clinical study for this indication.

Future technology breakthroughs in the field may include "closed-loop system" neurostimulators that continually monitor and stimulate the nervous system to preemptively detect and treat the underlying disorder, as well as integrated treatment methods in which drugs help to target neurostimulation to specific cells.

REFERENCES

1. Urinary Incontinence Guideline Panel. Urinary Incontinence in Adults: Clinical Practice Guidelines. Rockville, MD: Agency for Health Care Policy and Research, Public Health Service, U.S. Department of Health and Human Services, 1992, AHCPR Publication No. 92-00338.
2. Schmidt RA, Tanagho EA. Clinical use of neurostimulation. Urologe 1990; 29:191–195.
3. Tanagho EA. Principles and indications of electrostimulation of the urinary bladder. Urologe 1990; 29:185–190.
4. Schmidt RA, Doggweiler R. Neurostimulation and neuromodulation: a guide to selecting the right urologic patient. Eur Urol 1998; 34(suppl):23–26.
5. Fowler CJ, Swinn MJ, Goodwin RJ, Oliver S, Craggs M. Studies of the latency of pelvic floor contraction during peripheral nerve evaluation show that the muscle response is reflexly mediated. J Urol 2000; 163:881–883.
6. Dijkema HE, Weil EHJ, Mijs PT, Janknegt RA. Neuromodulation of sacral nerves for incontinence and voiding dysfunctions. Clinical results and complications. Eur Urol 1993; 24:72–76.

7. Bosch JLHR, Groen J. Treatment of refractory urge urinary incontinence with sacral spinal nerve stimulation in multiple sclerosis patients. Lancet 1996; 348:717–719.
8. Scheepens WA, Weil EH, Van Koeveringe GA, Rohrmann D, Hedlund HE, Schurch B, Ostardo E, Pastorello M, Ratto C, Nordling J, Van Kerrebroeck PE. Buttock placement of the implantable pulse generator: a new implantation technique for sacral neuromodulation-a multicenter study. Eur Urol 2001; 40:434–438.
9. Janknegt RA, Weil EHJ, Eerdmans PH. Improving neuromodulation: technique for refractory voiding dysfunctions: two-stage implant. Urology 1997; 358–362.
10. Hohenfellner M, Schultz-Lampel D, Dahms S, Matzel K, Thuroff JW. Bilateral chronic sacral neuromodulation for treatment of lower urinary tract dysfunction. J Urol 1998; 160:821–824.
11. Thon WF, Baskin LS, Jonas U, Tanagho EA, Schmidt RA. Neuromodulation of voiding dysfunction and pelvic pain. World J Urol 1991; 9:138–141.
12. Dijkema HE, Weil EH, Mijs PT, Janknegt RA. Neuromodulation of sacral nerves for incontinence and voiding dysfunctions. Clinical results and complications. Eur Urol 1993; 24(1):72–76.
13. Koldewijn EL, Rosier PF, Meuleman EJ, Koster AM, Debruyne FM, Van Kerrebroeck PE. Predictors of success with neuromodulation in lower urinary tract dysfunction: results of trial stimulation in 100 patients. J Urol 1994; 152:2071–2075.
14. Shaker HS, Hassouna M. Sacral nerve root neuromodulation: an effective treatment for refractory urge incontinence. J Urol 1998; 159(5):1516–1519.
15. Weil EH, Ruiz-Cerda JL, Eerdmans PH. Clinical results of sacral neuromodulation for chronic voiding dysfunction using unilateral sacral foramen electrodes. World J Urol 1998; 16:313–321.
16. Schmidt RA, Jonas U, Oleson KA, Janknegt RA, Hassouna MM, Siegel SW, Van Kerrebroeck PE. Sacral nerve stimulation for treatment of refractory urinary urge incontinence. Sacral Nerve Stimulation Study Group. J Urol 1999; 162:352–357.
17. Janknegt RA, Hassouna MM, Siegel SW, Schmidt RA, Gajewski JB, Rivas DA, Elhilali MM, Milam DC, Van Kerrebroeck PE, Dijkema HE, Lycklama a Nyeholt AA, Fall M, Jonas U, Catanzaro F, Fowler CJ, Oleson KA. Long-term effectiveness of sacral nerve stimulation for refractory urge incontinence. Eur Urol 2001; 39:101–106.
18. Hassouna MM, Siegel SW, Nyeholt AA, Elhilali MM, Van Kerrebroeck PE, Das AK, Gajewski JB, Janknegt RA, Rivas DA, Dijkema H, Milam DF, Oleson KA, Schmidt RA. Sacral neuromodulation in the treatment of urgency-frequency symptoms: a multicenter study on efficacy and safety. J Urol 2000; 163:1849–1854.
19. Jonas U, Fowler CJ, Chancellor MB, Elhilali MM, Fall M, Gajewski JB, Grunewald V, Hassouna MM, Hombergh U, Janknegt R, van Kerrebroeck PE, Lycklama a Nijeholt AA, Siegel SW, Schmidt RA. Efficacy of sacral nerve stimulation for urinary retention: results 18 months after implantation. J Urol 2001; 165:15–19.

36

Physical Exam and Assessment of Pelvic Support Defects

Steven Swift
Medical University of South Carolina, Charleston, South Carolina, U.S.A.

I. INTRODUCTION

Prior to examining and describing pelvic organ support defects in the female, all clinicians should have several tools in mind that will aid in providing a comprehensive and accurate diagnosis. These tools should include an understanding of what represents normal pelvic organ support versus pathologic prolapse, an inventory of symptoms that can be attributed to pelvic organ prolapse, and a reliable method of describing the physical findings during the exam. While the first two tools may seem unnecessary in the subject who has an obvious vaginal bulge that protrudes 4–5 cm beyond the vaginal opening and complaints of inability to completely empty her bowels or bladder, they are crucial in evaluating the subject who has a cystocele and no or minimal symptoms.

Until recently these tools were not readily available, and it is only within the past decade that investigators have begun to study these aspects of pelvic organ support defects. Three articles, all published in the past 5 years, have attempted to describe the normal distribution of pelvic organ support, but despite this, there remains a lack of consensus as to what is normal support versus pathologic prolapse. The recent development of quality of life (QOL) tools, specific to pelvic organ prolapse, are providing us with a reliable inventory of symptoms attributable to this condition, but there are still some misconceptions regarding symptoms of milder forms of prolapse. Finally, there has also been significant progress in standardizing the description of pelvic organ support. The publication of the Pelvic Organ Prolapse Quantification (POPQ) system in 1996 provided the first universally recognized and reliable system to codify pelvic organ support and prolapse.

This chapter will discuss how to approach the physical assessment of a patient with pelvic organ support defects from the standpoint of investigating symptoms and physical findings. This should allow the clinician to better manage and appreciate the subtleties of pelvic organ support defects.

II. NORMAL SUPPORT VERSUS PATHOLOGIC PELVIC ORGAN PROLAPSE

Pelvic organ prolapse is something that when present or absent is obvious, but the point at which an individual goes from normal support to pathologic prolapse cannot be defined. When the

497

leading edge of the prolapse extends well beyond the limits of the introitus, there is obvious pathology that all clinicians recognize. When there is little to no movement of any vaginal walls with Valsalva, the absence of pelvic organ prolapse is apparent, but the patient with pelvic organ support somewhere in between these extremes often presents a dilemma. Distinguishing age appropriate normal pelvic support from abnormal prolapse is often a very subjective clinical decision. This stems from the paucity of data in the literature regarding the normal distribution of pelvic organ support in women. Several recent studies have begun to explore this, but the findings are not consistent. One thing that is apparent is that as the patient ages, her pelvic organs begin to relax into the vaginal canal. What is normal support in 55-year-old women may be early signs of impending pelvic organ prolapse in 19-year-old women.

There are three studies in the literature that reported the normal distribution of pelvic organ support in populations of women. The first looked at all women between the ages of 18 and 59 in a small Swedish city (1). They found that only 2% of women had pelvic organ prolapse described as the leading edge of the prolapse being at or beyond the vaginal introitus. These women with prolapse were all in the top quartile of the age range investigated. In the second study, a group of perimenopausal women taking soy supplements for hormone replacement therapy were investigated and they found very few women with any degree of pelvic relaxation (2). In contrast, another study of women between the ages of 18 and 81 presenting for annual exams found a wide range of pelvic organ support with a much greater degree of pelvic relaxation than noted in previous studies (3). These authors demonstrated that as women age the leading edge of their pelvic organs descends into the vaginal canal such that by the time they reach the sixth decade of life the leading edge of their pelvic organs is often at the level of the introitus (Fig. 1). These studies give some information on the normal distribution of pelvic organ support; however, they do not define what is normal and what is pathologic pelvic organ support. One of the drawbacks to these studies is that subjects examined were not always questioned regarding their symptoms to determine at what level of support women begin experiencing symptoms of pelvic organ prolapse. Since pelvic organ prolapse is often a QOL issue, determining the degree of symptoms experienced by subjects with varying degrees of support would help us understand what represents symptomatic pelvic organ prolapse.

Every patient should serve as her own control. If a patient is asymptomatic and has some evidence of a pelvic organ support defect on physical exam, then the clinician may want to follow that patient over time to see if her support worsens. Alternatively, if the subject has new symptoms attributable to prolapse, then she should be thoroughly investigated and treated regardless of her degree of support. What is an asymptomatic degree of support in one subject may lead to symptoms in another. The data presented above on the normal distribution of pelvic organ support can aid in counseling subjects with minor degrees of relaxation who have concerns. This information may reassure some patients that they have age-appropriate support.

The definition of pelvic organ prolapse seems obvious but is often extremely complicated. Instead of relying on any one physical finding or stage of support as a definition, the clinician should put the physical findings in the context of a patient's symptoms and the distribution of normal support for her age. The clinician should be able to provide relief for their symptomatic patients without being overly aggressive in asymptomatic individuals.

III. SYMPTOMS OF PELVIC ORGAN PROLAPSE

The vaginal vault is surrounded by the bladder and urethra anteriorly, the uterus and small intestines superiorly, and the rectum and lower sigmoid posteriorly. Therefore, it is not surprising that when the vaginal support is abnormal, the function of these surrounding

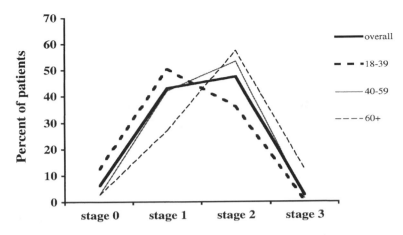

Figure 1   Distribution of pelvic organ support by POPQ stage in 487 women presenting for annual gynecologic healthcare. Note how the peak of the age range curves shifts to the right as the age increases.

structures is compromised. The symptoms commonly attributed to pelvic organ prolapse are a vaginal bulge, low back pain, sense of pelvic pressure and fullness, constipation, urinary and/or fecal incontinence, and the inability to empty the bladder and/or rectum (4). While it appears that this list is complete and all of these symptoms could be anticipated in subjects with pelvic organ prolapse, the only symptom that is consistently acknowledged by patients with severe prolapse is the presence of a vaginal bulge that can be seen or felt (5). This is often accompanied by a sense of pelvic pressure and fullness that is worse late in the day, with any prolonged standing or during physically demanding activities. However, the sense of pelvic fullness or pressure can also be a result of vaginal irritation from atrophy or vaginitis in a patient with otherwise excellent pelvic organ support. In postmenopausal women, complaints of pelvic pressure and a sense of something "wanting to fall out" of the vagina are often a symptom of severe urogenital atrophy particularly if the subject denies the presence of a vaginal bulge. In the only study to compare symptoms in subjects with and without objective pelvic organ prolapse, the symptom of heaviness in the lower abdomen was reported in 9.7% of subjects with any degree of prolapse and in 7.5% of subjects with no prolapse (1).

While it seems counterintuitive, the presence of urinary or fecal incontinence is generally not encountered in subjects with more severe degrees of pelvic organ prolapse. It has long been noted that urinary incontinence often improves as a patient's prolapse worsens and subjects with more severe degrees of prolapse register complaints more obstructive in nature. Therefore, it is not surprising from organ prolapse QOL questionnaires that the symptoms of urinary and fecal incontinence play a minor role in pelvic organ prolapse. The King's College Prolapse Quality of Life tool (P-QOL) leaves out any reference to stress urinary or fecal incontinence but has multiple questions regarding difficulty emptying the bladder and rectum (6). There are a few questions regarding urge incontinence and irritative voiding symptoms. The common lower urinary and intestinal tract symptoms involve the patient having to manually reduce her vaginal prolapse or bulge in order to fully empty either her rectum or her bladder. This symptom is much more prevalent than incontinence in women with genital prolapse.

Stress urinary incontinence can commonly become symptomatic when severe prolapse is reduced either surgically or with a pessary. This is often referred to as potential, latent, or occult stress incontinence and occurs in anywhere from 15% to 80% of subjects (7,8). It should be sought out during physical exam, particularly if contemplating surgical correction of the prolapse.

The symptoms of pelvic pain and or pressure are fairly nonspecific and do not specifically point to a diagnosis of pelvic organ prolapse. The symptom of low back pain is common to a multitude of conditions, and while often present in women with pelvic organ prolapse, it is not specific.

When identifying and discussing signs and symptoms of pelvic organ prolapse, the practitioner should focus on the patient's report of a vaginal bulge along with obstructive urinary and fecal symptoms. These are the more common symptoms that can be relieved when the prolapse is reduced. While symptoms of urinary and fecal incontinence are uncommon, if present, they should be explored.

IV. PELVIC ORGAN SUPPORT DEFECTS

There are countless systems for codifying pelvic organ support in the literature that date back to the late 1800s. They have been proposed by some of the fathers of modern gynecology (Professor Scanzoni, Dr. Keustner, and Dr. Howard Kelley), and while all have gained regional notoriety, no one system attained universal acceptance. In addition, none of these early systems were studied to determine their intra- or interexaminer reliability (9–11). The extent of this problem was documented in a review of over 100 articles and 15 textbooks that used or described various classification systems for pelvic organ prolapse (12). They found no consensus in how pelvic organ support defects were classified and in all but a few instances found no detailed description of any system being used.

The first system to gain widespread acceptance in the United States was the Baden and Walker "half-way" system that was introduced in 1972 and updated in 1992 (13,14). In this system, the vagina is divided up into six areas that are described separately, the anterior wall or urethrocele and cystocele, the posterior vaginal wall or rectocele, the apex or enterocele, the cervix, and the perineal body. The system then describes support for each of these segments based on the concept of half-way. If the segment being described descends no more than half-way to the introitus, it is said to be stage 1. If the segment descends into the lower half of the vagina but not through the introitus, it is stage 2. If it descends through the introitus but is less than half-way to completely prolapsed, then it is stage 3, and any prolapse greater than this is stage 4. This system was recently studied and demonstrated good intra-examiner reliability.

As described, the system is somewhat difficult to understand. For example, the anterior and posterior vaginal walls are continuous structures that begin at the introitus and extend up to the cervix and posterior fornix, respectively, or the cuff scar in the hysterectomized woman. Therefore, it can be difficult to decide what portion or aspect of the anterior and posterior walls to describe as descending into the lower half of the vaginal canal, as the lower half of each wall is already part of the lower half of the vaginal canal. Despite this, most clinicians find this system simple to use and it has demonstrated good interexaminer reliability (13).

In 1996, the International Continence Society's Committee on Terminology devised a classification system to recommend for international use (15). Out of this meeting came the Pelvic Organ Prolapse Quantification (POPQ) system. Similar to the "half-way" system, it divides the vagina up into several points that are each described independently. There are a total of nine points (eight if the women has had a hysterectomy) that are measured and reported in a 3×3 grid (Fig. 2). Instead of using vague terms to describe which aspect of the prolapsing organ or vaginal wall is to be judged, the POPQ requires that specific points on the vaginal walls and cervix be measured in 0.5-cm increments. In addition, the measurements are made around the fixed point of the hymenal remnants instead of the more vague introitus. If the point being described remains above the hymen, its position is recorded, in centimeters, as a negative number. If the point being described descends to the level of the hymen, its position is recorded

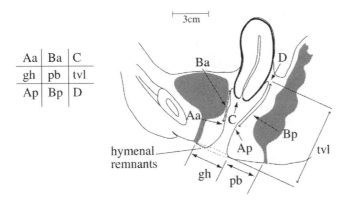

Aa	Ba	C
gh	pb	tvl
Ap	Bp	D

Figure 2 Diagrammatic representation of the nine points of the POPQ and the 3 × 3 grid used for reporting.

as 0. If the point passes beyond the hymen, its position is recorded, in centimeters, as a positive number. One overall stage is assigned for the patient as the most dependent or the most prolapsed point. The anterior, posterior, apical vaginal walls and cervix are not assigned individual stages.

The POPQ is a relatively complex system, and the document describing the technique for obtaining the nine measured points is seven pages in length, requiring a very thorough reading to understand how certain measures are derived. The A points of the anterior (Aa) and posterior (Ap) vaginal wall are determined by measuring 3 cm proximal to the urethral meatus for the Aa and 3 cm proximal to the hymenal remnent at the posterior fourchette for Ap (Fig. 4). Point B anterior (Ba) and posterior (Bp) are usually the most difficult to appreciate. They are the only points that are not fixed. They are used to designate the most dependant segments of the anterior and posterior vaginal walls that are between point Aa and point C anteriorly and point Ap and point D posteriorly (or point C posteriorly if the patient has had a prior hysterectomy). Point C represents the cervix or cuff scar (after hysterectomy). Point D represents the posterior fornix or apex of the vagina and is not measured if the patient has had a hysterectomy. These points on the vaginal wall are then observed as the patient performs either a cough or Valsalva. Where they

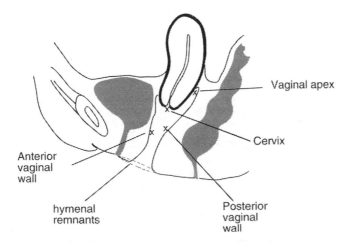

Figure 3 Diagrammatic representation of the four point of the simplified POPQ.

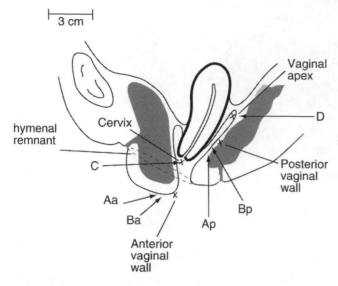

Figure 4   Diagrammatic representation of a stage 3 anterior vaginal wall prolapse identifying both the POPQ points and the simplified POPQ points. The POPQ points Aa, Ba, C, D, Ap, and Bp are all associated with lines ending with an arrowhead. The simplified POPQ points are represented by lines ending in x's.

descend in relation to the hymen is recorded in centimeters as either zero, a positive number, or a negative number, as described above. The genital hiatus (GH) is a measurement from the urethral meatus to the hymenal remnant at the posterior fourchette. This may be a misleading terms as the genital hiatus is actually the opening in the levator ani muscle that the vagina perforates. The perineal body (PB) is a measurement from the hymenal remnant at the posterior fourchette to the middle of the anus. The total vaginal length (TVL) is a measure of the total vaginal length from the hymeneal remnant to the vaginal apex. This is the only number recorded with the patient at rest. Once all of the numbers are obtained, a stage is assigned and a vaginal profile can be drawn. The staging system is described in Table 1. The easiest way to remember the staging system is to

Table 1   Ordinal Staging System of the POPQ

Stage	Leading edge of points Aa, Ba, Ap, Bp	Leading edge of point C and/or D
0	All 4 points are 3 cm above the hymenal remnants (value $= -3$)	Points C and D are at a position above the hymenal remnants that is equal to or within 2 cm of the total vaginal length (values $\geq -(tvl^a - 2)$)
1	All points are >1 cm above the hymenal remnants (value ≤ -1)	
2	Leading edge of the prolapse protrudes to a point to or above 1 cm above the hymenal remnants but no more than 1 cm beyond the hymenal remnants (value ≥ -1 to $\leq +1$)	
3	Maximal prolapse protrudes at least 1 cm beyond the hymenal remnants but <2 cm the total vaginal length (value $\geq +1$ to $+(tvl - 2)$)	
4	Maximal prolapse protrudes to within 2 cm of the total length of the vaginal tube (value $\geq (tvl - 2)$)	

[a]tvl = total vaginal length.

focus on the limits of stage 2 support. If the prolapsing organ being described comes to within 1 cm of the hymenal remnants, either above or through, then it is stage 2. If there is some movement of the vaginal wall but it does not descend to the limits of stage 2, then it is stage 1. If the prolapsing vaginal wall is >1 cm past the hymenal remnants, then it is stage 3. If there is no movement of the vaginal points, then it is stage 0, and complete uterovaginal prolapse is stage 4.

The POPQ, while difficult to learn initially, has several advantages over the other systems that rely on stages instead of specific measures. This is particularly apparent in following a patient over time to determine if the patient's pelvic support is changing or is stable. Instead of using stages, which are relatively gross descriptions of support that encompass a wide range of possible positions, the POPQ gives specific measures to within 0.5 cm. For example:

A subject presents in referral for evaluation of an anterior vaginal wall defect that is relatively assymptomatic. On exam her point Aa and Ba are at −1 cm (1 cm above the hymenal remnants) with Valsalva. She has stage 2 support. She is followed for 6 months and on return her point Aa and Ba are now at +1 cm (1 cm past the hymenal remnants). She still has stage 2 support but has obviously progressed, and the clinician may now consider an intervention. If she were followed by the gross description of stage, then her progression would be less apparent.

Alternatively, a patient presents with a mild anterior vaginal wall defect such that her point Aa and Ba are at −1.5 cm (1.5 cm above the introitus). She has stage 1 support. On reevaluation 6 months later, her point Aa and Ba are at −1 cm and she is now stage 2. This patient has had almost no progression, but without the specific measures of the POPQ it would appear she has had a one full stage progression.

The use of stages is adequate for describing populations, but a more descriptive system like the POPQ has more clinical applicability for evaluating and following individual patients. In

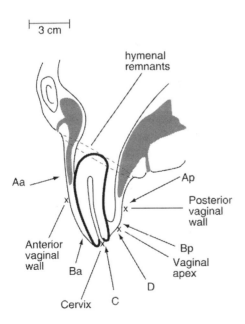

Figure 5 Diagrammatic representation of a stage 4 prolapse identified both the POPQ points and the simplified POPQ points. The POPQ points Aa, Ba, C, D, Ap, and Bp are all associated with lines ending with an arrowhead. The simplified POPQ points are represented by lines ending in x's.

addition, the POPQ system was the first to undergo extensive testing and was shown to have excellent intra- and interexaminer reliability (16–19).

The International Federation of Gynecologists and Obstetricians (FIGO) in 1998 became interested in endorsing a pelvic organ prolapse classification system for worldwide use. It initially considered the POPQ but found the system to be too complex to endorse for worldwide use by nonspecialists. Therefore a simplified version of the POPQ was developed with the International Urogynecological Association (IUGA) (20). This simplified version retained the staging system of the POPQ but eliminated stage 0 (Fig. 4). Stages 1–4 remained essentially identical to the POPQ. If the simplified version is adopted by FIGO, it will allow for crossover so that research employing the POPQ system can be translated into clinically useful information that doctors could use in their practice.

In the simplified version there are only four points measured instead of nine as with the POPQ; anterior vaginal wall, posterior vaginal wall, the cervix (if present), and posterior fornix. In describing the anterior vaginal wall, a point half-way between the hymenal remnants or urethral meatus and the cervix or cuff is identified. This is done by gently retracting the posterior vaginal wall with a Sims speculum, disarticulated Graves speculum, or two fingers to fully expose the anterior vaginal wall. The subject is then asked to Valsalva, and where that point on the vaginal wall descends to, in relation to the hymenal remnants, is documented as the stage for the anterior vaginal wall. A similar technique is employed to describe the stage of the posterior vaginal wall except that a point is chosen half-way between the hymenal remnants and the posterior fornix or cuff scar. Practitioners should be able to identify when the leading edge of the prolapse is >1 cm above or past the hymenal remnants with close inspection. Therefore, no specific measuring device is necessary. In addition, while the use of the descriptors of anterior vaginal wall, posterior vaginal wall, and apical vaginal segments is encouraged, the older terms of cystocele, rectocele, and enterocele are deemed acceptable. In the POPQ system these terms are disallowed.

This system was studied at one institution and its interexaminer reliability was deemed excellent (21). The modified IUGA/FIGO system was compared to the POPQ, and there was excellent agreement between the two systems for staging the various segments as well as for the overall stage. The simplified POPQ is still undergoing testing at various centers throughout the world to further study its inter- and intraexaminer reliability as well as to document its agreement with the POPQ. Prior to its adoption by FIGO it must also prove to be a simple and easy-to-use tool in clinical practice.

The three systems for describing and codifying pelvic organ support have their own advantages and disadvantages. The Baden and Walker "half-way" system and the simplified

Table 2 Ordinal Staging System for the Simplified POPQ

Stage	Leading edge of anterior and posterior vaginal wall, cervix, apex or posterior fornix (or cuff scar in the hysterectomized women). Each of the four segments (three in the hysterectomized women) is graded independently.
1	Prolapse that remains at least 1 cm above of the hymenal remnants.
2	Prolapse that descends to the introitus, defined as 1 cm above or below the hymenal remnants.
3	Prolapse that descends past the introitus, but does not represent complete vaginal vault eversion or complete procidentia uteri.
4	Complete vaginal vault eversion or complete procidentia uteri. (If one segment is stage 4 then all segments are stage 4.)

POPQ appear to be easy to use but lack specificity for describing subtle changes. The POPQ, while excellent at describing the detail of all aspects of pelvic organ support, can be cumbersome to employ in a busy clinical setting and requires practice and continued use to become comfortable using.

V. CONDITIONS FOR PERFORMING THE EXAM

There are many opinions regarding how to exam the subject with suspected pelvic organ prolapse. Some authors advocate always examining subjects in the standing position; others state that subjects should be examined with an empty bladder or only late in the afternoon, after they have been on their feet for several hours. While all of these recommendations seem appropriate, few have been studied to determine if they really allow the clinician to better determine the full extent of the subjects prolapse. Only patient positioning during the exam has been investigated. It has been demonstrated that exams in the dorsal lithotomy and standing position are equivalent (22). The authors concluded that patient positioning was not important, and they suggested the physician allow the patient to confirm her exam. This can be done by having the patient feel the bulge during the exam or use a mirror to visually confirm your findings. If you cannot reproduce the subjects complaints, then examining the subject more upright or having her come back late in the day for a follow-up exam may be indicated.

Another area, which is somewhat controversial, involves examining for the presence of occult or potential stress urinary incontinence. This involves reducing the prolapse during the exam and testing for the presence of stress incontinence. As previously mentioned, it is uncommon for subjects with severe anterior vaginal prolapse to have complaints of stress urinary incontinence. However, when the prolapse is corrected, either surgically or with a pessary, stress incontinence is unmasked in up to 80% of patients. It is felt that the anterior vaginal wall prolapse "kinks" the urethra leading to obstruction. Correcting this "kink" then reveals stress incontinence. This can be assessed during the examination by doing provocative testing with the patient's prolapse reduced. The provocative testing can range from a simple cough stress test with the bladder symptomatically full to stress testing during a multichannel urodynamic exam. Several techniques have been advocated for reducing the prolapse. This can be done with a pessary, disarticulated speculum directed into the sacrum, a vaginal pack, large cotton swab stick or two fingers placed in the vagina to support the apex. Regardless of the technique, it is important not to obstruct the urethra by compressing it against the posterior aspect of the pubic bone. If stress incontinence is only demonstrated with the prolapse reduced, then potential or occult stress incontinence is diagnosed. There are many ways to address this at the time of intervention but those will be discussed elsewhere.

VI. SUMMARY

Defining and describing pelvic organ prolapse is often more difficult than clinicians think. Obvious severe prolapse can be recognized by even the most junior health care provider as pathology. It is the more subtle forms of support defects that require a thorough understanding. By understanding the variations of normal support, the symptoms attributable to pelvic organ support defects, and the systems used to describe the prolapse, the practicing clinician will be better able to determine appropriate and well-timed interventions.

REFERENCES

1. Samuelsson EU, Victor FTA, Tibblin G, Svardsudd KF. Signs of genital prolapse in a Swedish population of women 20 to 59 years of age and possible related factors. Am J Obstet Gynecol 1999; 180:299–305.
2. Bland DR, Earle BB, Vitolins MZ, Burke G. Use of the pelvic organ prolapse staging system of the International Continence Society, American Urogynecologic Society, and the Society of Gynecologic Surgeons in perimenopausal women. Am J Obstet Gynecol 1999; 181:1324–1328.
3. Swift SE. The distribution of pelvic organ support in a population of women presenting for routine gynecologic healthcare. Am J Obstet Gynecol 2000; 183:277–285.
4. American College of Obstetricians and Gynecologists. Pelvic Organ Prolapse. ACOG Technical Bulletin 214. Washington, DC: ACOG, 1995.
5. Elkermann RM, Cundiff GW, Bent AE, Nihira MA, Melick C. Correlation of symptoms with location and severity of pelvic organ prolapse. Abstract presented at the 25th Annual Meeting of the International Urogynecology Association, Rome, Italy, Oct 22–25, 2000.
6. Digesu GA, Khullar V, Cardozo L, Robinson D, Salvatore S. P-QOL: a validated quality of life questionnaire for symptomatic assessment of women with uterovaginal prolapse. Abstract presented at the 25th Annual Meeting of the International Urogynecology Association, Rome, Italy, Oct 22–25, 2000.
7. Weil A, Gianoni A, Rottenberg RD, Krauer F. The risk of postoperative urinary incontinence after surgical treatment of genital prolapse. Int Urogynecol J 1993; 4:74–79.
8. Zivkovic F, Taumissimo K, Michelitsch L, Haas J. Urethral profilemetry in women with uterovaginal prolapse. Int Urogynecol J 1995; 6:10–13.
9. Kelly HA. Operative Gynecology. New York: Appleton & Co., 1898.
10. Scanzoni FW. Senkung und Vorfall des uterus und der scheide. In: Scanzoni FW, ed. Lehrbuch der Krankheiten der weiblichen geschlechstorgane. 5th ed. Vienna: Braumueller, 1875:654–664.
11. Kuestner O. Prolapsus uteri et vaginea. In: Kuestner O, Bumm E, Doederlein A, Kroenig B, Menge C, eds. Kurzes Lehrbuch der Gynaekologie. Jena: G Fischers, 1912:159–181.
12. Brubaker L, Norton P. Current clinical nomenclature for description of pelvic organ prolapse. J Pelvic Surg 1996; 2:257–259.
13. Baden WF, Walker TA. Genesis of the vaginal profile: a correlated classification of vaginal relaxation. Clin Obstet Gynecol 1972; 15:1048–1054.
14. Baden WF, Walker TA. Physical diagnosis in the evaluation of vaginal relaxation. Clin Obstet Gynecol 1972; 15:1055–1069.
15. Bump RC, Mattiasson A, Bo K. The standardization of terminology of female pelvic organ prolapse and pelvic organ dysfunction. Am J Obstet Gynecol 1996; 175:10–17.
16. Kobak WH, Rosenberger K, Walters MD. Interobserver variation in the assessment of pelvic organ prolapse. Int J Urogynecol Pelvic Floor Dysfunc 1996; 7:121–124.
17. Hall AF, Theofrastous JP, Cundiff GC, Harris RL, Hamilton LF, Swift SE, Bump RC. Interobserver and intraobserver reliability of the proposed International Continence Society, Society of Gynecologic Surgeons, and American Urogynecologic Society pelvic organ prolapse classification system. Am J Obstet Gynecol 1996; 175:1467–1469.
18. Athanasiou S, Hill S, Gleeson C, Anders K, Cardozo L. Validation of the ICS proposed pelvic prolapse descriptive system. Neurourol Urodyn 1995; 14:414–415. Abstract.
19. Schussler B, Peschers U. Standardisation of terminology of female genital prolapse according to the new ICS criteria: inter-examiner reliability. Neurourol Urodyn 1995; 14:437–438. Abstract.
20. Swift SE, Freeman R, Petri E, Scotti R, Dwyer P, Ulmsten U. Proposal for a world-wide, user-friendly classification system for pelvic organ prolapse. 16th FIGO World Conference, Washington DC, September 4, 2000.
21. Swift SE, Morris SA. Inter-examiner reliability of a simplified pelvic organ prolapse quantification system. Abstract presented at the 26th Annual Scientific Meeting of the International Urogynecologic Society, Melbourne, Australia, 2001.

37

Radiographic Evaluation of Pelvic Organ Prolapse

Craig V. Comiter
University of Arizona Health Sciences Center, Tucson, Arizona, U.S.A.

I. INTRODUCTION

Pelvic organ prolapse and pelvic floor relaxation are common problems in older multiparous women, affecting ~16% of women aged 40–56 (1). A detailed knowledge of pelvic anatomy is paramount for the proper evaluation and management of such patients. Pelvic support defects result from both neurophysiologic and anatomic changes (2) and often occur as a constellation of abnormal findings. Although a thorough pelvic examination is always indicated, even experienced clinicians may be misled by the physical findings, having difficulty differentiating among cystocele, enterocele, and high rectocele by physical examination alone. Depending on the position of the patient, strength of Valsalva maneuver, and modesty of the patient, the surgeon may be limited in his or her ability to accurately diagnose the components of pelvic prolapse. Furthermore, with uterine prolapse, the cervix and uterus may fill the entire introitus, making the diagnosis of concomitant pelvic prolapse even more difficult. Regardless of the etiology of the support defect, the surgeon must identify all aspects of vaginal prolapse and pelvic floor relaxation for proper surgical planning. Accurate preoperative staging should reduce the risk of recurrent prolapse. *Radiographic evaluation plays an important role in the identification of these defects, and should be used as an extension of the physical examination.*

II. ANATOMY

The female pelvis can be divided into three compartments: anterior, middle, and posterior. No longer are these compartments the domains of the urologist, gynecologist, and coloproctologist, respectively. On the contrary, urologists and gynecologists are increasingly working together in treating pelvic prolapse, and many specialized "female urologists" and "urogynecologists" are now quite adept at taking care of all aspects of pelvic prolapse and the often associated voiding dysfunction.

A. Bony and Musculofascial Support

The bony pelvis is a scaffold from which the intrapelvic structures draw their support. The tendinous arc, a linear fascial condensation arising from the obturator internus muscle, extends from the ischial spine to the lower portion of the pubic symphysis, and represents the insertion point for the levator muscles, providing the musculofascial support for a large portion of the *anterior pelvis* (3). The sacrospinous ligaments arise from the posterior aspect of the ischial spines and insert onto the anterolateral sacrum and coccyx, providing a broad support for the *posterior pelvis*.

The pelvic diaphragm is the superior layer of striated muscle and fascia, which provides the inferior support for the pelvic viscera. The levator ani muscle group, composed of the pubococcygeus and iliococcygeus, forms a hammock upon which the bladder, proximal vagina, and intrapelvic rectum lie. The vagina, rectum, and urethra traverse the pubococcygeus through a funneled hiatus. The anterior muscular decussation forms the external sphincter of the urethra. The medial fibers of the pubococcygeus (puborectalis), which travel posteriorly along the urethra, vagina, and rectum, fuse anterior to the rectum, forming part of the perineal support deep to the perineal body. Reflex contraction of this *levator sling* elevates and compresses the urethra, vagina, and rectum during straining maneuvers.

The "fascial" covering of the levator muscles provides a major part of the normal pelvic visceral support. The levator fascia consists of two leaves—the endopelvic fascia (abdominal side), and the pubocervical fascia (vaginal side). The urethra, bladder, vagina, and uterus are all enveloped within these two layers. The two leaves are made of a fibrofatty connective tissue which fuses laterally, inserting in the tendinous arc of the obturator internus. Specialized condensations of this levator fascia in the areas of the midurethra, bladder neck, bladder body, and cervix play a major role in pelvic organ support.

B.   Anterior Vaginal Wall Support

The *pubourethral ligaments* span from the midportion of the female urethra to the inferior pubis. Laxity of theses structures permit posterior and inferior movement of the midurethra, contributing to stress incontinence (4). The *urethropelvic ligaments* support the urethra and bladder neck to the tendinous arc. The *vesicopelvic ligaments* support the bladder base and anterior vaginal wall by attaching laterally to the tendinous arc of the obturator fascia. Tears in these ligaments lead to a lateral defect cystocele, and weakness of the midline pubocervical fascia leads to a central defect cystocele.

C.   Uterine Support

The cardinal ligaments are the most posterior condensations of the levator fascia, attaching the lateral aspects of the cervix to the ischial spines, thereby supporting the cervix and upper vagina. By supporting the vaginal vault, they form the base of the levator fascial rectangle responsible for bladder support as well (5). The uterosacral ligaments run from the posterolateral cervix and vaginal fornices to the insert at the second, third, and fourth sacral vertebrae (S2–S4) (4). Weakness of these ligamentous structures contributes to uterine prolapse or, in the absence of a uterus, can lead to vault prolapse, enterocele, and apical cystocele formation.

D.   Posterior Vaginal Support

The rectovaginal septum, a fibrous continuation of the cul-de-sac, is composed of the fused posterior vaginal connective tissue and prerectal connective tissue, which insert into the perineal body caudally (5). This rectovaginal septum acts to prevent anterior herniation of the rectum into the posterior vagina. The proximal relation of the rectovaginal septum to the sacrouterine-cardinal complex also contributes to vaginal apical support.

Normally, the distal vagina forms an angle of inclination of 45° from the vertical, while the proximal vagina lies more horizontally over the levator plate, pointing toward S2-S3 (6). The upper vagina is held over the levator plate by the cardinal and uterosacral ligaments, and this angulation is maintained by a strong levator plate and anterior traction of the levator sling. Normally intra-abdominal pressure may be displaced, and the downward pressure of the uterus and cervix is directed toward the posterior vaginal wall and levator plate. However, when the normal proximal vaginal orientation is altered and the vaginal axis becomes more vertical (pelvic floor relaxation), rectocele formation is likely. Moreover, with levator laxity and anterior proximal vaginal rotation, the cul-de-sac assumes a dependent position, open to the direct impact of intra-abdominal forces, potentially predisposing to enterocele formation and vault prolapse.

E. Perineal Support

The bulbocavernosus muscles, superficial and deep transverse perineal muscles, external anal sphincter, and central perineal tendon comprise the urogenital diaphragm. This muscular sheet, which lies caudal to the levator ani, provides additional pelvic support.

III. PHYSIOLOGIC EVALUATION

One in three patients presenting with prolapse also suffer from urinary or fecal incontinence (7). Multichannel urodynamics is clearly the gold standard for assessing voiding dysfunction and complex incontinence, which often accompany pelvic prolapse. A detailed urodynamic evaluation includes measurement of postvoid residual volume and bladder compliance, as well as documentation of the presence or absence of unstable detrusor contractions, bladder outlet obstruction, and the degree of sphincteric function/dysfunction. By combining radiographic imaging and direct cystoscopic visualization of the bladder, a comprehensive evaluation of the incontinent patient will often lead to a precise diagnosis with logical treatment options.

Anorectal physiologic testing is often used for assessment of anorectal neural integrity, nerve conduction, and muscular performance. Rectal manometry may detect abnormalities in rectal and anal pressures, while pudendal nerve terminal motor latency dysfunction is often related to stretch-induced injury following childbirth (8). Needle electromyography (EMG), by measuring electrical activity and quality, can reveal denervation and reinnervation injuries. Prior to endoanal ultrasonography, EMG was the only reliable method to preoperatively identify external sphincter tears (9). While few of these tests are absolutely diagnostic, these techniques provide valuable complementary information when considered together with symptoms, clinical findings, and imaging results (10).

IV. IMAGING TECHNIQUES

Radiographic imaging plays an important adjunctive role to the physical examination in the evaluation of pelvic organ prolapse and pelvic floor relaxation.

A. Intravenous Urography

An intravenous urogram (IVU) is often utilized for the evaluation of hematuria, for the purpose of identifying a renal mass, renal or ureteral stone, upper tract urothelial filling defect, and hydroureteronephrosis. Furthermore, the functional nature of the IVU often allows the physician to distinguish between obstructive and nonobstructive hydronephrosis.

The most common reasons for obtaining an IVU in a woman with pelvic organ prolapse are to detect hydronephrosis and to evaluate for ureteral obstruction from previous pelvic surgeries (11). Hydronephrosis secondary to uterine prolapse was first reported nearly a century ago (12), and, depending on the series presented, the prevalence of hydronephrosis with uterine prolapse varies from 0% to 100% (13,14). Moreover, while ureteral injuries during hysterectomy occur in 0.1–2.5% of cases (15), it has never been shown that routine preoperative IVU in patients with pelvic prolapse reduces the incidence of ureteral injury (16). In two contemporary series of patients with pelvic organ prolapse and no known malignancy, the prevalence of hydronephrosis on routine preoperative IVU was 7% (11,16), with 1% of patients rated as having severe dilatation. While the incidence of hydroureteronephrosis was low, it did increase with worsening pelvic prolapse and was more common with uterine prolapse than with vault prolapse. Serum creatinine levels were neither sensitive nor specific for predicting hydronephrosis, and knowledge of preoperative anatomy did not change the incidence of ureteral injury during surgery (11,16).

Approximately 3% of patients will have a significant adverse reaction to the IVU (16). At the University of Arizona Division of Urology, we do not routinely utilize any radiographic study to image the upper tracts in patients with normal renal function and pelvic prolapse. With the routine use of intravenous indigo carmine for determination of ureteral patency, there have been no instances of ureteral injury in more than 300 cases of transvaginal repair of pelvic organ prolapse over a 3-year period.

B. Fluoroscopy

Fluoroscopy is an excellent and time-tested technique for investigating pelvic organ prolapse. By instilling contrast material into the bladder (anterior compartment), vagina (middle compartment), or rectum (posterior compartment), the dynamic relationships among the pelvic organs may be viewed in real time.

1. Levator Myography

Levator myography is an outdated method of visualizing the pubococcygeus and iliococcygeus via direct injection of contrast solution into the levator muscles. Originally described in 1953 (17), this technique permits the preoperative visualization of the position and supportive role of these muscle groups. Widening of the levator or genital hiatus, which often follows traumatic childbirth and predisposes to pelvic floor relaxation and visceral prolapse, can be demonstrated with levator myography. Today, this information may be obtained noninvasively with computed tomography (CT) (18) and magnetic resonance imaging (MRI) (19,20).

2. Cystography

Lateral cystography allows for a static view of the bladder and bladder outlet in relation to the pubic bony structures. Early investigators utilized a bead chain cystourethrogram to aid with the analysis of the posterior urethrovesical angle (2,21,22). Voiding cystourethrography (VCUG) is mainly utilized for demonstrating a cystocele, evaluating bladder neck hypermobility, and demonstrating an open bladder neck at rest (sphincteric incompetence). Dynamic lateral fluoroscopy at rest and during straining is an important adjunct to the urodynamic evaluation, useful for demonstrating the presence of and degree of urethrovesical hypermobility and cystocele

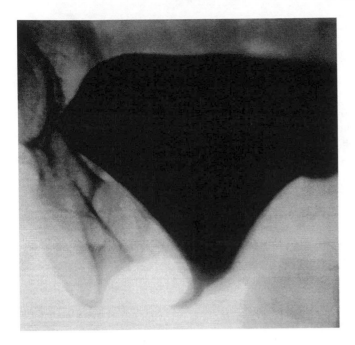

Figure 1 Cystogram demonstrating bladder neck descent and funneling in a patient with stress urinary incontinence.

formation (Fig. 1). While the radiographic findings do not always correlate well with urodynamic findings (23,24), in the incontinent patient with cystographic and/or cystoscopic evidence of an open bladder neck at rest and a low leak point pressure, the diagnosis of sphincteric incompetence is more certain (Fig. 2). Other pathologic conditions detected by VCUG include vesicoureteral reflux, vesicovaginal fistula, and urethral diverticular disease.

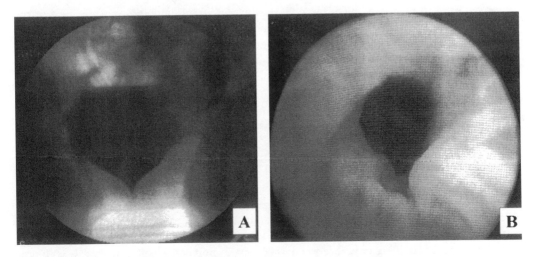

Figure 2 (A) Cystogram demonstrating open bladder neck, consistent with intrinsic sphincter dysfunction. (B) Cystoscopic view confirms radiographic findings.

3. Defacography

Defacography, or evacuation proctography, is used for evaluating the posterior (anorectal) compartment. Commonly measured variables include rectal volume, rectal emptying, perineal and pelvic floor muscle function, and anal sphincter function (2,18,25–27). Although the clinical value of defacography in the evaluation and management of constipation is not well proven (2,28), the presence of an obvious anatomic abnormality in a fecally incontinent patient such as a large rectocele, severe intussusception, or prolapse, supports surgical intervention.

Evacuation proctography relies on opacification of the rectal vault with barium paste (25–27,29) Instilling the paste is quite cumbersome, requiring a large-caliber enema similar to a caulking gun. Typically, 80–300 cc of paste is instilled, often confounded by reflux into the sigmoid colon (30,31). Fluoroscopic images are recorded with the patient relaxed and while performing active contraction of the pelvic floor; this should result in elevation of the pelvic floor musculature. The patient is then examined during cough and during a maximal straining maneuver, noting any pelvic floor descent or fecal incontinence. Finally, defecation is accomplished, and note is made of any rectocele, incomplete emptying, or need for digital assistance with evacuation.

In the cooperative patient, dynamic proctography allows precise identification and quantification of a rectocele, measured as the maximum extent of an anterior rectal bulge beyond the expected line of the rectum (31). Intussusception may be visible as a circumferential invagination of the rectal wall, presenting as mucosal prolapse through the anus in its most severe form. Limitations of this examination are the cumbersome and potentially painful instillation of rectal barium paste, lack of correlation between the viscosity of the paste and the individual patient's stool, and the inability of many patients to defecate on command. Modesty makes this a difficult technique for many individuals. Additionally, the presence of a rectocele in and of itself may be of limited concern, as previous studies have shown that an anterior rectal bulge is commonly demonstrated in nulliparous asymptomatic patients (31). Furthermore, the presence of or size of a rectocele does not correlate well with the completeness of barium evacuation (32).

4. Colpocystourethrography

First introduced in France in 1965, the colpocystourethrogram combines opacification of the bladder, urethra, and vagina (33). Modified and made popular in the mid-1970s, the colpocystourethrogram is a dynamic study of pelvic support and function (34). The anatomical relationships among the bladder, urethra, and vagina may be demonstrated, and when combined with proctography may be even more useful in outlining the anatomy of the normal pelvis and of complex pelvic organ prolapse.

Any insult that alters the normal anatomic relationships, such as hysterectomy, pelvic floor relaxation, or bladder neck suspension, may predispose to enterocele formation. In the case of pelvic floor relaxation, as often occurs in the multiparous woman, widening of the levator hiatus leads to a diminution in the pubococcygeal contraction in response to straining. This results in insufficient vaginal angulation, with the proximal vagina becoming more vertically oriented. Similarly, bladder neck suspension without proper repair of concomitant pelvic floor relaxation results in anterior displacement of the vagina. The cul-de-sac is left unprotected and exposed to increases in intra-abdominal pressure, predisposing to enterocele formation. An enterocele, defined as herniation of the peritoneum and its contents at the level of the vaginal apex, may be appreciated during straining or defecation during colpocystoproctography, seen as widening of the rectovaginal space (35). Dynamic fluoroscopy has been shown to be more accurate than physical examination in demonstrating an enterocele (32,36).

The accuracy of dynamic colpocystoproctography is even further enhanced by opacifying the small bowel. The patient drinks oral barium 2 h prior to the examination. With the vagina, bladder, small intestine, and rectum opacified, the vaginal axis may be measured at rest and with straining, and any prolapse of the anterior, middle, or posterior vaginal compartment is evident. Moreover, the examiner should be able to distinguish among various organs that may prolapse into a widened rectovaginal space, differentiating enterocele from sigmoidocele, further refining the operative approach.

Some investigators have advocated the use of positive-contrast peritoneography (37,38). By instilling water-soluble contrast medium directly into the peritoneal cavity, the pelvic peritoneal recesses may be imaged during relaxation, straining, voiding, and defecation. However, it is the author's opinion that this practice is unnecessarily invasive, risking peritonitis.

C. Ultrasound

Sonography offers a convenient, inexpensive, and radiation-free technique. Anorectal endosonography is a standard method for staging and following anal and rectal cancers, and for evaluating benign anorectal conditions such as anal sphincter defects, perianal abscesses, and fistulae (39). The integrity of the anal sphincter muscles may be assessed with a high-frequency (>7 MHz) transducer that produces a panoramic image (40,41). Defects in the internal sphincter generally appear as an echogenic discontinuity in the hypoechoic muscle between the vagina and rectum. On the other hand, external sphincteric injuries appear as hypoechoic lesions in a normally echogenic structure (40,41). Sonographic findings predict intraoperative diagnosis with a 95% accuracy (42–44). The recent advent of 3D sonography promises to further increase our understanding of anal sphincteric dysfunction (45). Moreover, a thickened sonographic appearance is indicative of sphincteric spasm or hypertrophy, which is often observed with obstructed defection (46).

Similar to fluoroscopy, a dynamic component may be added to sonography. In particular, dynamic ultrasound allows identification of an enterocele. A sagittal view probe is positioned in the rectum and directed against the ventral rectal wall. A 7.5-MHz radial rotating axial endoprobe is recommended (47). During a straining maneuver, widening of the rectovaginal septum, diminution of the peritoneal-anal distance, and herniation of bowel contents into the cul-de-sac may be observed (47). This technique can also accurately distinguish between small intestine and sigmoid colon loops which may enter the cul-de-sac.

Ultrasound is also useful for demonstrating vesicourethral anatomy (48) via abdominal, rectal, vaginal, or perineal transducer (49–51). Abdominal sonography has the advantage of being the least invasive, but has the disadvantage of potential interference from bony structures. Transabdominal ultrasound with a lower-frequency probe (<5.0 MHz) allows adequate resolution without pubic bone shadowing (52). Bladder neck descent may be measured during straining maneuvers (53). Vaginal ultrasound is the most commonly used and best-studied approach (54,55). Careful technique permits the examiner to avoid elevating the bladder neck with the probe, and the measurement of bladder neck hypermobility has been shown to be reproducible in experienced hands (54). While a urethral catheter is useful for identifying the bladder neck, it is not necessary (56). Transperineal sagittal sonography provides a reproducible method for measuring resting and straining angles of the vesicourethral junction and for identifying cystoceles (57).

"Contrast" sonography utilizes echogenic material that can settle into the bladder neck region with gravity, and can demonstrate bladder neck funneling with straining (58). This dynamic method of ultrasonic visualization offers two distinct advantages over the bead chain cystourethrogram: minimizing invasiveness, and eliminating the use of ionizing radiation.

Ostrzenski et al. have introduced a novel method for diagnosing paravaginal defects using contrast ultrasonography (59). A water-filled condom is placed intravaginally, and transabdominal pelvic ultrasound is performed with attention directed at the paravaginal spaces. In their study, paravaginal defects were identified in women with cystoceles and stress urinary incontinence with 100% accuracy (confirmed by laparoscopy). Furthermore, follow-up ultrasound revealed resolution of the defects in all patients postoperatively. This innovative technique should prove useful in the preoperative assessment of anterior vaginal prolapse, and may be used as an objective method for determining the success of surgical repair (59). Contrast ultrasonography is a safe, noninvasive, and simple office-based technique.

Overall, the information obtained from sonography is comparable to that from cystography, but avoids the ionizing radiation and the need for urethral catheterization (60). Both techniques provide the surgeon with reproducible information with either static or dynamic examination. With the use of vaginal, rectal, abdominal, and perineal probes, dynamic ultrasonography may be a reasonable substitute for dynamic fluoroscopy, obviating the need for opacification of the bladder, small bowel, and large bowel, and avoiding the radiation exposure.

D.   Computed Tomography

Computerized axial tomography (CT) has not been shown to be particularly useful in the evaluation of pelvic organ prolapse. This radiological method has the disadvantage of imaging structures which lie in the axial plane via an axial imaging technique. The components of the levator plate and urogenital diaphragm are better seen in the coronal plane or sagittal view. While CT images can be reconstructed into a coronal view using cumbersome and expensive computer software, poor image quality and distorted special resolution have limited the utility of this presentation technique (18).

Various groups have demonstrated the accuracy of CT pelvimetry (61,62). While debate remains over the utility of pelvimetry with regard to the risk of pelvic organ prolapse, this technique has been shown to be a simple, reproducible, and accurate method to measure pelvic dimensions and the capacity of the birth canal, with acceptably low-dose radiation exposure.

E.   Magnetic Resonance Imaging

The development of fast-scanning MRI techniques has improved our ability to describe and quantify anatomical changes that may cause pelvic floor relaxation. Fast-scan Valsalva imaging formated in a pseudokinematic cine-loop, provides a dynamic way to study the anatomical changes that occur with prolapse. MRI offers a method to noninvasively evaluate the female pelvis without ionizing radiation. Organ descent may be simultaneously evaluated in all three pelvic compartments. Kelvin's group has utilized "triphasic" dynamic MRI, consisting of a cystographic, proctographic, and posttoilet phase to facilitate the recognition of prolapsed organs that may be obscured by other organs that remain unemptied (32). Additionally, MRI has been shown to be useful for measuring levator muscle thickness (63) (Fig. 3), urethral length, and the thickness and integrity of periurethral muscle ring (19). The addition of 3D imaging has the advantage of quantification of muscle volume, which may give a more accurate representation of the relationships among pelvic floor structures, thereby potentially improving surgical planning (63).

Yang et al. were the first to popularize dynamic fast magnetic resonance imaging for the evaluation of pelvic organ prolapse (19). Since then, other investigators have shown that MRI is more sensitive than physical examination for defining pelvic prolapse (20,64,65). While some advocate the use of contrast opacification of the bladder, vagina, and rectum (32,66), others have

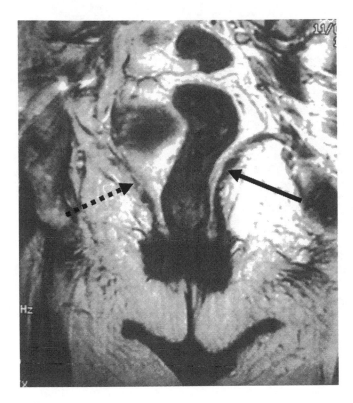

Figure 3 MRI demonstrating asymmetry of levator muscles. Note that atrophied right-sided pubococcygeus (dashed arrow) is thinner than normal left-sided muscle (solid arrow).

shown that the vagina, rectum, bladder, urethra, and peritoneum are adequately visualized without any contrast administration (64,65) (Fig. 4). By avoiding instrumentation of the vagina or urethra, iatrogenic alteration of the anatomy is minimized (20).

The group from UCLA recently published their experience using dynamic half Fourier acquisition, single-shot turbo spin-echo (HASTE sequence) T2-weighted MRI using a 1.5-Tesla magnet with phased array coils (Siemens), or single-shot fast spin echo (SSFSE, General Electric) for evaluating the female pelvis (64,65). Midsagittal and parasagittal resting and straining supine views were obtained for the purpose of identifying the midline and for evaluating the anterior pelvic compartment (anterior vaginal wall, bladder, urethra), posterior compartment (rectum), and middle compartment (uterus, vaginal cuff), as well as the pelvic floor muscles, adnexal organs, and intraperitoneal organs. Images were looped for viewing on a digital station as a cine stack and for measuring the relationship of pelvic organs to fixed anatomical landmarks. The first set of images are volumetric sagittal cuts from left to right, used to locate the midsagittal plane and to survey the pelvic anatomy. The second set of images are obtained with four cycles of repeated relaxation and Valsalva maneuver (64,65). Total image acquisition time is 2.5 min, and total room time is 10 min per study. The charge for each study (including interpretation) is only $540.

This dynamic MRI technique has been shown to be useful for grading pelvic organ prolapse and pelvic floor relaxation in a simple and objective manner (65). The size of the levator hiatus and degree of muscular pelvic floor relaxation and organ prolapse were measured. The "H-line" (levator hiatus width) measures the distance from the pubis to the posterior

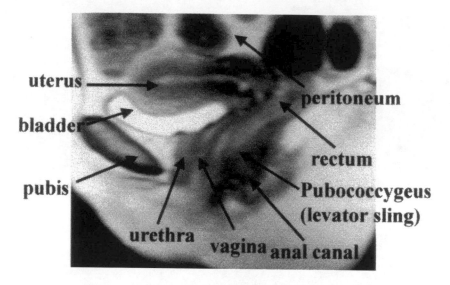

Figure 4   Midsagittal MRI demonstrating normal female anatomic structures.

anal canal. The "M-line" (muscular pelvic floor relaxation) measures the descent of the levator plate from the fixed pubosacral line. The pubosacral line spans the distance from the pubis to the sacrococcygeal joint (Fig. 5). The "O" classification (organ prolapse) describes the degree of visceral prolapse beyond the H-line. The degree of cystocele, rectocele, enterocele, and uterine descent were graded as 0, 1, 2, or 3 (none, mild moderate, severe; Fig. 6).

In a group of women with symptomatic prolapse, the H-line was significantly wider than in a control group (7.5 $\pm$ 1.5 cm vs. 5.2 $\pm$ 1.1 cm, $P < .001$). Similarly, the levator muscular descent (M-line) was greater in the prolapse groups than in the control group (4.1 $\pm$ 1.5 cm vs. 1.9 $\pm$ 1.2 cm, $P < .001$) (65). These objective findings fit well with our knowledge of the

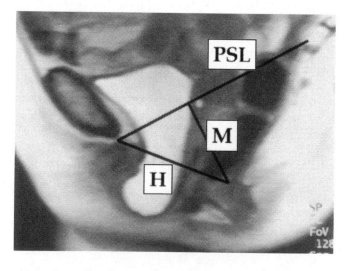

Figure 5   MRI, sagittal view in a patient with pelvic prolapse. The "H-line" (levator hiatus width) measures the distance from the pubis to the posterior anal canal. The "M-line" (muscular pelvic floor relaxation) measures the descent of the levator plate from the pubosacral line (PSL).

pathophysiology of pelvic prolapse. Trauma to the pubococcygeus and iliococcygeus, usually from childbirth, results in widening of the levator hiatus and laxity of the musculofascial support structures (67). This results in a sloping levator plate, with the more vertically oriented vagina and rectum tending to slide down through the widened hiatus. Therefore, the H and M lines

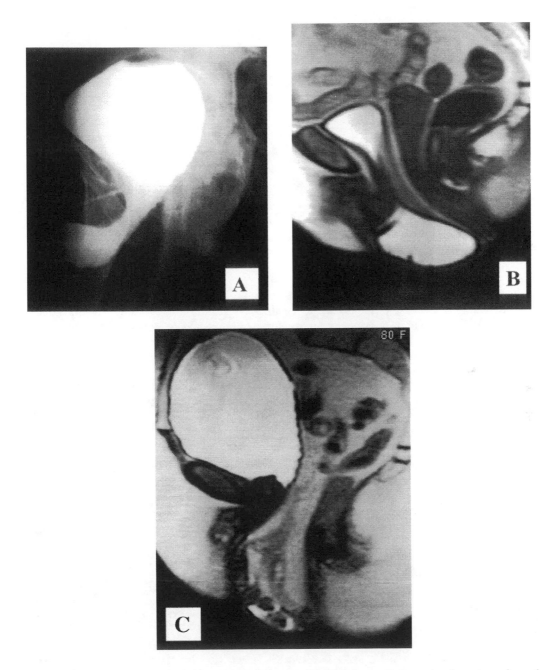

Figure 6   (A) Cystogram demonstrates cystocele only. (B) MRI demonstrates cystocele, enterocele, and vault prolapse. (C) Enterocele with minimal pelvic floor relaxation. (D) Combined cystocele, enterocele, rectocele, and significant pelvic floor relaxation.

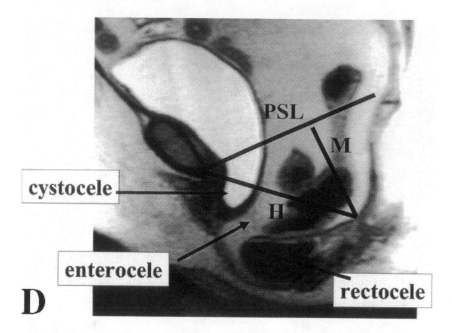

Figure 6 Continued.

both increase with pelvic floor relaxation relaxation. This in turn leads to organ prolapse (O classification). Because of the excellent visualization of fluid-filled viscera and soft tissues, MRI can differentiate among cystocele, enterocele, and high rectocele, which may be difficult by physical examination alone (Fig. 6).

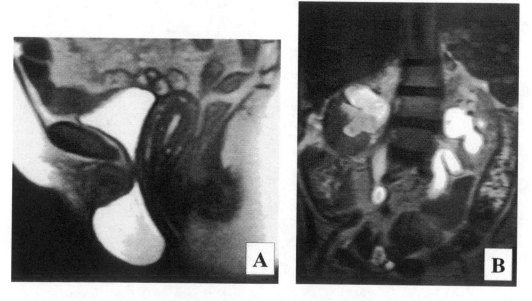

Figure 7 (A) Sagittal MRI. (B) MR urogram. Large cystocele and uterine prolapse, causing bilateral ureteral obstruction, with resulting hydroureteronephrosis.

MRI findings were compared to physical examination and intraoperative findings. HASTE-sequence MRI was more accurate than physical examination in identifying cystoceles, enteroceles, vault prolapse, and pelvic organ pathology such as uterine fibroids, urethral diverticula, ovarian cysts, and Nabothian and Barholin's gland cysts (64). Comiter et al. found that with dynamic MRI, surgical planning was altered in >30% of cases, most often because of occult enterocele not appreciated on physical examination (68).

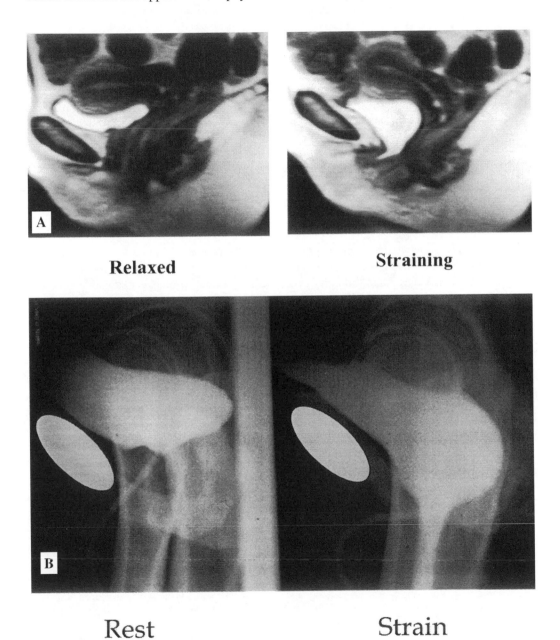

Figure 8 (A) Dynamic MRI (relaxed and straining) demonstrates bladder neck funneling and stress urinary incontinence. (B) Similar demonstration with lateral cystogram.

In patients with severe prolapse, especially with renal insufficiency, the surgeon must rule out obstructive hydroureteronephrosis. This may be accomplished by MR urogram, adding only 30 sec of examination time and no additional morbidity (Fig. 7). MRI may also be useful for the radiographic evaluation of stress incontinence. Hypermobility of the proximal urethra and bladder neck descent are important pathological features in the diagnosis of genuine stress urinary incontinence (69,70). Measurement data on dynamic MRI for the bladder neck position and the extension of cystocele at maximal pelvic strain are comparable with lateral cysto-urethrogram data (71) (Fig. 8).

The disadvantage of MRI is that the study must be performed supine, as no upright MRI machines are currently available. However, dynamic MRI with relaxing and straining views has been shown to adequately demonstrate organ prolapse during straining in the supine position (68,72,73). Competition among prolapsing organs filling a finite introital space may also limit MRI, just as it may limit physical examination and dynamic fluoroscopy. This is especially true for identification of a rectocele (64). Additionally, claustrophobic patients and those with cardiac pacemakers or sacral nerve stimulators cannot enter the enclosed magnet. Despite these limitations, dynamic MRI has become the study of choice at our institution for evaluating pelvic organ prolapse and pelvic floor relaxation.

V. SUMMARY

A detailed working knowledge of normal and abnormal female pelvic anatomy is necessary for the proper evaluation of pelvic organ prolapse. However, even the most experienced gyne-cologist or urologist may have difficulty distinguishing among prolapsing organs competing for introital space. Accurate identification of all aspects of vaginal prolapse and pelvic floor relaxation are vital not only to permit adequate surgical planning, but also to reduce the risk of recurrent prolapse. Radiographic evaluation of the woman with pelvic organ prolapse and pelvic floor relaxation should be viewed as a valuable extension of the physical examination. Urography, voiding cystography, dynamic colpocystodefacography, sonography, and MRI are each useful for the evaluation of pelvic prolapse and pelvic floor relaxation. MRI will continue to play an increasingly important role owing to its superior visualization of fluid-filled viscera and soft tissues, and the ability to simultaneously visualize all important pelvic organs without the need for patient preparation, instrumentation, or exposure to ionizing radiation.

REFERENCES

1. Hagstad A, Janson PO, Lindstedt G. Gynaecological history, complaints, and examinations in a middle-aged population. Maturitas 1985; 7:115–128.
2. Brubaker L, Heit MH. Radiology of the pelvic floor. Clin Obstet Gynecol 1993; 36:952–959.
3. Richardson AC, Lyon JB, Williams NL. A new look at pelvic relaxation. Am J Obstet Gynecol 1976; 126:568–573.
4. Zacharin RF. The anatomic supports of the female urethra. Obstet Gynecol 1968; 21:754–761.
5. Comiter CV, Vasavada S, Raz S. Anatomy and physiology of stress urinary incontinence and pelvic floor prolapse. In: Raz S, ed. Atlas of the Urologic Clinics of North America — Vaginal Surgery. Baltimore: Williams and Wilkins, 2000:1–22.
6. Comiter CV, Vasavada S, Raz S. Transvaginal culdosuspension: technique and results. Urology 1999; 54:819–824.
7. Hording U, Pedersen KH, Sidenius K, Hedegaard L. Urinary incontinence in 45-year-old women: an epidemiological survey. Scand J Urol Nephrol 1986; 20:183–186.

8. Snooks SJ, Setchell M, Swash M, Henry MM. Injury to innervation of pelvic floor sphincter musculature in childbirth. Lancet 1984; 2:546–550.

9. Sultan AH, Kamm MA, Talbot IC, Nicholls RJ, Bartram CI. Anal endosonography for identifying external sphincter defects confirmed histologically. Br J Surg 1994; 81:463–465.

10. Stoker J, Halligan S, Bartram OI. Pelvic floor imaging. Radiology 2001; 218:621–641.

11. Beverly CM, Walters MD, Wever AM. Prevalence of hydronephrosis in patients undergoing surgery for pelvic organ prolapse. Obstet Gynecol 1997; 90:37–41.

12. Brettauer J, Ruben JC. Hydroureter and hydronephrosis: a frequent secondary finding in cases of prolapse of the uterus and bladder. Am J Obstet Gynecol 1923; 6:696–709.

13. Wallingford AJ. The changes of the urinary tract associated with prolapse of the uterus. Am J Obstet Gynecol 1939; 38:489–494.

14. Stabler J. Uterine prolapse and urinary tract obstruction. Br J Radiol 1977; 50:493–498.

15. Solomons E, Levin EJ, Bauman J. A pyelographic study of ureteric injuries sustained during hysterectomy for benign conditions. Surg Gynecol Obstet 1960; 111:41–46.

16. Piscitelli JT, Simel DL, Addison A. Who should have intravenous pyelograms before hysterectomy for benign disease? Obstet Gynecol 1987; 69:541–545.

17. Berglas B, Rubin IC. Study of the supportive structures of the uterus by levator myography. Surg Gynecol Obstet 1953; 97:677–692.

18. Weidner AC, Low VHS. Imaging studies of the pelvic floor. Obstet Gynecol Clin North Am 1998; 25:825–848.

19. Yang A, Mostwin, JL, Rosenshein NB. Pelvic floor descent in women: dynamic evaluation with fast MR imaging and cinematic display. Radiology 1991; 179:25–33.

20. Goodrich MA, Webb MJ, King BF. Magnetic resonance imaging of pelvic floor relaxation: dynamic analysis and evaluation of patients before and after surgical repair. Obstet Gynecol 1993; 82:883–891.

21. Green TH. Urinary stress incontinence: pathophysiology, diagnosis and classification. In: Buchsbaum HJ, Schmidt JD, eds. Gynecologic and Obstetric Urology. Philadelphia: Saunders, 1982:199–224.

22. Raz S. Evaluation of urinary incontinence. In: Buchsbaum HJ, Schmidt JD, eds. Gynecologic and Obstetric Urology. Philadelphia: Saunders, 1982:225–238.

23. Kelvin FM, Maglinte DD, Hale D, Benson JT. Voiding cystourethrography in female stress incontinence. AJR 1996; 167:1065–1066.

24. Pelsang RE, Bonney WW. Voiding cystourethrography in female stress incontinence. AJR 1994; 166:561–565.

25. Whitehead WE, Schuster MM. Anorectal physiology and pathophysiology. Am J Gastroenterol 1987; 82:487–497.

26. Ott DJ, Donati DL, Kerr RM. Defecography: results in 55 patients and impact on clinical management. Abdom Imaging 1994; 19:349–353.

27. Mahieu P, Pringot J, Bodart P. Defecography. II. Contribution to the diagnosis of defecation disorders. Gastrointest Radiol 1984; 9:253–261.

28. Freimanis MG, Wald A, Caruana B. Evacuation proctography in normal volunteers. Invest Radiol 1991; 26:581–585.

29. Hiltunen KM, Kolehmainen H, Matikainen M. Does defecography help in diagnosis and clinical decision-making in defecation disorders? Abdom Imaging 1994; 19:355–360.

30. Maglinte DDT, Kelvin FM, Hale DS. Dynamic cystoproctography: a unifying diagnostic approach to pelvic floor and anorectal dysfunction. AJR 1997; 169:759–762.

31. Shorvon PJ, McHugh S, Diamant NE. Defecography in normal volunteers. Results and implications. Gut 1989; 30:1737–1740.

32. Kelvin FM, Maglinte DDT, Hornback JA, Benson JT. Pelvic prolapse: assessment with evacuation proctography (defacography). Radiology 1992; 184:547–551.

33. Bethoux A, Bory S, Huguier M, Sheao SL. Le colpocystogramme. J Chir (Paris) 1965; 8:809–828. (In French.)

34. Lazarevski M, Lazarov A, Novak J, Dimcevski D. Colpocystography in cases of genital prolapse and urinary stress incotnnience in women. Am J Obstet Gynecol 1975; 122:704–716.

35. Shorvon PJ, Stevenson GW. Defaecography: setting up a service. Br J Hosp Med 1989; 41: 460–467.

36. Altringer WE, Saclarides TJ, Dominguez JM. Four-contrast defecography: pelvic "flooroscopy". Dis Colon Rectum 1995; 38:695–699.

37. Bremmer S. Peritoneocele. A radiological study with defaeco-peritoneography. Acta Radiol Suppl 1998; 413(suppl):1–33.

38. Halligan S, Bartram CI. Evacuation proctography combined with positive contrast peritoneography to demonstrate pelvic floor hernias. Abdom Imaging 1995; 5:442–445.

39. Phang PT, Wong WD. The use of endoluminal ultrasound for malignant and benign anorectal diseases. Curr Opin Gastroenterol. 1997; 13:47–53.

40. Schafer, Anck P, Furst G. Anatomy of the anal sphincters: comparison of anal endosonography to magnetic resonance imaging. Dis Colon Rectum 1994; 37:777–781.

41. Gantke B, Schafer A, Enck P. Sonographic, manometric, and myographic evaluation of the anal sphincters morphology and function. Dis Colon Rectum 1993; 36:1037–1041.

42. Law PJ, Kamm MA, Bartram CI. Anal endosonography in the investigation of faecal incontinence. Br J Surg 1991; 78:312–314.

43. Deen KI, Kumar D, Williams JG. Anal sphincter defects: correlation between endoanal ultrasound and surgery. Ann Surg 1993; 218:201–205.

44. Sentovich SM, Wong WD, Blatchfent GJ. Accuracy and reliability of transanal ultrasound for anterior anal sphincter injury. Dis Colon Rectum 1998; 41:1000–1004.

45. Gold DM, Bartram CI, Halligan S, Humphries PN, Kamm ME, Kmiot WA. Three dimensional endoanal sonogrpahy in assessing anal canal injury. Br J Surg 1999; 86:365–370.

46. Nielsen MB, Rasmussen OO, Pedersen JF. Anal endosonographic findings in patients with obstructed defecation. Acta Radiol 1993; 34:35–42.

47. Karaus M, Neuhaus P, Weidenmann B. Diagnosis of enteroceles by dynamic anorectal endo-sonography. Dis Colon Rectum 2000; 43:1683–1688.

48. Gordon D, Pearce M, Norton P, Stanton SL. Comparison of ultrasound and lateral chain cystourethrography in the determination of bladder neck descent. Am J Obstet Gynecol 1989; 160:12–18.

49. Bergmann A, Ballard CA, Platt LD. Ultrasonic evaluation of urethro-vesical junction in women with stress urinary incontinence. J Clin Ultrasound 1988; 16:295–300.

50. Mouritsen L, Rasmussen A. Bladder neck mobility evaluated by vaginal ultrasonography. Br J Urol 1993; 71:166–171.

51. Kohorn E, Scioscia AL, Jeaty P, Hobbins JC. Ultrasound by perineal scanning for the assessment of female stress urinary incontinence. Obstet Gynecol 1986; 68:269–272.

52. Kohorn EL, Sciscia AL, Jeanty P. Ultrasound cystoruethrography by perineal scanning for the asssessment of female stress urinary incontinence. Obstet Gynecol 1986; 68:269–272.

53. Peschers U, Schaer G, Anthuiber C. Changes in vesical neck mobility following vaginal delivery. Obstet Gynecol 1996; 88:1001–1006.

54. Mouritsen L, Strandberg C, Frimodt-Moller C. Bladder neck anatomy and mobility, effect of the vaginal ultrasound probe. Br J Urol 1994; 74:749–752.

55. Mouritsen L. Techniques for imaging bladder support. Acta Obstet Gynecol Scand 1997; 166(suppl):48–49.

56. Mouritsen L, Bach P. Ultrasonic evaluation of bladder neck position and mobility. The influence of urethral catheter, bladder volume and body position. Neurourol Urodyn 1994; 13:637–646.

57. Bader W, Degenhardt F, Kauffels W, Nehls K, Schneider J. Ultrasonographic parameters for the assessment of emale urinary stress incontinence. Ultraschall Med 1995; 16:180–185.

58. Schaer GN, Koechli OR, Schuessler B. Improvement of perineal sonographic bladder neck imaging with ultrasound contrast medium. Obstet Gynecol 1995; 86:950–954.

59. Ostrzenski A, Osborne NG, Ostrzenska K. Method for diagnosing paravaginal defects using contrast ultrasonographic technique. J Ultrasound Med 1997; 16:673–677.

60. Mouritsen L, Strandberg C. Vaginal ultrasonography versus colpocystourethrography in the evaluation of female urinary incontinence. Acta Obstet Gynecol Scand 1994; 73:338–342.

61. Sze EHM, Kohli N, Miklos JR, Roat T, Karram MM. Computed tomography comparison of bony pelvis dimensions between women with and without genital prolapse. Obstet Gynecol 1999; 93:229–232.

62. Federle MP, Cohen HA, Rosenwein MR, Brant-Zawadzki MN, Cann CE. Pelvimetry by digital radiography: a low dose examination. Radiology 1982; 143:733–735.

63. Fielding JR, Dumanli H, Schreyer AG, Okuda S, Gering DT, Zou KH, Kikinis R, Jolesz FA. MR-based three dimensional modeling of the normal pelvic floor in women: quantification of muscle mass. AJR 2000; 174:657–660.

64. Gousse AE, Barbaric ZL, Safir MH, Madjar S, Marumoto AK, Raz S. Dynamic half Fourier acquisition, single shot turbo spin-echo magnetic resonance imaging for evaluating the female pelvis. J Urol 2000; 164:1606–1613.

65. Comiter CV, Vasavada SP, Barbaric ZL, Gousse AE, Raz S. Grading pelvic prolapse and pelvic floor relaxation using dynamic magnetic resonance imaging. Urology 1999; 54:454–457.

66. Kelvin FM, Maglnte DDT, Hale DS, Benson JT. Female pelvic organ prolapse: a comparison of triphasic dynamic MR imaging and triphasic fluoroscopic cystocolpoproctography. AJR 2000; 174:81–88.

67. Babiarz JW, Raz S. Pelvic floor relaxation. In: Raz S, ed. Female Urology. Philadelphia: Saunders, 1996:445–456.

68. Comiter CV, Vasavada S, Raz S. Preoperative evaluation of pelvic prolapse using dynamic magnetic resonance imaging. 29th Annual International Continence Society, Denver, CO, August 1999.

69. Jeffcoate TN, Roberts H. Observation on stress incontinence of urine. Am J Obstet Gynecol 1952; 64:721–738.

70. Enhorning G. Simultaneous recording of intravesical and intraurethral pressure. Acta Chir Scand 1956; 276(suppl):1–68.

71. Gufler H, DeGregorio G, Allman K-H, Kundt G, Dohnicht S. Comparison of cystourethrography and dynamic MRI in bladder neck descent. J Comput Assist Tomogr 2000; 24:382–388.

72. Lienemann A, Anthuber CJ, Baron A. Dynamic MR colpocystorectogrpahy assessing pelvic floor descent. Eur Radiol 1997; 7:1309–1317.

73. Lienemann A, Anthuber CJ, Baron A. Dynamic MR colpocystorectography. A new method for evaluating pelvic floor descent and genital prolapse. Aktuell Radiol 1996; 6:182–186.

38

Surgical Therapy of Uterine Prolapse

Karyn Schlunt Eilber,* Nirit Rosenblum,† and Shlomo Raz
University of California, Los Angeles, California, U.S.A.

I. INTRODUCTION

Uterine prolapse is a relatively common, disabling condition and often requires surgical intervention. Hysterectomy is the second most commonly performed gynecological surgery in the United States after cesarean section with ~600,000 procedures done each year (1). In a review by the National Center for Health Statistics for the years 1988–1990, 16.3% of hysterectomies were performed for pelvic prolapse (2). Thus, almost 100,000 hysterectomies are performed each year for prolapse. Although over 70% of hysterectomies are performed transabdominally, the transvaginal approach is preferred when there is associated vaginal prolapse (3). By understanding the female pelvic anatomy and maintaining control of the uterine vascular pedicles, a transvaginal hysterectomy can effectively be performed with minimal morbidity.

II. UTERINE ANATOMY

The uterus is a viscous muscular organ located between the bladder and rectum and is usually in an anteverted position. The superior portion of the uterus, the fundus, is covered anteriorly and posteriorly by the peritoneum. Uterine support is mainly provided by the pelvic floor musculature and two sets of ligaments: the uterosacral and the cardinal (Mackenrodt's) ligaments. The body of the uterus is enclosed between the double-layered broad ligaments. Each broad ligament extends from the lateral aspect of the body of the uterus and contains a Fallopian tube, the round and ovarian ligaments, and the uterine and ovarian vessels (4–6). The broad ligaments do not contribute greatly to uterine support.

The uterosacral and cardinal ligaments pass from the cervix to the sacrum and arcus tendineus, respectively. These ligaments are localized thickenings of the endopelvic fascia and fuse at the cervix to provide the major uterine and apical vaginal support (6–8). Anterior to the vagina the endopelvic fascia is referred to as the pubocervical fascia and posteriorly is termed the rectovaginal fascia, or Denonvillier's fascia (7). These layers consist of fibrofatty tissue and do not represent a true fascia. The fusion of the cardinal and uterosacral ligaments becomes

*Current affiliation: Memorial Sloan-Kettering Cancer Center, New York, New York, U.S.A.
†Current affiliation: NYU School of Medicine, New York, New York, U.S.A.

clinically significant when performing a transvaginal hysterectomy, as will become apparent in the subsequent description of the technique.

The pelvic floor musculature that provides significant uterine support includes the levator ani muscle group (pubococcygeus, iliococcygeus, puborectalis) and the coccygeal muscles (5). Other anatomic structures that contribute uterine and vaginal support include the bony pelvis, the urogenital diaphragm, and the perineal body (6).

III. PATHOPHYSIOLOGY OF PROLAPSE

The pathophysiology of uterine prolapse can be more easily understood when considering the interactions of the ligamentous support of the uterus and the pelvic floor. DeLancey described pelvic support in terms of levels (9): Level I support refers to support of the upper vagina and cervix by the cardinal-uterosacral complex; level II support is that of the midportion of the vagina to the arcus tendineus; and level III support involves the fusion of the anterior, lateral, and posterior vagina to the urethra, levator ani, and perineal body, respectively.

Uterine prolapse is the result of a defect in level I support. Some theorize that attenuation of the cardinal-uterosacral ligament complex may occur because of trauma (childbirth), chronic elevations in abdominal pressure or, possibly atrophy, allowing the cervix to descend and move anteriorly. The uterus then begins to rotate posteriorly such that the intraabdominal pressure is directed on the anterior surface of the uterus. The uterus becomes progressively more retroverted until the axis of the uterus is in an essentially vertical position at which time prolapse occurs (7,10,11).

The exact etiology of pelvic prolapse is still unclear. Abnormalities in sacral nerve function or collagen have been suggested. Predisposing factors for the development of prolapse include increasing age, multiparity, maximal infant birth weight, postmenopausal status, chronic constipation, prior surgery for prolapse, and decreased pelvic floor muscle strength (9,12,13).

IV. CLINICAL EVALUATION

The clinical evaluation of the patient with uterine prolapse includes a complete history and physical examination as well as a limited number of ancillary tests. Considerations such as symptomatology, associated prolapse, pathology of other pelvic organs, urinary incontinence, reproductive status, and sexual function all influence the choice of management.

A. History

The most common presentation of uterine prolapse is a patient complaining of a mass or bulge at the introitus. Other presenting complaints include perineal pressure, dyspareunia, or difficulty walking (14–16). When concomitant prolapse of other organs is present, urinary retention, urinary incontinence, or constipation may also occur. Less commonly, a patient presents simply because uterine prolapse was incidentally found on routine physical examination. Symptoms are classically aggravated by standing and may improve when the patient resumes a recumbent position.

It is important to determine whether the patient has had a previous hysterectomy. Occasionally what is assumed to be uterine descent is only cervical descent after a prior supracervical hysterectomy. Also of importance is any known history of uterine disease such as fibroids or endometriosis, symptoms of urinary incontinence, sexual function, bowel function, and the overall health status of the patient.

B. Physical Examination

Physical examination should be performed both in the supine and standing positions, as the severity of prolapse is not always evident in the recumbent position. When in the supine position, the patient needs to perform a Valsalva maneuver in order to fully appreciate the prolapse. Uterine examination includes determination of the level of cervical descent, uterine size, uterine mobility, and any abnormal gross pathology. The anterior, posterior, and apical vaginal walls are examined separately with the aid of a half-speculum. Speculum examination is useful to assess the remainder of the pelvic floor for other prolapse such as cystocele, rectocele, or enterocele and also to assess the presence of urethral hypermobility. The size of the introitus and vaginal canal should also be noted as this may limit transvaginal delivery of an enlarged uterus. Rectal and pelvic floor tone are also assessed. At the time of surgery the physical examination should be repeated. The degree of uterine descent and other prolapse may become more pronounced with the patient under general anesthesia.

C. Diagnostic Tests

A urinalysis and postvoid residual urine volume are obtained for all patients. For patients with uterine prolapse and no history of stress or urge incontinence and normal residual urine, we do not routinely perform a urodynamic evaluation. However, for patients with the above symptoms or with elevated residual urine, we recommend assessment of the lower urinary tract with urodynamic studies and cystoscopy. Stress incontinence that is masked by the prolapse may manifest itself after correction of the prolapse (16,17). Furthermore, as many patients with prolapse are elderly, detrusor instability associated with obstruction versus hyperreflexia secondary to an occult neurologic condition must be identified. Cystoscopy is useful to rule out any intrinsic urethral or bladder abnormalities that may be causing lower urinary tract symptoms.

Imaging of the upper urinary tracts is also recommended as patients with uterine prolapse are more likely to have associated hydronephrosis as compared to other vaginal prolapse and may be severe enough as to cause renal failure (18,19). Our preferred imaging test to assess the presence of hydronephrosis as well as other pathology is the dynamic magnetic resonance imaging (MRI). A dynamic MRI of the pelvis not only identifies the presence of hydronephrosis, but it also allows for evaluation of the uterus and adnexa for abnormal pathology that might preclude a vaginal hysterectomy. The dynamic MRI is a relatively simple, noninvasive test that takes only minutes to complete. There is no need for intravesical contrast as the bladder is quite distinct on the MRI. Sagittal images are taken of the pelvis with the patient at rest and then with a Valsalva maneuver. Pelvic organ prolapse and other pathology are readily identified with this imaging modality (Fig. 1). Advantages include its ability to accurately determine uterine and ovarian pathology as well as the presence and degree of associated prolapse.

V. CLASSIFICATION

The pelvic organ prolapse quantification (POP-Q) is a validated staging system for defining vaginal prolapse. This staging system separately addresses the vaginal compartments (anterior, posterior, apical) and defines the extent of prolapse in relation to the hymen. Stage 0 indicates no prolapse, stage 1 implies that the most distal portion of the prolapsed organ is >1 cm above the hymenal ring, stage 2 defines prolapse within 1 cm of the hymen (proximal or distal), stage 3 denotes prolapse >1 cm distal to the hymen, and stage 4 implies complete vaginal eversion (20).

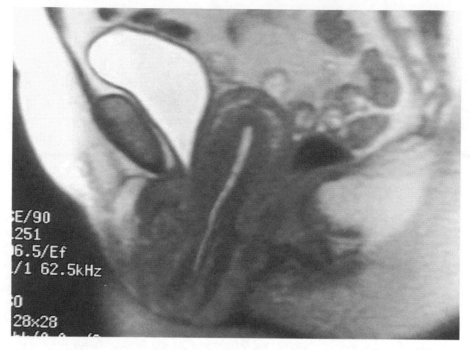

Figure 1   MRI of the pelvis. Dynamic MRI of the pelvis demonstrating uterine prolapse.

As we routinely obtain a dynamic pelvic MRI for patients with uterine prolapse, we classify uterine prolapse based on this study. Prolapse is classified in reference to the puborectalis hiatus (sling) which is formed by the puborectalis muscle (the most inferior part of levator ani) and includes the urethra, vagina, and rectum. The degree of prolapse is based on 2-cm increments: mild uterine prolapse is between 0 and 2 cm below the hiatus, moderate prolapse is 2–4 cm, and severe prolapse is >4 cm below the hiatus (21).

VI. THERAPEUTIC OPTIONS

When choosing the type of treatment for uterine prolapse, several considerations must be made. The degree of prolapse and the patient's symptomatology are the main considerations. Patients with minimal prolapse and/or mild symptoms often require no therapy. For patients in their reproductive years, it is of paramount importance to determine whether childbearing is desired. Current and expected sexual function must be discussed. The size of the uterus and uterine pathology must also be taken into account as well as associated prolapse of other organs. Lastly, but not least important, the overall health status of the patient must be considered.

A. Conservative Treatment

The primary nonsurgical treatment for uterine prolapse involves the use of a pessary. This option is reserved mainly for patients who are not surgical candidates or who do not wish surgical intervention. Efficacy of this treatment relies on the adequacy of perineal outlet support, which is often lacking in this patient population.

Complications secondary to pessary use include mechanical irritation or ulceration of the vaginal mucosa. Topical estrogen cream may alleviate these symptoms. In extreme cases the pessary may become embedded or erode into the vaginal wall, requiring surgical intervention for removal. Erosion of a pessary through the anterior vaginal and bladder walls has been reported (22).

Another use of a pessary is for diagnostic purposes. Patients with symptoms that do not necessarily correlate with the degree of prolapse may wear a pessary for a few weeks to determine whether the symptoms are indeed secondary to prolapse.

B. Surgical Treatment

The basic tenet of surgical repair of uterine prolapse is that the defect is not with the uterus itself but with the pelvic support. Thus, hysterectomy alone is not sufficient to treat pelvic prolapse. Every effort must be made to restore normal pelvic anatomy with adequate support and create a functional vaginal vault.

1.   Uterine Sparing Procedures

Many women choose to avoid hysterectomy because of a delay in childbearing to a later age, a belief that the uterus plays a role in sexual satisfaction, or more effective medical treatment of menorrhagia (23–25). For women desiring uterine preservation, the more commonly performed procedures include the Manchester operation, the Gilliam suspension, sacrospinous hysteropexy (cervix to the sacrospinous ligament), and sacral hysteropexy (cervix to sacrum) (11,26–28). More recently a laparoscopic approach to hysteropexy has been described (29). For the rare cases of patients who are not sexually active and who might otherwise use a pessary, colpocleisis is another alternative.

a. Manchester Operation. The Manchester operation is a transvaginal uterine suspension reserved for the patient with combined uterine prolapse and cystocele. The goal of this surgery is to bring the cardinal and uterosacral ligaments anterior to the lower uterine segment in order to restore the uterus to an anteverted position (30). In this procedure the cervix is amputated and the cardinal and uterosacral ligaments are sutured to the anterior, lower uterine segment (30,31). This repair is followed by a standard anterior repair and/or Kelly plication (30). The problems with this repair include a >20% prolapse recurrence within months of surgery, a decrease in fertility, and difficulty with future cervical sampling for cytologic analysis (32,33).

b. Gilliam Suspension. The Gilliam suspension is another technique when attempting to preserve childbearing potential. In this procedure the round ligaments are sutured to the rectus sheath via the internal inguinal ring (11). This may be performed either through a lower abdominal incision or laparoscopically. There are no adverse sequelae for subsequent pregnancies, although some patients report transient round ligament pain (11). Gordon reported a 93% success rate with this procedure (34). However, this procedure is not effective in the long run as it does not address the basic condition of weakness of the pelvic floor and the cardinal-uterosacral ligament complex.

c. Hysteropexy. Sacrospinous hysteropexy and sacral hysteropexy involve fixation of the cervix to the sacrospinous ligament or sacrum, respectively. Sacrospinous vaginal fixation has been found to be effective in 64–97% of cases while sacral colpopexy has an 84–98% success rate (35,36). Unfortunately, these repairs rely on nonphysiologic support of the upper vagina and may result in prolapse of other organs (29). Potential complications include bleeding, sciatic nerve injury, and rectal laceration (36,37). Furthermore, dissection to remove the cervix from the sacrospinous ligament or sacrum is difficult if a hysterectomy is required subsequent to one of these procedures.

　　d. Laparoscopic Hysteropexy.　Recently a laparoscopic suture hysteropexy has been described which involves plication of the uterosacral ligaments which are then reattached to the cervix. The reported success rate in 43 women was 81%, and two women subsequently completed term pregnancies without recurrence of prolapse (29). Complications included a uterine artery laceration in one patient that required a laparotomy and ureteral kinking in two patients which required only a relaxing incision in the peritoneum.

　　e. Colpocleisis.　Colpocleisis as described by LeFort involves excision of anterior and posterior vaginal flaps proximal to the prolapsed cervix to the level of the introitus. The denuded areas are then approximated (31). Disadvantages of this procedure are loss of sexual function, inability to perform cytologic cervical analysis, and urinary incontinence in up to 24% of patients (38). However, Ahranjani et al. reported no recurrence of prolapse in a series of 30 patients (39).

2. Hysterectomy

A multitude of approaches to hysterectomy have been described such that it is impossible to include a description of them all. This chapter will focus on the technique of vaginal hysterectomy and provide a brief overview of other approaches to hysterectomy.

　　a. Subtotal Hysterectomy.　Subtotal or supracervical hysterectomy is a procedure that was largely discarded in the past but has recently made a slight resurgence. Advocates of the subtotal hysterectomy propose that it preserves posthysterectomy bladder and sexual function (40–43). The procedure involves separation of the uterine body from the cervix, and the cervical stump is left remaining.

　　The most common short-term complications are infection (1.0–5.0%), hemorrhage (0.7–4.0%), and adjacent organ injury (0.6–1.0%) (44). These rates are comparable to those for total hysterectomy. Ewies and Olah reported that the most common long-term complication following subtotal hysterectomy was regular menstruation (45). No study has proven any superiority of subtotal hysterectomy over total hysterectomy in terms of operative complications or sexual function, and thus total hysterectomy remains the procedure of choice for most women.

　　b. Abdominal Hysterectomy.　The great majority of hysterectomies performed in the United States are abdominal. Indications for using the abdominal approach include surgeon preference, known or suspected pelvic adhesions or endometriosis, leiomyoma, adnexal pathology, the need to remove adnexal structures and the absence of pelvic relaxation. The possibility of oophorectomy should be determined preoperatively.

　　The operation is performed through either a low midline or Pfannenstiel incision. Although many techniques for abdominal hysterectomy have been described, typically the round ligament on one side of the uterus is ligated then transected and the leaves of the broad ligament are separated. The infundibulopelvic or utero-ovarian ligaments are then mobilized above the ureter, ligated and cut. Care should be taken to clearly disect out the ureter on the medial leaf of the broad ligament. After the bladder is dissected off the lower uterine segment, the uterine vessels are clamped and suture is ligated. The ipsilateral cardinal ligament and uterosacral ligament are also clamped and the suture ligated. The uterus is then dissected from the vaginal wall, and, depending on surgeon preference, the vaginal cuff is left open or closed after bleeders are controlled (30,46).

　　Bladder and ureteral injury occur in 0.5% and 0.5–1.0% of cases, respectively (47). A multicenter, prospective, nonrandomized study of 1851 patients reported a perioperative death rate of 0.1% after abdominal hysterectomy (48).

　　c. Laparoscopic Hysterectomy.　With the increasing popularity of minimally invasive surgical techniques, descriptions for the technique of laparoscopic hysterectomy have emerged.

The terms "laparoscopic hysterectomy" and "laparoscopic-assisted vaginal hysterectomy" both refer to a variety of procedures that include a portion of the operation performed vaginally. Compared to the traditional abdominal approach, the laparoscopic approach has the benefits of shorter hospital stay and decreased convalescence. However, no benefit has been found for the laparoscopic approach compared to the vaginal approach (49). When added anesthesia time and the cost of disposable instruments are considered, the cost of laparoscopic surgery is ~$3000 more when compared to the vaginal approach (50).

Laparoscopic hysterectomy has been classified into four types: a type I procedure includes dissection up to but not including the uterine arteries, a type II procedure involves division of the uterine artery pedicle, a type III procedure is performed when the cardinal-uterosacral ligament complex is partially dissected, and complete division of this complex constitutes a type IV procedure (51). A Finnish report on 3928 women who underwent a laparoscopic hysterectomy from 1995 to 1996 reported major complications in 2.2% and one death secondary to a massive pulmonary embolus (52). The complications of ureteral injury, vesicovaginal fistula, intestinal injury, and cystotomy occurred in 1.2%, 0.4%, 0.4%, and 0.18% of cases respectively.

d. Vaginal Hysterectomy. Vaginal hysterectomy has the advantage of avoiding the morbidity associated with an abdominal incision, but several important relative and absolute contraindications to vaginal hysterectomy exist: size disproportion (enlarged uterus and vaginal stenosis), obliteration of the cul-de-sac, adnexal tumor, pelvic tumor, pelvic inflammatory disease, and malignancy of the uterus or ovaries (10). A history of endometriosis of unknown extent is also considered a contraindication (53).

C. Technique

Prophylactic quinolone antibiotics are administered preoperatively. Following administration of adequate anesthesia, the patient is placed in the dorsal lithotomy position. If no contraindication exists, we prefer the use of spinal anesthesia. The suprapubic area, vagina, and external genitalia are prepped with an iodine-based solution. Sutures are used to retract the labia laterally. A weighted speculum is inserted for vault exposure. If a bladder neck suspension or cystocele repair is planned, a Lowsley retractor may be used to place a suprapubic catheter. The bladder is emptied via a catheter. A ring retractor with elastic stays is placed for exposure, and two Lahey clamps are used to grasp the cervix. Using electrocautery, a circumferential incision is made approximately 1 cm from the cervical os (Fig. 2). Sharp dissection is used to dissect the uterus from the bladder and develop the vesicoperitoneal space (Fig. 3). This dissection is facilitated by placing gentle traction on the tenacula and pointing the scissors toward the uterus. A Heaney retractor is used to retract the bladder anteriorly. Maneuvers to avoid an inadvertent cystotomy include dissection in the midline of the uterus and remaining parallel to the glistening white surface of the uterus.

At this point attention is turned toward the posterior dissection. The posterior peritoneal fold is exposed in a similar fashion to the vesicoperitoneal fold, and the posterior peritoneum is opened sharply. The cul-de-sac is inspected for adhesions or other pathology. A Heaney retractor is placed in the posterior peritoneum. If difficulty is encountered when attempting to expose the cul-de-sac, the hysterectomy may be initiated in an extraperitoneal fashion by severing the uterosacral ligament and caudal portions of the cardinal ligament close to the cervix. This maneuver allows descent of the uterus to provide better visualization.

Division of the ligamentous attachments is now performed. With the cervix under slight traction, a right-angle clamp is introduced into the cul-de-sac alongside the cervix. The cardinal and uterosacral ligaments are sequentially isolated first with a large right-angle then with a Phaneuf clamp and divided with electrocautery (Figs. 4,5). The stumps are ligated with

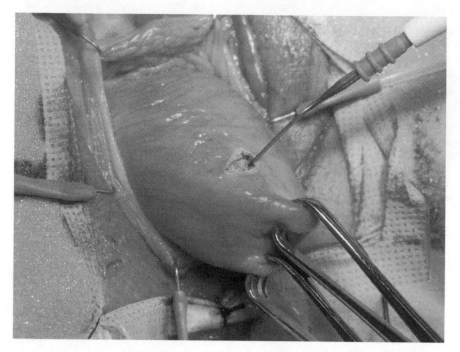

Figure 2   Incision. A circumferential incision is made ~1 cm from the cervical os with electrocautery.

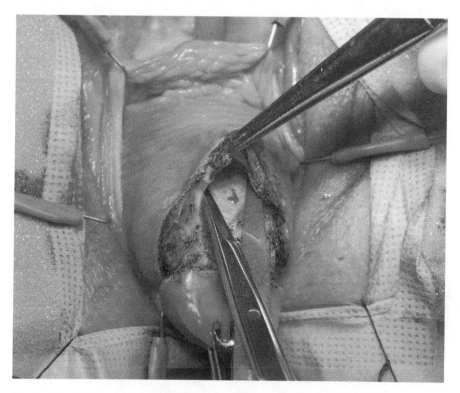

Figure 3   Exposure of anterior uterus. Sharp dissection is used to expose the anterior uterus and develop the vesicoperitoneal space.

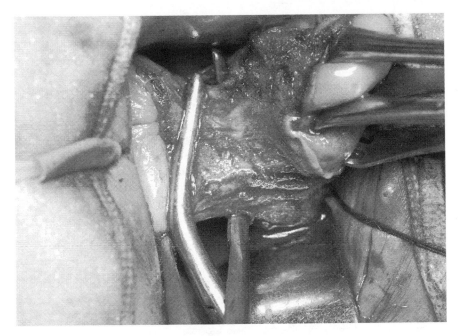

Figure 4 **Isolation of cardinal-uterosacral ligaments.** Right-angle and Phaneuf clamps are used in succession to better delineate the cardinal-uterosacral complex.

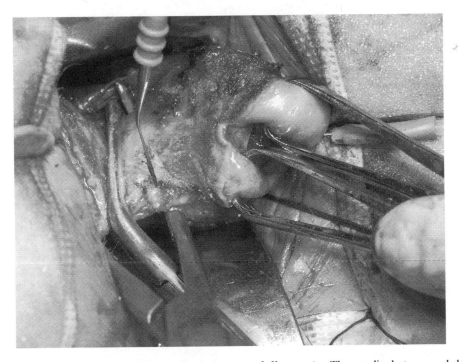

Figure 5 **Transection of cardinal-uterosacral ligaments.** The cardinal-uterosacral ligaments are transected using electrocautery.

figure-of-eight suture ligatures (of a delayed absorbable suture). These sutures are left long and placed in the grooves of the retractor ring. Anterior retraction of the bladder exposes the vesicoperitoneal fold (Fig. 6). At this point the uterus can be everted and brought outside the introitus (Fig. 7). Safe entry into the anterior peritoneum can be made by placing a finger through the cul-de-sac and up over the fundus to tent the peritoneum. Electrocautery can then be used to incise the peritoneum overlying the surgeon's finger. Now the broad ligament is exposed and ligated as above (Fig. 8). If the adnexae are not removed, their attachments are also now divided. The utero-ovarian ligament, Fallopian tube, and round ligament are visible from anterior to posterior and are sequentially divided and ligated. The uterus is finally removed. A circular arrangement of the six ligated pedicles and their attached sutures remains (Fig. 9).

Two methods are used to provide vault support and vaginal depth: perivesical and prerectal fascia are approximated in order to close the cul de sac; and a modified McCall culdoplasty is performed. The culdoplasty sutures are placed first. Starting outside the vaginal wall toward the peritoneal cavity (in the area of the ligated cardinal-uterosacral complex), bilateral figure-of-eight sutures of 0-Vicryl are used to incorporate the area lateral to the rectum and the uterosacral ligaments as they cross the iliococcygeus muscle in the posterolateral pelvic wall (Figs. 10,11). These sutures are ~8–10 cm from the vaginal cuff. They are tagged at this time and will not be tied until after the cuff is closed. Exposure is facilitated by packing the peritoneal cavity with moist laparotomy sponges.

Two pursestring sutures of 0-Vicryl are now placed to close the cul-de-sac. These sutures incorporate the prerectal fascia, the cardinal-uterosacral ligament complex, the broad ligaments,

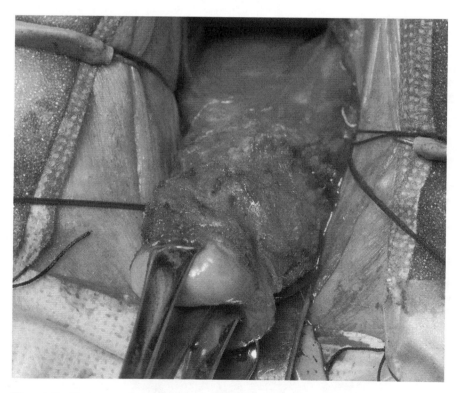

Figure 6   **Exposure of vesicoperitoneal fold.** Anterior retraction of the bladder exposes the peritoneal cavity.

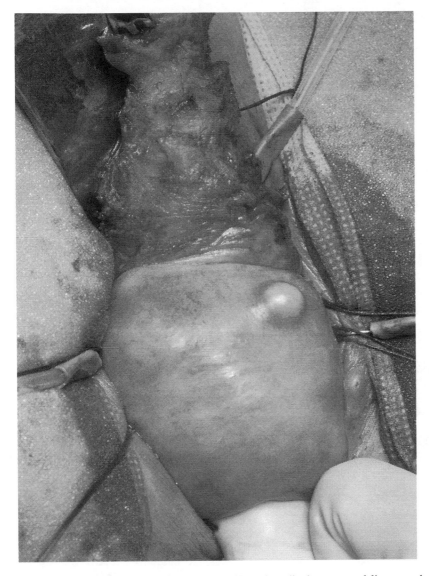

Figure 7   Eversion of uterus. After the bilateral cardinal-uterosacral ligaments have been ligated, the uterus is manually everted (note leiomyoma).

and the perivesical fascia (Fig. 12A, B). It is extremely important to stay in the midline when incorporating the perivesical fascia as sutures placed too lateral may cause ureteral injury. The purse-string sutures are also tagged and not tied at this time. The sutures of the previously ligated pedicles of the broad ligaments and the cardinal-uterosacral ligament complex are identified on each side and approximated in the midline. The purse-string sutures are now tied. If simultaneous repair of other prolapse or bladder neck suspension is planned, it is now performed. Finally, the culdoplasty sutures are tied. Vaginal depth is restored with tying of the culdoplasty sutures (Fig. 13). Excess vaginal wall is excised before closure with a running absorbable suture (Figs. 14 and 15).

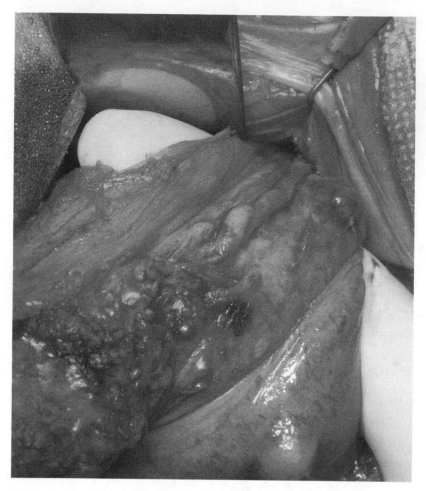

Figure 8   Division of broad ligament. The surgeon's index finger is inserted into the peritoneal cavity and hooked around the uterine vessels (broad ligament), which are ligated in the same fashion as the cardinal-uterosacral ligaments.

D.   Complications

Short-term complications common to both the abdominal and vaginal approaches include hemorrhage, infection, and adjacent organ injury, although these complications occur less frequently with the vaginal technique (44,48,54). Ileus may also occur with the abdominal approach but responds well to conservative treatment. Interestingly, bladder and ureteral injury occurs less commonly during vaginal hysterectomy than during abdominal hysterectomy. It has been proposed that traction applied to the cervix in combination with anterior retraction of the vesicouterine peritoneal fold provides sufficient displacement of the ureters (55). An important point to remember is that as long as the uterus is freely mobile, the technical difficulty of hysterectomy increases with increasing degrees of prolapse owing to the inconsistent anatomy (10). In a recent 10-year review by Varol et al., the overall complication rate was 44% for abdominal hysterectomy compared to 27.3% for vaginal hysterectomy (3). Furthermore, the abdominal hysterectomy group was four times more likely

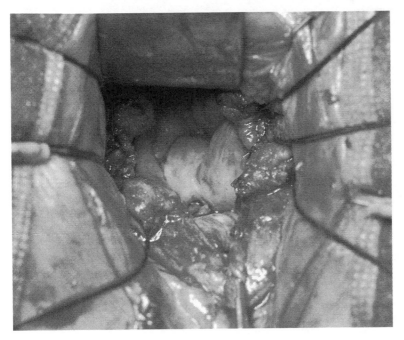

Figure 9   Transected uterine pedicles. Arrangement of the transected pedicles of the cardinal, uterosacral, and broad ligaments before approximation.

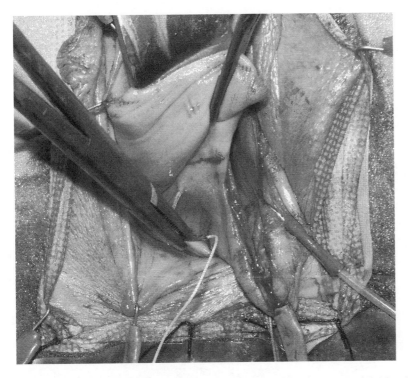

Figure 10   Origin of culdoplasty sutures. The culdoplasty sutures are initiated outside the vaginal wall and brought into the peritoneal cavity.

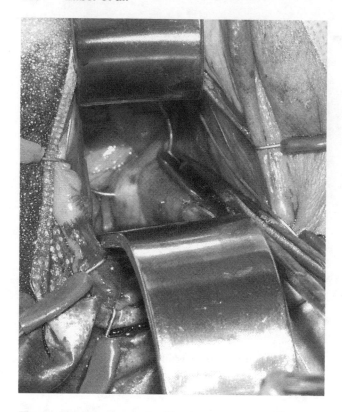

Figure 11   Placement of culdoplasty sutures. Inside the peritoneal cavity, a figure-of-eight culdoplasty suture approximates the area lateral to the rectum and the uterosacral ligaments as they cross the iliococcygeus muscle.

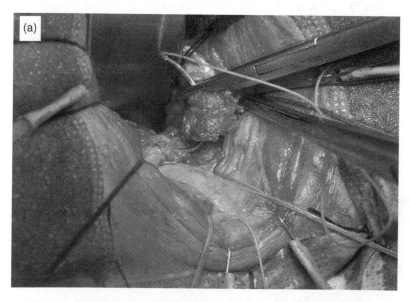

Figure 12   Placement of purse-string suture. The purse-string suture is shown incorporating the transected cardinal-uterosacral complex (a) and the perivesical fascia (b).

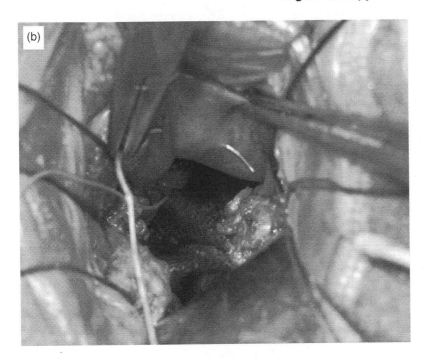

Figure 12   Continued.

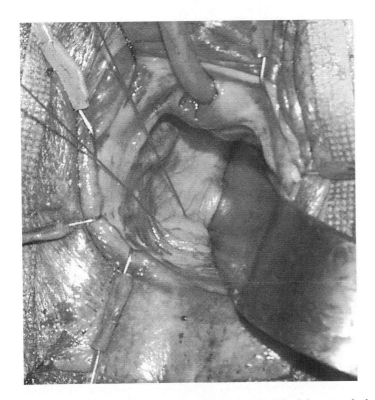

Figure 13   **Restoration of vaginal depth.** Vaginal depth is restored when the culdoplasty sutures are tied.

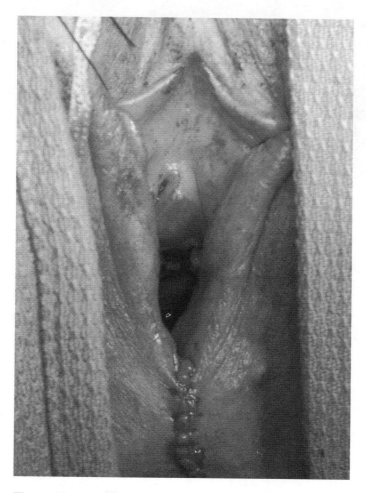

Figure 14   Postoperative result. Postoperative result following transvaginal hysterectomy.

to require surgical intervention at readmission and had a higher febrile morbidity and minor complication rate.

Long-term complications include recurrent prolapse and urinary fistula. The majority of vault prolapse involves only the upper vagina and is asymptomatic. More significant prolapse is uncommon. Prolapse that develops following hysterectomy may be an enterocele that occurred because of insufficient closure and/or support of the cuff. Enterocele may also develop postoperatively if concurrent pelvic floor relaxation was not repaired. Absence of the normal posterior vaginal axis may promote further prolapse of the cuff.

Ureterovaginal and vesicovaginal fistulas occur in 0.09–0.5% and 0.6% of cases, respectively (10). With adequate anterior retraction of the bladder, ligation of the pedicles close to the cervix and avoidance of lateral placement of the purse-string sutures in the perivesical fascia, bladder, and ureteral injury can be avoided. In regard to overall lower urinary tract function, Vierhout concluded that there is minimal to no effect of nonradical hysterectomy on lower urinary tract function (56).

Sexual function has always been a concern following hysterectomy; however, recent data indicate that hysterectomy actually improves sexual functioning and overall quality of life.

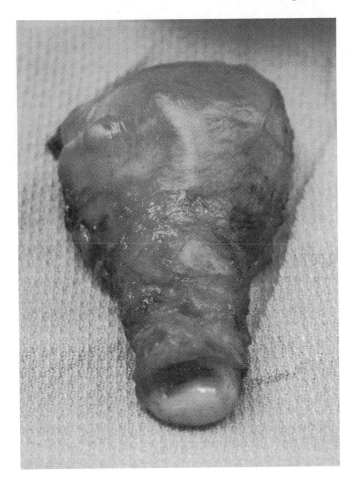

Figure 15   Pathologic specimen. The uterus is removed intact with surgical margins in close proximity to the uterus, which facilitates avoidance of ureteral injury.

Rhodes and associates found that after hysterectomy, the occurrence of sexual relations and orgasm increased and the rates of dyspareunia and low libido decreased (57). Similarly, researchers from the Maine Medical Assessment Foundation concluded that hysterectomy relieved pelvic pain, fatigue, depression, and sexual dysfunction and improved quality of life 1 year postoperatively (58).

VII.   CONCLUSION

Uterine prolapse is a condition that, depending on severity of prolapse and symptoms, can be treated conservatively or surgically. Surgical treatment includes uterine sparing procedures and hysterectomy. Hysterectomy can be performed by the traditional abdominal approach, laparoscopically, or vaginally. Considerations such as surgeon preference, uterine size, uterine and/or adnexal pathology, and fertility must be taken into account before choosing therapy.

542 **Eilber et al.**

REFERENCES

1. Bren L. Alternatives to hysterectomy: new technologies, more options. FDA Consum 2001; 35:1–9.
2. Graves EJ, Kozak LJ. Detailed diagnoses and procedures, National Hospital Discharge Survey, 1996. Vital Health Stat 1998; 13:1.
3. Varol N, Healey M, Tang P, Sheehan P, Maher P, Hill D. Ten-year review of hysterectomy morbidity and mortality: can we change direction? Aust N Z J Obstet Gynaecol 2001; 41:295–302.
4. Hacker NF, Moore JG. Essentials of Obstetrics and Gynecology. 2nd ed. Philadelphia: W.B. Saunders, 1992:6–7.
5. Moore KL. Clinically Oriented Anatomy. 2nd ed. Baltimore: Williams & Wilkins, Baltimore, 1985:373–376.
6. Wahle GR, Young GPH, Raz S. Anatomy and pathophysiology of pelvic support. In: Raz S, ed. Female Urology. 2nd ed. Philadelphia: W.B. Saunders, 1996:60–62.
7. Adam RA. Enterocele and massive vaginal eversion. eMedicine Journal 2000; 2:1–21.
8. De Lancey JOL. Surgical anatomy of the female pelvis. In: Rock JA, Thompson JD, eds. Te Linde's Operative Gynecology. 8th ed. Philadelphia: J.B. Lippincott, 1997:63–93.
9. De Lancey JOL. Anatomic aspects of vaginal eversion after hysterectomy. Am J Obstet Gynecol 1992; 166:1717–1724.
10. Chopra A, Stothers L, Raz S. Uterine prolapse. In: Raz S, ed. Female Urology. 2nd ed. Philadelphia: W.B. Saunders, 1996:457–464.
11. Thompson JD. Retrodisplacement of the uterus. In: Rock JA, Thompson JD, eds. Te Linde's Operative Gynecology. 8th ed. Philadelphia: J.B. Lippincott, 1997:941–949.
12. Swift SE. The distribution of pelvic organ support in a population of female subjects seen for routine gynecologic health care. Am J Obstet Gynecol 2000; 183:277–285.
13. Samuelsson EC, Arne Victor FT, Tibblin G. Signs of genital prolapse in a Swedish population of women 20 to 59 years of age and possible related factors. Am J Obstet Gynecol 1999; 180:299–305.
14. Kobashi KC, Leach GE. Pelvic prolapse. Urology 2000; 164:1879–1890.
15. Winters JC, Cespedes RD, Vanlangendonck R. Abdominal sacral colpopexy and abdominal enterocele repair in the management of vaginal vault prolapse. Urology 2000; 56(suppl 6A):55–63.
16. Stanton S, Hilton P, Norton C, Cardozo L. Clinical and urodynamic effects of anterior colporrhaphy and vaginal hysterectomy for prolapse with and without incontinence. Br J Obstet Gynaecol 1982; 89:459–463.
17. Fianu S, Kjaeldgaard A, Larsson B. Preoperative screening for latent stress incontinence in women with cystocele. Neurol Urodynam 1985; 4:3–8.
18. Gemer O, Bergman M, Segal S. Prevalence of hydronephrosis in patients with genital prolapse. Eur J Obstet Gynecol Reprod Biol 1999; 86:11–13.
19. Churchill DN, Afridi S, Dow D, McManamon P. Uterine prolapse and renal dysfunction. J Urol 1980; 124:899–900.
20. Bump RC, Mattiasson A, Bo K, Brubaker LP, DeLancey JO, Klarskov P, Shull BL, Smith AR. The standardization of terminology of female pelvic organ prolapse and pelvic floor dysfunction. Am J Obstet Gynecol 1996; 175:10–17.
21. Barbaric ZL, Marumoto AK, Raz S. Magnetic resonance imaging of the perineum and pelvic floor. Top Magn Reson Imaging 2001; 12:83–92.
22. Goldstein I, Wise GJ, Tancer ML. A vesicovaginal fistula and intravesical foreign body. A rare case of the neglected pessary. Am J Obstet Gynecol 1990; 163:589–591.
23. Wilcox LS, Koonin LM, Pokras R, Strauss LT, Xia Z, Peterson HB. Hysterectomy in the United States. Obstet Gynecol 1994; 83:549–555.
24. Masters WH, Johnson V. Human Sexual Response. Boston: Little, Brown, 1966:238.
25. Barrington JW, Bowen-Simpkins P. The Levonorgestrel intrauterine system in the management of menorrhagia. Br J Obstet Gynaecol 1997; 104:614–616.
26. Thomas AG, Brodman ML, Dottino PR, Bodian C, Friedman F, Bogursky E. Manchester procedure vs. vaginal hysterectomy for uterine prolapse. J Reprod Med 1995; 40:299–304.

27. Cruikshank SH, Cox IN. Sacrospinous fixation at the time of vaginal hysterectomy. Am J Obstet Gynecol 1991; 164:1072–1076.

28. Costantini E, Lombi R, Micheli C, Parziani S, Porena M. Colposacropexy with Gore-Tex mesh in marked vaginal and uterovaginal prolapse. Eur Urol 1998; 34:111–117.

29. Maher CF, Carey MP, Murray CJ. Laparoscopic suture hysteropexy for uterine prolapse. Obstet Gynecol 2001; 97:1010–1014.

30. Wheeless CR. Atlas of Pelvic Surgery. 2nd ed. Philadelphia: Lea & Febiger, 1988.

31. Thompson JD. Surgical techniques for pelvic organ prolapse. In: Rock JA, Thompson JD, eds. Te Linde's Operative Gynecology. 8th ed. Philadelphia: J.B. Lippincott, 1997: 969–979.

32. Williams BFP. Surgical treatment in uterine prolapse in young women. Am J Obstet Gynecol 1966; 95:967–972.

33. Naya y Sanchez RM, Velasco VR, Garcia TL. Manchester operation: late complications and obstetric future. Ginecol Obstet Mex 1973; 33:457–459.

34. Gordon SF. Laparoscopic uterine suspension. J Reprod Med 1992; 37:615–616.

35. Sze EH, Karram MM. Transvaginal repair of vault prolapse: a review. Obstet Gynecol 1997; 89: 466–475.

36. Hardiman PJ, Drutz HP. Sacrospinous vault suspension and abdominal colposacropexy: success rates and complications. Am J Obstet Gynecol 1996; 175:612–616.

37. Nichols DH. Sacrospinous fixation for massive eversion of the vagina. Am J Obstet Gynecol 1982; 142:901–904.

38. Ridley JH. Evaluation of the colpocleisis operation: a report of 58 cases. Am J Obstet Gynecol 1972; 113:1114–1119.

39. Ahranjani M, Nora E 2nd, Rezai P, Bujewski S. Neugebauer-LeFort operation for vaginal prolapse. J Reprod Med 1992; 37:959–964.

40. Munro MG. Supracervical hysterectomy: a time for reappraisal. Obstet Gynecol 1997; 89:133–139.

41. Dennerstein L, Wood C, Burrows GD. Sexual response following hysterectomy and oophorectomy. Obstet Gynecol 1977; 49:92–96.

42. Kilkku P. Supravaginal uterine amputation versus hysterectomy: effects of coital frequency and dyspareunia. Acta Obstet Gynecol 1983; 62:141–145.

43. Kilkku P, Gronroos M, Hirvonen T, Rauramo L. Supravaginal uterine amputation vs hysterectomy: effects on libido and orgasm. Acta Obstet Gynecol Scand 1983; 62:147–152.

44. Scott JR, Sharp HT, Dodson MK, Norton PA, Warner HR. Subtotal hysterectomy in modern gynecology; a decision analysis. Am J Obstet Gynecol 1997; 176:1186–1191.

45. Ewies AA, Olah KS. Subtotal abdominal hysterectomy: a surgical advance or a backward step? Br J Obstet Gynaecol 2000; 107:1376–1379.

46. Miyazawa K. Technique for total abdominal hysterectomy: historical and clinical perspective. Obstet Gynecol Surv 1992; 47:433–447.

47. Parker WH. Total laparoscopic hysterectomy. Obstet Gynecol Clin North Am 2000; 27:431–440.

48. Dicker RC, Greenspan JR, Strauss LT, Cowart MR, Scally MJ, Peterson HB, DeStefano F, Rubin GL, Ory HW. Complications of abdominal and vaginal hysterectomy among women of reproductive age in the United States. The collaborative review of sterilization. Am J Obstet Gynecol 1982; 144: 841–848.

49. Harkki-Siren P, Sjoberg J, Toivonen J, Tiitinen A. Clinical outcome and tissue trauma after laparoscopic and abdominal hysterectomy: a randomized controlled study. Acta Obstet Gynecol Scand 2000; 79:866–871.

50. Summitt RL Jr, Stovall TG, Lipscomb GH, Ling FW. Randomized comparison of laparoscopy-assisted vaginal hysterectomy with standard vaginal hysterectomy in an outpatient setting. Obstet Gynecol 80:895–901.

51. Munro M, Parker W. A classification system for laparoscopic hysterectomy. Obstet Gynecol 1993; 82:624–629.

52. Harkki-Siren P, Sjoberg J, Kurki T. Major complications of laparoscopy: a follow-up Finnish study. Obstet Gynecol 1999; 94:94–98.

53. Kursh ED, McGuire E. Female Urology. Philadelphia: J.B. Lippincott, 1994.

54. Gitsch G, Berger E, Tatra G. Trends in thirty years of vaginal hysterectomy. Surg Gynecol Obstet 1991; 172:207–210.
55. Hofmeister FJ, Wolfgram RL. Methods of demonstrating measurement relationships between vaginal hysterectomy ligatures and the ureters. Am J Obstet Gynecol 1962; 83:938–948.
56. Vierhout ME. Influence of nonradical hysterectomy on the function of the lower urinary tract. Obstet Gynecol Surv 2001; 56:381–386.
57. Rhodes JC, Kjerulff KH, Langenberg PW, Guzinski GM. Hysterectomy and sexual functioning. JAMA 1999; 282:1934–1941.
58. Carlson KJ, Miller BA, Fowler FJ Jr. The Maine Women's Health Study. I.: Outcomes of hysterectomy. Obstet Gynecol 83:556–572.

39

Vaginal Hysterectomy and Other Operations for Uterine Prolapse

Paul M. Fine and Dallas Johnson
Baylor College of Medicine, Houston, Texas, U.S.A.

I. HISTORICAL PERSPECTIVE

A. Prolapse

Uterine prolapse was an ancient affliction. It was described by the Egyptians 2000 years BC. The uterus had been described by Aristotle as "the seat of womanhood" and was considered an indispensable and vital organ that somehow embodied the spirit of the woman. It is therefore not surprising that ancient practitioners tried or suggested multiple therapies of every imaginable type to correct prolapse without removing this vital organ of womanhood (1). Succession therapy and vaginal pessaries were two popular nonsurgical treatments for genital prolapse. Succussion therapy, described by Hippocrates (460–377 BC.), involved securing the patient to a frame with ropes then inverting her to a head-down position. The entire frame was then moved up and down in a shaking motion to allow gravity to return the uterus to its normal pelvic position. This was followed by placement of an object in the vaginal canal to prevent recurrence of the prolapse. A widely used object was half of a pomegranate soaked in vinegar as recommended by Diocles of Carystos in the 4th century BC (2).

Over the centuries many objects of various sizes and shapes were utilized as pessaries. There are many ancient writings describing pelvic discomfort, foul-smelling vaginal discharge, and bleeding. There were sporadic reports of vaginal amputation of the prolapsed part from as early as 100 AD by Soranos (3) through the early 19th century. The prolapsed part was ligated as high as possible, followed by excision with the knife or cautery, or allowing the ligated organ to slough over a period of weeks (4). Genital prolapse was the first recorded indication for hysterectomy (5).

B. Anesthesia

The discovery of general anesthesia using chloroform and ether was a medical milestone. There is debate as to who was the first to use chloroform as an anesthetic. The German chemist Justus von Liebig discovered chloroform in 1831 (6). Simpson used chloroform fumes to lessen the pain of labor in 1847 (7). The subsequent discovery of ether as a general anesthetic agent was an important American contribution to medicine. Crawford Long, a practitioner in rural Georgia, first used ether as a general anesthetic in 1842 and published his results in 1849. Oliver Wendell Holmes first suggested the name "anesthesia" (6).

C. Antisepsis and Asepsis

The discovery of general anesthesia opened the door to the rapid progress in pelvic surgery, but the discovery of antisepsis and asepsis was equally important. Semmelweis proved the contagiousness of puerperal fever at the Vienna Krankenhaus and published it in 1845. His insistence of asepsis by thoroughly scrubbing of the hands in the delivery room caused him to be ridiculed and persecuted by his colleagues, eventually forcing him into an insane asylum, where he died at the age of 47 (8). Joseph Lord Lister devised a method of antisepsis by sterilizing of the operating room and operating field with carbolic spray in 1865 (9).

D. Hysterectomy

Oslander reported eight partial vaginal hysterectomies in 1808. His first such procedure in 1801 for cervical cancer required traction on a nonprolapsed uterus. He used a speculum to aid in visualization then, with traction, sharply excised the cancerous cervix with a knife and curved scissors (10). In 1842, Charles Clay of Manchester removed a fibroid uterus. He had opened the abdomen to remove an ovarian tumor and encountered a large fibroid uterus. He then performed a supracervical hysterectomy. Unfortunately, the patient died on postop day 15. The first successful removal of a fibroid uterus occurred in 1853 by Dr. Walter Burnham of Lowell, MA. He was forced to remove the uterus without intending to do so. The abdomen had been opened to remove what was thought to be an ovarian cyst when the patient suddenly vomited and extruded the fibroid uterus through the incision. He was unable to replace it and was forced to perform the hysterectomy. He was encouraged by colleagues to attempt further hysterectomies. Of his next 15 attempted hysterectomies, only three survived. Gilman Kimball, also of Lowell, was the first to correctly diagnose uterine fibroids preoperatively, and performed an abdominal hysterectomy for that indication in September 1853 (11).

Between 1800 and 1875, cervical cancer provided the impetus in vaginal surgery. In 1810, Wrisberg delivered a prize-winning essay to the Vienna Royal Academy of Medicine advocating vaginal hysterectomy for cervical cancer. Paleta, an Italian surgeon, in 1812 reported the removal of the entire uterus vaginally, although he had intended to remove only the cancerous cervix and lower uterine segment (12). Conrad Langenbeck of Gottingen, Germany, performed the first planned successful vaginal hysterectomy in 1818 and reported it in 1819. The patient had cervical cancer and prolapse. She was 50 years of age at the time of surgery and lived until the age of 76. It is remarkable that Langenbeck performed this successful surgery without an assistant, anesthesia, antisepsis, hemostatic clamps, and blood transfusion and without opening the peritoneum (13). The first reported American vaginal hysterectomy was by J.F. Warren in 1829 (14). This was not a complete hysterectomy, as the fundus was not removed.

Blood loss and infection were the major causes of death from early hysterectomy. By 1880, the operative mortality from vaginal hysterectomy was under 40% compared to a 70% mortality following abdominal hysterectomy. Wilhelm Freund in Breslau, Germany (1881), developed the technique of placing hemostatic clamps ("compression forceps") on the broad ligament rather than ligation or cautery during abdominal hysterectomy. He left them in place for several days prior to removing them (15). Pean, a French surgeon, reported in 1889 the technique of combined clamping and suturing. His mortality rate was only 2% for vaginal hysterectomy. Pean also first described the morcellation technique for vaginal removal of fibroid uterus in 1886 (16).

II. HISTORICAL OPERATIONS FOR UTERINE PROLAPSE

The *Manchester-Fothergill operation*, first performed by Duncan of Manchester in 1879 (17), consists of cystocele and rectocele repairs, if necessary, amputation of the cervix and suture of the cervical ligaments in front of the cervix to draw the cervix up into the vagina. The *Watkins transposition operation* was first performed by Thomas J. Watkins in 1898. It was used to correct cystocele and uterine prolapse with generally satisfactory results. It has also been referred to as the *interposition operation*. The technique involved repositioning or interposing the uterine fundus between the anterior vaginal wall and urethra/bladder (18). The *Spalding-Richardson procedure* was described in 1937 by Edward H. Richardson (19). Spalding had independently described a nearly identical procedure earlier in 1919 (20). The procedure consists of removal of the cervix and corpus of the uterus and utilization of the isthmic portion of the uterus with its broad and uterosacral ligament attachments into which the cystocele repair may be anchored. This procedure allowed for the removal of the diseased vaginal portion of the cervix, removal of the uterine corpus with the tubes and ovaries if indicated, destruction or excision of the remaining endocervical canal, retention and use of a well vascularized uterine isthmus with proven supporting structures, and the pubocervical and rectovaginal fascial attachments. This procedure is more difficult to perform than a vaginal hysterectomy. Should disease develop in the retained portion of the uterus, surgery to remove it may be complicated. The *LeFort colpocleisis* was first described by Leon LeFort in 1877 for the treatment of total procidentia (21). It is still used today in selected patients. It has the advantage of high success rates (>95%) in the cure of advanced procidentia combined with relatively quick operating time and avoidance of general anesthesia in often medically compromised patients. It is described in detail below.

A. LeFort Colpocleisis

There are various modifications of the original technique described. The basic technique is to denude a rectangular area of anterior and posterior vaginal mucosa from the level of the cervix to the urethrovesical crease and then to suture these "mirror image" denuded areas together anteroposteriorly, creating a permanent internal pessary. Care is taken to leave sufficient vaginal mucosa bilaterally to allow formation of bilateral canals for drainage of cervical secretions. Care is also taken to remove only the vaginal epithelium, preserving the underlying fibromuscular or "fascial" layer. This allows for better vaginal support, better vascularity, and deeper placement of sutures with less risk of bowel or bladder injury. Injection with a dilute pitressin solution may facilitate this dissection. Scoring with the knife or marking with a pen outlines the rectangular areas on the anterior and posterior vaginal mucosa to be excised. Smith-Pratt clamps are useful in grasping the vaginal mucosa for counter traction during this dissection.

The epithelial edges below the cervix are reapproximated with interrupted absorbable sutures (0 or 00 Vicryl or Dexon). Beginning at the top (near the cervix), interrupted rows of sutures (also 0 or 00 Vicryl or Dexon) are placed between the anterior and posterior denuded vaginal wall. The prolapse is gradually reduced by these rows of sutures. Generally, these rows are placed 1–1.5 cm apart with the interrupted sutures of each row ~1.0 cm apart laterally. Once the prolapse has been reduced, the outer vaginal epithelial edges are reapproximated with interrupted sutures (0 or 00 Vicryl or Dexon). Perineorraphy should then be performed with midline plication to reduce the genital hiatus and increase the thickness of the perineal body. Obviously, the LeFort colpocleisis is intended for use in the elderly and frail woman whose future sexual activity is not a concern. It is advisable to perform a dilatation and curettage prior to LeFort colpocleisis to rule out occult endometrial malignancy. Preoperative testing for occult stress urinary incontinence can be performed with prolapse reduction stress testing (pessary stress test). Minimally invasive anti-incontinence procedures such as tension-free vaginal tape (TVT) can be performed concurrently in patients with preoperative complaints of stress urinary incontinence, or demonstration of urinary stress incontinence with the prolapse reduction stress test. The LeForte colpocleisis can also be performed for posthysterectomy vaginal vault prolapse with similar indications for patient selection. Creation of bilateral vaginal tunnels is less important in these patients since there will not be any uterine or cervical secretions to drain.

B. Gilliam Uterine Suspension

First described by D.T. Gilliam in 1900, the Gilliam uterine suspension is still occasionally used. This procedure involves exteriorizing a knuckle of round ligament transperitoneally and lateral to the rectus muscle bilaterally. This exteriorized knuckle of round ligament is then attached to the anterior rectus fascia using permanent sutures. This procedure converts a prolapsed or retroverted uterine fundus to an anteflexed and more well-supported position (22). The procedure can be done by open laparotomy or by laparoscopic technique. It was often done concurrently with infertility surgical procedures in order to elevate the adnexae out of the cul-de-sac in the hope of reducing future adnexal adhesions. High recurrence rates of uterine prolapse have been reported following Gilliam suspension. This is due to restretching of the round ligament. In addition, fewer fertility surgeries are performed today because of higher pregnancy rates with assisted reproductive technology. Enhancement of fertility or reduction of adnexal adhesions with concurrent Gilliam suspension was also never demonstrated.

III. HYSTERECTOMY

A. Contemporary Practice and Incidence

Generally, women today with symptomatic uterine and pelvic organ prolapse are advised to complete childbearing prior to undergoing reconstructive pelvic surgery. Although the addition of hysterectomy does not enhance the success of operations for stress urinary incontinence, hysterectomy is frequently performed for standard gynecological indications. Gynecological indications for hysterectomy include severe dysmenorrhea (painful menses), menorrhagia (heavy menses), menometrorrhagia (frequent and heavy menses), endometriosis, high-grade cervical intraepithelial neoplasia (dysplasia), and atypical adenomatous hyperplasia of the endometrium. Fibroids and uterine prolapse remain the most common indication for hysterectomy in the United States. Hysterectomy is currently the second most common surgical procedure performed in the United States (cesarean section is first), with almost 600,000 performed in 1997. Of these 63% were done abdominally and only 37% vaginally or with the laparoscopic approaches (23). As the population ages, the estimated number of hysterectomies will increase. Using 1987 age-specific hysterectomy rates and population projections from the Census Bureau, over 823,000 hysterectomies will be performed in 2005 (24). Vaginal or abdominal hysterectomy is frequently performed in combination with other pelvic reconstructive procedures.

B. Vaginal or Abdominal?

The choice of a vaginal or abdominal approach for hysterectomy will depend on several factors. Uterine enlargement greater than a 12- to 14-week pregnancy may require an abdominal approach. Morcellation techniques are currently a "dying art," but in trained hands allow for vaginal removal of an 18- to 20-week-size uterus (to the umbilicus). Many younger gynecologists are unfamiliar or uncomfortable with this technique. The presence of adnexal pathology including large pelvic masses, suspected pelvic malignancy, or probable pelvic adhesions such as those following myomectomy or pelvic abscess, may favor an abdominal approach. Desired removal of tubes and ovaries is not generally an indication for abdominal approach since bilateral salpingo-oophorectomy can be safely accomplished vaginally in >90% of cases. The requirement of an abdominal incision for a concurrently planned Burch urethropexy or abdominal sacrocolpopexy may also favor an abdominal approach for hysterectomy. Some would argue that the need for an abdominal incision in a Burch would justify an abdominal approach to hysterectomy. Others would argue that the Burch urethropexy following vaginal hysterectomy requires a smaller incision with less invasion of the peritoneal cavity and no bowel packing. Prior cesarean section was once considered a relative contraindication for vaginal hysterectomy. Several recent studies, including one from our institution, have demonstrated the safety and efficacy of vaginal hysterectomy in patients with one or multiple prior cesarean sections (25). Benson compared the abdominal approach for pelvic reconstructive surgery to the vaginal approach and found less evidence of neuropathy, as measured by pudendal nerve terminal motor latency studies, than with the abdominal approach (26). Pudendal terminal motor latency measurements do not necessarily correlate with denervation of the pelvic floor and a definitive answer to this question awaits more randomized controlled clinical trials.

Obviously, the decision regarding the route of hysterectomy will depend on the above factors as well as surgeon preference. Vaginal hysterectomy has been performed in the same-day surgery setting in selected patients, and has been shown to be less expensive in direct costs than either abdominal or laparoscopic hysterectomy. Discussion of laparoscopic hysterectomy is beyond the scope of this chapter. Obviously there is a steep learning curve to become proficient in laparoscopic assisted or total laparoscopic hysterectomy. Concurrent repair of pelvic organ prolapse of anterior, posterior, or apical vaginal defects can also be accomplished vaginally. Obesity may favor the choice of the vaginal route.

A nulliparous patient may also be a candidate for a vaginal hysterectomy. However, a nulliparous and obese patient with little uterine descent, a narrow pubic arch, and upper thigh and gluteal obesity may prove a challenge, even to the most experienced vaginal surgeon. These patients are also technically difficult from an abdominal perspective owing to the thick abdominal wall, and a deep and narrow bony pelvis. Finally, any orthopedic condition preventing positioning in the dorsal lithotomy position would contraindicate a vaginal approach.

C. Risks: Vaginal Versus Abdominal Hysterectomy

There is an incidence of complications following hysterectomy in the range of 15%. This is more easily understood by considering the anatomy and technical details. Opening the vaginal cuff contaminates the peritoneal cavity with upper vaginal flora. The bowel, bladder, and ureters are close to the lines of incision, clamping, and suturing. Pelvic surgery also predisposes to thromboembolism. Obviously many factors influence risk including patient's age and general health, the indication for hysterectomy, the urgency (emergency or planned), the use of suction drainage and prophylactic antibiotics, the experience and training of the surgeon, and the choice of vaginal versus abdominal approach.

Comparative risks of vaginal and abdominal hysterectomy were assessed by the Collaborative Review of Sterilization (CREST) study conducted by the Centers for Disease Control (CDC) between 1978 and 1981. This study included women aged 15–44 who had nonemergency, nonradical hysterectomies at nine institutions for all indications excluding pregnancy and cancer. One thousand eight hundred fifty-one patients were analyzed for 568 vaginal and 1283 abdominal procedures. The overall complication rate was 24.5 per 100 women who had vaginal hysterectomy and 42.8 per 100 women who underwent abdominal hysterectomy. Thus, the risk for one or more complications was 70% higher in the abdominal hysterectomy group than in the vaginal hysterectomy group (relative risk of 1.7). The risk of infection was 2.1 times higher and the risk of transfusion was 1.9 times higher for the abdominal hysterectomy patients (27). A smaller but more recent study has shown similar trends but significantly lower complication rates. The complications following vaginal hysterectomy were 10.4% versus 13.6% for abdominal hysterectomy. The decrease in hematocrit was 5.7% for vaginal and 6.5% for abdominal hysterectomy. Hospital stay was 2.1 days for vaginal and 2.7 days for abdominal hysterectomy (28).

IV. VAGINAL HYSTERECTOMY

A. Technique

There are numerous classical descriptions and illustrations of the technique of vaginal hysterectomy. Most are derived from the technique described by Heaney. We will emphasize modifications of technique especially as it relates to prevention of future pelvic floor dysfunction. The decision to inject vasoconstrictors diluted with saline into the pericervical tissues is optional. The author prefers to use a solution of 20 units of pitressin diluted with 20 cc saline injected 360° around the cervical/vaginal tissues. A short Auvard weighted speculum is placed in the vagina, and the bladder is drained with a red rubber catheter. The cervix is grasped on the anterior and posterior lip with Lahey thyroid or "Massachusetts" traction forceps. Care must be taken to grasp only the outer (more distal) cervix, as the bladder may be relatively lower on the cervix in elderly patients with anterior wall prolapse or prior cesarean section. The choice of a sharp knife or angled Bovie tip is optional, but we prefer sharp knife dissection to better identify the proper tissue planes and to minimize tissue necrosis. Classically, a circumferential incision is made at the cervicovaginal junction. This incision transects the full thickness of the vaginal epithelium. However, since the posterior cul-de-sac is entered first, we prefer a U-shaped incision starting from three and continuing to the 9 o'clock position. In this manner, the cul-de-sac peritoneum can be entered and the uterosacral ligaments divided before any anterior cervicovaginal incision is needed. There is no reason to start potential bleeding in the anterior area until dissection into the vesicouterine space is necessary as the blood only runs downward obscuring the posterior operative field. In addition, initial division of the uterosacral ligaments allows for better mobilization of the uterus downward with traction and, therefore, better visualization and access.

With countertraction and a gauze-wrapped forefinger, the cul-de-sac peritoneum is identified and entered by sharp dissection with the curved Metzanbaum or Harrington scissors. In patients with uterine prolapse, this peritoneal reflection is often more distal from the cervix, and the posterior vaginal incision is therefore made lower into the cul-de-sac. A rectal finger may aid in clarifying this altered anatomy. Once the posterior cul-de-sac peritoneum is entered, the uterine fundus and adnexae are palpated to exclude unexpected uterine or adnexal pathology. A decision can then be finalized regarding the technical feasibility of continuing with the vaginal approach if any doubt had existed.

Conversion to an abdominal approach at this point can easily be accomplished. In the event of excessive bleeding from the posterior colpotomy, a running locking suture can be placed. Prior injection of vasoconstrictors eliminates the need for this. At this point, the short-bladed Auvard weighted speculum is replaced with the long-bladed weighted speculum with the blade inserted into the peritoneal cavity through the posterior colpotomy. This facilitates the visualization of the posterior compartment and pelvic sidewall.

Attention is now given to the anterior dissection. Using the scalpel or angled Bovie tip, an inverted "U" incision is made on the anterior cervix, from 9 to 3 o'clock, with care being taken to stay on the distal cervix in patients with anterior wall prolapse or prior cesarean. Traction on the cervix with countertraction with an anterior right-angled retractor will aid in identifying the correct tissue plane because the vagina will retract when cut to the correct full-thickness depth. If this does not occur, the cut anterior vaginal wall may be grasped with Allis tissue forceps and pulled anteriorly under tension. Sharp dissection with curved Metzanbaum scissors, tip down and staying close to the cervix, will facilitate entry into the vesicouterine space. Once the cleavage plane of the vesicocervical space is reached, gentle dissection with the finger will lift the bladder off the cervix. If the bladder pillars are prominent, they can be cross-clamped close to the cervix, transected, and ligated to provide better lateral exposure. The location of the peritoneal reflection is palpable as the two slippery mesotheleal surfaces sliding on one another. The peritoneum can then be elevated with a Sarot artery forceps and transected. The forefinger is placed through the peritoneal opening, and a Haney right-angle retractor is placed below this forefinger to guide its placement into the peritoneal cavity.

Visualization of bowel and omentum confirms correct intraperitoneal entry. An opposing right-angle retractor may facilitate visualization of bowel and/or omentum. In cases with an enlarged and well-supported uterus or prior cesarean section, this peritoneal reflection may be higher up and technically difficult to enter. In this case, the transverse cervical ("cardinal" or "Mackenrodt") ligament may be safely divided first to allow further descent of the uterus and better visualization of the anterior peritoneal reflection. A curved uterine sound can also be passed from the cul-de-sac around the uterus anteriorly to help identify the proper tissue plane. In cases where difficulty has been encountered in entering the anterior peritoneum, the bladder integrity can be tested by transurethral instillation of methylene blue or sterile milk into the bladder.

Once the anterior and posterior peritonea have been entered, the ureter can often be palpated to determine its position prior to shortening and transecting the uterosacral and cardinal ligaments. Shortening of these ligaments prior to reattachment is important for apical cuff support. Only if the ligaments are shortened will the vaginal cuff be held at a level higher than that of the prolapsed cervix, unless some other type of apical cuff suspension is planned such as a sacrospinous ligament fixation. To palpate the ureter, a retractor is placed in the lateral vaginal fornix and a finger in the anterior cul-de-sac. Because the ureter must pass under the uterine artery and enter the bladder anterior to the examining finger, it can be palpated against the retractor blade. The characteristic snap of the ureter permits its identification. It can be followed for some distance by moving the retractor and examining finger anteriorly and posteriorly.

At this point, the uterosacral ligaments are palpated and cross-clamped with Heaney-type hysterectomy forceps if not already divided as described above. If significant shortening of the uterosacral ligament is planned, this step is done after the anterior peritoneum is opened in order to palpate the ureter first. Placement of this clamp more laterally and more distal from the uterus will shorten the uterosacral pedicle and assist in better apical support of the vaginal cuff later when reattached to the vaginal cuff. The uterosacral pedicles are not cut flush with the clamp. Instead, an extra 2 mm of tissue is left to aid in future identification and to facilitate later resuturing of these pedicles to the angles of the vaginal cuff. In addition, transfixion suturing is used to avoid the tie coming loose when traction is placed on this pedicle later. These pedicles are tagged with a curved hemostat. We use 0 Dexon or Vicryl synthetic absorbable suture throughout the hysterectomy utilizing "popoff" CT-1 size tapered needles. The transverse cervical (cardinal or Mackenrodt) ligaments are similarly grasped by swinging the Heaney forceps out laterally to shorten this pedicle, and a transfixion suture is placed. These pedicles are also not cut flush with the clamp as described above; rather they are rather tagged with a straight hemostat. If a long cervix makes visualization or access to the uterine fundus difficult, all or part of the cervix may now be amputated (Fig. 1A) and the remaining lower uterine segment regrasped (Fig. 1B) prior to division of the uterine arteries. The uterine artery is bilaterally cross-clamped with the Heaney forceps placed perpendicular to the lateral uterus, making sure that the pedicle includes the peritoneum anteriorly and posteriorly. This assures the complete purchase of the uterine vessels. These vascular pedicles are not transfixed to avoid hematoma or held with tags that might cause slippage. The lower broad ligament is then bilaterally clamped and divided.

At this point, the uterine fundus can usually be delivered through the posterior colpotomy site by grasping it with a single toothed tenaculum and using gentle traction. This exposes the remaining connections between the uterus and adnexal structures (round ligament, Fallopian tube, and utero-ovarian vessels). These uteroadnexal structures are then divided using a variety of techniques. We prefer to first place a free ligature with the digital flip placement (Fig. 2) followed by clamping with Heaney forceps distal to the free tie. A transfixion suture distal to the free tie is then placed (Fig. 3). This allows for a double tie on this rather large pedicle and the benefit of a transfixion suture without risk of hematoma (29). The uterus is thus removed. These utero-ovarian pedicles are then tagged until hemostasis of all pedicles has been confirmed.

When the uterus is enlarged by fibroids, delivery of the fundus may not be possible. At the point where the uterine arteries have been successfully divided and ligated, various morcellation techniques can be utilized with minimal blood loss. The uterus may be divided sagitally and one-half of the uterus pushed cephalad while the other half is now accesssable for division of the uteroadnexal structures. Then, the remaining hemiuterus is brought down to complete the hysterectomy. Myomectomy can be utilized to reduce the size of the bulky fundus. The fundus may also be "cored" sequentially to facilitate lateral access for clamping. If, however, the uterine arteries are unable to be divided because of anatomical or technical difficulty, the vaginal approach should be abandoned in favor of an abdominal approach. Attempted morcellation prior to division and ligation of the uterine arteries will result in excessive blood loss, poor visualization, and "blind clamping."

Following removal of the uterus, all pedicles are examined for hemostasis with gentle traction on the tagged ligatures as needed. A moistened sponge stick is useful as both a bowel retractor and blotting instrument. If necessary, two 4 × 4 gauzes can be placed in the ring forceps to create a "double sponge stick" where more deflection of bowel is required.

The adnexae are now visualized and palpated. If adnexectomy is planned or indicated by unexpected pathology it is now performed. The adnexa is better mobilized by first dissecting it free from the remaining round ligament. The tissues under the proximal remaining round ligament are serially cross-clamped and ligated with 00 synthetic absorbable suture. The adnexa is then grasped with Babcock forceps and gently pulled medially exposing the infundibulopelvic ligament and vessels (Fig. 4). The prior separation of the round ligament from the adnexa greatly facilitates this, especially when the adnexae are relatively high in the pelvis. The infundibulopelvic structures are clamped, usually with a Sarot or Mixter right-angled forceps, divided, and ligated. Transfixion sutures are not used because of the risk of hematoma. This pedicle may, however, be doubly ligated by flashing the clamp or by placement of two sandwiched clamps if space permits. The pelvic sidewalls are carefully examined for hemostasis. Several large series have demonstrated the efficacy (>90% success) and safety in performing transvaginal bilateral salpingo-oophorectomy. In our opinion, however, because of the potentially increased risk of postoperative ovarian abscess

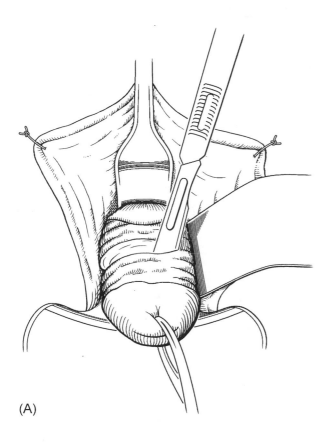

(A)

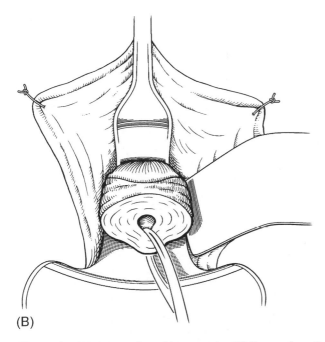

(B)

Figure 1   (A) Amputation of long cervix. (B) Regrasping of cervical stump.

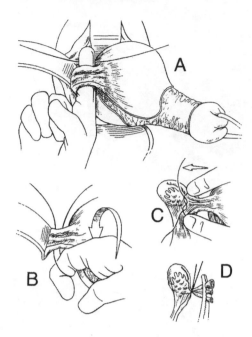

Figure 2   (A, B, C, D) Digital flip placement of utero-ovarian tie.

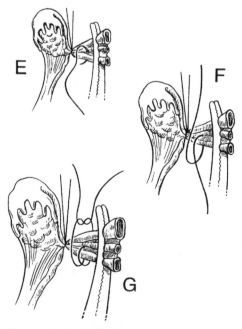

Figure 3   (E, F, G) Transfixion suture placed distal to digital flip free tie.

Round Ligament

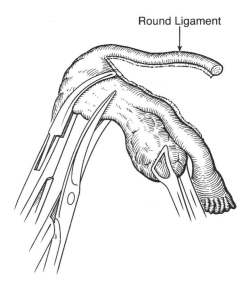

Figure 4   Separation of round ligament facilitating adnexal removal.

due to contamination from the vaginal field, an ovary with a ruptured functional cyst should be removed. This complication may occur despite the use of prophylactic antibiotics.

Culdoplasty, if indicated, may now be performed by a variety of techniques that are described elsewhere in this textbook. Although the need for closure of the pelvic peritoneum is controversial, it is our opinion that it should be closed when the adnexae are conserved in premenopausal women. This avoids prolapse of the distal tube through the vaginal cuff. Once hemostasis of the pedicles has been confirmed, this peritoneal closure is begun. The anterior peritoneum is grasped with a long Allis forceps. Sweeping a SpongeStick downward on the anterior peritoneum will bring the anterior peritoneal edge into plain view. The long-bladed Auvard weighted speculum is replaced with the short-bladed Auvard. The posterior vaginal wall is grasped with another long Allis forceps. Utilizing a non-pop-off synthetic absorbable 0 or 00 suture, the pelvic peritoneum is closed with a purse-string suture taking care not to place the suture too deep anteriorly avoiding the bladder, and to avoid the uterine artery pedicles laterally. The peritoneum is closed as high as possible. Care should be taken to not incorporate the adnexal pedicle into this suture. Such incorporation would bring the adnexa into opposition with the vaginal cuff and potentially cause later deep thrust dyspareunia. The patient is placed in Trendelenberg position and the assistant's forefinger is placed into the peritoneal cavity while the purse-string suture is tied. This avoids trapping of intra-abdominal contents in the suture. The finger is withdrawn as the suture is snugged down. Irrigation of the vagina is then performed.

Now the shortened uterosacral ligament and transverse cervical ligament pedicles are reattached to the lateral vaginal cuff bilaterally. This is an important step in reestablishing proper apical support of the post-hysterectomy vaginal vault. These pedicles had been tagged and purposefully cut to leave a large and easily identifiable pedicle. There are numerous techniques to reattach these pedicles directly with interrupted sutures. We prefer the "lasso" technique where the uterosacral and transverse cervical pedicles are placed under tension by gentle traction, and a suture of 0 Vicryl or Dexon is placed in the vaginal mucosa from outside to inside entering just below these ligaments. This suture is then brought around both of these pedicles ("lassoing" them), and then brought from inside to outside (Fig. 5). The lateral vagina is grasped

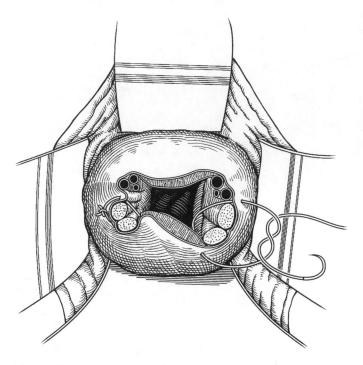

Figure 5   Fixation of uterosacral and transverse cervical ligament pedicles to lateral vaginal cuff for apical support.

with an Allis forceps and brought downward during tying of this suture above the Allis. With this technique, the angle sutures are placed more cephalad on the vaginal cuff, maximizing apical support. This lasso technique is more effective in controlling bleeding that might occur between the uterosacral and transverse cervical pedicles or for bleeding that might result from direct suture placement through the pedicle itself.

At this point the vaginal cuff is closed with either interrupted or a continuous locking suture. One or two layers may be utilized. The proper closure of the full thickness of anterior and posterior vagina reapproximates the anterior pubocervical fascia with the posterior rectovaginal fascia. This is an important step in minimizing the potential for later enterocele formation. Nonclosure of the vaginal cuff, as might occur with "whip-stitching" of the vaginal cuff, leaves an apical transverse "fascial" defect through which the bowel can later herniate to form an enterocele. With the use of prophylactic preoperative antibiotics and careful hemostatic technique, there are few indications to whip-stitch the vaginal cuff for drainage in our opinion. There is also no need to leave the vaginal cuff open to start the incision for colporraphy if one is planned. To do so results in a "T"-type incision at the vaginal cuff that is inherently weaker. Additional bleeding from the vaginal cuff during colporraphy is also avoided.

The bladder is now drained with a red rubber catheter if anterior colporraphy is planned; otherwise, a Foley to gravity drainage is placed. The presence of clear urine without hematuria is reassuring. It is debatable whether cystoscopy and ureteral evaluation with IV dye is required routinely following vaginal hysterectomy. However, we would recommend it be performed in cases of advanced uterine prolapse, concurrent culdoplasty, high uterosacral suspension of the vaginal cuff, difficult entry into the anterior peritoneum including prior cesarean section, and difficult morcellation cases. It should also be performed where bleeding has occurred following adnexectomy, and additional suture placement in the pelvic sidewall was required to secure hemostasis. Obviously, cystoscopy can be performed earlier following any of the above stages in the procedure rather than waiting until the end.

Once the weighted speculum is removed, adequate vaginal cuff support will be evidenced by visualization of lateral dimples where the uterosacral and transverse cervical ligaments had been reattached. Additionally, the vaginal length will be equal to or greater than the surgeon's finger (generally >7 cm). If vaginal cuff support is inadequate at this point, additional cuff suspension may be indicated including vaginal or abdominal techniques including sacrospinous ligament fixation or abdominal sacral colpopexy. Patients with significant preoperative uterine prolapse to or beyond the hymeneal ring should always be consented for these possible procedures.

B.   Complications

Although performed occasionally in an outpatient surgical setting, vaginal hysterectomy should be considered a major surgical procedure with the risks usually associated with such procedures. The complications unique to vaginal hysterectomy are discussed in this section.

1.   Intraoperative Complications

Cystotomy may occur during attempt to enter the vesicouterine peritoneal space. This occurs more frequently in patients with prior cesarean section with scarring in this area. These cystotomies are at the base of the bladder and generally above the trigone. Because the dependant portion of the bladder is involved, care must be taken to close the cystotomy in several layers and test for a watertight repair with sterile milk or Methylene Blue dye instilled transurethrally. Cystoscopy with IV Indigo Carmine dye should also be performed to confirm bilateral ureteral patency following such repair. The bladder should be drained for 7–10 days postoperatively.

Ureteral injury may occur during any hysterectomy. Patients with prolapse have distorted anatomy and the ureter may lie <0.5 cm lateral to the cervix (15). Care should be taken to place the clamps close to the uterus. Cystoscopic evaluation with IV Indigo Carmine dye may be helpful to confirm bilateral ureteral integrity and should be performed in cases of advanced pelvic organ prolapse.

GI injury may occur as a laceration of the rectum. Small defects may be repaired with a simple two-layer closure with synthetic absorbable suture while large lacerations may require a diverting colostomy following repair.

2.   Postoperative Complications

Vaginal cuff cellulitis or abscess can occur following either abdominal or vaginal hysterectomy. The vagina is a bacterially contaminated area despite preoperative douching or prolonged prepping in the OR. Cuff cellulitis generally presents on the second or third postoperative day with fever in the 101° range with excessive tenderness and induration of the vaginal cuff. Spiking fevers may be indicative of a vaginal cuff abscess. A palpable, fluctuant, and tender mass in the vaginal cuff may be palpated. The formation of a vaginal cuff hematoma may predispose to abscess formation. Ultrasonic evaluation is helpful in delineating the size and location since pelvic exam is limited owing to tenderness. Transvaginal drainage in the operating room is performed for palpable cuff abscesses. Radiology-guided needle drainage may be required for nonpalpable pelvic abscesses. These infections are polymicrobial, and intravenous broad-spectrum antibiotics covering gram-positive, gram-negative, and anaerobic bacteria are needed.

Urinary retention. The Foley catheter is normally removed on the morning of the first postoperative day, and most patients have no difficulty in resumption of voiding. However, occasionally, patients may require Foley drainage for an extra day or two. This is more common in patients with multiple prior cesarean sections where separation of the bladder off the uterus was more difficult. It may also be more common with prolonged anterior vaginal retraction in technically difficult cases.

Vesicovaginal fistula. This relatively rare complication may occur days to several weeks postoperatively. The patient generally complains of continuous vaginal leakage of urine. Diagnosis may be confirmed by transurethral installation of Methylene Blue dye in the bladder with a tampon placed into the vagina. Transvaginal leakage of the dye through the fistula will result in blue staining of the inner portion of the tampon. These fistulas are more common following recognized cystotomy with repair, or may occur following undiagnosed cystotomy or inadvertent passage of a suture into the bladder during closure of the pelvic peritoneum or vaginal cuff. Generally, the vesicovaginal fistula repair is delayed for 3 months to allow complete resolution of induration and swelling. Occasionally a small fistula may spontaneously heal during this prolonged catheter drainage. A vaginal repair can be accomplished by the Latzko procedure, which is essentially an upper vaginal colpocleisis without excision of the fistulous tract (30). Other surgeons, and most urologists, prefer the abdominal approach.

Vaginal prolapse is a rare complication of hysterectomy that may be avoided if proper attention is paid to vaginal vault support during the procedure (31,32). Suspension of the vault from the uterosacral-cardinal ligament complex provided they are of adequate strength, or colpopexy should prevent this complication.

C. Recuperation

Patients generally have a faster recovery following vaginal compared to abdominal hysterectomy. Lack of an abdominal incision facilitates early ambulation and fewer respiratory complications. Without the need for bowel packing, there is quicker return of normal bowel function, typically on the first postoperative day. It should be remembered that the synthetic absorbable sutures used, typically Dexon or Vicryl, are hydrolyzed and predictably lose >70% of their strength within 4 weeks. Patients are often relatively pain-free at 3 weeks postop and, accordingly, return to full activity. Studies have shown that wound tensile strength at 3 weeks postoperatively is only 25% as compared to preoperatively and rarely more than 50% at 6 weeks postoperative (33). Patients therefore must be cautioned to refrain from heavy lifting (>20–30 lb) and refrain from intercourse until after the 6-week postoperative visit. Proper healing of the vaginal cuff, including the newly reattached apical lateral ligamentous support (transverse cervical and uterosacral ligaments) and the midline fascial suture line (pubocervical and perirectal), requires 6–8 weeks at a minimum. As the synthetic absorbable sutures hydrolyze, the patient may notice a vaginal discharge, possibly blood tinged. She may even notice pieces of suture passed transvaginally. This is normal. She should refrain from tampon use during the 6-week post-operative period. Physiological estrogen replacement therapy may be begun or restarted upon full ambulation. Patients previously on combined estrogen-progestagen regimens may be switched to an estrogen only formulation.

REFERENCES

1. Benrubi GI. History of hysterectomy. J Fla Med Assoc 1988; 75:533.
2. Temkin OS. Gynecology. Baltimore: Johns Hopkins University Press, 1956.

3. Blain AW. Present status of vaginal hysterectomy. Surg Gynecol Obstet 1942; 75:307–313.

4. Kennedy JW, Campbell AD. Vaginal Hysterectomy. Philadelphia: F.A. Davis Co, 1942.

5. Emge LA, Durfee RB. Pelvic organ prolapse. Four thousand years of treatment. Clin Obstet Gynecol 1966; 9(4):997.

6. Miller RD. Anesthesia, 5th ed. Philadelphia: 2000:2–4.

7. Chestnut DH. Obstetric Anesthesia, Principles and Practice. St. Louis: Mosby, 1994:3–4.

8. Speert H. Obstetric and Gynecologic Milestones Illustrated. New York: Parthenon Publishing, 2000.

9. Lister JB. The antiseptic principle in the practice of surgery. BMJ 1867; 11:246.

10. Cianfrani T. A Short History of Obstetrics and Gynecology. Springfield, IL: Charles C. Thomas, 60:341–351.

11. Copeland LJ. Textbook of Gynecology. Philadelphia: W.B. Saunders, 1993:780.

12. Pichevin R. Vaginal hysterectomy. Br Gynaecol J 1896–1897; 11:566–574.

13. Lagenbeck CJM. Geschichte einer von mir glukich verrichteten extirpation der ganzen gebarmutter. N. Biblioth f Chir Ophthalm 1819–1820; 1:551.

14. Warren JP. Extirpation of cancer of the uterus. Am J Med Soc 1829; 4:536–537.

15. Gray LA. Vaginal Hysterectomy. Springfield, IL: Charles C. Thomas, 1983:135–173.

16. Pean J. De l'hysterectomie vaginale totale appliquee au traitement des tumeurs fibreures multiples de l'uterus; morcellement des tumeurs; pincement definitive des ligaments larges; absence de fermeture du vagin. Gaz Hop Paris 1886; 59:950.

17. Duncan WA. Two cases of vaginal extirpation of the uterus. BMJ 1885; 1:283.

18. Watkins TJ. The treatment of cystocele and uterine prolapse after the menopause. Am Gynecol Obstet J 1899; 15:420–423.

19. Richardson EH. An efficient composite operation for uterine prolapse and associated pathology. Am J Obstet Gynecol 1937; 34:814–827.

20. Spalding AB. A study of frozen sections of the pelvis with description of an operation for pelvic prolapse. Surg Gynecol Obstet 1919; 29:529–536.

21. Le Fort L. Nouveau procede pour la guerison du prolapsus uterin. Bull Gen Therap 1877; 92:337–344.

22. Gilliam DT. Round-ligament ventrosuspension of the uterus: a new method. Am J Obstet Gynecol 1900; 41:299.

23. Farquhar CM, Steiner CA. Hysterectomy rates in the United States 1990–1997. Obstet Gynecol 2002; 99:229–234.

24. Pokras R. Hysterectomy: past, present and future. Stat Bull Metrop Insur Co 1989; 70:12.

25. Poindexter YM, Sangi-Haghpeykar H, Poindexter AN, Young RL, Fine PM, Miller HJ. Previous cesarean section: a contraindication to vaginal hysterectomy? J Reprod Med 2001; 46:840–844.

26. Benson JT, McClellan E. The effect of vaginal dissection on the pudendal nerve. Obstet Gynecol 1993; 82:387–390.

27. Dicker RC, Scally MJ, Greenspan JR. Hysterectomy among women of reproductive age: trends in the United States, 1970–1978. JAMA 1982; 248:323.

28. Doucette RC, Sharp HT, Alder SC. Challenging generally accepted contraindications to vaginal hysterectomy. Am J Obstet Gynecol 2001; 184(7):1386–1391.

29. Fine PM, Thomakos N, Young RL. Digital flip placement of free ligatures in hysterectomy. J Gynecol Tech 1998; 4:51–53.

30. Gershenson DM, DeCherney AH, Curry SL, Brubaker L. Operative Gynecology. Philadelphia: W.B. Saunders, 2001:404.

31. Symmonds RE, Williams TJ, Lee RA, Webb MJ. Posthysterectomy enterocele and vaginal vault prolapse. Am J Obstet Gynecol 1981; 140:852.

32. Webb MJ, Aronson MP, Ferguson LK, Lee RA. Posthysterectomy vaginal vault prolapse: primary repair in 693 patients. Obstet Gynecol 1998; 92:10.

33. Orr JA, Shingleton JM. Complications in Gynecologic Surgery: Prevention, Recognition, and Management. Philadelphia: J.B. Lippincott, 1994:171–178.

34. Hurd WW, Chee SS, Gallagher KL, Ohl DA, Hurteau JA. Location of the ureters in relation to the uterine cervix by computed tomography. Am J Obstet Gynecol 2001; 184:336–339.

40

Advanced Anterior Vaginal Wall Prolapse (Stage III and IV)

Christina H. Kwon and Peter K. Sand
Evanston Continence Center, Evanston, Illinois, U.S.A.

I. INTRODUCTION

Anterior vaginal wall prolapse is a common finding, especially in parous women. While often secondary to a cystocele (loss of support of the posterior wall of the bladder), anterior vaginal wall prolapse may also be secondary to an enterocele (herniation of the peritoneum through the endopelvic connective tissue). Anterior vaginal wall prolapse is best defined as a relaxation of the anterior vaginal wall supports. Histologic studies have determined that the vagina is made up of three layers: the epithelium, muscularis, and adventitia (1). The frequently used term "endopelvic fascia" is a misnomer and should be abandoned, as there is no vaginal "fascia." Support for the vagina is supplied by the levator ani muscles and the lateral attachments of the endopelvic connective tissue layers to the arcus tendineus fasciae pelvis ("white line").

White proposed three theories in 1912, derived from his historic cadaveric dissections on the etiology of these support defects (2). The first was that support defects occurred from overstretching of the vaginal wall and thinning of the supporting tissue. The second theory attributed this to stretching of the attachment of the bladder to the uterus. Finally, he proposed that stretching of the ligamentous suspension of the bladder led to prolapse. In 1976, Richardson proposed the concept of site-specific defect repair, with lateral, transverse, and midline defects in the pubocervical connective tissue (3). Historically it has been difficult to surgically obtain optimal repair of the anterior compartment prolapse. In a review of his surgical outcomes after sacrospinous ligament suspension, Shull et al. declared that "the anterior segment provides the greatest challenge to restoration of normal anatomy" (4).

In 1995, the International Continence Society, the American Urogynecologic Society, and the Society of Gynecologic Surgeons formally adopted a standardized system of terminology for the description of female pelvic organ prolapse and pelvic floor dysfunction (5). This system uses the hymen as a fixed point of reference for a quantitative prolapse description. In stage III, the most distal portion of the prolapse is >1 cm beyond the plane of the hymen but protrudes no farther than 2 cm less than the total vaginal length. Stage IV is reserved for essentially complete eversion of the lower genital tract or complete procidentia. This chapter focuses on stage III and IV anterior vaginal wall prolapse.

II. PATHOPHYSIOLOGY OF SEVERE ANTERIOR VAGINAL WALL PROLAPSE

A. Anatomic Supports and Histology

As mentioned previously, the vagina histologically is composed of three layers: the epithelium (often referred to as the mucosa, despite the absence of mucous secretory glands); muscularis; and adventitia. The vaginal epithelium is composed of a nonkeratinizing squamous epithelium overlying a thin connective tissue layer, the lamina propria. The vaginal muscularis is primarily composed of smooth muscle with smaller amounts of collagen and elastin. The adventitia is a connective tissue layer of collagen and elastin that lies between the vaginal muscularis and the bladder. At the level of the urethra, this adventitial layer is less distinct, with fusion of the muscular layers of the vagina and urethra.

Laterally the anterior vagina is attached by fibrous connections to the parietal fascia overlying the levators, which forms the arcus tendineus fasciae pelvis. The arcus tendineus extends from the inferior aspect of the pubis at the level of the pubic tubercle to the ischial spine. These lateral fibrous attachments, in conjunction with the levator ani, protect the anterior vaginal wall from downward forces generated intra-abdominally. The top one-third of the vagina is also supported by the uterosacral-cardinal ligament complex by its suspension bilaterally to the fascia overlying the sacrum.

The top two-thirds of the vagina are supported by the levator ani, which is composed of three muscles: the puborectalis, the ischiococcygeus, and the iliococcygeus. These muscles work in conjunction with the coccygeus muscle to form the pelvic diaphragm. The levator ani muscles separate in the midline anteriorly to form the urogenital hiatus that allows passage of the urethra, vagina, and rectum. The levator ani maintain a constant basal tone that keeps this potential space almost completely closed. Posterior to the rectum, the levator ani muscles meet in the midline to form the levator plate. The levator plate is responsible for absorbing and responding to sudden increases in intra-abdominal pressure, often likened to a trampoline-type effect (6). The tonic contraction of the pelvic diaphragm is normally reflexively increased in response to increased intra-abdominal pressure in a fraction of a second (7).

The endopelvic connective tissue also plays a major role in the support of the vagina. This connective tissue contains fibrous elements such as collagen, and elastin, a viscoelastic matrix made up of proteoglycans. The inherent strength of a tissue is dependent on its collagen content. More than 19 different types of collagen have been identified, but two types of fibers predominate in determining tensile strength. Type I collagen, the most abundant type, is composed of two chains of $\alpha1(I)$ and one $\alpha2(I)$ chain. These are cross-striated fibrils that are found in a large variety of tissues. Type III collagen fibers are smaller and more randomly organized than type I. They are composed of three identical chains called $\alpha1(III)$. Type III collagen is found in large amounts in blood vessels and in small amounts in tissues containing type I collagen (8).

With increasing age, collagen turnover becomes slower (9). Following menopause this decrease in the turnover rate leads to tissue with a higher collagen content with changes in cross-linking (10). In women with genital prolapse, this change in collagen metabolism leads to a significant reduction in the type I : III collagen ratio (11). The result is tissue that has increased load-bearing potential, but with decreased elasticity (12).

After surgical repair, collagen is essential for wound healing. Although the exact mechanisms underlying wound healing are still being explored, fibroblasts synthesize and secrete collagen. The more flexible type III collagen is the primary type found during the early healing phase. As the scar matures, the stronger type I collagen gradually replaces the type III collagen. Tissue can approach but will never reach its original strength. Other factors in tissue healing certainly seem to have an effect but have not been fully elucidated. For example, cigarette smoking has been shown to impair collagen production in wound-healing processes (13).

B. Predisposing Factors

It is generally accepted that vaginal delivery is a predisposing factor toward the development of prolapse, although the exact etiology is unclear. During childbirth, downward expulsive efforts of the mother as well as compression from the presenting part of the fetus combine, exposing the pelvic floor to great amounts of potential compression injury. This can cause direct damage to the endopelvic connective tissue and the vaginal walls as well as indirect injury to the pelvic musculature by potential nerve compromise, either caused by direct compression or by a neuropathic stretch injury. EMG studies have shown that vaginal delivery causes partial denervation of the pelvic floor (14). Invesigators have found an association between weakening of the pelvic floor postpartum and the degree of lacerations and incisions of the perineum during vaginal delivery (15,16).

Although the exact mechanism is unclear, vaginal delivery clearly has a significant effect on the pelvic floor muscles. When the pelvic diaphragm does not maintain an adequate basal resting tone, the genital hiatus widens. The pelvic viscera become increasingly reliant on their ligamentous supports and their inherent tissue strength as the support from the levator plate lessens. Repetitive stress and tension from increases in intra-abdominal pressure can eventually cause separation or attenuation of these connective tissue supports. Denervation injury from vaginal childbirth can contribute to this loss of tone. Conditions such as muscular dystrophy, myelodysplasia, and trauma, which affect spinal cord pathways and pelvic nerve roots, are associated with pelvic organ prolapse resulting from flaccid paralysis of the pelvic floor musculature (17).

Connective tissue also plays a major role in the support of the pelvic viscera. Collagen deficiency or imbalance can contribute to pelvic organ prolapse. Women undergoing surgery for pelvic organ prolapse have significant changes in their endopelvic connective tissue with a decreased number of fibroblasts and an increase in the amount of abnormal collagen when compared to samples taken from women having hysterectomy without pelvic organ prolapse (18). Women with joint hypermobility have also been found to be at increased risk for the development of pelvic organ prolapse as a result of their underlying connective tissue disorder (19). As mentioned earlier, cigarette smokers have been found to have impaired collagen production in wound healing (13), which may also be compounded by repetitive and chronic coughing. This may explain the increased rate of stress urinary incontinence in current and former smokers (20).

III. CONSERVATIVE THERAPIES FOR ADVANCED PELVIC ORGAN PROLAPSE

Pessaries are the most common nonsurgical way to support pelvic organ prolapse. A pessary is an object that is placed into the vagina to support the anterior, posterior, and apical vaginal walls. There is evidence that pessaries have been used as early as the 5th century BC (21). A wide variety of items and materials have all been used as pessaries in the past, such as wood, rags, and even various fruits. Today pessaries are most commonly made of latex rubber, silicone, or acrylic. Pessaries come in multiple shapes and sizes. They are available by prescription after examination and fitting by a health care provider. Pessaries are very useful in those patients who cannot or choose not to undergo surgery. They can also play a vital role in delaying surgery to a more favorable time, such as in a young woman who has not yet completed her childbearing.

Fitting a pessary is an educated trial and error process. Various types of pessaries are available for use (Fig. 1). A digital vaginal examination allows one to have a general idea of the length and depth of the vagina. It is often easiest to begin with the largest pessary that can be accommodated in the vaginal introitus but does not protrude from the orifice. If a woman has signs of urogenital atrophy, using a local estrogen cream nightly for a 2-week period prior to attempting a pessary fitting may improve her comfort level during the fitting. The pessary should be moistened with water or a small amount of lubricant to decrease the friction on insertion. Once it has been inserted into the vagina, the pessary should not cause discomfort to the patient and should not be extruded on Valsalva. If this is successful, the patient should stand and walk around the exam room. She should cough, Valsalva, and bend down with the pessary in place. If the pessary is not expelled by these efforts and is not uncomfortable for the patient, then the fitting is successful. If the pessary falls out, it is either too small or of an improper shape to maintain support in the vagina. If the pessary causes discomfort or irritation, it is too large. If the pessary causes urinary obstruction or retention, it is also too large. A different size or an alternative shape can be tried.

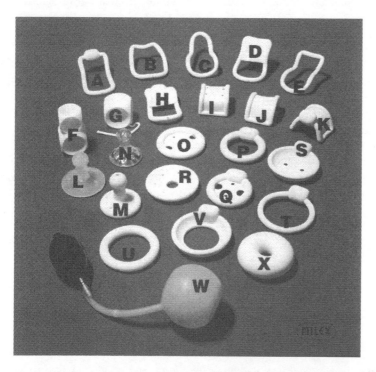

Figure 1   Various types of pessaries. **A,** Hodge with knob (silicone); **B,** Risser (silicone); **C** Smith (silicone); **D** Hodge with support (silicone); **E** Hodge (silicone); **F** Tandem cube (silicone); **G** Cube (silicone); **H** Hodge with support knob (silicone); **I** Regula (silicone); **J** Gehrung (silicone); **K** Gehrung with knob (silicone); **L** Gellhorn 95% rigid (silicone); **M** Gellhorn flexible (silicone); **N** Gellhorn rigid (acrylic); **O** Ring with support (silicone); **P** Ring with knob (silicone); **Q** Ring with support + knob (silicone); **R** Shaatz (silicone); **S** Incontinence dish with support (silicone); **T** Ring incontinence (silicone); **U** Ring (silicone); **V** Incontinence dish (silicone); **W** Inflatoball (latex); **X** Donut (silicone).

Ideally, the patient should be able to remove and insert the pessary on the daily basis. If she is unable to do this herself, she should come back to the office at 2- to 3-month intervals for removal and cleansing, although this interval should be tailored for the individual patient and the pessary type. The vagina should be systematically inspected for any abrasions or pressure ulcers. The pessary should be cleansed with regular soap and water. Regular use of a vaginal estrogen cream is advocated if there is no contraindication in the postmenopausal patient, especially if the pessary is not removed on a daily basis. If estrogen is contraindicated in the patient, Trimo-San (Milex Products, Inc., Chicago, IL) vaginal gel is helpful in maintaining proper vaginal pH to prevent bacterial vaginosis.

Pessaries can be associated with complications as well. Abrasions or ulcers of the vagina can cause vaginal bleeding. The pessary should be removed and the vagina carefully inspected. Application of silver nitrate can help stop vaginal bleeding in ulcerated areas. The pessary should not be replaced into the vagina until the ulcer has healed. Vaginal estrogen cream can be used to help heal and prevent future ulcerations. Vaginal discharge and odor may come from bacterial overgrowth. More frequent removal and cleansing usually resolves the problem. Recurrent ulceration and persistent discharge are common reasons why patients discontinue pessary use. Pessaries may also become less supportive as prolapse worsens, or the patient may develop urinary incontinence, recurrent infections, vaginal pain, or rectal pressure.

Incarceration of the pessary may also occur, usually because of neglect and failure to have removal performed for a prolonged period of time. Using topical estrogen cream regularly prior to attempted removal can often be helpful. In some cases, patients may need regional or general anesthesia to allow for adequate pelvic relaxation to permit removal. In rare cases, a fistula can result, usually in cases of extreme neglect with a rigid pessary.

Poor posterior introital support usually requires the use of a Gellhorn or cube pessary. Specially designed pessaries may also be useful for concurrent stress incontinence. Although it is truly a trial-and-error process, finding a correctly fitting pessary provides an alternative to surgical correction for some patients with vaginal prolapse, and can have great impact on their quality of life. With an increasingly aging population, pessaries will continue to be useful in managing pelvic organ prolapse.

IV. SURGICAL REPAIR TECHNIQUES

Two different surgical approaches to anterior vaginal support defects are available. The anterior colporrhaphy aims to excise or plicate weakened or redundant endopelvic connective tissue via a vaginal approach. Vaginal tissue can also be excised abdominally to repair a cystocele (22). An alternative procedure is the paravaginal repair. This procedure aims to reattach isolated lateral defects between the endopelvic connective tissue and smooth muscle of the anterior lateral vaginal wall to the arcus tendineus fasciae pelvis.

A. Anterior Colporrhaphy

The anterior colporrhaphy aims to plicate the vaginal muscularis and adventitia underlying the bladder to reduce redundancy and protrusion of the bladder and vaginal wall into the vagina and beyond (Fig. 2A–G). The patient is placed in the dorsal lithotomy position. The vagina and perineum should be sterilely prepped and draped. A Foley catheter should be inserted to drain the bladder as well as to assist in identification of the bladder neck. Hydrodissection using sterile saline with or without vasopressin can facilitate identification of the plane of dissection and decrease bleeding.

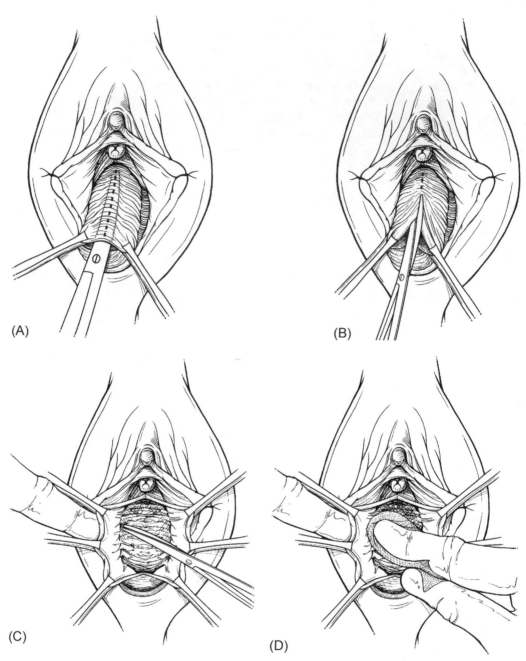

(A)

(B)

(C)

(D)

Figure 2 Technique of anterior colporrhaphy. (A) Dissection of the vaginal epithelium from the underlying endopelvic connective tissue. (B) Cutting epithelium in the midline to expose endopelvic connective tissue overlying bladder. (C) Sharp dissection of the endopelvic connective tissue off of the vaginal epithelium flaps. Care should be taken to preserve the endopelvic connective tissue overlying the bladder by dissecting this tissue deep enough off of the vaginal flaps to reach the relatively avascular plane just beneath the vaginal epithelium. Bracing the tissue behind the scissor tips helps prevent cutting through the vaginal epithelium. (D) Once a plane has been established, blunt dissection can also be performed using a gauze sponge. Again, bracing the tissue behind the traction point can help prevent tearing. (*continued*)

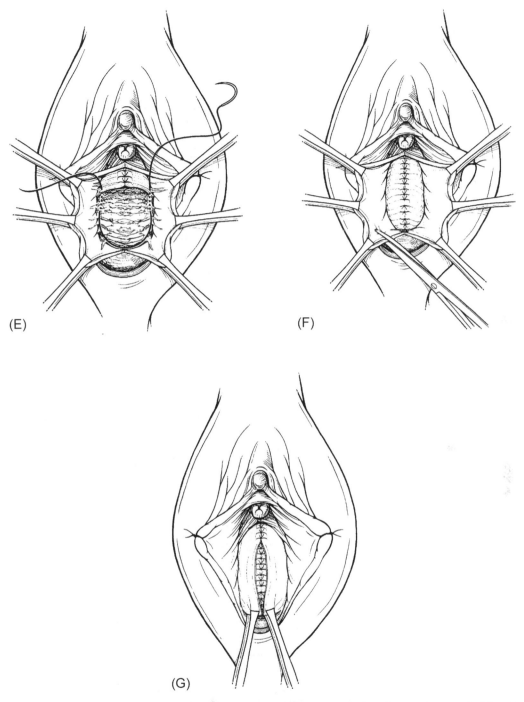

(E)

(F)

(G)

Figure 2 (*continued*) (E) Plication of redundant endopelvic connective tissue using no. 0 delayed-absorbable vertical mattress suture at the lateral borders of the mobilized endopelvic connective tissue. (F) Tying the sutures in the midline corrects the redundancy, repairing the cystocele. The excess vaginal epithelium is trimmed. (G) The trimmed vaginal epithelium edges are approximated in the midline using interrupted or a running locked suture of no. 2-0 delayed-absorbable suture to complete the anterior colporrhaphy.

If the anterior colporrhaphy is being performed concomitantly with a vaginal hysterectomy, the anterior cut edge of the vaginal apex should be grasped to the right and left of midline with Allis clamps, Kocher clamps or the hooks of a self-retaining vulvar retractor. If the patient has previously had a hysterectomy or is preserving her uterus, the most inferior edge of the anterior vagina or the anterior fornix should be grasped with Allis clamps lateral to the midline. A horizontal incision should be made between these clamps. Using Metzenbaum scissors, a vertical T-shaped incision should then be extended from the midline of the vagina up to the level of the urethrovesical junction. Allis clamps, Kocher clamps, or hooks should be placed along these cut vertical edges and held out laterally. The endopelvic connective tissue is then sharply and bluntly dissected off of these vaginal flaps out laterally, taking care to preserve as much endopelvic connective tissue on the bladder. The lateral extent of the dissection should be the medial borders of the descending pubic rami bilaterally.

Vertical mattress sutures of delayed absorbable or permanent sutures are placed along the lateral edges of the endopelvic connective tissue and tied to plicate the tissues in the midline. The importance of preserving as much endopelvic connective tissue upon the bladder becomes apparent during this step, as having adequate tissue prevents intravesical sutures and adds to the strength of the repair. These sutures also should not be placed on the vaginal tissue. Alternatively, specific defects in the endopelvic connective tissue may be identified during the initial dissection. These may be directly repaired in a site-specific fashion in the midline, laterally, or transversely with interrupted or running delayed absorbable sutures. When the anterior endopelvic connective tissue has been supported, the vaginal epithelium should be trimmed and closed using a running, locked, absorbable suture.

B. Paravaginal Defect Repair

Richardson et al. popularized the idea of the site-specific defect repair for the anterior compartment (3). Using careful physical examination, isolated defects in the connective tissue supports of the anterior quadrant of the pelvis can be identified. Lateral defects were most commonly detected, and are described as unilateral or bilateral defects in the fascia laterally or near its attachment to the levator insertion at the lower margin of the superior pubic ramus. The fibrous connections forming the lateral attachment of the vagina to the arcus tendineous fasciae pelvis (ATFP) may have torn, leading to a left, right, or bilateral paravaginal defect. Classically these are described as maintaining the ruggae in the anterior vaginal wall, as stretching or thinning of the tissue is not the etiology for the relaxation. In theory, if the lateral attachments are torn, plication of redundant tissue in the midline could actually exacerbate the problem by placing greater medial tension on the already compromised paravaginal separation from the arcus tendineus. For these deficiencies, a paravaginal repair is advocated. From the level of the urethrovesical junction to near the vaginal apex, the vaginal muscularis and adventitia are reapproximated to the ATFP. This repair can be performed via a retropubic abdominal or a vaginal approach (23). One must also be cautious not to neglect a concurrent central defect as this may be worsened by paravaginal lateral tensioning of the anterior vaginal wall. This is often missed at the time of surgery when paravaginal sutures may be placed medial to the anterior lateral vaginal sulcus, hiding this defect by stretching out the anterior vaginal wall without correcting the central defect in the endopelvic connective tissue.

C. Abdominal Paravaginal Repair

Abdominally, a Pfannensteil skin incision can be used to access the retropubic space. After the rectus fascia is incised sharply, the rectus muscles are separated laterally. The space of Retzius is then accessed medial to the pubic ramus on both sides. The loose areolar tissue should be cleared from the pubic bone using blunt dissection. The arcus tendineous fasciae pelvis extends from the posterior aspect of the pubis (at the level of the pubic tubercle) to the ischial spine. The bladder and the urethra may be gently retracted medially using a "daisy sponge," made of several folded 4 × 4 sponges placed in a ring forcep. Care should be taken not to reflect the bladder off the anterior vaginal surface, as this may disrupt its venous supply from the inferior vesical plexus and cause exuberant bleeding. The ATFP is easiest to identify at its insertion at the back of the pubic bone. Its course should be followed as it extends to the ischial spine.

Similar to performing an abdominal retropubic urethropexy, the operator's nondominant hand is placed into the vagina and used to elevate the periurethral and perivesical tissue. Using nonabsorbable sutures, a series of interrupted or "figure of eight" sutures are placed along the length of the ATFP to the detached vaginal muscularis and adventitia at the anterior lateral vaginal sulcus from the level of the urethrovesical junction to the ischial spine. Three to six sutures per side will likely be needed to reapproximate the length of the defect. Fewer sutures are needed if a Burch retropubic urethropexy is performed concomitantly. Bleeding that may be encountered from the venous plexuses of the vagina is usually controlled after tying the sutures.

D. Vaginal Paravaginal Repair

When using the vaginal approach to this repair, the goal continues to be reapproximation of the detached vaginal muscularis and adventitia laterally to the arcus tendineous. A vaginal approach requires more technical skill than the open retropubic approach. Patient selection is important in choosing this procedure, as a narrow pubic arch will limit exposure to the retropubic space, making an open retropubic approach a better choice in these patients.

The patient should be placed in dorsal lithotomy position and the bladder drained prior to starting the procedure. Marking sutures are placed through the vaginal epithelium at the level of the urethrovesical junction ~1 cm to the right and left of midline. If the patient has had a previous hysterectomy, marking sutures are placed at the vaginal apices. If a concomitant vaginal hysterectomy and culdoplasty are performed, the culdoplasty sutures should be left untied until all paravaginal sutures have been placed. Allis clamps should be placed at the lateral edges of the vaginal apex. If a concomitant central defect is to be repaired or a sling placed, a midline incision should be made in the vaginal epithelium up to the level of the urethrovesical junction. The endopelvic connective tissue should be dissected off of the vaginal epithelium sharply to the medial border of the descending pubic ramus laterally. Metzenbaum scissors are placed against the pubic ramus at the level of the urethrovesical junction, and the scissors are pushed toward the ipsilateral shoulder to enter the space of Retzius. The index finger can then be used to extend this space along the inferior pubic ramus toward the ischial spine. Alternatively, if only a paravaginal or bilateral paravaginal defect exists, the initial incision may be made in the anterior lateral vaginal sulci. This allows for the vaginal sutures to be placed in an undissected vaginal wall and limits blood loss. The arcus tendineous fascia pelvis can then be followed from the back of the pubic ramus to the ischial spine by retracting the bladder and urethra medially using a Briesky-Navratil retractor. Allis clamps or retractor hooks can be placed laterally to retract the vaginal epithelium. Using permanent suture, the first stitch should be placed just anterior to the ischial spine through the arcus tendineous (or through the obturator internus fascia if the arcus tendineous is too attenuated). The suture line is started here, as traction on this first stitch can facilitate placement of the subsequent sutures. A series of three to six sutures should be placed and tagged sequentially, starting from the ischial spine and moving anteriorly along the arcus tendineous to the level of the urethrovesical junction, leaving the needles intact on the sutures. It is helpful to have a marking system on the series of tagging clamps (such as small pieces of tape or placing sutures into a horse's comb) so the sutures do not become disordered.

Beginning with the most distal suture, the needle is placed through the endopelvic connective tissue at the level of the urethrovesical junction and then through the undersurface of the vaginal epithelium at the level of the previously placed distal marking suture. This sequence is continued posteriorly, with the most proximal suture anterior to the ischial spine being placed through the undersurface of the vaginal epithelium at the level of the apex marking sutures. Care should be taken when placing the sutures through the medial vaginal edge that an adequate margin is left on the cut medial edge to allow for subsequent vaginal closure. The sutures should be left untied. The process is repeated on the other side. The stitches are then tied sequentially in a distal to proximal direction, alternating from one side to the other. If a central defect exists, traditional anterior colporrhaphy sutures can then be placed to plicate the redundant endopelvic connective tissue. The vaginal epithelial flaps can be trimmed once all sutures have been placed and tied, and can be closed using a running suture of a delayed absorbable suture.

E. Adjunctive Materials to Enhance Long-Term Success of the Repair

The ideal biomaterial, natural or man-made, would be able to perform, augment, or replace a natural function (24). The ideal adjunctive material must be mechanically strong, cause no inflammatory reaction, be sterilizable, be resistant to modification by the body tissue, and be convenient to use. There currently exists no adjunctive material that meets all of these criteria. General surgeons first popularized the use of synthetic biomaterials by applying them to the repair of abdominal wall hernias. This approach has also been used in the repair of anterior vaginal wall prolapse, although there is a lack of data that prove their efficacy. In 1996, Julian published results on using Marlex polypropylene mesh in the repair of recurrent vaginal prolapse (25). A trapezoidal piece of synthetic mesh was sewn from the urethrovesical junction anteriorly to the vaginal apex posteriorly and to the levator fascia laterally. None of the patients who received the mesh had recurrence of anterior vaginal wall prolapse, although 25% of these patients had mesh-related complications postoperatively. This approach was not advocated as a primary procedure for the repair of anterior vaginal wall prolapse; rather, it was recommended only for those patients with two or more reparative failures.

Other observational studies have subsequently been published in the literature describing the usually successful experience of using a synthetic mesh, most often Marlex polypropylene, in reducing recurrence of anterior vaginal wall prolapse (26–29). These studies are most often limited by their small numbers of patients and lack of long-term follow-up.

Many physicians have begun using xenografts and allografts to enhance outcomes following anterior vaginal wall repairs. Theoretically these materials have the advantage of possibly being better tolerated by the vagina than synthetic material, although they too have been associated with minor erosions. These materials are quite expensive, however, and there is no published literature proving their benefits or efficacy.

One prospective randomized controlled trial was performed using polyglactin 910 mesh to prevent recurrent anterior vaginal wall prolapse by Sand et al. (30). This mesh is absorbable, and instead of being used as an overlay, it was used as a bulking material folded into the anterior colporrhaphy stitches. The approach is thought to enhance scarring just anterior to the suture line, providing greater protection to an area potentially more vulnerable to direct intra-abdominal downward forces. Patients with anterior vaginal wall prolapse to or beyond the hymenal ring were eligible for the study. At 1 year postoperatively, 30 of 70 (43%) women who did not receive mesh had recurrent anterior vaginal wall prolapse to the midvaginal plane versus 18 of 73 (25%) women who did receive polyglactin 910 mesh ($P = 0.02$). Prolapse to the hymenal ring occurred in 8 of 70 (11.4%) controls and in 2 of 73 (2.7%) women with mesh ($P = 0.04$). No patients had recurrent prolapse past the hymenal ring.

One randomized study of three different treatments of anterior vaginal wall prolapse has been performed. Weber et al. compared the effects of "standard anterior colporrhaphy" (muscularis plication in the midline without tension), versus "ultralateral anterior colporrhaphy" (dissection laterally to the limits of the pubic rami with plication of the muscularis in the midline under tension), versus "standard anterior colporrhaphy plus mesh" (polyglactin 910 mesh placed over the plication and anchored at the lateral limits of the dissection). Over 50% of the women enrolled in their study had stage III anterior vaginal wall prolapse or greater. At 1 year, 10 of 33 patients (30%) of the standard anterior colporrhaphy group had satisfactory or optimal anatomic outcome, versus 11 of 26 (42%) of the standard plus mesh group, versus 11 of 24 (46%) of the ultralateral anterior colporrhaphy group. No significant differences among the three different techniques were detected, although the sample sizes for each group were small, allowing for the possibility of type II error in the conclusions. The authors acknowledged that although the percentages for "successful" anatomic outcomes were relatively low, all three techniques provided excellent symptomatic relief from vaginal protrusion with no clinically significant differences among the groups (31).

F. Effect of Concomitant Operations on Anterior Compartment Prolapse

There also exists evidence that concomitant procedures at the time of anterior vaginal wall prolapse repair may affect long-term outcomes. Kohli et al. reported a significantly higher incidence of recurrent anterior prolapse if concomitant needle bladder neck suspension was performed with an anterior colporrhaphy (32). This effect was also seen in a randomized, prospective comparison of needle colposuspension versus endopelvic fascia plication in women undergoing vaginal reconstruction for stage III or IV pelvic organ prolapse (33). Especially when combined with a sacrospinous vaginal vault suspension, those patients randomized to receive concomitant needle suspension developed a relatively high incidence of early, advanced, recurrent, anterior vaginal prolapse. The needle suspension also increased the short-term complications without providing additional protection from the development of de novo genuine stress incontinence.

Sacrospinous vaginal vault suspension has also been associated with recurrent anterior segment prolapse theoretically because of the exposure of the anterior segment to increased pressure caused by the fixed retroversion of the vagina (34,35). Conversely, concomitant suburethral slings at the time of reconstructive vaginal surgery have been shown to significantly reduce the recurrence of anterior vaginal wall prolapse. The presence of any type of suburethral sling was associated with a 54.8% reduction in anterior prolapse recurrence (36). This finding should be taken into consideration when planning a surgical repair for the woman with concurrent prolapse and genuine stress incontinence. The same group also showed a significantly higher long-term risk of anterior vaginal wall prolapse associated with a traditional posterior approach to the sacrospinous vaginal vault suspension, whereas an anterior approach to the sacrospinous vaginal vault suspension (37) was associated with no such risk.

The available literature on repair of the anterior vaginal wall is surprisingly sparse, with the majority of these publications usually being descriptive outcome studies. Our ability to surgically correct this condition can be enhanced if we can predict those for whom progression or recurrence of their prolapse is most likely. As our understanding of the etiology of pelvic organ prolapse improves, we will improve our treatment of the condition and may ultimately be better able to prevent its occurrence.

REFERENCES

1. Weber AM, Walters MD. Anterior vaginal prolapse: review of anatomy and techniques of surgical repair. Obstet Gynecol 1997; 89:311–318.
2. White GR. An anatomic operation for the cure of cystocele. Am J Obstet Dis Women Child 1912; 65:286–290.
3. Richardson AC, Lyon JB, Williams NL. A new look at pelvic relaxation. Am J Obstet Gynecol 1976; 126:568–573.
4. Shull BL, Capen CV, Riggs MW, Kuehl TJ. Preoperative and postoperative analysis of site-specific pelvic support defects in 81 women treated with sacrospinous ligament suspension and pelvic reconstruction. Am J Obstet Gynecol 1992; 166(6 Pt 1):1764–1768.
5. Bump RC, Mattiasson A, Bo K, Brubraker LP, DeLancey JO, Klarskov P, Shull BL, Smith AR. The standardization of terminology of female pelvic organ prolapse and pelvic floor dysfunction. Am J Obstet Gynecol 1996; 175:10–17.
6. Gill EJ, Hurt WG. Pathophysiology of pelvic organ prolapse. Obstet Gynecol Clin North Am 1998; 25(4):757–769.
7. Rosenzweig BA, Bhatia NN. Temporal separation of cough-induced urethral and bladder pressure spikes in women with urinary incontinence. Urology 1992; 39(2):165–168.
8. Prockop DJ, Kuivaniemi H, Tromp G. Inherited disorders of connective tissue. In: Fauci A, Braunwald E, Isselbach K, Wilson J, Martin J, Kasper D, et al. Harrison's Principles of Internal Medicine. New York: McGraw-Hill, 1998.
9. Mays PK, McAnilty RJ, Campa JS, Laurent GJ. Age-related changes in collagen synthesis and degradation in rat tissue. Importance of degradation of newly synthesized collagen in regulation of collagen production. Biochem J 1991; 276:307–313.
10. Falconer C, Ekman-Ordeberg G, Ulmsten U. Changes in paraurethral connective tissue at menopause are counteracted by estrogen. Maturitas 1996; 24:197–204.
11. Norton P, Boyd C, Deak S. Collagen synthesis in women with genital prolapse or stress urinary incontinence. Neurourol Urodyn 1992; 11:300–301.
12. Vogel KG, Paulsson M, Heinegard D. Specific inhibition of type I and type II collagen fibrillogenesis by the small proteoglycan of tendon. Biochem J 1984; 223:587–597.
13. Jorgensen LN, Kallehave F, Christensen E, Siana JE, Gottrup F. Less collagen production in smokers. Surgery 1998; 123:450–455.
14. Allen RE, Hosker GL, Smith ARB, Warrell DW. Pelvic floor damage and childbirth: a neurophysiological study. Br J Obstet Gynaecol. 1990; 97(9):770–779.
15. Rockner G, Jonasson A, Olund A. The effect of mediolateral episiotomy at delivery on pelvic floor muscle strength evaluated with vaginal cones. Acta Obstet Gynecol Scand 1991; 70:51–54.
16. Klein MC, Gauthier RJ, Robbins JM, Kaczoroswki J, Jorgensen SH, Franco ED, Johnson B, Waghorn K, Gelfand MM, Guralnick MS. Relationship of episiotomy to perineal trauma and morbidity, sexual dysfunction, and pelvic floor relaxation. Am J Obstet Gynecol 1994; 171:591–598.
17. Loret de Mola JR, Carpenter SE. Management of genital prolapse in neonates and young women. Obstet Gynecol Surv 1996; 51:253–260.
18. Makinen J, Soderstrom KO, Kiilholma P, Hirvonen T. Histological changes in the vaginal connective tissue of patients with and without uterine prolapse. Arch Gynecol 1986; 239(1): 17–20.
19. Norton PA, Baker JE, Sharp HC, Warenski JC. Genitourinary prolapse and joint hypermobility in women. Obstet Gynecol 1995; 85(2):225–228.
20. Bump RC, McClish DK. Cigarette smoking and urinary incontinence in women. Am J Obstet Gynecol 1992; 167:1213–1218.
21. Miller DS. Contemporary use of the pessary. In: Sciarra JJ, ed. Gynecology and Obstetrics. Vol. 1. Philadelphia: J.B. Lippincott, 1995:1–12.
22. Macer GA. Transabdominal repair of cystocele, a 20 year experience, compared with the traditional vaginal approach. Am J Obstet Gynecol 1978; 131:203–207.

23. Shull BL, Benn SJ, Kuehl TJ. Surgical management of prolapse of the anterior vaginal segment: an analysis of support defects, operative morbidity, and anatomic outcome. Am J Obstet Gynecol 1994; 171:1429–1439.

24. Cervigni M, Natale F. The use of synthetics in the treatment of pelvic organ prolapse. Curr Opin Urol 2001; 11:429–435.

25. Julian TM. The efficacy of Marlex mesh in the repair of severe, recurrent vaginal prolapse of the anterior midvaginal wall. Am J Obstet Gynecol 1996; 175:1472–1475.

26. Nicita G. A new operation for genitourinary prolapse. J Urol 1998; 160:741–745.

27. Flood CG, Drutz HP, Waja L. Anterior colporrhaphy reinforced with Marlex mesh for the treatment of cystoceles. Int Urogynecol J 1998; 9:200–204.

28. Migliara R, De Angelis M, Madeddu G, Verdacchi T. Tension-free vaginal mesh repair for anterior vaginal wall prolapse. Eur Urol 2000; 38:151–155.

29. Canepa G, Ricciotti G, Introini C, Vigliercio G, Puppo P. Horseshoe-shaped Marlex mesh for the treatment of pelvic floor prolapse. Eur Urol 2000; 39(suppl 2):23–26.

30. Sand PK, Koduri S, Lobel RW, Winkler HA, Tomezsko J, Culligan PJ, Goldberg R. Prospective randomized trial of polyglactin 910 mesh to prevent recurrence of cystoceles and rectoceles. Obstet Gynecol 2001; 184:1357–1364.

31. Weber AM, Walters MD, Piedmont MR, Ballard LA. Anterior colporrhaphy: a randomized trial of three surgical techniques. Am J Obstet Gynecol 2001; 185:1299–1306.

32. Kohli N, Sze EHM, Roat TW, Karram MM. Incidence of recurrent cystocele after anterior colporrhaphy with and without concomitant transvaginal needle suspension. Am J Obstet Gynecol 1996; 175:1476–1482.

33. Bump RC, Hurt WG, Theofrastous JP, Addison WA, Fantl JA, Wyman JF, McClish DK. Randomized prospective comparison of needle colposuspension versus endopelvic fascia plication for potential stress incontinence prophylaxis in women undergoing vaginal reconstruction for stage II or IV pelvic organ prolapse. Am J Obstet Gynecol 1996; 175:326–333.

34. Bonney V. The principles that should underlie all operations for prolapse. J Obstet Gynaecol Br Commonw 1934; 41:669–683.

35. Holley RL, Varner RE, Gleason BP, Apffel LA, Scott S. Recurrent pelvic support defects after sacrospinous ligament fixation for vaginal vault prolapse. J Am Coll Surg 1995; 180:444–448.

36. Goldberg RP, Koduri S, Lobel RW, Culligan PJ, Tomezsko JE, Winkler HA, Sand PK. Protective effect of suburethral slings on postoperative cystocele recurrence after reconstructive pelvic operation. Am J Obstet Gynecol 2001; 185:1307–1313.

37. Winkler HA, Tomezsko JE, Sand PK. Anterior sacrospinous vaginal vault suspension for prolapse. Obstet Gynecol 2000; 95:612–615.

41

Anterior Vaginal Wall Prolapse: Mild/Moderate Cystoceles

Harriette M. Scarpero and Victor W. Nitti
New York University School of Medicine, New York, U.S.A.

I. INTRODUCTION

Pelvic organ prolapse is a common disorder affecting millions of women worldwide. The lifetime risk of undergoing surgery for prolapse by age 80 is 11.1% (1). Correction of anterior compartment relaxation, specifically cystocele and cystourethrocele, comprises a significant proportion of the procedures done for prolapse. Within a large cohort of HMO participants, 384 patients underwent one or more surgeries for correction of prolapse. Of these, 154 (40.1%) were performed on the anterior compartment. Another 60 (15.6%) procedures were done for correction of combined anterior and posterior compartment prolapse.

Anterior vaginal wall prolapse may involve the urethra, manifesting as urethral hypermobility and/or the bladder, cystocele. In many cases, small and moderate degrees of anterior vaginal wall prolapse are asymptomatic and do not require treatment. However, cystoceles may be associated with pelvic discomfort, sexual dysfunction, recurrent urinary tract infections, difficulty voiding, difficulty defecating, or incontinence. Stress urinary incontinence may occur as part of the clinical condition of prolapse associated with urethral hypermobility and lack of urethral support. It may also be associated with intrinsic sphincter deficiency. Patients with cystocele can also experience urinary incontinence secondary to detrusor instability which may, or may not, be related to the cystocele itself (2). Anterior vaginal wall prolapse is often associated with prolapse of other vaginal compartments: apical (uterine or enterocele) and posterior (rectocele or posterior enterocele).

The annual direct cost to society of pelvic organ prolapse procedures is significant. In 1997 the direct costs were $1012 million, with $74.2 million (7%) spent on the correction of cystoceles (3). An additional $279 million (28%) were spent on combined cystocele and rectocele repair. As the population ages and life expectancy increases, the number of cases performed for pelvic organ prolapse will certainly increase, translating into an even greater cost burden on society. A better understanding of the condition, its causes, and how to diagnose it accurately will improve the cost-effectiveness of our treatment and hopefully patient satisfaction.

575

II. ANATOMY

The anterior compartment of the female pelvis is composed of the bladder and urethra. Prolapse of this compartment may manifest as varying degrees of cystocele, urethral hypermobility, or intrinsic sphincteric deficiency (4). These defects may be seen alone or, more commonly, in combination with each other or with defects of the apical compartment (enterocele, uterine prolapse) or posterior compartment (rectocele, posterior enterocele). Any discussion of anterior compartment prolapse requires a basic understanding of its supporting anatomy.

The pelvic organs are suspended over the pelvic floor by the endopelvic fascia (EPF). This fascia is not like the tough ligamentous fascia of the rectus abdominous. Rather, it is a thinner condensation of smooth muscle fibers, blood vessels, connective tissue, and nerves; yet it is important to the stability of the pelvic organs and support of the vagina in particular (5). It is the first mechanism of defense against forces causing genital prolapse. Also of paramount importance to pelvic support are the levator ani muscles, which constrict the lumen of the vagina to prevent prolapse and produce a solid support on which the organs can rest. The levators are intimately connected to the EPF by virtue of their fascial covering, which merges into the adjacent EPF. A third source of support is a flap valve mechanism which results from the first two anatomic arrangements (6). In the flap valve mechanism, as abdominal pressure is placed on the suspended upper vagina, which has a horizontal axis in its natural state, the force pins the vagina against the levator muscles rather than everting it (6).

Delancey described three levels of vaginal support (Fig. 1) (6). The upper vagina, level 1, is supported by the parametrium, a term given to the EPF that attaches the vagina to the pelvic

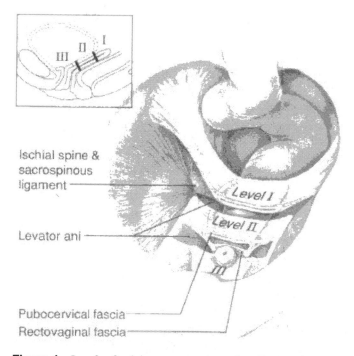

Figure 1   Levels of pelvic organ support as described by DeLancey. In level I the paracolpium *suspends* the vagina from the lateral pelvic walls. Fibers from level I extend vertically and posteriorly towards the sacrum. In level II the vagina is *attached* to the arcus tendineus fasciae pelvis and support fascia of the levator ani. [From Ref. (6).]

sidewall in that region. The cardinal and uterosacral ligaments are contained within the parametrium and support the uterus, cervix, and upper vagina. The cardinal ligaments, which primarily support the cervix, also provide support for the bladder base as it fuses with the EPF in that region, known as the pubocervical fascia. In cases of uterine prolapse, the cardinal ligament is lax, displacing the pubocervical fascia laterally and predisposing to cystocele formation. At midvagina, level 2, the EPF attaches to the vagina more laterally and stretches it transversely between the bladder and rectum. Level 2 EPF is termed the paracolpium. As the EPF approaches the bladder and urethra, it splits into two sheaths and envelops both the abdominal side and vaginal side of these structures. The abdominal side is still referred to as endopelvic fascia while the vaginal side is termed the periurethral or pubocervical fascia. Other names for condensations of EPF may be found in the literature. For example, the band or hammock of fascial support that extends from the arcus tendineus has been described as the pubovesical ligament (7) and the urethropelvic ligament in the urological literature (7,8). More proximally, where it supports the bladder, this condensation has been called the vesicopelvic ligament. Anteriorly, a condensation of (levator fascia/EPF) forms the pubourethral ligament, which is a pair of dense connective tissue bands. The pubourethral ligament arises from the vaginal wall and periurethral tissue and is attached to the undersurface of the symphysis pubis (6,9). The distal vagina, level III, is securely fixed by direct attachment to adjacent structures. It is not subject to the same risk of laxity as levels I and II.

The support of the anterior vaginal compartment (bladder and urethra) is dependent on the integrity of the EPF and its attachments to the pelvic sidewall at the arcus tendineus (Fig. 2). Breaks in the integrity of these structures produce defects that result in particular forms of cystocele: central and lateral (Fig. 3) (10). A central defect occurs by an attenuation or tear in the enveloping pubocervical fascia between bladder and vaginal wall. A lateral defect occurs when the EPF separates from its side wall attachment at the arcus tendineus (11). Lateral defects

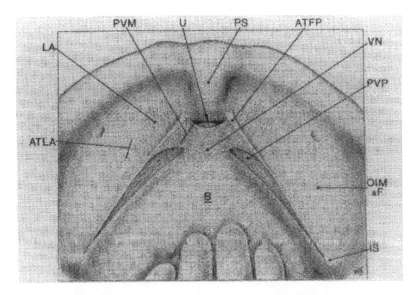

Figure 2 Retropubic view of bladder neck and urethral support drawn from cadaver dissections according to DeLancey. The pubovesical muscle (PVM) can be seen going from the vesical neck (VN) to the arcus tendineus fasciae pelvis (ATFP) and running over the paraurethral vascular plexus (PVP). ATLA, arcus tendineus levator ani; b, bladder; IS, ischial spine; LA, levator ani muscles; OIM&F, obturator internus muscle and fascia; PS, pubic symphysis; U, urethra. [From Ref. (7).]

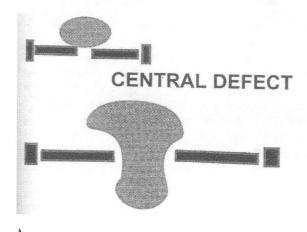

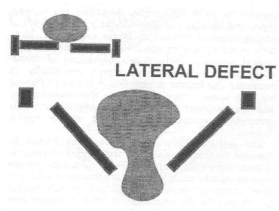

Figure 3 (A) Central defect cystocele. Note the break in the pubocervical fascia causing central herniation (Normal support shown in inset). (B) Lateral defect cystocele. Note the laxity or break in the attachment of the endopelvic fascia to the arcus tendineus fasciae. [From Ref. (10).]

are not thought to be caused by attenuation of the EPF at this area, only true separation (12). Separation may occur on one or both sides. Isolated lateral defects are fairly common while isolated central defects comprise <10% of cystoceles (13). Combinations of central and lateral fascial defects are very common especially in larger symptomatic cystoceles.

III. GRADING SYSTEMS

This chapter addresses mild to moderate cystoceles specifically. The designation of mild or moderate is subjective and must be translated into an accepted grading scale. Several grading systems have been used for cystocele and prolapse in general. One common system is the half-way system described by Baden and Walker, which uses the hymen as a reference point (Table 1) (14). Although this system is widely used, it has been criticized for lacking reproducibility and specificity (15).

An attempt to standardize the terminology of female pelvic organ prolapse was adopted by the International Continence Society (ICS) and other groups in 1995 (16). They recommended

Table 1 Baden and Walker Grading System

Grade	Definition
0	Normal position for bladder
I	Descent halfway to the hymen
II	Descent to the hymen
III	Descent halfway past the hymen
IV	Maximum possible descent for bladder

that terms such as cystocele, rectocele, enterocele, or urethrovesical junction be avoided because these terms imply an unrealistic certainty as to what structures inhabit the vaginal bulge. This concern is particularly appropriate in women who have undergone prior prolapse surgery. In the ICS grading system, Pelvic Organ Prolapse Quantification (POP-Q), the hymenal ring is the fixed anatomic landmark of reference. Six sites of the vagina and perineal body are measured in centimeters from the hymen. Two points of reference are given to the anterior aspect, posterior, and apical vagina. Measurement of the genital hiatus, perineal body, and total vaginal length are also included (Fig. 4). The intraobserver and interobserver reliability of this system has been shown to be very good, and it allows for a very accurate measurement of distances (17). The disadvantage of this system is that it is cumbersome and better suited for evaluating radiographic images of the pelvic floor than performing in vivo measurements. In clinical practice this system seems particularly useful when describing surgical outcomes. For example, it is much more informative to describe the leading edge of a prolapse as 2 cm inside the hymenal ring as compared to a preoperative finding of 0.5 cm outside the hymenal ring, instead of describing the same situation as a prolapse reduction from grade 3 to grade 1.

IV. PREOPERATIVE EVALUATION

It is difficult to determine whether a patient's symptoms are directly caused by the cystocele alone. Shull has advocated pelvic organ support must be related to pelvic organ function, and thus every specific defect should be repaired to give the best opportunity for resolution of symptoms and reduction of the risk of new defects (18). If this is true, and this can only be determined by defining a clear set of outcome parameters that would include certain visceral functions, then it would be argued that any degree of prolapse, even small or asymptomatic, is clinically significant and should be corrected. Additionally, in patients with a cystocele, symptoms of stress urinary incontinence cannot be attributed solely to it. Urethral dysfunction from intrinsic sphincteric incontinence may coexist (2,4).

A careful physical examination is necessary in evaluating patients with pelvic prolapse. We prefer to examine the patient with a full bladder in the dorsal lithotomy position. The vaginal mucosa is first inspected for any signs of mucosal atrophy. Spreading the labia for better visualization of the urethral meatus, the patient is asked to cough and Valsalva to test for stress incontinence, urethral mobility, and anterior vaginal wall prolapse. The lower blade of a Graves speculum is used to retract the posterior vaginal wall and gain better visualization of the anterior vaginal wall. The patient is asked to Valsalva and any descensus of the anterior vaginal wall is graded. Although not pathognomonic, central defects classically produce a bulge in the anterior vaginal wall that causes disappearance of the normal vaginal rugae. In postmenopausal women with significant atrophy of the vaginal tissues, the rugae may be absent from lack of

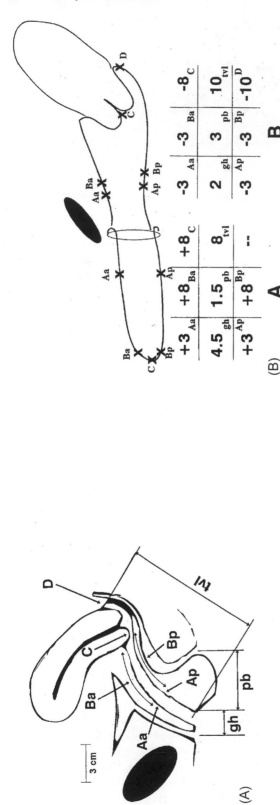

(A)

(B)

-3 Aa	-3 Ba	-8 C
2 gh	3 pb	10 tvl
-3 Ap	-3 Bp	-10 D

B

+3 Aa	+8 Ba	+8 C
4.5 gh	1.5 pb	8 tvl
+3 Ap	+8 Bp	--

A

Figure 4 (A) Six sites (points Aa, Ba, C, D, Bp, and Ap), genital hiatus (gh), perineal body (pb), and total vaginal length (tvl) used for pelvic organ support quantification. Point Aa = point located in the midline of the anterior vaginal wall 3 cm proximal to the external urethral meatus. Point Ba = point that represents the most distal (dependent) position on any part of the upper anterior vaginal wall. Point C = point that represents either the most distal (dependent) edge of the cervix or leading edge of the vaginal cuff after hysterectomy. Point D = point that represents the location of the posterior fornix in a woman with a cervix. It is omitted if patient has had a hysterectomy. Point Bp = point that represents the most distal (dependent) postion of any part of the upper posterior vaginal wall from the vaginal cuff or posterior vaginal fornix to point Ap. (−3 cm by definition if no prolapse). Point Ap = point located in the midline of the posterior vaginal wall 3 cm proximal to the hymen. (range of position of point Ap relative to hymen is −3 to +3 cm by definition). Genital hiatus = measurement of distance in cm from middle of the external urethral meatus to the posterior midline hymen. Perineal body = measurement of distance in cm from the posterior margin of the genital hiatus to the midanal opening. Total vaginal length = greatest depth of the vagina in cm when point C or D is reduced to its full normal position (eccentric elongation of prolapsed vaginal wall should not be included in the measurement of total vaginal length). (B) (a) Grid and line diagram of complete eversion of vagina. The most distal point of anterior wall (point Ba), vaginal cuff scar (point C), and most distal point of the posterior wall (point Bp) are all at the same position (+8) and points Aa and Ap are maximally distal (both at +3). Because total vaginal length equals maximum protrusion, this is stage IV prolapse. (b) Normal support. Points Aa and Ba and points Ap and Bp are all −3 because there is no anterior or posterior wall descent. Lowest point of the cervix is 8 cm above the hymen (−8) and posterior fornix is 2 cm above this (−10). Vaginal length is 10 cm and genital hiatus and perineal body measure 2 and 3 cm, respectively. This represents stage 0 support. [From Ref. (15).]

estrogen instead. Lateral defects have been detected on exam by palpating the break in the EPF on bimanual exam and by identifying movement of the lateral sulcus. It has also been described that using a ring forceps to elevate the lateral sulcus, the lateral defect cystocele is corrected (19). The sensitivity and negative predictive value of this method of clinical assessment of paravaginal defects are good. Specificity and positive predictive value of this diagnostic pearl are poor (20).

If the patient has not undergone a hysterectomy, the uterus should be evaluated for prolapse and movement. In posthysterectomy patients, support of the vaginal vault must be assessed. An enterocele may appear as a high continuation of the rectocele bulge in the posterior vaginal wall. They can be differentiated by palpation of the rectovaginal septum. The examiner's index finger is placed in the rectum and his/her thumb in the vagina. The patient is then instructed to cough or bear down. An increased thickness in the rectovaginal septum may indicate a loop of small bowel insinuating itself between the vagina and rectum (enterocele).

If stress urinary incontinence with cough or Valsalva is not seen initially, the prolapse is reduced with either the speculum blade, a pessary, or packing. The patient is asked to cough and Valsalva again. Occult stress incontinence is diagnosed if leakage is seen with the prolapse reduced. It may be necessary to evaluate the patient in the standing position to demonstrate leakage. We routinely examine women in the standing position in addition to in lithotomy because it provides a more realistic impression of the degree of prolapse experienced during daily activity. The patient is asked to elevate one foot on a step, which separates the legs and provides better visualization of the perineum and vagina. The vagina is examined for any prolapsing mass at rest and with Valsalva. If there is any question of the degree of uterine descensus or from which compartment the prolapse originates, the same maneuver is performed with two of the examiner's fingers within the vagina.

It is important to assess bladder emptying preoperatively, which can be done at the time of physical examination with bladder ultrasound or catheterization. We routinely perform preoperative urodynamics on patients to assess for any bladder dysfunction or voiding abnormality that may not have been suggested in the patient's history. It also provides a baseline for comparison should the patient develop any new lower urinary tract symptoms postoperatively. Women with occult stress incontinence can be identified with careful preoperative examination and urodynamic evaluation with reduction of the prolapse. We routinely perform simultaneous anti-incontinence surgery in all patients with clinical or occult stress incontinence. We have found no significant added morbidity from the addition of a pubovaginal sling to transvaginal prolapse repair.

In the case of mild to moderate cystoceles (grades 1, 2, and 3), the addition of radiographic studies to the preoperative evaluation is likely of less yield than in cases of severe prolapse. In significant prolapse, even that of the anterior vaginal wall, it may be harder to tell what structures are actually included in the bulging mass. A voiding cystourethrogram (VCUG) in the anteroposterior view can define a cystocele well and demonstrate how far the bladder base descends below the inferior margin of the pubic symphysis during straining (21). Lateral views are required to assess the urethra and bladder neck descent fully (22). Fluoroscopy during videourodynamic studies may also be used to obtain a VCUG. The benefits of preoperative urodynamics in the detection of occult stress urinary incontinence or other voiding dysfunction has been espoused elsewhere in this chapter. When one has the capabilities of fluoroscopy during the urodynamic study, there is the added benefit of being able to elucidate the anterior vaginal wall anatomy. It also provides objective evidence of stress incontinence, an estimation of residual volume, and an assessment of any urethral pathology such as diverticulum.

Magnetic resonance imaging (MRI) of the pelvis is another method of detecting the components of prolapse. It offers the advantage of being noninvasive, rapid, and free of ionizing radiation, and it provides superior soft-tissue differentiation. Structures can also be evaluated in multiple planes without any distortion of image quality as in reconstructing computed tomography images. Arguably, however, it is expensive, and its utility may be greater in cases of enterocele and vault prolapse than in anterior vaginal wall prolapse. In complicated cases of severe prolapse, MRI is ideal for objective radiographic evaluation. It lends itself well to simple objective grading for quantifying pelvic floor prolapse (23).

Preoperative cystoscopy is helpful to evaluate the bladder for trabeculation, foreign body, or other pathology. In the absence of an abnormal urinalysis however, the yield of cystoscopy may be low. We typically perform a quick cystoscopic inspection of the bladder at the start of surgery.

V. NONSURGICAL MANAGEMENT

Cystoceles may be treated nonsurgically with pelvic floor exercises or pessaries and surgically with a variety of procedures depending on the specific defect involved. When comparing nonsurgical to surgical treatment or comparing methods of surgical repair, it is important to realize that the outcome parameters used in evaluation of these options differ considerably. There are no established guidelines for what outcome parameters to use in evaluating results, nor are the definitions of terms such as cured, improved, or failed standardized (Table 2).

Table 2 Reported Surgical Outcomes of Anterior Vaginal Wall Prolapse Repair

Type of procedure	Lead author	No. of patients	Mean F/U	Results at F/U (%) (refers only to cure of cystocele)	Type of graft used
Anterior colporrhaphy	Walter (48)	86	14 m	Cured (100)	N
	Porges (49)	299	31 m	Cured (97)	N
	Colombo (32)	33	60 m	≤Gr I (97)	N
	Gardy (2)	45[a]	24 m	Cured (95)	N
	Kohli (50)[b]	27	13 m	Cured (93)	N
		40	13 m	Cured (67)	N
Vaginal Paravaginal	Chesson (30)	32	9 m	Cured (97)	AFL/CFL
	Shull (51)	62	1.6 y	Cured (73)	N
	Benson (52)	48	2.5 y	Cured (29)	N
Four-corner bladder neck suspension	Raz (38)	120	24 m	Cured (98)	N
	Dmochowski (53)	47	37 m	Cured (43)	N
Other vaginal procedures	Raz (40)	51	34 m	Cured (88)	N
	Julian (54)	24	2 y	Cured (66) vs. (100)	N vs. S
	Migliari (41)	15	23 m	Cured (93)	S
	Kobashi (42)	50	6 m	Cured (100)	CFL
	Nicita (43)	44	13.9 m[c]	Cured (100)	S
Retropubic paravaginal	Bruce (33)	52	17 m	Cured/improved (85)	N
	Shull (31)	149	6–48 m	Cured (95)	N
	Richardson (12)	213	2–8 y	Cured (92)	N
	Benson (52)	40	2.5 y	Cured (58)	N

[a]17 patients subtracted from total number of patients because they had urethral suspension alone for mild cystocele.
[b]Divided into those that underwent anterior colporrhaphy alone (27) and those that underwent anterior colporrhaphy and transvaginal needle bladder neck suspension (40).
[c]Median rather than mean. m, months; y, years; N, none; S, synthetic; AFL, autologous fascia lata; CFL, cadaveric fascia lata.

Not all studies include quality-of-life (QOL) evaluations, and when used there is no uniformity in which QOL instrument is employed. These differences make comparison of various studies difficult.

This section will highlight the treatment options and techniques that are recognized and reported in the literature. The descriptions of various surgical techniques are not meant to be as detailed as could be obtained from a surgical atlas or from the original article. When learning the technique, the original source should be consulted for a detailed description.

"Watchful waiting" is an option with any form of prolapse except the most severe that is causing such serious complications as erosion of vaginal skin, threatened evisceration, or hydronephrosis. However, if the mild to moderate cystocele is not repaired surgically, there is certainly a chance of progression and the risk of developing other associated pelvic floor defects. Patients should be apprised of these risks when considering watchful waiting. In asymptomatic cases, patients may reasonably choose not to intervene, yet they may also inquire as to whether there is anything they can do to help lower the risk of progression of their prolapse.

Pelvic floor exercises have been studied as a treatment for rehabilitation of the pelvic floor musculature. As originally described by Kegel in 1948, the exercises could help strengthen the pelvic support after childbirth (24). Most recent studies have focused exclusively on its efficacy in the treatment of urinary incontinence, not prolapse, and there are no good data in the literature to suggest that the exercises slow or arrest the progression of pelvic organ prolapse.

Pessaries used most commonly for more severe pelvic organ prolapse can also be used for the symptomatic moderate cystocele. In most cases pessaries are reserved for patients who either do not want surgery or who are not surgical candidates; however, no strict indication for pessary exists. In a survey of the American Urogynecologic Society, 77% used pessaries as first-line therapy for prolapse, whereas 12% reserved pessaries for women who were not surgical candidates (25). A pessary was used more commonly for anterior defect (89%) than any other specific defect (posterior, apical, or complete procidentia).

No strict contraindications to pessary use exist, either. Some conditions that place a woman at higher risk for complication with pessary include vaginal mucosal atrophy that results from low estrogen status and radiation, as well as the inability to independently change and clean the pessary (26). Reported complications include vaginal wall ulceration, fistula formation, and bowel herniation (27,28). In order to avoid complication it is necessary to choose a pessary that fits well without excessive pressure on the vaginal mucosa. In women with vaginal mucosal atrophy, the use of estrogen either topically or systemically should be encouraged. Patients should also be taught to remove and clean the pessary frequently. No consensus exists as to how frequently to change the pessary, usually every 1–2 months. Some physicians have the patient return to the office for frequent pessary changes. Each time the pessary is changed, the vagina should be inspected closely with a full speculum to determine if any vaginal erosion is occurring. The pessary should be discontinued at any sign of such erosion.

Not all women are able to use a pessary successfully. Some patient characteristics and habits make pessary use more difficult. A patient with a large introitus may not be able to retain a pessary. In the patient with occult stress urinary incontinence, the use of a pessary will render them incontinent and thus may worsen their quality of life. Sexual activity does not preclude pessary use, but the patient must be able to remove it herself.

VI. SURGICAL MANAGEMENT

All cystocele repairs revise the pubocervical fascia in some manner. They may be performed vaginally (e.g., anterior colporrhaphy) or retropubically (e.g., paravaginal repair). Combined central and lateral defects may require a combination of methods. The advent of minimally invasive surgery had led to the application of laparoscopy in retropubic repair.

Whether to repair an asymptomatic mild or moderate cystocele is controversial. Some advocate surgical repair only if performing other vaginal surgery such as hysterectomy or an anti-incontinence procedure. If undergoing surgery for incontinence such as a pubovaginal sling or urethropexy, it is reasonable to repair an asymptomatic small to moderate cystocele since fixation of the urethra and bladder neck may promote progression of the remainder of the anterior vaginal wall. Others suggest repair any detected prolapse. Most patients with a grade 3 or higher cystocele will require treatment.

VII. REPAIR OF CENTRAL DEFECTS

Anterior colporrhaphy consists of plication of the pubocervical fascia and is the most common method of central defect repair. This approach alone is not recommended in combined central and lateral defects because it does not correct the lateral component. When performing an anterior colporrhaphy, the patient is placed in the dorsal lithotomy position. Exposure of the anterior vaginal wall is facilitated by using an Allis clamp to grasp the prolapsing wall and stretch it cephalad. A weighted vaginal speculum in the vagina helps to reduce the posterior wall. A midline incision is made in the vaginal wall from the area of the cardinal ligament attachment to just distal to the bladder neck. The vaginal wall is then dissected off the bladder and underlying attenuated pubocervical fascia so the entire cystocele can be exposed. When full exposure is accomplished, the bladder is reduced with a finger or small packing of polyglycolic acid (PGA) mesh, so that the pubocervical fascia can be visualized clearly and reapproximated in the midline. The PGA mesh packing does not add strength to the repair, but we have found it useful to keep the bladder reduced.

After successful plication, it is not necessary to remove the mesh. Plication sutures used are 2-0 PGA and extend from the bladder neck to the cardinal ligaments (Fig. 5). The addition

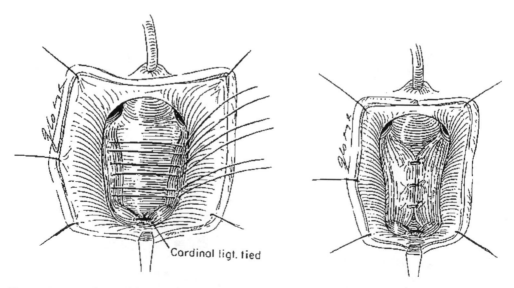

Cardinal ligt. tied

Figure 5   Anterior colporrhaphy. The vaginal wall is dissected off of the bladder and pubocervical fascia via a midline incision. The pubocervical fascia is reapproximated with 2-0 absorbable suture from the bladder neck to the cardinal ligaments, avoiding vaginal wall. [From Ref. (40).]

of a Kelly plication stitch to narrow the urethrovesical junction in cases of stress incontinence has been advocated by some authors. The Kelly plication was originally described as an anti-incontinence procedure. The pubocervical fascia at the bladder neck is plicated in order to reduce the diameter of the urethra at the site of funneling (29). We prefer to perform a formal anti-incontinence procedure, e.g., pubovaginal sling, when overt or occult stress incontinence is present. In cases in which the pubocervical fascia is too attenuated for adequate repair, a piece of synthetic mesh or allographic material may be employed to strengthen the repair and prevent suture pull-through (30). The graft is interposed between the pubocervical fascia and vaginal wall on one side, securing it to the inner side of one vaginal wall and pubocervical fascia laterally on each side. It is trimmed and stretched beneath the bladder to be interposed between the structures on the opposite side. After completion of the colporrhaphy, the vaginal wall is trimmed and closed with interrupted absorbable sutures.

Keeping in mind the discrepancies of technique, time to follow-up, definitions of cure and failure, and the incidence of concomitant procedures, the anterior colporraphy has a published failure rate of 0–20% (5).

VIII. REPAIR OF LATERAL DEFECTS

Lateral defects may be repaired retropubically or vaginally. The most anatomical repair is a paravaginal defect repair. The goal of paravaginal repair is to reattach the pubocervical fascia to the arcus tendineus, thus restoring support to the bladder, urethra, and anterior vaginal wall. The paravaginal repair was originally described as a retropubic route, which is ideal for isolated lateral defects. A vaginal paravaginal repair can easily be combined with a central defect repair for combined central and lateral defects.

Abdominal retropubic paravaginal repair can be accomplished via a low midline or transverse incision. The retropubic space is developed so that the bladder neck, symphysis pubis, endopelvic fascia, arcus tendineus, and obturator fascia can be clearly identified. Avulsion of the pubocervical fascia can be seen easily by placing two fingers of the nondominant hand in the vagina to elevate the vaginal wall and paravaginal fascia. This maneuver also facilitates correct placement of the sutures. The defect is repaired with multiple permanent sutures such as 0-Ethibond placed ∼1 cm apart along the superior lateral angle of the vagina to the arcus tendineus that runs from the lower edge of the symphysis to the ischial spine (12,31). The sutures should be placed through the paravaginal fascia, vaginal wall (excluding the epithelium), and the arcus tendineus (Fig. 6). In cases where the arcus cannot be clearly identified, sutures may be placed in the obturator fascia. The sutures are not tied until all have been placed. Some authors have recommended that a set of sutures be placed through Cooper's ligament, thus performing a combined Burch and paravaginal repair. We also perform this routinely and feel it should always be done in cases with concomitant type II stress incontinence.

Richardson, who is responsible for the popularization of the paravaginal defect repair, stated that the procedure was not intended as an operation for incontinence. As an incontinence procedure, the paravaginal defect repair falls short of Burch colposuspension. In a randomized comparison of the two procedures for the correction of stress urinary incontinence, Burch out performed paravaginal defect repair with a cure rate of 100% versus 72% (32). Bruce et al. found a 72% cure of incontinence at 17 months in patients who underwent paravaginal defect repair for type 2 stress urinary incontinence (33). The paravaginal repair distributes the weight-bearing suture line along a much greater length of vaginal wall. When Burch reported his urethrovaginal fixation to Cooper's ligament for stress incontinence, he described placing an additional three sutures from paravaginal fascia to the white line. He found that these additional sutures not only restored the normal anatomy of the bladder neck but also

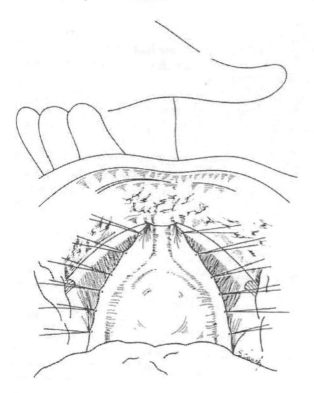

Figure 6   A finger is placed in vagina to help demonstrate the paravaginal defect. None of the sutures are tied until all have been placed. [From Ref. (31).]

resulted in "surprising correction of most of the cystocele" (34). In a group of 147 patients, Shull et al. reported a 95% cure rate of cystoceles after paravaginal defect repair (31). Five percent developed an enterocele postoperatively. Richardson reported his long-term results with the procedure in 1980. Of 233 repairs with a minimum of 2 years follow-up, 223 were cured of anterior wall prolapse, for a failure rate of 4.7% (12). A total of 188 were cured of incontinence. Others have reported a 3–14% failure rate with paravaginal defect repair (5).

Paravaginal repair performed through a vaginal approach is more technically challenging, but allows one to also perform a central defect repair in cases of combined defects. The goal of restoring vaginal and urethral support to the arcus remains the same. A midline incision is made in the vaginal wall then separated from the attenuated pubocervical fascia and bladder, all the way to the pubic bone bilaterally. It is important that the most distal portion of the cystocele be mobilized so that the entire bladder can be reduced to its normal anatomic position. The retropubic space is entered by sharply perforating the endopelvic fascia with Metzenbaum scissors at the level of the pubic bone. The lateral attachment of the endopelvic fascia is then completely taken down using blunt dissection. The bladder is retracted medially and the paravaginal space is identified. The arcus tendineus should be palpated and seen running between the ischial spine and the symphysis pubis. Care should be exercised to remain posterior and inferior the obturator nerve and vessels to prevent damage to them. Also of anatomic relevance are the internal pudendal vessels that run posterior and medial to the ischial spine. Knowledge of these anatomic relationships can help avoid complications from an errant suture. Permanent sutures are then placed through the arcus tendineus (or obturator fascia) and the pubocervical fascia, plus full thickness of vaginal wall, excluding the epithelium (Figs. 7, 8). Sutures should be placed

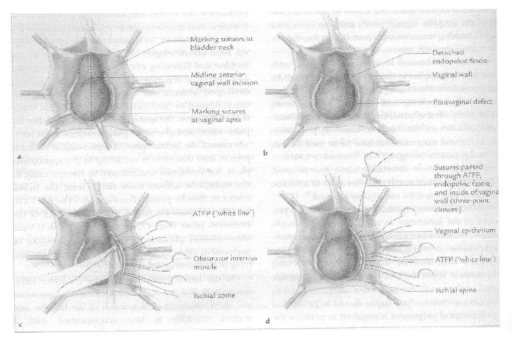

Figure 7 Technique of vaginal paravaginal defect repair. (a) The vagina is opened through a midline incision. (b) The opened vagina reveals bilateral paravaginal defects. (c) The bladder is retracted medially to expose the arcus tendineus. Permanent sutures are placed into the arcus tendineus or obturator fascia (see Fig. 8 below). Four to five sutures are placed from ischial spine to the pubic bone. (d) Each suture is then passed through the detached edge of the endopelvic fascia and in inside of the vaginal epithelium forming a three point closure. [From Ref. (36).]

laterally in the vaginal wall, although not so lateral as to preclude midline reapproximation (35). No sutures should be tied until all are placed on both sides. This procedure can be combined with a sacrospinous ligament fixation or other vault suspension, pubovaginal sling, anterior colporrhaphy, or pubovaginal sling. It may also be combined with graft interposition to correct both central and lateral defect (36).

Needle suspensions are another method of restoring lateral support based on the principles of the Raz bladder neck suspension (37). The four-corner bladder neck suspension was described for the treatment of moderate (grades 2 and 3) cystocele due to lateral defect only (38). In this procedure, an extra set of polypropylene suspension sutures is placed in the vaginal wall and pubocervical fascia, proximal to the bladder neck suspension sutures. Early results of this procedure were encouraging but unfortunately, this procedure, like needle suspensions for stress incontinence, did have a significant number of late failures. However, the principles developed were applied to other more durable procedures.

IX. LAPAROSCOPIC REPAIR OF THE ANTERIOR VAGINAL WALL

A variety of procedures for pelvic reconstruction can be performed laparoscopically but require proficiency in laparoscopic techniques and have a steep learning curve. The advantages of laparoscopy cited include better visualization deep in the pelvis due to the magnified view, smaller incisions, and possible reduced morbidity and reduced blood loss. These improvements generally lead to the

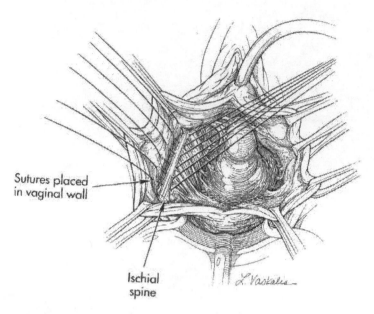

Sutures placed
in vaginal wall

Ischial
spine

Figure 8   Vaginal paravaginal repair; placement of sutures in the arcus tendineus. Sutures placed through the arcus tendineus fascia pelvis and the anterior vaginal wall, excluding the squamous epithelium. [From Ref. (35).]

expectation of faster patient recovery, shorter hospital stay, a decreased analgesia requirement, and quicker return to normal activities for the patient. Currently the majority of these procedures use laparoscopy as a mode of access and do not modify the conventional surgical approach (39).

Laparoscopic paravaginal repair is performed under general anesthesia in the dorsal lithotomy position. The vagina and perineum are prepped into the field, and a Foley catheter is placed. The first trocar (10 mm) is inserted through the umbilicus. Two other trocars (5 mm and 10 mm) are placed in the lower abdomen on left and right, respectively. Before dissection into the retropubic space is begun, the bladder is filled with 300 cc of normal saline to identify the bladder dome and thus facilitate the dissection. The parietal peritoneum is incised transversely ∼2 cm above the bladder dome. Dissection is then carried out bluntly toward the top of the pubic bone. Once in the retropubic space, the bladder is retracted medially to expose the arcus tendineus. If present, paravaginal defects can be seen clearly with this maneuver. If any Burch sutures are to be placed concomitantly, the paravaginal defect should be closed first. Just as in the open approach, the urethrovesical junction and vaginal wall adjacent to it are identified. Correct placement of the sutures can be aided by putting two fingers of the surgeon's nondominant hand into the vagina to elevate the lateral vagina and help sweep the urethra medially, away from the repair. A permanent suture on a CT 1 needle is used for intracorporeal suturing. Prospective randomized trials comparing the laparoscopic method to the classic open methods remain to be done before recommending it in place of traditional methods.

X. COMBINED CENTRAL AND LATERAL DEFECT REPAIRS

Based on the four-corner repair described above, Raz et al. later described a procedure utilizing the principals of needle suspension to fix larger cystoceles with combined central and lateral defects (Fig. 9) (40). A vertical incision is made in the anterior vaginal wall extending from

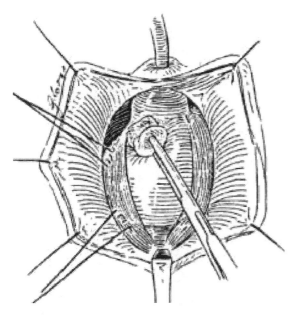

Figure 9 Grade IV cystocele repair. A midline incision is made in the anterior vaginal wall from the midurethra to base of bladder where anterior extensions of cardinal ligaments insert. The pubocervical fascia is identified laterally. After perforation of the endopelvic fascia into the retropubic space, two sets of No. 1 polypropylene suspension sutures are placed as described in the text. After transfer to the anterior abdominal wall, the central defect repair is performed as shown in Figure 3. [From Ref. (40).]

the midurethra to the posterior edge of the cystocele. Dissection is performed laterally in the avascular plane between the bladder and vaginal wall. The pubocervical fascia is exposed on both sides. Posteriorly, the dissection reaches the cervix or peritoneal fold, exposing the attenuated cardinal ligaments. If indicated, a hysterectomy or enterocele repair may be performed. At the level of the bladder neck, the retropubic space is entered sharply. The medial edges of the urethropelvic ligaments are exposed.

As described above for the four-corner bladder and bladder neck suspension, suspension sutures of No. 1 polypropylene are placed. However, the proximal sutures are placed under direct vision. These sutures are then transferred to the suprapubic region by needle suspension technique. Following transfer, a central defect repair is performed by plicating the pubocervical fascia across the midline using 2-0 PGA sutures as in Figure 3. The vaginal wall is trimmed and closed. Raz et al. reported excellent or good results in 88% with a mean follow-up of 34 months (40).

We have used the grade IV cystocele repair using an autologous fascial pubovaginal sling in place of the distal suspension sutures in cases where there is concomitant stress incontinence. Migilari and Usai described another similar procedure where a 5 × 5 cm synthetic mesh (60% polyglactin 910 and 40% polyester) is tailored to create an enclosure anteriorly to accommodate the urethra and the bladder base (41). The suspension sutures are then incorporated into the mesh's four corners. The sutures were then passed suprapubically and tied. Fourteen of 15 women (93%) who underwent this procedure for grade 4 cystocele were cured at a mean follow-up of 23 months.

Because of reported long-term recurrences of anterior vaginal prolapse, several new techniques using allographic and synthetic repairs have been described to improve long-term success rates. These procedures seem to make sense anatomically but await long-term results. Kobashi and Leach described a technique using allograft fascia lata (42). A midline anterior vaginal wall incision is made, extending from the distal urethra to the cystocele's apex. The bladder and urethra are dissected off of the anterior vaginal wall and the underside of the pubic bone is cleared. The bladder is mobilized medially away from the pubic bone, and the endopelvic fascia is perforated. A 6 × 8 cm segment of cadaveric fascia lata is incised into a T-shaped configuration with the top portion serving as the 2-cm sling. The corners of the sling portion are folded in triangular fashion to cross the fascial fibers, decreasing the risk of sutures pulling through the fascia. Bone anchors placed transvaginally anchor the sling to the pubic bone. The remainder of the fascial patch is secured to the medial edge of the levator muscles bilaterally with No. 0 polydioxanone suture and at the vaginal cuff or cervix with absorbable sutures to reduce the cystocele. Nicita described a similar procedure using polypropylene mesh sutured directly to the arcus tendineus bilaterally with polypropylene sutures (Fig. 10) (43).

As in the procedure described by Kobashi and Leach, the mesh is fashioned in such a way as to provide urethral support. We have recently started using a similar technique using allographic fascia because of the risk of erosion of synthetic material. A piece of fascia is sutured to the arcus

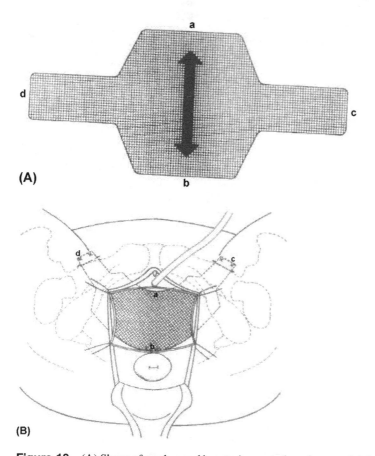

Figure 10   (**A**) Shape of mesh. a and b, anterior posterior edge. c and d, lateral wings. Distance between a and b is equal to anteroposterior dimension of cystocele. (**B**) Suture a fixes mesh to bladder neck. Suture b to cervix or cardinal ligaments, and sutures c and d to openings through pubic bone insertions of arcus tendineus of endopelvic fascia. [From Ref. (43).]

tendentious bilaterally, while a separate piece (or a single piece fashioned into a T-shape) is used as a pubovaginal sling. We prefer to secure the sling in the standard fashion (the pubovaginal sling extends into the retropubic space and is tied over the midline rectus fascia). The bladder sling portion of the fascia (or mesh) should also repair the central defect as the bladder is packed into its normal anatomic position. However, we prefer to also plicate the pubocervical fascia in the midline if possible as in an anterior colporrhaphy. These procedures should theoretically correct central and lateral defects as well as urethral hypermobility and intrinsic sphincter deficiency. The potential problem with such procedures involves the foreign material that must be used. Synthetic material is durable, but there is a risk of infection and erosion. Recent literature suggests that cadaveric fascia used as a pubovaginal sling may not have the durability of auto-logous fascia (44). Unfortunately, the amount of fascia required to perform a prolapse repair is too large to harvest easily from the rectus fascia or fascia lata. Therefore, until long-term data are available, such procedures should be done in select patients with informed consent.

XI. COMPLICATIONS

Paying careful attention to detail during surgery can minimize complications. In the absence of any bleeding diathesis, significant bleeding with cystocele repair is unusual. In one study of 52 retropubic paravaginal repairs, the mean estimated blood loss was 350 mL. Three patients required blood transfusion (33). Most bleeding in the retropubic space is due to the high vascu-larity of the vagina and the venous complex beneath the inferior pubic bone. During transvaginal procedures, bleeding may occur if dissection is carried out in the wrong plane. The vaginal wall should be taken off of the pubovesical fascia directly on its white shiny surface. Adherence to this principle may be difficult in cases of previous surgery and scarring, so bleeding is a higher risk in these patients. Perforation of the endopelvic fascia required in a vaginal paravaginal repair is another potential source of bleeding. The vessels responsible are usually difficult to visualize, but with the wider dissection and opening of EPF in this procedure, the bleeding site may be seen and can be overseen with a 2-0 PGA figure-of-eight stitch.

Bladder or ureteral injuries are rare, but can be discovered intraoperatively with the aid of cystoscopy and the administration of indigo carmine. Failure to see efflux of blue-stained urine after placement of sutures may signify kinking or ligation of a ureter. Before taking down the sutures, consider performing a retrograde pyelogram. In some cases the ureter is patent and the ipsilateral kidney is poorly functioning instead. If ureteral kinking or ligation is confirmed, the offending suture must be removed and replaced. The ureter may be prophylactically stented.

Bladder injuries should be closed in two layers. In retropubic procedures bladder injuries are easily closed in two layers with absorbable sutures. In transvaginal procedures injuries to the bladder most commonly occur when perforating into the retropubic space. The risk of this can be reduced by ensuring that the bladder is empty prior to perforation. Should inadvertent injury to the bladder occur, two-layer closure can usually be accomplished transvaginally. If the patient has a history of pelvic irradiation, an omental flap of labial fat pad interposition is recommended to prevent fistula formation (45,46). If a bladder injury is not detected until after surgery, a trial of conservative management with a Foley catheter may be tried.

Early postoperative complications of surgery for cystocele include wound infection, immediate postoperative retention, and irritative voiding symptoms. Retention is most likely in cases in which an anti-incontinence procedure has also been performed. In the study of results of retropubic paravaginal repair, Bruce et al. found that 32% of patients required clean intermit-tent catheterization (CIC) for ~2 weeks after repair, whereas 70% of patients who underwent paravaginal defect repair and sling required CIC for this length of time (33).

Long-term complications include postoperative voiding dysfunction such as stress incontinence, detrusor instability (frequency, urgency, urge incontinence), and incomplete voiding. Stress incontinence can be minimized with proper preoperative evaluation and performance of simultaneous anti-incontinence procedure, when indicated. De novo detrusor instability is a known complication of all bladder surgery and occurs in 5–7% of patients (38,40). However preexisting urge incontinence secondary to detrusor instability has been reported to resolve in 63% of cases (47). Incomplete emptying secondary to urethral obstruction (~1% of cases) may also occur and may require urethrolysis. When impaired emptying is due to poor contractility, this a condition that likely existed preoperatively and may require clean intermittent catheterization. Other complications include chronic pain, vaginal shortening or stenosis, and dyspareunia. Care should be taken not to aggressively excise excessive vaginal wall causing vaginal shortening. Finally, a missed or "potential" prolapse of other organs can result in clinical postoperative prolapse—for example, apical prolapse or enterocele.

XII. CONCLUSION

A number of surgical techniques have been described for repair of anterior vaginal prolapse. These techniques continue to evolve as our understanding of the anatomy and pathophysiology of prolapse improves. The mere evolution of new techniques is a sign that one "perfect" or standard technique does not exist, and no procedure is completely satisfactory for all patients. What has been established is that it is important to correct all identifiable defects both with relationship to the cystocele and to other areas of prolapse. Procedures will likely continue to be developed that emphasize a more minimally invasive approach with optimal long-term results and improvement in patient quality of life.

REFERENCES

1. Olsen AL, Smith VJ, Bergstrom JO. Epidemiology of surgically managed pelvic organ prolapse and urinary incontinence. Obstet Gynecol 1997; 89:501–506.
2. Gardy M, Kozminski M, DeLancey J. Stress incontinence and cystoceles. J Urol 1991; 145:1211–1213.
3. Subak LL,Waetjen LE, Van den Eeden S. Cost of pelvic organ prolapse surgery in the United States. Obstet Gynecol 2001; 98:646–651.
4. Kayigil O, Ahmed SI, Metin A. The coexistence of intrinsic sphincter deficiency with type II stress incontinence. J Urol 1999; 162:1365–1366.
5. Weber AM, Walters ME. Anterior vaginal prolapse: review of anatomy and techniques of surgical repair. Obstet Gynecol 1997; 89:311–818.
6. DeLancey JO. Anatomy and biomechanics of genital prolapse. Clin Obstet Gynecol 1993; 36:897–909.
7. DeLancey JO. Pubovesical ligament. A separate structure from the urethral supports: pubourethral ligaments. Neurourol Urodyn 1989; 8:53–61.
8. Klutke C, Golomb J, Barbaric Z. The anatomy of stress incontinence: magnetic resonance imaging of the female bladder neck and urethra. J Urol 1990; 143:563–566.
9. Mostwin JL. Current concepts of female pelvic anatomy and physiology. Urol Clin North Am 1991; 18:175–195.
10. Chopra A, Raz S, Stothers L. Pathogenesis of cystoceles-anterior colporrhaphy. In: Raz S, ed. Female Urology. Philadelphia: WB Saunders, 1996:338–343.

11. Richardson AC, Lyon JB, Williams NL. A new look at pelvic relaxation. Am J Obstet Gynecol 1976; 126:568.

12. Richardson AC, Edmonds PB, Williams NL. Treatment of stress urinary incontinence due to paravaginal fascial defect. Obstet Gynecol 1981; 57:357–362.

13. Rovner ES, Ginsberg DA, Raz S. Cystocele. In: Glenn's Urologic Surgery. 5th ed. Philadelphia: Lippincott-Raven, 1998:361–381.

14. Baden WF, Walker T. Evolution of the defect approach. In: Surgical Repair of Vaginal Defects. Philadelphia: J.B. Lippincott, 1992:13–17.

15. Bump RC, Mattiasson A, Bo K. The standardization of terminology of female pelvic organ prolapse and pelvic floor dysfunction. Am J Obstet Gynecol 1996; 175(1):10–17.

16. Bump RC, Mattiasson A, Bo K. The standardization of terminology of female pelvic organ prolapse and pelvic floor dysfunction. Am J Obstet Gynecol 1996; 175:10–17.

17. Hall AF, Theofrastous JP, Cundiff GW. Interobserver and intraobserver reliability of the proposed international continence society, society of gynecologic surgeons, and American urogynecologic society pelvic organ prolapse classification system. Am J Obstet Gynecol 1996; 175:1467–1471.

18. Shull BL. Pelvic organ prolapse: anterior, superior, and posterior vaginal segment defects. Am J Obstet Gynecol 1999; 181:6–11.

19. Shull BL. Clinical evaluation of women with pelvic support defects. Clin Obstet Gynecol 1993; 36:939–951.

20. Barber MD, Cundiff GW, Weidner AC. Accuracy of clinical assessment of paravaginal defects in women with anterior vaginal wall prolapse. Am J Obstet Gynecol 1999; 181:87–90.

21. Zimmern PE. The role of voiding cystourethrography in the evaluation of the female lower urinary tract. Prob Urol 1991; 5:23–41.

22. English SF, Amundsen CL, McGuire EJ. Bladder neck competency at rest in women with incontinence. J Urol 1999; 161:578–580.

23. Comiter CV, Vasavada SP, Barbaric ZL. Grading pelvic prolapse and pelvic floor relaxation using dynamic magnetic resonance imaging. Urology 1999; 54:454–457.

24. Kegel AH. Progressive resistance exercise in the functional restoration of the perineal muscles. Am J Obstet Gynecol 1948; 56:238–244.

25. Cundiff GW, Weidner AC, Visco AG. A survey of pessary use by members of the American Urogynecologic Society. Obstet Gynecol 2000; 95:931–935.

26. Cundiff GW, Addison WA. Management of pelvic organ prolapse. Obstet Gynecol Clin North Am 1998; 25:907–921.

27. Muram D, Summitt RL, Feldment N. Vaginal dilators for intermittent pelvic support: a case report. J Reprod Med 1990; 35:303–304.

28. Ott R, Richter H, Behr J. Small bowel prolapse and incarceration caused by a vaginal ring pessary. Br J Surg 1993; 80:1157–1159.

29. Kelly HA, Dumm WM. Urinary incontinence in women, without manifest injury to the bladder. Surg Gynecol Obstet 1914; 18:444–450.

30. Chesson RR, Schlossberg SM, Elkins TE. The use of fascia lata graft for correction of severe or recurrent anterior vaginal wall defects. J Pelvic Surg 1999; 5:96–103.

31. Shull BL, Baden WF. A six-year experience with paravaginal defect repair for stress urinary incontinence. Am J Obstet Gynecol 1989; 160:1432–1435.

32. Colombo M, Vitobello D, Proietti F. Randomised comparison of Burch colposuspension versus anterior colporraphy in women with stress urinary incontinence and anterior vaginal wall prolapse. Br J Obstet Gynecol 2000; 170:544–551.

33. Bruce RG, El-Galley RES, Galloway NTM. Paravaginal defect repair in the treatment of female stress urinary incontinence and cystocele. Urology 1999; 54:647–651.

34. Burch JC. Urethrovaginal fixation to Cooper's ligament for correction of stress incontinenc, cystocele, and prolapse. Am J Obstet Gynecol 1961; 81:281–290.

35. Veronikis DK. The paravaginal defect. In: Clarke-Pearson DL, ed. Gynecolgic, Obstetric, and Other Related Surgery. 2nd ed. St. Louis: Mosby, 2000:361–364.

36. Walters MD, Weber AM. Anterior vaginal prolapse with and without geuine stress incontinence. In: Cardozo L, Staskin D, eds. Textbook of Female Urology and Urogynecology. London: Isis Medical Media, 2001:587–597.
37. Raz S, Little NA, Juma S. Female urology. In: Walsh PC, Retik AB, Stamey TA, Vaughan ED, eds. Campbell's Urology. 6th ed. Philadelphia: W.B. Saunders, 1992:2782–2828.
38. Raz S, Klutke CG, Golomb J. Four-corner bladder and urethral suspension for moderate cystocele. J Urol 1989; 142:712–715.
39. Margossian H, Walters MD, Falcone T. Laparoscopic management of pelvic organ prolapse. Eur J Obstet Gynecol 1999; 85:57–62.
40. Raz S, Little NA, Juma S. Repair of severe anterior wall prolapse (grade IV cystourethrocele). J Urol 1991; 146:988.
41. Migliari R, Usai E. Treatment results using a mixed fiber mesh in patients with grade IV cystocele. J Urol 1999; 161:1255–1258.
42. Kobashi KC, Mee SL, Leach GE. A new technique for cystocele repair and transvaginal sling: the cadaveric prolapse repair and sling (CsPS). Urology 2000; 56:9–14.
43. Nicita G. A new operation for genitourinary prolapse. J Urol 1998; 160:741–745.
44. Fitzgerald MP, Mollenhauer J, Brubaker L. Failure of allograft suburethral slings. BJU Int 1999; 84:785–788.
45. Tancer ML. Urologic injuries: bladder and urethra. In: Schaefer G, Graber EA, eds. Complications in Obstetric and Gynecologic Surgery. New York: Harper and Row, 1981.
46. Kreder KJ. Female urethral diverticulum and urethral fistulae. In: Webster GD, Kirby R, Goldwasser B, eds. Reconstructive Urology. Oxford: Blackwell, 1993:861.
47. Nguyen JK, Bhatia NN. Resolution of motor urge incontinence after surgical repair of pelvic organ prolapse. J Urol 2001; 166:2263–2266.
48. Walter S, Olesen KP, Hald T. Urodynamic evaluation after vaginal repair and colposuspension. Br J Urol 1982; 54:377–380.
49. Porges RF, Smilen SW. Long-term analysis of the surgical management of pelvic support defects. Am J Obstet Gynecol 1994; 171:1518–1528.
50. Kohli N, Sze EHM, Roat TW. Incidence of recurrent cystocele after anterior colporrhaphy with and without concomitant transvaginal needle suspension. Am J Obstet Gynecol 1996; 175:1476–1482.
51. Shull BL, Benn SJ, Kuehl TJ. Surgical management of prolapse of the anterior vaginal segment: an analysis of support defects, operative morbidity, and anatomic outcome. Am J Obstet Gynecol 1994; 171:1429–1439.
52. Benson JT, Lucente V, McClellan E. Vaginal versus abdominal reconstructive surgery for the treatment of pelvic support defects: a prospective randomized study with long-term outcome evaluation. Am J Obstet Gynecol 1996; 175:1418–1422.
53. Dmochowski RR, Zimmern PE, Ganabathi LS. Role of the four-corner bladder neck suspension to correct stress incontinence with a mild to moderate cystocele. Urology 1997; 49:35–40.
54. Julian TM. The efficacy of Marlex mesh in the repair of severe, recurrent vaginal prolapse of the anterior midvaginal wall. Am J Obstet Gynecol 1996; 175:1472–1475.

42

Diagnosis and Treatment of the Stage IV Cystocele

Nancy B. Itano,* Fernando Almeida,*
Larissa V. Rodríguez, and Shlomo Raz
University of California, Los Angeles, California, U.S.A.

I. STAGE IV CYSTOCELE

A cystocele is defined as anterior vaginal wall (bladder) prolapse into the vagina, with or without urethral hypermobility. Cystoceles have been described by several different classification systems, and most commonly categorized by the degree of bladder descent and anatomic defect as in the Baden and Walker classification (1) (Table 1). More recently the International Continence Society (ICS) has accepted standardization of the terminology for pelvic organ prolapse quantification (POP-Q) (2). Using POP-Q, both the stages III (Ba) and IV (C, D) would be classified as grade IV cystoceles, according to the traditional nomenclature (Table 2). However, it is rare to see an isolated stage III or IV cystocele without concurrent pelvic organ prolapse. The focus of this chapter is the pathophysiology, diagnosis, and surgical treatment of severe bladder prolapse, which for simplicity will be referred to as stage IV cystocele.

The goals of surgery in patients with severe prolapse are correction of all anatomic defects and restoration of bowel and bladder function. Anatomic considerations include vaginal depth, restoration of vaginal axis, urethral hypermobility, and closure of the widened urogenital diaphragm and levator hiatus. Creating normal anatomy, however, does not ensure a return to normal bladder, bowel, and sexual function.

The natural history of a cystocele is a continuous progression from mild to severe prolapse (correlating to stages 0 to IV), but the actual risk of progression is unknown. In some patients, the progression is rapid; in others it can be insidious, taking many years. Most lesser degrees of prolapse (stage I and II) are asymptomatic, except when accompanied by urinary incontinence. Pelvic prolapse does not spontaneously regress and, often, does not become symptomatic until the descent reaches the introitus (3).

---

*Current affiliation: Mayo Clinic Scottsdale, Scottsdale, Arizona, U.S.A.

Table 1 Cystocele Classifications

By degree of bladder descent	
Grade 0	No prolapse
Grade I	Prolapse to proximal vagina with straining
Grade II	Prolapse to midvagina with straining
Grade III	Prolapse to introitus with straining
Grade IV	Prolapse to introitus at rest
By anatomic defect	
Central	Attenuation of midline pubocervical fascia; loss of rugae
Lateral	Loss of paravaginal support; rugae present

Proposed risk factors for the development of a cystocele have included difficult or prolonged vaginal deliveries, elevated body mass index (BMI), parity, menopause, and previous vaginal surgery.

II. ANATOMIC CONSIDERATIONS

To treat pelvic organ relaxation, one must gain an understanding of pelvic floor support. We will focus on the anterior compartment, in which laxity will present as a cystocele. In the treatment of vaginal prolapse, however, all levels of support must be addressed in order to produce a successful outcome.

Normally, in the standing position, the vagina forms a "banana" shape with two distinct vaginal angles. This can be demonstrated on a midsagittal pelvic magnetic resonance image in a patient with normal anatomy. The distal vagina forms a 45° angle from the vertical plane. The proximal vagina then lies almost horizontally over the posterior levator plate creating a 110° angle, which is maintained by the anterior pull of the pubococcygeus muscle (anterior segment of the levator plate).

This support is due to the connective tissue and muscular components of the pelvic floor. Superiorly, and adjacent to the pelvic organs, is the *pelvic diaphragm*. Inferiorly, and more superficial, is the *urogenital* (UG) *diaphragm*. The pelvic diaphragm, and its investing connective tissue, is the primary source of pelvic organ support (4–8). The UG diaphragm consists of the bulbocavernosus muscle on either side of the introitus and the external anal sphincter surrounding the anus. The transverse perinei (superficial and deep) inserts on the ischial tuberosities and fuses in the midline on the central tendon. The superior and inferior perineal fascia reinforces these muscles. Both muscle and fascia must be incorporated in a repair of the perineum.

Table 2 Standardized Pelvic Organ Prolapse (POP) Staging for Anterior Vaginal Wall Relaxation

Stage	Findings
0	No prolapse is demonstrated. (Aa, Ba are −3 cm.)
I	Most distal portion of the prolapse is >1 cm above the level of the hymen.
II	Most distal portion of the prolapse is ≤1 cm proximal to the hymen or distal to the hymen. (Aa and Ba are between −1 cm and +1 cm.)
III	Most distal portion of the prolapse is >1 cm below the hymen but protrudes no more than 2 cm less than the total vaginal length (cm).
IV	Complete eversion of the total length of the lower genital tract.

The pelvic diaphragm muscles consist of the levator ani and coccygeus. The levator ani can be subdivided into the *pubococcygeus* and the *iliococcygeus*. The pubococcygeus muscle is a thick, U-shaped muscle that arises from the pubic symphysis and fuses around the urethra, vagina, and anus, as the organs exit through the diaphragm. It creates a sling like hammock, pulling the organs anteriorly. The pubococcygeus (also referred to as the *pubovisceralis*) contracts to create anterior angulation of these organs, serving to prevent prolapse. The iliococcygeus creates a horizontal sheet that attaches laterally, creating the fibrous band *arcus tendineus levator ani* (ATLA) where the levator ani attaches to the pelvic sidewall and obturator internus muscle. The insertion of the ATLA to the sidewall divides the obturator internus into supralevator and infralevator segments. The levator plate (and ATLA) extends anteriorly to attach to the underside of the midpubic bone. The opening in the levators, in which the urethra, vagina, and rectum exit, is called the *urogenital* (UG) *hiatus*. The *arcus tendineus fascia pelvis* (ATFP) is the medially based fascia that directly envelops the organs as they pass through the pelvic diaphragm. The ATFP is an extension from the levators to the pelvic organs as they cross the levator hiatus. The ATFP attaches anteriorly to the pubic rami and expands to the ischial spines bilaterally. This fascial layer lies on the cephalad surface of the levator plate.

The pelvic diaphragm has investing connective tissue, which is less organized and distinct than traditional fascia. The top layer of connective tissue overlying the pelvic diaphragm is referred to as *endopelvic fascia*. The *paracolpium* is the connective tissue that attaches to the vagina, and the *parametrium* attaches to the uterus. Prominent folds of the paracolpium and parametrium are clinically referred to as the *cardinal ligaments*, which attach laterally to the pelvic sidewall and ischial spine, and the *uterosacral ligaments*, which attach posteriorly on the sacrum. DeLancey has described three levels of support (9) from this viscerofascial layer. Level I suspends the top two-thirds of the vagina to the posterior sidewall. These fibers include the uterosacral-cardinal ligament complex, which extend toward the sacrum. Level II attaches the midvagina to the sidewalls, ATFP, and ATLA. Most distally, level III, is local support as the "fascia" attaches the urethra to the pubic bone and vagina to the perineal body.

To better understand the surgical anatomy, we describe four areas of interest in the anterior compartment. When we describe ligaments, we are referring to the condensations of connective tissue that provide pelvic organ support: (a) The *pubourethral ligaments* support the midurethra to the inferior rami of the symphysis, and are analogous to the puboprostatic ligaments in the male. (b) The *urethropelvic ligaments* provide support of the proximal urethra to the lateral pelvic sidewall. They consist of both the periurethral and endopelvic fascia, as each envelops the proximal urethra. (c) The *vesicopelvic ligaments* provide support of the bladder to the ATFP. This includes the perivesical connective tissue, as seen in the vaginal exposure of the bladder, and the endopelvic fascia. (d) The *cardinal-sacrouterine ligament complex* attaches to the bladder base and cervix (or vaginal vault, if reapproximated during the hysterectomy). Microscopic studies suggest that these fascial layers encountered during vaginal surgery may be histologically indistinct from the deep vaginal wall, and not a separate "fascia" (10).

III. ETIOLOGY AND PATHOPHYSIOLOGY

Pelvic organ prolapse is prevented by several mechanisms. The pelvic floor musculature has basal resting tone, an involuntary reflex, and voluntary activity. At rest, there is static tone of the levator plate and UG diaphragm that creates the *anorectal angle* (normal range, 60–120°) and narrows the UG hiatus. This banana shape of the vagina is very important in preventing future prolapse. After surgery, the vaginal axis must recreate this alignment, so that increased abdominal pressures causes coaptation of the proximal vagina against the levator shelf. If the vaginal vault is not secured posteriorly, increases in abdominal pressure will cause the pelvic contents to be pushed out (telescoped) of the vagina (11). Increases in intra-abdominal pressure causes a reflexive arc that contracts the pelvic floor to further angulate the rectum anteriorly and narrow the levator hiatus. Similarly, there is a coordinated involuntary reflex to relax the pelvic floor, which occurs during defecation. This widens the UG hiatus and straightens the distal rectum to allow for evacuation of stool. The pelvic floor musculature is also under somatic control, so that the pelvic floor can be voluntarily contracted or relaxed. Pelvic floor muscles exercises (PFME) are an application of this capability. Loss of levator function will cause loss of normal support and the vaginal axis, making pelvic organ prolapse more likely.

Normal function of the levator ani requires functioning muscle fibers (primarily slow-twitch, type I fibers) and intact neural connections. Innervation of the muscles is primarily derived from the ventral roots of the second, third, and fourth sacral nerve roots via the pudendal nerve. There also may be direct innervation to the cranial surface of the levators through the third and fourth sacral motor nerve roots (8). The investing connective tissue layers provide static support.

Because of the complexity of pelvic organ support, vaginal prolapse is likely multifactorial. A cystocele results when there is damage to the level II supports and/or pelvic floor dysfunction. Traditionally, cystoceles have been categorized into central and lateral (paravaginal) defects. A central defect presents as midline weakness. This may be due to stretching of vaginal tissue beyond its capacity to recover, so that the vesicopelvic fascia covering the levator hiatus becomes attenuated and the vaginal wall thins (12). A lateral defect occurs when there is weakness or disruption of lateral attachments of the vagina (and ATFP) to the ATLA. Cysto-celes with an isolated central defect represent only 5–15% of all cystoceles, whereas a lateral paravaginal defect is present in 70–80% of patients. Stage IV cystoceles usually present with both defects.

Poor function of the levator ani muscles may be due to direct myopathic injury or from an abnormality of innervation. Loss of pelvic floor function will cause the UG hiatus to widen, increasing the risk of organ prolapse. Relaxation of the pubococcygeus will similarly decrease the angulation of the midvagina, so that the upper vagina does not lie flat against the pelvic floor plate. Instead of a banana configuration, the vagina would be vertically oriented, allowing for the pelvic contents to be pushed out of the vagina.

The reason for a neuropathy in a healthy woman is not clear. Childbirth has been suggested as the cause of pelvic denervation, but studies in this area have shown that uncomplicated child-birth creates transient neurological damage to the pelvic floor that is restored after 2 months (13). The pelvic floor neuropraxia related to vaginal delivery is associated with multiple births, prolonged labor, high birth weigh, and traumatic deliveries. Other risk factors for neurological damage are congenital abnormalities, loss of neuronal mass, aging, chronic constipation (abdominal straining), and perineal laxity (5,7). In a study of 50 women with prolapse, Sharf performed electromyography on the levator ani and found evidence of denervation in half of the patients (13). Other studies have confirmed evidence of neurological damage to the UG muscles in pelvic prolapse (14,15).

The connective tissue of the pelvic floor ("endopelvic fascia") can be described as a group of collagen fibers interlaced with elastin, smooth muscle cells, fibroblasts, and vascular struc-tures. These structures may be weakened due to pregnancy and parturition, lack of estrogen, aging, diet, chronic straining, and certain connective tissue disorders (Ehlers-Danlos and Marfan's syndrome) (6). Patients with vaginal prolapse have fewer fibroblasts and more collagen fibers in the pubocervical fascia than do controls (16). It has also been shown there may be a difference in collagen metabolism, with a reduction in type I:III collagen ratio. Type I collagen is less flexible than type III collagen, but has increased tensile strength (17). Intrinsic collagen abnormalities and other individual predisposition factors (genetics, differences in pelvic architecture, inherent quality of the pelvic musculature, and tissue response to injury) might also explain why patients with known risk factors do not develop prolapse and why many patients without any known risk factor do.

Risk factors for anterior vaginal wall prolapse include: neuropathy, myopathy, aging, hormonal, surgical trauma (especially previous vaginal hysterectomy), vaginal childbirth, and increased abdominal pressures (obesity, constipation, chronic cough).

Correction of a cystocele alone, without reconstructing the entire pelvic floor, may further alter the vaginal axis and increase the likelihood of uterine prolapse, enterocele and rectocele formation (18). Additionally, a severe cystocele rarely occurs in isolation. Michael et al. (19) observed a simultaneous enterocele in 35%, rectocele in 63%, and uterine prolapse in 38% of patients with grade IV cystoceles. Urethral hypermobility, coaptation, and function should also be addressed at the same time.

IV. CLINICAL PRESENTATION

A. Symptoms

Cystoceles are often asymptomatic until pelvic organ prolapse is severe. The most common complaint due to anterior compartment prolapse is vaginal bulging, with or without suprapubic pressure and pain. Other possible coexisting symptoms include urgency, frequency, urge incontinence, stress incontinence, recurrent urinary tract infections, back pain, renal failure, and urinary retention. Obstructive voiding symptoms are due to urethral kinking when the bladder descends beyond the pubic ramus but the urethra remains fixed. This is commonly seen in the setting of previous surgery (i.e., bladder neck suspension, urethropexy, sling) (19). Patients may describe using unusual positions to void, such as pelvic tilting, squatting, and standing. In contrast, patients with concomitant urethral dysfunction may present with stress urinary incontinence, especially when the cystocele is manually reduced.

B. Clinical Evaluation

There are some critical points in the evaluation of a stage IV cystocele that must be answered before treatment. The degree of cystocele and concurrent voiding dysfunction such as stress incontinence, detrusor overactivity, and ability to empty to completion should be investigated. Surgical planning is also affected by the need to preserve sexual function and vaginal depth. The overall health of the patient is considered as well as the impact of the symptoms on the patient's quality of life.

Preoperative planning demands an assessment of which pelvic organs are prolapsing and to what degree. Associated abnormalities of the perineum and levator hiatus should also be noted. It must be decided what should be done with the urethra, in the face of such severe pelvic floor relaxation. If the quality of the vaginal tissue is poor, it must be decided whether local estrogen replacement is needed.

C. Physical Examination

A thorough physical examination must be done with a full bladder, at rest, and with straining, in both the standing and supine positions. The goal of examination is to determine the degree of prolapse, the specific anatomic defects, and the presence of concomitant organ prolapse. Straining and standing should accentuate the degree of descent. In the supine position, we try to determine the origin of prolapse. Using a half-speculum blade we retract the posterior vaginal wall and ask the patient to strain, to evaluate the anterior defect. An isolated central defect is identified as bulging in the central region of the vagina (midline) with the lateral sulci high and well supported. Loss of vaginal rugae is due to smooth muscle atrophy of the vaginal wall, as is commonly seen in older patients, and is a nonspecific finding. A lateral defect is identified when there is loss of the lateral vaginal sulci, as the vesicopelvic fascia attenuates from the ATFP. There will be loss of the "M" vaginal profile (coronal view) and sliding herniation of the bladder into the vagina. After characterizing the anatomic defects, it is important to reduce the cystocele to elicit occult stress urinary incontinence and urethral hypermobility. Similarly, we retract the anterior vaginal wall to determine the presence of a posterior defect. A digital rectal exam assesses rectal tone, presence of impacted stools, attenuation of the prerectal fascia, and perineal laxity. Using both blades of speculum, the vaginal vault or cervix can be examined for uterine descent, vault prolapse, and enterocele.

To ensure consistency, examiners must note the conditions of the exam findings, such as rest, strain, or supine positioning. Using the POP-Q classification, stage III (Ba) is the most severe form of isolated anterior compartment prolapse. This is when the point that represents the most dependent position of the anterior vaginal wall descends >1 cm below the hymen but protrudes no further than 2 cm less than the total vaginal length (TVL-2). Stage IV is total vaginal eversion, with the most distal portion of prolapse descending a minimum of 2 cm less than the total vaginal length, and in most instances, the entire vaginal length. The cervix (C) or vaginal cuff is most commonly the leading point (2).

D.   Imaging Studies

In the setting of a large introital bulge, it may be difficult to differentiate a severe cystocele from an enterocele by only physical exam (20). Imaging studies can be helpful in assessing severe organ prolapse, especially when one compartment has such significant bulging that it acts as a space-occupying lesion.

An ideal imaging study should provide precise information about which structures are prolapsed, the presence of urinary retention and obstruction, urethral hypermobility and urinary incontinence.

1.   Cystourethrography

The patient should be upright and have a full bladder. Films should be taken during both rest and strain. This exam provides information about bladder position, bladder neck funneling, urethral mobility, stress incontinence, and postvoid residual. The presence of a rectocele can also be inferred when bowel gas is identified below the pubic symphysis. This exam is static and does not provide information about other pelvic organs or soft tissues of the pelvic floor.

2.   Dynamic Fluoroscopy (Colpocystodefecography, Vaginography)

This study relies on making the organs of interest radiopaque (bladder, vagina, rectum) and studying their positional changes with straining under fluoroscopy. This is a dynamic exam done with the patient upright. Standing recreates the setting in which the patient experiences maximal vaginal bulging. Unfortunately, contrast paste must be placed into the vagina and rectum, which can be uncomfortable.

3.   Ultrasonography

Ultrasound (US) is an attractive imaging modality because it is easy to perform, is minimally invasive, and avoids radiation exposure. Tubo-ovarian and renal disease can also be assessed during the same exam. There is evidence that US is useful in evaluating bladder neck hypermobility, but transvaginal imaging for pelvic prolapse does not provide adequate visualization of the soft tissues (21). Translabial ultrasound can be used to quantify prolapse, although it appears to be better for the anterior compartment and uterine descent than the posterior compartment (22).

4. Dynamic Magnetic Resonance Imaging

Recently, MRI has been used to evaluate pelvic prolapse. It is performed quickly, without contrast or ionizing radiation, and permits visualization of the soft tissues as well as the upper urinary tract. Gousse and colleagues have shown that in comparison with findings at surgery, MRI has a 100% sensitivity, 83% specificity and a positive predictive value of 97% when assessing cystoceles. When compared to colpocystodefecography, MRI does not require intravesical catheterization, does not require contrast, and is fast (5 min) and noninvasive. MRI may be less sensitive, underestimating the extent of apical and posterior compartment defects (23,24). Unfortunately, MRIs must be performed in the supine position, which diminishes the downward forces that can be generated with abdominal straining.

At our institution, pelvic MRI is done without endorectal or endovaginal coils, with the intention of being as noninvasive as possible (Fig. 1). The diagnostic value would be increased with the addition of water-soluble lubricant in the vagina and/or rectum.

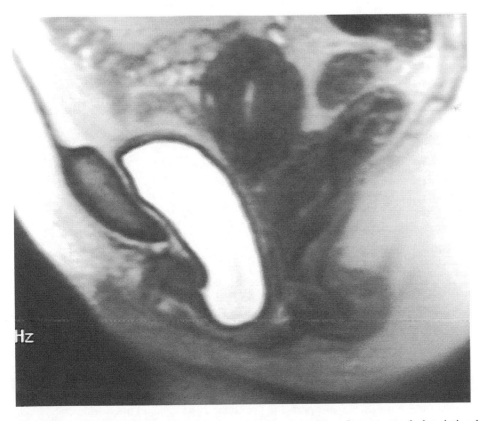

Figure 1 Midsaggital MRI (HASTE sequence) demonstrating a large cystocele herniating below the pubic symphysis.

E. Video Urodynamic Study

A urodynamic study (UDS) can be done with or without video assistance. Both methods provide information about bladder compliance, capacity, sensation of filling, detrusor instability, and contractility. An advantage in performing video urodynamics is the capability to correlate standing cystography (anatomic information) with simultaneous pressure-flow studies. Choosing to use fluoroscopy should be based on cost, availability, and familiarity with this method.

The importance of documenting the presence of urinary incontinence among patients with large cystoceles is controversial. The incidence of occult stress urinary incontinence is felt to be as high as 22–80% among patients with high stage vaginal vault prolapse (25). Owing to the masked urinary incontinence and the high incidence of postoperative de novo stress incontinence, many authors routinely perform a concomitant anti-incontinence surgery in all anterior vaginal reconstruction independent of continence status.

A recent study by Barnes et al. (26) retrospectively reviewed the charts of 38 women with grade 3–4 prolapse who did not have significant symptoms of stress incontinence. None of the patients demonstrated stress incontinence during physical exam or video urodynamic studies, until the prolapse was mechanically reduced. All patients subsequently had documented stress incontinence with a mean abdominal leak point pressure of 86 cmH$_2$O. All patients then underwent surgical repair of the prolapse and a pubovaginal sling. None of the patients developed permanent retention. Recurrent stress incontinence occurred in 5% of the patients. Conversely, Chaikin and colleges (27) evaluated 24 "continent" women with severe cystoceles. They used a pessary to reduce the cystocele during UDS and documented incontinence in only 58% of patients. The patients with overt incontinence received an anti-incontinence procedure, and the others did not. With a mean follow-up of 47 months, no patients treated only by colporrhaphy developed incontinence. They recommend concomitant anti-incontinence procedures in patients with overt leakage. In order to improve the sensitivity of the urodynamic test to reveal urinary incontinence, the use of a pessary or a vaginal pack can be used to reduce the cystocele (28,29).

Complete reduction of the vaginal prolapse is not always possible with a pessary if the prolapse is severe. Additionally, there has been no proven correlation between pessary reduction and the reduction obtained by surgery. Vaginal packing and pessaries can also artificially obstruct the urethra. It is our feeling that a nonobstructive anti-incontinence procedure to support the urethra should be done to restore urethral function and prevent incontinence.

Determining the presence of bladder instability is important in preoperative counseling because it can affect the postoperative result. In the majority of cases (60–80%), urgency may resolve after surgery (30). Some patients may have no change in urgency or even see their urgency exacerbated by sling placement and/or bladder neck elevation. UDS may also indicate urinary obstruction preoperatively with an elevated voiding pressure, low urinary flow, or radiologic evidence of urethral kinking.

F. Cystourethroscopy

This exam is performed to rule out concurrent pathology in the bladder and urethra, such as bladder carcinoma, urethral diverticulum, stones, or foreign bodies (such as suture material) from previous surgery. Cystoscopic illumination can also be used to differentiate an enterocele from a cystocele (31). A pelvic exam is performed with the cystoscope in the bladder. The bladder transilluminates through the anterior vaginal wall, so that the extent of the bladder prolapse is demarcated (Fig. 2).

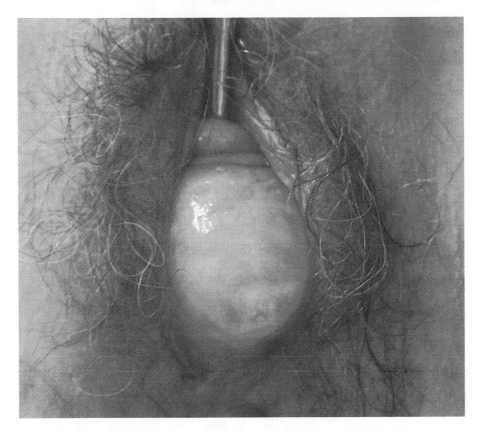

Figure 2 Cystoscopic transillumination of the cystocele. The illumination ends at the most proximal extent of the cystocele, demarcating the border between the cystocele and enterocele.

We assess bladder neck competence both at rest and during straining. It can also be used as a bedside urodynamic exam, assessing filling sensation, postvoid residual, and visual cystometrics for bladder contractions. With a full bladder, a supine Valsalva stress test can be performed to look for urethral leakage.

G. Upper Urinary Tract Evaluation

Patients with a stage IV cystocele should have upper tract imaging because there is a 4–7% incidence of moderate hydroureteronephrosis amongst patients with severe vaginal prolapse (32,33). This risk is greater in patients with procidentia. Ultrasound, excretory urography, computed tomography, or MRI can be used. An advantage of MRI is the ability to simultaneously evaluate the upper urinary tract, tubo-ovarian disease, and pelvic organ prolapse simultaneously.

H. Laboratory Evaluations

Patients must have sterile urine prior to proceeding with an operative procedure. In preparation for surgery, we routinely obtain a complete blood count, basic metabolic panel, and coagulation profile in addition to the urine culture.

V. TREATMENT

Treatment of the stage IV cystocele cannot be addressed in isolation but rather as a component of the entire pelvic floor, including restoration of vaginal depth and axis. Obviously, the superior and posterior compartments must be reconstructed, in addition to the UG hiatus and perineum. There are several approaches to surgery, including abdominal, laparoscopic, and/or vaginal repair.

A. Abdominal Approach

There are two classic abdominal techniques that have been used together in the treatment of anterior vaginal wall prolapse: the paravaginal defect repair (PVDR) by Richardson (34), and the Burch colposuspension (35). Most abdominal approaches are made with the patient in a low lithotomy position with a Pfannenstiel incision. A 16–18F urethral catheter is useful to isolate the bladder neck.

In Richardson's surgery, after the retropubic space has been dissected, the bladder neck, urethra, anterior vaginal wall, and ATLA are identified. The operator then inserts his nondominant hand into the vagina and using his finger, elevates the lateral sulcus of the vagina to the level of the bladder neck. The first permanent suture placed attaches the lateral vagina wall to the levator fascia and ATLA. Three additional sutures are passed anterior and posterior to the first stitch at intervals of 1–2 cm. Sutures are held, being tied only after the last suture has been placed.

Richardson (34), who first described the anatomic surgical repair for cystocele, emphasized that his technique was designed solely to correct the paravaginal defect and did not address the urethra. In fact, this procedure only repairs the level II lateral support, and does not address the vaginal axis, central defects, sacrouterine-cardinal ligament weakness, or urethral dysfunction.

In a follow-up of 2–8 years using this approach in properly selected patients, the overall success was 95% (34). Recently Bruce et al. (36), using the same technique, with a mean follow-up of 17 months showed an 80% cystocele cure rate and 72% cure of urinary incontinence.

Colposuspensions are well known among physicians that treat urinary incontinence. The difference between the Burch colposuspension and a PVDR is that the lateral vaginal wall is suspended to Cooper's ligament instead of the ATLA. Excessive tension must be avoided to prevent postoperative urinary retention. Although the Burch procedure has been initially described to treat anterior wall descent, it is used more commonly to treat urinary incontinence. Thus, there are limited data showing its success as solely a cystocele repair.

Modifications have been made, including various suture materials, location of suture placement, use of anchoring devices, and different graft materials. A recent randomized trial compared three anterior colporrhaphy techniques (37): standard plication colporrhaphy, standard colporrhaphy with polyglactin mesh, and an ultralateral anterior colporrhaphy. Preoperative and postoperative exams were standardized with the POP-Q staging system, as recommended by the International Continence Society. At a mean follow-up of 23 months, patients in all three groups had similar anatomic cure rates (standard, 30%; standard with mesh, 42%; ultralateral 46%). Symptomatology related to the prolapse also resolved without significant difference among the three groups.

Sullivan et al. (38), reported results with a modified sacrocolpopexy to treat complete pelvic organ prolapse. This group used several pieces of Marlex mesh (CR Bard Inc, Charlotte, NC) as a scaffold for support. The peritoneal sac is dissected off the vaginal apex in the treatment of the enterocele, and mesh is placed behind the vagina reinforcing the rectovaginal septum. It is attached to the perineal body with a two-pronged Cobb-Ragde needle passer. Polypropylene (Prolene: Johnson & Johnson, Cincinnati) is used to fix the mesh superiorly to the S1–2 periosteum. Lateral support is created with two additional strips of mesh, attached to the posterior mesh on either side of the vagina, and then suspended to Cooper's ligament bilaterally. If there is a prominent cystocele, an additional piece of bridging mesh is placed anterior to the vagina, sutured to the lateral mesh strips. There was a 5% mesh erosion rate and 4% rate of reoperation for small bowel obstruction. Specific outcomes of vault prolapse were not included in the outcome reporting, but 36% underwent corrective surgery for bladder-related symptoms and 28% underwent subsequent repair of anorectal mucosal prolapse or rectocele. Mean follow-up was >5 years. Because of the need for additional corrective surgery for bladder symptomatology and low posterior compartment defects, the authors feel that their total mesh repair is only a foundation for pelvic support. Rectocele repair and/or urethral support should be done concomitantly if needed, presumably through a vaginal and/or rectal approach. The widened levator hiatus itself is not repaired with this approach.

Despite good results with the abdominal approaches, it is not clear if these procedures should be used in all stages of cystocele. There have been a limited number of studies evaluating the anatomic result (prolapse) as the primary outcome measure. Abdominal procedures are an excellent option for patients with cystoceles who may require concurrent abdominal surgery (such as transabdominal hysterectomy or oophorectomy), have a isolated lateral defect, or have a narrow vagina that does not allow adequate surgical exposure. Besides the increased morbidity, a major disadvantage of any abdominal approach is that low posterior compartment abnormalities (rectocele or rectal mucosal prolapse), a widened levator hiatus, and urethral dysfunction are not corrected.

B. Laparoscopic Approach

The laparoscopic retropubic bladder neck suspension was first described in 1991 (39). Reported advantages include a shorter hospital stay, faster recovery, improved visualization, and decreased blood loss. With the increased training in laparoscopy and classic teaching from traditional abdominal approaches, some surgeons have begun treating urinary incontinence and anterior vaginal wall relaxation with a laparoscopic paravaginal repair. Because results with a paravaginal defect repair alone were less successful than with the Burch procedure, some authors began to repair the paravaginal defect together with the Burch bladder neck suspension with good results. The laparoscopic route can be transperitoneal or extraperitoneal (retropubic). The surgical procedure starts with the placement of the trocars, usually consisting of a 10-mm trocar at the umbilicus, which is used to house the camera. An additional two or three 5-mm trocars are placed in lower quadrants of abdomen. The dissection of the retropubic space is made, and after the anatomic structures have been visualized, sutures are placed as previously described.

There have been variations in suture placement, number of sutures, suture material, use of allograft or synthetic materials, and anchoring devices (40). In a retrospective study by El-Toukhy and Davies (41), patients with genuine stress incontinence underwent either an open Burch or a laparoscopic modified Burch colposuspension. The bladder neck was elevated using polypropylene mesh (2.5 × 5 cm) and titanium tacks. Two titanium coils were placed into the paravaginal tissue with the strip of mesh, and then the other end of the mesh was adhered to Cooper's ligament with two additional coils. This was then repeated on the contralateral side. Early results show that the laparoscopic route is equivalent to the open procedure for treatment of stress incontinence, but that with time, the laparoscopic approach is less durable ("cure" at >2 years, laparoscopic 62% versus open 79%, $P < 0.05$). Outcome of prolapse is not quantified.

Because laparoscopy allows the performance of similar procedures with minimal invasiveness, adherence to strict anatomic principles must remain. Sutures can be difficult to place and time-consuming to tie, so some laparoscopic surgeons have modified the technique to use fewer sutures. With each modification, there is a mandatory time lag to see if the results remain durable. However, if the laparoscopic approach is performed the same as open surgery, it would allow a more confident extrapolation of previously published outcomes to more contemporary series.

There is a lack of published data available regarding the success of laparoscopic surgery for the treatment of severe anterior vaginal prolapse. The majority of studies using a laparoscopic approach on the anterior vaginal wall are related to the treatment of urinary incontinence. The laparoscopic approach, as with the open abdominal approach, may be an option in patients whose prolapse can be addressed without vaginal reconstruction and who need concomitant abdominal surgery.

C. Vaginal Approach

Historically, in 1914, Kelly and Drum first described the anterior colporrhaphy as a treatment for stress incontinence (47). The continence results were disappointing, but repair of the anterior vaginal prolapse was successful, and this became a widely popularized treatment for cystoceles. The central pubocervical fascia defect is corrected by plicating the "fascia," imbricating the detrusor, and approximating the tissue in the midline. Because the goal of the initial "Kelly" plication was continence, the sutures were placed at the level of the proximal urethra and urethrovesical junction. Variations of the anterior colporrhaphy include the shape of the vaginal incision, extent of dissection, and which layers are plicated (4).

There have been numerous modifications to the anterior colporrhaphy, including the use of synthetic or allograft materials, suture placement, and anchoring techniques. Synthetic materials have been used to correct anterior vaginal wall prolapse since 1996, when Julian described the use of Marlex mesh to treat severe anterior prolapse (42). Currently, several materials are available for use, but the ideal biocompatible material should be chemically and physically inert, noncarcinogenic, durable, sterile, readily available, noninflammatory, and inexpensive.

Vaginal paravaginal repairs have also been popularized, either alone or in conjunction with an anterior colporrhaphy. The anatomic goal of the traditional abdominal approach (PVDR) is a reapproximation of the ATFP to the ATLA. From a vaginal approach, the objective is to reattach the anterolateral vaginal sulcus (ATFP) to the pubococcygeus muscle and fascia. Bone anchoring devices can also be used to place hardware to the underside of the pubic bone and/or Cooper's ligaments.

There have been successful reports of stage IV cystocele repair with cadaveric dermis (43) and cadaveric fascia lata (Tutoplast; Mentor Corp., Santa Barbara, CA) (44). These repairs address both the central and paravaginal defects, and incorporate allograft materials.

It would be ideal to use nonattenuated autologous fascia, but the size needed for complete vaginal reconstruction is prohibitive owing to the morbidity of harvest. One day genetic engineering may allow for the production of autologous materials for surgical use. We currently use polypropylene because it is nonabsorbable, macroporous, monofilamentous, flexible, and sterile. The large pore size (>75 μm) allows for the ingrowth of macrophages, fibroblasts, collagen, and blood vessels. This aids in rebuilding autologous tissue within the mesh and allows for the chemotaxis of macrophages in battling infection. Another theoretical advantage of monofilament mesh is that bacteria cannot infiltrate as they can with a multifilament composition (45). Stiffness is another important property that is related to pore size. A larger pore size confers greater flexibility, so that polypropylene (1500 μm) is more flexible than Marlex (600 μm). It is postulated that erosion is less likely with a larger pore size, because of the host tissue ingrowth and material flexibility.

VI. OUR TECHNIQUE

In the anterior compartment, we specifically address four defects: urethral hypermobility, lateral bladder support (paravaginal), perivesical fascia (central) support, and separation of sacrouterine ligaments. Options for surgical treatment include abdominal, laparoscopic, or vaginal approaches.

Four-Defect Repair of Stage IV Cystocele

1. Urethral hypermobility
2. Central defect (attenuation of perivesical fascia)
3. Paravaginal defect (attenuation of lateral vesicopelvic fascia)
4. Separation of the sacrouterine ligament complex

   With the patient in dorsal high-lithotomy position a 16F urethral catheter is placed to drain urine from the bladder. Exposure is maximized with a weighted vaginal speculum and a Scott ring retractor with six hooks (placed at the odd-numbered hands of a clock).

   If there is significant uterine prolapse, we proceed with hysterectomy and complete vault prolapse suspension prior to cystocele repair. The cuff is secured to the inferior edge of

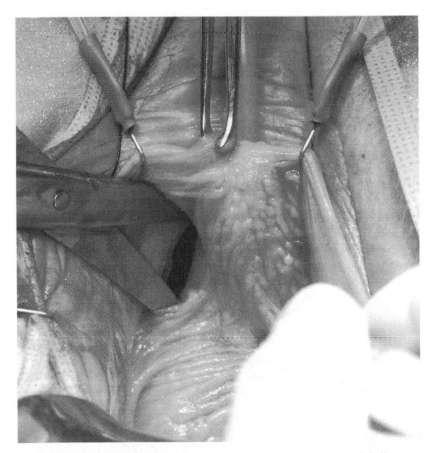

Figure 3   Metzenbaum scissors in the retropubic space. The urethropelvic ligament can be seen medially.

the uterosacral ligament complex bilaterally. If an enterocele is identified, we repair it prior to the cystocele repair, because these obliterative sutures will be used as the base of the cystocele repair. We close the cul-de-sac in purse-string configuration. These sutures distally incorporate the pararectal fascia, prerectal fascia, cardinal ligaments, and bladder wall within the peritoneum.

We initially perform a distal urethral prolene sling (DUPS) in all patients with stage IV cystoceles, as previously described (46). An Allis clamp is used to retract the urethra superiorly. Two oblique incisions are made in the distal vagina, carefully avoiding the inner labia. Metzenbaum scissors are used to expose the periurethral fascia. A small window is made in the retropubic space with the aid of a curved Mayo scissors directed to the patient's ipsilateral shoulder bilaterally. The medial edges of the urethropelvic ligaments are seen (Fig. 3). A tunnel between the vaginal wall and periurethral fascia is made at the level of the distal urethra with a fine right angle, ∼1.5 cm cephalad from the urethral meatus. A soft Prolene mesh sling, measuring 1 × 10 cm, is passed in through the superficial tunnel (Fig. 4). On each end there is a 0-polyglactin suture. The sling is positioned using the Raz double-pronged ligature carrier (Cook Urological, Spencer, IN) through a 1-cm midline transverse puncture. An Allis clamp is placed on each arm of the sling, on either side of the urethra, and held in a horizontal plane while tying down the sutures, to prevent tying the sling with too much tension. Additionally, the ties are only secured at the level of the superficial subcutaneous fat 3-mm below the skin. Incisions are closed with a running locking 3-0 polyglactin suture.

An Allis clamp is used to grasp the anterior vaginal wall at the point of greatest cystocele descent (about midway between the urethra and vaginal cuff) (Fig. 5). A vertical midline

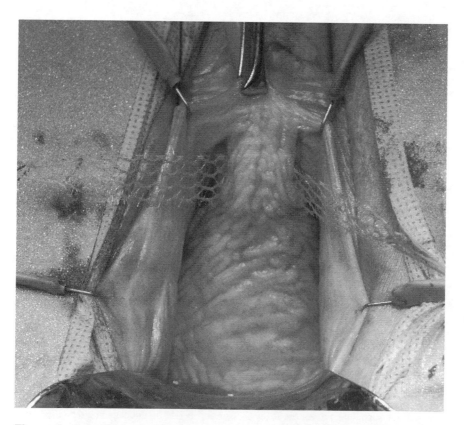

Figure 4   Superficial tunnel in the anterior vaginal wall for the distal urethral Prolene sling (DUPS).

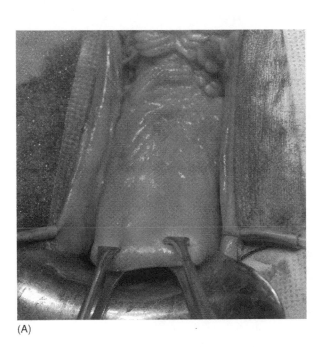

(A)

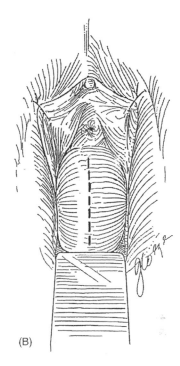

(B)

Figure 5 **(A)** Two Allis clamps are placed on the most distal anterior wall prolapse (correlating to point Ba). **(B)** A vertical incision will be made, extending proximally to the vaginal cuff.

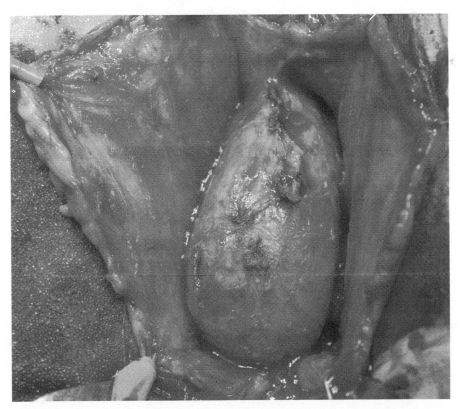

Figure 6 Exposure of the bladder and perivesical fascia utilizing the midline vertical incision.

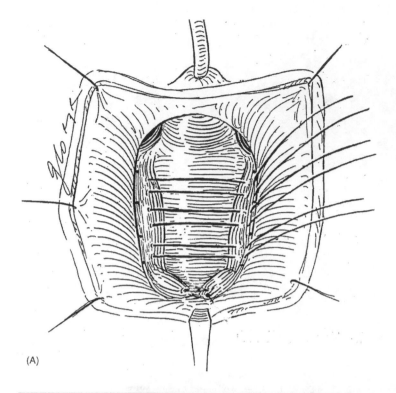

(A)

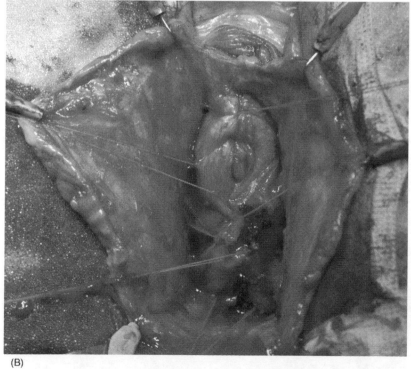

(B)

Figure 7 **(A)** Anterior colporrhaphy: interrupted sutures placed in the lateral perivesical fascia. **(B)** Horizontal mattress sutures imbricating the attenuated central defect (perivesical fascia).

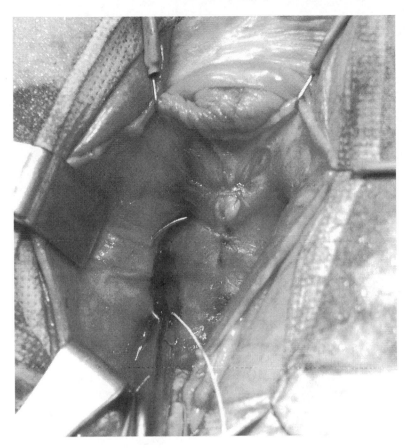

Figure 8   Vaginal paravaginal defect repair: lateral sutures placed in the infralevator obturator fascia just proximal to the descending pubic ramus.

incision is made in the anterior vaginal wall extending from the bladder neck to the vaginal cuff. The dissection is made laterally in the avascular plane between the vaginal wall and perivesical connective tissue. At the level of bladder, the lateral dissection exposes the vesicopelvic fascia to free the herniated bladder from the anterior vaginal wall (Fig. 6). The dissection is carried laterally until the descending ramus of the pubic bone is palpable bilaterally. This allows access to infralevator obturator "fascia" as it condenses on the pubic bone. This will be the basis of our vaginal paravaginal defect repair, as an immobile structure to secure the mesh. The vesicopelvic fascia can be identified and is noted to be thin medially, becoming thicker laterally toward the levator ani muscles. Posteriorly, the dissection will reach the peritoneal fold, exposing the attenuated and pathologically separated cardinal ligaments as they fuse with the pubocervical fascia. Sutures are placed through the cardinal ligaments and brought midline, to form the most proximal support of the bladder. If a hysterectomy or enterocele repair was done, we use the pursestring suture to mark the bladder base (sacrouterine ligaments).

The reconstruction starts with a central defect repair. Horizontal mattress sutures are placed in the lateral aspects of the perivesical fascia (3-0 polyglactin) from the bladder neck to the vaginal cuff (Fig. 7). Once all sutures have been placed, they can be tied in the anterior-to-posterior direction, after cystoscopy is done to ensure ureteral efflux and that the bladder is without injury. To correct the lateral defect, we place a 0-polyglactin suture through

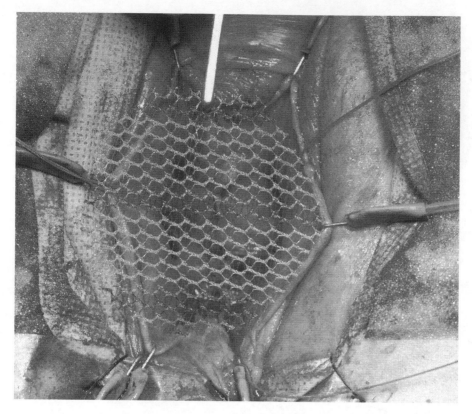

Figure 9 5 × 5 cm polypropylene mesh disk to be used in the four-defect cystocele repair. It will be secured to the plicated sacrouterine ligaments, obturator fascia, and vesicopelvic fascia at the level of the urethrovesical junction with 2-0 polyglactin.

the previously dissected infralevator obturator connective tissue (Fig. 8). After that, a circular soft Prolene mesh is cut in the shape of a disc (5 × 5 cm) (Fig. 9). This is secured to the previously plicated cardinal ligaments posteriorly and then the obturator fascias laterally. Two additional sutures are placed anteriorly, one on each side of the proximal urethra/bladder neck, to complete the fixation of the mesh.

If there was a vault repair, the colposuspension sutures (to the sacrouterine ligaments) are tied prior to trimming the excess vaginal wall. The vaginal incision is closed with a running 3-0 polyglactin suture. If a rectocele is present, we restore the rectovaginal "fascia," levator hiatus, and perineal defects. An antibiotic soaked vaginal pack is placed for 2–3 h. Most patients go home after 24 h of observation. The suprapubic tube is clamped and attempts at voiding are instituted prior to discharge.

The majority of patients void within 72 h, so placement of a suprapubic tube or urethral catheter (and possible preoperative teaching of intermittent catheterization) is the surgeon's preference. Because many of our patients are not local residents, we currently place a suprapubic tube and teach the patient how to remove it once postvoid residuals are <60 cc. We do keep the catheter for a minimum of 1 week to minimize possible urinary extravasation with its removal.

We have reported our promising results with the Prolene sling in treating stress urinary incontinence (46). We have had similar success in the treatment of prolapse and, importantly, have not had any cases of urinary obstruction or mesh erosion.

VII. CONCLUSION

The diagnosis and treatment of stage IV cystoceles is challenging, even to the most experienced pelvic surgeons. The etiology is multifactorial and most patients present with concomitant pelvic organ prolapse. A thorough preoperative evaluation allows one to address all pelvic floor anatomic defects at the time of surgery.

REFERENCES

1. Baden WF, Walker T. Surgical Repair of Vaginal Defects. Philadelphia: J.B. Lippincott, 1992.
2. Bump RC, Mattiasson A, Bo K. The standardization of terminology of female pelvic organ prolapse and pelvic floor dysfunction. Am J Obstet Gynecol 1996; 175(1):10–17.
3. Zimmern PE, Leach GE. The urological aspects of vaginal wall prolapse. Part I. Diagnosis and surgical indications. AUA Update Ser 1993 1993; 12(Lesson 25).
4. Weber AM, Walters MD. Anterior vaginal prolapse: review of anatomy and techniques of surgical repair. Obstet Gynecol 1997; 89(2):311–318.
5. Wall LL. The muscles of the pelvic floor. Clin Obstet Gynecol 1993; 36(4):910–925.
6. Norton PA. The role of fascia and ligaments. Clin Obstet Gynecol 1993; 36:926–938.
7. Babiarz JW, Raz S. Female urology. In: Pelvic Floor Relaxation. 2nd ed. Philadelphia: WB Saunders, 1996:445–456.
8. Strohbehn K. Normal pelvic floor anatomy. Obstet Gynecol Clin North Am 1998; 25(4):683–705.
9. DeLancey JO. Anatomy and biomechanics of genital prolapse. Clin Obstet Gynecol 1993; 36(4):897–909.
10. Farrell SA, Dempsey T, Geldenhuys L. Histologic examination of "fascia" used in colporrhaphy. Obstet Gynecol 2001; 98(5):794–798.
11. Nichols DH, Milley PS, Randall CL. Significance of restoration of normal vaginal depth and axis. Obstet Gynecol 1970; 36(2):251–255.
12. Shaw W. A study of surgical anatomy of the vagina, with special reference to the vaginal operations. BMJ 1947; 1:477–482.
13. Sharf B, Zilberman A, Sharf M, Mitrani A. Electromyogram of pelvic floor muscles in genital prolapse. Int J Gynecol Obstet 1976; 14:2–4.
14. Gilpin SA, Gosling JA, Smith ARB, Warrell DW. The pathogenesis of genitourinary prolapse and stress incontinence of urine: a histological and histochemical study. Br J Obstet Gynaecol 1999; 96:15–23.
15. Smith ARB, Hosker GL, Warrell DW. The role of partial denervation of the pelvic floor in the etiology of genitourinary prolapse and stress incontinence of urine: a neurophysiological study. Br J Obstet Gynaecol 1989; 96:24–28.
16. Makinen J, Kahari VM, Soderstrom KO, Vuorio E, Hirvonen T. Collagen synthesis in the vaginal connective tissue of patients with and without uterine prolapse. Eur J Obstet Gynaecol Reprod Biol 1987; 24:319–325.
17. Norton PA, Boyd C, Deak S. Collagen synthesis in women with genital prolapse or stress urinary incontinence. Neurourol Urodyn 1992; 11:300–301.
18. Dietz HP, Wilson PD. Colposuspension success and failure: a long term objective follow-up study. Int Urogynecol J Pelvic Floor Dysfunc 2000; 11(6):346–351.
19. Michael HS, Gousse AE, Rovner ES, Ginsberg DA, Raz S. 4-defect repair of grade 4 cystocele. J Urol 1999; 161:587–594.
20. Rodriguez LV, Raz S. Diagnostic imaging of pelvic floor dysfunction. Curr Opin Urol 2001; 11:423–428.
21. Gordon D, Pearce M, Norton PA, Stanton SL. Comparison of ultrasound and lateral chain urethrocystography in the determination of bladder neck descent. Am J Obstet Gynecol 1989; 160(1):182–184.
22. Dietz HP, Haylen BT, Broome J. Ultrasound in the quantification of female pelvic organ prolapse. Ultrasound Obstet Gynecol 2001; 18(5):511–514.

23. Kelvin FM, Maglinte DD, Hale DS, Benson JT. Female pelvic organ prolapse: a comparison of triphasic dynamic MR imaging and triphasic fluoroscopic cystocolpoproctography. AJR 2000; 174(1):81–88.

24. Vandbeckevoort D, Van Hoe L, Oyen R, Ponette E, DeRider D, Deprest J. Comparative study of colpocystodefecography and dynamic fast MR imaging. J Magn Reson 1999; 9:373–377.

25. Gallentine ML, Cespedes RD. Occult stress urinary incontinence and the effect of vaginal vault prolapse on abdominal leak point pressures. Urology 2001; 57(1):40–44.

26. Barnes NM, Dmochowski RR, Park R, Nitti VW. Pubovaginal sling and pelvic prolapse repair in women with occult stress urinary incontinence: effect on postoperative emptying and voiding symptoms. Urology 2002; 59:856–860.

27. Chaikin DC, Groutz A, Blaivas JG. Predicting the need for anti-incontinence surgery in continent women undergoing repair of severe urogenital prolapse. J Urol 2000; 163:531–534.

28. Ghoneim GM, Walters F, Lewis V. The value of the vagina pack test in large cystoceles. J Urol 1994; 152:931.

29. Bhatia NN, Bergman A. Pessary test in women with urinary incontinence. Obstet Gynecol 1985; 65:220.

30. Blaivas JG, Jacobs BZ. Pubovaginal fascial sling for the treatment of complicated stress urinary incontinence. J Urol 1991; 145:1214–1218.

31. Vasavada SP, Comiter CV, Raz S. Cystoscopic light test to aid in the differentiation of high-grade pelvic organ prolapse. Urology 1999; 54(4):1085–1087.

32. Beverly CM, Walters MD, Weber AM, Piedmonte MR, Ballard LA. Prevalence of hydronephrosis in patients undergoing surgery for pelvic organ prolapse. Obstet Gynecol 1997; 90:37–41.

33. Gemer O, Bergman M, Segal S. Prevalence of hydronephrosis in patients with genital prolapse. Eur J Obstet Gynecol Reprod Biol 1999; 86:11–13.

34. Richardson AC, Edmonds PB, Williams NL. Treatment of stress urinary incontinence due to paravaginal fascial defect. Obstet Gynecol 1981; 57:357–362.

35. Burch JC. Urethrovaginal fixation to Cooper's ligament for the correction of stress incontinence, cystocele, and prolapse. Am J Obstet Gynecol 1961; 88:281–290.

36. Bruce GR, El Galley R, Galloway N. Paravaginal defect repair in the treatment of female stress urinary incontinence and cystocele. Urology 1999; 54:647–651.

37. Weber AM, Walters MD, Piedmonte MR, Ballard LA. Anterior colporrhaphy: a randomized trial of 3 surgical techniques. Am J Obstet Gynecol 2001; 185(6):1299–1306.

38. Sullivan ES, Longaker CJ, Lee PYH. Total pelvic mesh repair. Dis Colon Rectum 2001; 44:857–863.

39. Vancaille TG, Schussler W. Laparoscopic bladder neck suspension. J Laparoendosc Surg 1991; 1:169–173.

40. Miklos JR, Kohli N. Laparoscopic paravagina repair plus Burch colposuspension: review and descriptive technique. Urology 2000; 56(6A):64–69.

41. El-Toukhy TA, Davies AE. The efficacy of laparoscopic mesh colposuspension: results of a prospective controlled study. BJU Int 2001; 88:361–366.

42. Julian TM. The efficacy of Marlex mesh in the repair of severe, recurrent vaginal prolapse of the anterior midvaginal wall. Am J Obstet Gynecol 1996; 175:1472–1475.

43. Chung SY, Franks M, Smith CP, Lee JY, Lu SH, Chancellor M. Technique of combine pubovaginal sling and cystocele repair using a single piece of cadaveric dermal graft. Urology 2002; 59:538–541.

44. Kobashi KC, Leach GE, Chon J, Govier FE. Continued multicenter followup of the cadaveric prolapse repair with sling. J Urol 2002; 168:2063–2068.

45. Cervigni M, Natale F. The use of synthetics in treatment of pelvic organ prolapse. Curr Opin Urol 2001; 11:429–435.

46. Rodriguez LV, Raz S. Polypropylene sling for the treatment of stress urinary incontinence. Urology 2001; 58(5).

47. Kelly HA, Dimm DM. Urinary incontinence in women without manifest injury to the bladder. Surg Gynecol Obstet 1914; 18:444–450.

43
Surgical Correction of Paravaginal Defects

Matthew D. Barber
Cleveland Clinic Foundation, Cleveland, Ohio, U.S.A.

I. INTRODUCTION

The durable surgical correction of pelvic organ prolapse remains a significant challenge for pelvic reconstructive surgeons. Prolapse of the anterior vaginal wall, usually in the form of a cystocele, is the most common form of pelvic organ prolapse (1). Recent studies suggest that, of the various segments of the vagina which may be involved in prolapse (anterior, posterior, or apical), the anterior vaginal wall is the segment most likely to demonstrate recurrent prolapse after reconstructive surgery (2). Additionally, normal anterior vaginal support plays an important role in supporting the urethra and loss of this support can contribute to the development of stress urinary incontinence (3). It is therefore important that the pelvic reconstructive surgeon understand the normal support mechanisms of the anterior vaginal wall and the full spectrum of techniques for correction of anterior vaginal prolapse and cystoceles.

In 1909, George R. White described a method of cystocele repair that consisted of "suturing the lateral sulci of the vagina to the white line of pelvic fascia" through a vaginal approach (4). His was the first known description of the paravaginal defect as a cause of anterior vaginal wall prolapse. As fortune would have it, Howard Kelly described his method of cystocele repair 4 years later and, perhaps owing to Kelly's renown and/or the relative simplicity of his operation, the Kelly plication and its modifications became the primary technique of cystocele repair for the next 70 years and White's concepts were largely forgotten (5). In 1976, Richardson et al. reintroduced the paravaginal defect repair, but described a technique of repair using an abdominal approach (6). They described isolated defects of the pubocervical "fascia" as the cause of anterior vaginal wall prolapse and, based on cadaveric dissections, concluded that the majority of cystoceles resulted from a detachment of the pubocervical fascia at or near its lateral attachment to the arcus tendineus fasciae pelvis (ATFP). Since this report, the paravaginal defect repair has become a widely used procedure for correcting anterior vaginal prolapse. Vaginal and laparoscopic techniques have also been described. This chapter will discuss the current understanding of anterior vaginal support and review the current concepts in diagnosis and surgical correction of paravaginal defects. Specifically, abdominal and vaginal paravaginal defect repairs will be discussed. Correcting paravaginal defects using the laparospcopic approach will be discussed in Chapter 44.

II. ANATOMY OF ANTERIOR VAGINAL SUPPORT

The vagina is a hollow, flattened fibromuscular tube lined with nonkeritinized stratified squamous epithelium. The longitudinal shape of the vagina resembles a trapezoid, being narrowest at the introitus and becoming progressively wider as you approach the vaginal apex and cervix. In the transverse dimension, the vagina is H-shaped at its distal end (toward the introitus) and flattened proximally (Figs. 1, 2). Underlying the vaginal epithelium is the vaginal muscularis, a well-developed layer made up primarily of smooth muscle along with collagen and elastin (7). Some have labeled this layer of the anterior vaginal wall *pubocervical fascia*. Although this term is widely used, the use of the term "fascia" is a misnomer, as it does not accurately reflect the histology of the vagina (7).

Normal, vaginal support is maintained by intact pelvic floor muscles and connective tissue supports. DeLancey described three levels of connective tissue support for the vagina (Fig. 2) (8). The cervix and top one-fourth of the vagina are suspended by the cardinal/uterosacral ligament complex (level I). The distal one-fourth is supported by fusion of the lower vagina to the urogenital diaphragm and perineal body (level III). The middle half (level II) is attached to the pelvic sidewall bilaterally. The lateral vagina attaches to the levator ani muscle on each side along a line from the anterior pubic rami to the ischial spine known as the "white line," or arcus tendineus fasciae pelvis (ATFP). The ATFP is formed from a condensation of the obturator internus and levator ani fascia and is composed primarily of organized fibrous collagen (9), making the lateral connective tissue attachment of the vagina more dense than the superior/apical connective tissue support of the cardinal and uterosacral complex (8). The distal aspect of the ATFP as it inserts into the inferior pubis can be found 35–55 mm below the pectineal line. The midportion of the ATFP is 25–50 mm directly below the obturator foramen, and its

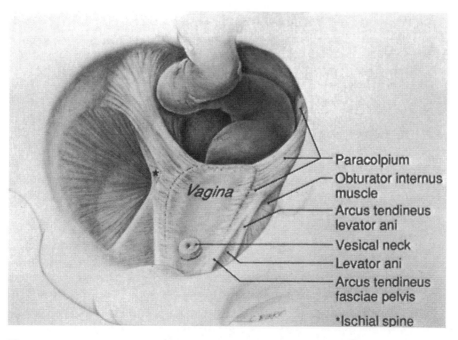

Figure 1   Vagina and supporting structure in a woman after hysterectomy. Bladder has been removed above vesical neck. (∗) indicates location of ischial spine. Note the lateral attachment of the vagina to the arcus tendinious fasica pelvis. (From Ref. (8).)

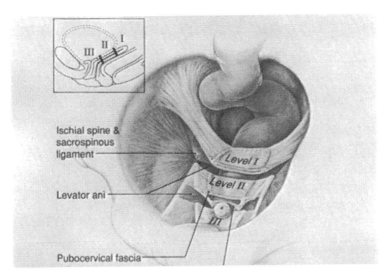

Ischial spine & sacrospinous ligament

Levator ani

Pubocervical fascia

Level I

Level II

III

III   II   I

Figure 2 Levels of vaginal support: level I, apical support from the cardinal/uterosacral ligament complex; level II, vagina is attached to arcus tendineus fascia pelvis (ATFP) laterally; level III, distal perineal fusion. Note that in the distal vagina, the vaginal cross section is H-shaped and in the proximal vagina, the vaginal cross section resembles a flattened tube. [From Ref. (8).]

proximal end predictably terminates at the ischial spine (10). DeLancey demonstrated, through careful cadaveric dissections, that transecting level I support results in apical prolapse, while detaching level II support results in anterior vaginal prolapse and cystoceles (8). The loss of lateral, or level II, support is often referred to as a paravaginal defect.

Strobehn and DeLancey conceptualized the paravaginal defect as similar to a semiadhesive note being peeled off a wall as described in Figure 3 (11). Shull has noted that paravaginal defects may occur in three forms: the entire arcus may remain attached to the pelvic sidewall with the lateral vagina breaking away from the arcus; the ATFP may pull away from the side of the pelvis but remain attached to the lateral vagina; or the ATFP may split with a portion of it remaining attached to the levator ani and a portion attached to the lateral vagina (12).

The anterior vaginal wall provides support to the urethra and may play an important role in urinary continence. The urethra lies on a hammocklike supportive layer composed of endopelvic connective tissue and anterior vaginal wall. DeLancey hypothesized that increased intra-abdominal pressure, as with a cough or sneeze, causes compression of the urethra against this hammocklike layer, thereby compressing the urethral lumen closed (3). The stability of the sub-urethral layer depends on the intact connection of the anterior vaginal wall and its connective tissue attachments to the ATFP and levator ani muscles. Detachment of the anterior vaginal wall from the pelvic sidewall, or relaxation of the anterior vaginal wall itself, can result in ure-thral hypermobility and genuine stress incontinence. With this in mind, some have advocated reattachment of the anterior vaginal wall to its lateral attachments (a paravaginal defect repair) as a treatment for genuine stress incontinence. Urethral support is not the only factor involved in urinary continence; competence of the urethral sphincter itself plays an important role. This may partially explain why paravaginal defect repair has had only modest success as an anti-incontinence procedure.

Anterior vaginal prolapse can result from loss of midline, lateral, and/or superior support. In Richardson's original study he reported loss of lateral support (paravaginal defects) in 67% of

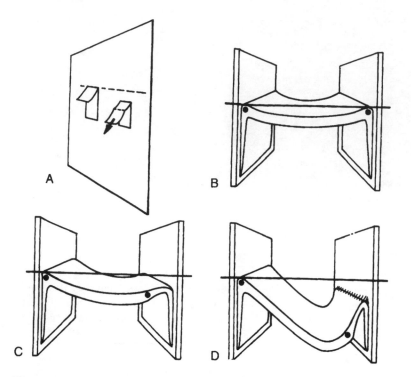

Figure 3   A semiadhesive note is an example of paravaginal defect of the vagina (A). Imagine a creased note pasted at a right angle to the wall, so that its free edge, representing the anterior vaginal wall, projects obliquely toward the floor (B). The crease of the note represents the pubocervical fascia that normally inserts at the arcus tendineus fascia pelvis overlying the fascia of the levator ani muscle, represented by the wall (C). As traction is applied to the note (the anterior vaginal wall), the note peels away from the wall (levator ani muscle) (D). [From Ref. (9).]

his 93 patients with "symptomatic anterior quadrant relaxation" (6). Three-quarters of his patients with paravaginal defects had unilateral loss of support, with the majority being right-sided. In contrast to this early study, some authors have found that in women with advanced anterior vaginal prolapse (ICS stage III or IV), paravaginal defects occur in fewer than half and that when they do occur, bilateral, rather than unilateral, loss of support is found most often (13,14).

III.   DIAGNOSIS OF PARAVAGINAL DEFECTS

A.   Physical Examination

A method for clinically identifying paravaginal defects in women with prolapse was originally described by Richardson in 1976 and utilized two tongue blades to mimic lateral vaginal support (6). Shull, using the original ideas of Richardson and subsequent work by Baden and Walker, later described a more standardized method to clinically evaluate anterior wall support defects (15). A curved ring forceps is placed in the lateral vaginal sulci and directed toward the ischial spines along the course of the ATFP to reproduce the lateral support of the vagina. A Sims speculum is placed posteriorly to expose the anterior vaginal wall and reduce any posterior prolapse. The patient is asked to strain maximally, and, if complete reduction of the anterior prolapse occurs with the ring forceps in this position, she is thought to have paravaginal defects. If, when she strains, the anterior vagina continues to bulge between the arms of the ring forceps without any evidence of reduction, this suggests a midline loss of support. If supporting the lateral vagina results in partial reduction of the prolapse, she is thought to have lost both midline and lateral support. Unilateral elevation of each vaginal sulcus allows differentiation of bilateral and unilateral paravaginal defects.

Current evidence suggests that this technique of physically assessing anterior vaginal support may not accurately reflect findings at the time of surgery, however. A study of 117 women found a discrepancy between the prevalence of paravaginal defects noted at a standardized preoperative clinical examination (63%) and the prevalence of discrete paravaginal detachment noted at surgery (42%) (13). The clinical finding of paravaginal defects in this study was sensitive (sensitivity 92%) but not specific (specificity 52%) and had an adequate negative predictive value (91%), but low positive predictive value (61%). Subjects in whom normal paravaginal support was found at physical examination usually had intact paravaginal support confirmed at surgery, but fewer than two-thirds of women who were thought to have paravaginal defects based on physical examination actually had them at the time of surgery. Accuracy of the clinical examination was not affected by previous anterior colphorraphy, previous hysterectomy, or stage of prolapse, but a significant decrease in examination accuracy was noted in patients who had undergone previous retropubic urethropexy (13).

B. Radiology

Several authors have used magnetic resonance imaging (MRI) to evaluate lateral vaginal support. Aronson et al. used a vaginally placed endoluminal coil coupled to a pelvic phased-array coil to image periurethral and paravaginal anatomy in four continent and four incontinent women (16). Lateral vaginal attachment was seen in all four of the continent women (Fig. 4). In two of the four incontinent women, paravaginal defects were suspected on clinical examination, and lateral detachment of the vagina from the levator ani muscles was clearly seen in both of these women. In another study, Huddleston et al. demonstrated bilateral paravaginal defects using MRI and a standard body coil in 12 women with genuine stress incontinence and clinically suspected paravaginal defects (17). The preoperative MRI findings were confirmed intraoperatively, and postoperative MRI revealed intact paravaginal attachment in 10 of 12 women after retropubic paravaginal defect repair. Although MRI appears promising for preoperative detection of paravaginal defects, it is expensive and not universally available. It is therefore unlikely that MRI will replace clinical examination as the preoperative assessment of choice for pelvic organ prolapse.

Ultrasonography is less expensive than MRI, more widely available, and commonly used to image pelvic organs. Unfortunately, studies investigating the use of ultrasound to diagnose paravaginal defects have shown mixed results. Ostrzenski et al. investigated the use of transabdominal ultrasonography for the detection of paravaginal defects (18,19). They placed a water-filled condom into the vagina as a contrast medium and made the ultrasound diagnosis of paravaginal detachment if the bladder appeared to sag on either side of the water-filled vagina. Using this technique, they found that paravaginal defects were present in all of 16 women with genuine stress incontinence and in two of the three primiparous continent women in their study. None of the five nulliparous continent patients in their study demonstrated paravaginal defects clinically or ultrasonographically (19). Surgery confirmed paravaginal defects in all of the patients with genuine stress incontinence. In contrast, Nguyen et al. found that the ultrasound appearance of paravaginal defects could be demonstrated in both patients with and without clinically apparent prolapse and that the size of the apparent defect directly correlated with the amount of water

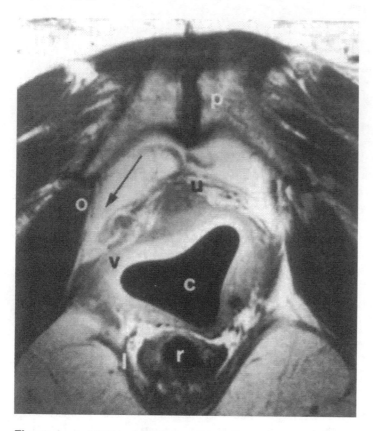

Figure 4   Axial T1-weighted image from a 57-year-old woman with genuine stress urinary incontinence, showing full field of view of paravaginal detachment (arrow) at level of urethrovesical junction. p, pubic symphysis; u, urethra; o, obturator internus muscle; v, vaginal wall; c, endovaginal coil; l, levator ani muscle; r, rectum. [From Ref. (16).]

in the vaginal balloon (20). They concluded that the appearance of lateral bladder sagging that suggested paravaginal detachment was actually an artifact created by the intravaginal water-filled balloon. Based on these findings, it appears that ultrasonography is not a useful tool for detecting paravaginal defects, at least using the only technique that has been described in the literature thus far.

It is important to understand the limitations of the clinical and radiographic assessment of pelvic relaxation. The preoperative evaluation for specific defects in pelvic support is important in planning the surgical repair of pelvic organ prolapse, but until better techniques are available, neither physical examination nor radiology can substitute for a careful intraoperative assessment of vaginal support defects.

IV. SURGICAL TECHNIQUES

The goal of the paravaginal defect repair is to correct anterior vaginal wall prolapse that results from loss of lateral support by reattaching the lateral vaginal sulcus to its normal attachment site along the ATFP. This can be performed abdominally (retropubically), vaginally, or laparoscopically. As many patients may have loss of midline and/or superior (level I) support in addition to loss of lateral support (paravaginal defects), the reconstructive pelvic surgeon may need to combine the paravaginal defect repair with an anterior colporraphy and/or a vaginal vault suspension in order to completely correct a patient's anterior vaginal prolapse.

A. Abdominal (Retropubic) Approach

The patient is placed in modified lithotomy position using low leg holders such as Allen stirrups, and is draped to allow both abdominal and vaginal access. The bladder is drained with a Foley catheter. The abdomen may be entered through either a transverse or vertical abdominal incision. While this procedure may be performed entirely retroperitoneally, entering the peritoneal cavity and packing the bowel out of the pelvis often provides better visualization of the retropubic space. Entering the peritoneal cavity also allows for concurrent hysterectomy or additional abdominal prolapse repairs that may be necessary. The retropubic space is entered, and the bladder is retracted medially to expose the lateral aspect of the retropubic space. The pubic bone, obturator muscle, obturator fossa, and neurovascular bundle identified. Blunt dissection is used to identify the lateral vagina, urethra, and ischial spine. A fluffed-up gauze and a medium malleable retractor can be useful to retract the bladder medially to expose these lateral structures. The normal site of lateral vaginal attachment on the pelvic sidewall from the interior aspect of the superior pubic ramus to the ischial spine is then identified. If the lateral vagina is avulsed from this attachment site, then a paravaginal defect is present. As physical examination is less than perfect in identifying paravaginal detachment, a bilateral assessment of paravaginal support should be made in all patients in whom paravaginal defects are suspected.

The surgeon's nondominant hand is the placed into the vagina and used to elevate the lateral superior vaginal sulcus to its site of normal attachment along the course of the ATFP. Typically, four to six simple interrupted stitches of nonabsorbable suture (No. 0 or 2-0) are used to reattach the lateral vagina to the ATFP. The first suture is placed through the full thickness (excluding the vaginal epithelium) of the lateral vaginal apex and then through the ATFP and the aponeurosis of the levator ani muscle just distal to the ischial spine. This suture is tied and cut. Additional sutures are placed at 1-cm intervals through the lateral vaginal wall and into the levator ani aponeurosis along the entire course of the ATFP. In patients with a cystocele and genuine stress incontinence, many surgeons combine an abdominal paravaginal repair with a Burch colposuspension (Fig. 5). At the end of the procedure, cystoscopy should be performed to document ureteral patency and the absence of intravesical sutures. Closed-suction drainage of the retropubic space is rarely indicated. Postoperatively, the bladder is drained with either a transurethral or suprapubic catheter until normal voiding occurs.

B. Vaginal Approach

Paravaginal defect repair using the transvaginal approach can be more challenging than the retropubic approach, but offers the advantage of avoiding an abdominal incision and facilitating a concurrent anterior colporrhaphy for those women with loss of midline as well as lateral anterior vaginal support. The technique begins similar to that of an anterior colporrhaphy. Patients are placed in dorsal lithotomy position. A Foley catheter is used to drain the bladder. A weighted speculum is placed into the vagina. A midline vertical incision is made through the vaginal epithelium from the midurethra to the vaginal apex. The vaginal epithelium is then sharply dissected off the underlying vaginal muscularis, and the dissection is continued laterally to the pelvic sidewall from immediately behind the pubic rami to the level of the ischial spine. Visualization of the adipose tissue of the retropubic space from this transvaginal approach confirms the presence of a paravaginal defect, as normal lateral attachment of the anterior vaginal

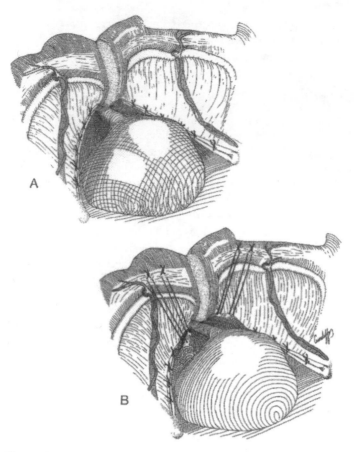

Figure 5   (**A**) Retropubic approach to the paravaginal defect repair. The avulsed vaginal sulcus has been sutured to the arcus tendineus fascia pelvis bilaterally. (**B**) The paravaginal repair has been combined with a Burch colposuspension to provide preferential support to the urethrovesical junction. [From Ref. (34).]

wall would preclude this. If visualization is limited, gentle palpation of the lateral attachment site can be used. The ability of the examining finger to enter the retropubic space indicates a paravaginal defect. Every precaution should be taken to avoid iatrogenic creation of paravaginal defects with dissection, palpation, or retractors.

Once a paravaginal defect is identified, the normal site of lateral attachment of the vagina should be clearly visualized. This can be facilitated by placing a gauze sponge through the paravaginal defect into the retropubic space and using a narrow deaver retractor to retract the sponge, underlying adipose tissue, and lateral bladder anteriorly. A Briesky-Navratil retractor can then be used to retract the remainder of the bladder medially, clearly exposing the levator ani muscle and the course of the ATFP from the ischial spine to the inferior aspect of the pubic ramus. Five to seven interrupted nonabsorbable sutures (No. 0 or 2-0) are placed at 1-cm intervals through the ATFP and the aponeurosis of the levator ani muscle from the level of the ischial spine to the pubic symphysis at 1-cm intervals and their needles left on. Once all of the stitches are placed through the ATFP, the sponge in the retropubic space is removed. Each stitch is then placed through the lateral edge of the detached vaginal muscularis (*pubocervical "fascia"*) at their corresponding level and then tied. Once paravaginal support has been assessed and, if necessary, restored on both sides, a midline plication of pubocervical "fasica" (anterior colporrhaphy), a bladder neck plication, or sling can be performed, as necessary. The vaginal epithelium is then trimmed and closed. If a vaginal hysterectomy is needed, this should be performed prior to the paravaginal defect repair. If a vaginal vault suspension or culdeplasty is necessary, these sutures should be placed prior to the paravaginal defect repair, but not tied until the paravaginal defect repair has been completed. As with the retropubic approach, cystoscopy should be performed at the end of the procedure to confirm ureteral patency and the absence of intravesical sutures. Transurethral or suprapubic bladder drainage should continue until normal voiding occurs (Figs. 6–9).

V. SURGICAL OUTCOMES

A. Genuine Stress Incontinence

Richardson et al. introduced the retropubic paravaginal defect repair in 1976 as an operation for correction of defects of lateral vaginal support that resulted in cystourethroceles and stress urinary incontinence (6). In this initial report, they described their experience treating 60 women with both anterior vaginal prolapse and "significant" stress urinary incontinence that resulted

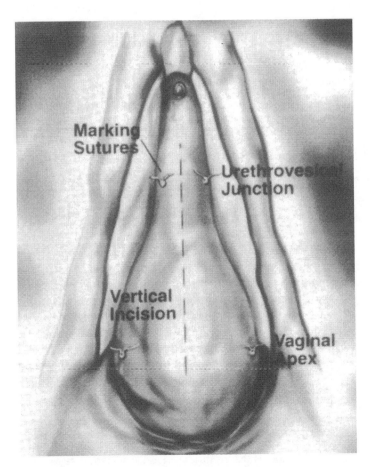

Figure 6 Vaginal paravaginal repair. Marking sutures placed at urethrovesical junction and vaginal apices. [From Ref. (32).]

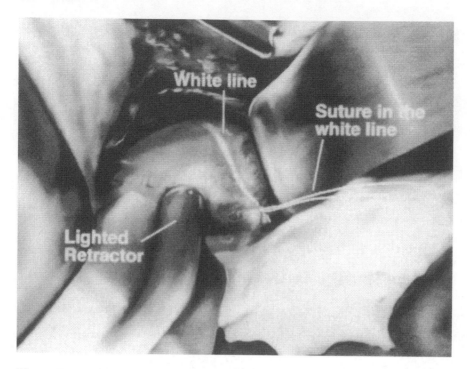

Figure 7 Vaginal paravaginal repair. A right-angle retractor is in the retropubic space, retracting the bladder medially. The suture is through the arcus tendineus fasciae pelvis ~2 cm ventral to the ischial spine. [From Ref. (32).]

from paravaginal defects. After an average of follow-up of 20 months, 86% of their patients were subjectively cured of their stress incontinence, and an additional 6% were improved. Additionally, all but two patients had satisfactory correction of their anterior vaginal prolapse. Over the next 15 years, a number of authors published the results of case series that demonstrated similar encouraging results with cure rates from 86% to 97%. Table 1 summarizes the results of studies in which the retropubic paravaginal defect repair was used as the sole anti-incontinence operation.

In spite of these encouraging early results, evidence suggests that paravaginal defect repair is not as effective as other standard anti-incontinence procedures such as the Burch or MMK retropubic urethropexies or the suburethral sling. In 1996, Colombo et al. published the results of a randomized trial comparing Burch colposuspension to paravaginal defect repair for treatment of genuine stress incontinence (21). This is the only randomized trial evaluating paravaginal defect repair as an anti-incontinence operation. They found that paravaginal defect repair was inferior to Burch colposuspension for treatment of genuine stress incontinence. The subjective cure rate for the Burch procedure in this trial was 100%, compared with 72% for paravaginal defect repair. Similarly, the objective (urodynamic) cure rates in this trial were 100% for Burch and 61% for paravaginal defect repair. These authors concluded that paravaginal defect repair should not be recommended for treatment of stress incontinence (21).

One reason why the paravaginal defect repair may be inferior to other anti-incontinence procedures is that it does not preferentially support the urethra or bladder neck, but rather provides equal support along the entire length of the anterior vaginal wall. In the Columbo et al. study, Burch urethropexy significantly increased the functional urethral length and pressure

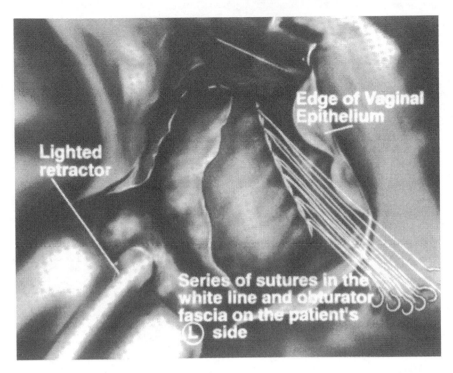

Figure 8 Vaginal paravaginal repair. A series of sutures has been placed in the arcus tendineus fasciae pelvis from a point ventral to the ischial spine to the back of the pubic bone. [From Ref. (32).]

transmission ratio measured in the proximal two-thirds of the urethra, whereas the paravaginal defect repair did not (21). Because of this, some surgeons have opted to combine the paravaginal defect repair with a retropubic urethropexy in order to gain the advantages of both operations. Thompson et al. refer to this combination as a "paravaginal plus," and found in a retrospective review of 454 patients that the combination of the paravaginal defect repair with a MMK procedure provided a higher cure rate for stress urinary incontinence than either urethropexy alone or paravaginal defect repair alone (22). In addition to its retrospective design, a weakness of this report is that the group who received the paravaginal defect repair alone was followed for over a year longer than the other two groups.

Paravaginal defect repair using the transvaginal approach has been used infrequently as an isolated procedure for treatment stress urinary incontinence. Current evidence suggests that it has less than satisfactory results when used in this capacity (Table 2). In a recent report by Mallipeddi et al., 57% of subjects with anterior vaginal prolapse and genuine stress incontinence treated with a vaginal paravaginal repair and a bladder neck plication had persistent urinary incontinence after an average of 1.6 years of follow-up (23). These authors concluded that while the vaginal paravaginal repair is safe and effective for correction of anterior vaginal prolapse, it has limited applicability in the surgical correction of genuine stress incontinence.

B. Anterior Vaginal Prolapse

The paravaginal defect repair has been widely used for correction of anterior vaginal prolapse thought to result from lateral vaginal detachment. Current evaluation of the success rate of this procedure for treatment of anterior vaginal prolapse is limited to case series and retrospective

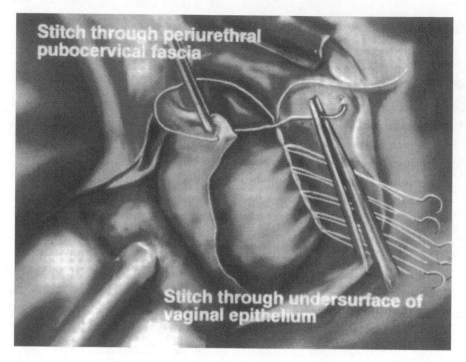

Figure 9 Vaginal paravaginal repair. The suture in the arcus tendineus faciae pelvis near the pubic bone is also sewn into the lateral margin of the pubocervical fascia periurethrally at the site of the marking suture at the urethrovesical junction. (From Ref. (32).)

reviews. Reports of retropubic paravaginal repair demonstrate anatomic success rates ranging from 92% to 97% (Table 3), and reports of vaginal paravaginal repair demonstrate success rates of 76–100% (Table 4) after variable lengths of follow-up. Failure or recurrence of anterior vaginal prolapse after paravaginal defect may occur laterally, centrally, or both. Elkins et al. reported a 8% lateral recurrence rate and a 22% central recurrence rate after transvaginal paravaginal defect repair in 25 patients with grade III or greater pelvic organ prolapse (24). At the time of the initial surgery, bulging of the midline bladder wall that was present after paravaginal repair was repaired with purse-string or imbricating sutures. Young et al. retrospectively evaluated 100 subjects who underwent vaginal paravaginal repair along with other reconstructive procedures for symptomatic pelvic organ prolapse (25). Subjects received an anterior colporraphy and a vaginal paravaginal repair if a midline cystocele was thought to be present in addition to paravaginal defects. They found a lateral anterior wall recurrence rate of 2% and a central anterior recurrence rate of 22% after an average of 11 months of follow-up (25). Other studies do not provide separate results of lateral versus central recurrence. To date there are no studies comparing paravaginal defect repair with or without midline anterior repair to traditional anterior colporraphy alone.

C. Complications

Complications after paravaginal defect repair are, for the most part, infrequent. Febrile morbidity occurs in 6–20% of patients and is most often self-limited. Lower urinary tract injury occurs in 0–4%, similar to other pelvic reconstructive procedures (26). In the randomized trial

Table 1 Outcomes of Abdominal Paravaginal Repair for Treatment of Genuine Stress Incontinence

| Study (year) | No. of patients | Study design | Follow-up | | Dry (%) | Improved (%) | Failed (%) |
			Mean	Range			
Richardson et al. (1976) (6)	60	Retrospective cohort	20 mo	3–48 mo	86	6	8
Richardson et al. (1981) (29)	233	Retrospective cohort	NR	2–8 yr	88	7	5
Baden and Walker (1987) (30)	215	Retrospective cohort	NR	2–15 yr	85	NR	15
Shull and Baden (1989) (14)	149	Retrospective cohort	48 mo	0.5–6 yr	97	0	3
Colombo et al. (1996) (21)[a]	18	Randomized trial	2.2 yr	1–3 yr	72	5	22
Thompson et al. (1998) (22)[b]	130	Retrospective cohort with controls	39.5 mo	NR	49	31	20
Bruce et al. (1999) (28)[c]	25	Retrospective cohort with control	17 mo	NR	72	12	16

NR, not reported.
[a]Randomized trial of Burch colposuspension ($n = 18$) versus abdominal paravaginal repair ($n = 18$). Subjective cure rate for Burch group (100%) was significantly higher than that of the paravaginal group (72%) ($P = 0.02$)
[b]Study retrospectively compared cure rates of paravaginal repair ($n = 130$; dry, 49%; improved, 31%; failure, 20%), retropubic urethropexy ($n = 194$; dry, 64%; improved, 20%; failure, 16%) and paravaginal repair combined with retropubic urethropexy ($n = 130$; dry, 78%; improved, 14%; failure, 8%).
[c]Study retrospectively reported cure rates of paravaginal repair for stress urinary incontinence with bladder neck hypermobility ($n = 25$; dry, 72%, improved, 12%; failure, 16%) and of paravaginal repair with rectus muscle sling for stress urinary incontinence due to intrinsic sphincteric deficiency ($n = 27$; dry, 85%, improved, 8%, failure, 7%).

performed by Columbo et al., paravaginal defect repair resulted in a quicker return to normal voiding and a lower long-term catheterization rate than the Burch cystourethropexy (11% vs. 17%, respectively). The rate of irritable bladder symptoms postoperatively was low in both groups (0% and 5%, respectively) (21). While paravaginal repair through the vaginal approach

Table 2 Outcomes of Vaginal Paravaginal Repair for Treatment of Genuine Stress Incontinence

| Study (year) | No. of patients | Study design | Follow-up | | Cure (%) | Failed (%) |
			Mean	Range		
Baden and Walker (1987) (30)	47	Retrospective cohort	NR	2–15 yr	77	33
Farrel and Ling (1997) (31)	27	Retrospective cohort	8 mo	NR	96	4
Mallipeddi et al. (2001) (23)	21	Retrospective cohort	20 mo	0.8–35 mo	43	57

NR, not reported.

Table 3 Outcomes of Abdominal Paravaginal Repair for Treatment of Anterior Vaginal Prolapse

Study (year)	No. of patients	Study design	Follow-up		Cure (%)	Failed (%)
			Mean	Range		
Richardson et al. (1976) (6)	60	Retrospective cohort	20 mo	3–48 mo	97	3
Richardson et al. (1981) (29)	233	Retrospective cohort	NR	2–8 yr	95	5
Shull and Baden (1989) (14)	149	Retrospective cohort	48 mo	0.5–6 yr	95	5
Bruce et al. (1999) (28)	52	Retrospective cohort	17 mo	NR	92	8
Scotti et al. (1998) (27)[a]	40	Prospective cohort	39 mo	7–52 mo	97	3

NR, not reported.

[a]Paravaginal attachment site included ischial periosteum and obturator membrane in addition to arcus tendinius fasciae pelvis.

offers some potential advantages over the retropubic approach including shorter recovery time, the ability to simultaneously correct midline anterior defects and the avoidance of an abdominal incision, it may have a higher rate of intraoperative hemorrhage and blood transfusion. Young et al. reported a 9% blood transfusion rate in their series of 100 vaginal paravaginal repairs, and three patients required intraoperative vascular surgery consultation (25). Similarly, 12% of patients received a blood transfusion in the Elkins et al. series of 25 patients who received a vaginal paravaginal repair (26). This is in contrast to a transfusion rate of 0–4% in series of

Table 4 Outcomes of Vaginal Paravaginal Repair for Treatment of Anterior Vaginal Prolapse

Study (year)	No. of patients	Study design	Follow-up		Cure (%)	Failed (%)
			Mean	Range		
White (1909) (4)	19	Retrospective cohort	NR	Up to 3 yr	100	0
Shull et al. (1994) (32)	62	Retrospective cohort	1.6 yr	0.1–5.6 yr	76	24
Farrell and Ling (1997) (31)	27	Retrospective cohort	8 mo	NR	80	20
Nguyen and Bhatia (1999) (33)	10	Retrospective cohort	1 yr	NR	100	0
Elkins et al. (2000) (24)	25	Retrospective cohort	NR	0.5–3 yr	76	24
Mallipeddi et al. (2001) (23)	35	Retrospective cohort	20 mo	8–35 mo	97	3
Young (2001) (25)	100	Retrospective cohort	11 mo	1–36 mo	78	22

NR, not reported.

abdominal paravaginal defect repair (6,14,21,27,28). The limited exposure and technical challenge of the vaginal approach likely explain this difference.

VI. CONCLUSION

Anterior vaginal prolapse commonly results from loss of lateral vaginal support. Paravaginal defect repairs appear to be effective in correcting this loss of lateral support and can be performed from abdominal, vaginal, or laparoscopic approaches. Although initially advocated as a treatment for genuine stress urinary incontinence, current evidence suggests that it is less effective than other standard anti-incontinence procedures. Studies evaluating the long-term efficacy of the paravaginal defect repair and studies comparing paravaginal defect repair with other procedures for treating anterior vaginal prolapse are necessary.

REFERENCES

1.   Samuelsson EC, Victor FTA, Tibblin G, Svardsud KF. Signs of genital prolapse in a Swedish population of women 20 to 59 years of age and possible related factors. Am J Obstet Gynecol 1999; 180:299–305.
2.   Shull BL, Bachofen C, Coates KW, Kuehl TJ. A transvaginal approach to repair of apical and other associated sites of pelvic organ prolapse with uterosacral ligaments. Am J Obstet Gynecol 2000; 183:1365–1373.
3.   DeLancey JOL. Structural support of the urethra as it relates to stress urinary incontinence: the hammock hypothesis. Am J Obstet Gynecol 1994; 170:1713–1723.
4.   White GR. Cystocele. JAMA 1909; 21:1707–1710.
5.   Kelly HA. Incontinence of urine in women. Urol Cutaneous Rev 1913; 17:291–293.
6.   Richardson AC, Lyon JB, Williams NL. A new look at pelvic relaxation. Am J Obstet Gynecol 1976; 126:568–571.
7.   Weber AM, Walters MD. Anterior vaginal prolapse: review of anatomy and techniques of surgical repair. Am J Obstet Gynecol 1997; 89:311–318.
8.   DeLancey JO. Anatomic aspects of vaginal eversion after hysterectomy. Am J Obstet Gynecol 1992; 166:1717–1724.
9.   Strohbehn K. Normal pelvic floor anatomy. Obstet Gynecol Clin North Am 1998; 25:683–705.
10.   Mauroy B, Goullet E, Stefaniak X. Bonnal JL, Amara N. Tendinous arch of the pelvic fascia: application to the technique of paravaginal colposuspension. Surg Radiol Anat 2000; 22:73–79.
11.   Strohbehn K, DeLancey JOL. The anatomy of stress incontinence. Oper Tech Gynecol Surg 1997; 2:5–16.
12.   Shull BL. How I do the abdominal paravaginal repair. J Pelvic Surg 1995; 1:43–46.
13.   Barber MD, Cundiff GW, Weidner AC, Coates KW, Bump RC, Addison WA. Accuracy of clinical assessment of paravaginal defects in women with anterior vaginal wall prolapse. Am J Obstet Gynecol 1999; 181:87–90.
14.   Shull BL, Baden WF. A six-year experience with paravaginal defect repair for stress urinary incontinence. Am J Obstet Gynecol 1989; 160:1432–1439.
15.   Shull BL. Clinical evaluation of women with pelvic support defects. Clin Obstet Gynecol 1993; 36:939–951.
16.   Aronson MP, Bates SM, Jacoby AF, Chelmow D, Sant GR. Periurethral and paravaginal anatomy: an endovaginal magnetic resonance imaging study. Am J Obstet Gynecol 1995; 173:1702–1708.
17.   Huddleston HT, Dunnihoo DR, Huddleston PM, Meyers PC. Magnetic resonance imaging of defects in DeLancy's vaginal support levels I, II, III. Am J Obstet Gynecol 1995; 172:1778–1782.

18. Ostrzenski A, Osborne NG, Ostrenska K. Method for diagnosing paravaginal defects using contrast ultrasonograpic technique. J Ultrasound Med 1997; 16:673–677.

19. Ostrzenski A, Osborne NG. Ultrasonography as a screening tool for paravaginal defects in women with stress incontinence: a pilot study. Int Urogynecol J 1998; 9:195–199.

20. Nguyen JK, Hall CD, Bhatia NN. Sonographic diagnosis of paravaginal defects: A standardization of technique. Int Urogynecol J 2000; 11:341-345.

21. Colombo M, Milani R, Vitobello D, Maggioni A. A randomized comparison of Burch colposuspension and abdominal paravaginal defect repair for female stress urinary incontinence. Am J Obstet Gynecol 1996; 175:78–84.

22. Thompson PK, Mooney RJ, Plummer A, Bahar VT. Paravaginal plus: a better incontinence operation? J Pelvic Surg 1998; 4:157–162.

23. Mallipeddi PK, Steele AC, Kohli N, Karram MM. Anatomic and functional outcome of vaginal paravaginal repair in the correction of anterior vaginal prolapse. Int Urogynecol J 2001; 12:83–88.

24. Elkins TE, Chesson RR, Videla F, Menefee S, Yordan R, Barksdale PA. Transvaginal paravaginal repair: a useful adjunctive procedure in pelvic relaxation surgery. J Pelvic Surg 2000; 1:11–15.

25. Young SB, Daman JJ, Bony LG. Vaginal paravaginal repair: one-year outcomes. Am J Obstet Gynecol 2001; 185:1360–1367.

26. Harris RL, Cundiff GW, Theofrastous JP, Yoon H, Bump RC, Addison WA. The value of intraoperative cystoscopy in urogynecologic and reconstructive pelvic surgery. Am J Obstet Gynecol 1997; 177:1367–1369.

27. Scotti RJ, Garely AD, Greston WM, Flora RF, Olson TR. Paravaginal repair of lateral vaginal wall defects by fixation to the ischial periosteum and obturator membrane. Am J Obstet Gynecol 1998; 179:1436–1445.

28. Bruce GR, El-Galley RES, Galloway NTM. Paravaginal defect repair in the treatment of female stress urinary incontinence and cystocle. Urology 1999; 54:647–651.

29. Richardson AC, Edmonds PB, Williams NL. Treatment of stress urinary incontinence due to paravaginal fascial defects. Obstet Gyencol 1981; 57:357–362.

30. Baden WF, Walker T. Urinary stress incontinence: evolution of paravaginal repair. Female Patient 1987; 12:89–105.

31. Farrell SA, Ling C. Currycombs for the vaginal paravaginal defect repair. Obstet Gynecol 1997; 90:845–847.

32. Shull BL, Benn SJ, Kuehl TJ. Surgical management of prolapse of the anterior vaginal segment: an analysis of support defects, operative morbidity and anatomic outcomes. Am J Obstet Gynecol 1994; 171:1429–1439.

33. Nguyen JK, Bhatia NN. Transvaginal repair of paravaginal defects using the Capio suturing device: a preliminary experience. J Gynecol Tech 1999; 5:51–54.

34. Cundiff GW, Addison WA. Management of pelvic organ prolapse. Obstet Gynecol Clin North America 1998; 25:914.

44

Paravaginal Repair: A Laparoscopic Approach

John R. Miklos and Robert Moore
Atlanta Urogynecology Associates, Atlanta, Georgia, U.S.A.

Neeraj Kohli
Harvard University, Boston, Massachusetts, U.S.A.

I. INTRODUCTION

The support of the anterior vaginal wall, with its overlying bladder and urethra, is dependent upon the inherent strength of the pubocervical fascia and its lateral attachment to the pelvic sidewalls. Specifically, the pubocervical fascia is attached to the arcus tendineus fascia pelvis (also termed "the white line"). The arcus tendineus fascia pelvis is a condensation of intervening connective tissue overlying the obturator internus muscle (Fig. 1). Upon vaginal inspection the anterior lateral vaginal sulcus shows excellent support when the pubocervical fascia and the arcus tendineus are intact (Fig. 2). Loss of the lateral vaginal attachment to the pelvic sidewall is called a paravaginal defect and usually results in a cystourethrocele, urethral hypermobility, and/or stress urinary incontinence (Fig. 3). Vaginal inspection in patients with bilateral paravaginal defects reveals loss of anterior vaginal wall support with detachment of the lateral sulci, resulting in a displacement cystocele (Fig. 4). White (1) first described the paravaginal repair in 1909, but it did not gain popularity until decades later, when Richardson (2,3) and Shull (4,5) described their abdominal and vaginal approaches to this type of anterior wall repair. Paravaginal defect repair has been described using not only vaginal and open abdominal approaches but also, more recently, via a laparoscopic approach (6–8).

II. OPERATIVE INDICATIONS

Laparoscopy should be considered as only a mode of abdominal access and not a change in the operative technique. The surgical repair of paravaginal defects should not be different whether the approach is vaginal, abdominal, or laparoscopic. Ideally, the indications for a laparoscopic approach to paravaginal defect repair should be the same as an open abdominal approach. The laparoscopic approach to paravaginal defect repair can be substituted for an open paravaginal repair in the majority of cases. Factors that might influence this decision include previous abdominal, pelvic or anti-incontinence surgery, the patient's weight, the need for concomitant surgery, and the surgeon's experience. The surgeon's decision to proceed with a laparoscopic paravaginal repair should be based on an objective clinical assessment that is consistent with a paravaginal defect cystocele or cystourethrocele, as well as the surgeon's own surgical skills. The paravaginal repair can be performed alone or in combination with a urethropexy procedure in patients with concomitant stress urinary incontinence.

631

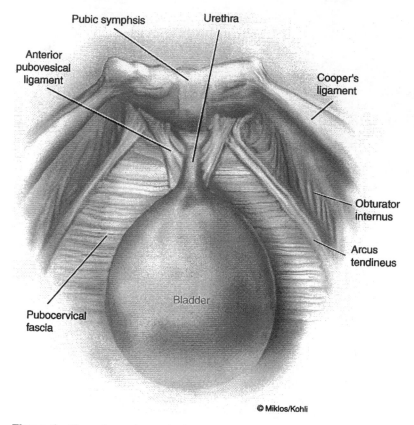

Figure 1 Normal anterior vaginal wall support (aerial view). The space of Retzius and normal anterior vaginal wall support.

III. PREOPERATIVE CONSIDERATIONS

A bowel preparation should be considered in any patient undergoing advanced reconstructive pelvic surgery. The authors recommend a full liquid diet 48 h prior to surgery, and a clear liquid diet and one bottle of magnesium citrate 24 h before surgery. This regimen appears to improve operative field visualization by bowel decompression and reduces the chance of contamination in case of accidental bowel injury. A single dose of prophylactic intravenous antibiotics is administered 30 min before surgery. Antiembolic compression stockings are routinely used. The patient is intubated, given general anesthesia, and placed in dorsal lithotomy position with both arms tucked to her side. A 16F three-way Foley catheter with a 5-mL balloon tip is inserted into the bladder and attached to continuous drainage. The authors find that a 30-cc balloon tip filled to capacity actually will hinder visualization and suture placement, especially paraurethrally.

IV. SURGICAL TECHNIQUE

The technique of abdominal entry and insufflation is a matter of surgeon's preference. The authors routinely perform open laparosocopy at the inferior margin of the umbilicus. A 10-mm access port is inserted to introduce the laparoscope. The abdomen is insufflated

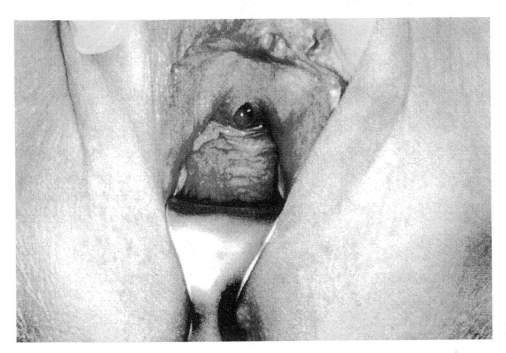

Figure 2 Normal anterior vaginal wall support (vaginal exam). The anterior vaginal wall is well supported with normal lateral fornix attachment.

with CO_2 to 15 mm Hg intra-abdominal pressure. Three additional ports are placed under direct vision (Fig. 5). The type of port, choice of port size, and placement depend upon the planned concomitant surgery as well as the surgeon's preference.

The bladder is filled in a retrograde fashion with 200–300 mL of sterile water, allowing identification of the superior border of the bladder edge. A harmonic scalpel is used to incise the peritoneum ~3 cm anterior to the bladder reflection, between the obliterated umbilical ligaments (Fig. 6). Identification of loose areolar tissue confirms a proper plane of dissection.

After the space of Retzius has been entered and the pubic ramus visualized, the bladder is drained to prevent injury. Using blunt dissection the retropubic space is developed by separating the loose areolar and fatty layers. Blunt dissection is continued until the retropubic anatomy is visualized. The pubic symphysis and bladder neck are identified in the midline and the obturator neurovascular bundle, Cooper's ligament, and the arcus tendineus fascia pelvis (white line) are visualized bilaterally along the pelvic sidewall (Fig. 1). The anterior vaginal wall and its point of lateral attachment from its origin at the pubic symphysis to its insertion at the ischial spine are identified. If paravaginal wall defects are present, the lateral margins of the pubocervical fascia will be detached from the pelvic sidewall at the arcus tendineus fascia pelvis. The lateral margins of the detached pubocervical fascia and the broken edge of the white line can usually be clearly visualized confirming the paravaginal defect. Unilateral or bilateral defects may be present (Fig. 3).

After identification of the defect, the repair is begun by inserting the surgeon's nondominant hand into the vagina to elevate the anterior vaginal wall and the pubocervical fascia to their normal attachment along the arcus tendineus fascia pelvis. A 2-0 nonabsorbable suture with attached needle is introduced through the 12-mm port and the needle is grasped using a laparoscopic needle driver.

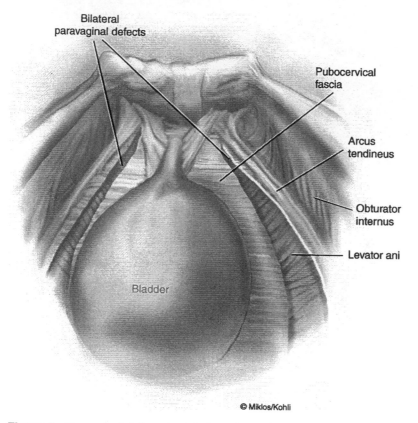

Bilateral
paravaginal defects

Pubocervical
fascia

Arcus
tendineus

Obturator
internus

Levator ani

Bladder

© Miklos/Kohli

Figure 3   Paravaginal defects (aerial view). Loss of lateral vaginal attachment at the arcus tendineus, resulting in a cystourethrocele.

The first suture is placed near the apex of the vagina through the paravesical portion of the pubocervical fascia. The needle is then passed through the ipsilateral obturator internus muscle and fascia around the arcus tendineus fascia at its origin 1–2 cm distal to the ischial spine. The suture is secured using an extracorporeal knot-tying technique. Good tissue approximation is accomplished without a suture bridge. Sutures are placed and tied sequentially along the paravaginal defects from the ischial spine toward the urethra. Usually a series of four to six sutures are required to repair the paravaginal defect unilaterally. The surgical procedure is then repeated on the opposite side if a bilateral paravaginal defect is present. Paravaginal defect repairs restore anterior vaginal wall lateral attachment and support (Fig. 6). However, paravaginal defect repair has little support in the literature for treatment of stress urinary incontinence. If a patient has concomitant stress urinary incontinence, a laparoscopic urethropexy procedure can be performed after the paravaginal repair.

The urethropexy will focus on the distal aspect of the anterior vaginal wall and the paravaginal repair will anatomically restore and support the proximal (bladder) portion of the anterior vaginal wall. Instead of placing four to six paravaginal sutures on each side as previously described, the proximal paravaginal repair, between the ischial spine and the urethrovesical junction, usually only requires two or three sutures on each side. This portion of the surgery should repair the cystocele but will do nothing to support the urethra and its coexisting stress urinary incontinence. The authors recommend coupling a Burch urethropexy with the

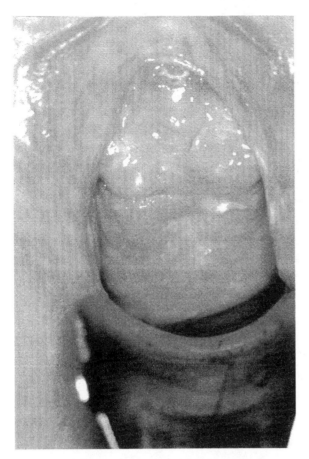

Figure 4 Paravaginal defects (vaginal exam). Loss of lateral vaginal attachment at the arcus tendineus, resulting in a cystourethrocele.

paravaginal repair to address the incontinence. A total of four sutures should be placed to complete the Burch urethropexy: two sutures bilaterally, one paraurethrally at the midurethra, and the other at the urethral vesical junction (Fig. 8). By coupling the Burch urethropexy with the paravaginal repair, the surgeon can address both the proximal cystocele and the distal urethral hypermobility and its coexisting stress urinary incontinence.

Upon completion of the Burch and/or paravaginal repair the intra-abdominal pressure is reduced to 10–12 mm Hg, and the retropubic space is inspected for hemostasis. Cystoscopy is performed to rule out urinary tract injury. The patient is given 5 mL of Indigo Carmine and 10 mL of furosemide intravenously, and a 70° cystoscope is used to the visualize the bladder mucosa, assess for unintentional stitch penetration and bladder injury, and confirm ureteral patency. After cystoscopy, attention is returned to laparoscopy. The authors recommend routine closure of the anterior peritoneal defect using an absorbable suture or a multifire hernia stapler. All ancillary trocar sheaths are removed under direct vision to ensure hemostasis and exclude iatrogenic bowel herniation. Excess gas is expelled and fascial defects of 10 mm or more are closed using delayed absorbable suture. Skin edges are closed using an absorbable suture. Postoperative bladder drainage and voiding trials are accomplished using a transurethral catheter, suprapubic tube, or intermittent self-catheterization.

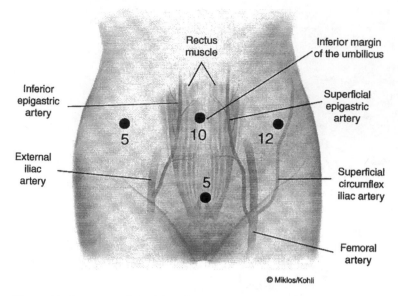

Figure 5   Laparoscopic incision sites. Port size and placement are illustrated.

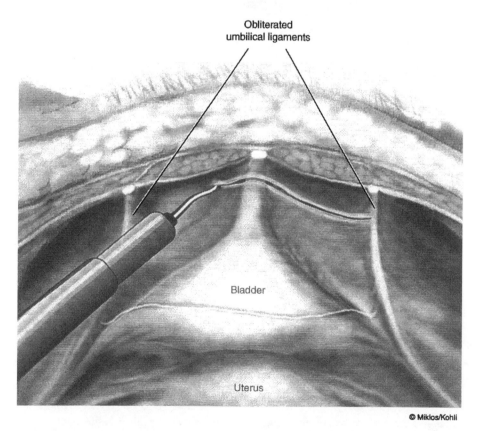

Figure 6   Peritoneal incision. Using a harmonic scalpel to incise the peritoneum between the obliterated umbilical ligaments and anterior to the bladder.

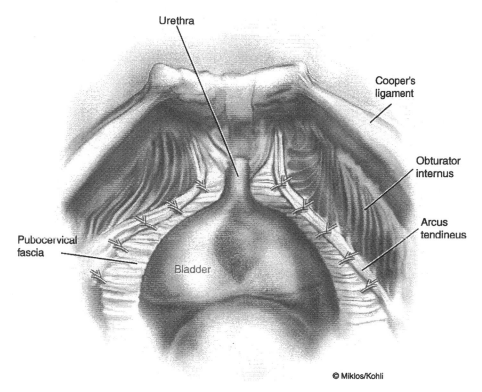

Urethra

Cooper's ligament

Obturator internus

Arcus tendineus

Pubocervical fascia

Bladder

© Miklos/Kohli

Figure 7 Paravaginal repair: conventional repair of paravaginal defects. Nonabsorbable suture is used to reapproximate the pubocervical fascia (i.e., anterior vaginal wall) back to its original point of lateral attachment, known as the arcus tendineus fascia pelvis (i.e., "white line").

V. CLINICAL RESULTS

Most studies reporting the efficacy of paravaginal repair in the treatment of genuine stress incontinence, whether performed vaginally or abdominally, lack appropriate outcome data and control groups. In a randomized prospective trial, Colombo et al. (12) performed Burch colposuspension on 18 patients and abdominal paravaginal repair on 18 patients with genuine stress incontinence. Patients undergoing Burch colposuspension had a significantly higher subjective (100% vs. 72%; $P = 0.2$) and objective (100% vs. 61%; $P = 0.04$) cure rates compared with patients undergoing paravaginal repair. The study was discontinued early because the authors no longer regarded it as ethical to propose paravaginal repair for the treatment of stress urinary incontinence (13). Specifically, data regarding the efficacy of laparoscopic paravaginal repair are also limited. Ostrzenski (14) performed laparoscopic paravaginal repair in 28 women with stress urinary incontinence. The subjective cure rate was 93% with follow-up ranging from 1 to 4.5 years. Pre- and postoperative urodynamic testing were not utilized. Given a patient has concomitant stress urinary incontinence with anterior vaginal wall prolapse due to paravaginal defects, the authors recommend coupling the paravaginal repair with a proven anti-incontinence operation such as a Burch urethropexy or a transvaginal sling.

Most surgeons utilize the paravaginal repair for the correction of anterior vaginal wall prolapse and do not rely on this operation for the treatment of stress urinary incontinence.

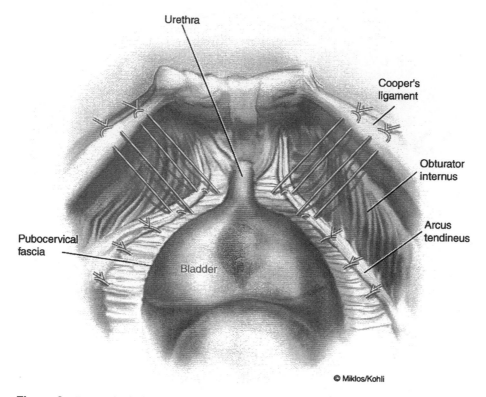

Urethra

Cooper's
ligament

Obturator
internus

Arcus
tendineus

Pubocervical
fascia

Bladder

© Miklos/Kohli

Figure 8 Paravaginal plus Burch urethropexy. The paravaginal sutures are placed to restore anatomy and correct the proximal cystocele, and four additional paraurethral suspension sutures (i.e., Burch urethropexy) are placed in patients diagnosed with stress urinary incontinence.

Paravaginal repair is an anatomically correct operation for the treatment of anterior vaginal wall prolapse due to paravaginal defects. As described above, the objective of the paravaginal repair is to reattach the anterolateral vaginal sulcus to the obturator internus muscles and fascia at the level of the white line. Anterior vaginal wall prolapse cure rates >95% have been reported utilizing the abdominal approach (2–4), and >90% utilizing the vaginal (5,9–11) approach to paravaginal repair. Literature concerning the efficacy of the laparoscopic paravaginal repair for the cure of anterior vaginal wall prolapse is lacking. A recent review of our experience (15) revealed that 130 of 171 patients had a Burch urethropexy and paravaginal repair, 23 of 171 patients a Burch urethropexy alone, and 18 of 171 patients a paravaginal repair alone. Of the authors' 171 patients, four (2.3%) had injury to the lower urinary tract during laparoscopic Burch urethropexy or paravaginal repair. All four injuries were cystotomies, two in patients with previous open retropubic urethropexies. No ureteral ligations or intravesical placement of suture was diagnosed. Other surgical parameters for the laparoscopic Burch urethropexy and paravaginal repair include an estimated blood loss of 50 mL, average hospital stay of <23 h, and an average operative time of 70 min. All patients had their surgery completed via laparoscopy.

Assuming that the paravaginal repair technique is not compromised by the abdominal approach utilized (laparoscopic vs. laparotomy), one should expect equal surgical efficacy.

VI. CONCLUSION

Defects in the lateral attachment of the pubocervical fascia to the arcus tendineus fasciae pelvis results in anterior vaginal wall prolapse and subsequent cystocele. The literature supports the use of paravaginal repair in the treatment of anterior vaginal wall prolapse but does not support its use for the treatment of stress urinary incontinence.

The authors support the use of the laparoscopic paravaginal repair in the treatment of cystocele or cystourethroceles in patients with lateral anterior vaginal wall defects. The laparoscopic approach to paravaginal defect repair can be substituted for an abdominal or transvaginal paravaginal repair in the majority of cases. Factors that might influence this decision include previous abdominal, pelvic or anti-incontinence surgery, patient's weight, the need for concomitant surgery, and the surgeon's experience. The paravaginal repair can be performed alone or in combination with a urethropexy procedure in patients with concomitant stress urinary incontinence.

REFERENCES

1. White GR. Cystocele, a radical cure by suturing lateral sulci of vagina to white line of pelvic fascia. JAMA 1909; 65:286–290.
2. Richardson AC, Lyon JB, Williams NL. A new look at pelvic relaxation. Am J Obstet Gynecol 1976; 126:568–573.
3. Richardson AC, Edmonds PB, Williams NL. Treatment of stress urinary incontinence due to paravaginal fascial defects. Obstet Gynecol 1981; 57:357–361.
4. Shull BL, Baden WF. A six year experience with paravaginal defect repairs for stress urinary incontinence. Am J Obstet Gynecol 1989; 160:1432–1437.
5. Shull BL, Benn SJ, Kuehl TJ. Surgical management of prolapse of the anterior vaginal sement: an analysis of support defects, operative morbidity and anatomic outcome. Am J Obstet Gynecol. 1994; 171:1429–1439.
6. Miklos JR, Kohli N. Paravaginal plus Burch procedure: a laparoscopic approach. J Pelvic Surg 1998; 4:297–302.
7. Miklos JR, Kohli N. Laparaoscopic paravaginal repair plus Burch colposuspension: review and descriptive technique. Urology 2000; 56:64–69.
8. Ross JW. Techniques of laparoscopic repair of total vault eversion after hysterectomy. J Am Assoc Gynecol Laparosc 1997; 4(2):173–183.
9. Elkins TE, Chesson RR, Videla F, Menefee S, Yordan R, Barksdale PA. Transvaginal paravaginal repair: a useful adjunctive procedure in pelvic relaxation surgery. J Pelvic Surg 2000; 6:11–15.
10. Young SB, Daman JJ, Bony LG. Vaginal paravaginal repair: one-year outcomes. Am J Obstet Gynecol 2001; 185:1360–1367.
11. Mallipeddi PK, Steele AC, Kohli N, Karram MM. Anatomic and functional outcome of vaginal paravaginal repair in the correction of anterior vaginal wall prolapse. Int Urogynecol J 2001; 12:83–88.
12. Colombo M, Milani R, Vitobello D. A randomized comparison of Burch colposuspension and abdominal paravaginal defect repair for female stress urinary incontinence. Am J Obstet Gynecol 1996; 175:78–84.
13. Nguyen JK. Current concepts in the diagnosis and surgical repair of anterior vaginal prolapse due to paravaginal defects. Obstet Gynecol Surv 2001; 56:239–246.
14. Ostrzenski A. Genuine stress urinary incontinence in women: new laparoscopic paravaginal reconstruction. J Reprod Med 1998; 43:466–482.
15. Speights SE, Moore RD, Miklos JR. Frequency of lower urinary tract injury at laparoscopic Burch and paravaginal repair. J Am Assoc Gyencol Laparosc 2000; 7(4):515–518.

45

Transvaginal Levator Myorraphy for Vaginal Vault Prolapse

Gary E. Lemack and Philippe E. Zimmern
University of Texas, Southwestern Medical Center, Dallas, Texas, U.S.A.

I. INTRODUCTION

The progressive development of vaginal pain or pressure in women with vaginal vault prolapse and the frequent presence of accompanying lower urinary tract symptoms or bowel symptoms often ultimately result in the desire for treatment. Proper repair of vault prolapse will not only restore vaginal position and function, but also result in an improvement of pelvic symptoms. Though conservative measures such as colpocleisis or pessaries may be appropriate to consider in a subset of women who are less fit for surgery, most active women desire an intervention that will not preclude or interfere with intercourse. Surgical procedures offer the best hope of a permanent correction, and several techniques have been described, including both abdominal (1,2) and vaginal approaches (3,4).

Both approaches for repairing vault prolapse appear to be equally efficacious. However, using vaginal approaches, recovery is expedited, and the morbidity occasionally associated with open abdominal procedures is minimized. While for years several authors have advocated sacrospinous fixation as a means of treating vaginal vault prolapse (5,6), the inherent dangers associated with possible damage to the adjacent vascular and neural structures make it a less favored approach for some. Additionally, vaginal axis often becomes altered with a unilateral fixation, and there may be an increased risk of secondary cystocele formation following traditional vaginal approaches (7). Therefore, an alternative vaginal approach was developed over 10 years ago, using the levator shelf to both recreate the pelvic floor and to anchor the upper vagina. The principles of this repair are based on an understanding of defects in the pelvic floor that have been addressed in previously described abdominal levator repairs for incontinence (8).

II. TECHNIQUE

A. Preoperative Evaluation

After performing a thorough history (with particular attention to previous attempts at repair), a physical examination is performed. Care is taken to assess each vaginal compartment so as to detect laxity posteriorly, anteriorly, and from the vault. Often, examination in the standing position may help to distinguish a rectocele from an enterocele associated with vault prolapse. If the patient is noted to have an atrophic or ulcerated vagina, she is given vaginal estrogen cream to administer topically, which may enhance wound healing postoperatively.

Since supine physical examination may underestimate the degree of prolapse present, we normally obtain a standing voiding cystourethrogram (VCUG) prior to proceeding with surgical correction. This study is performed largely from a lateral view with and without straining, both with a Foley catheter and then during voiding (9). The VCUG gives information about the presence and extent (central and/or lateral defects) of cystocele, degree of urethral hypermobility, presence of bladder wall trabeculations, urethral configuration during voiding, amount of post-void residual, and presence or absence of vesicoureteral reflux. Determining the severity of the anterior vaginal prolapse may impact on the type of surgical repair recommended in conjunction with the vault fixation, and impact the need for further renal imaging preoperatively. Currently, we obtain upper tract imaging in women who have grade 3 or 4 cystoceles (Baden classification) in order to evaluate for hydronephrosis and for the possible need for intraoperative ureteral stenting.

It is our practice to perform urodynamics both with and then without a vaginal pack to reduce the associated cystocele, which is frequently present. While still controversial, recent evidence suggests that correction of the prolapse during urodynamics may affect both pressure flow relationship during voiding and may unmask incontinence during testing (10). These findings, in turn, may influence the nature of the surgical repair, and play a role in preoperative counseling. If a hysterectomy is being considered, pelvic ultrasound is obtained to assess uterine size and endometrial lining, as well as to evaluate for ovarian abnormalities, since they are not always easily removed from a vaginal approach.

The overall goals of the procedure depend on the clinical scenario. When uterine prolapse is present, the levator myorraphy to fix the vault is coupled with vaginal hysterectomy, enterocele repair, and possible posterior repair. When an associated mild to moderate cystocele is present, an anterior vaginal wall suspension, which anchors the upper vagina to the cardinal ligaments bilaterally, is also performed. Larger cystoceles will normally require both central and lateral support. If the uterus has already been removed and an enterocele is present, vault fixation and enterocele repair are carried out. By closing the enterocele sac, recreating a strong levator plate and anchoring the upper vagina to that plate, a normal vaginal cavity with an adequate posterior axis is restored. Other times, the enterocele sac can be identified and purposefully not entered, but instead dissected proximally. Vault fixation and enterocele repair can still be carried out after a levator myorraphy is accomplished, though in this instance, the dissection remains extraperitoneal.

B. Technique of Vault Prolapse Repair After Hysterectomy

Patients are normally administered general anesthesia and given intravenous antibiotics at the start of the procedure. Pneumatic compression stockings are applied and the patient is placed in the dorsal lithotomy position. While the legs should be positioned fairly high, care should be taken not to overextend or overabduct the hips, overflex the knees, and to be sure that all joints are well padded. The perineum and suprapubic areas are completely trimmed and prepped since an associated bladder neck suspension is often also required. A critical step is the placement of a rectal pack (vaginal pack soaked with povidone iodine and surgical lubricant), which is inserted after the vagina, perineum, and lower abdomen have been prepped.

After placing the patient in Trendelenburg position, a Lone Star retractor (Lone Star, Inc., Houston, TX) is placed, exposing the vaginal bulge over the prolapsed vault (Fig. 1), which normally represents the position of the enterocele. Generally, panendoscopy is carried out, noting

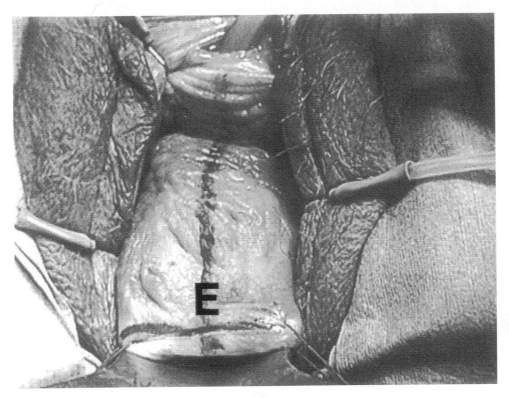

Figure 1   Vault prolapse. E, enterocele sac. This can be confirmed by simultaneous placement of rectal pack (to establish extent of rectocele), and catheter or cystoscope (to establish extent of cystocele).

the position of the ureters, and examining for bladder wall changes (trabeculations, diverticuli). For large prolapses, it is our practice to place a suprapubic tube at this point. Ureteral stents can be useful in case of hydronephrosis or in reoperations when trigonal anatomy has been distorted. A urethral catheter is then placed, leaving the bladder on drainage during the entire case. Two sutures are placed at the fornices of the vaginal vault for identification at the conclusion of the case, and the dimensions of the reduced vagina are measured. We normally place a weighted speculum at this point, but, owing to foreshortening associated with the exteriorization of the prolapse, it may not be able to be placed until later in the case.

After infiltrating the incision line with sterile saline, a midline incision is made overlying the area of prolapse extending from the vaginal apex as far distally as the associated rectocele is appreciated. Occasionally, if a large ulcerated area on the vaginal wall is present, this area will be excised superficially at the beginning of the procedure to ensure it is not incorporated in the closure. If there is any suspicion of its appearance, it is sent to pathology for frozen section analysis. Vaginal flaps are developed on both sides of the original incision, reapplying the hooks of the Lone Star retractor periodically to provide enhanced exposure. Often, a Deaver will be required to retract the bladder superiorly during this dissection.

After the vaginal flaps have been created and the dissection continued to the vaginal apex, the enterocele sac may be identified. It may be difficult to differentiate the enterocele sac from a large cystocele, and in these cases either a Van Buren sound or cystoscope placed into the bladder may aid in differentiating between the two. The peritoneal cavity is entered and small laparotomy pads are positioned to displace the bowels superiorly. Placing the patient in a more exaggerated Trendelenburg position may enhance exposure by allowing the peritoneal contents to gravitate away from the operative field. The levator musculature can then be identified bilaterally along the pelvic sidewall, just lateral to the rectum, which can easily be appreciated by the presence of the preplaced rectal pack (demonstrated from intraabdominal view in Fig. 2). A No. 1 absorbable suture is then placed into the levator musculature (which is covered by a thin layer of peritoneum), ~3 cm above the junction of the levator with the rectum, coming out just above the rectum within the body of the levator. This suture should be placed fairly deep into the body of the muscle, and then the same suture is used to secure the levator muscle on the contralateral side. This suture will later be tied across the midline to accomplish the levator myorraphy which is shown postplacement from a cephalad view within the pelvis in Figure 3. The entire pelvis should then be able to be rocked by tugging firmly on this suture. Another suture, similarly positioned into the body of the levator, is then placed 1 cm proximal to the last suture. Both are left on stay clamps until the next step, the closure of the enterocele sac, is accomplished.

Prior to securing these sutures each across the midline and completing the levator myorraphy, a purse-string suture is placed circumferentially to close the peritoneal cavity, taking care to remain superficial particularly along the peritoneal surface of the posterior bladder. The landmarks used for enterocele closure are prerectal fascia posteriorly, pelvic sidewall laterally (taking care to avoid the ovarian vessels which loom very close below the peritoneal surface), and peritoneal surface over the posterior bladder wall anteriorly (Fig. 4). One should take care to leave the ovaries within the peritoneal cavity if present, normal appearing, and not easily reached to be removed during hysterectomy. This purse-string suture is placed above the levator sutures, so as not to include them into the peritoneal cavity closure. After the peritoneal packs are removed and the purse-string suture cinched down, Indigo Carmine is administered intravenously and cystoscopy is carried out to insure ureteral patency. Any redundant portion of the enterocele sac is excised.

The two preplaced levator sutures are then tied sequentially across the midline, and final cystoscopic examination is performed. A strong, gushing efflux should be seen from both ureters. If there is any doubt as to their patency, the levator suture may need to be cut and replaced. If there is persistent decreased flow (no flow or very sluggish), then retrograde pyelograms and/or stenting may be required to assure ureteral patency. The levator sutures (proximal and distal) are then tagged with a hemostat. If the patient is sexually active, one should ensure at this point that there is not excessive tightening of the upper vaginal segment by inserting two or three fingers into the vaginal cavity. If this is the case, usually the more distal of the levator sutures can be removed without jeopardizing the strength of the repair. If an anterior repair or anti-incontinence procedure is required, it can now be carried out, followed by a rectocele repair with perineorraphy, if indicated.

Prior to closing the epithelial edges at the vaginal apex, one end of each of the proximal and distal levator myorraphy sutures from one side is threaded on a No. 6 curved Mayo needle and transfixed at the new vaginal apex from the inside out, separated by ~1 cm from each other. The ideal placement of these sutures is at the vaginal fornix, which had been marked by a stay suture at the start of the procedure. The same is carried out on the contralateral side, with one end taken from the more proximal of the levator sutures, and one from the more distal of the two. The former proximal and distal levator sutures are then secured to one another thereby firmly anchoring the upper vagina to the newly created levator plate. Figure 5 demonstrates the levator myorraphy sutures transfixed to the apex of the vagina, and Figure 6 shows the final appearance of the recreated vaginal floor with direct apposition of the vaginal apex to the rebuilt levator plate.

In some instances, entry into the enterocele sac may be unnecessary, particularly if the sac is located proximally, high at the vaginal vault. In these cases, it can often be dissected cranially,

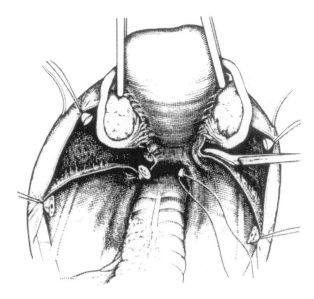

Figure 2 Classic abdominal approach to enterocele/prolapse repair during hysterectomy. Note the uterosacral ligaments, adjacent to the rectum, used for vaginal vault fixation and/or enterocele closure.

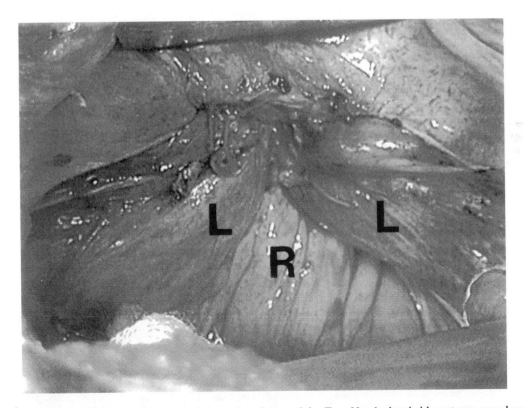

Figure 3 Placement of levator sutures, view from pelvis. Two No. 1 absorbable sutures are placed intraperitoneally into the body of the levator muscles bilaterally, and they are drawn together in the midline after being tied vaginally. L, levator muscles; R, rectum.

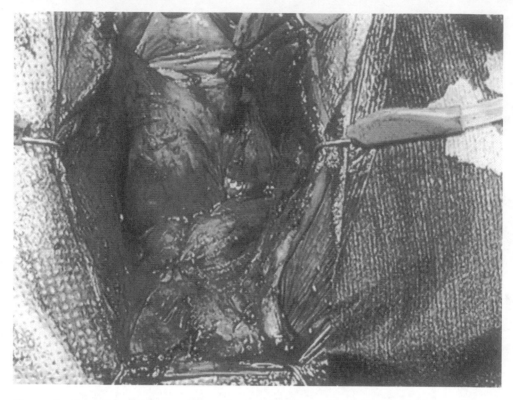

Figure 4   Extraperitoneal levator myorraphy. Levator muscles have been tied across the midline, while enterocele sac has not been entered. It has been dissected proximally and is now secured behind the midline myorraphy.

away from the rectocele, while leaving the sac intact. However, failure to repair an enterocele may lead to recurrent prolapse. The levator sutures can still be placed, tied, and secured to the vaginal vault, but they remain entirely extraperitoneal (Fig. 4).

After completion, an antibiotic-soaked vaginal pack is placed, and a Foley urethral catheter (and suprapubic tube if placed earlier) is left to drainage. The vaginal pack and urethral catheter are left in place for 24–48 h and then removed. Residuals are checked by ultrasound or suprapubic tube. If residuals are >100 mL, clean catheterization is performed, or, if a suprapubic tube has been placed, the tube is opened and residuals recorded until <100 mL. This occurs in generally less than 5 days.

III. RESULTS AND COMPLICATIONS

Postoperatively, most patients are hospitalized for 24–48 h. In our experience, no patients have experienced anesthetic complications. As with most vaginal procedures, there is very little need for postoperative analgesics, and all patients are ambulatory by the first postoperative day. Patients are advised to avoid sexual intercourse for at least 3 months postoperatively, to give the repair time to heal, and to allow time for all vaginal sutures to resorb.

A multicenter review of results using the levator myorraphy for repair of vaginal vault prolapse or for vaginal vault fixation in the setting of vaginal hysterectomy is under way. We

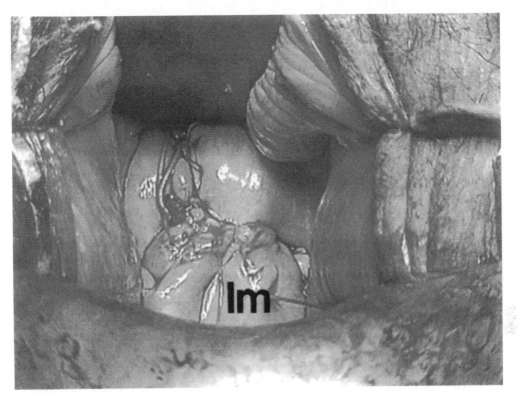

Figure 5 Vaginal vault has been fixed to levator myorraphy (lm) sutures (one on each side passed for this photo). Note closure of vaginal vault (sutures) just superior to the levator myorraphy sutures, with direct apposition of the vaginal vault to the rebuilt levator muscle complex beneath.

recently reported on 36 women who underwent levator myorraphy and vaginal vault fixation at the University of Texas Southwestern Medical Center over the last 4 years and who had at least 1-year follow-up and who completed a five-question telephone interview (mean follow-up 27.9 months, range 12–45 months) (11). Five patients required reoperation (four vaginal and one abdominal). One had a symptomatic cystocele, two had anterior enteroceles, and two had recurrent vault prolapse. Occasional urge urinary incontinence was reported in 20 of 36 women, though pad usage was rarely required, while stress urinary incontinence was noted by four women (present in eight preoperatively). On examination, mild to moderate cystoceles were noted in seven asymptomatic women.

Sexual function, while not a priority in many elderly patients undergoing prolapse surgery (12), may be important to younger women (13). Among the women answering the telephone questionnaire, 14 were sexually active with three (21%) reporting discomfort with intercourse. Among these 14 were three women unable to have intercourse preoperatively because of the extent of prolapse. In most women, there appeared to be no deleterious affect on sexual function, similar to our findings in women undergoing anterior vaginal wall suspension surgery for stress incontinence (14). Overall, when asked how satisfied they were with the results of the surgery, six women (17%) were dissatisfied with the results of their operation (<50% satisfied) and 17 were extremely satisfied (>90%).

The major complications associated with any repair of vaginal prolapse include hemorrhage requiring transfusion, ureteral injury, rectal injury, rectal pain upon defecation, vaginal narrowing affecting sexual function, and prolapse recurrence. In our hands, the risk of significant

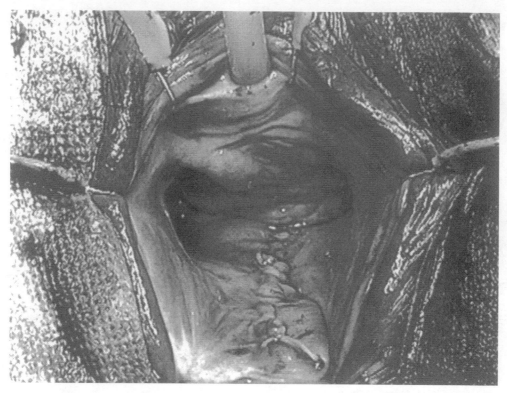

Figure 6   Final appearance of the posterior vaginal wall after completion of levator myorraphy. Vault fixed in high location. Posterior suture line extends from vault toward perineum. Vagina is capacious, with the natural 130° posterior axis preserved.

bleeding has been minimal, with only two patients requiring transfusion over a 10-year period of performing this procedure in over 120 patients. One patient with bilateral ureteral obstruction was noted to be anuric in the recovery room, and required reexploration with removal of one of the levator myorraphy sutures. One patient was noted to have flank pain and unilateral hydronephosis after repair, which permanently resolved after 3 months of ureteral stenting. We have had five cases where ureteral drainage was noted to decrease intraoperatively after tying one of the levator myorraphy sutures. Prompt return of urine flow was observed after removing one of the sutures, and we suspect that medial traction on the distal ureters resulted from tying the levator myorraphy stitch. Secondary anterior enterocele formation has been noted in two asymptomatic patients postoperatively, neither of whom has required revision or sacrocolpopexy as yet. Rectal pain is uncommon, but when present usually subsides within 4–6 weeks after the procedure and is best treated with stool softeners and warm Sitz baths.

IV.   CONCLUSION

The levator myorraphy repair for vaginal vault prolapse is minimally invasive, is well tolerated, requires no specific instrumentation, and is successful in the great majority of cases. Since no intra-abdominal exploration is required, postoperative hospital stay is minimized. Risks to the pudendal nerve and vessels are avoided using this technique, and therefore any pelvic surgeon comfortable with vaginal surgery should be able to complete this repair without difficulty. As with any enterocele and vault repair, ureteral injury is always a risk, and precautions should be taken throughout the procedure to guard against this possibility.

REFERENCES

1. Lane FF. Repair of posthysterectomy vaginal vault prolapse. Obstet Gynecol 1962; 126:590–596.
2. Timmons MC, Addison WA, Addison SB, Cavenar MG. Abdominal sacral colpopexy in 163 women with posthysterectomy vaginal vault prolapse and enterocele. J Reprod Med 1992; 37:322–327.
3. Winkler HA, Tomeszko JE, Sand PK. Anterior sacrospinous vaginal vault suspension for prolapse. Obstet Gynecol 2000; 95(4):612–615.
4. Goldberg RP, Tomezsko JE, Winkler HA, Koduri S, Culligan PJ, Sand PK. Anterior or posterior sacrospinous vaginal vault suspension: long-term anatomic and functional evaluation. Obstet Gynecol 2001; 98(2):199–204.
5. Nichols DH. Sacrospinous fixations for massive eversion of the vagina. Am J Obstet Gynecol 1982; 142:901–904.
6. Morley GW, DeLancey JOL. Sacrospinous ligament fixation for eversion of the vagina. Am J Obstet Gynecol 1988; 158:872–881.
7. Sze EH, Kohli N, Miklos JR, Roat T, Karram MM. A retrospective comparison of abdominal sacrocolpopexy with Burch colposuspension versus sacrospinous fixation with transvaginal needle suspension for the management of vaginal vault prolapse and coexisting stress incontinence. Int Urogynecol J 1999; 10(6):390–393.
8. Mouritsen L, Hansen PT, Kielmann J, Nielsen EL. Results of abdominal levator-muscle repair in urinary stress incontinence. Scand J Urol Nephrol 1987; 21:281–284.
9. Lemack GE, Zimmern PE. Voiding cystourethrography and magnetic resonance imaging of the lower urinary tract. In: Corcos J, Schick E, eds. The Urinary Sphincter. NY: Marcel Dekker, 2001:407–422.
10. Romanzi LJ, Chaikin DC, Blaivas JG. Effect of genital prolapse on voiding. J Urol 1997; 161:581–586.
11. Lemack G, Blander DS, Margulis V, Zimmern PE. Vaginal vault fixation and prevention of enterocele recurrence by high midline levator myorraphy (HMLM): physical examination and questionnaire-based follow-up. Eur Urol 2001; 40:648–651.
12. Holley RL, Varner RE, Gleason BP, Apfell LA, Scott S. Sexual function after sacrospinous ligament fixation for vaginal vault prolapse. J Reprod Med 1996; 41:355–358.
13. Weber AM, Walters MD, Schover LR, Mitchinson A. Sexual function in women with uterovaginal prolapse and urinary incontinence. Obstet Gynecol 1995; 85:483–487.
14. Lemack GE, Zimmern PE. Sexual function after vaginal surgery for stress incontinence: results of a mailed questionnaire. Urology 2000; 56:223–227.

46

Sacrospinous Ligament Suspension for Vaginal Vault Prolapse

Roger P. Goldberg and Peter K. Sand
Northwestern University Medical School, Evanston, Illinois, U.S.A.

I. INTRODUCTION

Sacrospinous vaginal vault suspension has been utilized for the repair of vaginal vault prolapse for several decades—first described in Europe in 1958 (1), and later introduced to the United States in 1971 (2). Long-term support of the vaginal apex can be achieved in 81–100% of cases (3–6) even in the presence of severely attenuated pelvic supports, with anatomic and sexual function effectively maintained in the vast majority of cases. Maintaining familiarity with variations of surgical technique, and key anatomical landmarks, will help the reconstructive surgeon to maximize the efficacy and safety of this operation.

II. INDICATIONS

A. Posthysterectomy Vault Prolapse

The most common indication for sacrospinous ligament suspension is resuspending a prolapsed posthysterectomy vaginal apex. For women with pelvic ligaments and connective tissue supports that are severely attenuated or absent, the sacrospinous ligament provides a consistently strong site for apical fixation. Sacrospinous ligament suspension carries the advantages of the trans-vaginal approach performed within the retroperitoneal rather than intra-abdominal space, involving relatively limited dissection beyond that which is performed for transvaginal enterocele, rectocele, and cystocele repair. After sacrospinous suspension, the vaginal apex is suspended posterolaterally to the ligament on either side or both sides.

B. Accompanying Vaginal Hysterectomy

Whereas the role of sacrospinous ligament suspension for posthysterectomy vault prolapse is widely accepted, its use as a "prophylactic" measure to prevent future apical prolapse—at the time of vaginal hysterectomy—has been a subject of debate. Some surgeons have advocated sacrospinous suspension as an adjunct to vaginal hysterectomy only when pelvic connective tissues are markedly weakened, as demonstrated either by advanced uterine prolapse

651

preoperatively or absent uterosacral ligaments intraoperatively (7). Cruikshank and Cox (8) performed sacrospinous ligament suspension on 48 of 135 such patients with lax or absent uterosacral ligaments at the time of vaginal hysterectomy; only one case of recurrent vaginal vault prolapse was noted postoperatively, with no apparent excess morbidity. The authors concluded that sacrospinous fixation is an appropriate adjunct to vaginal hysterectomy for cases involving significant connective tissue weakness. Smilen and Porges (9) reported a trend indicating that for severe uterine prolapse, adding that sacrospinous suspension to vaginal hysterectomy and colporrhaphy may reduce the odds of recurrent apical prolapse.

Other retrospective studies, however, have indicated that even in the presence of uterovaginal prolapse, sacrospinous ligament suspension at the time of hysterectomy is not routinely indicated (4,10,11). The use of McCall culdoplasty following vaginal hysterectomy, even in the presence of markedly attenuated uterosacral ligaments, has been supported by retrospective analyses (12,13), including Colombo et al., who evaluated 62 matched pairs of women undergoing hysterectomy with either sacrospinous ligament suspension or McCall culdoplasty (14). Operative time and average blood loss were greater in the sacrospinous group, and recurrent cystoceles were more likely at follow-up ranging from 4 to 9 years. No differences were found with respect to the rates of recurrent prolapse of the vaginal apex (5–8%), overall prolapse at any site, or sexual function (14). However, the potential for bias within a retrospective study design—due to the assignment of subjects to their "strongest available ligament" at the time of surgery—limits the conclusions that can be drawn. In actual practice, sacrospinous ligament suspension may occasionally represent the most reliable alternative for apical fixation at the time of vaginal hysterectomy, if no palpable uterosacral ligaments exist.

C. For Uterine Suspension

Finally, sacrospinous ligament suspension has been successfully utilized for women with symptomatic uterovaginal prolapse who wish to preserve their uterus and reproductive capacity. Kovac and Cruikshank (15) evaluated 19 women (average age 27) who underwent uterine-sparing sacrospinous ligament suspension, and reported that four of five of them who subsequently underwent a successful pregnancy and vaginal delivery did not have recurrent apical prolapse. The procedure entails fixation of the distal uterosacral ligaments to the sacrospinous ligament, often combined with uterosacral plication to reduce the risk of enterocele formation. Bilateral rather than unilateral suspension was performed in 15 of the 19 subjects in this series, to avoid lateral deviation of the uterus and any adverse effect it might have on reproductive capacity.

III. TECHNIQUES

A. Exposing the Ligament

Access to the sacrospinous ligament and coccygeus muscle can be achieved by several means. The most common approach, as described by Nichols (16), involves a posterior vaginal incision and posterior colporrhaphy dissection, facilitating perforation of the rectal pillar near the ischial spine. With blunt dissection of the pararectal space medial to the ligament, the coccygeus muscle and sacrospinous ligament are exposed. The "anterior" sacrospinous suspension technique (17), on the other hand, involves perforation into the retropubic space through an anterior colporrhaphy incision, and dissection of the ipsilateral paravesical and paravaginal area from the level of the bladder neck to the ischial spine. For cases involving mainly anterior compartment defects with no rectocele, the anterior approach facilitates suspension of the vaginal apex without a posterior vaginal incision. Finally, some surgeons approach the sacrospinous ligament by resecting a circumferential patch of excess epithelium at the most advanced portion of the prolapsed vaginal cuff—a region of the vaginal skin that overlies an enterocele in most cases. After repair of the enterocele, the ligament is exposed with posterolateral dissection within the retroperitoneal plane. Because this apical approach exposes both the anterior vaginal epithelium with underlying pubocervical fascia, and the posterior vaginal epithelium with rectovaginal fascia, sutures can be anchored through either or both of these cuff edges. Briesky-Navratil retractors are well suited for exposing the coccygeus muscle and sacrospinous ligament without obstructing the surgical field; some surgeons find retractors or suction devices mounted with a fiberoptic light source to be particularly useful for identifying the retroperitoneal anatomy.

B. Suture Placement

Various devices have been specifically designed for placing sutures into the sacrospinous ligament—including the Deschamps ligature carrier, Miya hook (18), and in-line "push and catch" suturing devices (19). With proper assistance, some surgeons find a standard long curved needle holder to be sufficient. The use of a "minimally invasive" device for transvaginal fixation of the vaginal apex to the sacrospinous ligament, without an incision, has been recently described (20). Among 12 women, the procedure appeared to be safe and well tolerated, with one case of recurrent vault prolapse reported at a mean follow-up of 16 months. Prospective, longer-term studies will be necessary to determine its safety and efficacy.

Suturing into the sacrospinous ligament should be performed with key anatomic landmarks in mind. The lateral suspension suture is placed through the ligament 1–2 fingerbreadths medial to the ischial spine to safeguard against injury to the pudendal vessels, though the risk of this particular complication may be commonly overestimated (44). Care must be taken to place sutures through the superficial portion of the ligament, rather than deep into or around it. Medially, the rectum represents the anatomic boundary for suture placement. During this stage of the operation, the primary surgeon must ensure that all retractors maintain their proper position. The traumatic insertion of retractors beyond the ligament, or excessive medial traction against the rectum and presacral area, is a potential source of operative complications. Medial rather than lateral placement of sutures in the ligament also allows for a more cephalad suspension of the vaginal vault.

Fixation of the vaginal wall at the apex is most commonly performed with permanent monofilament sutures; other surgeons prefer synthetic absorbable material to reduce the theoretical risk of suture erosion and granulation tissue formation. Preparation of the vaginal apex for fixation can involve either full cuff closure, or a circumferential "whip stitch" for securing hemostasis followed by apposition of the open cuff against the ligament. Medial and lateral anchoring sutures are secured to the undersurface of the posterior vaginal cuff epithelium (for the posterior approach), or anterior vaginal cuff epithelium (for the anterior approach), or both (for the apical approach). Although scarring and fibrosis at the interface of the ligament and new vaginal apex may theoretically eliminate the need for sutures after the initial healing phase, the relative advantages of permanent versus absorbable sutures have not been scientifically evaluated.

Regardless of the type of suture used or anatomic approach to the ligament, a few principles for suture placement appear to be universally important. First, the surgeon should take care to avoid the creation of a "suture bridge" between the vagina and ligament; the use of pulley stitches, which attach one end of each suture to the vaginal cuff epithelium, may help in applying the vagina directly against the ligament. Secondly, maintaining a width of at least two centimeters between the medial and lateral fixation sutures will minimize the risk of constriction at the vaginal apex.

C. Unilateral Versus Bilateral

Sacrospinous ligament suspension is most commonly performed as a unilateral procedure on the patient's right side owing to the mechanical advantage afforded to right-hand-dominant surgeons, and the anatomic advantage resulting from the absence of the sigmoid colon on the right. Bilateral suspension was emphasized in early reports (21) and even recently has been advocated by some experienced surgeons (22). Pohl and Frattarelli (23) reported no recurrent apical prolapse among 40 women treated with bilateral sacrospinous ligament suspension after 6–40 months follow-up. Cespedes (24) reported good success following bilateral sacrospinous fixation by the anterior vaginal approach; at 17 months, no recurrent vault prolapse was seen in 27 of 28 women with grade 3–4 prolapse. However, there is little evidence to suggest that bilateral suspension improves outcomes compared with the unilateral approach (4). Moreover, in comparison to the unilateral sacrospinous ligament suspension, the bilateral procedure entails more extensive dissection and requires generous width at the vaginal apex to avoid causing tension between fixation points. Because of these additional challenges and its lack of clear advantage, the bilateral technique is utilized far less often than unilateral fixation.

D. Pre- and Perioperative Considerations

The decision to proceed with sacrospinous ligament suspension may be influenced by a patient's specific anatomic features or medical history. For women with prior intra-abdominal surgery, pelvic adhesions, or other contraindications to abdominal surgery, the fully retroperitoneal nature of sacrospinous ligament suspension may confer advantages with respect to surgical risk, operative time, and speed of recovery. Preoperative evaluation should also include assessment of bony and soft tissue pelvic anatomy. Markedly foreshortened bony pelvic dimensions—such as a true "platypoid" pelvis—may limit the surgeon's ability to preserve adequate vaginal length, and weigh against the choice of sacrospinous suspension for sexually active patients. With respect to soft tissue, the length of the vaginal vault should be sufficient to avoid tension following sacrospinous fixation, which may predispose to suture pullout, anatomic distortion, and possibly even an "unmasking" of potential urinary incontinence due to posterior displacement of the urethra from the pubic bone (9). In the absence of adequate length, operative revision of the cuff, or suspension to a more anterior or distal structure such as iliococcygeus fascia (25), may be performed. Consideration of concomitant sacrospinous vaginal suspension on the right, with an iliococcygeal suspension on the left at a slightly more distal point, may lead to improved apical support and diameter.

Preoperative planning should include assessment of estrogen status for postmenopausal women, and consideration of systemic or local estrogen therapy before surgery if the vaginal cuff epithelium appears thin or poorly vascularized. Estrogen improves vaginal vascularization and supports an improved epithelium and connective tissue. A well-estrogenized vaginal epithelium should therefore facilitate healing at the site of suture fixation and reduce the likelihood of subsequent surgical failure resulting from suture "pullout" from the vaginal side.

At the time of surgery, coexisting pelvic floor support defects need to be recognized and repaired. An unrecognized enterocele, in particular, is often to blame for the rare case of recurrent apical prolapse following sacrospinous suspension. As with all reconstructive operations, appropriate patient selection and flexibility in the operating room will maximize the odds of success.

IV. ANATOMIC OUTCOMES

A. Support of the Vaginal Apex

The long-term efficacy of sacrospinous ligament suspension for resuspending a prolapsed vaginal cuff has been borne out by several clinical series. The success rates of the larger reports, with mean follow-up intervals, are listed in Table 1. Although the majority of outcomes reported for the sacrospinous ligament suspension have referred to either the posterior or apical approach, recent reports evaluating the anterior sacrospinous ligament suspension have found similar rates of success. Furthermore, based on one retrospective analysis of 168 women following either anterior (n = 76) or posterior (n — 92) sacrospinous vault suspension, no measurable differences appeared to exist with respect to apical support, vaginal caliber according to maximum dilator size, or angle of the vaginal vault (26).

Following sacrospinous ligament suspension, the apex of the vagina is retroverted and laterally positioned—anatomic changes that appear to have no functional consequences. Morley and DeLancey proposed that this asymmetry might even confer a functional benefit postoperatively by positioning the vaginal vault away from the urogenital hiatus and over the levator muscles, lessening the intra-abdominal pressures applied to the vaginal apex. Narrowing of the vaginal apex into a cylindrical shape, due to the excision of excess anterior and/or posterior vaginal epithelium, is felt by some to be a desired anatomic consequence of unilateral sacrospinous suspension (27). Following bilateral suspension, a T-shaped or Y-shaped (with concomitant enterocele repair) vaginal apex will often be appreciable by examination, but appears to confer no functional disadvantage.

One matched case control study compared sacrospinous suspension to iliococcygeus fixation for prolapse of the vaginal apex, and reported higher "patient satisfaction" scores among the sacrospinous group at a mean follow-up of 20 months. Nonsignificant trends

Table 1 Suspension of the Vaginal Apex: Sacrospinous Ligament Suspension

Study	No. of subjects	Mean follow-up (months)	Success: apical support (%)
Richter and Albrich, 1981 (47)	81	not reported	100
Nichols, 1982 (48)	163	≥ 24	97
Morley and DeLancey, 1988 (4)	71	≥ 12	96
Shull et al., 1992 (25)	41	≥ 48	98
Pasley, 1995 (30)	156	35	94.4
Hardiman and Drutz, 1996 (5)	125	6–60[a]	97.6
Paraiso et al., 1996 (35)	243	73.6	93
Meschia et al., 1999 (51)	91	≥ 12	85
Winkler et al., 2000 (17) (*anterior approach*)	75	8.5	93
Cespedes, 2000 (37) (*anterior bilateral approach*)	28	17	96.4
Lantzsch et al., 2001 (41)	123	57	96.7

[a]Follow-up reported as range; mean interval not specified.

indicated better support after the sacrospinous approach, according to both subjective and objective outcomes (28).

B. Anterior Vaginal Wall Support

The anterior vaginal compartment appears to represent a particularly vulnerable site following sacrospinous vaginal vault suspension, perhaps a consequence of vaginal retroversion predisposing to a compensatory abnormality. Several clinical series, but not all (29), have demonstrated an elevated risk of cystocele formation following sacrospinous ligament suspension. Recurrent cystoceles have been reported in 7.6–92% (4,30,36,47) of women after sacrospinous ligament suspension, depending on the other specific procedures performed concurrently.

Although early series found recurrent cystoceles in 6% of women who had satisfactory support at the apex (4), Paraiso (35) reported significant anterior wall defects in 26.7% of women after sacrospinous ligament suspension. Another retrospective series, comparing 122 sacrospinous suspensions to a variety of other reconstructive procedures performed by a single surgeon, reported that sacrospinous suspension had no association with subsequent anterior compartment defects.

Sze et al. (3) reported on 96 women who had pelvic organ prolapse to or beyond the hymen, and compared women who underwent sacrospinous ligament suspension with and without concomitant transvaginal needle suspension. An overall 33% rate of recurrent prolapse was observed when the two procedures were performed in tandem, compared with 19% in women who underwent sacrospinous suspension only. The difference, however, did not reach statistical significance. Barber et al. (50) reported a 21% incidence of stage III cystoceles following sacrospinous ligament suspension, at a mean follow-up interval of 19 months. The incidence rose to 36% when sacrospinous suspension was performed in tandem with needle bladder neck suspension. Although the precise mechanisms leading to recurrent anterior vaginal wall prolapse have yet to be outlined, it has been proposed that posterior deflection of the vaginal vault after sacrospinous ligament suspension leads to increased "exposure" of the anterior compartment to intraperitoneal forces (31,32). Shull et al. (25) suggested that underestimation of the severity of anterior prolapse on preoperative examination—or overreliance on the apical suspension for compensation of anterior support defects—may also play a role. In their series, 16% of patients with anterior vaginal wall prolapse before surgery had no repair of the anterior vaginal wall performed during their initial surgery. Accurately identifying all areas of prolapse and tailoring the pelvic reconstruction according to intraoperative findings, represent key ingredients for a successful outcome.

C. Vaginal Anatomy and Sexual Function

Most studies of sacrospinous ligament suspension have focused on anatomic outcomes—specifically, the rates of recurrent apical and anterior vaginal prolapse. Fewer studies have addressed outcomes more directly relevant to function, such as vaginal length, caliber, axis, and sexual satisfaction. Morley and DeLancey reported vaginal stenosis in four of 78 women evaluated at least 1 year after sacrospinous ligament suspension, and one patient with vaginal foreshortening requiring subsequent vaginaplasty. Elkins et al. (33) and Given et al. (34) quantified postoperative vaginal anatomy in more detail, reporting an average vaginal length following sacrospinous ligament suspension of 8.3 cm, and 8.2 cm, respectively. Paraiso et al. (35) evaluated an even wider variety of outcomes following sacrospinous suspension at a mean interval of 98.8 months. Vaginal length averaged 8.0 cm, and vaginal caliber measured as less than two fingerbreadths in 17%; new-onset vaginal constriction was reported in 7.4%.

Sexual dysfunction following pelvic reconstruction with sacrospinous suspension was reported in 14% by Paraiso et al. (35); however, less than half represented de novo cases. Surprisingly, vaginal length and caliber, and the presence of specific support defects, were not associated with reported sexual activity in this series. Holley et al. (36), on the other hand, concluded that postoperative vaginal narrowing was a significant predictor of sexual activity following sacrospinous suspension and vaginal reconstruction, with 25% of patients reporting postoperative sexual dysfunction. When vaginal narrowing did not occur, sexually active partners reported either unchanged or improved sexual function. These authors, in agreement with other reports (14,36), concluded that vaginal narrowing and sexual dysfunction after sacrospinous ligament suspension is most often the result of anterior colporrhaphy and the repair of other concomitant defects rather than the sacrospinous suspension itself. Retroversion of the vaginal apex, and deviation after unilateral sacrospinous suspension, appear to have no adverse effects on coital function postoperatively.

Another retrospective analysis addressed sexual outcomes in 133 women following sacrospinous ligament suspension: 76 following posterior sacrospinous suspension, and 57 following anterior suspension, at a median interval of 41.3 months. Before surgery, 19 (33%) were sexually active in the anterior vault suspension group, and 0% reported dyspareunia; 28 (37%) were sexually active in the posterior vault suspension group, with nine (13%) reporting dyspareunia. At long-term follow-up, two subjects in the anterior vault suspension group and two in the posterior vault suspension group reported new onset dyspareunia; three of these four cases of de novo dyspareunia were referable to either severe atrophy or recurrent grade 3 prolapse, and none were attributed to vaginal narrowing or shortening. Sacrospinous ligament suspension itself thus appears to have minimal if any impact on sexual function postoperatively, and the choice of anterior or posterior technique has no discernable impact on sexual outcomes. Perhaps most encouragingly, five women in this series reported dyspareunia at their preoperative baseline visit, which resolved after vaginal reconstruction with sacrospinous ligament suspension.

D. Predictors of Success

The long-term success of sacrospinous ligament suspension depends on a multitude of factors, including the quality of endopelvic connective tissues, postoperative convalescence, lifestyle factors, and the repair of all coexisting pelvic floor support defects at the time of surgery. Clearly, over the years after vaginal reconstructive surgery, new risk factors may emerge along with changes in hormonal status and activity patterns; physical stresses, such as a chronic cough or constipation, may accumulate over time. Regardless of the multiple factors determining surgical success, it appears that a successful healing process in the short term may reflect strong odds for success over the long run. Shull et al. (25) reported that among 81 women treated with sacrospinous ligament suspension and pelvic reconstruction, the absence of any pelvic support defect at the 6-week postoperative visit was associated with only 3% likelihood that the patient would require subsequent reconstructive surgery within 2–5 years.

V. SAFETY AND COMPLICATIONS

Aside from the general risks accompanying transvaginal reconstructive surgery, specific potential risks associated with the sacrospinous should be addressed. Local neurological complications may include sacral neuropathy (11). Pudendal nerve entrapment may result in pain localizing in the buttocks or perineum, and may improve following replacement of lateral fixation sutures more medially (37). Gluteal pain or paresthesias may occur after sacrospinous suspension (3,38,39), possibly due to peripheral nerve trauma. Though these symptoms are nearly always transient and self-limited, they may persist for a period of weeks or even months postoperatively. Cruikshank found that 20 of 135 women experienced buttock pain after sacrospinous ligament suspension, with all cases resolving spontaneously by 6 weeks. Even in the absence of direct pudendal nerve injury, pain may still occur due to the wide distribution of nerve tissue throughout the ligament and apparently most concentrated in its medial portion (40). Sciatic nerve irritation after sacrospinous suspension has been described as a new-onset problem (41) and as an exacerbation of previous symptoms (4).

Serious vascular injury is a rare complication of sacrospinous ligament suspension, but can be life-threatening. Morley and DeLancey (4) reported a transfusion rate of only 4%, and one infected hematoma resulting in sepsis. Various other series have reported transfusion rates ranging from 2% to 28% (30,42). To effectively manage pelvic hemorrhage, familiarity with the surrounding anatomic landmarks is essential. Verdeja et al. (43) demonstrated that the pudendal neurovascular bundle ranges in location from 0.90 to 1.30 cm medial to the ischial spine; the sciatic nerve is located 3.10–3.30 cm medial to the spine. Based on these anatomical relationships, the sacrospinous ligament would appear to be most vulnerable along its lateral third. Yet another series of cadaver dissections, performed by Barksdale et al. (44), showed the pudendal neurovascular bundle to be relatively shielded from injury by the ischial spine and sacrospinous ligament. The inferior gluteal artery—with a more perpendicular course relative to the ligament—was the vascular structure whose location appeared most vulnerable to injury. The authors referred to three elements of the operation that may carry particular risk: suture placement along the posterior ligament, retractor placement beyond the ligament, and overly aggressive denuding of the ligament surface.

For the vast majority of cases involving significant bleeding, ligation with either sutures or surgical clips can be achieved under direct exposure with simple retraction; a rectal examining finger can be particularly useful for both tamponade and exposure of medial vessels. Systematic inspection of the superior, inferior, and lateral surfaces of the dissected space should be performed—with particular focus on the ligament and adjacent coccygeus muscle, right medial rectal surface, and endopelvic connective tissue adjacent to the perforation of the rectal pillar. Throughout a 16-year experience performing sacrospinous ligament suspension procedures at our center, hemorrhage from the ligament or coccygeus muscle has been observed as an exceedingly rare event. Far more commonly, bleeding encountered during the sacrospinous dissection results from the shearing of small vessels along the medial aspect of the rectum (3,45) due to overzealous medial retraction; less commonly, deeper vessels in the presacral area can be disrupted by the medial retractor. In this latter case, if an individual vessel cannot be visualized with adequate retraction and lighting, the use of prolonged pressure packing may become necessary. Selective arterial embolization may be considered in hemodynamically stable patients if a defect or injured vessel cannot be localized (44).

Although Hardiman and Drutz (5) reported a 10% incidence of febrile morbidity following vaginal reconstructive surgery that included sacrospinous ligament suspension, the risk of clinically significant infection resulting from the apical suspension itself appears to be low. The lack of a tissue graft eliminates the risk of foreign body infection, but suture abscesses can develop on rare occasion (46,47). Proctotomy has been reported (30,48); however, significant injuries to the bowel are rare. In contrast to uterosacral vault suspension techniques, ureteral injuries are also exceedingly rare, though bladder laceration has been reported (47).

VI. CONCLUSIONS

The "best" choice of operation for advanced prolapse of the vaginal apex remains a subject of debate. According to some surgeons, the correction of all anatomic defects and restoration of "normal anatomy" should be the overarching goal. Others regard a "compensatory" postoperative anatomy as acceptable and perhaps even preferable in certain cases, for achieving maximizing long-term function and minimizing the risk of recurrent or de novo prolapse. Whatever operation is chosen, its success should be evaluated according to how effectively it relieves symptoms and restores normal bladder, bowel, and sexual function. In experienced hands, it appears that a variety of suspension techniques for the vaginal apex—through both vaginal and abdominal routes—can restore a normal anatomy while preserving sexual function. Ideally, to achieve the optimal outcomes for each patient, given the specific strengths and limitations characterizing their pelvic floor anatomy, the reconstructive surgeon should maintain a high level of skill with several techniques.

Sacrospinous vaginal vault fixation offers a generally short operative time and recovery period, lack of an abdominal incision, avoidance of a graft, reliable strength even in the presence of severely weakened pelvic supports, and excellent postoperative function despite a new posterolateral position for the vaginal apex. Long-term support of the prolapsed vaginal apex appears comparable to abdominal colpopexy, with shorter operative time and avoidance of intraabdominal surgery. Advocates of abdominal sacral colpopexy, on the other hand, highlight a longer postoperative vagina on average (49), with a midline orientation. Suspension of the vaginal apex to the proximal uterosacral ligaments has been favored by some recently, and can indeed achieve an excellent anatomic and functional outcome. However, the uterosacral tissues will occasionally lack sufficient tensile strength for an effective vault suspension, and the risk of ureteral injury may be as high as 11% when multiple fixation sutures are placed into the uterosacral ligament (50). Based on the existing literature it appears that each of these operations, in experienced hands, can provide excellent long-term outcomes. Prospective comparison between sacrospinous ligament suspension and its alternatives will hopefully be the subject of future research.

For the surgical management of advanced prolapse of the vaginal apex, sacrospinous ligament suspension represents a highly reliable transvaginal alternative. Familiarity with the various methods for approaching the ligament and anchoring the vaginal apex will allow the surgeon to easily combine this operation with a variety of other vaginal reconstructive procedures. Adherence to fundamental anatomic and surgical principles will ensure that a functional vaginal anatomy is maintained, and that complications are minimized.

REFERENCES

1. Sederl J. Zur operation des prolapses der blind endigenden sheiden. Geburtshilfe Frauenheilkd 1958; 18:824–828.
2. Randall CL, Nichols DH. Surgical treatment of vaginal inversion. Obstet Gynecol 1971; 38:327–332.
3. Sze EHM, Karram MM. Transvaginal repair of vault prolapse: a review. Obstet Gynecol 1997; 89:466–475.
4. Morley GW, DeLancey JOL. Sacrospinous ligament fixation for eversion of the vagina. Am J Obstet Gynecol 1988; 158:872–881.
5. Hardiman PJ, Drutz HP. Sacrospinous vault suspension and abdominal colposacropexy: success rates and complications. Am J Obstet Gynecol 1996; 175:612–616.
6. Shull BL, Capen CV, Riggs MW, Kuehl TJ. Preoperative and postoperative analysis of site-specific pelvic support defects in 81 women treated with sacrospinous ligament suspension and pelvic reconstruction. Am J Obstet Gynecol 1992; 166:1764–1771.
7. Cruikshank SH. Sacrospinous fixation—should this be performed at the time of vaginal hysterectomy? Am J Obstet Gynecol 1991; 164:1072–1076.

8. Cruikshank SH, Cox DW. Sacrospinous ligament fixation at the time of transvaginal hysterectomy. Am J Obstet Gynecol 1990; 162:1611–1619.
9. Porges RF, Smilen SW. Long-term analysis of the surgical management of pelvic support defects. Am J Obstet Gynecol 1994; 171:1518–1528.
10. Scotti RJ. Prophylactic sacrospinous fixation discouraged [letter]. Am J Obstet Gynecol 1992; 166:1022–1023.
11. Carey MP, Slack MC. Transvaginal sacrospinous colpopexy for vault and marked uterovaginal prolapse. Br J Obstet Gynaecol 1994; 101:536–540.
12. Cruikshank SH. Preventing posthysterectomy vaginal vault prolapse and enterocele during vaginal hysterectomy. Am J Obstet Gynecol 1987; 156:1433–1440.
13. Sze EHM, Karram MM. Transvaginal repair of vault prolapse: a review. Obstet Gynecol 1997; 89:466–475.
14. Colombo M, Milani R. Sacrospinous ligament fixation and modified McCall culdoplasty during vaginal hysterectomy for advanced uterovaginal prolapse. Am J Obstet Gynecol 1998; 179(1):13–20.
15. Kovac SR, Cruikshank SH. Successful pregnancies and vaginal deliveries after sacrospinous uterosacral fixation in five of nineteen patients. Am J Obstet Gynecol 1993; 168:1778–1786.
16. Nichols DH. Sacrospinous fixation for massive eversion of the vagina. Am J Obstet Gynecol 1982; 142:901–904.
17. Winkler HA, Tomeszko JE, Sand PK. Anterior sacrospinous vaginal vault suspension for prolapse. Obstet Gynecol 2000; 95:612–615.
18. Miyazaki FS. Miya hook ligature carrier for sacrospinous ligament suspension. Obstet Gynecol 1987; 70:286–288.
19. Lind LR, Shoe J, Bhatia NN. An in-line suturing device to simplify sacrospinous vaginal vault suspension. Obstet Gynecol 1997; 89(1):129–132.
20. Giberti C. Transvaginal sacrospinous colpopexy by palpation—a new minimally invasive procedure using an anchoring system. Urology 2001; 57(4):666–668.
21. Richter K. Die chirurgische anatomie der vaginaefixatio sacrospinalis vaginalis. Geburtshilfe Frauenheilkd 1968; 28:321–327.
22. Nichols DH. Transvaginal sacrospinous colpopexy. J Pelvic Surg 1996; 2:87–91.
23. Pohl JF, Frattarelli JL. Bilateral transvaginal sacrospinous colpopexy: preliminary experience. Am J Obstet Gynecol 1997; 177:1356–1362.
24. Cespedes RD. Anterior approach bilateral sacrospinous ligament fixation for vaginal vault prolapse. Urology 2000; 56(6 suppl 1):70–75.
25. Shull BL, Capen CV, Riggs MW, Kuehl TJ. Preoperative and postoperative analysis of site-specific pelvic support defects in 81 women treated with sacrospinous ligament suspension and pelvic reconstruction. Am J Obstet Gynecol 1992; 166:1764–1767.
26. Goldberg RP, Tomezsko JE, Winkler HA, Koduri S, Culligan PJ, Sand PK. Anterior or posterior sacrospinous vaginal vault suspension: long-term anatomic and functional evaluation. Obstet Gynecol 2001; 98:199–204.
27. Nichols DH, Randall CL. Massive eversion of the vagina. In: Vaginal Surgery. 3rd ed. Baltimore: Williams & Wilkins; 1989:328–357.
28. Maher CF, Murray CJ, Carey MP, Dwyer PL, Ugoni AM. Iliococcygeus or sacrospinous fixation for vaginal vault prolapse. Obstet Gynecol 2001; 98(1):40–44.
29. Smilen SW, Saini J, Sallach SJ, Porges RF. The risk of cystocele after sacrospinous suspension. Am J Obstet Gynecol 1998; 179:1465–1471.
30. Pasley WW. Sacrospinous suspension: a local practitioner's experience. Am J Obstet Gynecol 1995; 173:440–448.
31. Elkins TE, Hopper JB, Goodfellow K, Gasser R, Nolan TE, Schexnayder MC. Initial report of anatomic and clinical comparison of the sacrospinous ligament fixation to the high McCall culdoplasty for vaginal cuff fixation at hysterectomy for uterine prolapse. J Pelvic Surg 1995; 1:12–17.
32. Shull BL. Pelvic organ prolapse: anterior, superior, and posterior vaginal segment defects. Am J Obstet Gynecol 1999; 181:6–11.

33. Elkins TE, Hopper JB, Goodfellow K, Gasser R, Nolan TE, Schexnayder MC. Initial report of ana-tomic and clinical comparison of the sacrospinous ligament fixation to the high McCall culdeplasty for vaginal cuff fixation at hysterectomy for uterine prolapse. J Pelvic Surg 1995; 1:12–17.
34. Given FT, Muhlendorf IK, Browning GM. Vaginal length and sexual function after colpopexy for complete uterovaginal eversion. Am J Obstet Gynecol 1993; 169:284–287.
35. Paraiso MF, Ballard LA, Walters MD, Chi Lee J, Mitchinson AR. Pelvic support defects and visceral and sexual function in women treated with sacrospinous ligament suspension and pelvic reconstruc-tion. Am J Obstet Gynecol 1996; 175:1423–1431.
36. Holley RL, Varner RE, Gleason BP, Apffel LA, Scott S. Sexual function after sacrospinous ligament fixation for vaginal vault prolapse. J Reprod Med 1996; 41:355–358.
37. Alevizon SJ, Finan MA. Sacrospinous colpopexy: management of postoperative pudendal nerve entrapment. Obstet Gynecol 1996; 88:713–715.
38. Guner H, Noyan V, Tiras MB, Yildiz A, Yildirim M. Transvaginal sacrospinous colpopexy for marked uterovaginal and vault prolapse. Int J Gynaecol Obstet 2001; 74(2):165–170.
39. Cespedes RD. Anterior approach bilateral sacrospinous ligament fixation for vaginal vault prolapse. Urology 2000; 56:70–75.
40. Barksdale PA, Gasser RF, Gauthier CM, Elkins TE, Wall LL. Intraligamentous nerves as a potential source of pain after sacrospinous ligament fixation of the vaginal apex. Int Urogynecol J Pelvic Floor Dysfunct 1997; 8(3):121–125.
41. Lantzsch T, Geopel C, Wolters M, Koelbl H, Methfessel HD. Sacrospinous ligament fixation for vaginal vault prolapse. Arch Gynecol Obstet 2001; 265(1):21–25.
42. Heinonen PK. Transvaginal sacrospinous colpopexy for vaginal vault and complete genital prolapse in aged women. Acta Obstet Gynecol Scand 1992; 71:377–381.
43. Verdeja AM, Elkins TE, Odoi A, Gasser R, Lamoutte C. Transvaginal sacrospinous colpopexy: anatomic landmarks to be aware of to minimize complications. Am J Obstet Gynecol 1995; 173:1468–1469.
44. Barksdale PA, Elkins TE, Sanders CK, Jaramillo FE, Gasser RF. An anatomic approach to pelvic hemorrhage during sacrospinous ligament fixation of the vaginal vault. Obstet Gynecol 1998; 91:715–718.
45. Morley GW. Discussion of: Cruikshank SH, Cox DW. Sacrospinous ligament fixation at the time of transvaginal hysterectomy. Am J Obstet Gynecol 1990; 162:1611–1619.
46. Porges RF, Smilen SW. Long-term analysis of the surgical management of pelvic support defects. Am J Obstet Gynecol 1994; 171:1518–1528.
47. Richter K, Albrich W. Long-term results following fixation of the vagina on the sacrospinous liga-ment by the vaginal route (vaginaefixatio sacrospinous vaginalis). Am J Obstet Gynecol 1981; 1412:811–816.
48. Nichols DH. Sacrospinous fixation for massive eversion of the vagina. Am J Obstet Gynecol 1982; 142:901–904.
49. Given FT, Muhlendorf IK, Browning GM. Vaginal length and sexual function after colpopexy for complete uterovaginal eversion. Am J Obstet Gynecol 1993; 169:284–287.
50. Barber MD, Visco AG, Weidner AC, Amundsen CL, Bump RC. Bilateral uterosacral ligament vaginal vault suspension with site-specific endopelvic fascia defect repair for treatment of pelvic organ prolapse. Am J Obstet Gynecol 2000; 183:1402–1411.
51. Meschia M, Bruschi F, Amicarelli F, Pifarotti P, Marchini M, Crosignani PG. The sacrospinous vaginal vault suspension: critical analysis of outcomes. Int Urogynecol J 1999; 10:155–159.

47

Surgical Treatment of Vaginal Apex Prolapse: Transvaginal Approaches

Mark D. Walters
Cleveland Clinic Foundation, Cleveland, Ohio, U.S.A.

Tristi W. Muir
Brooke Army Medical Center, Fort Sam Houston, Texas, U.S.A.

I. INTRODUCTION

In recent years, the problem of pelvic organ prolapse has been given much more attention. Many women are living longer, and there is more interest in maintaining self-image of femininity and the capacity of sexual activity beyond menopause. Although few data on the incidence or prevalence of various forms of pelvic organ prolapse exist, the incidence appears to be rising based on increased longevity of women.

The management of pelvic organ prolapse can be difficult. Several support defects often coexist, and simple anatomic correction of the various defects does not always result in normal function of the vagina and surrounding organs. To accomplish the goals of pelvic reconstruction, the surgeon must thoroughly understand normal anatomical support and physiological function of the vagina, bladder, and rectum. These goals are to restore anatomy, maintain or restore normal bowel and bladder function, and maintain vaginal capacity for sexual intercourse.

This chapter discusses the pathology and surgical correction of posthysterectomy apical prolapse via the vaginal route. Obliterative procedures, such as colpectomy, and the transabdominal and laparoscopic support procedures are described elsewhere in this text.

II. PATHOLOGY OF PELVIC ORGAN PROLAPSE

DeLancey (1) described the anatomy of vaginal vault eversion and divided vaginal support into levels I, II, and III. In level I, the cervix (in a woman who has her uterus in place) or the vaginal apex (in a woman who has previously had a hysterectomy) is suspended to the cardinal and uterosacral ligaments. In level II, the areas along the base of the bladder anteriorly and along the rectum posteriorly are attached to the arcus tendineus fasciae pelvis or to the fascia over the levator ani muscle. Level III, the area along the base of the hymen and perineum, is derived from the urogenital sinus and is an area of fusion to the perineal body. Richardson (2) believed that the connective tissue around the vaginal tube, generally called endopelvic "fascia," does not stretch or attenuate but rather breaks at specific definable points. By integrating the concepts of suspension of level I with breaks in pelvic connective tissue, one can conclude that enterocele and vaginal apex prolapse result from specific defects of the presacral endopelvic fascia (cardinal-uterosacral ligaments), where they connect to the apex of the vagina. The vaginal epithelium covering the connective tissue is not important in maintaining normal support.

Pelvic organ prolapse can result when normal pelvic organ supports are subjected chronically to increases in intra-abdominal pressure or when defective genital support responds to normal intraabdominal pressure. Individual organs that pass through the levator ani can lose support singly or in combination, resulting in various degrees and combinations of pelvic organ prolapse. This loss of support occurs as a result of damage to any of the pelvic supportive systems. These systems include the bony pelvis, to which the soft tissues ultimately attach; the pelvic diaphragm, with the levator ani muscles and their fibromuscular attachments to the pelvic organs; the subperitoneal retinaculum and smooth muscle component of the endopelvic fascia (the cardinal and uterosacral ligament complex); and the perineal membrane. The perineal body and the walls of the vagina can lose tone and weaken from pathologic stretching from childbirth and attenuating changes of aging and menopause.

Loss of support or integrity of the anterior and posterior vaginal walls results in cystocele and rectocele, respectively. Uterovaginal prolapse occurs with damage or attenuation of endopelvic fascia that supports the uterus and upper vagina over the pelvic diaphragm. Furthermore, when the muscles of the pelvic diaphragm weaken as a result of congenital factors, childbirth injury, pelvic neuropathy, and/or aging, the levator ani lose resting tone and fail to contract quickly and strongly with increases in intra-abdominal pressure. Muscle atrophy and a wider levator hiatus result; weak and less rapid muscle contractions with rises in intra-abdominal pressure contribute to related symptoms of urinary and fecal incontinence.

Apical enterocele is a common defect seen in women with prior hysterectomy. In this case, the anterior vaginal wall muscularis (pubocervical "fascia"), the rectovaginal "fascia" posteriorly, or both, have separated from the supportive endopelvic fascia (uterosacral ligaments) at the apex of the vagina. With apical and posterior enterocele a defect occurs at the superior or transverse portion of rectovaginal "fascia" allowing a peritoneal sac with intra-abdominal contents to herniate between the rectum and apex of the vagina. A poorly supported vaginal apex and/or posterior vaginal wall often prolapses with the enterocele, leading to concurrent apical prolapse and rectocele.

Etiologic factors for the development of pelvic organ prolapse are incompletely understood. In their case control study, Swift et al. (3) found that advancing age, increasing weight of infants delivered vaginally, a history of hysterectomy, and previous prolapse surgery were the strongest etiologic predictors of severe pelvic organ prolapse. Conditions and life situations that chronically increase intra-abdominal pressure also appear to increase the risk of uterine and vaginal prolapse. These factors include obesity (4), heavy lifting at work (5), and bowel dysfunction (6).

The normal vaginal axis of a nulliparous woman in the standing position is nearly horizontal and is directed toward S3 and S4 (7). Distortion of the normal vaginal axis during reconstructive pelvic surgery may predispose women to the development of pelvic organ prolapse at an anatomic site opposite to where the repair was performed. Examples of this are the development of posterior vaginal wall prolapse after colposuspension procedures for stress incontinence and the development of anterior vaginal wall prolapse after suspension of the vaginal apex to the sacrospinous ligament.

The true incidence and prevalence of vaginal prolapse are unknown. In a cross-sectional study of over 21,000 women attending a menopause clinic in Italy, uterine prolapse was found in 5.5%, the frequency increasing with age, number of vaginal births, and increased weight (4). Olsen et al. (8) determined that women have a 11% lifetime risk of undergoing a single operation for pelvic organ prolapse and urinary incontinence, and reoperation for these conditions was common.

III. GENERAL CONCEPTS OF SURGICAL REPAIR

When mild forms of isolated uterovaginal prolapse (descent of the cervix not beyond the mid-portion of the vagina) are present, vaginal hysterectomy and culdeplasty with anterior and posterior colporrhaphy are usually sufficient to relieve the patient's symptoms or restore normal vaginal function. Prophylactic measures performed at the time of hysterectomy (vaginal or abdominal) probably decrease the incidence of future vaginal vault prolapse and enterocele. These measures include routine reattachment of endopelvic fascia—cardinal and uterosacral ligaments—to the vaginal vault and routine use of culdeplasty sutures, cul-de-sac obliteration, or enterocele excision after removal of the uterus.

During the preoperative assessment of patients with prolapse, certain decisions must be made:

1.   If the uterus is still present, should hysterectomy be part of the surgical correction? The majority of patients require removal of the uterus. The techniques of vaginal and abdominal hysterectomy are sufficiently discussed in other texts and will not be mentioned further. If hysterectomy is not desired, then pessary use or LeForte partial colpocleisis should be considered. If surgical correction is needed and the patient desires fertility potential (or simply chooses to not have her uterus removed), the preferred surgical approach is controversial because few data exist. A review of the subject has been published by Nichols (9). Abdominal (or laparoscopic) approaches to such patients via modified sacral uterocolpopexy probably provide the most durable repair. Abdominal, laparoscopic, or vaginal uterosacral ligament uterine suspension are innovative and potentially effective approaches, but cure rates are unknown. Sacrospinous fixation with preservation of the uterus also has been shown to be effective in a small selected group of patients (10).

2.   Is the surgical correction intended to preserve a functional vagina? The operations discussed in this chapter are aimed at preservation of vaginal and coital function. For patients in whom future sexual function is not a goal or operative time and morbidity are best kept at a minimum, colpectomy with partial or complete colpocleisis may be indicated.

3.   Should the surgical correction be approached via a vaginal or abdominal route? Factors such as the patient's general medical condition and weight, the need for concurrent surgical procedures, and the preference and expertise of the surgeon influence this decision. A prospective randomized trial by Benson et al. (11) seems to indicate that an abdominal approach to prolapse provides a better anatomic and functional outcome when compared with a vaginal approach, although more studies are clearly needed.

4.   Does the patient have occult or potential stress urinary or fecal incontinence? When choosing the route of surgical correction, the surgeon always must consider the correction of lower urinary tract and lower gastrointestinal dysfunction. Preoperative reduction of the prolapse followed by urodynamic or rectal manometric tests will help the physician to answer this question and to determine which concurrent operations are required.

As previously mentioned, any reconstructive surgery should return the upper vagina to the normal near-horizontal axis. Failure to recognize an enterocele or failure to reconstruct a widened levator hiatus may predispose to postoperative recurrent vaginal prolapse. The length of the vagina is also an important factor for surgical success. The upper 3–4 cm of the vagina lies horizontally over the levator plate. Operations that shorten the vagina do not allow the upper vagina to lie over the levator plate and may predispose to recurrent vaginal prolapse.

Although many different techniques have been described to suspend the vagina, only the most popular techniques done via the vaginal route will be discussed.

IV. VAGINAL PROCEDURES THAT SUSPEND THE VAGINAL APEX

A. Sacrospinous Ligament Suspension: *Surgical Anatomy*

To perform this procedure correctly and safely, the surgeon must be familiar with pararectal anatomy as well as the anatomy of the sacrospinous ligament and its surrounding structures (Fig. 1) (12). The sacrospinous ligaments extend from the ischial spines on each side to the lower portion of the sacrum and coccyx. Nichols and Randall (13) described the sacrospinous ligament as a cordlike structure lying within the substance of the coccygeus muscle. However, the fibromuscular coccygeus muscle and sacrospinous ligament are basically the same structure and thus are called the coccygeus-sacrospinous ligament (C-SSL). The coccygeus muscle has a large fibrous component that is present throughout the body of the muscle and on the anterior surface, where it appears as white ridges. The C-SSL can be identified by palpating the ischial spine and tracing the flat triangular thickening posteriomedially to the sacrum. The fibromuscular coccygeus is attached directly to the underlying sacrotuberous ligament.

Posterior to the C-SSL and sacrotuberous ligament are the gluteus maximus muscle and the fat of the ischiorectal fossa. The pudendal nerves and vessels lie directly posterior to the ischial spine. The sciatic nerve lies superior and lateral to the C-SSL. Also superiorly lies an abundant vascular supply that include superior gluteal vessels and a hypogastric venous plexus (Fig. 1).

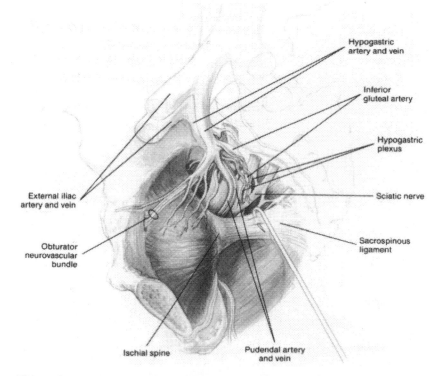

Figure 1 Anatomy of the coccygeus-sacrospinous ligament (C-SSL) complex and surrounding structures. Note close proximity of pudendal vessels, hypogastric plexus, inferior gluteal vessels, and sciatic nerve to C-SSL. (From Ref. 12.)

B.   Sacrospinous Ligament Suspension: *Surgical Technique*

Before this operation is initiated, one should have preoperatively recognized the ischial spine and C-SSL on pelvic examination. Preoperative estrogen replacement therapy should be given liberally, if appropriate. We prefer to use a vaginal estrogen cream for 4–6 weeks preoperatively.

Performance of this operation almost always requires simultaneous correction of the anterior and posterior vaginal walls and enterocele repair. Displacing the prolapsed vaginal apex to the sacrospinous ligament to see whether the anterior and posterior vaginal wall prolapse disappears, helps to determine whether cystocele and rectocele repairs are needed. The patient should be routinely consented for these repairs because many times it is difficult to discern the extent of the various defects preoperatively.

The technique of unilateral sacrospinous ligament fixation is as follows:

1.   The patient is placed in dorsal lithotomy position and the bladder is drained before the first incision. Prophylactic antibiotics are given routinely before the operation.

2.   The apex of the vagina is grasped with two Allis clamps, and downward traction is used to determine the extent of the vaginal prolapse and associated pelvic support defects. The vaginal apex is reduced to the sacrospinous ligament intended to be used, usually on the right. The apex is tagged with two sutures for its later identification.

3.   If the patient has complete eversion of the vagina and requires anterior vaginal wall repair and/or bladder neck suspension, we prefer doing this portion of the operation first. During this procedure one should dissect the bladder base away from the vaginal apex, thus lowering the risk of cystotomy. An anterior colporrhaphy with suburethral plication and/or sling is completed. The anterior vaginal wall epithelium is closed with a continuous running suture.

4.   The posterior vaginal wall is then incised. After a transverse perineal incision, a midline posterior vaginal wall incision is made just short of the apex of the vagina, leaving a small vaginal bridge 3–4 cm wide. In the majority of cases, an enterocele sac is present. This sac should be dissected off the posterior vaginal wall and closed with a high purse-string suture. Once the enterocele has been incised and ligated, one is ready to begin the sacrospinous ligament fixation.

5.   The first step is entry into the perirectal space. The rectal pillar separates the rectovaginal space from the perirectal space. The rectal pillar is areolar tissue that may contain a few small muscle fibers and blood vessels. In the majority of cases, entry into the perirectal space is best achieved by breaking through the fibroareolar tissue just lateral to the enterocele sac at the level of the ischial spine. This maneuver can usually be accomplished bluntly by mobilizing the rectum medially. The use of gauze on the index finger or a tonsil clamp may aide in breaking through into this space.

6.   Once the perirectal space is entered, usually on the right, the ischial spine is identified and, with dorsal and medial movement of the fingers, the C-SSL is palpated. Blunt dissection is used to further remove tissue from this area. The surgeon should take great care to ensure that the rectum is adequately retracted medially. At this time we recommend performing a rectal examination to ensure that no inadvertent rectal injury has occurred.

7.   Two techniques have been popularized for the actual passage of sutures through the ligament (Fig. 2). The first technique uses a long-handled Deschamps ligature carrier and nerve hook (Fig. 2A). Long straight retractors are used to expose the coccygeus muscle. Heaney retractors or Breisky-Navratil retractors are preferred. One must take great care not to let the tip of the medial retractor be pushed across the anterior surface of the sacrum, risking potential damage to nerves and vessels. If the right sacrospinous ligament is to be used, the middle and index fingers of the left hand are placed on the medial surface of the ischial spine and, under

direct vision, the tip of the ligature carrier penetrates the C-SSL at a point two fingerbreadths medial to the ischial spine. When pushing the ligature carrier through the body of the C-SSL, considerable resistance should be encountered; this must be overcomed by forceful yet controlled rotation of the handle of the ligature carrier. If visualization of the C-SSL is difficult, the muscle and the ligament can be grasped in a long Babcock or Allis clamp, which helps to isolate the tissue to be sutured. After suture passage, the fingers of the left hand are withdrawn. The retractor is suitably repositioned and the tip of the ligature carrier is visualized. Alternatively, sutures may be delivered under direct investigation without the placement of the left hand in the space and with use of lateral and medial Breisky-Navratil retractors and a posterior retractor. The suture is then grasped with a nerve hook (Fig. 2A). A second suture is similarly placed 1 cm medial to the first. To ensure that an appropriate amount of tissue has been obtained, one should be able to gently move the patient with traction of the sutures.

A second technique that has been popularized for passing the sutures through the C-SSL is the technique of Miyazaki (14) using a Miya hook ligature carrier (Fig. 2B). Several disposable instruments have since been developed to imitate this technique. The proposed advantage is that it is safer and easier to direct the ligature carrier into the C-SSL with palpation and then pull it down into the safe perirectal space below. In this modification, the surgeon uses the middle finger of one hand to palpate the C-SSL approximately two fingerbreadths medial to the ischial spine. The Miya hook with a suture attached is slid along the palmer surface of the hand that has palpated the ligament and the hook point pushed through the C-SSL from above downward (Fig. 2B). The handle of the instrument is closed and elevated and the posterior notched retractor is placed to visualize the posterior tip of the instrument. A nerve hook is used to retrieve the suture (Fig. 2B, inset). Again, this procedure can be performed with retractors, under direct vision as an alternative to the use of the operator's left hand.

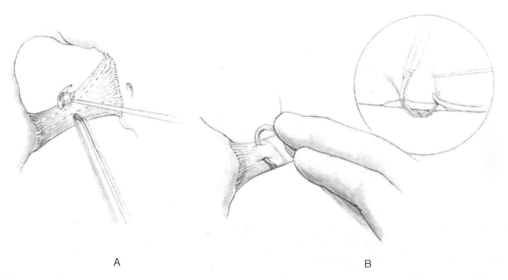

A   B

Figure 2   (A) Passage of Deschamps ligature carrier with suture through C-SSL. Note that needletip is passed in superior direction. Retrieval of suture is with nerve hook. (B) Passage of Miya hook through C-SSL. Note that needletip is passed inferiorly. Retrieval of suture is facilitated by using notched speculum. (From Ref. 12.)

8.   The surgeon is now ready to bring these stitches out to the apex of the vagina. If nonabsorbable sutures are used, then the sutures should be placed through the full-thickness fibromuscularis of the undersurface of the vaginal apex but not through the epithelium. The suture is placed and tied by a single half-hitch, while the free end of the suture is held long. Traction of the free end of the suture pulls the vagina directly onto the C-SSL. A square knot fixes it in place. Some surgeons prefer to use delayed absorbable suture and, in this case, the free end of the suspending sutures can be passed through the vaginal apex and tied. It is important that the vagina come into direct contact with the coccygeus muscle to facilitate scarring and to ensure that no suture bridge exists. While tying these sutures, it may be useful to perform a rectal examination to detect any suture bridges.

9.   After these sutures are tied, the posterior colpoperinorrhaphy is completed, as needed, and the vagina is packed with a moist gauze overnight.

The results of sacrospinous fixation are difficult to evaluate because few studies report long-term follow-up, and prospective randomized surgical trials utilizing this technique are rare. Karram et al. (12) reviewed the literature on cure rates for studies reported from 1981 to 1997. After 2 or more years of follow-up, objective cure rates ranged from 70% to 94%. Recurrent vaginal apex prolapse is relatively uncommon. The most common site for recurrent prolapse in nearly every series is the anterior vaginal wall, perhaps because the vagina is pulled in an exaggerated posterior direction, possibly exposing the anterior vaginal wall to excessive intra-abdominal forces.

One of the largest studies on surgical outcomes after sacrospinous ligament suspension and pelvic reconstruction was reported by Paraiso et al. (15). This study followed 243 patients for an average of 74 months. Recurrent vaginal support defects were found in the anterior, posterior, and apical segments in 37%, 14%, and 8% of patients, respectively. Defect-free survival rates at 5 and 10 years were 80% and 52%, respectively. In this study only 4.5% of patients underwent subsequent pelvic reconstructive surgery.

Although infrequent, serious intraoperative complications can occur with sacrospinous ligament fixation. Potential complications of the procedure include hemorrhage from the veins around the C-SSL complex, buttock pain, pudendal nerve injury, rectal injury, stress urinary incontinence, and vaginal stenosis (15).

C. Endopelvic Fascia Repair (Modified McCall Culdeplasty)

Webb et al. (16) reported on 660 women who underwent primary endopelvic fascia repair for posthysterectomy vault prolapse between 1976 and 1987. The technique of this repair is as follows:

1.   An elliptical wedge of vaginal epithelium is excised initially from the anterior and posterior walls of the prolapsed vagina to narrow the vault and to allow access to the lateral apical supports of the vagina and rectum. The width and length of the excised wedge are determined by the desired dimensions of the reconstructed vagina.

2.   The enterocele sac is isolated and excised, and the ureters are identified by palpation or dissection.

3.   Up to three modified McCall stitches are placed. Each suture incorporates a full thickness of the posterior vaginal wall, the cul-de-sac peritoneum, the remnants of the uterosacral-cardinal ligament complex laterally, and the fascial tissue lateral and posterior to the upper vagina and rectum.

4.   Sutures are then tied, resulting in fixation of the prolapsed vaginal vault to the uppermost portion of the endopelvic fascia as well as high closure of the cul-de-sac peritoneum.

Webb et al. (16) reported results of 660 women, most of whom were followed up with a questionnaire. Information about recurrent prolapse was available on 504 women (76%). Fifty-eight patients (9%) complained of a "bulge" or "protrusion" at the time of questioning. The question about satisfaction with the operation was answered by 385 patients, and 82% indicated that they were satisfied. Forty-two (22%) of 189 sexually active women complained of dyspareunia.

D.   Iliococcygeus Fascia Suspension

In 1963, Inmon (17) described bilateral fixation of the everted vaginal apex to the iliococcygeus fascia just distal to the ischial spines in three patients with atrophied uterosacral ligaments. The technique of this repair is as follows:

1.   The posterior vaginal wall is opened in the midline as for a posterior colporrhaphy, and the rectovaginal spaces are dissected widely to the levator ani muscles bilaterally. The dissection is extended bluntly toward the ischial spines.

2.   With the surgeon's nondominant hand pressing the rectum downward and medial, an area 1–2 cm caudad and posterior to the ischial spine in the iliococcygeus muscle and fascia is exposed (Fig. 3). A single No. 0 delayed absorbable suture is placed deeply into the levator muscle and fascia. Both ends of the suture are passed through the ipsilateral posterior section of vaginal apex and held with a hemostat. This is repeated on the opposite side.

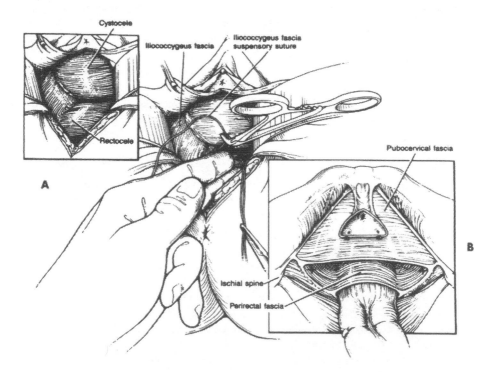

Figure 3   Iliococcygeus fascia suspension. (A) With the surgeon's finger pressing the rectum downward, the right iliococcygeus fascia suture is placed. *Inset:* view of the dissected vagina. (B) Abdominal view of the endopelvic fascia. *Plus marks* show the approximate location of the iliococcygeus fascia sutures. (From Ref. 19.)

3.   The posterior colporrhaphy is completed and the vagina closed. Both sutures are tied, elevating the posterior vaginal apices. This repair is probably most effective when done in conjunction with a culdeplasty or uterosacral ligament suspension.

From 1981 to 1993, Shull et al. (18) and Meeks et al. (19) used the Inmon technique to treat 152 patients with posthysterectomy vault prolapse or total uterine procidentia. There were four intraoperative complications, including one rectal and one bladder laceration and two cases of hemorrhage requiring transfusion. Thirteen (8%) patients developed recurrent pelvic support defects at various sites 6 weeks to 5 years after the initial procedure; two had vault prolapse, eight had anterior vaginal wall relaxation, and three had posterior wall defects.

In a more recent retrospective study, Maher et al. (20) compared the results of iliococcygeus fascia suspension to sacrospinous ligament suspension in 128 patients. Objective cure (defined as no vaginal prolapse beyond the halfway point of the vagina) was found in 53% of patients after iliococcygeus fascia suspension, and in 67% after sacrospinous ligament suspension. As with other studies, most recurrences of prolapse were in the anterior vaginal wall.

E.   High Uterosacral Ligament Suspension With Fascial Reconstruction

A technique for vaginal apex prolapse and enterocele repair—high uterosacral ligament suspension with fascial reconstruction—can be performed either transvaginally, transabdominally, or laparoscopically. The approach is not as important as are the concepts involved. This operation closely follows the principles of hernia surgery used in the management of umbilical, ventral, and inguinal hernias: the identification of a "fascial" defect, reduction of intraabdominal contents, closure and reinforcement of the defect. The enterocele must be closed and both the anterior and posterior vaginal walls must be reliably suspended at the apex. In a woman with normal support, the vaginal apex is suspended by the cardinal and uterosacral ligaments; these same structures are used in most operations for prolapse and enterocele repair. The technique of this repair is as follows:

1.   The patient is placed in dorsal lithotomy positon, and the bladder is drained before the first incision. Prophylactic antibiotics are given routinely before the operation.

2.   We attempt to identify the limits of the enterocele by physical examination, looking for demarcation of rugae along the anterior and posterior walls of the vagina near the apex. The absence of rugae implies deficient or absent connective tissue and, by inference, defines the borders of the enterocele itself. Occasionally, an enterocele is not present and entry into the peritoneal cavity is not possible. In this case, an extraperitoneal suspension to uterosacral ligaments or an iliococcygeus fascia suspension or sacrospinous ligament suspension is done.

3.   The vaginal epithelium at the apex is grasped with Allis clamps and a vasoconstricting solution is injected submucosally. The vaginal epithelium is incised with a scalpel vertically or in a diamond shape (Fig. 4), the enterocele is identified, and the edges of the vaginal epithelium are dissected sharply away from the enterocele sac.

4.   The enterocele sac is opened by sharp dissection, and the abdominal cavity is inspected for the presence of adhesions or other pathology. A large, moist, soft pack is placed in the posterior cul-de-sac and hollow of the sacrum. A wide Deaver or Breisky-Navratil retractor is used to elevate the pack and the intestines out of the operative field.

5.   The ischial spines are palpated. The remnants of uterosacral ligaments are found posterior and medial to the ischial spines. They can be identified more easily by using Allis or Kocher clamps attached to the vaginal epithelium at approximately 4 o'clock and 8 o'clock (at the old hysterectomy scar) to place tension on structures in the lateral wall of the pelvis

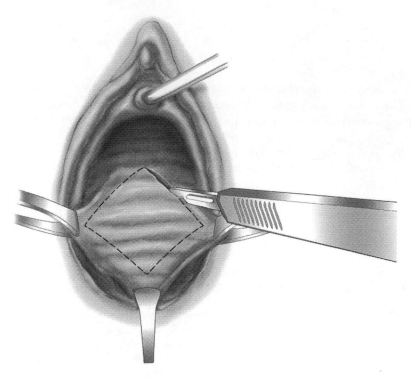

Figure 4 High uterosacral ligament vaginal suspension. To identify the enterocele sac, a diamond-shaped incision is made at the vaginal apex, and the epithelium is dissected away to facilitate identification of the enterocele.

(Fig. 5). The clamp is elevated and pulled straight upward; when tension is placed with the clamp, the contralateral index finger is used to palpate the connective tissue condensations along the side of the pelvis (uterosacral ligaments).

6.   A series of interrupted nonabsorable (or delayed absorbable) sutures then are placed in each uterosacral ligament beginning at approximately the level of, but posterior and medial to, the ischial spine. The needle is driven from a lateral to medial position each time. Care should be taken to avoid the ureter with these sutures. After the first suture has been placed, the second is placed in a more cephalad and medial position (toward the sacrum). The third is placed cephalad and medial to the second (Fig. 6).

7.   After the suspensory sutures have been placed, the gauze pack and retractors are removed, and the surgeon should perform any required cystocele repair and/or bladder neck suspension or sling, as needed. The suspensory sutures in the uterosacral ligaments are then systematically placed into the most apical portions of the pubocervical and rectovaginal "fasciae." The most superior suspensory sutures (closest to the sacrum) are sewn to the most medial portions of the pubocervical and rectovaginal fasciae, as shown in Figure 6. This suture can be nonabsorbable or delayed absorbable. The suture next to that one is placed more laterally into the pubocervical and rectovaginal fasciae. The most caudal (delayed absorbable) suture then is placed most laterally into the pubocervical and rectovaginal fasciae and passed out the vaginal epithelium laterally at 3 o'clock and 9 o'clock.

8.   The patient is given intravenous Indigo Carmine, and the suspensory sutures are tied sequentially. Once the suspensory sutures have been tied properly, the apex of the vagina

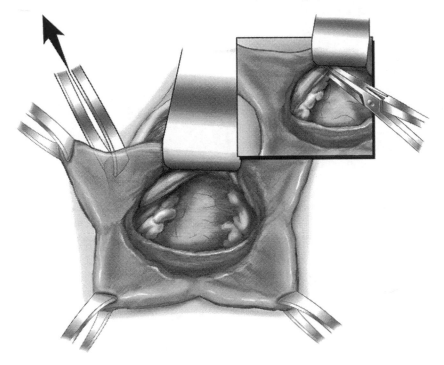

Figure 5 High uterosacral ligament vaginal suspension. To identify the uterosacral ligament, an Allis clamp is placed on the vaginal epithelium at the right apex and pulled straight upward (arrow). The right uterosacral ligament, now on tension, is visible in the pelvis. *Inset:* A long Allis clamp is used to grasp the right uterosacral ligament.

should be in the hollow of the sacrum and the connective tissue tube closed at the vaginal apex.

    9.   Cystoscopy is performed to ensure ureteral patency. If no flow of urine is seen from one of the ureters, the sutures are removed on that side one at a time from lateral to medial. This usually restores ureteral patency. If not, then cul-de-sac exploration and ureteral stent placement may be necessary.

    10.   The vaginal epithelium is assessed and tailored to the contour of the vagina by excising excess tissue. The epithelial incision is closed vertically or horizontally with an absorbable suture.

    This technique of vaginal vault suspension, and enterocele repair also can be done laparoscopically or transabdominally. Figure 7 shows the approximation of the vaginal cuff to uterosacral ligaments, in conjunction with an anterior colporrhaphy. In the case of a woman who has vaginal apex prolapse and urodynamic stress incontinence, our preference would be to perform a sling in conjunction with the procedure. When appropriate, a perineorrhaphy is performed at the completion of the procedure.

    Several studies have described outcomes of series of patients with vaginal prolapse after uterosacral ligament vaginal suspension. No prospective trial comparing this operation with others has been done. Shull et al. (21) described the results of 302 consecutive women who underwent uterosacral ligament vaginal suspension. Eighty-seven percent of women had optimal anatomic outcomes with no prolapse at any site in the vagina at follow-up examination. Only 5% of patients had development of stage II or greater prolapse at any site and most recurrences were

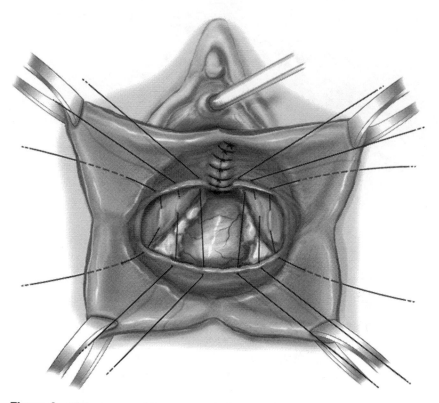

Figure 6 High uterosacral ligament vaginal suspension. Three sutures are placed from lateral to medial in each uterosacral ligament. The arms of the sutures are brought through the vaginal muscularis anteriorly (pubocervical fascia) and posteriorly (rectovaginal fascia). The most lateral suture on each side is absorbable, and is passed through the vaginal epithelium at the apex.

in the anterior wall. A 1% rate of intraoperative ureteral injury or obstruction and a 1% rate of blood transfusion were reported (21).

Barber et al. (22) performed uterosacral ligament vaginal suspension on 46 women with pelvic organ prolapse. At follow-up examination, 23% of patients had stage II prolapse, usually a recurrent cystocele or rectocele. Two patients (5%) developed stage III apical prolapse with enterocele and required another operation. Importantly, five of 46 patients (11%) were found to have ureteral obstruction intraoperatively after the apex suspension sutures were tied. This observation underscores the need to assess ureteral patency in every patient at the completion of this procedure and to remove any offending sutures if a ureter is obstructed.

V. CONCLUSION

The prevalence of vaginal prolapse appears to be increasing. This may be because of the increased longevity of women, but also is probably a result of inadequate recognition and repair of pelvic organ support defects when pelvic surgery has been performed. The standard use of

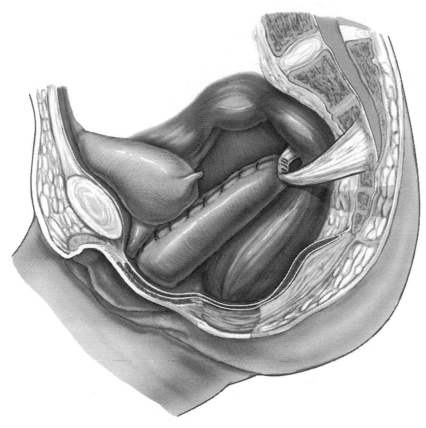

Figure 7 Completed uterosacral vaginal vault suspension and anterior colporrhaphy.

cul-de-sac plication (McCall culdeplasty) at every hysterectomy and urethropexy would probably decrease the likelihood of iatrogenic enterocele. Finally, more education and research in
the principles of pelvic and vaginal reconstructive surgery are needed to improve care to all
affected women.

REFERENCES

1. DeLancey JO. Anatomic aspects of vaginal eversion after hysterectomy. Am J Obstet Gynecol 1992;
    166:1717–1724.
2. Richardson AC. The anatomic defects in rectocele and enterocele. J Pelvic Surg 1995; 1:215.
3. Swift SE, Pound T, Dias JK. Case-control study of etiologic factors in the development of severe
    pelvic organ prolapse. Int Urogynecol J 2001; 12:187–192.
4. Progetto Menopausa Italia Study Group. Risk factors for genital prolapse in non-hysterectomized
    women around menopause. Results from a large cross-sectional study in menopausal clinics in
    Italy. Eur J Obstet Gynecol Reprod Biol 2000; 93:135–140.
5. Jorgensen S, Hein HO, Gyntelberg F. Heavy lifting at work and risk of genital prolapse and herniated
    lumbar disc in assistant nurses. Occup Med (Oxf) 1994; 44:47–49.

6. Spence-Jones C, Kumm MA, Henry MM, Hudson CN. Bowel dysfunction: a pathogenic factor in uterovaginal prolapse and urinary stress incontinence. Br J Obstet Gynaecol 1994; 101:147–152.
7. Funt MI, Thompson JD, Birch H. Normal vaginal axis. South Med J 1978; 71:1534–1535.
8. Olsen AL, Smith VJ, Bergstrom JO, Colling JC, Clark AL. Epidemiology of surgically managed pelvic organ prolapse and urinary incontinence. Obstet Gynecol 1997; 89:501–506.
9. Nichols DH. Fertility retention in the patient with genital prolapse. Am J Obstet Gynecol 1991; 164:1155–1158.
10. Kovac RS, Cruikshank SH. Successful pregnancies and vaginal deliveries after sacrospinous uterosacral fixation in five of nineteen patients. Am J Obstet Gynecol 1993; 168:1778–1790.
11. Benson JT, Lucente V, McClellan E. Vaginal versus abdominal reconstructive surgery for the treatment of pelvic support defects: a prospective randomized study with long-term outcome evaluation. Am J Obstet Gynecol 1996; 175:1418–1421.
12. Karram MM, Sze E, Walters MD. Surgical correction of uterine and vaginal apex prolapse: vaginal, abdominal and obliterative procedures. In: Walters MD, Karram MM, eds. Urogynecology and Reconstructive Pelvic Surgery. 2nd ed. St. Louis: Mosby, 1999.
13. Nichols DH, Randall CL. In: Vaginal Surgery. 3rd ed. Baltimore: Williams & Wilkins, 1989.
14. Miyazaki FS. Miya hook ligature carrier for sacrospinous ligament suspension. Obstet Gynecol 1987; 70:286–288.
15. Paraiso MFR, Ballard LA, Walters MD, Lee JC, Mitchinson AR. Pelvic support defects and visceral and sexual function in women treated with sacrospinous ligament suspension and pelvic reconstruction. Am J Obstet Gynecol 1996; 175:1423–1431.
16. Webb MJ, Aronson MP, Ferguson LK, Lee RA. Posthysterectomy vaginal vault prolapse: primary repair in 693 patients. Obstet Gynecol 1998; 92:281–285.
17. Inmon WB. Pelvic relaxation and repair including prolapse of vagina following hysterectomy. South Med J 1963; 56:577–582.
18. Shull BL, Capen CV, Riggs MW, Kuehl TJ. Bilateral attachment of the vaginal cuff to iliococcygeus fascia: an effective method of cuff suspension. Am J Obstet Gynecol 1993; 168:1669–1674.
19. Meeks GR, Washburne JF, McGehee RP, Wiser WL. Repair of vaginal vault prolapse by suspension of the vagina to iliococcygeus (prespinous) fascia. Am J Obstet Gynecol 1994; 171:1444–1452.
20. Maher CF, Murray CJ, Carey MP, Dwyer PL, Ugoni AM. Iliococcygeus or sacrospinous fixation for vaginal vault prolapse. Obstet Gynecol 2001; 98:40–44.
21. Shull BL, Bachofen C, Coates KW, Kuehl TJ. A transvaginal approach to repair of apical and other associated sites of pelvic organ prolapse with uterosacral ligaments. Am J Obstet Gynecol 2000; 183:1365–1374.
22. Barber MD, Visco AG, Wiedner AC, Amundsen CL, Bump RC. Bilateral uterosacral ligament vaginal vault suspension with site-specific endopelvic fascia defect repair for treatment of pelvic organ prolapse. Am J Obstet Gynecol 2000; 183:1402–1410.

48

Abdominal Sacrocolpopexy for the Correction of Vaginal Vault Prolapse

J. Christian Winters and Richard Vanlangendonck
Ochsner Clinic Foundation, New Orleans, Louisiana, U.S.A.

R. Duane Cespedes
Wilford Hall Medical Center, Lackland AFB, Texas, U.S.A.

I. INTRODUCTION

Prolapse of the vaginal vault is one of the most challenging conditions encountered by pelvic surgeons. A comprehensive knowledge of the anatomy and function of female pelvic organs is essential to achieve optimal outcome. Vaginal vault prolapse is reported to occur in ~20% of all women with prolapse (1). As the life expectancy of the population increases and awareness of this condition improves, a greater number of patients with this condition will be detected.

Vaginal vault prolapse occurs as a loss of apical support, which is a result of detachment or excessive stretching of the cardinal and uterosacral ligaments from the vagina. Factors predisposing to this form of pelvic floor relaxation include multiparity, enterocele, trauma occurring during labor and delivery, postmenopausal atrophy, obesity, connective tissue abnormalities, and strenuous physical activity. Vaginal vault prolapse is usually accompanied by a cystocele, rectocele, enterocele, or a combination of these defects (2). Richter reported that 72% of patients with vault prolapse had a combination of other pelvic floor defects (3).

Ideally, treatment of vaginal vault prolapse should recreate almost normal vaginal anatomy by preserving vaginal depth and axis to create a functional vagina with durable pelvic support. This should be performed utilizing procedures with minimal morbidity and a low recurrence rate.

There are many procedures to correct vaginal vault prolapse, and several factors must be considered when selecting therapy. Proper evaluation should encompass identification of all anatomic defects, assessment of urethrovesical, anal sphincter and sexual function, and the medical condition of the patient. Once these factors are considered, optimal selection of treatment is possible for each individual. In this chapter we will describe how to diagnose vaginal vault prolapse, and review the use of the most common abdominal approach to repair this pelvic floor defect, the abdominal sacral colpopexy.

II. EVALUATION OF VAGINAL VAULT PROLAPSE

A patient with vaginal vault prolapse often complains of vaginal protrusion and pressure, dyspareunia, difficulty walking, pelvic pain, and urinary or anal incontinence. Difficulty voiding, recurrent urinary tract infections, and inability to empty the bladder are associated symptoms. Some women present with isolated complaints of urinary incontinence and no local symptoms related to the prolapsed vaginal vault. Patients with complete vaginal vault eversion or uterine procidentia may develop hydronephrosis due to angulation of the ureters (4). The psychological impact of this problem on females can be significant.

Meticulous examination is important not only to establish the diagnosis, but also to uncover the other disorders of pelvic floor dysfunction that frequently occur with vaginal vault prolapse. Support of the anterior vaginal wall, vaginal apex (or uterus), posterior vaginal wall, and perineum should be separately evaluated. During examination of the anterior vaginal wall, the urethral support should be assessed. In many cases, the lack of support and hypermobility of the urethra are obvious with straining; however, a sterile cotton swab test may be employed with a well-lubricated cotton swab placed at the level of the bladder neck in equivocal exams. During straining, a deflection of the cotton swab >30° signifies urethral hypermobility (5). If a cystocele is present, it should be determined if the loss of support is in the midline ("central defect") or paravaginal, caused by a "lateral defect" separation of the vagina from its attachment to the pelvic side wall at the arcus tendineus. This is done simply by placing sponge forceps into the lateral fornices of the vagina to reapproximate the lateral vaginal walls to the arcus. If this completely reduces the prolapse, an isolated lateral defect exists. However, if prolapse of the anterior wall still occurs during support of the lateral vaginal wall, a central defect exists. If apical support with the forceps completely reduces the cystocoele, a transverse defect due to separation from the apical paracervical support of the anterior vaginal wall may exist. With half the speculum displacing the anterior vaginal wall, the posterior wall of the vagina is assessed. It is important to distinguish the etiology of prolapse high in the posterior vaginal wall as either enterocele or high rectocele. This is accomplished by bimanual rectovaginal examination in the supine and/or standing position to detect an enterocele. If a sac or bowel can be palpated during this exam, this indicates the presence of an enterocele. If no enterocele sac or bowel is palpated between the rectum and vagina, this defect is most likely a high rectocele. A high rectocele can be confirmed by transvaginal palpation of the examiner's finger in the rectum without intervening tissue between the rectum and the vaginal wall.

The assessment of apical support of the vagina is easiest when the cervix is present, as it is a well-defined landmark of the vaginal apex. With straining, the descent of a well-supported uterus should not occur, and is noted by an absence of cervical descent. The descent of the cervix half-way to the hymenal ring indicates a moderate loss of uterine support. In posthysterectomy patients, defining the true vaginal apex can be more difficult. This is a difficult aspect of the pelvic examination that warrants attention to detail, as apical prolapse can be hidden by large anterior or posterior compartment prolapse or partially reduced by the examining speculum. The cuff scar will denote the apex, and "dimples" at the lateral aspects of the apex of the vagina usually represent attachments of the uterosacral ligaments. When the cuff and apex of the vagina extend half-way to the hymenal ring with straining, these patients have significant prolapse of the vaginal vault. Many patients may need to be evaluated in the standing position with the examiner's fingers placed at the vaginal apex. If the examiner's fingers descend half-way to the hymenal ring or more with straining, significant vault prolapse exists. However, women may be symptomatic with even lesser degree of apical prolapse. When it is difficult to identify the exact pelvic floor defects present, dynamic evaluation of the pelvic floor can be accomplished with magnetic resonance imaging (6,7).

It is essential for the clinician to also detect any functional abnormalities of the lower urogenital tract by assessing lower urinary tract and colorectal function. Stress incontinence may develop after correction of prolapse (8,9), most likely as a result of "unmasking" occult stress urinary incontinence after the bladder support is restored. A stress test with reduction of the vaginal prolapse by a pessary or vaginal packing should be performed. Care should be taken to not occlude the urethra during packing, as a false-negative result may occur. Many of these women have concomitant urethral sphincteric deficiency, so the authors prefer urodynamics with vaginal packing to assess abdominal leak-point pressures to evaluate urethral function. This is an accurate way to assess abdominal leak-point pressures in patients with significant prolapse (10,11), and allows selection of the most appropriate stress incontinence procedure. All patients should be carefully screened for colorectal dysfunction. Although the vast majority of patients complain of constipation, symptoms of fecal incontinence and/or rectal prolapse should be completely evaluated. Rectal ultrasonography and/or sphincter manometry with electromyography testing should be considered in patients complaining of fecal incontinence.

After evaluation of pelvic floor defects and pelvic organ function, treatment options can be based on the patient's age, medical condition, coexisting vaginal support defects, previous surgical procedures, and the desire for sexual activity. There is not one procedure for vaginal vault prolapse correction that is optimal for all patients. The patients should be individualized, and the pelvic surgeon should be proficient in several procedures to achieve correction of vaginal vault prolapse. In the young female who desires a fully active lifestyle and sexuality, or a patient who has failed a transvaginal approach to vaginal vault suspension, the abdominal sacral colpopexy is an excellent procedure to achieve durable support to the vaginal apex while restoring a functional vagina.

III. ABDOMINAL SACRAL COLPOPEXY: SURGICAL TECHNIQUE

Pelvic surgeons should be familiar with many of the surgical principles to achieve a most successful outcome. Important details to successfully complete this procedure are cul-de-sac closure, fixation of the vaginal apex to the sacrum with graft interposition, and correction of any paravaginal defects. To just suspend the apex of the vagina with mesh and not complete these associated repairs, places a patient at significant risk for recurrent enterocele or cystocele.

Postmenopausal women with ovaries remaining are counseled about the risks and benefits of oophorectomy at the time of surgical intervention. All patients are administered a mechanical bowel preparation. Thromboembolic elimination stockings and sequential compression devices are utilized. The patients are positioned in the low lithotomy position, providing both transvaginal and transabdominal access. A low midline abdominal incision is preferred to allow exposure of the sacral promontory. A Pfannenstiel incision may also be chosen in younger patients, although exposure may be slightly more difficult. If anterior colporrhaphy or pubovaginal sling is needed, these procedures should be performed initially as access may be more difficult following colpopexy. When a sling is performed, the authors complete the vaginal dissection but do not perforate the endopelvic fascia until after a paravaginal repair is performed. Venous bleeding into the retropubic space can complicate exposure of the arcus tendineus on the pelvic sidewall. We commonly perform the anterior repair and place sutures to secure the sling into position initially. After the abdominal sacral colpopexy and abdominal enterocele repair are completed, the paravaginal repair is performed. When the retropubic space is exposed, the endopelvic fascia is perforated and the sling is positioned using the previously placed sutures.

The operation begins by entry into the peritoneal cavity and removal of adhesions within the pelvis. Packing of the small intestine and sigmoid colon is performed above the level of the sacral promontory to complete exposure. An incision is made in the posterior peritoneum over the sacral promontory, extending into the cul-de-sac along the right lateral aspect of the rectum. Electrocautery is utilized when dividing the fatty tissue over the promontory. Excessive blunt dissection is avoided in this area as shearing of presacral veins with severe bleeding may occur. Care is taken to avoid the middle sacral vein traversing over the promontory. The anterior sacral ligament is visualized. Two or three permanent sutures (authors use No. 1 Ethibond, MO-7 needle [Ethicon Inc, Johnson & Johnson, Somerville, NJ]) are placed into the ligament and periosteum over the sacral promontory (insert) (Fig. 1). These sutures are safely secured for later placement into the graft. The peritoneum over the vaginal cuff is incised, and the peritoneum is dissected off of the apex of the vagina (Fig. 2). Large EEA (end-to-end anastomosis) sizers are useful to provide exposure of the vaginal apex and facilitate suture placement. Spongesticks are to be avoided as retained sponge material can occur during suture placement (12). A 2.0-cm-wide segment of graft is sutured to the exposed vaginal cuff utilizing six permanent sutures (authors use 2-0 Ethibond). The graft is secured to the vagina by folding it over the cuff of the vagina and allowing the long end of the graft to exit posteriorly and extend to the sacrum (Fig. 3). After placing an obturator in the vagina, the enterocele sac (if present) is identified and elevated with an Allis clamp. Several permanent purse-string sutures are placed into the enterocele sac to obliterate it (Fig. 4). A Halban culdeplasty is performed by placing linear sutures (2-0 Ethibond) into the posterior peritoneum on the anterior surface of rectum up to the graft on the vaginal cuff. The central sutures are placed through the obliterated enterocele sac to prevent recurrence of enterocele (Fig. 5). Upward retraction of the graft will assist in exposing the cul-de-sac. Usually four to six sutures are utilized to complete adequate cul-de-sac closure. After closure of the cul-de-sac, the graft is secured to the sacral promontory with the preplaced permanent sutures. The proper length of the graft is established by placing the obturator all the way into the vagina, but not pushing the vagina upward. The graft is placed around the right lateral aspect of the rectum. A space of two fingerwidths between the graft and the rectum prevents

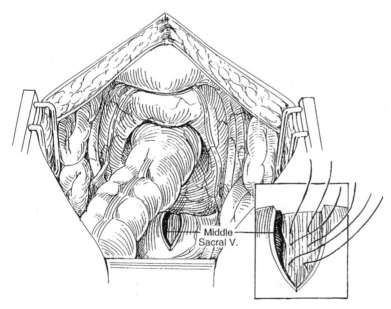

Figure 1   An incision is made in the posterior peritoneum over the sacral promontory, and sutures of No. 1 Ethibond (MO-7 needle) are placed into the ligament and periosteum over the sacral promontory (insert).

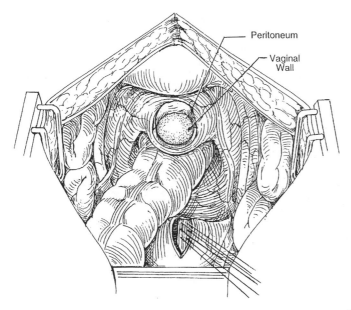

Figure 2   The peritoneum is dissected off the apex of the vagina. The peritoneum is preserved as a flap for later placement over the graft. Dissection is facilitated by placing an EEA sizer in the vagina.

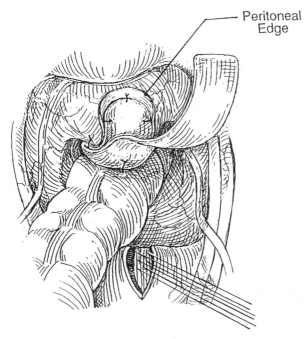

Figure 3   The graft is sutured to the exposed vaginal cuff utilizing six sutures of 2-0 Ethibond.

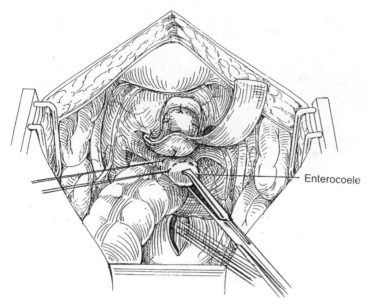

Figure 4   Purse-string sutures of 2-0 Ethibond are placed into the enterocele sac to obliterate it.

compression of the rectum over the graft (Fig. 6). The excessive length of the graft is trimmed after fixation to the sacrum. The graft is positioned in the retroperitoneal space by closing the presacral peritoneum over the graft, and covering the graft on the vagina with the superior edge of the peritoneum flap over the vagina. (Figure 7 demonstrates the completed repair in sagittal view.) Note the completed culdeplasty obliterating the cul-de-sac and the vaginal cuff supported by the suspensory graft. When properly performed, the reoccurrence of enterocele

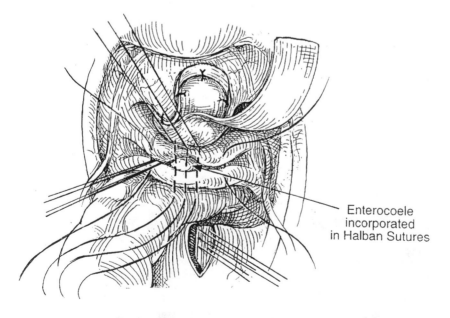

Figure 5   Step 5. A Halban culdeplasty is performed by placing linear sutures (2-0 Ethibond) through the posterior peritoneum and on the outer surface of rectum up to the vaginal cuff.

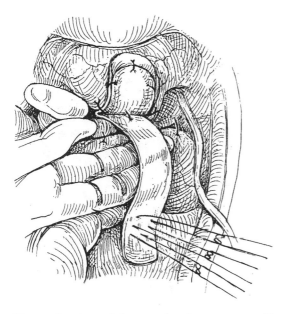

Figure 6 The graft is secured to the promontory. Note two fingers between graft and rectum to prevent excess tension.

and vault prolapse should be minimal. Paravaginal repair and stress incontinence procedure are then performed if indicated. The patient is then examined to determine if posterior repair is needed.

A. Results

The sacral colpopexy has been consistently documented as an excellent method to correct vaginal vault prolapse with success rates of 85–100%. Minimal failure rates are reported in numerous series (Table 1).

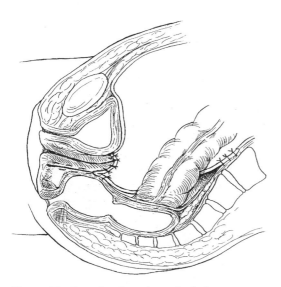

Figure 7 Completed repair, sagittal view.

Table 1   Failure (Recurrent Vaginal Vault Prolapse) Rates and Complications After Abdominal Sacral Colpopexy

Author	No. of patients	Mean age	Mean follow-up (months)	Concomitant surgery	Failure N (%)	Graft material	Complications and/or recurrent prolapse
Addison (13)	54	58.4	39	6 A/P repairs	2 (3.7)	Mersilene	Hemorrhage 1
Fox (14)	29	57	14	N/A	0 (0)	Teflon	Mesh infect. 1 Cystotomy 1 Foot palsy 1
Patsner (15)	75	62	36	25 radical hyst	2 (2.7)	Marlex	Mesh erosion 1
Snyder (16)	116	62	43	N/A	8 (6.7)	PTFE Dacron	Mesh erosion 4 Cystocele and rectocele 24
Diana (7)	15	57	20	N/A	0 (0)	Prolene	None
Virtanen (18)	30	60.7	36	N/A	4 (13.3)	LyoDura Gore-Tex	Mesh erosion 1 Cystocele (18%) Rectocele (15%)
Benson (19)	40	66.2	30	12 anterior rep 20 posterior rep 19 culdeplasty	1 (2.5)	N/A	Cystocele 4 Enterocele 2
Cowan (20)	39	54.5	30	N/A	1 (2.6)	Mersilene Prolene	Mesh erosion 2
Winters (21)	20	67	11.3	Anterior rep 1 Posterior rep 5 PV sling 9 Burch 7	0 (0)	Marlex	Cystocele 3 Rectocele 3

B.   Abdominal Sacral Colpoperineopexy

Cundiff and associates have described a technique to incorporate the correction of posterior compartment defects and perineal descent associated with vaginal vault prolapse (22). The rationale is to decrease the incidence of recurrent enterocele, rectocele, and perineal body descent by incorporating the posterior vaginal fascia and perineal body into the suspensory procedure. This is done by extending the mesh all the way down the posterior vaginal wall to the perineal body or the portion of the posterior vaginal fascia that is contiguous with the perineal body. In the initial 19 patients, excellent reduction in prolapse and perineal descent was achieved. The procedure evolved into a combined abdominal and vaginal approach with either perineal fixation sutures or mesh transferred abdominally through a vaginal incision (23). Although excellent reduction in prolapse was achieved, the incidence of mesh erosion was higher in the procedures that required transvaginal passage of suture or mesh. In the abdominal sacral colpoperineopexy procedures done entirely abdominally, the incidence of mesh erosion was low. Studies comparing the result of traditional sacral colpopexy and posterior repair with colpoperineopexy are needed.

C. Abdominal Sacral Colpopexy: Graft Material

When selecting appropriate graft interposition material for use in colpopexy procedures, one should consider a graft with significant strength and durability. Additionally, this material should elicit minimal inflammatory or foreign body reaction, and not serve as a nidus for infection. The length of the segment needed varies depending on vaginal depth; often the length is too long to consider the use of autologous fascia. Cadaveric fascia lata may be used. Sizes are available to complete most colpopexy procedures, and the risk of erosion appears low. Concern that a lack of strength of this material precipitated early failure of pelvic reconstructive procedures (24,25) has prompted most pelvic surgeons to use synthetic graft material. The most commonly utilized synthetic materials are: Marlex (26) (CR Bard, Cranston RI), Mersilene (13) (Ethicon, Somerville, NJ), Prolene (27) (Ethicon, Somerville, NJ), and Gore-Tex (28) (WR Gore, Flagstaff, AZ). All of these materials have been utilized with excellent success rates.

The major concern when utilizing synthetic mesh material during pelvic reconstruction is infection and/or erosion of the material into the vagina. In a review of the literature, Iglesia et al. reported on the incidence of mesh erosion for abdominal sacral colpopexy. This review comprised procedures utilizing Marlex, Prolene, Mersilene, and Gor-Tex graft materials. Marlex and Mersilene had minimal erosion complications, and Gore-Tex had the highest incidence of erosion. The overall incidence of erosion of all types of graft materials in sacral colpopexy procedures was 9% (29). The likelihood of encountering a mesh complication when utilizing Marlex or Mersilene appears to be <5%. If the mesh is exposed vaginally, the incidence of erosion is much higher. This implies that bacterial contamination does have a role in promoting mesh erosion. Additionally, avoiding excessive tension is an important step to reduce erosion. Compression can decrease blood flow to the area of the vagina where the mesh is attached, promoting ischemia and tissue breakdown.

In summary, the incidence of mesh erosion after colpopexy is very low, particularly if using Marlex or Mersilene. Exposure of the mesh to the vaginal flora and excessive compression of the mesh are factors that increase the risk of mesh complications. If one performs an abdominal sacral colpopexy with attention to detail, the use of synthetic material is durable providing long-lasting support with minimal risk of infection or erosion.

IV. DISCUSSION

The first abdominal sacral colpopexy was reported by Lane in 1962 (30). He expressed concern that many procedures to correct vaginal vault utilized the already weakened, tenuous supporting "fascia" for reconstruction. The repairs mainly consisted of the reapproximation of weak tissue to provide support. His modification of existing suspensory procedures included placement of a supporting vascular graft on the vaginal apex and suspending it to the sacrum utilizing a stainless-steel staple. The use of the vascular graft arose out of concern over the amount of tension frequently required to suture the vaginal apex directly to the promontory. Eventually the graft was secured to the sacrum by permanent sutures, replacing the staple. He concluded, "The advantages of this procedure are that vaginal function is maintained, difficult dissection is not required, and an indestructible plastic replaces the inadequate supporting structures which were factors in the production of the prolapse" (30). These principles described by Lane still apply today.

The abdominal sacral colpopexy maintains a functional vagina; it restores maximum vaginal length and durable support by securing the vaginal apex to the periosteum of the sacrum.

This surgical approach demands excellent exposure of the pelvis, which facilitates more complete reduction of the enterocele, and cul-de-sac obliteration. Several modifications in technique have been described using autologous fascia (31,32) and synthetic mesh (33,34) in different configurations, and results appear to be comparable. Timmons and Addison observed only three recurrences in 250 patients treated with abdominal sacral colpopexy over 20 years (35). Many reports demonstrate minimal failure rates (Table 1).

Most previous reports have defined treatment success after colpopexy as an absence of prolapse to the hymen or lack of symptoms related to prolapse. The incidence of site-specific pelvic defects occurring after colpopexy is not clearly reported. The incidence of "de novo" anterior wall defects (anterior wall defects not diagnosed before or during the operation for which no anterior colporrhaphy was performed) has been reported to be ~18% after sacrospinous fixation (36). In the authors' experience, the incidence of recurrent central cystocele and recto-cele after abdominal sacral colpopexy is not uncommon, and similar to the reported incidence of recurrent defects after sacrospinous fixation. The completion of a colpopexy with a paravaginal repair does not correct central cystocele or rectocele defects. Extension of the graft posteriorly may help prevent rectocele formation. Careful examination should be carried out in an attempt to determine if a significant anterior central defect exists. If present, one should consider anterior colporrhaphy prior to colpopexy. More study is needed to identify site-specific defects occurring after colpopexy and to determine the clinical significance of these defects.

The most significant complication of sacral colpopexy is life-threatening hemorrhage from disruption of the presacral vessels. The risk of significant bleeding has been reported from 1.2– 2.6% and may be controlled with the use of stainless steel thumbtacks if encountered (37). Addison described a modification of technique securing the mesh to the sacral promontory to reduce the risk of bleeding from presacral vessels (38). Since employing this technique, he has not encountered significant bleeding. The authors have not encountered significant blood loss, utilizing fixation of the graft high on the sacral promontory. Mesh erosion into the sigmoid colon has not been observed, and we believe this complication is prevented by assuring a space between the mesh and sigmoid that will accept two fingers and by meticulous retroperitoneal placement of the mesh. In addition, positioning of the mesh loosely around the bowel will prevent postoperative bowel obstruction.

As in other major pelvic operations postoperative ileus can occur, and this is the most common bowel dysfunction encountered postoperatively. Mesh infection and/or erosion into the vagina has been reported to occur in ~9% of all cases (29). However, Timmons et al. (33), Hardimann et al. (39), and Benson and colleagues (19) had no mesh complications in a combined 281 patients. Podratz and colleagues removed mesh in two out of 50 patients for erosion or infection (40), and recurrent vaginal vault prolapse did not occur after mesh removal. Simultaneous pubovaginal sling procedures and abdominal sacral colpopexy have been performed by the authors. Although there is a concern about abdominal mesh infection occurring with pubovaginal sling procedures, the authors have not encountered this problem.

Comparative studies of colpopexy to transvaginal vault suspension procedures are rare. Benson et al. (19) reported the results of a randomized controlled trial comparing vaginal and abdominal correction of vaginal vault prolapse. In the vaginal group, the surgical outcome was optimal in 29%, satisfactory in 38%, and unsatisfactory in 33%. In the abdominal group, surgical outcome was optimal in 58%, satisfactory in 26%, and unsatisfactory in 16%. There was no significant difference between the groups in morbidity, complications, hemoglobin change, dyspareunia, pain, or hospital stay. They concluded that the correction of vaginal vault prolapse was more effective with an abdominal approach (19). By providing more normal restoration of vaginal axis and preserving maximal depth, the sacral colpopexy restores a func-tional vagina. These factors should be considered when planning operative correction in the sexually active patient. Given (41) found sacral colpopexy to be superior to sacrospinous fixation in terms of vaginal length. After colpopexy an 11.3-cm length of functional vagina was measured versus 8.2 cm in length after sacrospinous fixation. Angulo and Kligman (42) observed normal return to sexual activity without recurrent prolapse with a follow-up period of 36 months in 18 patients.

Since 1962, the correction of vaginal vault prolapse by abdominal sacral colpopexy has undergone modifications. Consistently superior rates of success have been achieved largely as a result of adhering to the basic principles described by Lane: closure of the cul-de-sac and suspension of the vaginal vault by a strong mesh material. Laparoscopic transabdominal sacral colpopexy has been performed in an effort to provide less invasive surgery and shorter hospitalization (43). At present, limitations of this modality include a steep learning curve, cumbersome laparoscopic knot tying, and possibly longer operative times (44). Laparoscopic repair of vaginal vault prolapse will become more widely used as technology develops better suturing and anchoring devices. With continued adherance to the basic principles of the procedure, these modifications should also provide durable support of the vaginal apex while decreasing the overall morbidity of the procedure.

V. CONCLUSION

Abdominal sacral colpopexy is an excellent procedure to correct vaginal vault prolapse. The procedure can be performed with minimal complications. Because of its durability and preservation of a functional vagina, this procedure should be considered not only for those women who have failed a previous transvaginal suspension procedure, but also as a primary approach in young females with vaginal vault prolapse.

Pelvic surgeons are especially suited to master the techniques essential to perform a successful colpopexy and incorporate this procedure into their armamentarium for pelvic floor reconstruction.

REFERENCES

1. Duton CJ, Mikuta JJ. Posthysterectomy vaginal vault prolapse. Postgrad Obstet Gynecol 1988; 8:1–6.
2. Herbst A, Mishell D, Stenchever M, Droegemueller W. Disorders of the abdominal wall and pelvic support. In: Stenchever MA, ed. Comprehensive Gynecology. 2d ed. Philadelphia: Mosby Year Book, 1992:594–612.
3. Richter K. Massive eversion of the vagina: pathogenesis, diagnosis and therapy of the true prolapse of the vaginal stump. Clin Obstet Gynecol 1982; 25:897–912.
4. Delaere K, Moonen W, Debruyne F, Jansen T. Hydronephrosis caused by cystocele. Treatment by colpopexy to sacral promonotory. Urology 1984; 24:364–365.
5. Karram M, Bhatia N. The Q-Tip test: standardization of the technique and its interpretation in women with urinary incontinence. Obstet Gynecol 1988; 71:807–811.
6. Yang A, Mostwin JL, Rosenshein NB, Zerhouni EA. Pelvic floor descent in women: dynamic evaluation with fast MR imaging and cinematic display. Radiology 1991; 179:25–33.
7. Dohke M, Mitchell D, Vasavada S. Fast magnetic resonance imaging of pelvic organ prolapse. Tech Urol 2001; 7:133–138.
8. Fianu S, Kjaeldgaard A, Larsson B. Preoperative screening for latent stress incontinence in women with cystocele. Neurourol Urodyn 1985; 4:3–8.
9. Stanton S, Hilton P, Norton P, Cardozo L. Clinical and urodynamic effects of anterior colporrhaphy and vaginal hysterectomy for prolapse with or without incontinence. Br J Obstet Gynaecol 1982; 89:459–463.

10. Gallentine M, Cespedes R. Occult stress urinary incontinence and the effect of vaginal vault prolapse on leak point pressures. Urology 2001; 57:40–44.

11. Ghoniem G, Walters F, Lewis V. The value of the vaginal pack test in large cystoceles. J Urol 1994; 152:931–934.

12. Hemelt B, Finan M. Abdominal sacral colpopexy resulting in a retained sponge. A case report. J Reprod Med 1999; 44:983–985.

13. Addison W, Livengood C, Sutton G, Parker R. Abdominal sacral colpopexy with Mersiliene mesh in the retroperitoneal position in the management of posthysterectomy vaginal vault prolapse and enterocele. Am J Obstet Gynecol 1985; 153:140–146.

14. Fox S, Stanton S. Vault prolapse and rectocele: assessment of repair using sacrocolpopexy with mesh interposition. Br J Obstet Gynaecol 2000; 107:1371–1375.

15. Patsner B. Abdominal sacral colpopexy in patients with gynecologic cancer: report of 25 cases with long-term followup and literature review. Gynecol Oncol 1999; 75:504–508.

16. Snyder T, Krantz K. Abdominal-retroperitoneal sacral colpopexy for the correction of vaginal prolapse. Obstet Gynecol 1991; 77:944–949.

17. Diana M, Zoppe C, Mastrangeli B. Treatment of vaginal vault prolapse with abdominal sacral colpopexy using prolene mesh. Am J Surg 2000; 179:126–128.

18. Virtanen H, Hirvonen T, Makinen J, Kiilholma. Outcome of thirty patients who underwent repair of post-hysterectomy prolapse of the vaginal vault with abdominal sacral colpopexy. J Am Coll Surg 1994; 178:283–287.

19. Benson J, Lucente V, McClellan E. Vaginal vs. abdominal reconstructive for the treatment of pelvic floor defects. A randomized study with long term outcome evaluation. Am J Obstet Gynecol 1996; 175:1419–1422.

20. Cowan W, Morgan H. Abdominal sacral colpopexy. Am J Obstet Gynecol 1980; 138:348–350.

21. Winters J, Cespedes R, Vanlangendonck R. Abdominal sacral colpopexy and abdominal enterocele in the management of vaginal vault prolapse. Urology 2000; 56(6 suppl 1):55–63.

22. Cundiff G, Harris R, Coates K, Low V, Bump R, Addison WA. Abdominal sacral colpoperineopexy: a new approach for correction of posterior compartment defects and perineal descent associated with vaginal vault prolapse. Am J Obstet Gynecol 1997; 177:1345–1355.

23. Visco A, Weidner A, Barber M. Vaginal mesh erosion after abdominal sacral colpopexy. Am J Obstet Gynecol 2001; 184:297–302.

24. Fitzgerald M, Mollenhauer J, Bitterman P, Brubaker L. Functional failure of fascia lata allografts. Am J Obstet Gynecol 1999; 181:1339–1346.

25. Carbone J, Kavaler E, Hu J, Raz S. Pubovaginal sling using cadaveric fascia and bone anchors: disappointing early results. J Urol 2001; 165:1605–1611.

26. Kohli N, Walsh P, Roat T, Karram M. Mesh erosion after abdominal sacrocolpopexy. Obstet Gynecol 1988; 92:999–1004.

27. Baker K, Beresford J, Campbell C. Colposacropexy with prolene mesh. Surg Gynecol Obstet 1990; 171:51–54.

28. Iosif C. Abdominal sacral colpopexy with the use of synthetic mesh. Acta Obstet Gynecol Scand 1993; 72:214–217.

29. Iglesia C, Fenner D, Brubaker L. The use of mesh in gynecologic surgery. Int Urogynecol J 1997; 8:105–115.

30. Lane F. Repair of posthysterectomy vaginal-vault prolapse. Obstet Gynecol 1962; 20:72–77.

31. Beecham CT, Beecham JB. Correction of prolapsed vagina or enterocele with fascia lata. Obstet Gynecol 1973; 42:542–546.

32. Ridley JH. A composite vaginal vault suspension using fascia lata. Am J Obstet Gynecol 1976; 126:590–596.

33. Timmons MC, Addison WA, Addison SB, Cavenar MG. Abdominal sacral colpopexy in 163 women with posthysterectomy vaginal vault prolapse and enterocele: evolution of operative techniques. J Reprod Med 1992; 37:323–327.

34. Menefee SA, Miller KF, Wall LL. Abdominal sacral colpopexy: description of a technique using polyester mesh in the treatment of posthysterectomy vaginal vault prolapse. J Pelvic Surg 1998; 4:130–136.

35. Addison WA, Timmons MC, Wall LL, Livengood CH. Failed abdominal sacral colpopexy: observations and recommendations. Obstet Gynecol 1989; 74:480–483.

36. Smilen S, Saini J, Wallach S, Porges R. The risk of cystocele after sacrospinous fixation. Am J Obstet Gynecol 1998; 179:1465–1472.

37. Timmons MC, Kohler MF, Addison WA. Thumbtack use for control of presacral bleeding with description of an instrument for thumbtack application. Obstet Gynecol 1991; 78:313–315.

38. Addison WA, Livengood CH, Parker RT. Vaginal vault prolapse with emphasis on management by transabdominal sacral colpopexy. Postgrad Obstet Gynecol 1998; 8:1–7.

39. Hardiman P, Drutz HP. Sacrospinous vault suspension and abdominal colposacropexy: success rates and complications. Am J Obstet Gynecol 1996; 175:612–615.

40. Podratz K, Ferguson L, Hoverman V, Lee R, Symonds R. Abdominal sacral colpopexy for post-hysterectomy vaginal vault descensus. J Pelvic Surg 1995; 1:18–23.

41. Given FT. Vaginal length and sexual function after colpopexy for complete uterovaginal eversion. Am J Obstet Gynecol 1993; 169:284–287.

42. Angulo A, Kligman I. Retroperitoneal sacrocolpopexy for correction of prolapse of the vaginal vault. Surg Gynecol Obstet 1992; 169:319–323.

43. Dorsey JH, Sharp HT. Laparoscopic sacral colpopexy and other procedures for prolapse. Baillieres Clin Obstet Gynecol 1995; 9:749–756.

44. Liu CY, Reich H. Correction of genital prolapse. J Endourol 1996; 10:259–265.

49

Laparoscopic Abdominal Sacral Colpopexy

Marie Fidela R. Paraiso
Cleveland Clinic Foundation, Cleveland, Ohio, U.S.A.

I. INTRODUCTION

Laparoscopic treatment of vaginal apex prolapse has not become as popular as laparoscopic hysterectomy and Burch colposuspension most likely owing to vaginal route preference by many gynecologic surgeons and the technical difficulty of laparoscopic suturing. Since Nezhat et al. (1) reported a small series of laparoscopic sacral colpopexies in 1994, there have been few subsequent case series on surgical procedures for pelvic organ prolapse.

The reported advantages of laparoscopic prolapse surgery are: (a) the improved visualization of the anatomy of the presacral space, rectovaginal space, and peritoneal cavity due to laparoscopic magnification and improved hemostasis; (b) shortened hospitalization; (c) decreased postoperative pain; (d) rapid recovery and return to work; and (e) cosmetic appearance of smaller incisions. Disadvantages of laparoscopic abdominal sacral colpopexy include: (a) technical difficulty in acquiring suturing skills; (b) increased operating time early in the surgeon's experience especially if concomitant procedures are performed; (c) necessity of a highly skilled laparoscopic assistant; and (d) increased hospital cost secondary to increased operating room time and the use of disposable surgical instruments (2).

When performing laparoscopic procedures for repair of vaginal apex prolapse, the laparoscopic operation must be identical to conventional pelvic reconstructive procedures, and cure rates must be similar to those performed by other routes. The goals of the surgery to relieve symptoms, correct anatomic defects, and restore or maintain urinary, bowel, and sexual function should not be compromised when operating by the laparoscopic route.

II. INDICATIONS

The indications for laparoscopic sacral colpopexy are identical to those for the open abdominal route. A patient should desire maintenance or restoration of sexual function or vaginal preservation. Surgeon and patient preference and the laparoscopic skill of the surgeon determine the choice of laparoscopic route. Additional factors that should be considered include history of previous pelvic or anti-incontinence surgery, previous failed vaginal apex suspensions, a small or foreshortened vagina, severe levator muscle weakness and atrophy, severe abdomino-pelvic adhesions, advanced patient age and weight, chronically increased abdominal pressure, need for concomitant pelvic surgery, and patient ability to undergo general anesthesia. Some surgeons choose to perform laparoscopic sacral colpopexy only in cases of isolated apical segment defects because of the increased operative time.

Laparoscopic sacral colpoperineopexy (3) involves the attachment of a graft material that spans from perineal body to the sacrum and incorporates the length of the posterior vaginal wall. This extensive modification of the sacral colpopexy is indicated in patients who have vaginal apex prolapse and concomitant perineal descent (4). This graft may be attached to the perineum by the laparoscopic route or by the vaginal route prior to laparoscopic fixation to the sacrum.

III. ANATOMY

When considering the repair of pelvic organ support, a surgeon needs to keep in mind the three levels of support of the vagina described by DeLancey in 1992 (5). The top fourth of the vagina (level I) is suspended by the cardinal/uterosacral complex; the middle half (level II) is attached laterally to the arcus tendineus fasciae pelvis and the medial aspect of the levator ani muscles; and the bottom fourth (level III) is fused to the perineal body. The endopelvic connective tissue (referred to as the pubocervical fascia anteriorly) contributes to the integrity of the anterior vaginal wall. The rectovaginal "fascia" contributes to the support of the posterior wall of the vagina. All pelvic support defects, whether anterior, apical, or posterior, usually represent a break in the continuity of the endopelvic "fascia" and/or a loss of its suspension, attachment, or fusion to adjacent structures. The goals of pelvic reconstructive surgery are to correct all defects, thus reestablishing vaginal support at all three levels and to maintain and/or restore normal visceral and sexual function.

The key anatomic landmarks of sacral colpopexy are the middle sacral artery and vein, sacral promontory with anterior longitudinal ligament, the aortic bifurcation and vena cava at the L4-5 level, the right common iliac vessels and right ureter at the right margin of the presacral space, and the sigmoid colon at the left margin. The left common iliac vein is medial to the left common iliac artery and can be damaged during dissection or retraction as discussed in Chapter 48.

Additional anatomic landmarks of laparoscopic sacral colpoperineopexy are the rectovaginal septum comprised of Denonvilliers' "fascia" and its lateral attachment to the medial aspect of the levator ani muscles and fusion to the perineal body. Denonvilliers' "fascia" is the endopelvic connective tissue which is attached to the uterosacral cardinal ligament complex superiorly, the superior fascia of the levator ani muscles laterally, and the perineal body inferiorly. The rectovaginal septum is the posterior point of attachment of the sacral colpopexy mesh. Rectovaginal "fascia," rectovaginal septum, and Denonvilliers' "fascia" are synonymous terms. The pubocervical "fascia" is the anterior point of mesh attachment during sacral colpopexy.

IV. OPERATIVE TECHNIQUE OF LAPAROSCOPIC
SACRAL COLPOPEXY

In addition to the infraumbilical port for the laparoscope, one 10/12-mm trocar should be placed in the lower quadrants bilaterally for suture introduction. Two 5-mm ports are placed at the level of the umbilicus, lateral to the rectus muscle for retraction. After the ancillary ports are placed, anterior dissection taking care to avoid damage to the bladder is performed (Fig. 1). The bladder may be filled with 200–300 cc of sterile water to aid the dissection. A vaginal obturator,

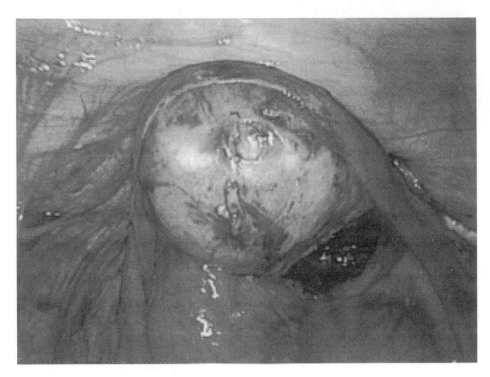

Figure 1 Dissection of the pubocervical and rectovaginal fasciae. Manipulators have been placed in the vagina and rectum.

SpongeStick, or equivalent vaginal manipulator (EEA sizer by U.S. Surgical Corp., Norwalk, CT, or the CDH by Ethicon Endo-Surgery Inc., Cincinnati, OH) is used for delineation of the vaginal apex and/or rectum. In order to delineate the rectovaginal fascia, the vaginal EEA sizer is directed anteriorly while the rectal EEA sizer is directed cephalad (Fig. 2). Dissection of the peritoneum off the posterior vaginal apex and use of electrocautery are avoided to decrease risk of vaginal erosion. Sharp dissection is performed with scissors into the avascular space until the inferior point of mesh fixation is reached. In cases of laparoscopic sacral colpoperineopexy, dissection is carried down to the perineal body. Vaginal palpation or transillumination is helpful to ensure that the dissection to the perineum has been achieved.

The peritoneum overlying the sacral promontory is incised longitudinally and extended to the cul-de-sac. A laparoscopic blunt tipped instrument or suction irrigator is used to expose the periosteum of the sacral promontory (Fig. 3). If blood vessels are encountered during the dissection, coagulation or clip placement is used to achieve hemostasis. If exposure of the sacral promontory and presacral space is not adequate, the patient should be tilted to her left and/or a snake retractor (Genzyme Corporation, Cambridge, MA) placed through an ancillary port.

A 15 × 2.5 cm piece of autologous fascia lata, freeze-dried nonradiated cadaveric fascia lata, polypropylene, Mersilene mesh, or xenograft (porcine dermis, porcine intestinal submucosa, or bovine pericardium) is introduced through the 10/12-mm port. Use of synthetic materials should be considered if the integrity of the pelvic floor muscles and their nerve supply are poor. When a T-shaped mesh is used, a 5×2.5 cm mesh is sutured to the larger piece of mesh with No. 0 nonabsorbable suture. In order to construct the T-shaped mesh in one piece, a surgeon may fold a 15 × 5 cm piece of mesh in half, incise the mesh 10 cm longitudinally, and stitch it with No. 0 polypropylene suture at the apex of the incision (Fig. 4). This technique results in

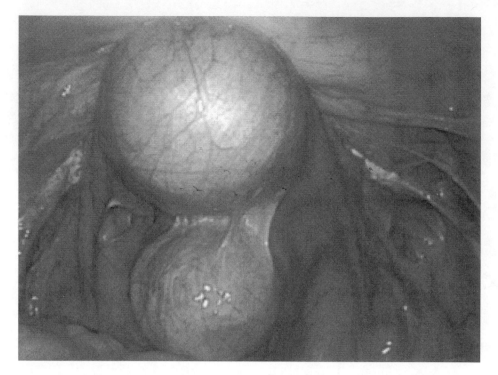

Figure 2   Delineation of the rectovaginal septum after placement of EAA sizers into the vagina and rectum.

a doubled layer at the base of the T. The shortest arm of the mesh is sutured to the vaginal apex anteriorly with two or three pairs of No. 0 nonabsorbable sutures (Fig. 5) and to the posterior vaginal apex and rectovaginal septum with three or more similar rows of suture (Fig. 6). When using a T-shaped mesh, it is easier to suture the anterior portion first so that the cephalad portion of the mesh may be retracted anteriorly while the posterior rows of sutures are being placed. The sutures are tied extracorporeally as they are placed.

The technique we currently use, involves suturing two pieces of mesh separately. I believe that this modification places less tension on the anterior vaginal wall thus resulting in fewer mesh erosions. The shorter piece of mesh (10 × 2.5 cm) is sutured to the anterior wall. A larger piece (15 × 2.5 cm) is sutured to the posterior vaginal wall. Care is taken to place the stitches through the entire thickness of the vaginal wall excluding the epithelium. The surgeon stitches the mesh to the longitudinal ligament of the sacrum with two or three stitches of No. 0 nonabsorbable suture. Titanium tacks or hernia staples may also be utilized to attach the mesh to the longitudinal ligament (Fig. 7). No undue tension is placed on the mesh. The redundant portion of the mesh is excised. The peritoneum is re-approximated over the mesh with No. 2-0 polyglactin suture (Fig. 8). If the mesh remains exposed, sigmoid epiploic fat may be sutured over it.

If a graft is secured by vaginal route, an introital incision and dissection of the vaginal epithelium off the underlying vaginal muscularis are performed. This dissection extends to the medial aspect of the levator ani muscles and superiorly into the enterocele sac. The mesh is stitched laterally to the iliococcygeus and pubococcygeus fasciae and muscles with three No. 2 braided polyester sutures. The stitch placed most cephalad is at the level of the ischial spine. Use of an allograft or xenograft may result in less infection and erosion. Visco et al. have reported a 40% rate of synthetic mesh erosion and shorter time to erosion when sutures

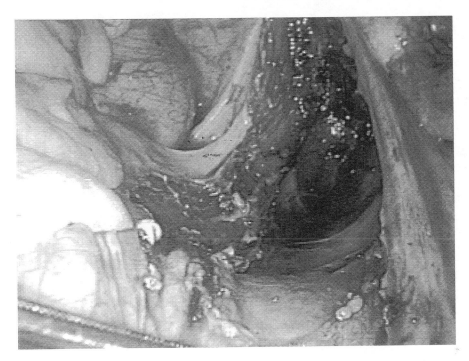

Figure 3 Incision of the peritoneum from sacral promontory to cul-de-sac and dissection of the presacral space.

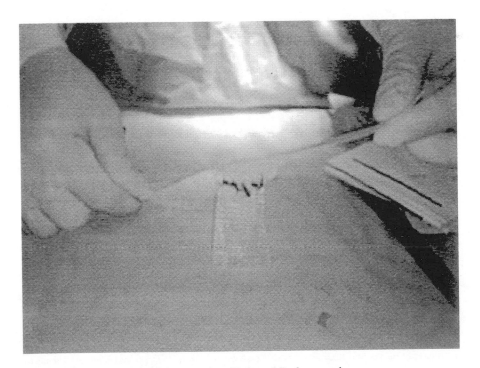

Figure 4 Configuration of the one-piece T-shaped Prolene mesh.

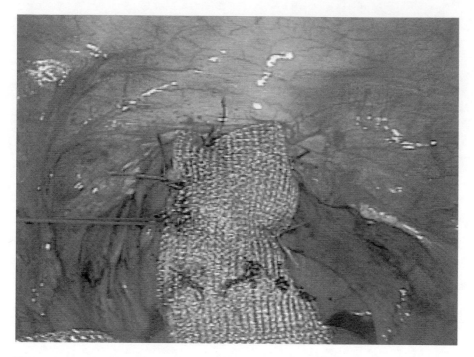

Figure 5   Attachment of the short arm of the T-shaped Prolene mesh to the anterior vagina.

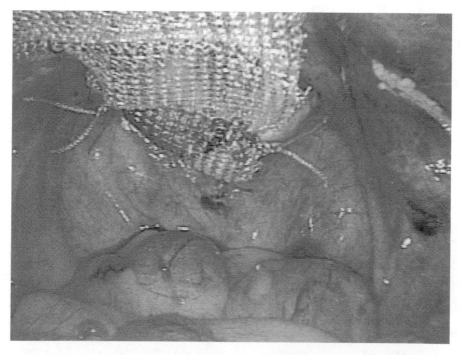

Figure 6   Attachment of one of the long arms of the T-shaped mesh to the perineal body and posterior vaginal wall.

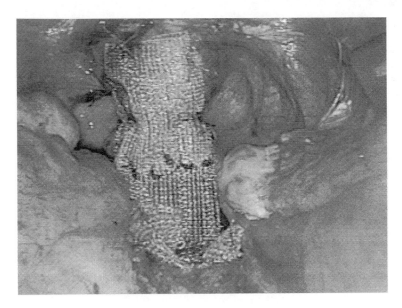

Figure 7 Titanium tacks secure the mesh to the anterior longitudinal ligament of the sacrum with no tension.

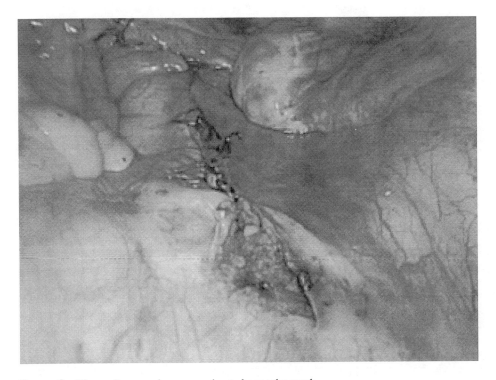

Figure 8 The peritoneum is reapproximated over the mesh.

or mesh were placed vaginally and brought into the abdominal field when comparing vaginal-abdominal sacral colpoperineopexy with abdominal sacral colpopexy (6). We recommend placement of a fascial graft, allograft, or xenograft vaginally and stitching a synthetic graft over the proximal portion of the graft laparoscopically in order to complete the vaginal-laparoscopic sacral colpoperineopexy.

A concomitant laparoscopic colposuspension is performed if the patient has genuine stress incontinence. A paravaginal defect repair may also be performed, if needed, to prevent compensatory anterior defects or repair coexisting paravaginal defects. If rectal prolapse is present, a rectopexy may be performed laparoscopically. We perform these combined cases with our colorectal surgery colleagues.

A concomitant culdeplasty may be performed prior to laparoscopic attachment of the posterior mesh to the vagina and sacrum (Fig. 9). The Moschcowitz procedure is performed laparoscopically exactly as during laparotomy. A No. 0 nonabsorbable 36-in suture is stitched in the peritoneum around the cul-de-sac in a purse-string fashion and subsequently tied extracorporeally. Additional sutures are placed as needed. The ureters should be carefully examined during and after the Moschcowitz procedure. The peritoneum medial to the ureters may be incised in order to prevent ureteral kinking.

Alternatively, the Halban procedure may be performed by suturing No. 0 nonabsorbable suture starting at the posterior vagina and proceeding longitudinally over the cul-de-sac peritoneum and then over the anterior inferior sigmoid serosa. These sutures are tied as they are placed. Sutures should be ~1 cm apart. There is little risk of ureteral compromise with this procedure; however, it is important to visualize the ureters after all sutures are tied. Outcome data for Moschcowitz and Halban procedures do not exist.

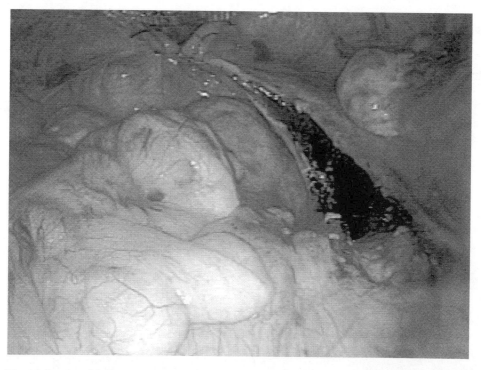

Figure 9 A culdeplasty incorporating the uterosacral ligaments has been performed after posterior attachment of the graft.

V. CLINICAL OUTCOME OF LAPAROSCOPIC SACRAL COLPOPEXY

The current gynecologic literature for laparoscopic pelvic reconstruction is sparse and consists of descriptive studies with short-term follow-up. Nezhat et al. (1) reported a series of 15 patients who underwent laparoscopic sacral colpopexy in whom the mean operative time was 170 min (range 105–320 min) and mean blood loss was 226 mL (range 50–800 mL). The mean hospital stay was 2.3 days, excluding the case converted to laparotomy for presacral hemorrhage. The cure rate for apical prolapse was 100% at 3–40 months. Lyons (7) reported four laparoscopic sacrospinous fixations and 10 laparoscopic sacral colpopexies with operative times comparable to vaginal and abdominal approaches. He reported less intra- and postoperative morbidity with the laparoscopic route, which was attributed to a superior anatomic approach and better visualization of anatomic structures. Nezhat et al. (1) and Lyons (7) both used mesh and suture and at times stapled the mesh into the longitudinal ligament of the anterior sacrum rather than suturing it.

Ross (8) evaluated 19 patients with posthysterectomy vaginal apex prolapse prospectively with extensive preoperative and post-operative testing including multichannel urodynamics and transperineal ultrasound. All patients underwent sacral colpopexy, Burch colposuspension, and modified culdeplasty. Paravaginal defect repair and posterior colporrhaphy were added as indicated. The author reported seven complications: three cystotomies, two urinary tract infections, one seroma, and one inferior epigastric vessel laceration. Five patients had recurrent defects which were all less than grade 2 (two paravaginal defects and three rectoceles). Vaginal length ranged from 10.8 to 12.1 cm, and no sexually active patients reported sexual dysfunction. All but four patients voided spontaneously, and no one required more than 4 days of catheterization. All were discharged within 24 h. The cure rate at 1 year was 100% for vaginal apex prolapse and 93% for genuine stress incontinence, although two patients were lost to follow-up.

Cosson et al. in the French literature (9) have reported the largest series of 83 women undergoing laparoscopic sacral colpopexy. Six cases required conversion to laparotomy; thus, 77 women underwent successful procedures with 60 of them having concomitant supracervical hysterectomy. Two strips of synthetic mesh were placed. Operative time decreased from 292 to 180 min as the surgeon gained experience. Three patients required reoperation, one for recurrent prolapse and two for recurrent stress incontinence.

Our first 18 patients who underwent laparoscopic sacral colpopexy had a 100% cure of the apical vaginal prolapse, with 13% of patients having recurrent anterior vaginal prolapse and 13% having posterior vaginal wall prolapse (10). One patient who was undergoing concomitant rectopexy required conversion to laparotomy. The majority of patients underwent concomitant laparoscopic Burch and paravaginal defect repairs. I have noted that with increased experience, time for sacral colpopexy alone has decreased to 90 min. To date we have performed over 80 of these procedures.

There are several reports of laparoscopic rectopexy in the colorectal surgery literature, which is beyond the scope of this chapter. We have performed seven combined laparoscopic sacral colpopexy and rectopexy cases to date. One patient underwent laparoscopic sigmoid resection. In that case, cadaveric fascia was used for sacral colpopexy to avoid infection of synthetic mesh.

VI. CONCLUSION

The principles of laparoscopic reparative procedures for vaginal apex prolapse, enterocele, and concomitant perineal descent are not new; it is the route by which they are performed that is different. Laparoscopic sacral colpopexy and colpoperineopexy are feasible and safe. Adequate laparoscopic suturing skills are essential when performing these procedures. The increase in operative time may elevate the cost of the procedure early in a surgeon's experience. The laparoscopic route offers many advantages to women who require abdominal sacral colpopexy. Prospective clinical trials and long-term follow-up are warranted from experienced laparoscopic surgeons prior to universal application of laparoscopy for the repair of pelvic organ prolapse.

REFERENCES

1. Nezhat CH, Nezhat F, Nezhat C. Laparoscopic sacral colpopexy for vaginal vault prolapse. Obstet Gynecol 1994; 84:885–888.
2. Paraiso MR, Falcone T, Walters MD. Laparoscopic surgery for genuine stress incontinence and pelvic organ prolapse. In: Walters MD, Karram MM, eds. Urogynecology and Reconstructive Pelvic Surgery. 2d ed. Chicago: Mosby, 1998.
3. Paraiso MFR, Tulikangas PK. Laparoscopic sacral colpoperineopexy with control of a presacral bleed. Proceedings of the 21st American Urogynecologic Society Conference 2000, Hilton Head, SC, and the 24th American Association of Gynecologic Laparoscopists Conference 2000, Orlando, FL.
4. Cundiff GW, Harris RL, Coates K, Low VH, Bump RC, Addison WA. Abdominal sacral colpoperineopexy: a new approach for correction of posterior compartment defects and perineal descent associated with vaginal vault prolapse. Am J Obstet Gynecol 1997; 177:1345–1353.
5. DeLancey JO. Anatomic aspects of vaginal eversion after hysterectomy. Am J Obstet Gynecol 1992; 166:1717–1728.
6. Visco AG, Weidner AC, Barber MD, Myers ER, Cundiff GW, Bump RC. Vaginal mesh erosion after abdominal sacral colpopexy. Am J Obstet Gynecol 2001; 184:297–302.
7. Lyons TL. Minimally invasive treatment of urinary stress incontinence and laparoscopically directed repair of pelvic floor defects. Clin Obstet Gynecol 1995; 38:380–391.
8. Ross JW. Apical vault repair, the cornerstone of pelvic vault reconstruction. Int Urogynecol J 1997; 8:146–152.
9. Cosson M, Bogaert E, Narducci F, Querleu D, Crepin G. Laparoscopic sacral colpopexy: short-term results and complications in 83 patients. J Gynecol Obstet Biol Reprod 2000; 29:746–750.
10. Paraiso MFR, Margossian H, Tulikangas PK, Walters MD. Laparoscopic sacral colpopexy and pelvic reconstruction. J Am Assoc Gynecol Laparosc 200; 7(3):S46. Abstract.

50

Colpocleisis for the Treatment of Severe Vaginal Vault Prolapse

R. Duane Cespedes
Wilford Hall Medical Center, Lackland AFB, Texas, U.S.A.

J. Christian Winters
Ochsner Medical Foundation, New Orleans, Louisiana, U.S.A.

I. INTRODUCTION

Pelvic prolapse conditions have plagued women for thousands of years; however, it is only recently that procedures have been developed that safely and effectively treat these conditions. Even today, pelvic prolapse conditions remain a challenging problem, with vault prolapse remaining the most difficult problem to treat because multiple support defects usually coexist. A thorough understanding of pelvic anatomy, pathophysiology, and urodynamics and experience in selecting the appropriate surgical techniques are required to treat vault prolapse with minimal morbidity or treatment failures. Although the goal of a vault prolapse procedure is to restore normal anatomy and function in most cases, this is not always possible or necessary. For the elderly, the medically unstable, and sexually inactive individual, it may be preferable to simply "close off" the vagina to maximize long-term results and minimize operative complications. These procedures, including colpocleisis and partial colpocleisis, are thought of as "destructive" procedures and are currently unpopular; however, these procedures can be extremely helpful in certain situations and should be in every reconstructive surgeon's armamentarium.

The traditional approach to colpocleisis has been to simply "invert" the vagina using purse-string sutures after removing the vaginal epithelium. While simple to perform, after repairing referred treatment failures who used this approach, we began to utilize a different approach, which emphasizes the strength of an anterior repair and extensive posterior repair which is then sutured together. This vaginal closure is then reinforced with a strong perineorrhaphy. The purpose of this chapter is to discuss the indications, procedural aspects, and results of performing a multicompartment colpocleisis and partial colpocleisis for total vault prolapse in elderly females.

The opinions contained herein are those of the authors and are not to be construed as reflecting the views of the Air Force or the Department of Defense.

II. PATHOPHYSIOLOGY AND INDICATIONS

All pelvic prolapse conditions result from weakness or damage to the normal pelvic support systems (1). Many etiologies have been proposed for pelvic floor relaxation including multi-parity, advanced age, prior pelvic surgery, hormonal insufficiency, obesity, neurological disorders, connective tissue disorders, and strenuous physical activity (2,3). Vaginal vault prolapse, the most severe form of pelvic prolapse, can occur after a hysterectomy if the vault is not adequately resuspended to the cardinal and uterosacral ligaments (4). The incidence of vault prolapse after hysterectomy is reported to be as high as 18.2% and is accompanied by significant prolapse in other areas in at least 72% of patients (5,6).

A complete vaginal colpocleisis is an appropriate option for the treatment of severe, symptomatic vaginal vault prolapse in women who have been sexually inactive for many years and do not desire continued sexual function. This procedure is especially useful in elderly women with multiple medical problems in whom a definitive procedure with little risk of recurrence and minimal associated morbidity is desired (7).

Partial colpocleisis is indicated when retention of a prolapsing uterus is desired. As partial colpocleisis usually precludes future coital function and examination of the cervix is virtually impossible, most women with a prolapsing uterus are probably better served by vaginal hysterectomy followed by a colpocleisis or one of the standard vault suspensions. As noted by Ridley, "Any operation less than a complete colpocleisis has an increased incidence of failure," and therefore we rarely utilize a partial colpocleisis (8). The ideal candidate for partial colpocleisis is a frail, elderly female with a documented normal cervix and uterus who has failed a trial with a pessary and is a poor surgical risk for a vaginal hysterectomy. In many of these patients, the risk of hysterectomy outweighs the risk of symptomatic prolapse recurrence because these patients are usually not physically active, which reduces the risk of subsequent recurrence.

III. EVALUATION

A. History

Patients with high-grade vaginal vault prolapse commonly complain of a mass prolapsing through the introitus with a feeling of vaginal fullness. When severe, the prolapse can cause difficulty walking and low back pain that worsens with activity and are relieved by lying flat. Patients frequently complain of associated voiding dysfunction. Stress urinary incontinence can be caused by either urethral hypermobility (a sequela of pelvic relaxation) or from intrinsic sphincter deficiency (ISD) (9). Most candidates for colpocleisis are elderly, and ISD is much more common in this age group. It is important to distinguish between these two causes of stress urinary incontinence (SUI) as suspension procedures are associated with a higher failure rate in patients with ISD. Some patients complain of frequency and urgency due to incomplete emptying from urethral obstruction, which may result from rotation of the cystocele around a partially fixed urethra. Many patients do not complain of SUI due to this urethral obstruction, and leak only when the prolapse is reduced while lying flat or upon urodynamic testing. Recurrent urinary tract infections may also occur from the incomplete emptying.

Bowel complaints, especially "constipation," are common in this group of elderly patients; however, constipation alone is not specific for a rectocele or pelvic prolapse. "Splinting" (i.e., applying finger pressure to the posterior vaginal wall to effectively empty the bowels) is relatively specific for a rectocele but may not always respond to surgical correction (10).

B. Physical Examination and Studies

In the severe cases of prolapse for which colpocleisis is indicated, the diagnosis is generally straightforward with a pelvic exam demonstrating total prolapse of the vaginal vault (Fig. 1). Any associated conditions such as cystocele, enterocele, or rectocele will be repaired by the colpocleisis. In severe prolapse cases, radiographic studies should be considered to rule out possible ureteral obstruction from the severe ureteral angulation that can occur. If ureteral obstruction is demonstrated, a ureteral stent should be placed if the procedure cannot be performed expeditiously (11).

We have found that it is easier to perform the vaginal exam at the same time as the urodynamics evaluation. Urodynamics should be performed on all patients to unmask "occult" SUI. Significant pelvic prolapse can cause urethral obstruction; therefore, the prolapse must be reduced during the stress maneuvers to create the situation that will exist after the procedure. The easiest way to reduce the prolapse and not alter the leak-point pressure measurement is to pack the vagina with lubricated gauze and hold the vault in place with the lower blade of a vaginal speculum taking care not to obstruct the urethra (12) (Fig. 2). A Pap smear and

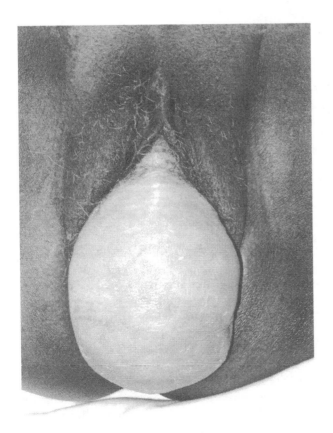

Figure 1   Severe vaginal vault prolapse in an elderly patient.

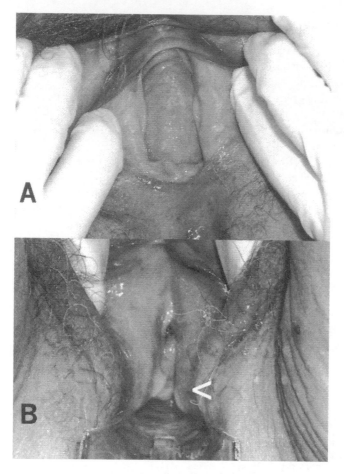

Figure 2 (**A**) A patient with moderate-grade prolapse without stress incontinence demonstrates the severe urethral hypermobility usually associated with vault prolapse. The urethra is noted to be directed vertically with mild straining. (**B**) After packing of the vagina with gauze and supporting the vault with a speculum, the urethra is now directed horizontally, and occult incontinence was demonstrable with coughing. At the arrow, the bladder neck and urethra are shown to be unobstructed.

endometrial biopsy and/or dilatation and curettage should be performed if a partial colpocleisis is considered, as access to the uterus will be impossible after the procedure (13).

C. Stress Incontinence: Techniques of Repair

Almost all women who require a colpocleisis will also have significant urethral hypermobility, and some will complain of SUI. The choice of an anti-incontinence procedure is difficult in this elderly population, who are more likely to suffer the adverse consequences of anti-incontinence procedures than younger patients. The prevention of postoperative SUI must be balanced with the avoidance of disabling detrusor instability or urinary retention, as medical therapy may not improve symptoms, and a urethrolysis after colpocleisis can be quite difficult.

Incontinence associated with urethral hypermobility can be treated with a sling or one of the suspension procedures; however, the authors do not perform transabdominal incontinence procedures in these patients because of the additional morbidity and similar rates of voiding dysfunction as sling procedures. A Kelly plication of the bladder neck may be considered in two patient groups (14). If SUI cannot be demonstrated with the prolapse reduced, a Kelly plication can be used to provide additional support at the bladder neck. If an elderly, debilitated patient has minimal SUI and cannot perform clean intermittent catheterization (CIC) then a Kelly bladder neck plication or minimally invasive sling may be performed. Minimally invasive sling techniques include a vaginal wall sling without perforation of the endopelvic fascia, or a paravaginal sling secured bilaterally to the arcus tendineus using a Capio needle driver (Boston Scientific, Natick, MA). These slings are minimally obstructive and CIC is rarely necessary (15). Transurethral collagen injections can be used if the patient develops significant SUI postoperatively (16).

If ISD is detected on urodynamic testing, a sling procedure or collagen injection is preferentially used (17,18). Pubovaginal slings are ordinarily used in patients with ISD, and cadaveric fascia or dermal grafts are utilized in most sling procedures to minimize the morbidity of autologous fascia harvest (19,20). Transient retention is common in this elderly group of patients, and all patients undergoing sling procedures should be instructed on CIC techniques preoperatively. Debilitated patients who cannot perform CIC may undergo a minimally invasive sling or Kelly plication with collagen injections if the SUI is not adequately treated.

IV. SURGICAL TECHNIQUES

A. Total Colpocleisis

Colpocleisis is performed with the patient in standard lithotomy position. A 16F Foley catheter is placed into the bladder for continuous drainage, and labial retraction sutures and a weighted vaginal speculum provide the necessary exposure.

An anti-incontinence procedure and anterior colporrhaphy are performed first. A midline vaginal incision is made on the anterior wall 1–2 cm proximal to the urethral meatus and extending just beyond the site of the proposed new vaginal cuff. In most cases, the vagina will only be 2–4 cm long when the colpocleisis is complete. The vaginal epithelium and smooth muscle are dissected off the pubocervical "fascia" in the usual manner, and multiple interrupted absorbable sutures are ordinarily used to perform the anterior repair (21,22). The extent of the anterior repair depends on which anti-incontinence procedure is performed. The anti-incontinence procedure is then performed and the epithelium closed.

The posterior vaginal wall and perineum are then repaired. A triangular perineoplasty incision is made and the epithelium defined by this incision is excised. Injectable saline is infiltrated into the posterior vaginal wall to aid dissection. Caudal retraction with an Allis clamp placed on the edge of the perineoplasty incision greatly facilitates the dissection of the epithelium from the posterior vaginal wall. The previously closed incision on the anterior vaginal wall defines the proximal extent of the posterior vaginal wall dissection (Fig. 3). Lateral dissection is continued to the posterior lateral sulcus. Dissection of the epithelium from the enterocele sac is usually slow and tedious, especially at the cuff; however, unlike a vault suspension, the enterocele sac is not opened or ligated (23). A colpocleisis obliterates the vaginal canal, so an enterocele has no place to recur (24). In addition, we have seen redundant bladder, small bowel, and rectum misidentified as "the sac" and mistakenly opened. If the enterocele can be manually reduced into the abdomen, the enterocele can be left alone. If the enterocele will not remain reduced, purse-string absorbable sutures incorporating the sac and uterosacral remnants can be used to reduce the sac. If these sutures are placed, cystoscopy should be performed after intravenous administration of Indigo Carmine to ensure ureteral patency. The foundation of the repair is the creation of multiple strong tissue layers which will resist the enterocele and pelvic prolapse. Basically, an extensive posterior repair and perineoplasty are used to create this

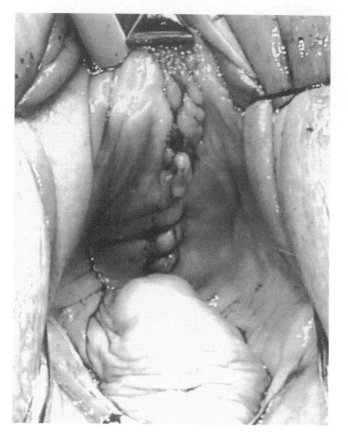

Figure 3   The incontinence procedure and anterior repair have been completed. The gaping introitus and severe apical and posterior wall defects can be clearly seen.

barrier. In most cases, two or three sequential layers of pararectal and levator fascia are brought together in the midline using a combination of permanent and absorbable interrupted sutures (Figs. 4–6). Two sequential purse-string sutures incorporating the completed anterior repair and the extensive posterior repair ensures a permanent closure of the vagina. As seen in Figure 7, after redundant posterior vaginal epithelium is excised, the lateral wall vaginal epithelium is dissected free and "rolled" anteriorly to form the new posterior vaginal wall. Generally, the vagina is 2–4 cm deep after the colpocleisis is completed. The remaining posterior vaginal edges are brought together in the midline using a running chromic catgut suture. An extensive perineoplasty is the final step in the procedure. This is performed by placing multiple O-Vicryl sutures deeply into the central tendon and bulbocavernosus muscles using a horizontal mattress sutures. The perineal skin is then closed with an absorbable suture. It is important that the perineorrhaphy not be extended too far anteriorly or the urethral meatus will be obstructed. The final result can be seen in Figure 8.

B.   Our Results Using Total Colpocleisis

Our experience using this colpocleisis procedure in 44 patients (mean age 78, range 68–91) has been favorable (25). All 44 patients underwent a multicompartment vaginal colpocleisis

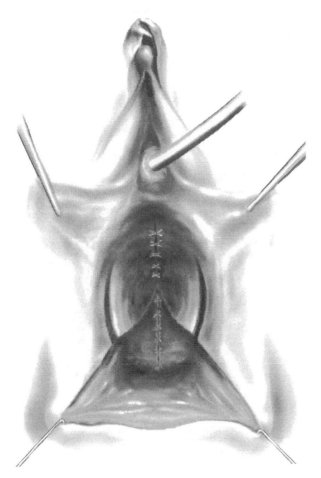

Figure 4 The first layer has been closed on the posterior wall, and the lateral vaginal wall incisions later used to form the new posterior vaginal wall have been made.

for either grade 3 or grade 4 vault prolapse accompanied by associated enteroceles, cystoceles, and rectoceles. Thirty-seven patients demonstrated SUI: seven patients underwent a pubovaginal sling, four had a modified vaginal wall sling, and 26 had a paravaginal sling. Seven had a Kelly plication as incontinence could not be demonstrated. At a mean follow-up of 27 months (range 1–62), all 44 patients are cured of vaginal vault prolapse, and there have been no recurrences of rectoceles or enteroceles. Three patients who underwent a Kelly plication and three who underwent a paravaginal sling have mild SUI, with four successfully treated with collagen injections. The other two patients have not desired further therapy. One patient who underwent a pubovaginal sling had large postvoid residuals and urge incontinence requiring a urethrolysis. The mean estimated blood loss for the entire procedure (including incontinence procedures) was ~175 mL and operating time 140 min. There were no significant complications, and all patients were satisfied with the results of the colpocleisis; however, two patients remain unsatisfied with their continence status owing to persistent urge incontinence. No patient has regretted the loss of sexual function.

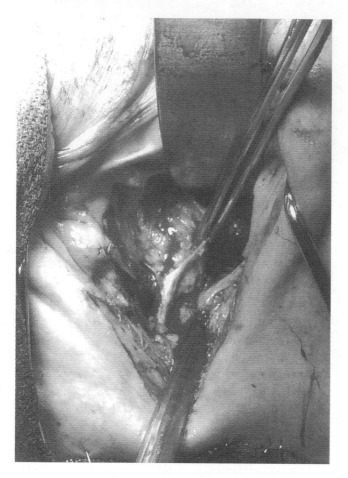

Figure 5   An intraoperative photograph showing the second layer (held by the forceps) on the posterior wall to be repaired. The strength of the posterior fascial layers used to close the vagina can be clearly seen. The diminishing size of the vagina is also evident.

C.   Partial Colpocleisis

Many surgeons have published variations of LeFort's original description of partial colpocleisis (26). The Goodall and Power modification of the LeFort operation limits the LeFort closure of the medial vagina to the proximal third of the vagina (27). This modification was designed to permit continued coital function. If preservation of sexual function is a goal, then a vaginal hysterectomy with vault suspension is a better option. Miklos and Karram recently published a paper demonstrating that the LeFort partial colpocleisis can be safely performed using a combination of pudendal nerve block, local anesthetic infiltration, and intravenous sedation if necessary (28).

The partial colpocleisis is initiated by excising a rectangular strip of epithelium from both the anterior and posterior vaginal walls (Fig. 9). The distal extent of the anterior incision is located 3–4 cm from the urethral meatus and the proximal extent of the incision is 2–3 cm from the cervix. The cervix is pushed into the depths of the vagina as the exposed anterior and posterior vaginal walls are sutured together using multiple interrupted O-Ethibond sutures. We place a 14F Red-Robinson catheter along the vaginal sidewalls to assist in the formation of

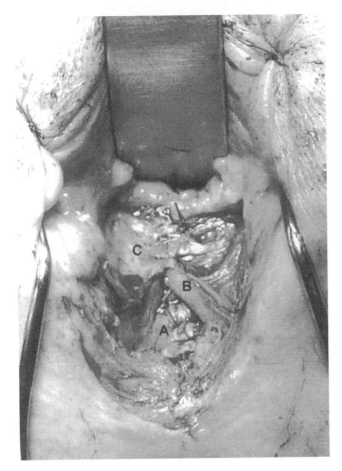

Figure 6 The last layer has been closed on the posterior wall. The three-layer closure can be seen with the three separate layers marked by A, B, and C. The anterior repair and posterior repair will be subsequently sutured together (not shown) to create a strong barrier, which will prevent future vault prolapse and enterocele formation.

mucosal drainage canals (Figs. 10, 11). The vaginal epithelium overlying the supported cervix is then closed, and a tight perineal body closure is performed to lend overall strength to the repair (Fig. 12). The Robinson catheter is removed on postoperative day 4 in most cases.

As for the total colpocleisis, prevention of postoperative incontinence depends on a careful preoperative urodynamic assessment. Many patients will require an anterior repair in addition to an incontinence procedure. For ISD, a pubovaginal or paravaginal sling is used in most cases. Transurethral collagen is used to treat any patients with postoperative incontinence.

V.   OUTCOMES AND COMPLICATIONS

The long-term risk of prolapse recurrence following total colpocleisis is not well documented in the recent literature (29). DeLancey and Morley, using a purse-string inversion technique, reported one recurrence in 33 patients after a mean follow-up of 3 years (24). Over the past

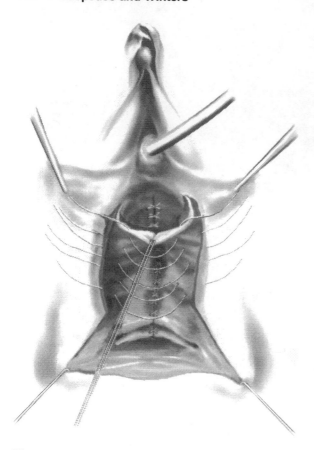

Figure 7   The lateral vaginal wall epithelial flaps are dissected free from the side walls and "rolled" anteriorly to form the new but much shorter posterior vaginal wall.

3 years, we have seen two of these inverted purse-string-type colpocleisis procedures performed elsewhere present to us with recurrent prolapse and subcutaneous enteroceles. This led us to develop a different approach that emphasizes the strength of an anterior and extensive posterior repair which is then sutured together. This vaginal closure is then reinforced with a strong perineorrhaphy to provide additional support. The authors noted that in the time it takes to perform an inverted purse-string-type colpocleisis repair, an anterior and multilayer posterior repair can be completed. The results of this modified colpocleisis have been very good, with no recurrences in 44 patients with a mean follow-up of 27 months. The only other contemporary report is from Ridley, who performed a modified LeFort colpocleisis in 41 patients. No postoperative failures were noted in this 1971 series with a maximum follow-up of 6 years (8).

The morbidity associated with these procedures appears to be quite low, especially in light of the advanced age and medical instability in most of these patients. This can probably be attributed to the shorter operating times and decreased blood loss associated with a partial colpocleisis as compared to a definitive vault suspension. The loss of sexual function has not been a problem in any of our patients or in DeLancey and Morley's report; however, these patients must be carefully selected to avoid this potential problem (24).

Partial colpocleisis, while historically yielding good results, can be problematic in some patients because the uterus and cervix are concealed from examination. With admittedly

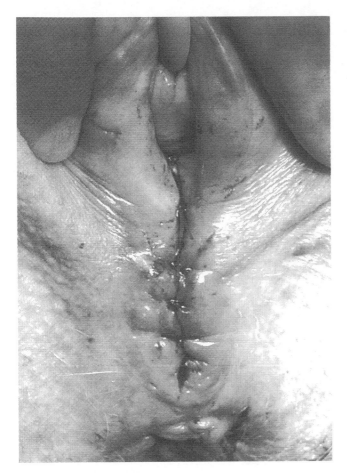

Figure 8 A postoperative photograph demonstrating the completed repair after the extensive perineal body closure has been performed.

small numbers, we have not yet seen a patient return with vaginal bleeding following partial colpocleisis, and only four cases of cancer developing in these patients have ever been reported (8). Therefore, we recommend that this procedure be reserved for high-risk patients and that a careful preoperative assessment (including Pap smear and uterine biopsy if necessary) be performed to prevent any problems.

Ureteral obstruction with resulting hydronephrosis occurs in 8% of patients undergoing surgery for pelvic prolapse (30). Patients with severe prolapse have a higher incidence, with up to 34% of patients demonstrating hydronephrosis on preoperative upper urinary tract imaging. In almost all cases, mild to moderate hydronephrosis related to pelvic prolapse resolves following surgical repair. In most cases in which surgical repair is imminent, preoperative imaging rarely changes the surgical management; however, patients with severe pelvic prolapse in which nonoperative therapy is pursued or surgical therapy will be delayed should undergo upper urinary tract imaging with stenting if obstruction is found.

Stress urinary incontinence that develops after a prolapse repair is performed has been called iatrogenic, latent, or, most commonly, occult incontinence. Reports have demonstrated that up to 50% of women with vault prolapse who do not complain of SUI will have leakage

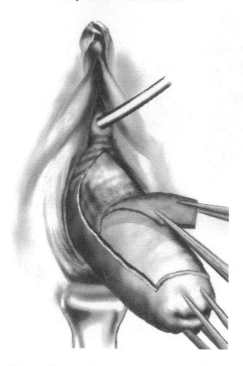

Figure 9   The first step in a LeFort partial colpocleisis. A rectangular segment of epithelium from the anterior and posterior vaginal walls is incised and subsequently removed.

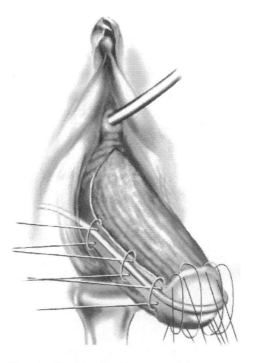

Figure 10   The anterior and posterior incised vaginal edges are sewn together using a catheter to help form the drainage channels.

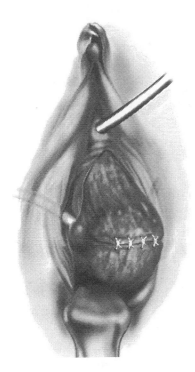

Figure 11   The first layer of the anterior to posterior wall closure has been completed. Subsequent layers are then closed until the cervix is deep within the vagina.

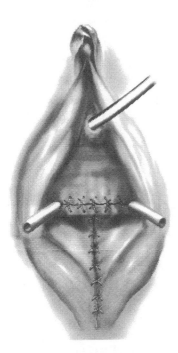

Figure 12   The final appearance of a LeFort partial colpocleisis after an extensive perineal body and distal rectocele closure used to strengthen the repair.

with the prolapse reduced and up to 75% will have a component of ISD (31,32). Ridley noted a 11% incidence of occult incontinence in his 47 patients, whereas DeLancey and Morley did not report any cases of occult incontinence (8,24). In our series, three patients who had incontinence only when the prolapse was reduced declined a formal incontinence procedure, and they required collagen injections postoperatively for SUI. Currently, the potential for postoperative incontinence can be accurately predicted *before* the procedure by reducing the prolapse when performing the pelvic exam and during urodynamics. This preoperative evaluation also allows the incontinence procedure to be tailored to the patient's specific problem and decreases the risk of postoperative incontinence.

VI. SUMMARY

The goal of reconstructive pelvic surgery is to restore normal anatomy and function; however, this is not always possible or necessary. For the elderly, medically unstable, and sexually inactive individual with severe symptomatic vault prolapse, partial or total colpocleisis may be the preferred procedure because of the low incidence of morbidity and consistently durable results. Accordingly, these colpocleisis procedures should be in every reconstructive surgeon's armamentarium.

REFERENCES

1. DeLancy JOL. Anatomic aspects of vaginal eversion after hysterectomy. Am J Obstet Gynecol 1992; 166:1717–1722.
2. Norton PA. Pelvic floor disorders: the role of fascia and ligaments. Clin Obstet Gynecol 1993; 36:926–938.
3. Wall LL. The muscles of the pelvic floor. Clin Obstet Gynecol 1993; 166:910–914.
4. Berglass B, Rubin IC. Study of the supportive structures of the uterus by levator myography. Surg Gynecol Obstet 1953; 97:677–692.
5. Herbst AL, Mishell DR, Stenchever MA, Droegemueller W. Disorders of the abdominal wall and pelvic support. In: Stenchever MA, ed. Comprehensive Gynecology. 2d ed. Philadelphia: Mosby Year Book, 1992:594.
6. Richter K. Massive eversion of the vagina: pathogenesis, diagnosis and therapy of the true prolapse of the vaginal stump. Clin Obstet Gynecol 1982; 25:89–92.
7. Morley GW. Vaginal approach to treatment of vaginal vault prolapse. Clin Obstet Gynecol 1993; 36:984–994.
8. Ridley JH. Evaluation of the colpocleisis operation: a report of fifty-eight cases. Am J Obstet Gynecol 1972; 113:1114–1119.
9. McGuire EJ, Cespedes RD, O'Connell HE. Leak-point pressures. Urol Clin North Am 1996; 23:253–262.
10. Siproudhis L, Lucas RJ, Raoul JL. Defecatory disorders, anorectal disorders and pelvic floor dysfunction: a polygamy? Int J Colorectal Dis 1992; 7:102–106.
11. Zimmern PE. The role of voiding cystourethrography in the evaluation of the female lower urinary tract. Prob Urol 1991; 5:23–33.
12. Ghoniem GM, Walters F, Lewis V. The value of the vaginal pack test in large cystoceles. J Urol 1994; 152:931–934.
13. Karram MM, Sze EHM, Walters MD. Surgical treatment of vaginal vault prolapse. In: Walters MD, Karram MM, eds. Urogynecology and Reconstructive Pelvic Surgery. 2d ed. St. Louis: Mosby, 1999:235–256.

14. Pelusi G, Bacchi P, Demaria F, Rinaldi A. The use of the Kelly plication for the prevention and treatment of genuine stress urinary incontinence in patients undergoing surgery for genital prolapse. Int Urogynecol J 1990; 1:196–200.

15. Couillard D, Deckard-Janatpour K, Stone A. The vaginal wall sling: a compressive suspension procedure for recurrent incontinence in elderly patients. Urology 1994; 43:203–207.

16. O'Connell HE, McGuire EJ, Aboseif S. Transurethral collagen injection therapy in women. J Urol 1995; 154:1463–1466.

17. Haab F, Zimmern PE, Leach GE. Diagnosis and treatment of intrinsic sphincter dysfunction in females. AUA 1996; Update Lesson 35 Vol 15.

18. O'Connell HM, McGuire EJ, Usui A. Pubovaginal slings in 1994. J Urol 1995; 153:525A, Abstract 1186.

19. Cespedes RD, Cross CA, McGuire EJ. Pubovaginal fascial slings. Tech Urol 1997; 3:195–201.

20. Blaivas JG, Jacobs BZ. Pubovaginal sling in the treatment of complicated stress incontinence. J Urol 1991; 145:1214–1218.

21. Beck RP, McCormick S, Nordstrum L. A 25 year experience with 519 anterior colporrhaphy procedures. Obstet Gynecol 1991; 78:1011–1015.

22. Kohli N, Sze EHM, Roat TW, Karram MM. Incidence of recurrent cystocele after anterior colporrhaphy with and without concomitant transvaginal needle suspension. Am J Obstet Gynecol 1996; 175:1476–1481.

23. Nichols DH, Randall CL. Enterocele. In: Nichols DH, Randal CL eds. Vaginal Surgery. 4th ed. Baltimore: Williams & Wilkins, 1996:345.

24. DeLancy JOL, Morley GW. Total colpocleisis for vaginal eversion. Am J Obstet Gynecol 1997; 176:1228–1235.

25. Cespedes RD, Winters JC, Ferguson KH. Colpocleisis for the treatment of vaginal vault prolapse. Tech Urol 2001; 7:152–160.

26. LeFort L. Nouveau procede pour la guerison du prolapsus uterin. Bull Gen Ther 1877; 92:337–346.

27. Goodall JR, Power RM. A modification of the LeFort operation for increasing its scope. Am J Obstet Gynecol 1937; 34: 968–971.

28. Miklos JR, Sze EHM, Karram MM. Vaginal correction of pelvic organ relaxation using local anesthesia. Obstet Gynecol 1995; 86:922–926.

29. Smale LE, Smale CL, Mundo NG, Rivera R. Vaginectomy: profile of success in treating vaginal prolapse. Medscape Womens Health 1997; 2(3):5.

30. Beverley CM, Walters MD, Weber AM, Piedmonte MR, Ballard LA. Prevalence of hydronephrosis in patients undergoing surgery for pelvic organ prolapse. Obstet Gynecol 1997; 90:37–41.

31. Gallentine ML, Cespedes RD. Occult stress urinary incontinence and the effect of vaginal vault prolapse on abdominal leak point presses. Urology 2001; 57:40–44.

32. Romanzi LJ, Chaikin DC, Blaivas JG. The effect of genital prolapse on voiding. J Urol 1999; 161:581–587.

51
Rectocele Repair/Posterior Colporrhaphy

Nirit Rosenblum,* Karyn S. Eilber,† and Larissa V. Rodríguez
University of California, Los Angeles, California, U.S.A.

I. INTRODUCTION

Damage to or anatomical changes in the posterior vaginal compartment may not be as clinically apparent as anatomic alterations in the anterior vaginal compartment, yet these abnormalities in pelvic floor support are clinically relevant in vaginal reconstructive surgery. Identification of posterior vaginal wall defects during routine gynecologic or urologic evaluation is critical in planning a definitive therapeutic approach to pelvic reconstruction. While the presence of posterior vaginal wall relaxation, or rectocele, may not necessarily be symptomatic, restoration of posterior vaginal wall support helps to restore both vaginal axis and function. The normal horizontal position of the proximal half of the vagina is restored, recreating a posterior curvature to the vaginal axis, thereby preventing progression of pelvic organ prolapse. Changes in intra-abdominal pressure will allow coaptation and closure of the vaginal vault, providing restored pelvic floor support for the pelvic organs. Thus, identification and repair of concomitant posterior vaginal wall defects are important in the treatment of symptomatic patients with other defects in pelvic floor support.

II. ANATOMY AND PATHOPHYSIOLOGY OF PELVIC FLOOR RELAXATION

In a normal female, the levator plate functions as a broad horizontal support mechanism on which the rectum and proximal vagina rest. This anatomic positioning is important during increases in intra-abdominal pressure, allowing two compensatory mechanisms to take place. First, there is reflex contraction of the levator musculature, pulling the midvagina forward while pushing the proximal vagina posteriorly; these active mechanisms increase the midvaginal angle and prevent pelvic organ prolapse. Secondly, the reflex contractions of the levator ani and urogenital diaphragm muscles narrow both the genital hiatus in the levator muscle and the vaginal introitus, further narrowing the defect through which pelvic organ prolapse occurs (1,2).

Many factors, including childbirth, aging, loss of estrogen stimulation, chronic abdominal straining and heavy labor, weaken the pelvic floor and its associated support structures. Child-

**Current affiliation*: NYU School of Medicine, New York, New York, U.S.A.
†*Current affiliation*: Memorial Sloan-Kettering Cancer Center, New York, New York, U.S.A.

birth causes stretching of the prerectal and pararectal "fasciae," with detachment of the prerectal "fascia" from the perineal body, allowing rectocele formation (3). In addition, childbirth damages and weakens the levator musculature and its fascia, attenuating the decussating prerectal levator fibers and the attachment of the levator ani to the central tendon of the perineum. The result is a convex sagging of the levator plate with a loss of the normal horizontal vaginal axis (2) (Fig. 1). The vagina becomes rotated downward and posteriorly, no longer providing horizontal support. These anatomic changes allow downward herniation of the pelvic organs along this new vaginal axis (4). Enterocele formation is caused by intra-abdominal pressure transmission to the pouch of Douglas. Widening of the anogenital hiatus and damage to the urogenital diaphragm and central tendon further facilitates pelvic prolapse by preventing the normal compensatory narrowing of the vaginal opening (Fig. 2). Varying degrees of perineal tears contribute to widening of the vaginal introitus.

There are several critical components of pelvic floor relaxation that are associated with rectocele formation. Loss of the normal horizontal axis of the levator plate and vagina, weakness of the urogenital and pelvic floor diaphragms, detachment of the levator ani from the central tendon of the perineum, and widening of the anogenital hiatus allow intra-abdominal forces to be transmitted directly to pelvic organs without normal underlying compensatory mechanisms. In addition, the rectovaginal septum becomes attenuated, allowing anterior displacement of the rectum (5). Isolated breaks in the rectovaginal septum facilitate rectocele formation.

Generally, there are several areas along the rectovaginal septum where breaks are commonly found. The most common site is a transverse separation immediately above the attachment of this septum to the perineal body, resulting in a low rectocele (seen just inside the introitus). A midline vertical defect is equally common, and apical transverse breaks have

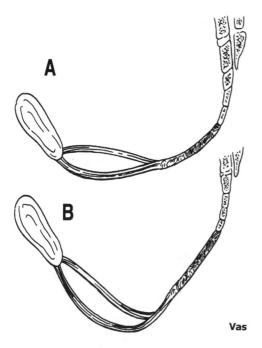

Vas

Figure 1 **(A)** Schematic diagram of a normal levator ani muscular sling. **(B)** Schematic diagram of a damaged and attenuated levator ani muscular sling, resulting in a convex sagging of the pelvic floor and loss of the normal horizontal vaginal axis.

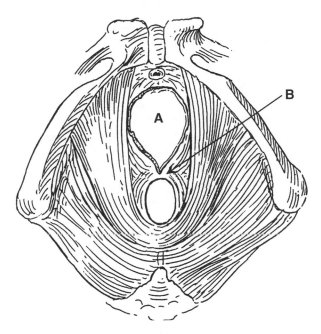

Figure 2 Schematic diagram of a widened levator hiatus, including damage to both the genital hiatus (**A**) and the central tendon of the perineum (**B**).

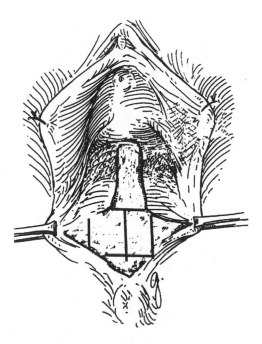

Figure 3 Schematic diagram of locations in the rectovaginal septum where segmental breaks commonly occur, contributing to rectocele formation. The lines represent the most common locations of breaks in the rectovaginal septum.

also been described, which may represent a poorly repaired or poorly healed episiotomy (Fig. 3). Rarely, one can see lateral separation on one side (6). Therefore, each of these components of pelvic floor relaxation must be addressed at the time of rectocele or posterior vaginal wall repair. Identification of this pathophysiology is critical when evaluating female patients with symptoms or signs of pelvic floor relaxation, including stress incontinence associated with urethral hypermobility and/or intrinsic sphincter deficiency. Correction of anterior wall prolapse and bladder neck hypermobility alone further predisposes the patient to subsequent uterine prolapse as well as enterocele and rectocele formation. Maintenance of the normal horizontal vaginal axis is an important goal of surgical repair of pelvic floor relaxation, in order to allow compensatory mechanisms to be re-established. Corrective surgery should include correction of the rectocele by reinforcement of the prerectal and pararectal "fasciae," repair of the levator muscle defect to restore the levator hiatus, restoration of the horizontal supporting plate of the proximal vagina, and repair of the perineum (5).

III. RECTOCELE CLASSIFICATION AND PREVALENCE

Classification of posterior vaginal wall prolapse is based on physical assessment, which has been recently standardized by the International Continence Society. Using this system, vaginal and perineal measurements are made at different sites, providing quantification of prolapse affecting discrete vaginal components. All measurements are made in centimeters relative to the hymen as the reference point. Negative values represent positions above the hymen; positive values represent points beyond or outside the hymen. Physical examination should include the staging of prolapse as previously described, as well as a rectovaginal and anal sphincter examination, an assessment of pelvic muscle contraction as well as a screening pelvic neurologic exam (7).

The grading of rectocele on physical examination was previously subjective and based on the location and degree of posterior vaginal wall protrusion (Table 1) (8). The rectal examination includes elevation of the rectum into the vagina to assess the degree of anterior rectal wall displacement and to assess the thickness and integrity of the perineal body. Evaluation of the rectovaginal septum performed during a bimanual examination may identify the presence of a sac of tissue in the rectovaginal septum (an enterocele), as well as attenuation of the rectovaginal septum (9).

Perineal tears are graded on a scale of I to IV, based on the posterior extent of the injury (Table 2) (10). Rectoceles are further classified based on their anatomic position: low, mid, or high. Low rectoceles result from childbirth causing disruption of the prerectal "fascia" and levator musculature from their attachments to the central tendon. In addition, direct damage to the central tendon itself will contribute to formation of a low rectocele. Midvaginal rectoceles are the most common and result from attenuation and stretching of the perirectal and prerectal

Table 1 Classification of Rectocele Based on Physical Examination

Grade	Physical examination findings
I	Posterior vaginal wall protrusion, saccular in nature, at level of hymenal ring with associated depression of perineum
II	Posterior vaginal wall protrusion at the level of the levator hiatus (more proximal)
III	Posterior vaginal wall protrusion outside or beyond the level of the introitus

Source: Ref. (8).

Table 2   Classification of Perineal Tears

Grade	Location of perineal tear
I	Tear limited to hymenal ring
II	Tear involving the perineal body but not the anal sphincter
III	Tear involving the anal sphincter
IV	Tear extending into the anal mucosa

Source: Ref. (10)

"fasciae." High rectoceles are often associated with enteroceles due to weakening of the upper portion of the rectovaginal septum or breaks in the prerectal "fascia."

The prevalence of rectoceles depends on the population of women studied. The incidence of rectoceles in the general population ranges between 20% and 80% (11). Clearly, there is a high incidence of women with asymptomatic rectoceles. In a cohort of patients with stress urinary incontinence, Raz et al. found a significant percentage of patients with rectocele and this incidence increased with the degree of associated prolapse (12,13). Severe anterior vaginal wall prolapse is often associated with significant posterior wall prolapse. In patients with defecatory dysfunction, the incidence of rectocele varies between 27% and 61%. A rectocele >2 cm in size is more likely to correlate with the presence of symptoms, making it more clinically significant (14).

IV. SYMPTOMATOLOGY

Posterior vaginal wall relaxation can lead to a variable degree of symptomatology, depending on rectocele size and generalized bowel habits. Constipation is a common complaint, reportedly found in 75–100% of patients with rectoceles (11). Despite the correlation of constipation to the presence of a rectocele, there are many other factors that can contribute to constipation. Other rectal symptoms include incomplete emptying, a sensation of rectal pressure, a vaginal bulge, and fecal straining. Furthermore, the need for either vaginal digitalization or manual perineal pressure to facilitate defecation may be necessary (15–17). A variety of nonspecific symptoms such as rectal pain, bleeding, fecal or flatal incontinence, low back pain associated with the upright position, and dyspareunia are also associated with rectoceles (9). On the other hand, many patients with rectoceles will be completely asymptomatic. The relationship between anatomic abnormalities and clinical symptoms is not clear, and often the correlation is poor (18).

V. EVALUATION

A. History

Questions pertaining to both bowel and sexual function symptoms associated with rectocele or posterior vaginal wall defects should be addressed and subjectively quantified. Many middle-aged and older women will complain of constipation that may or may not be related to the presence of a rectocele. There are many factors involved in bowel function that must be taken into consideration; if severe, referral to a gastroenterologist or colorectal surgeon may be appropriate.

B.   Physical Examination

Assessment of the posterior vaginal compartment should be a routine component of any patient being examined for incontinence or pelvic organ prolapse. This includes inspection for the presence of enterocele, rectocele, and perineal weakness. Generally, posterior compartment evaluation is performed by placing half of a vaginal speculum to displace the anterior vaginal wall and allow complete visualization of the posterior wall during straining. Digital examination with one finger in the vagina and one finger in the rectum allows for assessment of the recto-vaginal septum, which is often quite attenuated with large rectoceles, and may contain an enterocele sac. Physical examination may not reliably distinguish an enterocele from a high rectocele. Furthermore, inspection of the rectovaginal septum for isolated breaks, typically found near its attachment to the perineal body or in the midline, is performed by placing a finger in the rectum and lifting up the posterior vaginal wall. Finally, inspection of the perineal body is performed to identify a defect associated with a widened introitus and a shortened perineum. In cases of severe prolapse, combined defects of posterior vaginal wall support at the level of the pelvic floor and the perineum often occur.

The assessment of vaginal axis is achieved by digital examination. In a nulliparous woman with a well-supported pelvic floor, there will be a posterior curvature of the proximal vagina ("banana-shaped"). In a patient with pelvic floor relaxation, the vaginal axis will be horizontal in the lithotomy position. Restoration of this posterior vaginal axis helps prevent further development or recurrence of pelvic organ prolapse. Increases in abdominal pressure will cause vaginal coaptation when the normal banana-shaped axis has been restored.

The final portion of the posterior compartment examination involves assessment of the anal sphincter, including resting tone, voluntary activity, and reflex activity. Defects in the external anal sphincter may be associated with symptoms of fecal and flatal incontinence. Digital examination is performed during rest, strain, cough, and voluntary contraction.

C.   Radiographic Examination

The reported sensitivity of pelvic examination for the diagnosis of rectocele ranges from 31% to 81% (19–23). In addition, physical examination cannot reliably distinguish an enterocele from a high rectocele. For these reasons, imaging modalities have been used to aid in the diagnosis of a rectocele. Plain upright pelvic radiography, often obtained prior to voiding cystourethrography, may demonstrate an enterocele, a rectocele, or both. The hallmark is the presence of radiolucent gas 3–4 cm below the pubococcygeal line. Additional imaging can be performed by use of evacuation proctography, or defecography. However, the correlation between defecography and symptomatology in guiding patient selection for repair has been limited (20,22–25).

Magnetic resonance imaging (MRI) is a very useful tool in identifying and quantifying the presence of a rectocele as well as associated pelvic floor dysfunction, pelvic organ pathology, and pelvic organ prolapse. Static images are obtained in both sagittal and parasagittal planes from left to right across the pelvis. These are followed by a set of dynamic images in the mid-sagittal plane acquired during the resting and straining states. This particular set of dynamic images is helpful in identifying pelvic floor descent and pelvic organ prolapse. The pubococcygeal line and posterior puborectalis muscle sling are fixed anatomic reference points, used to quantify organ prolapse and pelvic floor dysfunction. Organ prolapse is defined as any protrusion through the puborectalis hiatus. Specifically, a rectocele is easily identified when filled with gas, fluid or gel (26,27) (Fig. 4). Although MRI without the use of a rectal contrast agent is relatively poor in diagnosing rectoceles in comparison with the detection rates of other forms of prolapse,

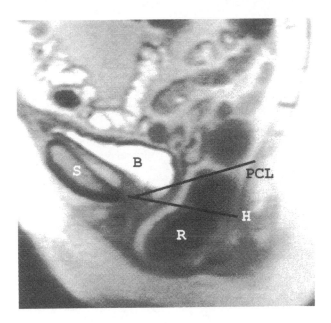

Figure 4   Magnetic resonance image of the pelvis in the sagittal plane during the straining state. A large, gas-filled rectocele (R) is seen protruding beyond the puborectalis hiatus. Bladder (B), symphysis (S), pubococcygeal line (PCL), puborectalis hiatus (H).

we currently rely primarily on MRI as a diagnostic tool in the evaluation of women with pelvic floor relaxation and organ prolapse.

D.   Identification of Perineal Laxity

In addition to posterior vaginal wall prolapse, the presence of perineal laxity is an important component of pelvic floor dysfunction. The urogenital diaphragm, made up of bulbocavernosus, superficial, and deep transverse perinei muscles and external anal sphincter musculature, joins with the levator ani to form the central tendon of the perineum (28). Attenuation of these structures along with detachment from the central tendon results in perineal laxity. On physical examination, there is an outward convexity of the perineum with straining and an increased distance between the posterior vaginal fourchette and the anus. Often, this defect will be present in association with rectocele. Specific symptoms associated with perineal laxity include severe constipation and the need to apply perineal pressure in order to evacuate the rectum. In addition, the patient may notice a bulging of the perineum during straining, or increases in abdominal pressure.

VI.   INDICATIONS FOR RECTOCELE REPAIR

In general, the repair of posterior vaginal wall prolapse is undertaken together with associated pelvic floor relaxation and organ prolapse. Surgical correction of cystocele, uterine prolapse, or enterocele often includes rectocele repair, as pelvic floor laxity usually affects all vaginal compartments (20). Rectocele repair during prolapse surgery helps to restore normal vaginal axis and introital diameter, thereby preventing future prolapse recurrence. Symptoms of a significant rectocele include difficult evacuation, sensation of a vaginal bulge, constipation, the need to splint the vagina in order to empty the rectum, fecal straining, and dyspareunia. These complaints are considered relative indications for surgical treatment, although the indications for repair of asymptomatic pelvic floor laxity at the time of incontinence surgery are less well defined and accepted.

Surgical repair of anterior vaginal wall prolapse or of incontinence alone leaves a portion of the vaginal hernia uncorrected, thereby exposing it to increased abdominal forces and facilitating further weakening of the pelvic floor with time (29). Repair of the posterior vaginal wall restores the normal horizontal vaginal axis, decreasing the likelihood of recurrent prolapse postoperatively (28). Furthermore, restoration of posterior vaginal wall support creates a backboard against which the urethra and bladder neck can be compressed, possibly improving the outcome of anti-incontinence surgery. Thus, we recommend simultaneous repair of asymptomatic moderate or severe pelvic floor weakness with anti-incontinence surgery in order to achieve these aforementioned goals.

VII. INDICATIONS FOR PERINEAL REPAIR

Generally, repair of the perineal body is performed at the time of rectocele repair to restore vaginal axis, recreate the anchoring of the levator ani muscle to the central tendon of the perineum, and restore the normal urogenital diaphragm. When there is specific herniation of the perineum and an increased distance between posterior fourchette and anus, a formal perineonhaphy should be undertaken. Indications for this type of repair are based on the patient's defecatory dysfunction, such as severe constipation and the need to provide manual perineal pressure in order to defecate effectively.

VIII. SURGICAL TECHNIQUE OF RECTOCELE REPAIR

The surgical repair of a rectocele incorporates three goals: rectocele reduction by plication of prerectal and pararectal "fascia," or endopelvic connective tissue, reconstruction of the levator hiatus by reapproximation of the prerectal levator fibers, and repair of the perineal body. These steps result in reconstruction of the rectovaginal septum as well as restoration of the horizontal levator plate. The perineal body repair reanchors the muscles of the lower vagina and perineum, restoring the urogenital diaphragm. A variety of surgical techniques have been described for the correction of posterior vaginal wall relaxation: posterior colporrhaphy with plication of the pararectal and prerectal "fascia"; traditional posterior colporrhaphy with levator ani approximation; and segmental repair of the rectovaginal septal defects. Each of these techniques will be described in addition to their associated complications and outcomes.

Preoperative preparation includes a lower bowel preparation with oral laxatives, such as bisacodyl, taken the two nights prior to surgery. In addition, a clear-liquid diet is advised for 48 h prior to surgery. Broad-spectrum intravenous antibiotics are administered the day of surgery to cover anaerobes, gram-negative bacilli, and group D enterococcus. We routinely utilize a fluoroquinolone antibiotic, unless contraindicated.

A. Plication of Prerectal and Pararectal Fasciae with Levator Reconstruction

The patient is placed in the dorsal lithotomy position with thorough perineal and vaginal preparation. A Betadine-soaked laparotomy pad is inserted as a rectal packing, followed by draping; care is taken to isolate the rectum from the operative field by double draping with adherent membranes. The drapes are then affixed to the perineum with sutures and the labia majora are retracted superiorly and laterally with stay sutures. A Foley catheter is placed, and anti-

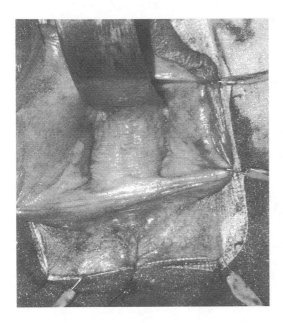

Figure 5   Photograph of rectocele following intraoperative exposure of posterior vaginal wall.

incontinence surgery, cystocele repair, vaginal hysterectomy, or enterocele repair is performed first. Surgical repair of the posterior vaginal wall is then performed.

A Scott ring retractor is utilized to provide lateral exposure of the vaginal vault (Fig. 5). Upward retraction of the anterior vaginal wall with a Heaney retractor improves visualization and prevents inadvertent narrowing of the vagina by excessive excision of vaginal wall tissue. Two Allis clamps are placed along the posterior fourchette at the 5-o'clock and 7-o'clock positions (Fig. 6). A V-shaped incision is made, creating a triangular flap of skin that is subsequently excised, exposing the attenuated perineal body (Figs. 7, 8). Two Allis clamps are then used to grasp the posterior vaginal wall overlying the rectocele, approximately 3 cm apart. An inverted V-shaped incision is made in the epithelium overlying the midportion of the rectocele, with its apex at the proximal most portion of the rectocele (Figs. 9, 10). Sharp dissection with Metzenbaum scissors aids in developing the plane between the posterior vaginal wall and the herniated rectal wall, thereby exposing the attenuated prerectal "fascia" (Fig. 11). It is important to maintain dissection along the vaginal wall as to avoid injury to the rectum. The dissection extends laterally to expose the pararectal "fascia" and is carried out along the midline to the level of the apex of the vagina. The isolated triangle of vaginal wall overlying the rectocele is then excised (Fig. 12).

Reconstruction of the posterior pelvic floor is performed next. A Heaney retractor is used to retract the rectum downward, reducing the rectocele and facilitating reapproximation of the pararectal and prerectal fascia. A running, interlocking 2-0 Vicryl suture begins at the apex of the vagina and is continued to the level of the levator hiatus (Fig. 13A). The first apical suture incorporates the uterosacral ligaments as well as the prerectal and pararectal "fascia." The running suture incorporates the edges of the vaginal epithelium with generous, deep bites of the right and left pararectal "fascia" as well as prerectal "fascia" (Fig. 13B). The levator musculature is incorporated in the distal one-third of the posterior vaginal wall closure with a figure-of-eight suture, to the level of the perineal incision. This last suture results in reapproximation of the levator hiatus, restoring the normal caliber of the introitus. It is important to pay

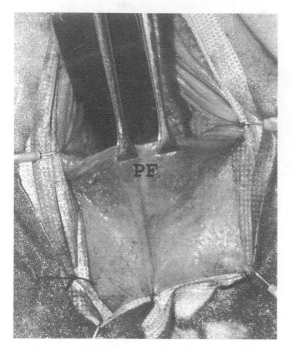

Figure 6 Intraoperative photograph of posterior vaginal fourchette (PF), seen held by two Allis clamps, with anterior vaginal wall retracted by Heaney retractor.

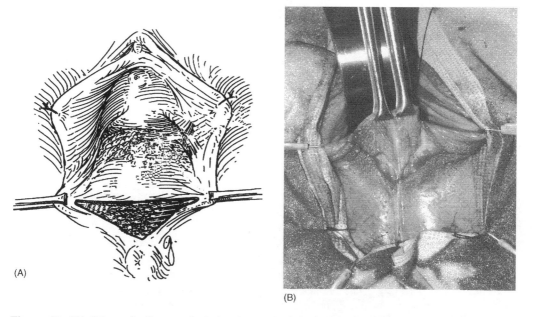

(A)

(B)

Figure 7 **(A)** Schematic diagram depicting inverted triangular incision of posterior fourchette during rectocele repair. **(B)** Photograph of triangular incision of posterior fourchette.

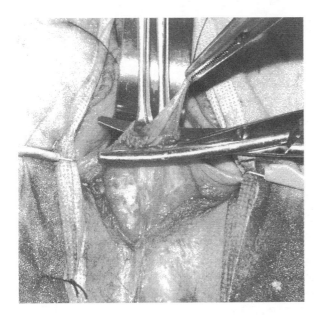

Figure 8 Photograph of excision of posterior fourchette epithelium and underlying tissue.

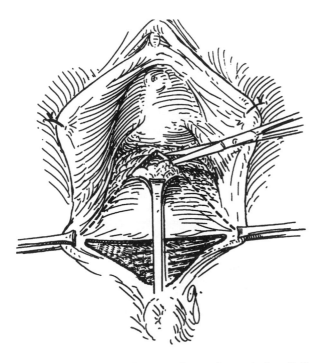

Figure 9 Schematic diagram of posterior vaginal wall dissection overlying rectocele, in a triangular fashion, from the level of the levator ani musculature to the posterior fourchette incision.

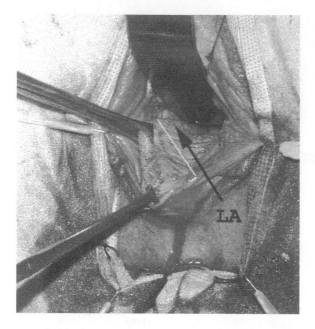

Figure 10   Photograph of two Allis clamps grasping posterior vaginal wall overlying rectocele, with proximal clamp at level of levator ani (LA) musculature. Line represents incision of vaginal epithelium on either side of Allis clamps. Arrowhead at level of levator ani hiatus.

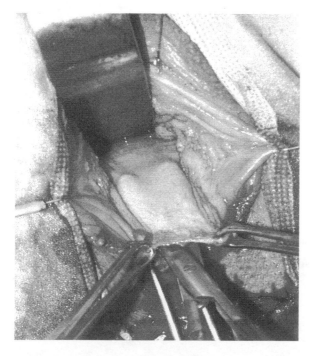

Figure 11   Photograph depicting dissection under posterior vaginal wall epithelium using Metzenbaum scissors from posterior fourchette to vaginal cuff or cervix in the midline.

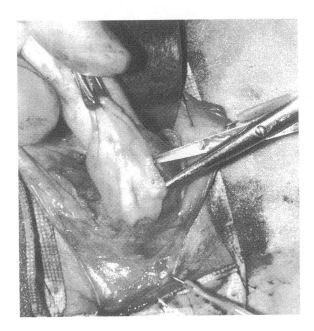

Figure 12 Photograph depicting excision of posterior vaginal wall epithelium at the level of the levator hiatus.

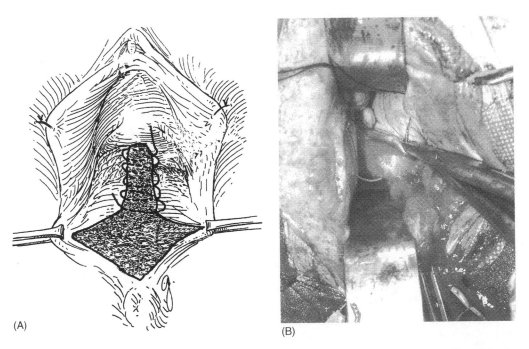

(A)

(B)

Figure 13 **(A)** Schematic diagram of rectocele repair suture line from level of vaginal cuff to posterior fourchette. Absorbable suture material is used in a running, interlocking fashion with incorporation of pararectal and prerectal fascia beneath vaginal epithelium. **(B)** Photograph depicting suture placement incorporating posterior vaginal epithelium and underlying pararectal fascia.

close attention to the creation of a smooth posterior vaginal wall, without the creation of painful ridges (28,30).

Repair of the perineum is then carried out by reapproximating the central tendon. Vertical mattress sutures of 2-0 Vicryl are placed in the perineum to reapproximate the bulbocavernosus muscles, the transverse perineal muscles and the levator complex. Finally, the overlying perineal skin is reapproximated with a running suture of Vicryl. An antibiotic-impregnated vaginal packing is placed at the completion of the procedure to aid in hemostasis. Patients are discharged home on stool softeners for 1 month.

Vasavada et al. reviewed the outcomes of 380 patients who underwent this method of rectocele repair with a mean follow-up of 22 months. Thirty-one percent of patients (117) had symptomatic posterior pelvic floor relaxation while 69% (263) were asymptomatic, the majority presenting with concomitant stress urinary incontinence, anterior vaginal wall prolapse, or uterine prolapse. One of the primary complaints related to rectocele was constipation, in 26%. Following posterior vaginal wall repair and levator reconstruction, 67% reported improvement in constipation. Furthermore, 95.7% are free of recurrent rectocele on physical examination at follow-up. Four percent exhibited recurrence of rectocele, grade II or higher, some with associated symptoms (31).

B. Traditional Posterior Colporrhaphy

The patient is again placed in the dorsal lithotomy position, and the vagina and perineum are prepped in the usual sterile fashion, as previously described. A triangular incision along the posterior fourchette is performed, and an additional incision is made in the midline of the posterior vaginal wall from the posterior fourchette to the apex of the rectocele. The vaginal epithelium is dissected free from the underlying perirectal "fascia" to the level of the rectocele apex. This dissection is also carried out laterally on either side of the incision line. A finger is then used to retract the rectocele downward, allowing identification of the levator ani muscles laterally. Heavy absorbable sutures are then placed through the levator ani margins in order to reapproximate the muscular defect in the midline along the entire length of the exposed rectum. The perirectal "fascia" is then closed with interrupted absorbable suture in the midline, as a second layer of repair. Excess posterior vaginal wall epithelium is excised followed by closure of the posterior vaginal wall with an uninterrupted, absorbable suture. A formal reconstruction of the hymenal ring is then carried out in addition to closure of the perineal body (32). This method of posterior colporrhaphy, as opposed to the aforementioned technique, involves more extensive lateral dissection, entrance into the pararectal space, and exposure of the levator musculature. Thus, the levator ani musculature is plicated along the entire length of the posterior vaginal wall incision.

Kahn et al. retrospectively reviewed the outcomes of 231 women who underwent traditional posterior colporrhaphy in order to determine both anatomical cure and effects on both bowel and sexual function. Mean follow-up was 42.5 months. Sixty-one percent of patients underwent follow-up physical examination and interview, while 13% underwent a telephone interview alone. The only symptom that was decreased postoperatively following posterior colporrhaphy was that of a lump or sensation of intravaginal pressure. The symptoms of incomplete bowel emptying, constipation, fecal incontinence, and sexual dysfunction increased postoperatively. Sixty-two percent of women reported improvement in their bowel symptoms, while 12% experienced more difficult defecation. A significant number of women in this study reported de novo symptoms of incomplete bowel emptying (22%), constipation (23%), fecal incontinence (8%), and sexual dysfunction (16%). The overall anatomical cure rate based on follow-up physical examination was 76% (35). The conclusions of this study are somewhat limited by its retrospective nature and lack of a standardized postoperative questionnaire. However, this study confirms that constipation and bowel dysfunction are not always associated with the presence of a rectocele. Despite anatomical correction of posterior wall prolapse, a significant number of these women continued to experience bowel dysfunction in follow-up. This point emphasizes the multifactorial nature of bowel dysfunction that must be taken into consideration when counseling patients prior to surgery for pelvic prolapse.

C. Defect-Specific Rectocele Repair

More recently, several authors have recommended a modified, discrete defect rectocele repair with attention given to the rectovaginal "fascia" as a separate layer (6,18). Cadaveric and surgical dissections confirmed the presence of this layer and its role in the development of a rectocele (6). The rectovaginal septum begins at the cul-de-sac, superiorly, and extends to the perineal body. This tissue layer consists of dense collagen fibers, smooth muscle, and dense elastin. Overdistention during childbirth causes tearing and separation within this septum, resulting in formation of a linear rectocele. This septum can become detached from the perineal body as well as from the deep endopelvic connective tissue. Adequate assessment of this defect is performed with one finger in the rectum and several fingers in the vagina, especially with the patient in an erect posture during Valsalva maneuvers. A similar bimanual examination is done intraoperatively to identify specific defects in the rectovaginal septum that will be repaired (33).

Repair of discrete defects in the rectovaginal septum is carried out by placing the nondominant index finger in the rectum and bringing it forward to distinguish areas of uncovered rectal muscularis from those covered by the semitransparent rectovaginal septum. Allis clamps are placed on surrounding connective tissue to facilitate repair of specific defects. Interrupted 2-0 sutures are used to plicate over the exposed rectal wall (11). Cundiff et al. (34) describe an avascular plane between the vaginal epithelium and rectovaginal "fascia." Thus, bleeding during this dissection generally originates from the underlying rectal muscularis, providing further clues to the areas of rectovaginal septum disruption. These authors do not routinely plicate the levator ani muscles during defect-specific rectocele repair.

Porter et al. (36) reviewed the outcomes of 125 women who underwent defect-specific rectocele repair, either alone or in conjunction with other pelvic procedures. Patients were examined postoperatively and given questionnaires addressing quality of life, sexual function and bowel function. The site-specific method of rectocele repair was performed, without plication of the levator ani musculature. In the majority of these cases (79 of 125), surgical correction was performed for a symptomatic rectocele. Anatomic correction was achieved in 82% with a mean follow-up of 18 months. Quality-of-life symptoms improved in all respects following surgery. Furthermore, bowel symptoms improved significantly following repair; specifically, 55% reported improvements in deflection difficulties, 73% in pelvic pain or pressure, 74% in sensation of a vaginal mass, and 65% in the need to splint. Fecal incontinence and constipation were not significantly altered by surgical repair. Overall, 44% reported improvement or cure in their constipation. Reported dyspareunia significantly improved or was cured postoperatively in 73%, worsened in 19%, and arose de novo in 3% (11).

Cundiff et al. (34) reported a similar series of 69 women who underwent discrete defect rectocele repair and were followed with objective physical examination as well as subjective symptom questionnaires. Preoperative symptoms related to rectocele included sexual dysfunction (36%) and defecatory dysfunction (71%). Postoperative questionnaires were given at a median of 24 months following surgery, and revealed a statistically significant improvement in rectocele symptoms. Dyspareunia in sexually active women improved from 29%

preoperatively to 19% at long-term follow-up. Constipation decreased significantly from 46% preoperatively to 13% following surgery. The need for splinting was eliminated in 63% of women, and fecal incontinence improved in 56% of women (34).

IX. OUTCOMES FOLLOWING RECTOCELE REPAIR

The main goals of posterior compartment reconstruction include restoration of bowel and sexual function, repair of a widened vaginal hiatus, and restoration of the normal vaginal axis. However, overcorrection can lead to significant vaginal narrowing and dyspareunia.

Outcomes following rectocele repair, whether it be traditional posterior colporrhaphy or defect-specific repair of the rectovaginal septum, are not entirely conclusive based on current studies. Bowel dysfunction is a complex, multifactorial process that may or may not be associated with the presence of a rectocele or perineal hernia. Rectocele repair helps to restore normal vaginal anatomy and pelvic support, which may facilitate complete rectal evacuation with appropriate transmission of intra-abdominal pressures. The effect of posterior colporrhaphy on sexual dysfunction postoperatively has not been clearly demonstrated. Future studies with validated sexual function questionnaires are needed to adequately assess any impact of rectocele repair on sexual function, taking into consideration the impact of concomitant pelvic surgery.

REFERENCES

1. Sturmdorf A. Gynoplastic Technology. Philadelphia: F.A. Davis, 1919.
2. Berglas B, Rubin IC. Study of the supportive structures of the uterus by levator myography. Surg Gynecol Obstet 1953; 97:677.
3. Kuhn RJ, Hollycock VE. Observations on the anatomy of the rectovaginal pouch and septum. Obstet Gynecol 1982; 59:445.
4. Nichols DH, Milley PS, Randall CL. Significance of restoration of normal vaginal depth and axis. Obstet Gynecol 1970; 36:251.
5. Raz S, Little NA, Juma S. Female urology. In: Walsh PC, Retik AB, Stamey TA, Vaughan ED Jr, eds. Campbell's Urology. Philadelphia: W.B. Saunders, 1992:2782–2829.
6. Richardson AC. The rectovaginal septum revisited: its relationship to rectocele and its importance in rectocele repair. Clin Obstet Gynecol 1993; 36:976–983.
7. Weber AM, Abrams P, Brubaker L, Cundiff G, Davis G, Dmochowski RR, Fischer J, Hull T, Nygaard I, Weidner AC. The standardization of terminology for researchers in female pelvic floor disorders. Int Urogynecol J 2001; 12:178–186.
8. Beecham CT. Classification of vaginal relaxation. Am J Obstet Gynecol 1980; 136:957.
9. Walters MD. Pelvic organ prolapse: cystocele and rectocele. In: Walters MD, Karram MM, eds. Clinical Urogynecology. St. Louis: Mosby, 1993:225–235.
10. Baden WF, Walker TA, Lindsey JH. The vaginal profile. Tex Med 1968; 64:56.
11. Mollen RM, Van Larrhoven CJ, Kuijpers JH. Pathogenesis and management of rectoceles. Semin Colon Rectal Surg 1996; 7:192–196.
12. Raz S, Sussman EM, Erickson DB, Bregg KJ, Nitti VW. The Raz bladder neck suspension: results in 206 patients. J Urol 1992; 148:845–850.
13. Raz S, Little NA, Juma S, Sussman EM. Repair of severe anterior vaginal wall prolapse (grade IV cystourethrocele). J Urol 1991; 146:988–992.
14. Mimura T, Roy AJ, Storrie JB, Kamm MA. Treatment of impaired defecation associated with rectocele by behavioral retraining (biofeedback). Dis Colon Rectum 2000; 43:1267–1272.
15. Mellegren A, Anzen B, Nilsson BY, Johansson C, Dolk A, Gillgren P, Bremmer S, Holmstrom B. Results of rectocele repair: a prospective study. Dis Colon Rectum 1995; 38:7–13.

16. Karlbom U, Graf W, Nilsson S, Pahlman L. Does surgical repair of a rectocele improve rectal emptying? Dis Colon Rectum 1996; 39:1296–1302.
17. Murthy VK, Orkin BA, Smith LE, Glassman LM. Excellent outcome using selective criteria for rectocele repair. Dis Colon Rectum 1996; 39:374–378.
18. Van Laarhoven CJ, Kamm MA, Bartram CI, Halligan S, Hawley PR, Phillips RK. Relationship between anatomic and symptomatic long-term results after rectocele repair for impaired defecation. Dis Colon Rectum 1999; 42:204–211.
19. Kelvin FM, Maglinte DD. Dynamic cystoproctography of female pelvic floor defects and their interrelationships. AJR 1997; 169:769–774.
20. Kelvin FM, Hale DS, Maglinte DD, Hale DS, Benson JT. Female pelvic organ prolapse: diagnostic contribution of dynamic cystoproctography and comparison with physical examination. AJR 1999; 173:31–37.
21. Siproudhis L, Ropert A, Vilotte J, Bretagne JF, Heresbach D, Raoul JL, Gosselin M. How accurate is clinical examination in diagnosing and quantifying pelvirectal disorders? A prospective study in a group of 50 patients complaining of defecatory difficulties. Dis Colon Rectum 1993; 36:430–438.
22. Altringer WE, Saclarides TJ, Dominguez JM, Brubaker LT, Smith CS. Four-contrast defecography: pelvic 'floor-oscopy'. Dis Colon Rectum 1995; 38:695–699.
23. Cundiff GW, Nygaard I, Bland DR, Versi E. Proceedings of the American urogynecologic society multidisciplinary symposium on defecatory disorders. Am J Obstet Gynecol 2000; 182:S1–S10.
24. Takano M, Hamada A. Evaluation of pelvic descent disorders by dynamic contrast reontography. Dis Colon Rectum 2000; 43:205–212.
25. Kelvin FM, Maglinte DD, Hale DS, Benson JT. Female pelvic organ prolapse: a comparison of triphasic dynamic MR imaging and triphasic fluoroscopic cystocolpoproctography. AJR 2000; 174:81–84.
26. Rodriguez L, Raz S. Diagnostic imaging of pelvic floor dysfunction. Curr Opin Urol 2001; 11:423–428.
27. Barbaric ZL, Marumoto AK, Raz S. Magnetic resonance imaging of the perineum and pelvic floor. Top Magn Res Imag 2001; 12:83–92.
28. Babiarz JW, Raz S. Pelvic floor relaxation. In: Raz S, ed. Female Urology. Philadelphia: W.B. Saunders, 1996:445–456.
29. Nichols DH, Randall CL. Vaginal Surgery. 3d ed. Baltimore: Williams and Wilkins, 1989.
30. Raz S, Stothers L, Chopra A. Vaginal reconstructive surgery for incontinence and prolapse. In: Walsh PC, Retik AB, Vaughan ED Jr, Wein AJ, eds. Campbell's Urology. Philadelphia: W.B. Saunders, 1998:1059–1094.
31. Vasavada SP, Eilber K, Freedland S, Kristo B, Berman J, Rodriguez LV, Comiter CV, Raz S. A contemporary approach to posterior pelvic floor relaxation: the UCLA experience. (Submitted for publication).
32. Wheeless CR. Atlas of Pelvic Surgery. 2d ed. Philadelphia: Lea & Febiger, 1988.
33. Grody MH. Posterior compartment defects. In: Rock JA, Thompson JD, eds. Te Linde's Operative Gynecology. Philadelphia: Lippincott Williams and Wilkins, 1997:1044–1059.
34. Cundiff GW, Weidner AC, Visco AG, Addison WA, Bump RC. An anatomic and functional assessment of the discrete defect rectocele repair. Am J Obstet Gynecol 1998; 179:1451–1457.
35. Kahn MA, Stanton SL. Posterior colporrhaphy: its effects on bowel and sexual function. Br J Obstet Gynaecol 1997; 104:82–86.
36. Porter WE, Steele A, Walsh P, Kohli N, Karram MM. The anatomic and functional outcomes of defect-specific rectocele repairs. Am J Obstet Gynecol 1999; 181:1353–1359.

52

Evaluation and Management of Rectoceles

Jeffrey L. Segal and Mickey M. Karram
Good Samaritan Hospital, Cincinnati, Ohio, U.S.A.

I. INTRODUCTION

Pelvic organ prolapse accounts for 10–20% of all major gynecologic surgeries according to one epidemiologic study (1). Approximately 11% of American women require surgery for pelvic organ prolapse and/or urinary incontinence, and of these, about 25–30% require a second procedure for recurrence (2). A rectocele is a form of pelvic organ prolapse in which there is herniation or bulging of the posterior vaginal wall, with the anterior wall of the rectum in direct apposition to the vaginal epithelium. Although the true prevalence of rectoceles is unknown, Olsen et al. noted that 76% of women with documented pelvic organ prolapse had a rectocele (2).

In the past, the surgical repair of rectoceles was generally successful in "fixing" the vaginal bulge. However, owing to a general lack of understanding of the correlation between anatomic support and functional derangement, functional outcomes have not been thoroughly addressed. Today, as the elderly population continues to grow and become more active, the outcome measures of surgery should include not only the success of restoring anatomy, but also quality-of-life issues, including the relief of symptoms related to prolapse and the maintenance or restoration of visceral and sexual function. The goals of this chapter are to review the anatomy and pathophysiology of rectoceles as well as the recent developments in diagnosis and management.

II. PELVIC ANATOMY

During the late 1800s it was believed that the main support of the uterus was the vagina, which in turn was supported by the insertion of the levator muscles into the perineal body. Today, based largely on the work of DeLancey, three basic levels of support for the vagina are described: level 1 consists of support of the cervix and upper vagina over the levator plate by the cardinal-uterosacral complex; level 2 reflects support of the mid-vagina by lateral connections to the arcus tendinous fascia pelvis; and level 3 reflects support of the lower vagina by connections to the perineal membrane anteriorly and the perineal body posteriorly (3,4). Defects in these various levels of support can result in the formation of a rectocele at anatomic sites that correspond to the level of the defect. High rectoceles, which are often due to stretching or disruption of the top third of the vaginal wall and the cardinal-uterosacral ligament complexes, are associated with loss of uterine support and genital descensus. Middle rectoceles, which are often influenced by parturition, are associated with separation of the rectovaginal septum and loss of pelvic floor support. Low rectoceles are associated with disruption of the perineal body and are thought to be secondary to an inadequately repaired obstetric injury or overdistension during childbirth (5).

Despite earlier controversy regarding the existence of the rectovaginal septum, surgical and cadaveric dissections (6) as well as histologic specimens (7) have confirmed a layer of dense tissue between the rectum and the vagina, consisting of collagen, smooth muscle and elastin fibers (6,7). This layer of fascia, which was first described in men by Denonvilliers in 1839, is known as rectovaginal fascia, Denonvillier's fascia, prerectal fascia, vaginal fascia, and the rectogenital septum (7). It extends from the sacrum to the perineum and laterally merges into the fascial covering of the iliococcygeus and pubococcygeus muscles. Richardson (6) demonstrated five types of isolated tears in the rectovaginal septum in patients with a rectocele. The most common was a transverse break above its attachment to the perineal body, resulting in a low rectocele, followed by a midline vertical defect, resulting in a midvaginal rectocele, and finally a lateral separation down one of the sides of the fascia. An L- or U-shaped defect was also described, in which there is a combination of a lateral separation down one side and a transverse separation from the perineal body (6). Figure 1 illustrates the five types of defects (8). These contributions by DeLancey, Nichols, and Richardson have resulted in a better understanding of the anatomy of rectoceles as well as a change in the surgical approach used to repair them.

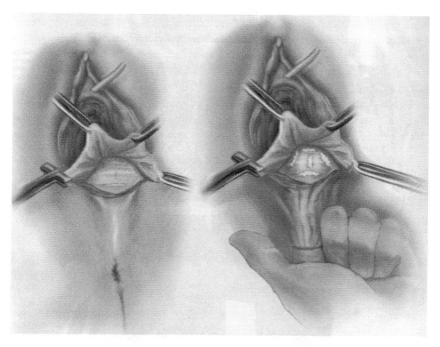

Figure 1   Five types of isolated tears in the rectovaginal septum in patients with a rectocele. (From Ref. 8.)

III. ETIOLOGY OF RECTOCELES

Although the true etiology of rectoceles is unclear, childbirth is a known risk factor. Childbirth has been shown to result in stretching and distension of the pelvic floor as well as tearing of the endopelvic fascia, including the rectovaginal septum. Prolonged straining during labor and descent of the presenting part also can result in traction and pressure of the pudendal nerve as it courses along the pelvic side wall causing partial denervation of the levator ani muscles. These changes lead to widening of the genital hiatus, perineal laxity and descent, and pelvic floor relaxation. During straining, because the vaginal opening can no longer completely close, the posterior vaginal wall is subjected to a higher pressure gradient.

Additionally, defecation disorders, such as chronic constipation and nonrelaxing puborectalis syndrome, which are associated with excessive straining, can also cause peripheral neuropathies as well as stretching and tearing of connective tissues. Chronic increased intra-abdominal pressure related to straining, resulting in a pudendal neuropathy with associated denervation of the pelvic diaphragm and external anal sphincter, can also lead to the development of fecal incontinence (9). Fecal incontinence, however, when associated with a rectocele, can have a multifactorial etiology, including occult rectoanal intussusception, complete rectal prolapse, physiologic dysfunction, decreased anorectal sensation, and frank sphincter disruption or atrophy. In determining the cause-and-effect relationship between rectoceles and defecatory dysfunction, one needs to better determine whether prolonged straining results in a rectocele or whether a rectocele results in stool trapping and prolonged straining. It is likely that a combination of both of these factors, and others, are causes (10). Table 1 lists coexisting causes of defecatory dysfunction (11).

Table 1   Coexisting Causes of Defecatory Dysfunction

---

1. Physiologic pelvic outlet obstruction (associated with contraction of the puborectalis and external anal sphincter during attempted defecation)
     Anismus
     Paradoxical puborectalis contraction
     Spastic pelvic floor
     Puborectalis dyssnergia
2. Anatomic pelvic outlet obstruction
     Rectoanal intussusception—infolding of the rectum into but not beyond the anal verge, which can induce a sensation of incomplete evacuation
     Solitary rectal ulcer syndrome—a benign condition caused by straining and associated with rectal bleeding, mucous discharge, pain, and difficult evacuation
     Rectal prolapse—full-thickness intussusception of the rectum toward or through the anal canal associated with straining, constipation, mucous discharge, bleeding, and soiling
     Rectocele—herniation or bulging of the posterior vaginal wall, with the anterior wall of the rectum in direct apposition to the vaginal epithelium
     Sigmoidocele—due to collapse of the rectal wall from extrinsic compression of the hernia contents and stasis of the sigmoid loop
3. Colonic inertia (slow transit throughout the colon)
4. Combined outlet obstruction and colonic inertia
5. Other
     Perineal descent—perineal descent below the ischial spines during rest and with straining, which may be associated with a pudendal neuropathy secondary to persistent straining
     Fecal incontinence—often associated with sphincter disruption or denervation, but may also be due to reflex relaxation of the anal sphincter when a large rectocele is filled with feces

---

Source: Ref. 11.

Other predisposing factors include postmenopausal status, connective tissue disorders, hysterectomy, and previous colposuspension and prolapse surgery. It has been suggested that a hysterectomy results in pelvic denervation, which can contribute to the later development of a rectocele (12). Retropubic colposuspension is felt to antevert the vagina and thus predispose women to posterior vaginal wall defects. Abnormalities may also arise when the rectovaginal fascia is not securely reattached to the perineal body during an episiotomy repair (13).

IV. SYMPTOMS

The majority of patients with an isolated rectocele are asymptomatic. In fact, Shorvon et al. found that 76% of asymptomatic nulliparous volunteers had small rectoceles on defecography studies (14). However, symptoms can gradually arise as a rectocele progresses due to the bulge or mass that a patient may feel in the vagina, which can cause pelvic pain or pressure, dyspareunia, and low back pain. These symptoms relating to pressure and a feeling of heaviness are typically worse at the end of the day after a patient has spent a prolonged period of time on her feet, and generally improve when the patient lies down. Symptoms are also often related to stool becoming trapped within the rectal bulge. Other related symptoms, as listed in Table 2, may include incomplete rectal emptying, difficulty with defecation requiring the need to splint, aching after a bowel movement, and postevacuation fullness. Although there are no published studies describing the natural history of rectoceles, current opinion suggests that they progress slowly over the years, and that functional difficulties tend to wax and wane, but progress slowly over time (13).

As noted in the previous section, constipation and other forms of defecatory dysfunction, such as fecal incontinence and paradoxical sphincter reaction, may coexist with rectoceles. The degree of posterior vaginal wall prolapse, however, does not correlate well with bowel dysfunction. Although they may frequently coexist, they do not necessarily have a causal relationship (10). Therefore one should appropriately counsel a potential surgical candidate who, for example, presents with a symptomatic rectocele and constipation, that repair of the rectocele may relieve symptoms related to stool trapping, but may not effectively relieve constipation. Because many of the symptoms of a rectocele overlap other pelvic floor disorders, it is imperative to rule out other treatable causes of symptoms, such as rectal intussusception or prolapse,

Table 2   Symptoms Associated with a Rectocele

Symptoms that may be directly related to rectocele	Symptoms that may overlap other pelvic floor disorders
Feeling of vaginal mass/bulge	Constipation
Pelvic or rectal pain/pressure	Fecal incontinence
Dyspareunia	Fecal urgency
Low back pain	Stool clustering
Incomplete rectal emptying	Outlet obstruction
Need to splint or insert fingers into vagina, rectum, or perineal support to facilitate defecation	
Aching after a bowel movement	
Postevacuation fullness	

perineal descent, and dyskinetic puborectalis syndrome (15) prior to surgically correcting posterior vaginal wall prolapse.

V. EVALUATION AND DIAGNOSIS

A. Physical Exam

The patient is examined first in the lithotomy position. All segments of vaginal support should be assessed in a site-specific fashion using the split blade of a Graves speculum or a Sims speculum. To visualize the posterior vaginal wall best, the speculum is used to displace the anterior vaginal wall. The patient is then asked to perform a Valsalva maneuver or cough vigorously, and if bulging of the posterior vaginal wall is noted, then a rectocele should be suspected. To better assess the extent of the prolapse, the patient should be reexamined in the standing position. A rectovaginal exam should be performed to assess the rectovaginal fascia as well as to rule out an enterocele, which can often occur in conjunction with a rectocele. An enterocele can be identified as a separate bulging sac arising from a higher point in the vagina. During the rectal exam the index finger should push toward the posterior vaginal wall in order to better assess the integrity of the rectovaginal fascia. A rectal exam may also be useful to assess the integrity of the external anal sphincter, especially for patients with symptoms of fecal incontinence. It can also be helpful in identifying other causes of defecatory dysfunction, such as a posterior rectocele, intussusception, skin tags, and mucosal prolapse (16).

The severity of a rectocele can be quantified either using the Baden-Walker grading system (17) or the Pelvic Organ Prolapse Quantification (POP-Q) system (18). Although it provides more precise information than the halfway system and may be useful for comparing anatomical changes following surgery, it does not identify structures behind the vaginal wall and does not quantify the size of the rectocele from the rectal side (16).

One should also look for perineal body defects. Perineal body defects are associated with a widened introitus with straining, and a decreased distance between the posterior margin of the vaginal introitus and the anterior margin of the anus. Measurements of the perineal body and genital hiatus are included as standard measurements in the POP-Q system. Routine evaluation of pelvic floor muscle function should also be performed by asking the patient to selectively contract and relax the pelvic floor muscles with the examiner's fingers in the vagina.

B. Adjunctive Studies

Ancillary studies, which include both radiologic and physiologic investigations as listed in Table 3, are being used to identify concomitant pathology, explain pathophysiology, provide objective outcome criteria and predict patients who will benefit most from surgery (11,19). However, there is no gold standard in diagnosing rectoceles, and the usefulness of these adjunctive studies in improving functional outcome is limited owing to the complex neuromuscular, physiological, and mechanical interactions that contribute to anorectal dysfunction (16). In general, rectoceles that are not associated with defecatory dysfunction do not require additional ancillary tests.

C. Defecating Proctography

For women with functional disorders of the pelvic floor, several recent studies have shown a limited role for proctography and dynamic MRI in characterizing posterior vaginal wall prolapse prior to surgery (20–22). The advantage of defecating proctography over physical examination is that in addition to providing a two-dimensional quantification of rectal parameters to diagnose

Table 3 Ancillary Studies for Women with Functional Disorders of the Pelvic Floor

Test	Purpose	Parameters	Usefulness
Defecating proctography	To evaluate dynamics of evacuation by visualizing the anorectum fluoroscopically after filling the rectum with liquid barium and barium paste. To provide structural information.	During resting/squeezing/straining phases, anorectal angle, anal canal length, puborectalis length, and perineal descent are evaluated. By measuring barium trapping, time and completeness of evacuation are estimated.	Useful in detecting size of rectocele. Can detect other anatomic abnormalities that may cause overlapping pelvic symptoms, including anorectal intussusception, sigmoidoceles, rectoceles, rectal prolapse, and perineal descent. Some use barium trapping as a criterion for rectocele repairs, but overall not a useful predictor of clinical outcome after rectocele repair.
Dynamic MRI	Combines dynamic visualization of rectal evacuation and fast-sequence examination of the pelvis to detect anatomic and functional abnormalities.	NA	Provides global view of all intrapelvic compartments. Aids in the differentiation of complex combined pelvic floor disorders.
Endoanal ultrasonography	Provides morphologic assessment of the internal and external anal sphincters, the puborectalis muscle, and the rectovaginal septum.	NA	Useful in detecting an anatomic defect associated with fecal incontinence.
Anorectal manometry	Sensory devices are used to quantitatively assess resistance to spontaneous evacuation by the anorectal mechanism. Using balloon distension, sensory capabilities of the rectum to provide a feeling of imminent emptying are also assessed.	Resting and squeeze anal pressures, including high-pressure zone, and anal canal length. Rectal sensory threshold, sensation of fullness, maximum tolerable volume, and rectal capacity. Rectoanal inhibitory reflex and anocutaneous reflex.	Useful in determining the physiologic components of fecal incontinence and constipation.

Electromyography.	To assess the neuromuscular integrity of the anal canal, using concentric needle electrodes or cutaneous surface electrodes which record motor unit action potentials generated by the EAS and puborectalis muscles at rest and with contraction. To assess the functional activity and presence of neurologic damage of the anal sphincter and pelvic floor muscles.	Electric activity in muscles of continence during anorectal function. Impaired recruitment or evidence of denervation Sphincter mapping Fiber density and nerve latency Measure striated muscle function	Useful in detecting muscular and neurogenic damage in fecal incontinence and inappropriate muscle activity in pelvic outlet obstruction. Useful in determining degree of denervation and conduction defects.
Pudendal nerve terminal motor latency.	Provides evaluation of pelvic floor neuromuscular integrity by measuring the length of time required for a fixed electrical stimulus to travel along the pudendal nerve between the ipsilateral ischial spine and the anal verge.	NA	Useful in determining neurogenic cause of fecal incontinence Useful for predicting outcome after anterior overlapping sphincteroplasty
Colonic transit study	Radiopaque markers are ingested and the percentage that are passed within a specified time as well as their distribution is measured.	NA	Useful in determining pelvic outlet obstruction and colonic inertia. Slow colonic transit may be predictive of poor outcome of a rectocele repair.
Mucosal electro-sensitivity and thermal sensitivity tests.	Uses electrode to pass current or probes which provide hot and cold stimuli to assess the sensory function of the anorectum.	NA	Useful to detect sensory impairment in patients with fecal incontinence.

Source: Refs. 11,16,19.

a rectocele, it can detect other anatomic abnormalities such as enteroceles, sigmoidoceles, perineal descent, and internal rectal prolapse. More importantly, defecating proctography also provides functional information regarding the efficiency of rectal emptying by enabling patients to mimic their defecating abnormalities in a physiologic manner.

However, the normal range of motion of the rectovaginal axis has not been determined, and cut-off values for diagnosing a rectocele are merely arbitrary numbers (13). Many reports define rectoceles ≥ 2.0–3.0 cm as being significant and indicative of patients who may benefit from operative repair (23,24), while others report that retention of contrast medium at defecography should be part of the selection criteria in determining who should undergo surgery. Preoperative size or grade of emptying, however, has not been shown to correlate well with symptoms (25,26).

Some have also advocated defecography as means of better detecting unsuspected rectoceles. Studies have shown, however, that physical examination alone has a 91–94% sensitivity in detecting a rectocele compared with proctography (27). Overall, rectoceles and other anatomic abnormalities may be easily and objectively diagnosed by defecating proctography, but its usefulness in the clinical evaluation of a rectocele and its ability to predict clinical outcome after a repair is limited (28).

D. Dynamic MRI Defecography

Dynamic MRI defecography has been considered superior compared to traditional defecating proctography because it is noninvasive, does not require ionizing radiation, and can provide a global view of all intrapelvic compartments (21). The study combines dynamic visualization of rectal evacuation with fast-sequence MRI examination of the pelvis. It helps determine complex, combined pelvic floor disorders such as rectoceles, enteroceles, rectal intussusception or prolapse, descending perineum, and dyskinetic puborectalis syndrome in association with defecation abnormalities, such as fecal incontinence, urgency, stool clustering, or outlet obstruction (22). Matsuoka et al. have shown, however, in comparing the two modalities, that despite costing 10-fold more than videoproctography, dynamic pelvic MRI has not been shown to change clinical decision making (29).

E. Physiologic Anorectal Studies

Anorectal studies can include anorectal manometry, electromyography, pudendal nerve terminal latency studies, and colonic transit studies as described in Table 3. In reviewing anorectal function tests, however, there are no physiologic findings that are specific for a rectocele (28). Although pudendal nerve terminal motor latency times are often increased in patients with perineal descent and chronic straining (31), prolonged latency is not consistently associated with rectoceles (32), and is not a good predictor of outcome after a rectocele repair (33). Those with an irritable rectum often feel an urge to defecate at small volumes and may experience symptoms of incomplete emptying and fecal incontinence. It is thought that a rectocele repair may worsen these symptoms by reducing rectal volume; anorectal manometry may prove helpful in this instance (16).

Van Dam et al., in a prospective study (34), evaluated the prognostic value of clinical and physiologic tests, such as defecography, pelvic floor electromyography, anorectal manometry, and balloon expulsion studies in women with obstructed defecation undergoing rectocele repair. They found that slow colonic transit studies were the only useful predictors of poor outcome in relieving obstructive symptoms after a combined posterior colporrhaphy and transanal repair. They also showed that women without a daily urge to defecate or a stool frequency of less than once per week or both, also had a worse postoperative outcome. The usefulness of colonic transit studies as part of the routine preoperative evaluation was later confirmed in separate prospective studies by Lopez et al. and Mellgren et al. (35,36). Mellgren also found through electrophysiologic analysis that two out of three patients with preoperative paradoxical sphincter reaction did not improve after a rectocele repair (36). However, the sample size was small, and a prospective study by Van Dam et al. found that paradoxical sphincter contraction did not affect the outcome of a rectocele repair (37).

F. Operative Criteria

Owing to the large prevalence of small rectoceles among healthy women, the association of rectoceles with defecatory dysfunction, and the varied results of rectocele repair reported among different investigators, it has become a challenge to decide who will most benefit from a surgical repair of a rectocele. As a result, various groups have tried to establish preoperative criteria to predict surgical outcome (38,39). Because gynecologists have traditionally evaluated a rectocele repair by its effects on vaginal function and coloproctologists have traditionally evaluated its effect on bowel function, different operative criteria and surgical techniques have evolved.

Rosato (39) and Murthy et al. (38) each describe strict criteria in determining which patients with a rectocele to select for surgery, as can be seen in Table 4. In accordance to his selection process, Murthy et al. recommended a rectocele repair for only 25 out of 132 patients with a confirmed rectocele who were evaluated for functional pelvic complaints. Besides defecography, they did not find any physiologic studies useful for recommending a repair (38).

Watson et al. require for operation demonstration of a large rectocele on evacuation proctography and a history of defecation aided by vaginal digitation (33). They, like others, believe that the preoperative need for vaginal digitalization for complete rectal evacuation is a significant test for predicting good outcomes of a rectocele repair. Other studies have also shown that many women with rectoceles do not need to splint, while some women without rectoceles do use manual pressure to assist in defecation (12,23,40). The feeling of incomplete emptying is not specific for rectoceles and can be due to many other disorders of the pelvic floor, including

Table 4 Criteria of Patient Selection for Rectocele Repair

Rosato's criteria[a]
1. Rectocele ≥ 4 cm in diameter as measured during defecography
2. Nonemptying or partial emptying of rectocele during evacuation phase of defecography
3. Rectal or vaginal symptoms present for longer than 12 months
4. Persistence of rectal or vaginal symptoms for at least 4 weeks, despite increased dietary fiber (35 g/d)
5. Need of rectal or vaginal digitation or perineal support maneuver to facilitate rectal evacuation

Murthy's criteria[b]
1. Sensation of a vaginal mass or bulge that required digital support and/or rectal digitizing for evacuation that was confirmed to be a rectocele
2. Demonstration on defecography of contrast retention in the rectocele
3. The presence of a very large rectocele associated with anterior rectal wall prolapse

[a]At least three of the five criteria should be present.
[b]Only one criteria required.

irritable rectum, enterocele, sigmoidocele, rectal intussusception, descending perineum syndrome, and slow transit constipation.

Coexisting causes of constipation, such as those listed in Table 1, could be predictors of a poor outcome following a rectocele repair due to the possibility that the rectocele is only a secondary condition. Paraiso et al. (41), in evaluating anatomic and functional outcomes utilizing a traditional posterior colporrhaphy, compared pre- and postoperative symptoms in women with successful versus unsuccessful outcome. Although not statistically significant, those with an unsatisfactory outcome were more likely to have persistent straining after surgery.

VI.   TREATMENT

It is generally agreed that only symptomatic rectoceles require treatment. However, for patients with asymptomatic rectoceles who are undergoing reconstructive repair of other pelvic organ defects, current expert opinion recommends concomitant surgical correction of the rectocele (13).

A.   Nonsurgical Approaches

Conservative therapy typically consists of pelvic floor rehabilitation for small degrees of prolapse and the initiation of oral or topical estrogen for those whose vaginal tissue is noted to be atrophic. A pessary can also be utilized as a temporizing measure for those with larger degrees of prolapse who are high surgical risks, or it can also be used to simulate a surgical repair to see if associated symptoms improve. Because surgical approaches have had mixed results in their efforts to relieve rectal emptying, it is important to treat underlying defecation disorders first. Biofeedback would be an appropriate first line of treatment for dyssnergic defecation, and constipation can initially be treated with a fiber-enriched diet and bulk-forming agents (28). The use of botulinum toxin has potential promise to inhibit paradoxical puborectalis contractions based on a limited study of 14 patients with symptomatic anterior rectoceles and outlet obstruction (42).

B.   Surgical Approaches

There are several different procedures with many variations to surgically correct rectoceles, which include transvaginal, transperineal, endorectal, transabdominal, and laparoscopic approaches. All share similar goals: to relieve symptoms, to restore anatomy, and to maintain or restore visceral and sexual function. To date there are no controlled studies comparing the different types of repair.

C.   Traditional Posterior Colporrhaphy

In 1867 Simon first described the term posterior colporrhaphy as a means to support the uterus when it was prolapsed (43), and in 1870, Hegar introduced the colpoperineorrhaphy, which was used to treat all forms of pelvic organ prolapse at that time (44). The traditional posterior colpoporrhaphy consists principally of reinforcing the rectovaginal fascia with a side-to-side plication, and oftentimes, the levator ani muscles are then plicated over the rectum in the midline. A perineorrhaphy is typically then performed by placing deep sutures into the perineal muscles and fascia to build up the perineal body. The incorporation of the levator plication may have arisen from observations of widening of the levator hiatus in patients with uterine prolapse (16). Plication of the levator ani muscles strengthened uterine support because it was believed that the levators supported the vagina, which in turn supported the uterus (44).

Using this approach the fascia is typically oversewn without ever identifying the defects. Because the normal vaginal anatomy is not properly restored, symptoms related to defecatory and sexual dysfunction are not adequately relieved. The traditional posterior colpoperineorrhaphy combined with a levator ani plication often results in increased dyspareunia due to constriction of the vaginal tube, partial closure of the genital hiatus, a transverse ridge created in the posterior vaginal wall, and atrophy and scarring of the levator muscles.

Francis and Jeffcoate in 1961 reported a 50% rate of dyspareunia following posterior colporrhaphy, which was thought to be secondary to overnarrowing of the introitus by means of a tight levator ani plication (45). Kahn and Stanton reported an increase in sexual dysfunction from 18% preoperatively to 27% postoperatively following a traditional posterior colporrhaphy, which they attributed to levator muscle atrophy and scar formation (46). In a prospective observational study of 108 patients using a traditional approach, Paraiso et al. found significant improvement in the severity of bowel symptoms and vaginal prolapse symptoms, but also noted increased dyspareunia (41). Another prospective study by Mellgren et al. of 25 patients showed similar findings. These authors, however, still support incorporating the levator ani muscles as part of their repair, citing better restoration of a firm rectovaginal septum with good functional results (36).

D. Defect-Specific Repair

Based largely on the findings of Richardson and Nichols, we prefer a defect-specific rectocele repair, which entails reapproximation of fascial breaks without performing a levator plication. Our technique for performing a defect specific repair is as follows:

The desired size of the introitus, which is typically three fingerbreadths, is first approximated by placing Allis clamps bilaterally on the labia minora and bringing them together along the midline. A finger of the nondominant hand is then inserted in the rectum, and a diamond-shaped wedge of perineal skin is removed, which again is tailored to the desired size of the introitus. The width and length of the perineal incision is dependent on the epithelium needed for restoration of the perineal body. Sharp dissection is utilized to make a plane in the rectovaginal space and to completely mobilize the posterior vaginal wall away from the anterior rectal wall up to the vaginal apex, laterally to the tendinous arch of the levator ani and inferiorly to the perineal body (see Figs. 2, 3).

Care is taken to leave as much fascia as possible on the rectum. Any pararectal fascia adherent to the posterior vaginal wall is mobilized, and redundant vaginal mucosa is trimmed along the midline if deemed appropriate. The finger in the rectum is used to elevate the anterior rectal wall to help delineate any fascial tears. Durable fascia is then plicated over the entire anterior rectal wall with interrupted 2-0 delayed absorbable sutures to resupport any segments that had been torn or attenuated. The following diagrams illustrate various defect-specific closures: Figure 4 shows a low transverse defect between the perineum and the distal edge of the rectovaginal fascia with a defect-specific closure using interrupted sutures, while Figure 5 illustrates a midline longitudinal defect. After reapproximating the vaginal mucosa along the posterior vaginal wall with a layer of 3-0 delayed absorbable running suture, a perineorrhaphy is performed if the perineal body is deficient or if the patient has a large genital hiatus. It is also utilized to add posterior vaginal length for a patient with postoperative vaginal shortening. Photographs delineating the surgical steps can be found in Appendix.

If at the completion of the defect-specific repair one cannot comfortably admit three fingers in the vagina, relaxing incisions are made through the full thickness of the vagina.

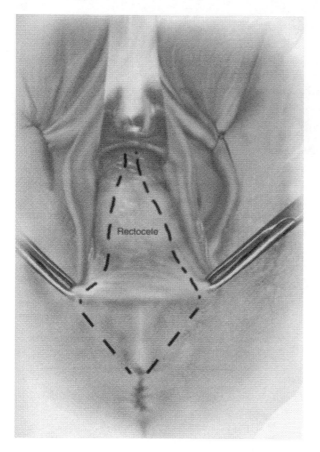

Figure 2 The dashed line outlines the area of perineal skin and posterior vaginal wall to be excised. (From Ref. 8.)

One should take into consideration that the levator ani and perineal muscles are relaxed from general anesthesia and that they will contract postoperatively. Vaginal scarring and postmenopausal atrophy could account for further narrowing in the future.

In three retrospective reviews of a defect-specific rectocele repair, recurrence rates varied from 18% to 23% with a mean follow-up between 12 and 18 months (47–49). Bowel and sexual function were subjectively improved. Cundiff et al., in a series of 69 patients undergoing a defect specific repair, reported constipation improved in 84%, dyspareunia improved in 66%, and fecal incontinence improved in 56% (48). This study noted the site-specific defect repair reestablishes the integrity of the rectovaginal fascia and at the same time repairs perineal descent, which may explain improved anorectal function. Outcomes, however, were not as good for fecal incontinence and constipation in the other studies (47,49). In Kenton et al.'s series of 66 patients at 1-year follow-up after a site-specific repair, constipation was clinically unchanged, and 64% returned to their preoperative practice of splinting (49). This study theorizes that perhaps the need for manual evacuation represents a rectocele of advanced stage in which chronic overdistension of the rectal wall results in physiologic abnormalities that are not amenable to surgical repair (49).

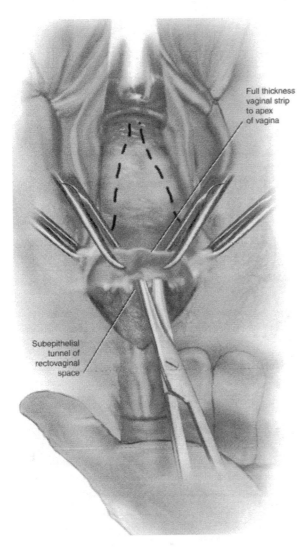

Full thickness
vaginal strip
to apex
of vagina

Subepithelial
tunnel of
rectovaginal
space

Figure 3 With a finger in the rectum, the posterior vaginal wall is sharply dissected from the anterior vaginal wall. (From Ref. 8.)

In a prospective study evaluating the defect-specific repair on 67 patients with a follow-up of only 3 months, Glavind et al. found no recurrences, an 85% cure for those with difficulties evacuating the rectum, and resolution of dyspareunia in six of eight sexually active patients. Two, however, developed de novo dyspareunia (50).

E. Transanal Repair

Low rectoceles with weakened rectovaginal septums are often repaired endorectally by colo-rectal surgeons in an effort to simultaneously treat anorectal pathology, such as hemorrhoids, fissures, papillae, and anal stenosis (51). This anorectal approach developed over time from the perceived failure of a vaginal repair to correct a ballooning anterior rectal wall. In 1965

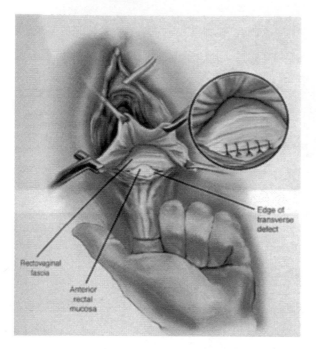

Figure 4   A low transverse defect between the perineum and the distal edge of the rectovaginal fascia, closed in a defect-specific fashion with interrupted sutures. (From Ref. 8.)

Redding recognized that rectoceles could be a cause of anorectal symptoms (52), and in 1967, Marks reported that only focusing on the vaginal deformity does not adequately relieve symptoms (53). Under the assumption that the loose inner lining of the rectocele following a posterior colporrhaphy was associated with an urge to defecate, he recommended a combined vaginal repair with a transanal resection of redundant rectal mucosa. This technique, however, resulted in a large number of recurrences and rectovaginal fistulas.

Based on Sullivan et al.'s initial description of an endorectal repair of a rectocele (54), today the colorectal surgeon's approach typically involves an endorectal plication using obliterative sutures to reduce the rectal luminal size. This may be indicated for patients with outlet obstruction or rectal herniation associated with thinning of the rectal submucosa and increased rectal reservoir size (55). It is inappropriate, however, for patients with high rectoceles and associated enteroceles. As described by Nichols, the redundant mucosa and submucosa of the weakened anterior rectal wall is first identified after inserting a rectal retractor. Two obliterative layers are then placed incorporating the full thickness of the rectal wall starting at the mucocutaneous junction (9). Others have also described incising the rectal mucosa above the dentate line in a transverse direction and then, depending on the size of the rectocele, excising a rectangular portion of mucosa (28).

Overall, transanal repairs have been shown to reduce the size of rectoceles on proctography. Although having inconsistent effects on anal pressures, they tend to improve rectal sensation, resulting in an urge to defecate at lower volumes and improving constipation and incontinence (16). In a prospective evaluation utilizing a transanal approach, Murthy et al. found improvements in constipation, incontinence, and symptoms of a vaginal mass (38). In a retrospective comparison, however, Arnold et al. found no significant difference between a

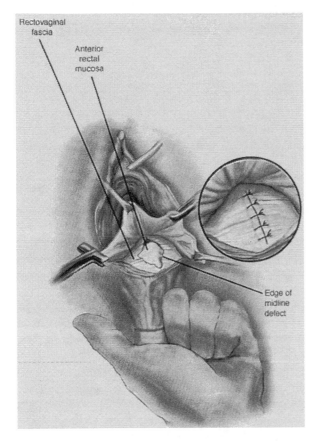

Rectovaginal fascia

Anterior rectal mucosa

Edge of midline defect

Figure 5 A midline longitudinal defect with a defect-specific closure using interrupted sutures. (From Ref. 8.)

transanal approach and the traditional posterior colporrhaphy in regard to constipation, fecal incontinence, and dyspareunia (56). The only difference was a greater frequency of postoperative pain with the vaginal approach. A more recent prospective study confirmed these results (57).

F. Laparoscopic Rectocele Repair

The indications for a laparoscopic rectocele repair are the same as those utilizing a vaginal or transanal approach. Paraiso et al. suggests using electrocautery, harmonic scalpel, or laser to open the rectovaginal septum (58). Blunt and/or sharp dissection is used to open the rectovaginal space extending to the perineal body. The perineal body is sutured to the rectovaginal septum and the rectovaginal fascial defects are closed with No. 0 nonabsorbable suture. If the rectovaginal fascia is detached from the iliococcygeus fascia, it is reattached with No. 0 nonabsorbable suture. The medial aspects of the levator ani muscles may also be plicated. Lyons and Winer incorporate polyglactin mesh from the uterosacral ligament complex to the perineal body in their laparoscopic rectocele repairs. They prospectively evaluated 20 patients who had this repair for 1 year and found a 95% rate of symptom relief (59). Larger prospective randomized trials comparing a laparoscopic repair to a more traditional approach are needed, however, before any conclusions can be drawn regarding its efficacy.

G. Incorporation of Mesh

For patients with high rectoceles, recurrence of posterior vaginal wall prolapse, or little or no supportive tissue to use in a repair, the use of mesh has been suggested as a means to improve the strength of the repair. Mesh, however, has historically been associated with vaginal erosion, sinus formation, and infection (60). In 1981 Oster and Astrup incorporated a dermis graft in the rectovaginal space as part of a posterior colporrhaphy for large rectoceles in 15 patients, and reported good outcomes after a mean follow-up of 2.6 years (61).

Two recent studies, however, in which mesh was incorporated transabdominally have had suboptimal results: Sullivan et al. (62) reported their experience using what they describe as a total pelvic mesh repair on 236 patients who had failed previous reconstructive surgery or had rectal procidentia combined with genitourinary prolapse. Utilizing a transabdominal approach they incorporated a strip of Marlex mesh to reinforce the rectovaginal septum as part of their repair. During a median follow-up of 5.3 years, 10% of patients required reoperation secondary to complications specific to the repair, and 28% required postoperative surgical correction of anorectal mucosal prolapse or rectocele. Baessler and Schuessler (63), as part of an abdominal sacrocolpopexy, used Gore-Tex mesh to support the posterior vaginal wall. During a mean follow-up of 26 months, rectoceles recurred in 57% and the authors have since switched to a site-specific defect rectocele repair.

Sand et al. (64) performed a prospective, randomized controlled trial using polyglactin 910 mesh during primary or recurrent anterior and posterior colporrhaphy in women with central cystoceles and found no effect of the mesh on the success of the rectocele repair. However, the power of the study was limited owing to the low incidence of recurrent rectoceles. In a prospective study Watson et al. (32) utilized a transperineal approach with the placement of Marlex mesh to replace the rectovaginal septum in 9 patients requiring preoperative vaginal digitation. They found defecatory dysfunction improved in 88% without recurrence over 29 months. As with laparoscopic rectocele repairs, more research is needed before a conclusion can be reached on the efficacy of mesh as part of the rectocele repair. It does seem apparent, however, from the transabdominal studies, that in addition to incorporation of mesh, repair of the fascial defects is required.

Table 5 compares the anatomic and functional outcomes following these various approaches to a rectocele repair.

VII. COMPLICATIONS

Complications of vaginal surgery in general include bleeding, infection, vaginal shortening, and vaginal wall inclusion cyst formation. Complications particular to a rectocele repair include incidental proctotomy and subsequent development of a rectovaginal fistula, which has been reported in up to 5% of patients. Urinary retention is a frequent but temporary complication, occurring in 12.5% of patients. The incidence of dyspareunia, which had been reported to occur in up to 30% of patients, has decreased in incidence in more recent studies (65). Early recurrence is thought to be caused by a failure to identify and repair all support defects, while late recurrence is probably caused by further weakening of supportive tissue related to aging, chronic straining, neurologic deficits associated with pelvic floor injury, estrogen deficiency, or significant alteration of the vaginal access.

Table 5 Summary of Anatomic and Functional Outcomes

Investigators	Paraiso et al. (41)		Mellgren et al. (36)		Kahn and Stanton (46)		Glavind and Madsen (50)	
Study type	Retrospective		Prospective		Retrospective		Prospective	
Year	2001		1995		1997		2000	
Type of repair	Traditional		Traditional		Traditional		Defect-specific	
Sample size	108		25		231		67	
Recurrence rate	12%		20%		24%		0%	
Mean follow-up (mos)	9.9		12		42.5		3	
Symptoms	Preop	Postop	Preop	Postop	Preop	Postop	Preop	Postop
Constipation/straining	76%	45%	96%	52%	22%	33%	—	—
Splinting/manual evacuation	45%	8%	48%	0%	—	—	—	—
Incomplete emptying	—	—	—	—	27%	38%	40%	15%
Fecal incontinence	10%	2%	8%	8%	4%	11%	—	—
Feeling lump/pressure	—	—	—	—	64%	31%	—	—
Dyspareunia	2%	12%	6%	18%	18%	27%	12%	6%

(continued)

Table 5 Summary of Anatomic and Functional Outcomes

Investigators	Porter et al. (47)		Cundiff et al. (48)		Kenton et al. (49)		Watson et al. (32)		Murthy et al. (38)	
Study type	Retrospective		Retrospective		Retrospective		Prospective		Retrospective	
Year	1999		1998		1999		1996		1996	
Type of repair	Defect-specific		Defect-specific		Defect-specific		Transperineal with Marlex mesh		Transanal	
Sample size	125		69		66		9		33	
Recurrence rate	18%		18%		23%		0		—	
Mean follow-up (mos)	18		12		12		29		31	
Symptoms	Preop	Postop	Preop	Postop	Preop	Postop	Preop	Postop	Preop	Postop
Constipation/ straining	60%	50%	46%	13%	41%	23%	—	—	35%	16%
Splinting/manual evacuation	24%	14%	39%	25%	30%	15%	100%	11%	—	—
Incomplete emptying	—	—	—	—	—	—	—	—	—	—
Fecal incontinence	24%	21%	13%	8%	30%	—	—	—	29%	12%
Feeling lump/ pressure	38%	14%	—	—	86%	9%	—	—	61%	12%
Dyspareunia	67%	46%	29%	19%	28%	2%	33%	—	—	—

VIII.   CONCLUSION

Over the past several decades, a better understanding of the anatomic relationships of the pelvic floor and posterior vaginal wall has altered the way we approach rectoceles, which has resulted in improved anatomic and functional postoperative outcomes. However, we have clearly been less successful in treating defecatory disorders associated with rectoceles. Although a surgical repair may reduce the dimensions of a rectocele, it does not alleviate rectal emptying difficulties that may be caused by other factors. Future research should better address (a) the relationship between defecatory dysfunction and rectoceles, and (b) preoperative studies that can be useful predictors of outcome regarding defecatory dysfunction following a rectocele repair. Additionally, prospective randomized trials are needed to compare the various surgical approaches to repair rectoceles. Both objective and subjective findings need to be described pre- and postoperatively in order to better determine surgical outcomes. Although the incidence of postoperative dyspareunia has decreased, it still remains an associated complication. Routine levator ani plication is no longer advocated, but dyspareunia may still result from vaginal scarring and narrowing as well as from the development of a vaginal constriction ring. The goal of the reconstructive pelvic surgeon should be to restore the normal vaginal axis and caliber as well as to maintain vaginal length, and, at the same time, to maintain or restore visceral and sexual function. To do so one must have a clear and thorough understanding of the pelvic anatomy as well as mechanisms of pelvic support.

APPENDIX

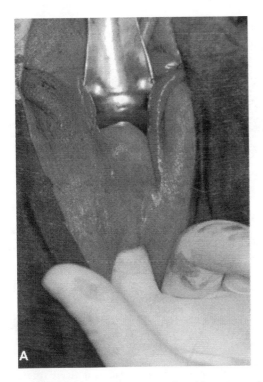

Appendix A   A distal rectocele with attenuated perineum.

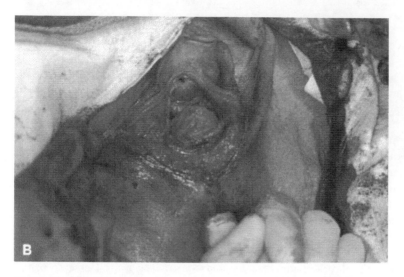

Appendix B   The initial wedge of perineal skin has been removed.

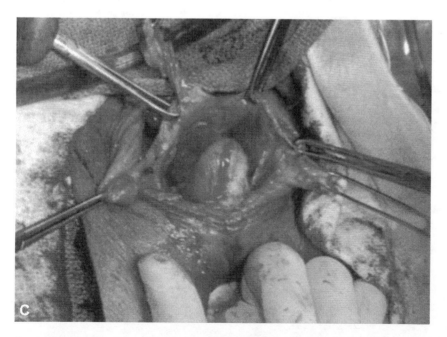

Appendix C   The posterior vaginal wall is completely mobilized from the anterior rectal wall using sharp dissection. Note that a narrow piece of vagina has been dissected in the midline. The width of this segment of vagina is determined by estimating the amount of vagina that will need to be trimmed.

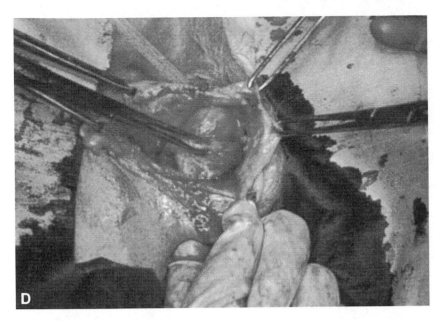

Appendix D   Identification of fascia to be utilized for plication over the anterior rectal wall.

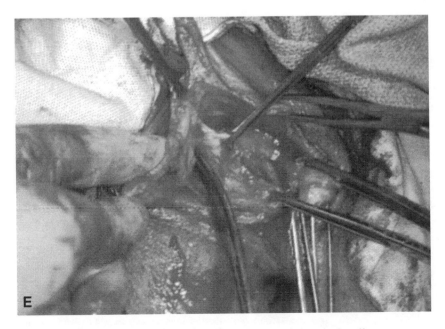

Appendix E   Mobilization of the fascia off the posterior vaginal wall.

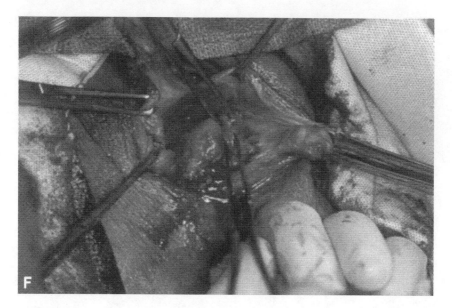

Appendix F   The fascia has been completely mobilized off the right vaginal wall. Note that the midline wedge of vaginal skin has no underlying fascia, confirming a midline-type defect.

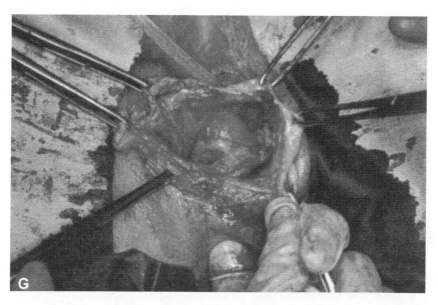

Appendix G   A high transverse defect is demonstrated. Note the fascia is present over the distal anterior rectal wall.

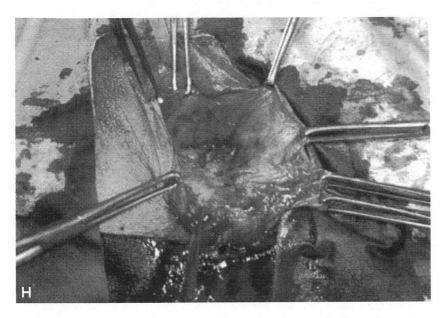

Appendix H   Completed fascial defect repair. Durable fascia has been plicated over the entire anterior wall (From Ref. 8.).

REFERENCES

1. Mant J, Painter R, Vessey M. Epidemiology of genital prolapse: observations from the Oxford family planning association study. Br J Obstet Gynaecol 1997; 104:579–585.
2. Olsen AL, Smith VJ, Bergstrom JO. Epidemiology of surgically managed pelvic organ prolapse and urinary incontinence. Obstet Gynecol 1997; 104:501–506.
3. Delancey JO. Anatomic aspects of vaginal eversion after hysterectomy. Am J Obstet Gynecol 1992; 166:1717–1728.
4. DeLancey JO. Structural anatomy of the posterior pelvic compartment as it relates to rectocele. Am J Obstet Gynecol 1999; 180(4):815–823.
5. Zbar AP, Beer-Gabel M, Aslam M. Rectoanal inhibition and rectocele: physiology versus categorization. Int J Colorectal Dis 2001; (5):307–312.
6. Milley PS, Nichols DH. A correlative investigation of the human rectovaginal septum. Anat Rec 1969; 163:443–452.
7. Richardson AC. The rectovaginal septum revisited: its relationship to rectocele and its importance in rectocele repair. Clin Obstet Gynecol 1993; 36(4):976–983.
8. Baggish MS, Karram MM. Atlas of Pelvic Anatomy and Gynecologic Surgery. Philadelphia: W.B. Saunders, 2001.
9. Nichols DH, Randall CL. Posterior colporrhaphy and perineorrhaphy. In: Nichols DH, Randall CL, eds. Vaginal Surgery. 4th ed. Baltimore: Williams & Wilkins, 1996:257–289.
10. Weber AM, Walters MD, Ballard LA. Posterior vaginal prolapse and bowel function. Am J Obstet Gynecol 1998; 179(6):1446–1450.
11. Rotholtz NA, Wexner SD. Surgical treatment of constipation and fecal incontinence. Gastroenterol Clin North Am 2001; 30(1):131–166.
12. Siproudhis L, Dautreme S, Ropert A. Dyschezia and rectocele—a marriage of convenience? Dis Colon Rectum 1996; 36:1030–1036.
13. Brubaker L. Rectocele. Curr Opin Obstet Gynecol 1996; 8(5):376–379.
14. Shorvon PJ, McHugh S, Diamant NE. Defaecography in healthy volunteers: results and implications. Gut 1989; 30:1737.

15. Kelvin FM, Maglinte DD, Benson JT. Evacuation proctography (defecography): an aid to the investigation of pelvic floor disorders. Obstet Gynecol 1994; 83:307–314.

16. Kahn MA, Stanton SL. Techniques of rectocele repair and their effects on bowel function. Int Urogynecol J 1998; 9:37–47.

17. Baden W, Walker T. Surgical Repair of Vaginal Defects. Philadelphia: J.B. Lippincott, 1992.

18. Bump RC, Mattiasson A, Bo K. The standardization of terminology of female pelvic organ prolapse and pelvic floor dysfunction. Am J Obstet Gynecol 1996; 175(1):10–17.

19. Giordano P, Wexner SD. The assessment of fecal incontinence in women. J Am Coll Surg 2001; 193(4):397–406.

20. Jorge JM, Habr-Gama A, Wexner SD. Clinical applications and techniques of cinedefecography. Am J Surg 2001; 182(1):93–101.

21. Dohke M, Mitchell DG, Vasavada SP. Fast magnetic resonance imaging of pelvic organ prolapse. Tech Urol 2001; 7(2):133–138.

22. Rentsch M, Paetzel C, Lenhart M. Dynamic magnetic resonance imaging defecography: a diagnostic alternative in the assessment of pelvic floor disorders in proctology. Dis Colon Rectum 2001; 44(7):999–1007.

23. Siproudhis L, Ropert A, Lucas J. Defecatory disorders, anorectal and pelvic floor dysfunction: a polygamy? radiologic and manometric studies in 41 patients. Int J Colorectal Dis 1992; 7:102–107.

24. Delemarre JB, Kruyt RH, Doornbos J. Anterior rectocele: assessment with radiographic defecography, dynamic magnetic resonance imaging and physical examination. Dis Colon Rectum 1994; 37:249–259.

25. Kelvin FM, Maglinte DD, Hornback JA. Pelvic prolapse: assessment with evacuation proctography (defecography). Radiology 1992; 184:547–551.

26. Halligan S, Bartram CI. Is barium tapping in rectoceles significant? Dis Colon Rectum 1995; 38:764–768.

27. Siproudhis L, Robert A, Vilotte J. How accurate is clinical examination in diagnosing and quantifying pelvirectal disorders? A prospective study in a group of 50 patients complaining of defecatory difficulties. Dis Colon Rectum 1993; 36:430–438.

28. Felt-Bersma RJ, Cuesta MA. Rectal prolapse, rectal intussusception, rectocele, and solitary rectal ulcer syndrome. Gastroenterol Clin North Am 2001; 30(1):199–222.

29. Matsuoka H, Wexner SD, Desai MB. A comparison between dynamic pelvic magnetic resonance imaging and videoproctography in patients with constipation. Dis Colon Rectum 2001; 44(4):571–576.

30. Kiff ES, Barnes PRH, Swash M. Evidence of pudendal neuropathy in patients with perineal descent and chronic straining at stool. Gut 1983; 25:1279–1282.

31. Kiff ES. Barnes PRH, Swash M. Evidence of pudendal neuropathy in patients with perineal descent and chronic straining at stool. Gut 1983; 25:1279–1282.

32. Johansson C, Nilsson BY, Homstrom B, Dolk A, Mellgren A. Association between rectocele and paradoxical sphincter response. Dis Colon Rectum 1992; 35:503–509.

33. Watson SJ, Loder PB, Halligan S. Transperineal repair of symptomatic rectocele with marlex mesh: a clinical, physiological and radiologic assessment of treatment. J Am Coll Surg 1996; 183(3):257–261.

34. Van Dam JH, Hop WC, Schouten WR. Analysis of patients with poor outcome of rectocele repair. Dis Colon Rectum 2000; 43(11):1556–1560.

35. Lopez A, Anzen B, Bremmer S. Durability of success after rectocele repair. Int Urogynecol J 2001; 12(2):97–103.

36. Mellgren A, Bo Anzen, Bengt-Yngve N. Results of rectocele repair: a prospective study. Dis Colon Rectum 1995; 38(1):7–13.

37. Van Dam JH, Schouten WR, Ginai AZ, Huisman WM, Huikeshoven FJM, Hop WC. The influence of ansimus on the final outcome of rectocoele repair: a prospective study. Second United European Gastroenterology Week, 1993. Abstract.

38. Murthy V, Orkin B, Smith LE, Glassman LM. Excellent outcome using selective criteria for rectocele repair. Dis Colon Rectum 1996; 39(4):374–378.

39. Rosato G. Rectocele and perineal hernias. In: Beck DE, Wexner SD, eds. Fundamentals of Anorectal Surgery. 2nd ed. London: W.B. Saunders, 1998:189–197.

40. Spence-Jones C, Kamm MA, Henry MM, Hudson CN. Bowel dysfunction: a pathogenic factor in uterovaginal prolapse and urinary stress incontinence. Br J Obstet Gynaecol 1994; 101:147–152.
41. Paraiso MF, Weber AM, Walters MD. Anatomic and functional outcome after posterior colporrhaphy. J Pelvic Surg 2001; 7(6):335–339.
42. Maria G, Brisinda G, Bentivoglio AR. Anterior rectocele due to obstructed defecation relieved by botulinum toxin. Surgery 2001; 129(5):524–529.
43. Simon G. Prag Viertelgahrsch 1867; 3:112–114.
44. Jeffcoate TN. Posterior colpoperineorrhaphy. Am J Obstet Gynecol 1959; 77:490–502.
45. Francis WJ, Jeffcoate TN. Dyspareunia following vaginal operations. J Obstet Gynaecol Br Emp 1961; 68:1–10.
46. Khan MA, Stanton SL. Posterior colporrhaphy: its effects on bowel and sexual function. Br J Obstet Gynaecol 1997; 104:882–886.
47. Porter WE, Steele A, Walsh P. The anatomic and functional outcomes of defect-specific rectocele repairs. Am J Obstet Gynecol 1999; 181(6):1353–1358.
48. Cundiff GW, Weidner AC, Visco AG. An anatomic and functional assessment of the discreet defect rectocele repair. Am J Obstet Gynecol 1998; 179(6):1451–1457.
49. Kenton K, Shott S, Brubaker L. Outcome after rectovaginal fascia reattachment for rectocele repair. Am J Obstet Gynecol 1999; 181(6):1360–1364.
50. Glavind K, Madsen H. A prospective study of the discrete fascial defect rectocele repair. Acta Obstet Gynecol Scand 2000; 79:145–147.
51. Khubchandani IT, Sheets JA, Stasik JJ, Hakki AR. Endorectal repair of rectocele. Dis Colon Rectum 1983; 26:792–796.
52. Redding MD. The relaxed perineum and anorectal disease. Dis Colon Rectum 1965; 8:279–282.
53. Marks MM. The rectal side of the rectocele. Dis Colon Rectum 1967; 10:387 388.
54. Sullivan ES, Leaverton GH, Hardwick CE. Transrectal perineal repair: an adjunct to improved function after anorectal surgery. Dis Colon Rectum 1968; 11:106–114.
55. Nichols DH, Genadry RR. Pelvic relaxation of the posterior compartment. Curr Opin Obstet Gynecol 1993; 5(4):458–464.
56. Arnold MW, Stewart WR, Aguitar PS. Rectocele repair: four years experience. Dis Colon Rectum 1990; 33:684–687.
57. Kahn MA, Stanton SL, Kumar DA. Randomized prospective trial of posterior colporrhaphy vs. transanal repair or rectocele: preliminary findings. In: Proceedings of the Eighteenth Annual Meeting of the American Urogynecologic Society; September 1997; New Orleans, LA. New Orleans: The Society, 1997.
58. Paraiso MFR, Falcone T, Walters MD. Laparoscopic surgery for enterocele, vaginal apex prolapse and rectocele. Int Urogynecol J 1999; 10:223–229.
59. Lyons TL, Winer WK. Laparoscopic rectocele repair using polyglactin mesh. J Am Assoc Gynecol Laparosc 1997; 4(3):381–384.
60. Graul E, Hurst B. An alternative approach to the repair of cystoceles and rectoceles. Obstet Gynecol 2001; 97(4 suppl 1):S48.
61. Oster S, Astrup A. A new vaginal operation for recurrent and large rectocele using dermis transplant. Acta Obstet Gynecol Scand 1981; 60:493–495.
62. Sullivan ES, Longaker CJ, Lee PY. Total pelvic mesh repair. Dis Colon Rectum 2001; 44(6):857–863.
63. Baessler K, Schuessler B. Abdominal sacrocolpopexy and anatomy and function of the posterior compartment. Obstet Gynecol 2001; 97(5):678–684.
64. Sand PK, Koduri S, Lobel RW. Prospective randomized trial of polyglactin 910 mesh to prevent recurrence of cystoceles and rectoceles. Am J Obstet Gynecol 2001; 184(7):1357–1364.
65. Rovner ES, Ginsberg DA. Posterior vaginal wall prolapse: transvaginal repair of pelvic floor relaxation, rectocele and perineal laxity. Tech Urol 2001; 7(2):161–168.

53

Vesicovaginal Fistula: Complex Fistulae

Karyn Schlunt Eilber,* Nirit Rosenblum,† and Larissa V. Rodríguez
David Geffen School of Medicine at UCLA, Los Angeles, California, U.S.A.

I. INTRODUCTION

In 1672, the first vesicovaginal fistula (VVF) repair was reported in which quills were used to approximate wound edges with silk threads (1). Since then, techniques utilizing abdominal, vaginal, and combined abdominal and vaginal approaches with and without tissue interposition have been described. This chapter will discuss the current concepts in evaluation and management of this potentially devastating condition.

The true incidence of vesicovaginal fistulae is unknown but has been estimated at 0.3–2% (1–3). The various etiologies of VVF are listed in Table 1. In developed countries, hysterectomy is the main cause of VVF, while in some areas of Africa and Asia obstetric trauma is the predominate cause (4,5). Obstetrical VVFs result from necrosis of the vaginal wall and bladder secondary to pressure from the fetal head during prolonged labor, and usually involve a large area of tissue damage. Associated injuries may include total urethral loss, urethrovaginal fistula, cervical destruction, and rectovaginal fistula (6). The focus of this chapter will be on VVF secondary to causes other than prolonged labor.

Vesicovaginal fistula after hysterectomy is most common after a laparoscopic approach (2.2/1000) followed in decreasing order by total abdominal hysterectomy (1.0/1000) and vaginal hysterectomy (0.2/1000) (3). The Mayo Clinic also reviewed causes of VVF and found that 82% were due to gynecologic surgery, 8% to obstetrical procedures, 6% to pelvic radiotherapy, and 4% to trauma or fulguration (7). Because in developed nations the majority of VVFs are a complication of hysterectomy, risk factors, and preventive measures need to be considered. Prior pelvic surgery including cesarean section, cervical conization, radiation therapy, and endometriosis may predispose patients to development of a VVF (8).

II. DIAGNOSIS

A. History

An individual with a VVF typically presents with continuous leakage of urine shortly after a pelvic operation or procedure. The temporal relationship of the onset of symptoms and pelvic trauma (surgery or vaginal delivery) must be ascertained. A history of radiation, prior treatments

*Current affiliation: Memorial Sloan-Kettering Cancer Center, New York, New York, U.S.A.
†Current affiliation: NYU School of Medicine, New York, New York, U.S.A.

Table 1   Etiology of Vesicovaginal Fistula

Congenital (rare)
Acquired
  Surgical
    Gynecologic procedures
      Hysterectomy
      Bladder neck suspension
      Anterior colporrhaphy
      Colposuspension
    Urologic procedures
      Sling
      Injectable bulking agents
    Other pelvic surgery
  Obstetric
    Prolonged labor
    Cesarean section
  Radiation
  Malignancy
  Infection
  Trauma
  Foreign body

or attempts at repair, infection of the vaginal cuff, and the patient's general state of health must also be determined. Depending on the size and location of the fistula, leakage may range from an occasional vaginal discharge between normal voiding per urethra to continuous leakage that prevents the patient from storing a volume of urine adequate for volitional voiding. Radiation therapy–induced VVF may present months to years following the treatment. A case has been reported in which a large vesicovaginal fistula developed 38 years after a radical hysterectomy and radiation (9).

When a patient presents with constant vaginal urinary leakage, the differential diagnosis includes VVF, ureterovaginal fistula, urethrovaginal fistula, and uterovesical fistula. History, physical examination, and selected diagnostic tests allow the diagnosis to be made with certainty.

B.   Physical Examination

During physical examination, the vagina needs to be evaluated for depth, diameter, mobility, prolapse of other organs, and evidence of vaginal atrophy. When a fistula is detected, the size, number (multiple/single), and location need to be noted. Finally, the patient needs to be evaluated for urethral hypermobility and incontinence.

Meticulous inspection of the vagina using a speculum facilitates visualization of the fistulous tract. The quality and quantity of the surrounding vaginal tissue should be assessed. Most fistulae that develop after hysterectomy are located at the vaginal cuff. For fistulous tracts that are not easily seen, the bladder can be filled with diluted Methylene Blue and the vagina inspected for leakage of the blue fluid. If the fistula is still not demonstrated, the vagina can be packed with gauze or a tampon. After the patient is allowed to ambulate for a short time, the gauze or tampon can be inspected for blue staining. Another method of demonstrating the presence of a VVF involves oral phenazopyridine, which causes orange discoloration of the urine. Phenazopyridine is administered a few hours before packing the vagina. Orange staining of the vaginal packing implies that the vaginal fluid is urine. A positive oral phenazopyridine test in the presence of a negative Methylene Blue bladder instillation implies the presence of a ureterovaginal fistula. Retrograde pyelography should be performed in anyone with a strong suspicion of ureterovaginal fistula.

If the diagnosis of VVF is in doubt, the fluid draining from the vagina must first be proven to be urine. The diagnosis can be confirmed if an adequate amount of fluid is collected and analyzed for creatinine. The creatinine measurement should be manyfold that of serum creatinine. If the creatinine measurement is similar to or less than that of the serum creatinine measurement, other sources of the fluid such as peritoneal fluid, lymphatic fluid, Fallopian tube secretions, or vaginal discharge must be considered (10). The phenazopyridine test can also be used to differentiate between urine and other secretions.

C. Diagnostic Tests

Cystoscopy must be performed in all patients in whom there is a suspicion or diagnosis of VVF. Cystoscopy may identify the location of the fistula, and is necessary to identify the location of the ureteral orifices in relation to the fistula, the size and number of fistulous tracts, to evaluate the bladder capacity, and to rule out the presence of any foreign body within the bladder or fistulous tract. Biopsy of the fistulous tract must be performed in any patient with a history or suspicion of malignancy.

A voiding cystourethrogram (VCUG) should also be performed in all patients to objectively demonstrate the fistula and evaluate for any evidence of prolapse or stress urinary incontinence (Fig. 1). VCUG is also useful to image fistulae to the uterus or rectum. The reported incidence of iatrogenic ureteral injuries following gynecologic surgical procedures ranges from 0.05% to 1% (11,12). Vesicovaginal and ureterovaginal fistulae coexist in up to 25% of

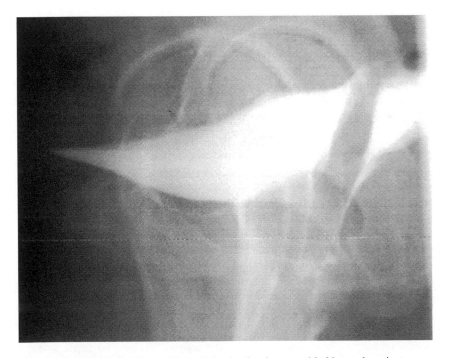

Figure 1   VCUG demonstrating communication between bladder and vagina.

cases (13–16). As such, routine examination of the upper urinary tract by means of intravenous pyelography, retrograde pyelography, or computed tomography (CT) is essential when evaluating a patient with a VVF to rule out concomitant ureteral injury and/or obstruction. Retrograde pyelography must be performed if there is a strong suspicion that a ureterovaginal fistula is present that is not demonstrated by intravenous pyelography.

III. CONSERVATIVE MANAGEMENT

Conservative measures including prolonged catheter drainage of the bladder or fulguration of the fistulous tract may be considered for small, well-vascularized, nonirradiated fistulae or for patients who have a small tract following prior repair. Although spontaneous resolution of VVF after prolonged catheter drainage (19–54 days) has been reported, this is a relatively rare event (17–20). Surgical reconstruction must be considered if resolution is not seen after 4 weeks of catheterization (15). The degree of tissue atrophy secondary to hormone deficiency or chronic infection may affect the rate of spontaneous closure. Therefore, in addition to catheter drainage, the use of antibiotic therapy and estrogen replacement therapy may also facilitate spontaneous closure (21,22).

Stovsky et al. reported a 73% success rate following electrocoagulation of vesicovaginal fistulae <3.5 mm in size (23). Successful ablation of small fistulous tracts by the use of the Nd-YAG laser has also been reported (24). Although small VVFs may respond to these conservative measures, there is little utility in delaying repair for a trial of conservative therapy for larger, complex, or radiation-induced fistulae.

IV. OPERATIVE MANAGEMENT

General considerations for the management of vesicovaginal fistulae are listed in Table 2. Several principles are essential to ensure a successful VVF closure. It is necessary to obtain adequate exposure of the fistulous tract and have healthy tissues available for the repair. The closure should be multilayered, watertight and tension free. Overlapping suture lines should be avoided. Also, it is essential to have maximal urinary drainage during the healing process. In many cases, tissue interposition is a useful adjunct to the above techniques.

A. Timing of Surgery

There has been much debate over the timing of surgical repair of vesicovaginal fistulae (Table 3). Early interventions usually involve repairs done only a few weeks after injury while delayed repairs refer to the traditionally described waiting period of 3–6 months following the injury. The rationale for delayed repair is to allow resolution of the acute inflammatory response and tissue edema. Although there are no randomized studies comparing the outcomes, several authors have described similar success rates of early and late repair (14,25–32). Successful fistula repair as early as 10 days after the injury has been reported (32).

Owing to the distressing nature of this condition, we advocate early (2–3 weeks) repair following recognition of the injury. Contraindications to early repair include VVF resulting from radiation injury or obstetrical trauma or prior failed repair, when associated tissue necrosis requires several months to fully delineate the extent of the injury. We also advocate waiting several months after a failed fistula repair to allow the postoperative inflammatory process to

Table 2   General Considerations in Management of VVF

Etiology of fistula
Timing of surgery
Abdominal vs. vaginal approach
Excision of fistulous tract
Postoperative drainage
Tissue interposition
Concomitant procedures
   Treatment of stress urinary incontinence
   Augmentation cystoplasty
Sexual function
Adjuvant treatment
   Antibiotic therapy
   Hormone replacement therapy
   Anticholinergic therapy

subside. Each case should be considered on an individual basis so as not to compromise surgical success for the sake of social convenience.

In developed nations, the majority of vesicovaginal fistulae are complications of clean gynecologic procedures. For most of these cases immediate repair should be attempted unless infection of the vaginal cuff or pelvic infection is present (23). When an abdominal approach is planned and the fistula is the result of an abdominal hysterectomy, we recommend a delayed repair. Aside from these circumstances, no additional risks or compromise of surgical success have been documented when instituting a short waiting period (14,22,25–31).

B. Abdominal Versus Vaginal Approach

The main consideration when choosing between the vaginal and abdominal approach to the repair of vesicovaginal fistulae should be the surgeon's level of comfort with each technique.

Table 3   Timing and Success of VVF Repair

Reference	No. patients	% Success	Timing of repair	Approach
Elkins et al. (26)	23	91	2–3 mos	Vaginal
Wang and Hadley (27)	16	94	7 < 3 mos, 9 > 3 mos	Vaginal
Collins et al. (31)	38	72	29 < 4 wks, 9 < 8 wks	Vaginal
Blaivas et al. (30)	24	96	14 < 3 mos, 10 > 3 mos	15 vaginal, 8 abdominal, 1 spontaneous closure
Persky et al. (32)	7	86	< 10 wks	6 abdominal, 1 vaginal
Blandy et al. (28)	25	100	12 < 6 wks, 13 > 6 wks	Abdominal
Diaz Calleja et al. (44)	6	100	> 3 mos	Abdominal
Motiwala et al. (39)	68	81	3 mos	58 transvesical, 10 abdominal
Nesrallah et al. (40)	29	100	6 wks to 48 mos (median 8 wks)	O'Conor technique

We support the adage that the best operation is the first operation, and thus the approach chosen should be that with which the surgeon is most experienced and familiar.

We prefer the vaginal approach for the repair of most VVF because it avoids the morbidity of an abdominal incision and cystotomy. A long or a narrow vagina is not a contraindication to the vaginal approach. A relaxing episiotomy can be done to facilitate exposure in an individual with a narrow introitus. The abdominal approach should be considered when concomitant abdominal procedures need to be performed (augmentation cystoplasty for a noncompliant bladder or repair of associated ureteral injury or other abdominal pathology).

C. Excision of Fistulous Tract

Historically, VVF repair has included wide excision of the fistulous tract to ensure approximation of healthy tissue. A number of surgeons have advocated repairing vesicovaginal fistulae without excision of the tract (23,27,29,30). A disadvantage of tract excision is that during repair of a small fistula, excision of the fistulous tract may increase the size of the fistula and make the repair more complex. Furthermore, hemorrhage encountered during an attempt to excise the fistulous tract may require the use of coagulation and result in the creation of more nonviable tissue, which could decrease the patient's chance for cure. The fistulous tract need not be excised, as it provides good anchoring tissue for the sutures of the first layer of the repair. An additional advantage of not excising the tract occurs when the fistula is in close proximity to the ureteral orifices. By not excising the fistula in this setting, ureteral stents may be used to identify the ureteral orifices and the fistula simply closed, avoiding injury to the trigone and ureters and the need for ureteral reimplantation.

D. Postoperative Drainage

Continuous, uninterrupted postoperative urinary drainage is essential to prevent bladder distension, which can create tension on suture lines and urinary extravasation. Urethral and suprapubic catheters are used whether a vaginal or abdominal approach is used. Additional pelvic drainage with a Penrose or Jackson-Pratt drain is recommended when a using a transvesical approach. Anticholinergic therapy is also essential to help prevent involuntary detrusor contractions.

E. Tissue Interposition

All vesicovaginal fistulae are repaired with a multilayer approach. Fistulae secondary to radiation or those with poor-quality tissue after a prior attempted repair have a higher rate of success when tissue interposition is used (19,23,26,27,29,33). Recently, Evans et al. reported on the use of interposition flaps in transabdominal repairs of VVF (34). The surgical success rate was 100% when an interposition flap was used, compared to only 64% success rate without interposition. Omentum is commonly used with the abdominal approach. Several options are available with the transvaginal approach including the Martius flap, peritoneum, rotational labial flap, gluteal flap, and gracilis flap.

F. Stress Incontinence

During the preoperative evaluation, the presence of stress urinary incontinence (SUI) prior to the development of the fistula must be determined. The reported incidence of SUI occurring following VVF repair ranges from 7% to 27% (35–37). Simultaneous correction of stress incontinence during fistula repair avoids the need for a separate surgical procedure and the psychologic distress of incontinence following an otherwise successful fistula repair.

G. Sexual Function

Preoperative determination of the patient's current and future expectation of sexual function is of paramount importance. For patients who are sexually active, attempts at preservation of a functional vagina must be made. Local or systemic estrogen replacement should be considered in patients who show signs of vaginal atrophy. For patients who are not sexually active and present with large fistulae, partial colpocleisis could be considered in order to maximize tissue coverage of the repair (23).

V. SURGICAL APPROACHES

Prior to any repair, adequate time must be allowed for all evidence of infection to subside. All fistula repairs should include the use of a broad-spectrum antibiotic prior to surgery. Preoperative urine cultures may aid in the choice of antibiotic. Additionally, pre- and postoperative hormone replacement may facilitate healing.

A. Vaginal Approach

The vaginal technique for uncomplicated vesicovaginal fistulae is a five-step process that results in a three-layer fistula repair (23). Many modifications exist, the main variable being that of fistula excision.

Step 1: Patient Preparation

Padded boots are placed on the patient before placing her in the high lithotomy position. The suprapubic area and external genitalia are shaved and then prepped with an iodine-based wash. Sutures are placed to retract the labia. Ureteral stents are placed at this time if preoperative cystoscopy indicated the fistulous tract to be in close proximity to the ureteral orifices. A urethral catheter is used to fill the bladder with normal saline, and a curved Lowsley retractor is used to place a suprapubic catheter via a small puncture wound in the suprapubic area. Vaginal packing may be necessary to occlude the fistulous tract during filling of the bladder. A ring retractor with elastic stays and a weighted speculum are used to gain exposure. Posterolateral episiotomies may need to be performed for a narrow vagina in order to gain maximum exposure of the vaginal vault.

Step 2: Isolation of Fistula

The fistula is catheterized with an 8 or 10F Foley catheter (Fig. 2A). Before insertion of the catheter, the tract may need to be dilated with metal sounds. Traction may be placed on the catheter to bring the fistula closer to the surgeon. If the fistula cannot be catheterized, an abdominal approach should be considered. To aid in catheterization, Methylene Blue is instilled into the bladder, and the tract may be visualized and catheterized. In the rare case that catheterization is still not possible, the repair can be performed under vision of Methylene Blue. After catheterization, a circumferential incision in the vaginal mucosa around the fistulous tract is made (Fig. 2B). The incision is then extended in an asymmetric "J" or inverted "J," depending on the location of the fistula. This allows for development of anterior or posterior vaginal flaps, which later will be used to cover the repair (Fig. 2C).

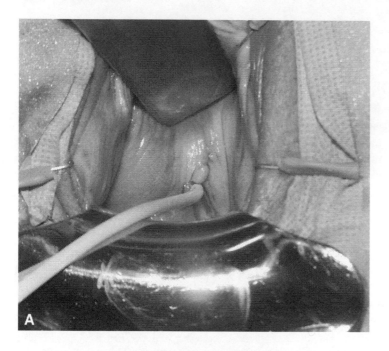

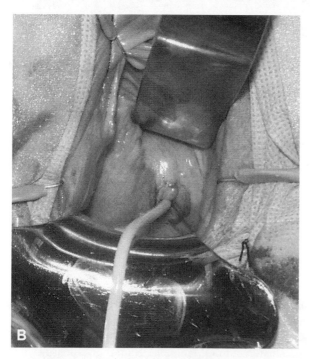

Figure 2   (A) Catheterization of fistulous tract with Foley catheter. (B) A circumferential incision around the fistulous tract with a margin of several millimeters is indicated. (C) Development of a vaginal wall flap. (D) First layer of repair: transverse approximation of the edges of the fistulous tract. (E) Second layer of repair: imbrication of first layer with perivesical fascia. (F) Third layer of repair: advancement of vaginal flap.

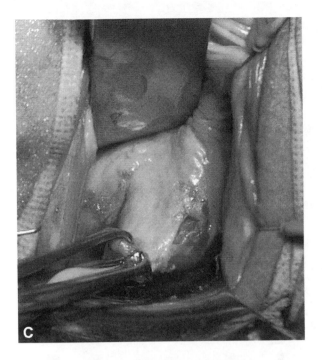

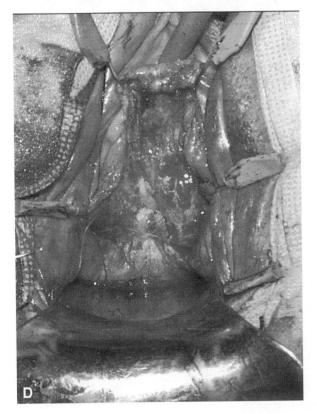

Figure 2 *Continued.*

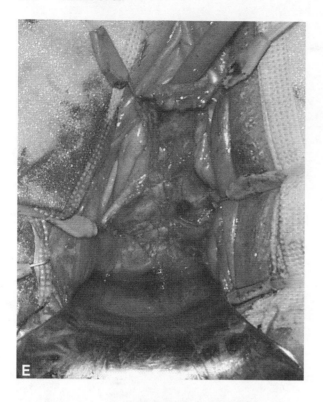

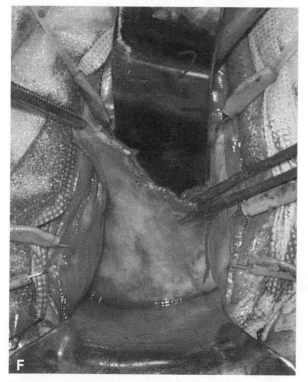

Figure 2 *Continued.*

Step 3: Creation of Flaps

Creation of anterior and posterior flaps is begun in healthy tissue away from the opening of the fistulous tract. The tissue circumscribing the fistulous tract is left intact. This technique avoids enlargement of the fistulous tract. Each flap is dissected for several centimeters from the fistula to expose the perivesical fascia.

Step 4: Closure of Fistula

The *first layer* of the repair is created by approximating the edges of the fistulous tract and a few millimeters of surrounding tissue with interrupted 3-0 absorbable sutures (Vicryl or Dexon) in a transverse fashion (Fig. 2D). These sutures incorporate the bladder wall and the fistulous tract itself. The *second layer* of perivesical fascia imbricates the prior layer also using interrupted, absorbable sutures (Fig. 2E). Before proceeding to the next layer, the integrity of the repair is tested by filling the bladder with Methylene Blue dyed saline. The *third layer* of the repair is advancement of the vaginal flap at least 3 cm beyond the fistula closure (Fig. 2F). Excess tissue from the flap is excised. The vaginal wall is then closed with a running, locking absorbable suture.

Step 5: Postoperative Care

The vagina is packed with a triple sulfa- or iodine-soaked gauze. The packing is removed 2 h postoperatively and the patient is discharged home. The urethral and suprapubic catheters drain to a single collection bag via a "Y" connector and are removed 2–3 weeks postoperatively. Oral antibiotics are continued until the catheters are removed, and anticholinergics are used as needed. It is important to avoid bladder spasms during the healing phase to avoid tension on the suture lines and urinary extravasation. Patients are instructed to avoid sexual intercourse for 3 months after surgery.

B. Abdominal Approach

The indications for an abdominal approach have been discussed previously and include the surgeon's preference and the need for concomitant abdominal procedures such as repair of ureteral injury or ureteral reimplantation. A previous failed vaginal approach does not preclude another transvaginal attempt (27). The same preoperative considerations for the vaginal approach must be taken into account, including the use of antibiotics, hormone replacement, and catheter drainage as well as the need for bowel preparation when augmentation cystoplasty is planned.

The patient is positioned supine with the lower extremities slightly abducted in order to provide access to the vagina. The vagina and lower abdomen are prepared and a suprapubic catheter is placed using a Lowsley retractor. A urethral catheter is also placed. A Pfannenstiel or low-midline incision is made, and the space of Retzius is developed. In general, efforts should be made to remain extraperitoneal unless omentum will be needed for tissue interposition. In these cases, a small peritoneal window can be made at the end of the repair, and the omentum mobilized.

The bladder is retracted cephalad with Allis clamps, and, starting laterally, the plane between the bladder and vagina is developed. Identification of the fistula may be facilitated by filling of the bladder with diluted Methylene Blue. After the bladder is completely dissected free and the fistulous tract is identified, the fistula may be catheterized toward the vagina to facilitate dissection of the bladder base. The bladder and vaginal defects are then each repaired in two layers using interrupted, absorbable sutures. An omental or peritoneal flap is placed between the bladder and vagina (Fig. 3). Urethral and suprapubic catheters are used for bladder drainage. Pelvic drainage is unnecessary unless the transvesical approach is used.

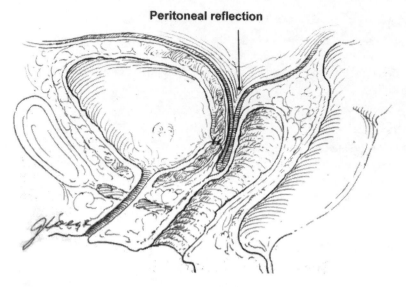
Peritoneal reflection

Figure 3   Tissue interposition between bladder and vagina. (From Ref. 61.)

C. Transvesical Approach

O'Conor and Sokol originally described the transvesical approach for the repair of vesicovaginal fistulae (38). This technique involves creating a cystotomy in the sagittal plane, both anterior and posterior, until the fistula is reached. Once the fistula is identified, the plane between the vagina and bladder is developed, and each is closed in two layers of absorbable sutures. Omentum is usually interposed between the bladder and vagina. Success rates with this technique range from 87% to 100% (39–42).

D. Success Rates

Multiple factors, including cure rate, patient morbidity, and patient satisfaction, must be considered when gauging the success of a procedure. A prospective, randomized study comparing the outcome of the vaginal versus abdominal approach to VVF repair has not been reported; however, there are multiple modern series reporting success rates from 90% to 100% with both approaches (29,43–45). As mentioned previously, the approach that is most successful is the one with which the surgeon is most experienced.

E. Complications

For both the vaginal and abdominal approaches, the two most worrisome potential intraoperative complications are hemorrhage and ureteral injury. Meticulous hemostasis should be achieved as hematoma formation may result in disruption of the suture line and recurrent fistula formation. The use of electrocautery should be minimized. Excessive bleeding encountered during dissection of the vaginal flaps should be controlled with absorbable sutures. When ureteral injury is in question, Indigo Carmine should be administered intravenously and cystoscopy performed to identify efflux of urine from the ureteral orifices. Early postoperative complications such as bleeding, infection, or bladder spasms should be treated aggressively, as any of these may weaken the repair. Ileus is often encountered following the abdominal approach.

Late complications of any approach include unrecognized ureteral injury or fistula recurrence. In the immediate postoperative period, ureteral obstruction or extravasation should be treated with percutaneous nephrostomy drainage. Retrograde procedures such as pyelography or ureteroscopy should be avoided, as these may result in disruption of the repair. Fistula recurrence may be repaired transvaginally with the use of tissue interposition. A delayed complication specific for the abdominal approach is bowel obstruction, which is usually successfully treated with conservative measures. Finally, a potential late complication of the vaginal approach is vaginal shortening or stenosis, which may require vaginoplasty.

VI. COMPLEX FISTULAE

We consider complex fistulae those that are the result of radiation therapy, large fistulae (>1 cm), obstetrical fistulae associated with other injuries, recurrent fistulae, fistulae high in the vaginal vault, and those associated with poor-tissue quality due to either hormone deficiency or ischemia. Special surgical techniques to provide tissue interposition are required for the repair of complex fistulae. The use of flaps increases the chance of surgical success by filling in dead space and providing an added layer of well vascularized tissue to the repair.

A. Radiation Fistulae

Special consideration must be given when dealing with radiation fistulae. The incidence of VVF after radiation therapy for cervical cancer ranges from 0.6% to 3% depending on disease stage and dosimetry (46). Unfortunately, modifications in mode of delivery and dosimetry have not decreased this incidence (47–49).

A fistula is usually the result of ischemic tissue injury secondary to obliterative endarteritis (46). The site of fistula formation is typically the trigone because, unlike the rest of the bladder, which changes position with filling and emptying, it is a relatively immobile area, making it vulnerable to higher radiation exposure. Nevertheless, all surrounding tissue is susceptible to radiation injury. Not uncommonly the bladder becomes a fibrotic, small-capacity, noncompliant organ following radiation therapy. Thus, when dealing with radiation-induced VVF, it is imperative to evaluate bladder capacity. Fistula repair is likely to fail if a high-pressure, noncompliant bladder is not augmented owing to increased pressure on the suture line. If augmentation cystoplasty is necessary, a nonirradiated bowel segment should be used to minimize complications with the vasculature to the augment or the bowel anastomosis.

B. Tissue Interposition

1. Martius Flap

The Martius flap is a fibrofatty labial flap first described by Heinrich Martius in 1928 (50). This flap has been used for the repair of a variety of fistulae involving the pelvic floor: urethrovaginal, peritoneovaginal, perianal, and vesicovaginal (51–53). Anatomical studies have demonstrated that the flap is composed of fibroadipose tissue from the labia majora and receives its blood supply anteriorly from the external pudendal artery and posteriorly from the internal pudendal artery (26). Branches of the obturator artery and vein enter the lateral aspect of the flap adjacent to the ischiopubic ramus but are sacrificed during harvest of the flap (23,26). The clinical importance of the blood supply is that the flap may be divided at either the superior or inferior margin and mobilized depending on the individual needs.

Preparation of the flap begins with a longitudinal incision over the labia majora. The medial, lateral, and posterior borders of dissection are the labiocrural fold, the labia minora and bulbocavernosus muscle, and the urogenital diaphragm, respectively (23,26). A Penrose drain is used to encircle the entire thickness of the fibrofatty flap, and gentle downward traction is applied as it is freed from the surrounding tissues (Fig. 4A). The superior or inferior portion is then clamped and transected, and the free end is now transferred from the labial area to the fistula site (Fig. 4B). Fixation of the flap is done with interrupted, absorbable sutures in a tension-free manner (Fig. 4C). Finally the vaginal flap is advanced over the Martius flap, and the wound is closed. Excellent hemostasis is important, and a small Penrose or Jackson-Pratt drain is left in the labial incision as well as a light-pressure dressing. Ice packs placed on the labia during the immediate postoperative period are also useful to prevent edema and hematoma formation.

The morbidity associated with the use of a Martius flap is minimal, but deep dissection into the erectile tissue of the vestibular bulb can cause serious hemorrhage (26). Overall, success rates have been good with most series reporting >90% success in fistula repairs utilizing a Martius flap (26,33,51).

2. Peritoneal Flap

The ease of preparation and location makes the peritoneal flap well suited for fistulae high in the vaginal vault. The posterior peritoneum, including the preperitoneal fat, is isolated using sharp dissection (Fig. 5). The flap is then advanced over the first two layers of the fistula repair. Interrupted, absorbable sutures are used to anchor the peritoneum without tension. The vaginal wall flap is advanced as the final layer. In their original description of the use of a peritoneal flap for the transvaginal repair of vesicovaginal fistulae, Raz and associates reported success in nine of 11 patients (82%) (54). Since then the success rate for 83 patients has improved to 96%, with 77% of those having failed a prior repair (55).

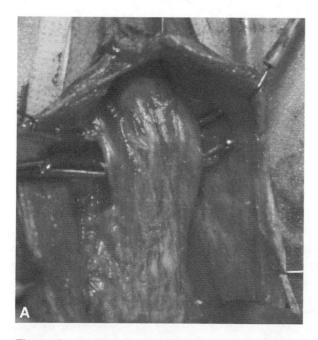

Figure 4   (A) Mobilization of Martius flap from superior attachments. (B) Transfer of Martius flap from donor site to fistula repair. (C) Fixation of Martius flap.

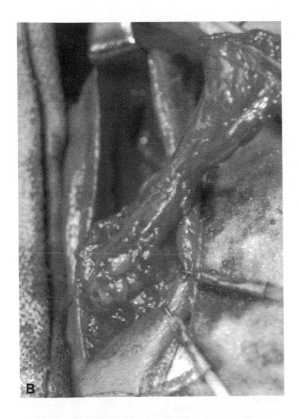

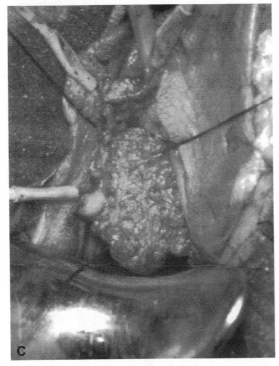

Figure 4 *Continued.*

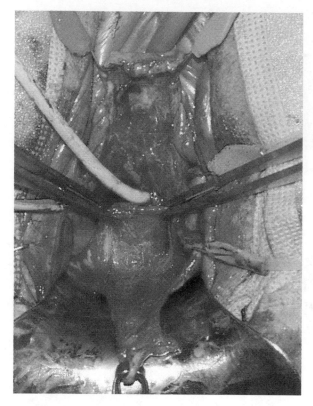

Figure 5   Development of peritoneal flap.

Inadvertent peritoneotomy is the most common complication of a peritoneal flap. A peritoneotomy can easily be repaired without compromise of the peritoneal flap. The use of a peritoneal flap is reserved for fistulae high in the vaginal canal, and we do not recommend its use in reconstruction of distal defects.

3.   Omental Interposition

The omentum is an ideal tissue for interposition because of its ability to establish neovascularity. This makes it particularly useful for the repair of complex fistulae. It can be used in the abdominal approach for fistula repair or in the vaginal approach if it was mobilized into the pelvis during a prior procedure. Cure rates of 93% have been reported when omental interposition is used during complex fistula repair (60).

The blood supply to the omentum arises from the right and left gastroepiploic arteries. These then give rise to the right and left omental arteries which extend inferiorly to form a "U." In approximately one-third of patients, no mobilization is required to bring the flap to the pelvis. Another third require division of the left gastroepiploic artery and lateral splenorenal ligaments. The remainder of patients require complete mobilization of the omentum by separating the attachments to the transverse colon and mesocolon and ligating the short gastric vessels (56–59).

Omental interposition is used almost exclusively with the transabdominal approach to vesicovaginal fistulae. Previous surgery and/or radiation therapy may affect the amount of omentum available and its mobility.

4. Full-Thickness Labial (Martius) Flap

For situations in which there is insufficient vaginal epithelium to achieve primary closure, a full-thickness labial (Martius) flap may be rotated to cover the defect. This flap provides a well-vascularized fibrofatty layer as well as full-thickness skin coverage. Following closure of the fistula, a "U" incision is made 1 cm lateral to the labia majora with the base at the level of the posterior fourchette (Fig. 6). The flap is dissected from the fascia covering the pubic bone and includes the labial skin and fibrofatty tissue. The flap is rotated to cover the repair, and the edges are sutured in place with absorbable sutures (61).

Margolis et al. reported an initial 100% flap survival in four patients who had undergone repair of VVF. One ultimately developed delayed recurrence (62). Carr and Webster also reported excellent results in four patients (63). Potential complications include an undesirable cosmetic result and reduced cutaneous sensation along the harvest site (61,63).

5. Gluteal Flap

Gluteal flaps are used mainly for patients with postradiation fistulae when there is paucity of vaginal tissue and no other viable skin source is available to provide skin coverage. Following closure of the first two layers as described for an uncomplicated VVF repair, an incision is made in the vaginal wall and continued toward the midportion of the labia majora. This incision is then extended toward the gluteal area (Fig. 7A). The skin is undermined and a flap is rotated and advanced into the vaginal canal to cover the first two layers of the fistula repair (Fig. 7B).

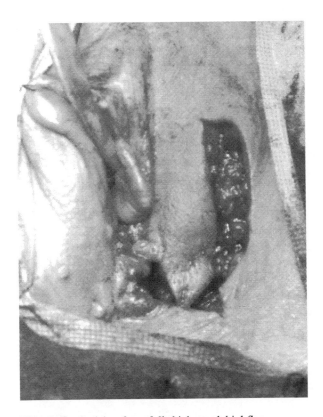

Figure 6   Incision for a full-thickness labial flap.

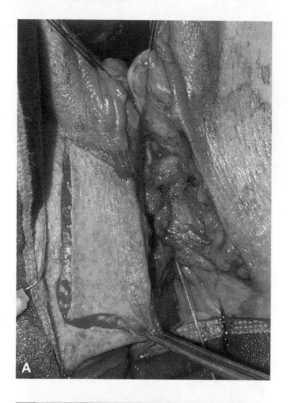

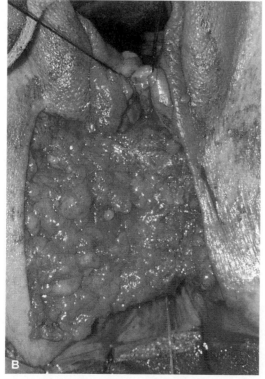

Figure 7   (A) Incision for a gluteal skin flap. (B) Transfer of gluteal flap to cover defect.

The flap is secured in place with interrupted, absorbable sutures, and finally the vaginal flaps are sutured to the edges of the flap (23). Potential complications of the gluteal flap are those common to all flaps, including wound infection and sloughing of the flap due to poor blood supply. Injury to the anal sphincter is a complication unique to the gluteal flap (64). Careful surgical technique must be employed to prevent this complication.

6. Gracilis Myocutaneous Flap

Both labial and gluteal flaps provide tissue coverage but do not provide for vaginal depth or restoration of sexual function. On the other hand, a myocutaneous flap is useful for complex, postradiation fistulae or vaginal vault deficiencies in which vaginal reconstruction is required. The gracilis muscle is a long, straplike muscle that extends from the inferior border of the symphysis pubis to the medial condyle of the femur. It is an accessory muscle for thigh adduction and knee flexion, and can be sacrificed without loss of function. The muscle alone can be used as an interposition, or a myocutaneous flap can be used to fill a large vaginal defect.

For gracilis flap harvest, an elliptical incision centered over the gracilis muscle is made on the medial aspect of the thigh (Fig. 8). The maximum skin island is 8 cm wide by 22 cm long and should not include the distal third of the muscle (59). The muscle is detached at its distal tendinous insertion point, and the flap is dissected until the vascular pedicle is identified. A tunnel is developed from the donor site to the vaginal introitus in order to transfer the flap to the vaginal area.

Although there are no large series reporting on the success of this flap, several authors report good outcomes when using the gracilis flap for the repair of VVF (64–66). The main complication is considerable scar formation, but there is usually no functional defect (19,67).

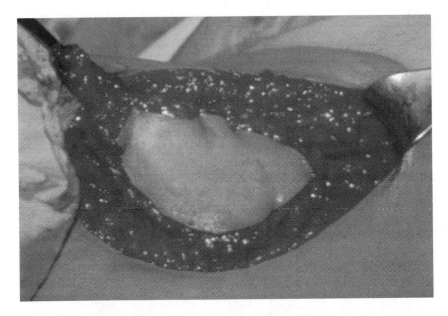

Figure 8 Gracilis myocutaneous flap. (From Ref. 61.)

VII.   CONCLUSION

Vesicovaginal fistula is a devastating complication resulting from various etiologies. With the proper preoperative evaluation and planning, the great majority of vesicovaginal fistulae can be repaired with the transvaginal approach. Complicated fistulae have a greater chance for success with the use of tissue interposition. Adequate drainage, anticholinergic therapy, and prophylactic antibiotic coverage postoperatively also increase the rate of surgical success.

REFERENCES

1. Mattingly RF, Thompson JD. Vesicovaginal fistulas. In: Te Linde's Operative Gynecology. Philadelphia: J.B. Lippincott, 1985.
2. Petri E, Friedberg V. Vaginaler oder abdominaler Verschluss von Blasenscheiden-fisteln. Gynakologe 1983; 16:231–237.
3. Harkki-Siren P, Sjoberg J, Tiitinen A. Urinary tract injuries after hysterectomy. Obstet Gynecol 1998; 92:113–118.
4. Kelly J. Vesico-vaginal and recto-vaginal fistulae. J R Soc Med 1992; 85:257–258.
5. Lawson J. Vaginal fistulae (editorial). J R Soc Med 1992; 85:254–256.
6. Arrowsmith S, Hamlin EC, Wall LL. Obstructed labor injury complex: obstetric fistula formation and the multifaceted morbidity of maternal birth trauma in the developing world. Obstet Gynecol Surv 1996; 51:568–574.
7. Lee RA, Symmonds RE, Williams TJ. Current status of genitourinary fistula. Obstet Gynecol 1988; 72(3 Pt 1):313–319.
8. Kursh ED, Morse RM, Resnick MI, Persky L. Prevention of the development of a vesicovaginal fistula. Surg Gynecol Obstet 1988; 166:409–412.
9. Kindt J, Retzke U, Ramthor W. Problems of late formation of a radiation-induced vesicovaginal fistula. Case report. Zentralbl Gynakol 1981; 103:313–317.
10. Muntz HG, Goff BA, Thor AD, Tarraza HM. Post-hysterectomy carcinoma of the Fallopian tube mimicking a vesicovaginal fistula. Obstet Gynecol 1992; 79:853–856.
11. Mariotti G, Natale F, Trucchi A, Cristini C, Furbetta A. Ureteral injuries during gynecologic procedures. Minerva Urol Nefrol 1997; 49:95–98.
12. Mattingly RF, Borkowf HI. Acute operative injury to the lower urinary tract. Clin Obstet Gynecol 1978; 5:123–149.
13. Lee RA, Symmonds RE. Ureterovaginal fistula. Am J Obstet Gynecol 1971; 109:1032–1035.
14. Goodwin WE, Scardino PT. Vesicovaginal and ureterovaginal fistulas: a summary of 25 years of experience. J Urol 1980; 123:370–374.
15. Miller EA, Webster GD. Current management of vesicovaginal fistulae. Curr Opin Urol 2001; 11:417–421.
16. Benchekroun A, Lachkar A, Soumana A, Farih MH, Belahnech Z, Marzouk M, Faik M. Uretero-vaginal fistulas. 45 cases. Ann Urol 1998; 32:295–299.
17. Davits RJ, Miranda SI. Conservative treatment of vesicovaginal fistulas by bladder drainage alone. Br J Urol 1991; 68:155–156.
18. Tancer ML. Observations on prevention and management of vesicovaginal fistula after total hysterectomy. Surg Gynecol Obstet 1992; 175:501–506.
19. Hilton P. Vesico-vaginal fistula: new perspectives. Curr Opin Obstet Gynecol 2001; 13:513–520.
20. Falk HC, Orkin LA. Nonsurgical closure of vesicovaginal fistulas. Obstet Gynecol 1957; 9:538–541.
21. Stothers L, Chopra A, Raz S. Vesicovaginal fistula. In: Raz S, ed. Female Urology. 2nd ed. Philadelphia: W.B. Saunders, 1996:490–506.
22. Leng WW, Amundsen CL, McGuire EJ. Management of female genitourinary fistulas: transvesical or transvaginal approach? J Urol 1998; 160:1995–1999.

23. Stovsky MD, Ignatoff JM, Blum MD, Nanninga JB, O'Conor VJ, Kursh ED. Use of electrocoagulation in the treatment of vesicovaginal fistulas. J Urol 1994; 152(5 Pt 1):1443–1444.

24. Dogra PN, Nabi G. Laser welding of vesicovaginal fistula. Int Urogynecol J Pelvic Floor Dysfunc 2001; 12:69–70.

25. Collins CG, Pent D, Jones FB. Results of early repair of vesico-vaginal fistula with preliminary cortisone treatment. Am J Obstet Gynecol 1960; 80:1005.

26. Elkins TE, DeLancey JO, McGuire EJ. The use of modified Martius graft as an adjunctive technique in vesicovaginal and rectovaginal fistula repair. Obstet Gynecol 1990; 75:727–733.

27. Wang Y, Hadley HR. Nondelayed transvaginal repair of high lying vesicovaginal fistula. J Urol 1990; 144:34–36.

28. Blandy JP, Badenoch DF, Fowler CG, Jenkins BJ, Thomas NW. Early repair of iatrogenic injury to the ureter or bladder after gynecological surgery. J Urol 1991; 146:761–765.

29. Zimmern PE, Hadley HR, Staskin DR, Raz S. Genitourinary fistulae: vaginal approach for repair of vesicovaginal fistulae. Urol Clin North Am 1985; 12:361–367.

30. Blaivas JG, Heritz DM, Romanzi LJ. Early versus late repair of vesicovaginal fistulas: vaginal and abdominal approaches. J Urol 1995; 153:1110–1112.

31. Collins CG, Collins JH, Harrison BR, Nicholls RA, Hoffman ES, Krupp PJ. Early repair of vesico-vaginal fistula. Am J Obstet Gynecol 1971; 111:524–528.

32. Persky L, Herman G, Guerrier K. Non-delay in vesicovaginal fistula repair. Urology 1979; 13:272–275.

33. Rangnekar NP, Imdad AN, Kaul SA, Pathak HR. Role of the Martius procedure in the management of urinary-vaginal fistulas. J Am Coll Surg 2000; 191:259–263.

34. Evans DH, Madjar S, Politano VA, Bejany DE, Lynne CM, Gousse AE. Interposition flaps in transabdominal vesicovaginal fistula repairs: are they really necessary? Urology 2001; 57:670–674.

35. Hassim AM, Lucas C. Reduction in the incidence of stress incontinence complicating fistula repair. Br J Surg 1974; 61:461–465.

36. Gray PH. Obstetric vesico-vaginal fistulas. Am J Obstet Gynecol 1970; 107:898–901.

37. Lavery DWP. Obstetrical vesico-vaginal fistulae. Med Proc 1960; 6:36–40.

38. O'Conor VJ, Sokol JK. Vesicovaginal fistula from the standpoint of the urologist. J Urol 1951; 66:579.

39. Motiwala HG, Amlani JC, Desai KD, Shah KN, Patel PC. Transvesical vesicovaginal fistula repair: a revival. Eur Urol 1991; 19:24–28.

40. Nesrallah LJ, Srougi M, Gittes RF. The O'Conor technique: the gold standard for supratrigonal vesicovaginal fistula repair. J Urol 1999; 161:566–568.

41. Cetin S, Yazicioglu A, Ozgur S, Ilker Y, Dalva I. Vesicovaginal fistula repair: a simple suprapubic transvesical approach. Int Urol Nephrol 1988; 20:265–268.

42. Udeh FN. Simple management of difficult vesicovaginal fistulas by anterior transvesical approach. J Urol 1985; 133:591–593.

43. Langkilde NC, Pless TK, Lundbeck F, Nerstrom B. Surgical repair of vesicovaginal fistulae: a ten-year retrospective study. Scand J Urol Nephrol 1999; 33:100–103.

44. Diaz Calleja E, Calatrava Gadea S, Caldentey Garcia M, Moreno Perez F, Lapuerta Torres E, Garcia Victor F. Surgical repair of vesico-vaginal fistulae with abdominal-transvesical approach. Comments on this technique with long-term results. Arch Esp Urol 1997; 50:55–60.

45. Frohmuller H, Hofmockel G. Transvaginal closure of vesicovaginal fistulas. Urologe A 1998; 37:102.

46. Perez CA, Grigsby PW, Lockett MA, Chao KS, Williamson J. Radiation therapy morbidity in carcinoma of the uterine cervix: dosimetric and clinical correlation. Int J Radiat Oncol Biol Phys 1999; 44:855–866.

47. Bottcher HD, Schutz J, Mathei B. Side effects of the treatment of cervix cancer. Strahlentherapie 1983; 159:334–343.

48. Perez CA, Breaux S, Bedwinek JM, Madoc-Jones H, Camel HM, Purdy JA, Walz BJ. Radiation therapy alone in the treatment of carcinoma of the uterine cervix. II. Analysis of complications. Cancer 1984; 54:235–246.

49. De Pree C, Popowski Y, Weber D, Nouet P, Rouzaud M, Kurtz JM. Feasibility and tolerance of pulsed dose rate interstitial brachytherapy. Int J Radiat Oncol Biol Phys 1999; 43:971–976.

50. Martius H. Die operative Wiedeherstellung der vollkommen fehlenden Harnrohare und des Schliess-muskels derselben. Zentralbl Gynakol 1928; 52:480–486.
51. Punekar SV, Buch DN, Soni AB, Swami G, Rao SR, Kinne JS, Karhadkar SS. Martius' labial fat pad interposition and its modification in complex lower urinary fistulae. J Postgrad Med 1999; 45:69–73.
52. Blander DS, Zimmern PE, Lemack GE, Sagalowsky AI. Transvaginal repair of postcystectomy peritoneovaginal fistulae. Urology 2000; 56:320–321.
53. Kay AR. Labial fat pad grafts (modified Martius graft) in complex perianal fistulas. Ann R Coll Surg Engl 1999; 81:143.
54. Raz S, Bregg KJ, Nitti VW, Sussman E. Transvaginal repair of vesicovaginal fistula using a peritoneal flap. J Urol 1993; 150:56–59.
55. Eilber KS, Rosenblum N, Rodríguez L, Raz S. 10-year experience of transvaginal vesicovaginal fistula repair utilizing a peritoneal flap. (Submitted.)
56. Woo HH, Rosario FJ, Chapple CR. The treatment of vesicovaginal fistulae. Eur Urol 1996; 29:1–9.
57. Turner-Warwick R. The use of the omental pedicle graft in urinary tract reconstruction. J Urol 1976; 116:341–347.
58. Turner-Warwick RT, Wynne EJC, Handley-Ashken M. The use of the omental pedicle graft in the repair and reconstruction of the urinary tract. Br J Surg 1967; 54:849–853.
59. Sirls LT, Leach GE. Repair of vesicovaginal fistula. In: Ehrlich RM, Alter GJ, eds. Reconstructive and Plastic Surgery of the External Genitalia. Philadelphia: W.B. Saunders, 1999:453–459.
60. Orford HJ, Theron JL. The repair of vesicovaginal fistulas with omentum. A review of 59 cases. S Afr Med J 1985; 67:143–144.
61. Raz S. Atlas of Transvaginal Surgery. Philadelphia: W.B. Saunders, 1992.
62. Margolis T, Elkins TE, Seffah J, Oparo-Addo HS, Fort D. Full-thickness Martius grafts to preserve vaginal depth as an adjunct in the repair of large obstetric fistulas. Obstet Gynecol 1994; 84:148–152.
63. Carr LK, Webster GD. Full-thickness cutaneous Martius flaps: a useful technique in female reconstructive urology. Urology 48:461–463.
64. Wang Y, Hadley HR. The use of rotated vascularized pedicle flaps for complex transvaginal procedures. J Urol 1993; 149:590–592.
65. Gerges DG, Mesfen W. Repair of a complex vesicovaginal fistula using a musculocutaneous flap of the gracilis muscle. J Urol (Paris) 1984; 90:491–493.
66. Ingelman-Sundberg A. Surgical treatment of urinary fistulae. Zentralbl Gynakol 1978; 100: 1281–1294.
67. Tolle E, Schmandt W, Beizai S, Drepper H. Closure of large vesico-urethro-vaginal defect with pedicled myocutaneous gracilis flap. Urologe A 1981; 20:274–277.

54

Vesicovaginal Fistula: Abdominal Approach

Martin B. Richman and Howard B. Goldman
Case Western Reserve University, University Hospitals of Cleveland, Cleveland, Ohio, U.S.A.

I. HISTORY

A vesicovaginal fistula (VVF) is an abnormal channel between the urinary bladder and the vagina that results in urinary leakage. Most of these fistulas occur in otherwise healthy women who undergo elective gynecologic surgery for benign disease, and as a result of the fistula, are completely incontinent of urine. This incontinence can have physical implications such as skin breakdown and infection as well as psychological sequelae such as depression and avoidance of social situations as the woman with a VVF is constantly wetting pads and is at risk of leaking onto her clothing and smelling from urine.

VVFs have been reported for hundreds of years, with the first description of repair by Van Roonhuyse in 1672 (1). However, the first modern description of VVF repair was by Sims in 1852, which emphasized the general principles of fistula repair, including adequate operative exposure, a tension-free closure, and adequate, continuous postoperative drainage to permit healing (2).

Modern-day VVF repair is performed by either an abdominal or vaginal approach, each with advantages and disadvantages. The next three chapters will describe the different techniques and applications of the abdominal and vaginal approaches for the management of vesicovaginal fistulae.

II. ETIOLOGY

Approximately 90% of VVFs in developed countries are due to prior pelvic surgery, with abdominal hysterectomy for benign disease accounting for 70% of these (3). The incidence of fistulas secondary to iatrogenic surgical trauma is reported as being between 0.1% and 2% (4,5). The remaining 10% of VVFs in developed countries are the result of radiation, infection, foreign bodies, and pelvic malignancies, including cervical, vaginal, and endometrial carcinomas (3) (Table 1). Fistulas resulting from radiation injury tend to be accompanied by extensive fibrosis and a compromised blood supply (4), making their management more complex and outcomes often less predictable.

In underdeveloped countries, most VVFs are the result of obstetrical trauma (6), particularly pressure necrosis of the bladder and vagina that occurs with compression of these structures between the infant's head and the pubic bone during prolonged labor (3). This mechanism results

Table 1   Etiology of Vesicovaginal Fistula

Iatrogenic injury from pelvic surgery
  Gynecologic surgery
  Obstetric surgery
  Urologic surgery
Radiation injury
Pelvic malignancy
Pelvic trauma
Obstetric trauma from prolonged labor
Vaginal or vesical foreign body

in morbidity for over 5 million women annually and is estimated to occur in three to four out of every 1000 deliveries (4). Tissue loss from ischemic injury may continue into the early postpartum period, and delay of repair must be considered until all sequelae of the trauma are evident. VVFs from obstetric trauma rarely occur in developed countries owing to the superior obstetric care available to the female population, including the use of early surgical delivery of the infant in complicated labor.

Most VVFs become evident at approximately the 10th postoperative day after pelvic surgery (7), although some are immediately evident in the first few postoperative hours or even while still in the operating room. The vaginal component of the fistula occurs at the suture line of the vaginal cuff. The bladder may become involved owing to a small posterior bladder laceration that occurs intraoperatively. Often this injury is unrecognized in the operating room. The bladder injury results in a pelvic urinoma that ultimately drains through the vaginal cuff suture line. Other mechanisms of intraoperative injury that can result in a VVF are due to ischemia from cautery use or injury due to an inadvertent suture placed in the bladder while attempting to control intraoperative bleeding. Either of these can lead to delayed necrosis and subsequent fistula formation. With any of these mechanisms of injury and ensuing fistula, the patient reports vaginal drainage that may or may not be continuous depending on the size of the fistula.

Radiation-induced necrosis causes 3% of all VVFs (8). Radiation therapy results in chronic regional tissue damage. These fistulas can occur months to years after the conclusion of therapy, and oftentimes repair is further complicated by the presence of prior abdominal surgery for the malignancy. Prior to the repair of fistulas related to cancer or the treatment of cancer, the recurrence of tumor should be ruled out with a biopsy of the fistula margin (6).

III. DIAGNOSIS

Though some fistulas may be easy to diagnose by a complete history and physical exam, many others will need further tests, including dye tests and radiographic imaging. Evaluation of a suspected VVF begins with a thorough medical history and physical examination. Past medical history is important to elucidate previous pelvic surgeries and malignancies with or without radiation therapy. Obtaining the underlying reason for fistula formation can be important in planning an operative technique for repair. It is important to elicit from the patient whether incontinence began immediately after pelvic surgery or whether it began days or weeks later. A woman with a VVF that was initially missed may present to the office with a diagnosis of stress or urge incontinence, and may have been having occasional leakage for months. Upon further evaluation, an association can be made between the onset of incontinence and a relatively remote pelvic surgery.

A pelvic exam is crucial in the evaluation of a potential fistula. The presence of urine in the vaginal vault is highly suspicious for a urinary-genital fistula. Other findings indicative of a VVF include observing a hole or an area of granulation tissue at the vaginal cuff or apex. With a large fistula, a defect may even be palpated during a digital vaginal exam.

A urinary-vaginal fistula also can be diagnosed by placing a vaginal packing or tampon in the vagina and giving the patient oral pyridium or intravenous Indigo Carmine. The presence of orange or blue discoloration on the vaginal pack or tampon indicates a fistula. The fistula can be further localized with the Double Dye Test (9,10). Classically, this test is performed by placing a vaginal packing or tampon in the vagina while the patient is in the lithotomy position. A Foley catheter is then placed and the bladder is filled with 1% carmine solution, a red dye. Next, 5 mL of Indigo Carmine solution is injected intravenously. This is normally excreted by the kidneys as a blue dye within 15 min (6). The vaginal packing is then examined for the presence of blue staining indicating an ureterovaginal fistula or red staining indicating a vesicovaginal fistula, or both. Red staining at the distal most part of the packing may indicate a urethral vaginal fistula. Today, this test is most commonly done with oral pyridium, which colors the urine orange, given for 24 h prior to the test, and then Indigo Carmine is instilled into the bladder during the test.

Radiographic imaging is also useful in the workup of a suspected urinary-vaginal fistula. In the presence of a VVF, a cystogram will almost always demonstrate contrast flowing from the bladder to the vagina (Fig. 1). On the other hand, a normal cystogram nearly rules out the possibility of a VVF. Computed tomography can be another useful modality. The presence of excreted contrast in the vaginal vault usually indicates a communication between the vagina and the urinary system, and the fistula may even be visualized with thin-cut images through the pelvis (Fig. 2). Intravenous or retrograde pyelography should be performed to exclude the possibility of concurrent ureterovaginal fistula or ureteral injury. With all radiographic studies, careful examination of the films is important, as the surgeon must have a complete understanding of the extent of the injury before attempting repair.

Cystourethroscopy and vaginoscopy may be important for diagnosis and evaluation of a VVF. During cystoscopy, the surgeon can look for one or more holes, which sometimes can be quite large and obvious. In the absence of a clear defect, irregularities of the mucosa may be suspicious for a fistula. Once a defect is found, cystoscopy can be useful for characterizing the location and size of the fistula, and how far it is from the ureteral orifices. Proximity of the fistula to one or both ureteral orifices may indicate the need for ureteral reimplantation during fistula repair. With vaginoscopy, one should look for small holes or areas of granulation signifying the location of a small fistula.

IV. TIMING OF REPAIR

The timing of repair of a VVF is controversial and has been debated extensively in the literature. Classically, surgeons waited 3–6 months after the injury to allow inflammation to decrease and to let surrounding tissues heal. In the past quarter-century, however, early repair of iatrogenic fistulas attributed to pelvic surgery has been advocated (11). Several authors report equivalent success rates of fistula closure with early repair for fistulas resulting from recent pelvic surgery (12,13). Most who advocate early repair mention the severe mental and physical distress a VVF presents to the usually otherwise healthy woman.

VVFs that are recognized in the immediate postoperative period have the best chance at successful repair if done as soon as the fistula is noted. However, early repair is not indicated

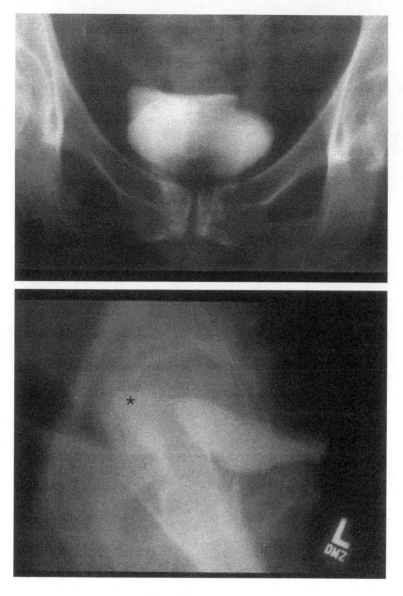

Figure 1   AP and lateral cystogram demonstrating filling of vagina (asterisk) with contrast after introduction of contrast into bladder. Diagnostic of a VVF.

in fistulas that result from obstetric trauma or from radiation therapy, since these injuries often result in ischemic injury and severe inflammation and one must let these processes stabilize prior to attempting a repair. A waiting period must also be considered in those with pelvic infection or infection of the vaginal cuff. Once acute local inflammation has subsided, either a vaginal or an abdominal approach can be utilized for successful early repair of a VVF (13).

If a waiting period before repair is necessary, a Foley catheter may be placed to diminish the amount of leakage and allow the patient a more normal lifestyle. Unfortunately, there may be persistent leakage of urine even with Foley catheter decompression (7).

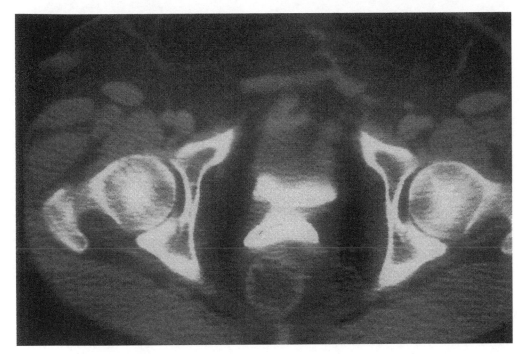

Figure 2   Computerized tomography image of contrast in both bladder and vagina suggestive of a VVF.

V.   ABDOMINAL APPROACH TO VVF REPAIR

A.   Indications for Abdominal Approach

There have been a few reports of successful resolution of VVF with conservative measures such as long-term bladder drainage or with fulguration of the fistulous tract (14,15). However, most fistulas require surgical repair. Many studies have shown that the best chance for successful surgical repair of a VVF is at the first attempt, and regardless of the method used, the basic principles of fistula repair must be followed (Table 2). These include a tension-free repair with tissue that has an adequate blood supply and is free of infection and inflammation. Avoidance of overlapping suture lines and the use of fine suture is recommended. Postoperative bladder drainage and decompression are essential for healing of the repair.

   VVFs can be repaired by either a vaginal approach or an abdominal approach. Each method has advantages and disadvantages for the patient. The route of repair that is most

Table 2   Principles for Successful Fistula Repair

Tension-free repair
Adequate tissue blood supply
Tissues free of infection and inflammation
Multiple-layer repair and/or interposition of other healthy
   tissue
Avoidance of overlapping suture lines
Postoperative rest for the repair site (bladder drainage and
   decompression)

comfortable to the surgeon based on training and experience is also an important factor in planning the operative approach. The vaginal approach often leads to less morbidity and a quicker recovery as the patient is spared an abdominal incision and bivalving of the bladder. This approach will be discussed in the subsequent chapter.

The abdominal approach to repair of VVF, which can be performed by either a transverse Pfannenstiel or a low-midline incision, affords the surgeon the opportunity to simultaneously treat other intra-abdominal pathology, including the repair of coexisting ureteral injury or fistula and bowel injury or fistula. This approach also permits augmentation cystoplasty for radiation-induced cystitis with a contracted bladder. Laparotomy also allows the opportunity to easily interpose omentum to reinforce a large or recurrent fistula. The abdominal approach to repair can also be done with an extraperitoneal technique if the above are not needed but the patient has vaginal stenosis or has comorbid musculoskeletal abnormalities that would prohibit positioning or adequate exposure with the vaginal approach. Finally, many surgeons may be more comfortable with an abdominal approach based on their personal training and experience.

B. Standard "O'Conor" Approach (Fig. 3)

The standard technique for abdominal approach of VVF repair was first described by O'Conor (16), and is the most common method of abdominal repair used today. The patient is placed in either the low lithotomy position or supine with the legs slightly separated and the knees abducted to allow intraoperative access to the vagina. A urethral Foley catheter is placed and a lower-midline or Pfannenstiel incision is made. If possible, the repair is performed from an extraperitoneal approach unless access to intraperitoneal structures is desired, in which case the peritoneum is opened and retracted from the dome of the bladder, packing the small bowel out of the way. Either way, the bladder is opened over the dome, and stay sutures are placed bilaterally. Surgeon choice and fistula location dictate the need for insertion of ureteral catheters.

The bladder wall is then bisected down to the edge of the fistula, and the fistula is excised from the bladder. Bladder exposure is improved by the placement of a self-retaining retractor with the lateral blades holding the lateral bladder walls. Mobilization of the bladder and vagina on either side of the fistula is performed to allow for proper closure of both structures in separate planes. We have found that placement of a metallic rectal dilator within the vagina allows for easier identification of the proper planes, and facilitates closure of the vaginal defect. The vaginal component of the fistula is completely excised as it becomes exposed. The vagina is then closed vertically or transversely with inverting interrupted synthetic absorbable sutures, taking care to avoid tension. More recently, the necessity of excising the fistulous tract has been questioned, and many surgeons just close the separate tissue layers without removal of the fistula tract.

The bladder epithelium and subepithelium are closed with 3-0 running chromic suture, and the muscularis and adventitia are reapproximated from the outside with 2-0 synthetic absorbable sutures. It is frequently easiest to begin the bladder closure by first closing the detrusor posteriorly and then closing the mucosa. Once the closure gets to the area of the dome, the mucosa can then be closed first and the detrusor second. Care must be taken to assure that the closure is tension free as the success of the repair is more dependent on the effectiveness of the bladder approximation than on the vaginal closure. Prior to bladder closure, the ureteral catheters are removed, or, if they were not placed, ureteral patency is assured by carefully watching for bilateral efflux of urine (this may be easier to see after intravenous injection of Indigo Carmine).

If a transperitoneal approach was undertaken, a peritoneal flap or omental graft can be mobilized and placed between the vagina and bladder and tacked into place. A large fistula or one resulting from radiation necrosis may be best managed with a myofascial flap such as

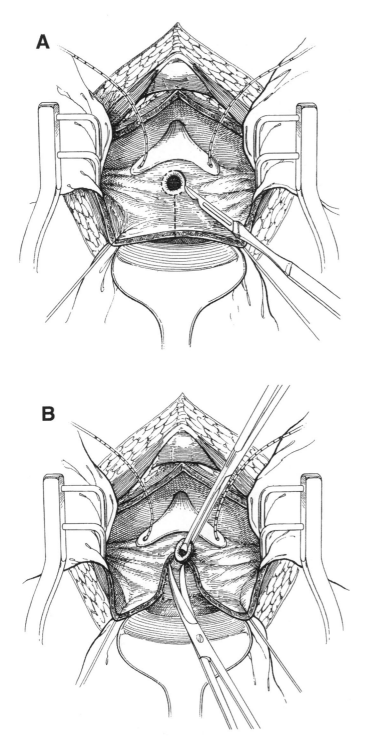

Figure 3 (A) The bladder is incised sagittally to the level of the fistula. (B) The fistulous tract is circumscribed and excised from surrounding tissue. (C) The vagina and bladder are closed separately. (D) Omentum is sutured down between the vagina and bladder.

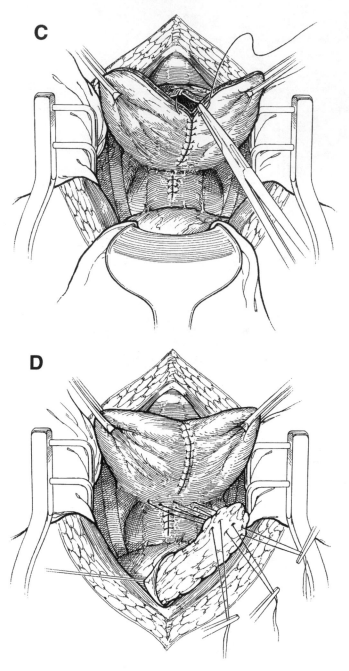

Figure 3 Continued.

one mobilized from the rectus abdominis muscle (8). Some recommend omental interposition for all fistula repairs (17), while others report excellent results with simple transvesical repair without the use of interposition grafts (18). Interposition of tissue is usually easy, and we recommend it for all cases. This is especially important with ischemic or recurrent fistulas. Our technique for omental interposition is to first place three 2-0 synthetic absorbable sutures into healthy tissue at the deep apex of the repair and then draw the needle through the omentum and use these sutures to seat the omentum into the pelvis to cover the repair.

Regardless of whether an interposition flap was utilized, the bladder must be adequately drained postoperatively with a urethral Foley catheter and/or a suprapubic catheter. At the time of repair, it is our practice to place a 24F Malecot suprapubic tube with two of the flanges excised to allow unobstructed drainage. We leave the urethral Foley catheter in as well and it is removed as soon as the urine clears.

C. Vesical Autoplasty

In addition to the classic suprapubic transvesical repair described above, other methods of abdominal repair have been reported. Gil-Vernet and colleagues described a technique of vesical autoplasty in recurrent VVFs to cover a large defect after excision of the fistulous tract (19). This modification can be used through a transperitoneal or extraperitoneal transvesical approach, and they reported a 100% success rate in a series of 42 patients with complex fistulas.

This technique involves mobilizing a full-thickness flap off the dome of the bladder to use for closure of the posterior bladder defect. The bladder is first incised transversely through the dome, and ureteral catheters are inserted. Stay sutures are then placed in the fistulous orifice and the surrounding fibrous tissues to simplify excision of a wider margin of affected tissue. The fistula and surrounding tissue are then excised until the well-vascularized, healthy bladder wall is encountered. After dissection and development of the tissue plane between the bladder and the vagina, a one-layer interrupted suture closure of the vaginal wall is completed. A flap of bladder wall is then formed through a bilateral, symmetrical incision of the superior edge of the resected defect toward the dome of the bladder until there is sufficient tissue to fill the defect. The flap is then approximated to the resection edges in one layer with interrupted 3-0 catgut sutures.

D. Free Mucosal Graft (Fig. 4)

Ostad and colleagues presented a technique of a free bladder mucosal graft during simple extraperitoneal repair of VVF (20). This modification eliminates any loss of bladder capacity as no detrusor muscle is excised, and success was 100% in their small study of six patients.

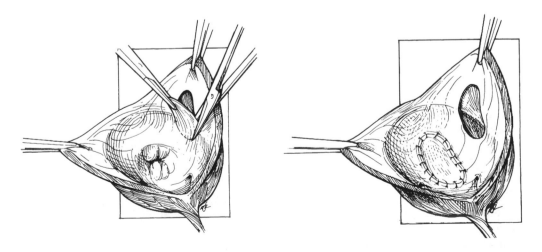

Figure 4 Free mucosal graft. (From Ref. 20.)

With an extraperitoneal approach, the bladder is opened through a small midline cystotomy, and the bladder mucosa surrounding the fistula is excised for a circumferential distance of 1 cm and discarded. No attempt is made to excise the fistulous tract from either the bladder or the vagina. Next, a free bladder mucosal graft is taken from the edge of the cystotomy line. This graft is placed over the fistula opening, replacing the excised surrounding mucosa, and sutured in place with interrupted 4-0 chromic catgut sutures. The mucosal harvest site is expected to reepithelialize in 4–6 weeks.

E. Laparoscopy

A laparoscopic approach to abdominal repair was described by von Theobald and colleagues (21). They presented a case where, via laparoscopic guidance, the bladder was dissected away from the vagina and the fistula was excised from the bladder. The bladder was closed in a single layer and an omental flap was dissected and placed between the bladder and vagina, with endostapling of the flap to the vagina. This procedure was successful at 6-month follow-up.

F. Interposition of Tissue

The interposition of translocated tissue between the bladder and the vagina in conjunction with the repair of a VVF is often recommended for complex and recurrent fistulas. Tissue that is used in VVF repair serves the purposes of a mechanical barrier to fistula recurrence and as a source of reperfusion of previously poorly vascularized tissue. This tissue must be highly vascular and easily mobilized with its blood supply.

The transperitoneal abdominal approach grants the surgeon the opportunity to use the omentum for this purpose. Walters first recommended the use of an omental flap in the repair of recurrent VVFs (22). He proposed suturing omentum between the vaginal and bladder closures to prevent the suture lines from overlapping. As described above, we do this by first placing three 2-0 synthetic absorbable sutures into healthy tissue at the deep apex of the repair and then placing the needles through the omentum and using these sutures to draw the omentum into the pelvis and cover the repair (Fig. 3D).

The omentum is usually sufficient to reach the pelvis with no or minimal alteration. However, if there is insufficient pelvic extension of the omentum, Turner-Warwick and colleagues described a method for creating and utilizing an omental pedicle graft (23). To extend the omentum to the pelvis, it must be mobilized with care to preserve an adequate blood supply. Since the left gastroepiploic artery is usually smaller than the right, it is often best to mobilize and divide the left side of the omentum along the greater curvature of the stomach and extend it to the pelvis based on the right gastroepiploic blood supply.

Eisen and colleagues described the use of a peritoneal flap interposition graft in VVF repair (24). Via a transperitoneal, transvesical approach, they formed a peritoneal flap from the lateral parietal pelvic peritoneum at the time the bladder was opened. The flap was then interposed between the vagina and bladder after fistula excision and primary closure of both components.

Brandt and colleagues proposed a technique of bladder mucosa autografting for interposition between the bladder and the vagina (25). After excision of the fistula tract and closure of both the bladder and the vagina, a free mucosal graft is taken from the dome of the bladder. The donor bed is fulgurated and left to reepithelialize. The graft is then placed between the bladder and vagina at the site of the repaired fistula with the mucosal surface facing the vagina, and both the vaginal serosa and posterior bladder wall are sutured to the graft. With this technique, they reported a 96% success rate in 80 women with VVFs that resulted from gynecologic surgery.

For large postradiation fistulas, Salup and colleagues proposed interposition of a rectus abdominis myofascial flap (8). They used a split right rectus abdominis flap based on the right deep inferior epigastric vessels. The muscle is divided from the pubis, placing the distal end of the myofascial flap in the pelvis for interposition.

We have found that any of these tissues serve as viable options and highly recommend interposition of tissue, as there is no downside and the benefit is significant reinforcement of the repair.

G. Postop Care

Postoperative bladder decompression is essential to permit adequate healing of the VVF repair. A urethral Foley catheter may or may not be placed. For low fistulas, the Foley balloon could place pressure on the repair site, leading to failure. A suprapubic drainage tube from the bladder should be placed in all cases. If both urethral and suprapubic catheters are placed, the urethral catheter may be removed as soon as the urine clears and the suprapubic tube should be kept to gravity drainage for at least 2–3 weeks. Smaller, simple fistula repairs heal quicker than large defects that contain ischemic tissues, and duration of bladder decompression should be based on the complexity of the fistula.

Low dose-prophylactic antibiotics may be used until the catheters are removed. Anticholinergic medications should be used to prevent bladder spasms that could cause suture line breakdown.

Routine cystography before removal of the suprapubic tube is probably unnecessary, as a persistent fistula will be readily noticeable when the tube is clamped prior to its removal. Nevertheless, many surgeons feel more comfortable obtaining a cystogram that shows no leak prior to removing the catheter.

H.   Results (Table 3)

Success rates for abdominal repair of VVFs are reported as 88–100% by all authors. The greatest successes are reported in patients with simple fistulas such as the 40 patients reported by Landes with a 100% success rate (18). Eisen and colleagues reported a 93% success rate in their series with a peritoneal flap interposition (24). O'Conor's cumulative results from three different studies showed a 91% success rate with a total of 77 patients (16,26). Bissada and McDonald reported a 100% success rate in seven patients with giant VVFs, which included radiation-induced and obstetrical fistulas (27). Wein and colleagues reported 88% success with 34 patients, although two of their patients who failed had fistulas related to the surgical treatment of malignancies and recurrent tumor was found at the site of fistula recurrence (28). Gil-Vernet and colleagues reported a 100% success in their study with vesical autoplasty in 42 patients with complex fistulas (19). Blandy and colleagues reported 100% success in their series of 25 patients with the same outcome in early or late repair (12). More recent studies reveal similar findings with success rates of 90%, 100%, and 92% with 11, 29, and 25 patients, respectively (29–31).

VI.   CONCLUSIONS

Vesicovaginal fistulas can develop as a complication of pelvic surgery, radiation necrosis, or obstetric trauma, and can be extremely debilitating to the affected woman. VVFs can be repaired

Table 3 Success Rates for Abdominal Repair of Vesicovaginal Fistula

Author	Year	Number of patients	Success rate	Comments
Landes (18)	1979	40	40/40 (100%)	Simple transvesical fistula repair
Eisen et al. (24)	1974	29	27/29 (93%)	Peritoneal flap interposition
O'Conor (16)	1973 1980	77	70/77 (91%)	
Bissada et al. (27)	1983	7	7/7 (100%)	"Giant" fistulas from radiation and obstetrics
Wein et al. (28)	1980	34	30/34 (88%)	Recurrent tumor found with 2 of 4 failures
Gil-Vernet et al. (19)	1988	42	42/42 (100%)	Vesicle autoplasty for complex fistulas
Blandy et al. (11)	1991	25	25/25 (100%)	Compared early vs. late repair
Leng et al. (29)	1998	11	10/11 (90%)	Compared to 30% success with vaginal repair in similar complexity of fistula
Nesrallah et al. (30)	1999	29	29/29 (100%)	
Langkilde et al. (31)	1999	25	23/25 (92%)	Compared to 42% success with vaginal repair in similar complexity of fistula

by either a vaginal approach or an abdominal approach. The abdominal approach to repair of VVF affords the surgeon the opportunity to simultaneously treat other intra-abdominal pathology and allows one the opportunity to interpose omentum to reinforce a large or recurrent fistula. It is also important to use the method of repair most comfortable to the surgeon, and often this is the abdominal approach.

Many studies have shown that the best chance for successful surgical repair of a VVF is the first attempt, and regardless of the timing of repair or method used, the basic principles of fistula repair must be followed. With good technique, one should expect a success rate of at least 90% when using an abdominal approach for vesicovaginal fistula repair.

REFERENCES

1. Zacharin RF. Grafting as a principle in the surgical management of vesicovaginal and rectovaginal fistulae. Aust N Z J Obstet Gynecol 1980; 20(1):10–17.
2. Sims JM. On the treatment of vesico-vagina fistula. Am J Med Sci 1852; 23:59–82.
3. Stothers L, Chopra A, Raz S. Vesicovaginal fistula. In: Raz S, ed. Female Urology. Philadelphia: W.B. Saunders, 1996:490–506.
4. Kreder K. The current trend in vesicovaginal fistula repair. Contemp Urol 1999; 34–43.
5. Thomas K, William G. Medicolegal aspects of vesicovaginal fistulae. Br J Urol 2000; 86:354–359.
6. Rackley RR, Appell RA. Vesicovaginal fistula: current approach. In: AUA Update Series. Houston: AUA Office of Education, 1998:162–167.

7. Carr L, Webster G. Abdominal repair of vesicovaginal fistula. Urology 1996; 48(1):10–11.
8. Salup RR, Julian TB, Liung MD, Narayanan K, Finegold R. Closure of large post-radiation vesico-vaginal fistula with rectus abdominis myofascial flap. Urology 1994; 44(1):130–131.
9. Raghavaiah NV. Double-dye test to diagnose various types of fistulas. J Urol 1974; 112(6):811–812.
10. O'Brien WM, Lynch JH. Simplification of the double-dye test to diagnose various types of vaginal fistulas. Urology 1990; 36(5):456.
11. Persky L, Herman G, Guerrier K. Nondelay in vesicovaginal fistula repair. Urology 1979; 13(3):273–275.
12. Blandy JP, Badenoch DF, Fowler CG, Jenkins BJ, Thomas NWM. Early repair of iatrogenic injury to the ureter or bladder after gynecological surgery. J Urol 1991; 146(3):761–765.
13. Blaivas JG, Heritz DM, Romanzi LJ. Early versus late repair of vesicovaginal fistulas: vaginal and abdominal approaches. J Urol 1995; 153(4):1110–1113.
14. Falk HC, Orkin LA. Nonsurgical closure of vesicovaginal fistulas. Obstet Gynecol 1957; 9(5):538–541.
15. Stovsky MD, Ignatoff JM, Blum MD, Nanninga JB, O'Conor VJ, Kursh ED. Use of electrocoagulation in the treatment of vesicovaginal fistulas. J Urol 1994; 152(5):1443–1444.
16. O'Conor VJ, Sokol JK, Bulkley GJ, Nanninga JB. Suprapubic closure of vesicovaginal fistula. J Urol 1973; 109(1):51–54.
17. Evans DH, Madjar S, Politano VA, Bejany DE, Lynne CM, Grousse AE. Interposition flaps in trans-abdominal vesicovaginal fistula repairs: are they really necessary? Urology 2001; 57(4):670–674.
18. Landes RR. Simple transvesical repair of vesicovaginal fistula. J Urol 1979; 122(5):604–606.
19. Gil-Vernet JM, Gil-Vernet A, Campos JA. New surgical technique for treatment of complex vesico-vaginal fistula. J Urol 1989; 141(3):513–516.
20. Ostad M, Uzzo RG, Coleman J, Young GPH. Use of a free bladder mucosal graft for simple repair of vesicovaginal fistulae. Urology 1998; 52(1):123–126.
21. Von Theobald P, Hamel P, Febbraro W. Laparoscopic repair of a vesicovaginal fistula using an omen-tal J flap. Br J Obstet Gynaecol 1998; 105:1216–1218.
22. Walters W. An omental flap in transperitoneal repair of recurring vesicovaginal fistulas. Surg Gynecol Obstet 1937; 64:74–75.
23. Turner-Warwick RT, Wynne EJC, Handley-Ashken M. The use of the omental pedicle graft in the repair and reconstruction of the urinary tract. Br J Surg 1967; 54(10):849–853.
24. Eisen M, Jurkovic K, Altwein J-E, Schreiter F, Hohenfellner R. Management of vesicovaginal fistulas with peritoneal flap interposition. J Urol 1974; 112(2):195–198.
25. Brandt FT, Lorenzato FR, Albuquerque CD. Treatment of vesicovaginal fistula by bladder mucosa autograft technique. J Am Coll Surg 1998; 186(6):645–648.
26. O'Conor VJ. Review of experience with vesicovaginal fistula repair. J Urol 1980; 123(3):367–369.
27. Bissada NK, McDonald D. Management of giant vesicovaginal and urethrovaginal fistulas. J Urol 1983; 130:1073.
28. Wein AJ, Malloy TR, Carpiniello VL, Greenberg SH, Murphy JJ. Repair of vesicovaginal fistula by a suprapubic transvesical approach. Surg Gynecol Obstet 980; 150:57–60.
29. Leng WW, Amundsen CL, McGuire EJ. Management of female genitourinary fistulas: transvesical or transvaginal approach? J Urol 1998; 160(6):1995–1999.
30. Nesrallah LJ, Srougi M, Gittes RF. The O'Conor technique: the gold standard for supratrigonal vesicovaginal fistula repair. J Urol 1999; 161(2):566–568.
31. Langkilde NC, Pless TK, Lundbeck F, Nerstrom B. Surgical repair of vesicovaginal fistulae: a ten-year retrospective study. Scand J Nephrol 1999; 33:100–103.

55

Urethrovaginal Fistula

John B. Gebhart and Raymond A. Lee
Mayo Clinic and Mayo Clinic College of Medicine, Rochester, Minnesota, U.S.A.

I. INTRODUCTION

The female urethra, because of its well-protected location, is rarely involved in injury. When injury does occur, it is usually related to childbirth or operation (1). Occasionally, the urethra sustains injury from penetrating trauma or undergoes avulsion from pelvic trauma resulting from a motor vehicle accident (2–5). When childbirth results in urethral injury, it is often caused by instrumentation or laceration. Obstructed birth or neglect of the second stage of labor, although not common in developed countries, continues to be a common cause of urethral and vaginal injury in underdeveloped countries (6).

The diagnosis of urethral injury can generally be made on careful inspection, which on occasion may require anesthesia. The integrity of the urethra and bladder neck can be assessed by physical examination and be greatly aided by cystourethroscopy or voiding cystourethrography. If trauma is detected but the urethra is intact, a urethral catheter can be inserted to ensure adequate drainage of the bladder. If a defect is noted, immediate operative repair can be accomplished by reconstructing the urethra, its supporting tissues, and the anterior vaginal wall with interrupted 4-0 delayed absorbable sutures. If there is a delay in diagnosis or there is significant edema, operative repair may be delayed.

II. ETIOLOGY

Prolonged labor continues to be a common cause of destruction of the urethra and the base of the bladder in patients in medically deprived countries (6–9), whereas anterior colporrhaphy and diverticulectomy are leading causes of urethrovaginal fistulas in the United States (10–13). The excision of friable, infected urethral diverticulum can be tedious and inexact (14,15). Despite meticulous efforts to reconstruct the urethral floor accurately, infection and edema may lead to imperfect healing and fistula formation. Overzealous plication of the urethra, inadvertent intramural placement of a suture (vaginal or retropubic needle suspension), or a suburethral sling placed under tension may produce a fistula of the urethra or a greater calamity—actual slough of the entire urethral floor and bladder neck (11). In addition, coital injury, malignancy, and radiation therapy may lead to urethral fistula.

III. CLINICAL PRESENTATION

Patients who experience trauma to the urethra from forceps or vacuum delivery or from auto-
mobile accidents have leakage immediately or within the first 24 h after damage. If a urethral
catheter was in place temporarily, after either delivery or trauma, catheter removal is generally
followed promptly by leakage of urine. In our experience, most urethrovaginal fistulas occur
after an operation for diverticulum or a procedure for cystocele or stress urinary incontinence
(SUI), such as an anterior colporrhaphy or pubovaginal sling. Patients who have undergone
these operations generally have a catheter in place for 2–7 days. Some of these patients may
have an unrecognized suture through the wall of the urethra, which generally results in necrosis
of the tissue and possibly associated hematoma formation or some degree of infection, the combination of which results in fistula formation and leakage of urine. The patient may initially be
continent, only to experience leakage 1–2 weeks postoperatively.

Patients who have had irradiation generally note the leakage sometime after the treatment,
generally within 2–4 months. Occasionally, a fistula develops as the result of long-term pressure
beneath the urethra that results in erosion. This is more likely to occur with synthetic sling
material, but it may occur with any graft material, especially if placed under too great a
tension (16).

Simple urethrovaginal fistula, depending on its location relative to the bladder neck, may
not produce urinary incontinence and may not necessitate operative repair. Fistulas located near
the bladder neck may be technically more difficult to repair. Even after what appears to be a
successful repair, the patient may experience stress urinary incontinence related to fibrosis, fixation, and poor contractility of the urethral musculature. One can consider performing an anti-
incontinence procedure at the time of fistula repair if SUI is also part of the symptom complex
(17). This decision should be individualized, and the consideration of additional procedures
should in no way compromise the success of the primary goal, which is resolution of the fistula.
A more complex problem is presented by patients who had a major slough resulting in a linear
loss of the floor of the urethra and frequently involving the bladder neck and base of the
bladder.

IV. OPERATIVE REPAIR

The basic phases of operative reconstruction consist of a linear incision, much like that for an
anterior colporrhaphy, and mobilization of the vaginal epithelium laterally off the underlying
pubocervical fascia (Fig. 1). This procedure must be accomplished in the proper bloodless tissue
plane sufficiently lateral to establish mobility so that a tension-free closure of the urethra can be
accomplished.

Once the fistula is completely mobilized and the scar tissue (fistula tract) is removed, the
fistula itself is closed with fine 4-0 delayed absorbable sutures placed extramucosally, and the
tissue edges are approximated free of tension and with excellent hemostasis (Fig. 2A). The presence of a small-caliber catheter within the urethra frequently assists in accurate placement of
the sutures to close the fistulous tract. This initial suture line is imbricated with a second set
of sutures, the most distal suture being just distal to the original suture line (Fig. 2B). Snug plication of the bladder neck by approximation, under the urethra, of the tissue (pubocervical
fascia) lateral to the urethra to create a tension-free second layer of sutures is mandatory for
a successful repair. A tension-free closure of the vaginal wall as a third layer (Fig. 3), or
when necessary for the obliteration of dead space and actual replacement of the anterior wall

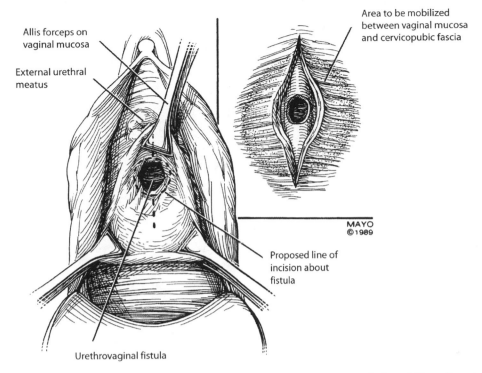

Figure 1 Incision and mobilization of fistula. (From Ref. 18. By permission of Mayo Foundation.)

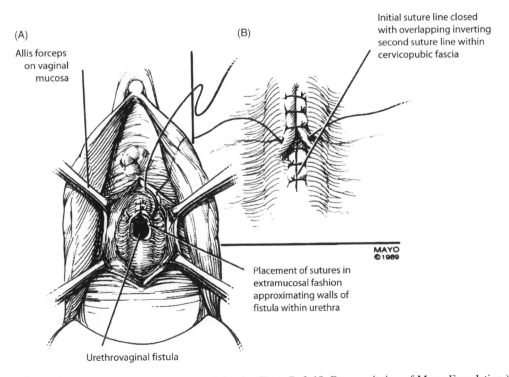

Figure 2 Multilayer closure of incised fistula. (From Ref. 18. By permission of Mayo Foundation.)

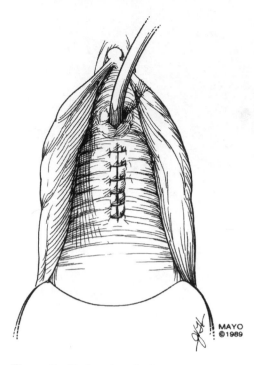

Figure 3   Enclosed vaginal suture line with Foley catheter in place. (From Ref. 18. By permission of Mayo Foundation.)

of the vagina with a pedicled skin, fibrofatty labial graft or Martius labial fat pad graft, may be indicated.

A second-stage retropubic urethrovesical suspension for patients who have a good anatomical result with an apparently intact urethra but who nevertheless remain incontinent (intact urethra with stress incontinence) may be necessary at a later date. Continence often cannot be predicted at the time of closure of the urethral fistula.

V. TRAUMATIC DISRUPTION OF URETHRA

Trauma is an infrequent cause of severe injury to the urethra. When it does occur, surgical repair usually can be undertaken once the patient is stabilized. In Figure 4, the urethra was traumatically disrupted from the bladder during operative vacuum extraction delivery. When catheterization was attempted, the catheter passed through the intact urethral meatus up the intact distal urethra, where it escaped into the vagina. Once the disrupted site was identified, the catheter could be passed through the bladder neck into the bladder. Reconstruction was begun by developing a flap of vaginal wall hinged posteriorly (Fig. 5). The reconstruction of the urethra begins with reanastomosis of the disrupted urethra to the bladder neck, with the initial suture placed in the 12 o'clock position. Each fine delayed absorbable suture is placed in an extramucosal position, reanastomosing the urethra to the bladder neck (Fig. 6). Once the urethra is reconstructed, the vaginal flap is placed in such a way that it avoids overlying suture lines (Fig. 7). A small urethral catheter (10F) is left in place for 5–7 days, after which it is removed and spontaneous voiding occurs.

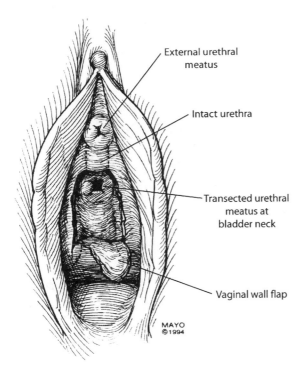

Figure 4   Traumatic disruption of the urethra. (From Ref. 19. By permission of Mayo Foundation.)

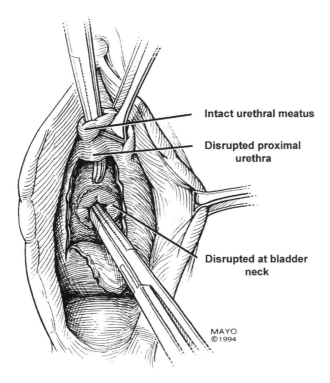

Figure 5   Vaginal flap exposing disrupted urethra at bladder neck. (From Ref. 19. By permission of Mayo Foundation.)

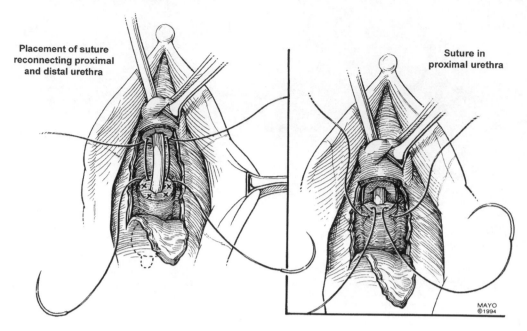

Figure 6 Reconstruction of urethra beginning with first suture at the 12 o'clock position. (From Ref. 19. By permission of Mayo Foundation.)

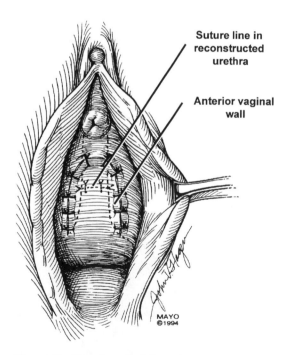

Figure 7 Closed vaginal flap with underlying closed urethra. (From Ref. 19. By permission of Mayo Foundation.)

VI. LINEAR URETHROVAGINAL FISTULA

In patients who have a linear urethrovaginal fistula, urethral reconstruction may be more difficult, and urinary continence, even in what appears to be a well-constructed urethral tube, may not be predictable. The basic principles of the repair are the same as those for simple urethrovaginal fistula. An incision is made in the anterior vaginal mucosa adjacent to the margin of the defect, with wide mobilization of the vaginal wall laterally to, or past, the descending pubic ramus (Fig. 8). The anatomical defect may appear to be rather extensive; however, the actual loss of urethral tissue and muscle may be minimal. The injury results in retraction of the uninvolved musculature into the urethral roof, which is usually intact in affected patients. After the vaginal mucosa is mobilized laterally, a small portion of the roof of the remaining urethra is mobilized in preparation for reconstruction of a new urethral tube (Fig. 9). The remaining urethral roof should provide the patient with a continent (albeit narrow) urethra.

Usually, a No. 8 or No. 10 urethral catheter is placed in the bed of the roof of the urethra; this permits accurate approximation of the freed edges of the roof of the urethra in reconstruction of the tube (Fig. 10A). The sutures are placed in an interrupted fashion with 4-0 delayed absorbable suture positioned extramucosally. This initial suture line reconstructing the urethra is inverted with a second layer approximating the periurethral tissues to aid in support of the initial suture line (Fig. 10B). The third layer of sutures is placed in the cervicopubic fascia to plicate the

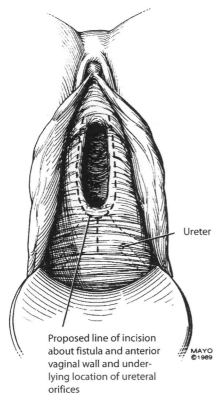

Ureter

Proposed line of incision
about fistula and anterior
vaginal wall and under-
lying location of ureteral
orifices

MAYO
©1989

Figure 8 Proposed line of incision about fistula and anterior vaginal wall. (From Ref. 18. By permission of Mayo Foundation.)

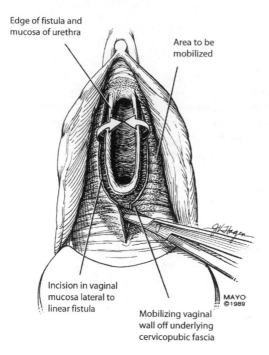

Edge of fistula and
mucosa of urethra

Area to be
mobilized

Incision in vaginal
mucosa lateral to
linear fistula

Mobilizing vaginal
wall off underlying
cervicopubic fascia

Figure 9   Mobilization of vaginal wall. (From Ref. 18. By permission of Mayo Foundation.)

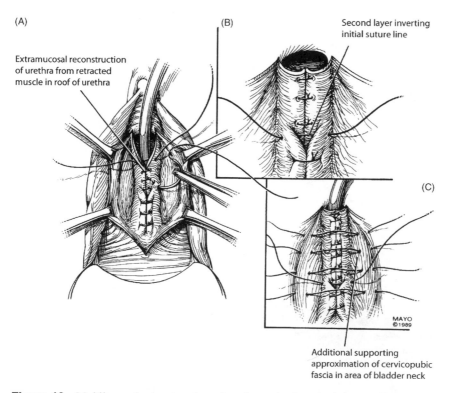

(A)

(B)

Extramucosal reconstruction
of urethra from retracted
muscle in roof of urethra

Second layer inverting
initial suture line

(C)

Additional supporting
approximation of cervicopubic
fascia in area of bladder neck

Figure 10   Multilayered reconstruction of urethra and suburethral tissues. (From Ref. 18. By permission of Mayo Foundation.)

urethra and bladder neck areas further (Fig. 10C). Figure 11A shows the third layer tied and closure of the vaginal wall, which in this case was approximated free of tension (Fig. 11B).

VII. SLOUGH OF URETHRAL FLOOR

In patients who have a slough of the entire floor of the urethra, including the bladder neck and the base of the bladder, reconstruction of a continent urethra may be more difficult. The surgical repair is initiated with a vertical incision in the anterior vaginal wall extending close to either edge of the defect, after which the vaginal mucosa is separated from the underlying cervicopubic fascia far laterally to provide for the possibility of reconstruction of a tension-free urethral tube (Fig. 12).

What later will be the second row of sutures is initially placed under direct vision to permit large, more secure portions of the supporting tissue to be obtained without fear of entering the urethra. The insertion of a finger into the open bladder neck ensures accurate identification and location of the ureters during the snug plication of the bladder neck (Fig. 13). Once these sutures are placed in the supporting tissues, they are tagged laterally.

The urethral tube is reconstructed in the manner already described, and care is taken to approximate the edges of the urethral mucosa accurately without entering the future urethral lumen. These sutures are then tied with a No. 4-0 delayed absorbable suture, after which the previously placed sutures are tied to result in a second layer of closure of the urethra (Fig. 14). If further supporting sutures of the cervicopubic fascia can be placed, this step is also accomplished at this time (Fig. 15).

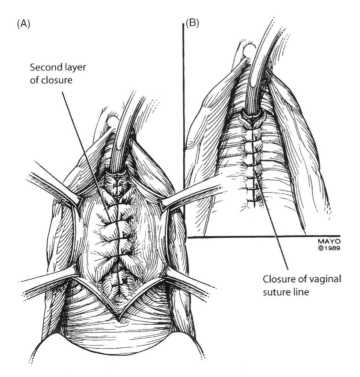

(A)

Second layer
of closure

(B)

MAYO
©1989

Closure of vaginal
suture line

Figure 11   Result with closure of vaginal mucosa. (From Ref. 18. By permission of Mayo Foundation.)

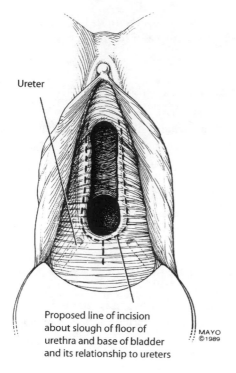

Ureter

Proposed line of incision
about slough of floor of
urethra and base of bladder
and its relationship to ureters

MAYO
©1989

Figure 12   Proposed incision. (From Ref. 18. By permission of Mayo Foundation.)

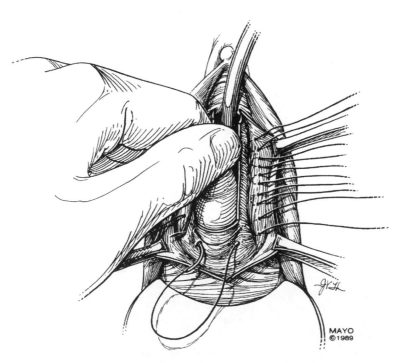

MAYO
©1989

Figure 13   Placement of second (deep) layer of sutures. (From Ref. 18. By permission of Mayo Foundation.)

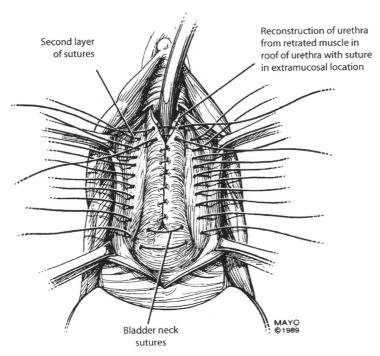

Figure 14 Primary reconstruction of urethral tube. (From Ref. 18. By permission of Mayo Foundation.)

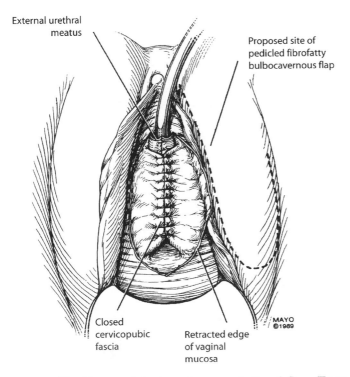

Figure 15 Closure of fascia and proposed site of flap. (From Ref. 18. By permission of Mayo Foundation.)

Occasionally, patients with linear loss of the urethral floor have loss of a significant portion of the anterior vaginal wall, and thus approximation of the wall of the vagina cannot be accomplished without undue tension (Fig. 15). In these cases, the size of the defect is accurately evaluated, and an appropriate tongue of tissue from the labium majus is identified to be incised and swung into the vagina to replace the anterior vaginal wall. This fibrofatty, bulbocavernous flap is usually hinged anteriorly, but it may be hinged posteriorly depending on the nature of the defect. The flap is developed, and the small venous bleeders in the subcutaneous tissues are suture-ligated or cauterized as necessary. The most distal portion of the flap (that deepest into the vagina) is secured initially with full-thickness interrupted 3-0 delayed absorbable sutures (Fig. 16). Care is taken to suture the labial flap to the edge of the vagina in an accurate way to promote primary healing. At the point at which the flap approximates the urethral meatus, it has a tendency to "hide" the meatus and may need to be tailored accordingly.

The site of the graft is closed with an initial layer of subcutaneous sutures, which permits closure of the skin edges of the labium with a No. 4-0 delayed absorbable suture in a tension-free fashion (Fig. 17). A small suction catheter has been placed under the reconstructed urethra. This is brought out through a stab wound laterally and usually is removed in 3–4 days. Despite adequate vesical neck plication and satisfactory elevation and support of the reconstructed urethra, what appears to be an anatomically sound urethra may not provide satisfactory urinary

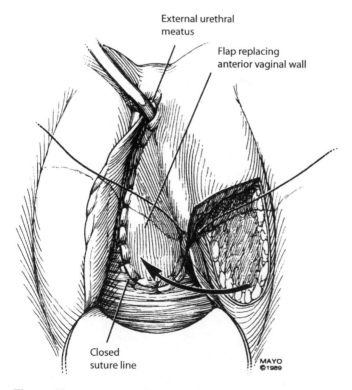

Figure 16   Mobilization of bulbocavernous flap. (From Ref. 18. By permission of Mayo Foundation.)

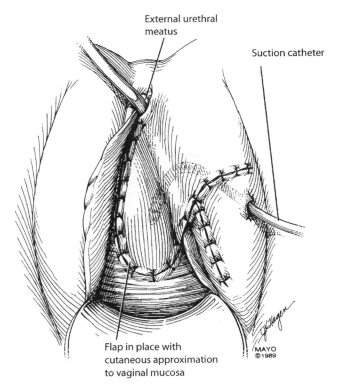

External urethral
meatus

Suction catheter

Flap in place with
cutaneous approximation
to vaginal mucosa

MAYO
©1989

Figure 17   Flap closure. (From Ref. 18. By permission of Mayo Foundation.)

control. In approximately 50% of patients, a delayed second-stage modified Marshall-Marchetti-Krantz type of bladder neck elevation may be required for urinary control.

REFERENCES

1. Lee RA, Symmonds RE, Williams TJ. Current status of genitourinary fistula. Obstet Gynecol 1988; 72:313–319.
2. Hemal AK, Dorairajan LN, Gupta NP. Posttraumatic complete and partial loss of urethra with pelvic fracture in girls: an appraisal of management. J Urol 2000; 163:282–287.
3. Turner-Warwick R. Prevention of complications resulting from pelvic fracture urethral injuries—and from their surgical management. Urol Clin North Am 1989; 16:335–358.
4. Parkhurst JD, Coker JE, Halverstadt DB. Traumatic avulsion of the lower urinary tract in the female child. J Urol 1981; 126:265–267.
5. Podesta ML, Jordan GH. Pelvic fracture urethral injuries in girls. J Urol 2001; 165:1660–1665.
6. Arrowsmith S, Hamlin EC, Wall LL. Obstructed labor injury complex: obstetric fistula formation and the multifaceted morbidity of maternal birth trauma in the developing world. Obstet Gynecol Surv 1996; 51:568–574.
7. Shigui F, Qinge S. Operative treatment of female urinary fistulas. Report of 405 cases. Chin Med J (Engl) 1979; 92:263–268.
8. Vanderputte SR. Obstetric vesicovaginal fistulae. Experience with 89 cases. Ann Soc Belg Med Trop 1985; 65:303–309.

9.   Hamlin RH, Nicholson EC. Reconstruction of urethra totally destroyed in labour. BMJ 1969; 1:147–150.
10. Gray LA. Urethrovaginal fistulas. Am J Obstet Gynecol 1968; 101:28–36.
11. Symmonds RE, Hill LM. Loss of the urethra: a report on 50 patients. Am J Obstet Gynecol 1978; 130:130–138.
12. Carlin BI, Klutke CG. Development of urethrovaginal fistula following periurethral collagen injection. J Urol 2000; 164:124.
13. Guerriero WG. Operative injury to the lower urinary tract. Urol Clin North Am 1985; 12:339–348.
14. Lee RA. Diverticulum of the female urethra: postoperative complications and results. Obstet Gynecol 1983; 61:52–58.
15. Ganabathi K, Leach GE, Zimmern PE, Dmochowski R. Experience with the management of urethral diverticulum in 63 women. J Urol 1994; 152:1445–1452.
16. Kobashi KC, Dmochowski R, Mee SL, Mostwin J, Nitti VW, Zimmern PE, Leach GE. Erosion of woven polyester pubovaginal sling. J Urol 1999; 162:2070–2072.
17. Blaivas JG. Treatment of female incontinence secondary to urethral damage or loss. Urol Clin North Am 1991; 18:355–363.
18. Lee RA. Atlas of Gynecologic Surgery. Philadelphia: W.B. Saunders, 1992: 273–279.
19. Lee RA. Management of genitourinary fistulas. In: Hurt WG, ed. Urogynecologic Surgery. 2nd ed. Philadelphia: Lippincott Williams & Wilkins, 2000:141–148.

56
Female Urethral Diverticula

Sandip P. Vasavada and Raymond R. Rackley
Cleveland Clinic Foundation, Cleveland, Ohio, U.S.A.

I. INTRODUCTION

The first description of a diverticulum of the female urethra was in 1805, and in the subsequent years only sporadic reports were noted (1). In the 1950s there was an increase in the incidence of diagnosis. Davis and Cian noted that as clinicians become more aware of the condition, the frequency of diagnosis increases (2). In one report, the compilation of 121 cases of urethral diverticula was the largest of its time, where 71 cases were diagnosed over 60 years, then a further 50 cases in the following 12 months (3). From this report the notion developed that in order to diagnose female urethral diverticula one must first suspect it. Investigators who described their experience with urethral diverticula stated that in order to identify patients with urethral diverticula, more general awareness of this condition must prevail (4).

Urethral diverticula can be difficult to diagnose; they are often overlooked as a source of recurrent urinary tract infections, chronic pelvic pain, and voiding dysfunction. These patients can be diagnostic challenges. The standard evaluation for all patients with acute and chronic pelvic disorders should include urethral diverticula in the differential diagnosis, so that the diagnosis and ultimate therapy will not be prolonged. Most patients present with a constellation of nonspecific irritative and obstructive voiding symptoms, making the correct diagnosis more challenging to identify; however, suspecting female urethral diverticula may ultimately lead to the correct diagnosis and treatment. It has been shown that there is often a significant delay in the diagnosis of female urethral diverticula in the majority of patients (5–8). Even now, there are likely many women who have had this diagnosis overlooked as a cause for their pelvic disorders, and many of these patients have seen more than one pelvic specialist, either urology or gynecology, for their symptoms. Changes in the standard evaluation of women with complaints of pelvic pain disorders should be instituted, so that with a thorough history, physical exam and appropriately selected radiologic imaging, an exact diagnosis of the correct urethral pathology can be made.

II. INCIDENCE

The true incidence of urethral diverticulum is unknown and the reported incidence varies. The incidence of urethral diverticula was examined in 1967; Andersen showed that of 300 women examined for cervical cancer nine patients were diagnosed with urethral diverticula, an incidence of 3% (9). The estimated incidence in the literature shows that urethral diverticula have been identified in 0.6–6% of women (6,10,11).

III. IDENTIFICATION AND EVALUATION

A. Etiology

The female urethra is a short tubular structure that is surrounded by multiple periurethral ducts and glands, the largest being the Skene's glands that are adjacent to the distal urethra and drain into the meatus (12). Congenital anomalies of the female urethra are quite rare. Infrequently obstructing urethral valves have been identified; more often, an ectopic ureter is identified within the urethra, which may masquerade as a urethral diverticular communication site (12). In one report an ectopic ureter was identified draining into a urethral diverticulum (13).

It is exceptionally rare to identify congenital urethral diverticula; however, suburethral cysts have been identified in the newborn (14). In those few instances, the urethral diverticula have been shown to be remnants of Gartner's ducts cysts, diverticula linked histologically to cloacal rests, and even diverticula confused as a possible urethral duplication (11,15). Nevertheless, the incidence of childhood female urethral diverticula is exceedingly low, and as such urethral diverticula are rarely diagnosed before the age of 20 years (2).

Female urethral diverticula are diagnosed most frequently in the third to fifth decades (6,10,11). Most diverticula are acquired, and a favored hypothesis regarding the etiology of female urethral diverticulum begins in the paraurethral glands. In accordance with anatomic studies by Huffman of the periurethral ducts and glands, most diverticula of the female urethra are located dorsally or laterally and distally (16). Female urethral diverticula are thought to arise from repeated infection, subsequent destruction of the paraurethral glands, and then abscess formation within the periurethral and urethral glands which lie in the mid to distal urethra along the posterolateral wall near the 3 and 9 o'clock positions. These obstructed glands then rupture into the urethral lumen and remain as outpouchings off the urethra, which eventually epithelialize becoming a true urethral diverticulum as opposed to a urethrocele or pseudodiverticulum (7).

Other possibilities to the etiology of female urethral diverticula include the formation of urethral diverticula resulting from obstetric trauma; however, there are significant numbers of diverticula diagnosed in nulliparous women, and urethral diverticula are no more common in women of high parity (2,15). Also cited as a possible source is trauma from urethral instrumentation, and postoperative urethral and vaginal surgery. Another rare, iatrogenic cause for urethral diverticulum has been described after collagen injection therapy for treatment of stress urinary incontinence, resulting in a noncommunicating diverticulum with obstruction of a periurethral gland and persistent accumulation of secretions (17). Noncommunicating urethral diverticula result when the communication site from the urethra to the diverticulum closes off.

Urethral diverticula are urothelial mucosa lined sacs that lie outside the urethra within the periurethral fascia which lack surrounding muscle. They are prone to urine stasis and repeated infections. Inflammation and chronic irritation due to the presence of urine and debris may lead to malignant degeneration into adenocarcinoma (18–24), transitional cell carcinoma (25), or squamous cell carcinoma. More commonly, the stasis of urine causes repeated urinary tract infection and possible calculus formation. Recurrent urinary tract infections are a frequent complaint of women with urethral diverticula, positive urine cultures (>100,000 colony-forming units per milliliter) will often grow strains of *Escherichia coli*, or other gram-negative bacilli, as well as gram positive species, such as *Streptococcus fecalis*. Peters and Vaughn showed that of the 32 women 19 (59%) had culture-proven urinary tract infections, and out of six asymptomatic women with diverticula, four (60%) had significant bacteriuria (26). They also noted an association that urethral diverticula are more common in patients with previous gonococcal infections, which in turn may contribute to its etiology in those women (26).

Urinary stasis may result in the formation of calculi. This has been clearly described before with renal calculi formation in the face of ureteropelvic junction obstruction, bladder calculi secondary to benign prostatic hypertrophy, and now urethral diverticular calculi. Case reports of urethral diverticulum with calculi have been found across all age ranges. A symptomatic pregnant woman was treated with incision and removal of the urethral diverticular calculi as an outpatient (27). A case report of an elderly woman with a firm vaginal mass was due to the presence of a large 5×6 cm stone in a urethral diverticulum (28). As such, calculi in diverticula are rare, with stone formation occurring in about 1.5–10%, usually as a result of stagnate urine, salt deposition, and mucus from the epithelial lining of the diverticula (28).

The location, number, and extent of urethral diverticula have an impact on the choice of treatment. A classification system for female urethral diverticula has been described by Leach, the LNSC3 (location, number, size, configuration, communication, and continence) (29). Providing an accurate description of the diverticulum under evaluation will in turn facilitate its subsequent treatment.

B. Presentation

Women will present to their physicians with a host of symptoms, and regrettably the patient's description of each complaint is not always textbook clear. Therefore, the task is left up to the doctor to identify, evaluate, and treat the pathology. A history of recurrent urinary tract infections, stress urinary incontinence, and incomplete voiding are some of the most common presenting symptoms in women with urethral diverticula (Table 1) (6,8,10,30–35). According to Hoffman, the single most important complaint is postmicturition-dribbling (30), and dysuria and dyspareunia complete the classic triad (11). These are all nonspecific complaints, however if the symptoms are also accompanied by urgency, urge incontinence, frequency, and a protruding vaginal mass, this is then more highly suggestive of a urethral diverticulum. If pus can be

Table 1 Most Common Initial Complaints in Women Who Present for Evaluation and Are Ultimately Found to Have Urethral Diverticula from 1964 to 2000

	Mean (%)	St dev	Range (%)
Recurrent urinary tract infections	47	±25	9–83
Stress urinary incontinence	46	±28	28–100
Incomplete voiding	33	±7	28–38
Dysuria	29	±21	4–58
Urgency	28	±11	18–47
Urge incontinence	27	±14	11–35
Frequency	26	±9	16–38
Postvoid dribbling	21	±22	4–65
Lower abdominal pain	20	±25	1–50
Pus per urethra	18	±28	3–50
Protruding vaginal mass	18	±14	7–17
Dyspareunia	13	±8	1–24
Hematuria	10	±5	5–18
Urine retention	10	±8	3–21
Difficulty voiding	8	±6	2–14

expressed out the meatus with manual compression of the anterior vaginal wall, then this strongly indicates the presence of a urethral diverticulum. Romanzi et al. reviewed their experience with diverse presentations of urethral diverticula and decided that when symptoms mimic other disorders and especially when they do not improve and respond with standard therapy, it is important to entertain the possibility that the source of the pathology is a urethral diverticulum (8).

Patients who have hematuria, difficulty voiding, and even frank urinary retention may have urethral diverticula, as well as a malignancy. In the patient who goes into acute urinary retention without any noted underlying neurologic, myopathic, pharmacologic, or pyschogenic cause, malignancy should be considered until it is excluded. As vertebral disk disease, spinal stenosis, spinal cord injury, transverse myelitis, radical pelvic surgery, postherpes zoster infection, and diabetes mellitus all can result in acute urinary retention in women, anatomic obstruction by carcinoma in a urethral diverticulum causing bladder outlet obstruction may also result in the inability to void.

Commonly patients are given an initial diagnosis after their preliminary evaluation, which is accompanied by the treatment of choice for that suspected condition (Table 2) (5,8,36,37). Many patients receive a variety of treatments that include antibiotics, anticholinergics, antidepressants, bladder hydrodistension, and urethral dilations for suspected pelvic disorders. Some of the more common presumed diagnoses are chronic cystitis, trigonitis, incontinence, vulvovestibulitis, sensory urgency, and psychosomatic disorders. We have seen patients mislabeled as interstitial cystitis/chronic pelvic pain syndrome (38), which carries the heavy burden of a chronic disease, when in fact these patients had true urethral pathology. Hence, the patients may at times express degrees of frustration and lack of hope because their symptoms have been longstanding. Therefore, a high index of suspicion is in order, as several patients may also not be overtly symptomatic upon initial evaluation. In summary, in any case of persistent lower urinary tract symptoms unresponsive to therapy, one should exclude a urethral diverticulum.

Table 2 Initial Diagnoses First Given to Patients and Their Subsequent Treatments Before the Diagnosis of Female Urethral Diverticulum

Diagnosis	Treatment
Chronic cystitis	Antibiotics
Trigonitis	Antibiotics
Cystitis cystica	Antibiotics
Stress urinary incontinence	Anti-incontinence surgery
Urge incontinence	Anticholinergic therapy
Interstitial cystitis	Hydrodistension
Idiopathic pain syndrome	DMSO instillation
	Tricyclic antidepressant therapy
Urethral syndrome	Urethral dilation
Vulvovestibulitis	Vaginal creams
	Antibiotic/antifungal
Cystocele	Surgery
Sensory urgency	Anticholinergics
Psychosomatic disorder	Psychotherapy
	Pharmacotherapy

C. Diagnosis

To establish the correct diagnosis in women with a myriad of symptoms it is critical to perform a thorough history and physical examination. Included in a standard history are questions relating to urinary control for stress urinary incontinence, urgency and urge incontinence, and pad usage. Irritative voiding symptoms such as, frequency, nocturia, urgency, dysuria, urinary tract infections, pyelonephritis, and hematuria should be noted. Obstructive voiding symptoms such as poor urine stream, difficulty voiding, hesitancy, and double voiding should also be noted. A complete obstetric history should be taken, noting the number of pregnancies, live births, and methods of delivery. A neurologic history and bowel patterns should be included in the questions. A complete medication list with allergies, and past medical and surgical histories are also important.

The physical exam should be performed in a warm room, with the patient in a hospital gown. The general exam of neck, thorax, back, and abdomen can be accomplished completely and quickly. A focused genitourinary exam is then performed with the patient in lithotomy position. A warmed half-speculum is gently placed into the vagina to expose the anterior abdominal wall. The urethra and bladder are well visualized, and the patient is asked to Valsalva and cough, performing a supine stress test to evaluation for hypermobility, stress urinary incontinence, and the presence of a cystocele. The cervix and posterior vaginal walls are then inspected, checking for discharge, inflammation, and masses. At this point, palpation of the anterior and posterior vaginal walls is performed. Careful attention is given to palpation of the urethra with attempts to express purulent material via the meatus and evaluation for suburethral masses or tenderness. Postvoid residuals can be accomplished with an office ultrasound, or with a red rubber catheter; the catheterized urine specimen should be sent for urine culture. If the patient had complaints of hematuria and irritative voiding symptoms, a urine cytology should be obtained.

Not all patients will present with a suburethral mass, and not all suburethral masses are urethral diverticula. The differential diagnosis of periurethral masses is extensive and includes: urethral diverticulum, urethrocele, Skene's gland abscess, Gartner's duct cyst, ectopic ureterocele, vaginal wall inclusion cyst, and other, less frequent diagnoses (Table 3) (31,39).

Table 3 Differential Diagnosis of Suburethral Masses

Urethral diverticulum
Urethrocele
Skene's gland abscess
Gartner's duct cyst
Ectopic ureterocele
Vaginal wall inclusion cyst
Urethral carcinoma
Vaginal carcinoma
Vaginal fibroma
Vaginal leiomyoma
Vaginal leiomyosarcoma
Hernangioma
Urethral varices
Endometriosis of the vagina
Sarcoma botryoides
Vaginal wall metastasis

The urethra may be tender, and on occasion a large diverticulum is evident as an anterior wall mass that may express pus and debris from the urethral meatus when compressed. Often, though, the physical exam is normal. Again, suspicions of a urethral carcinoma or calculi arise if a firm mass is palpated along the vaginal wall.

Urinary incontinence may be seen in patients suspected of having a urethral diverticulum. Examination for urethral hypermobility, stress incontinence, and pelvic organ prolapse are documented during the physical examination. Evidence of stress urinary incontinence may require urodynamic testing to assess the abdominal leak point pressure, and to determine a need for a simultaneous sling with the excision of the diverticulum and reconstruction of the urethra (7,32).

One must clinically suspect a urethral diverticulum in order to select the most appropriate procedures and imaging studies. Many patients with urethral diverticula will undergo urodynamic testing to evaluate their complaints of voiding dysfunction. Urodynamics provide information on bladder function, during both the storage and voiding phases, and electromyography (EMG) is utilized during some examinations when there is a history of complex voiding patterns and to assess for the presence of detrusor-sphincter dyssynergia. Not all patients will require urodynamic testing; however, it should be used in patients who have had previous pelvic surgery, recurrent stress urinary incontinence after bladder surgery, and urinary retention without any other known reason.

Urodynamics was performed in a patient who was ultimately diagnosed with a urethral diverticula-containing adenocarcinoma. Clearly, there is an obstructive pattern; from the exam one sees there is very high voiding pressure, and extremely low flow, which is especially noteworthy in a woman (Fig. 1). The bladder capacity was within normal limits with a maximal

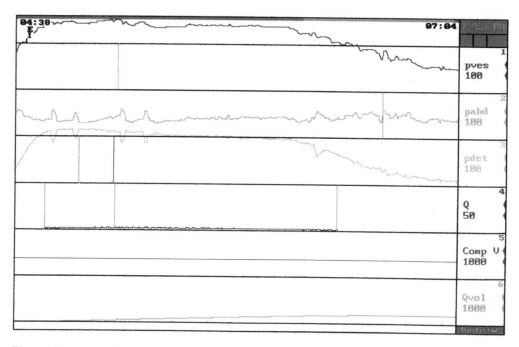

Figure 1   Pressure flow study. Voiding phase: the patient received total infusion volume of 367 cc. The maximum pressure (pDet) was 115 cmH$_2$O. Urinary flow rates were Q maximum, 3 mL/sec, Q average, 2 mL/sec. Pressure flow report shows minimal urination, requiring 97 sec, with extremely high voiding pressures. Cystometry phase of urodynamics not shown (there was no bladder instability).

infused volume of 369 mL, bladder pressures during cystometry showed a low normal pDet of 7 cmH$_2$O and a compliant bladder. The maximum pressure during voiding was 115 cmH$_2$O with a maximum flow rate of 3 mL/sec (Fig. 1).

Urethroscopy may help establish the diagnosis of urethral diverticula, as it is easily performed, has minimal morbidity, and will often produce a high yield of the correct diagnosis in experienced hands. Urethroscopy should be focused on the posterior wall in the 3 and 9 o'clock positions to try to identify the suspected communication sites. Properly performed urethroscopy under anesthesia was shown to be the best method to confirm the presence of a urethal diverticulum (34). In a study by Ganabathi, they were able to identify 53 of the 57 communication sites to the diverticula by cystourethroscopy (31). To supplement the pertinent history, a thorough physical examination, urodynamic testing, cystourethroscopy, and radiologic imaging have clearly enhanced the female urethral diverticular detection rate.

D. Radiologic Imaging

With suspicion of a female urethral diverticulum, the judicious selection of imaging techniques should correctly establish the diagnosis and provide details that aid in surgical excision. Traditionally, the evaluation to confirm the diagnosis of female urethral diverticula was performed with positive pressure urethrography (PPUG) and voiding cystourethrography (VCUG). There are currently several modalities available to identify and characterize female urethral diverticula: PPUG, VCUG, ultrasonography, and magnetic resonance imaging (MRI). There continue to be ongoing controversies as to which modality is the most accurate, while considering parameters such as cost, time, and patient comfort.

1. Positive Pressure Urethrography

In the female, a retrograde urethrogram is performed with a double balloon catheter (Trattner catheter). After catheterizing the urethra, both balloons were inflated with fluid, one inside the bladder, the other on the perineum (12). Contrast was then infused under pressure to fill out the urethral communications, while there was constant traction on the bladder balloon to occlude the bladder neck and prevent contrast from entering the bladder, thus leaving the contrast to exit through the side holes and fill the urethral cavity (12). When performing PPUG, the urethral diverticula were best seen when varying the concentration of contrast in both the proximal and distal balloon and then using undiluted contrast for the urethral injection (40). PPUG, in one study, was found to have the highest accuracy and sensitivity in detecting urethral diverticula when compared to all other imaging modalities (41). While there are diagnostic benefits to PPUG, there is often hesitation in ordering this study secondary to patient discomfort, invasiveness, and infrequent performance in the radiology departments. In another study, MRI was shown to be a more sensitive modality in detecting diverticula when compared to PPUG (42). Out of six patients with urethral diverticula, MRI identified four; however, PPUG identified only one diverticulum (42).

2. VCUG

Historically, voiding cystourethrography has been the radiologic study of choice, as it is easy to perform, and may identify the number and the location of female urethral diverticula. The technique in acquiring the x-ray films is important during a VCUG, for if the initial KUB does not show the inferior pubic rami, it is quite possible to miss the urethral pathology, as the urethra usually falls quite low on the KUB (Fig. 2). To obtain the best study, both lateral and AP (anteroposterior) views of the pelvis during voiding delineate the position and number of diverticula

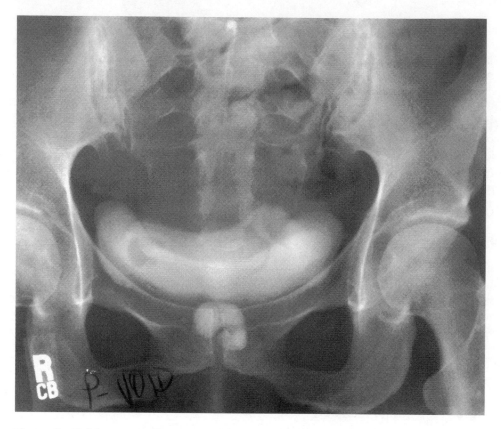

Figure 2   Voiding cystourethrogram demonstrates urethral diverticula. Postvoid film demonstrates urethral diverticula at the level of the pubic bone, as well as a moderate postvoid residual. No abnormalities were noted within the bony structures of the pelvis.

in relation to the urethra. As shown in Figure 3A and 3B, at least three diverticula are observed in the study, noting the position to be inferior to the urethra on the lateral view.

However, the success rates of VCUG vary when compared to PPUG and MRI. Wang reviewed a 3-year experience comparing VCUG and PPUG to evaluate for female urethral diverticula and found that the sensitivity for VCUG was 51.3%, which was significantly lower than with PPUG, sensitivity 84.6% (35). A recent study showed that in 22 of 30 cases the VCUG failed to demonstrate a female urethral diverticulum, but it was seen on PPUG (33). The costs of both tests were noted in the study, and they were found to be quite comparable, within only $5.00 of each other. A comparison between endoluminal MRI and VCUG demonstrated that VCUG missed 7% of the diverticula, and it underestimated their size and complexity (43).

3. Ultrasonography

The sonographic appearance of urethral diverticula was first described using a transabdominal approach (44). Transabdominal ultrasound is not considered an invasive test, and as an imaging modality it is frequently well tolerated. The development of higher-frequency probes and enhanced detection rates lead to the development of endovaginal, and the transperineal approaches. The noninvasive nature of transperineal ultrasound was considered advantageous in using this method as a screening technique for urethral diverticula (45).

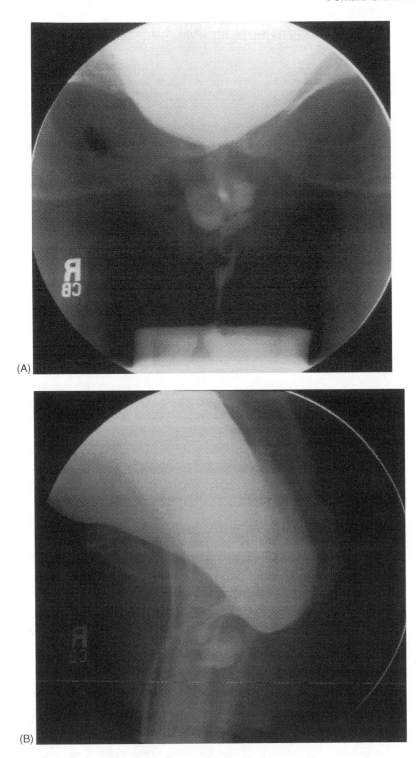

Figure 3 Voiding cystourethrogram demonstrates several urethral diverticula. (A) Anterior/posterior voiding phase view shows three urethral diverticula. (B) Lateral voiding phase view clearly shows the urethral communication to the diverticula and the inferior position of the diverticula in relation to the urethra.

Translabial ultrasonography (46), by placing the transducer against the labia minora and urethra, has also been described as a noninvasive approach to imaging the female urethra. An endorectal 5-MHz transducer has clearly shown the presence of a urethral diverticulum, which may differ from endovaginal transducers that will focus on the uterine neck not the anterior vaginal wall (47). The transperineal approach will be able to view both the sagittal and the coronal planes; however, there is often inadequate visualization of the urethra (47). The transrectal approach may be superior to the others to identify calculi, debris, or filling defects with diverticula. Evaluation of urethral diverticula can be done as a safe, accurate, and relatively inexpensive imaging modality by using the transrectal approach (48). Ultrasonography (transvaginal, transperineal, and endourethral) of urethral diverticula was investigated by Siegel in comparison to detection results with VCUG. Both ultrasound and VCUG identified 13 of the 15 urethral diverticula; however, ultrasonography provided more information on the extent and location of the communication site within the urethra (49).

Intraoperative monitoring can be accomplished with an endoluminal catheter-based ultrasound transducer to provide improved identification of the size, orientation, and characteristics of urethral diverticula and surrounding tissues (50). The endoluminal catheters used were 6F or 9F (12.5 or 20 MHz), and provided a 360-degree transaxial image, and were able to effectively differentiate fluid and solid components (50). The main limitation of ultrasonography as an imaging modality is that it is highly technician and operator dependent.

4. MRI

Magnetic resonance imaging (MRI) of the female urethra is very accurate. Over the previous years MRI has developed several methods by which to image the female urethra. There have been advances in the development of endoluminal (43), endovaginal (37), endorectal (5), and external coils for MRI. All methods clearly distinguish urethral disorders; a standard protocol used extensively requires an external coil, T2-weighted noncontrast study of the pelvis, which does not require premedication, instrumentation, or contrast opacification (51). The urine within the bladder has high signal intensity, bright white on T2-weighted images, and a fluid filled urethral diverticulum will also show a high signal intensity sac, and the soft tissue of the urethra has low signal intensity (52). Midsagittal and axial views (Fig. 4A and 4B) of the pelvis are requested with each study; MRI clearly identifies urethral pathology, which provides a superior examination for surgical planning by accurately delineating the extent of the diverticula (52). Figure 4a demonstrates an example of a large 3-cm "saddlebag" urethral diverticulum with an internal septation, from a MRI in the axial plane (53).

Urethral diverticula may contain debris, infected urine, calculi, and carcinoma. When additional lesions are suspected, tumors show enhancement with intravenous gadolinium (20). The multiplanar capability and excellent soft tissue contrast of MRI allow demonstration of periurethral and diverticular anatomy (54). MRI of urethral diverticular adenocarcinoma is shown in the midsagittal, and axial views of the pelvis (Fig. 5A and 5B) with an enhancing mass in the urethral diverticulum is evident.

Hricak showed that urethral diverticula were identified in all patients with the diagnosis (54). In a comparison of urethroscopy, PPUG and MRI of 20 women with voiding symptoms, MRI was shown to have a better sensitivity, and both positive and negative predictive values (55). Clearly, MRI of the female pelvis provides excellent visualization of urethral diverticula, in addition to identifying other pelvic pathology—for example, pelvic organ prolapse (51). Therefore, at present, MRI is often the procedure of choice for evaluation of suspected urethral diverticula.

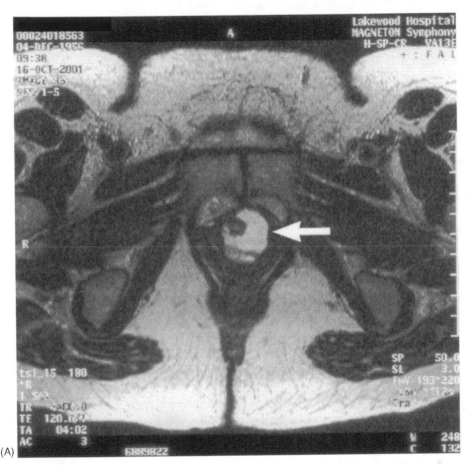

Figure 4   Axial and midsagittal MRI T2-weighted images were obtained through the pelvis. There is a large urethral diverticulum measuring approximately 3.0 × 2.0 × 2.5 cm. (A) Axial MRI shows portions of the diverticulum are seen to surround the urethra (arrow), as a "saddlebag" urethral diverticulum. The urethra has low intensity on MRI T2-weighted noncontrast images. (B) Midsagittal MRI T2-weighted image demonstrates a large urethral diverticulum (arrow) with high signal intensity, and a partially filled bladder with the same signal intensity as the diverticulum.

IV. URETHRAL AND URETHRAL DIVERTICULAR PATHOLOGY

A. Benign

Pathology reports of urethral diverticula most often reveal chronic inflammation within transitional cell epithelium, however, there will be times when other lesions are discovered. Vaginal leiomyoma are rare anterior vaginal wall masses that may mimic urethral diverticula (Table 3), and they may be removed during a vaginal exploration for a presumed urethral diverticulum. Careful histologic examination of the pathology specimen is needed to assure the benign nature of the entity and to rule out leiomyosarcoma (39). Case reports of benign pathology findings within urethral diverticula have shown calculi, Wegener's granulomatosis, and nephrogenic adenoma (56–59).

Nephrogenic adenomas arise from chronic irritation and infection of the transitional cell epithelium, creating a metaplastic response. These are more commonly reported from bladder biopsies in the trigone, posterior or lateral bladder walls, and the bladder dome (59). Histologically,

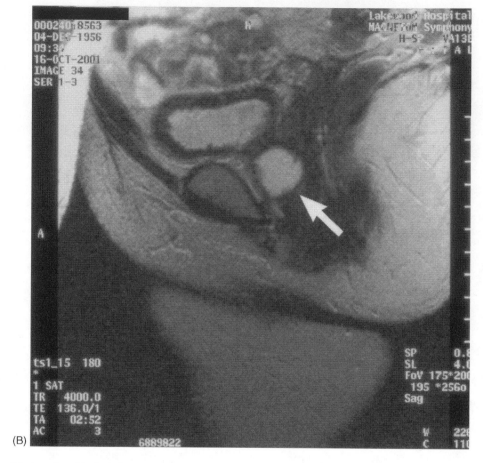

(B)

Figure 4 *Continued.*

nephrogenic adenoma is a benign lesion with no malignant potential, consisting of tubular structures with a single layer of cuboidal and columnar epithelium resembling renal tubules. Nephrogenic adenomas of the bladder will recur in a number of cases.

B. Malignant

Urethral diverticular malignancies are rare in women. Until 1993 only 53 cases had been reported, first in 1951 (24). The histology of malignancy within a urethral diverticulum confirms that adenocarcinoma is the most common (59%) followed by transitional cell carcinoma (30%), and the least common is squamous cell carcinoma (11%) (24). This histological pattern differs from malignancies of the urethra. The predominant cell type of malignancies of the urethra is most commonly squamous cell carcinoma. The most common presenting symptoms of patients with malignancy within a urethral diverticulum are dysuria, frequency, urethral bleeding, and outflow obstruction (Fig. 1).

Imaging of the female urethra is very accurate using MRI. Imaging of urethral adeno carcinoma is often best seen on pelvic MRI with and without intravenous gadolinium (20). T2-weighted images after gadolinium display increased signal intensity and tumors demonstrate enhancement (Fig. 5) (54).

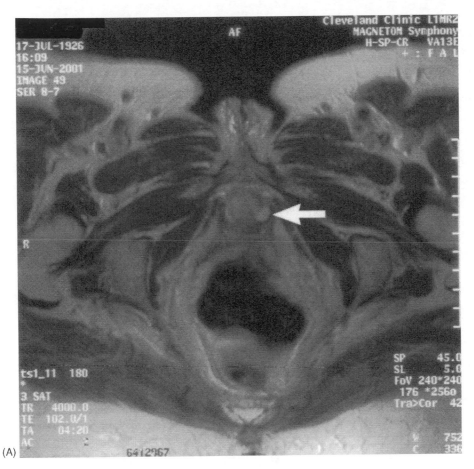

Figure 5 Axial and midsagittal MRI T2-weighted images were obtained through the pelvis. There is a urethral diverticulum with enhancement after intravenous gadolinium. (A) Axial MRI shows a high signal intensity urethral diverticulum (arrow) with an infiltrative central filling defect that enhances with gadolinium. (B) Midsagittal MRI T2-weighted images show a urethral diverticulum with a central filling defect (arrow).

Clear cell adenocarcinoma has been also called "mesonephric carcinoma" because of its morphologic resemblance to clear cell carcinoma of the kidney. Three theories to the origin of urethral diverticular carcinoma are periurethral gland changes, metaplastic changes of the transitional cell epithelium, and embryonic remnants that undergo malignant change (24). The predominance of adenocarcinoma as the most common malignancy in urethral diverticula may best be explained by the diverticula arising from periurethral glands (24). The cells of origin have been more recently studied. The female paraurethral ducts are thought to be embryologically homologous to the male prostate gland and are the likely origin for diverticular cancer of the urethra (60). Immunohistochemical staining analysis of endocrine cells in female paraurethral ducts noted a strongly positive staining for carcinoembryonic antigen (CEA) and a negative result for prostate-specific antigen (PSA). Further analysis revealed that the proximal and distal parts of the paraurethral ducts have different histology and that the cancer cell of origin may be from different parts within the paraurethral duct (61).

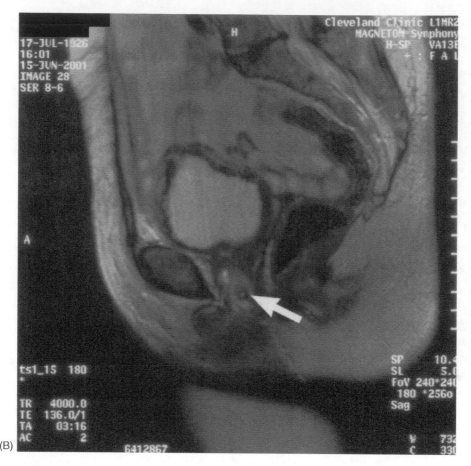

Figure 5   *Continued.*

The therapy of choice for malignancy within a female urethral diverticulum has been to perform an anterior pelvic exenteration (18,19,21–23). It is necessary to remove the bladder, urethra, anterior wall of the vagina, distal ureters, uterus, salpinx, ovaries, and pelvic lymph nodes, as well as create a urinary diversion. The urinary diversion is most often either an ileal conduit or a continent cutaneous diversion. Diverticulectomy alone is inadequate treatment secondary to the high rate of recurrence.

V.   MANAGEMENT OF FEMALE URETHRAL DIVERTICULA

A.   Nonsurgical

A number of patients who do not have significant symptoms from the diverticulum may be followed, treated with antibiotics and anticholinergics, and forego surgery if they remain asymptomatic (31). These small diverticula may be followed with conservative methods, which may include simple observation, manual postvoid decompression, aspiration, or even older methods of diverticular packing or injection therapy (41).

Female urethral diverticula identified during pregnancy should be managed conservatively during the antenatal period. Four cases of urethral diverticulum during pregnancy were all managed nonoperatively; three women underwent aspiration of their diverticulum for treatment of urethral symptoms, and one woman was treated with antibiotics alone, with excision performed postnatally (62). Aspiration can be performed easily using local anesthesia, gently inserting an 18-gauge needle into the diverticulum, and slow aspiration of diverticular fluid with a syringe (62).

Thus, nonsurgical management of urethral diverticula ought to be considered in all patients in whom the risk of surgery might outweigh the benefits, as in pregnancy. Hemorrhage and trauma of surgery in the vaginal and periurethral tissues could lead to wound breakdown, infection, and possible development of urethrovaginal fistula. Surgical management of female urethral diverticula might be best delayed until after the postnatal period, after antibiotic therapy has reduced inflammation, or in patients who are at the greatest risk for postoperative complications.

B. Surgical

1. Historical

The surgical techniques for the treatment of female urethral diverticulum have evolved as the incidence of this diagnosis has increased. Over the years the treatment options for symptomatic urethral diverticula have included incision and drainage with or without packing of the sac, marsupialization into the vagina, endoscopic electrofulgaration of the diverticular sac, and formal transvaginal open excision (10).

In an early technique, Ellik described draining and cleansing the diverticulum via a direct stab incision through the vaginal mucosa, then packing the diverticulum with strips of oxycel until it was a semisolid mass (63). The oxycel would obliterate the cavity and seal the urethral communication by "fibrotic assimilation" (63). The benefits of the technique in 1957 were noted to minimize surgical trauma and operating time, as well as expedite tissue healing and convalescence (63).

2. Marsupialization

Spence and Duckett advocated a "generous meatotomy"(4) to be employed for distal diverticulum, but could result in incontinence if performed in proximal to midurethral diverticula. This treatment was felt to be an effective treatment only for distal urethral diverticula, and required leaving the bladder neck area and proximal urethra completely untouched. The basic surgical technique involved incising along the floor of the urethra from the meatus to the diverticular ostia and trimming redundant tissue and saucerizing the sac into the vagina (4).

3. Endoscopic

Minimally invasive treatment options in the treatment of female urethral diverticula have evolved from cauterization of the exposed urethral wall to transurethral electrocoagulation, always using urethroscopy as an invaluable intraoperative aid to verify the location and number of diverticular ostia. Lapides, using electrocautery for the transurethral incision of the diverticular ostia, was the first to describe endoscopic treatment of urethral diverticula (64). In continued attempts to simplify the treatment of urethral diverticula, the transurethral incision of diverticula using a cold urethrotome in a longitudinal fashion both proximally and distally to widely open the roof of the diverticulum was employed (65). Transurethral diverticulotomy promotes drainage of diverticular contents into the urethra, noting that recurrent urethral diverticula may develop, as this was not considered a definitive cure as transvaginal diverticulectomy.

Transurethral electrocoagulation (34) was performed by insertion of the knife electrode through the diverticular ostia and elevating the resectoscope to invert the diverticula sac; then the tented roof was fulgarated as well as the wall of the diverticulum. This technique reminds us of the endoscopic treatment of bladder diverticula, where the sac is pulled into the bladder and then cauterized. Minimally invasive surgery for the treatment of urethral diverticula using an endoscopic approach is considered safe and effective regardless of the location, and in comparison to formal transvaginal diverticulectomy, has a shorter operative time and less risk of postoperative incontinence and urethrovaginal fistula (64).

4. Excision of Urethral Diverticula

Patients want definitive treatment for their urethral diverticula in most instances, especially patients with significant symptoms. A transvaginal formal excision of the urethral diverticula is our treatment of choice for symptomatic women. During the evaluation of a patient if there is a considerable amount of inflammation and infection, incision and drainage of an infected urethral diverticulum may be needed prior to excision. Also, stress urinary incontinence often coexists with urethral diverticula, and should be evaluated prior to surgery with urodynamics, in order to determine the need for concomitant pubovaginal sling surgery. Urodynamics that reveal detrusor instability may require anticholinergic therapy prior to surgery, to diminish the potential for high-pressure voiding, which could harm a new urethral reconstruction. Once a patient with a urethral diverticulum selects surgical excision, we proceed.

After the patient is prepped and draped a 16F Foley catheter is inserted and the bladder is filled with 200 cc normal saline. A suprapubic tube is placed using a Lowsley retractor through the lower midline anterior abdominal wall, and then placed on gentle traction to avoid irrigation extravasation. The urethral Foley is replaced once the Lowsley is removed, and a Scott ring with hooks and a weighted vaginal speculum is used for retraction. Exposure of the anterior vaginal wall reveals a cystic mass in the midurethra (Figs. 6, 7). An inverted U-incision is outlined with a marking pen, up to near the distal aspect of the urethral diverticulum and just proximal to the urethral meatus (Fig. 8). A prepared solution of 1 : 200,000 lidocaine with epinephrine is injected into the anterior vaginal wall to facilitate dissection and hemostasis.

A flap of the anterior vaginal wall is prepared and carefully dissected with Metzenbaum scissors (Fig. 9). Care should be taken to keep this dissection very superficial over the periurethral fascia, to avoid entrance into the urethral diverticula. The hooks are then advanced to retract the edges of the anterior vaginal wall (Fig. 10). The periurethral fascia should be opened transversally (Figs. 11, 12). It is imperative that the dissection be carried out precisely and that each layer be identified and preserved to assist in later reconstruction of the periurethral fascia and vaginal wall flaps (66). The periurethral fascia is dissected posteriorly, and the distal dissection of this fascia further exposes the wall of the diverticulum (Fig. 13). This dissection is easier while the diverticulum is still full of fluid; a full diverticular sac aids in identification of the edge of the sac and mobilization of the sac off the urethra and surrounding tissues. Another aid in the surgical dissection of a friable urethral diverticulum can be accomplished by placing a pediatric Foley into the diverticula, inflating the balloon, and distending a collapsed diverticula (40).

In an intact urethral diverticulum, the wall of the diverticulum is opened transversely, and a collection of pus and fluid is drained. The lumen of the diverticular sac is seen, and the thick wall of the sac is dissected free from the spongy tissue of the urethral wall (66). The diverticulum is excised flush to the point of entrance of the urethral wall (Fig. 14). The Foley balloon is taken down and the catheter is brought into the urethral lumen and irrigation of the urethra demonstrates the point of communication, the diverticular ostium (Fig. 15). The urethral communication site is identified and closed with fine synthetic absorbable suture in a longitudinal

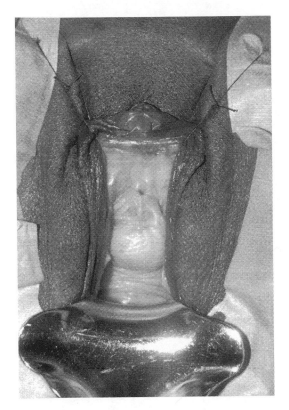

Figure 6 Intraoperative photograph demonstrate a suburethral swelling with labial sutures and a vaginal weighted speculum.

fashion and the periurethral fascia is reconstructed transversely and the sutures are applied in a figure-of-eight fashion and tied individually (Fig. 16). The two flaps of the periurethral fascia and muscular wall of the urethra are identified (Fig. 17). The defect in the periurethral fascia is sutured adjacent to the urethra in a vertical manner to close the dead space and prevent a recurrence of the diverticulum (67,68) (Fig. 18). The periurethral fascia is closed to avoid any overlapping suture lines, which could lead to a dehiscence. The catheter is partially removed and the urethra is irrigated to confirm a watertight closure. The transverse closure of the periurethral fascia and urethral wall has been completed (Fig. 19). If a Martius flap or a vaginal sling is necessary, it may be placed after the closure of the periurethral fascia, with the Martius fat pad graft most superficial, prior to closure of the anterior vaginal wall flap (7,32,69). A Martius labial fat pad graft can be used between the urethra and the vaginal wall when there is absence of adequate periurethral fascia for a second layer or when operating on recurrent diverticula (31,69).

The excess of vaginal wall is excised and the anterior vaginal wall is advanced forward in order to cover the area of the reconstruction. Running a 2-0 synthetic absorbable suture is used to complete the closure of the anterior vaginal wall (Fig. 20). An antibiotic or conjugated estrogen based pack is placed into the vagina, and the urethral and suprapubic catheters are left to gravity drainage.

When the urethral diverticulum is circumferential or a "saddlebag" (Fig. 4), it must be completely excised anterior to the urethra and behind the pubic rami. This dissection can be rather unwieldy, and visualization can be difficult. When a circumferential diverticulum is

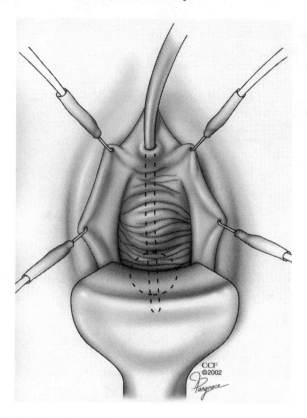

Figure 7   Anatomical representation demonstrates the vaginal exposure obtained with the Scott ring retractor, hooks, weighted speculum, urethral Foley catheter, and the approximate position along the Foley catheter of the urethral diverticulum.

encountered it may be necessary to completely divide the urethra, and excise a segment, in order to expose the dorsal wall of the diverticulum (70). Reconstruction of the urethra requires a tension-free end-to-end anastomosis; if the urethral ends will not meet the dorsal wall of the diverticulum, it can be tubularized to construct a "neourethra."

Surgical excision of female urethral diverticula is the standard therapy in symptomatic patients. Outstanding surgical results require absolute adherence to surgical principles and an understanding of the surgical anatomy of the layers of vaginal wall, periurethral fascia, and urethra. The most important factors in urethral diverticula operative success and avoidance of complications include a watertight anastomosis, precise dissection, anatomical closure of the urethral layers, and nonoverlapping suture lines.

5.   Excision of Urethral Diverticula and Concomitant Bladder Neck Suspension

Urethral diverticula may often present in women who have primary complaints of stress urinary incontinence (71 BASS). Between 28% and 100% (Table 1) of patients may present with bona fide stress urinary incontinence and a coexisting urethral diverticulum. Ganabathi performed transvaginal needle suspension in 48% of patients to treat stress urinary incontinence intraoperatively before proceeding with the urethral diverticular dissection; the needle suspension was performed first to prevent manipulation and compression of the diverticular sac (31). Continence rates from that study show that 45 of 56 (80%) of women were

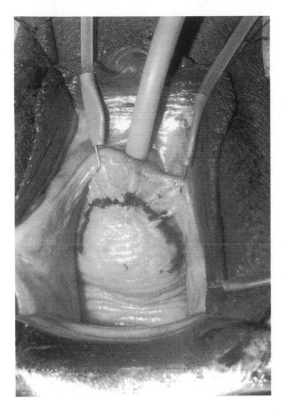

Figure 8   Intraoperative photograph demonstrates the placement of the inverted U-incision.

continent after surgery in those women who had a concomitant needle suspension and urethral diverticulum excision (31). Also reported was that the incontinence cure rate with needle suspension did not show long-lasting results; the recurrent stress incontinence rate was 20% (11/56). A concomitant pubovaginal sling showed improved continence rates postoperatively; Swierzewski showed that all patients were cured of their stress urinary incontinence during follow-up of a mean 17 months (72). Faerber has shown that 16 women were able to successfully perform simultaneous urethral diverticulectomy and pubovaginal sling safely, without erosion and with excellent continence rates (32). Pubovaginal sling can be successfully performed at the time of urethral diverticulectomy in patients with genuine stress incontinence.

6.   Postoperative Care

Patients who undergo surgery for urethal diverticula are discharged the same day as surgery or within 23 h, with both a urethral Foley and a suprapubic tube to gravity drainage. Antibiotics and anticholinergics are used while the catheters remain in place. A VCUG 2 weeks after surgery is obtained to rule out extravasation. If a small amount of extravasation is seen, the urethral Foley is removed and the suprapubic tube remains in place. A repeat VCUG is performed the following week to demonstrate the resolution of extravasation. The suprapubic tube is then plugged and voiding trials begin, until the patient can void with low postvoid residual urine volumes, at which point the suprapubic tube is removed.

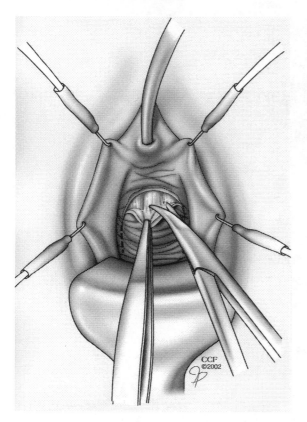

Figure 9 Anatomical representation demonstrates preparation of the anterior vaginal wall flap carefully dissected away from the periurethral fascia.

VI.   COMPLICATIONS

A.   Intraoperative Complications

During surgery it is always possible to encounter the unexpected complication. Most importantly, it is necessary to be prepared for the unexpected, recognize the error, and understand the anatomy; this will help hasten the correction and completion of a successful surgery. Rarely is excessive bleeding noted in vaginal surgery; however, this is usually controlled with judicious use of electrocautery and timely wound closure with vaginal packing for a tamponade effect.

If the urethral diverticulum was large and a large defect is noted in the urethra, this can be difficult to reapproximate. To close the urethral defect it may be necessary to expose more of the urethral wall and suture the edges over a smaller 8F catheter. Incomplete excision of the sac (65) should be noted intraoperatively; the sac would need to be completely excised to prevent recurrence of urethral diverticula or urethrovaginal fistula.

Patients with long-standing urinary tract infections often have diverticula that are significantly inflamed and infected, even if they have been on antibiotic therapy. This often leaves poor-quality tissue for the urethral reconstruction. A vascularized Martius fat pad graft placed between the periurethral fascia and the vaginal wall adds a protective layer, helping to minimize the occurrence of a urethrovaginal fistula (69). If a large periurethral abscess is seen on exploration, a staged procedure may be required. First incision and drainage of the abscess is needed, followed by the urethral diverticulum excision at a later date, after a period of healing.

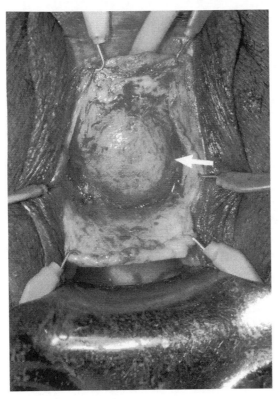

Figure 10 Intraoperative photograph demonstrates the anterior vaginal wall flap held by hooks and exposure of the periurethral fascia overlying the urethral diverticulum (arrow).

Large proximal urethral diverticula may extend into the trigone and bladder neck, which can be rather difficult to excise. The ureters lie in a position along the trigone and then out laterally; it is essential to identify them ahead of periurethral fascial closure. Bladder and ureteral injury can occur and should be recognized promptly and repaired. Intravenous injection of Indigo Carmine will assess both ureteral and bladder integrity (68,73).

B. Postoperative Complications

The most-recognized complications after urethral diverticular surgery are urethrovaginal fistula, urethral diverticula recurrence, and new-onset urinary incontinence. In a review of the literature before 1995, Ganabathi showed the most common postoperative complications were urethrovaginal fistula (mean 4.2%), recurrent diverticulum (mean 12.2%), stress incontinence (mean 8.5%), recurrent urinary tract infections (mean 11.7%), and urethral strictures (mean 2.1%) (31).

The urethrovaginal fistula formation is the most difficult and most dreaded complication of diverticular surgery, and should only be treated after a reasonable period of healing (66), usually 3 months. Inflammation must be reduced before attempted reconstruction to optimize the chance for a successful repair. In revision cases of vaginal surgery a Martius fat pad graft is often used over the repair to improve vascularity and postoperative healing.

Recurrent urethral diverticula have been shown in up to 12% of cases (31). Risk factors include active urethral infection at the time of surgery, difficult dissection, and excessive suture

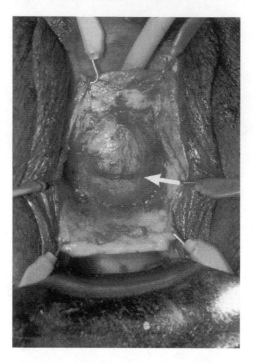

Figure 11   Intraoperative photograph demonstrates the transverse location (arrow) to make the incision of the periurethral fascia overlying the diverticulum.

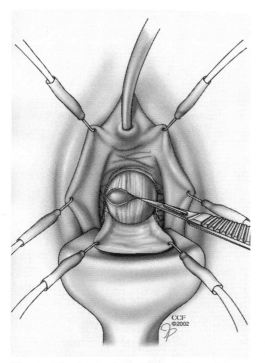

Figure 12   Anatomical representation of the transverse incision using a No. 15 blade to cut one tissue layer over the underlying urethral diverticulum.

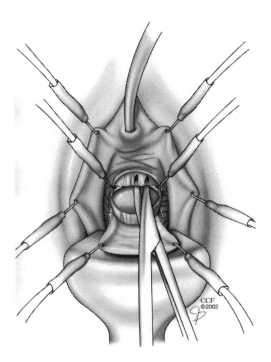

Figure 13   Anatomical representation of the diverticular dissection both proximally and distally with fine Metzenbaum scissors, used to carefully dissect the periurethral fascia off the diverticulum without entering it.

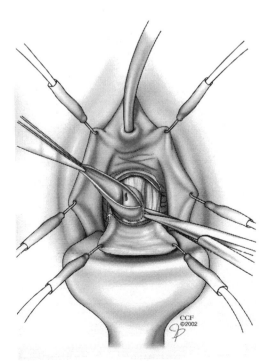

Figure 14   Anatomical representation of urethral diverticular excision flush with the urethral wall.

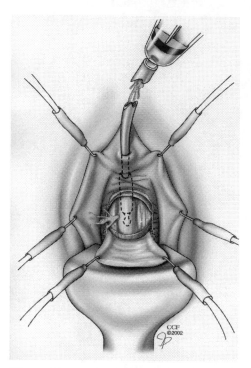

Figure 15 Anatomical representation demonstrating the communication site of the urethral diverticulum by taking down the Foley balloon, withdrawing the catheter into the lumen and flushing the catheter with normal saline.

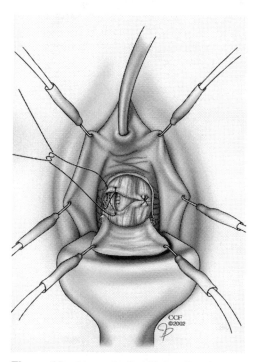

Figure 16 Anatomical representation demonstrates the urethral communication site is sutured using fine absorbable suture in a longitudinal fashion with care to avoid the urethral catheter and closure of the dead space in transverse figure of eight interrupted sutures.

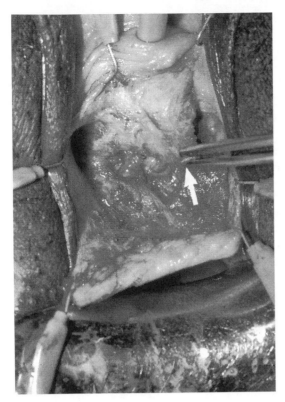

Figure 17 Intraoperative photograph demonstrates identification of the periurethral fascia (arrow) within the forceps in preparation of dead space closure.

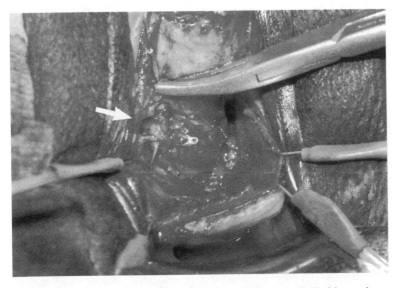

Figure 18 Intraoperative photograph shows Haney needle holder and suture vertically oriented and parallel to the urethra in order to close the adjacent dead space (arrow).

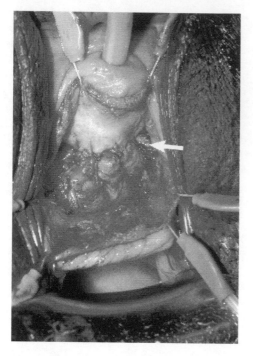

Figure 19 Intraoperative photograph demonstrates completion of the transverse periurethral fascia closure (arrow).

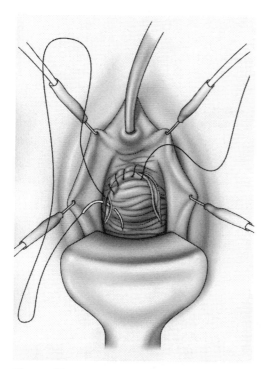

Figure 20 Anatomical representation demonstrates final closure of the anterior vaginal wall flap using running synthetic absorbable suture after excising excess vaginal wall tissue.

line tension. Care must be taken during the primary repair to avoid these risk factors, even if mobilization of the urethra is necessary.

Secondary stress urinary incontinence that was not present before surgery is rare, but may develop in women because of dissection of the urethral support mechanisms. A nonfunctional urethral sphincter mechanism may result in severe incontinence; extensive dissection of the urethral wall causes this damage. Postoperative stress incontinence may require treatment with a subsequent pubovaginal sling or periurethral injection therapy (66).

Once postoperative complications are recognized and identified, proper planning will lead to a cure. It may be necessary to delay a repair in order for tissues to heal from the primary surgery, and prevent subsequent failures. The curative strategy must be conveyed to the patient for her to develop accurate expectations.

VII. SUMMARY

It has been 50 years since T.D. Moore stated, "There is convincing evidence that this lesion is one of those conditions which is found in direct proportion to the avidity with which it is sought" (74). This observation holds true today; the single most important diagnostic instrument for the discovery of female urethral diverticula is a high index of suspicion (3). The key to successful treatment of female urethral diverticula is not only in the surgical management, but also in the identification and evaluation of the patients who present with a myriad of symptoms. Spence and Duckett noted that "recognition of this disorder is particularly gratifying" (4). It is our responsibility to include urethral diverticula in the differential diagnosis when evaluating women that appear to have urethral syndrome, interstitial cystitis, and urgency-frequency syndrome, before these labels are misplaced on these patients. The diagnosis may not be obvious, and the pathology not easily seen on physical exam; however, if the index of suspicion is high and the proper radiologic imaging studies are acquired, then the correct diagnosis will be made.

The evaluation of the female urethral diverticulum has evolved over the past 50 years, yet once the accurate diagnosis is identified, the management is mostly straightforward. Strict adherence to the principles of surgical reconstruction will eradicate the diverticulum and prevent complications and recurrences. The method of identification, evaluation, and management for female urethral diverticulum as well as some of the surgical technical points are described to help accomplish a successful reconstruction and avoid complications.

REFERENCES

1. Hey W. Practical Observations in Surgery. Philadelphia: J. Humphreys, 1805.
2. Davis HJ, Cian LG. Positive pressure urethrography: a new diagnostic method. J Urol 1956; 75:753–757.
3. Davis HJ, TeLinde RW. Urethral diverticula: an assay of 121 cases. J Urol 1958; 80:34–39.
4. Spence HM, Duckett JW. Diverticulum of the female urethra: clinical aspects and presentation of a simple operative technique for cure. J Urol 1970; 104:432–437.
5. Fortunato P, Schettini M, Gallucci M. Diverticula of the female urethra. Br J Urol 1997; 80:628–632.
6. Leng WW, McGuire EJ. Management of female diverticula: a new classification. J Urol 1998; 160:1297–1300.
7. Daneshgari F, Zimmern PE, Jacomides L. Magnetic resonance imaging detection of symptomatic noncommunicating intraurethral wall diverticula in women. J Urol 1999; 161:1259–1261.
8. Romanzi LJ, Groutz A, Blaivas JG. Urethral diverticulum in women: diverse presentations resulting in diagnostic delay and mismanagement. J Urol 2000; 164:428–433.

9. Andersen MJF: The incidence of diverticula in the female urethra. J Urol 1967; 98:96–98.

10. Leach GE, Bavendam TG. Female urethral diverticula. Urology 1987; 30:407–415.

11. Young GPH, Wahle GR, Raz S. Female urethral diverticulum. In: Raz S, ed. *Female Urology.* Philadelphia: W.B. Saunders, 1996:477–489.

12. Yoder IC, Papanicolaou N. Imaging the urethra in men and women. Urol Radiol 1992; 14:24–28.

13. Boyd SD, Raz S. Ectopic ureter presenting in midline urethral diverticulum. Urology 1993; 41:571–574.

14. Glassman TA, Weinerth JL, Glen JF. Neonatal female urethral diverticulum. Urology 1975; 5:249.

15. Bennett SJ. Urethral diverticula. Euro J Obstet Gynecol Reprod Biol 2000; 89:135–139.

16. Huffman JW. The detailed anatomy of the paraurethral ducts in the adult female urethra. Am J Obstet Gynecol 1948; 55:86.

17. Clemens JQ, Bushman W. Urethral diverticulum following transurethral collagen injection. J Urol 2001; 166:626.

18. Collado A, Algaba F, Caparros J. Clear cell adenocarcinoma in a female urethral diverticulum. Scand J Nephrol 2000; 34:136–138.

19. Mai KT, Yazdi HM, Perkins DG. Multicentric clear cell adenocarcinoma in the urinary bladder and the urethral diverticulum: evidence of origin of clear cell adenocarcinoma of the female lower urinary tract from Mullerian duct remnants. Histopathology 2000; 36:380–382.

20. Hickey N, Murphy J, Herschorn S. Carcinoma in a urethral diverticulum: magnetic resonance imaging and sonographic appearance. Urology 2000; 55:588–589.

21. Geisler E, Basu A, Abughaida A. Mesonephric carcinoma arising from a female urethral diverticulum. Br J Urol 1998; 81:637–638.

22. Seballos RM, Rich RR. Clear cell adenocarcinoma arising from a urethral diverticulum. J Urol 1995; 153:1914–1915.

23. Rajan N, Tucci P, Mallouh C. Carcinoma in female urethral diverticulum: case reports and review of management. J Urol 1993; 150:1911–1914.

24. Clayton M, Siami P, Guinan P. Urethral diverticular carcinoma. Cancer 1992; 70:665–670.

25. Catalano S, Jones I. Transitional cell carcinoma in a urethral diverticulum. Aust N Z J Obstet Gynaecol 1992; 32:85–86.

26. Peters WA, Vaughn ED. Urethral diverticulum in the female. Etiologic factors and postoperative results. Obstet Gynecol 1976; 47:549–552.

27. Wittich AC. Excision of urethral diverticulum calculi in a pregnant patient on an outpatient basis. J Am Osteopath Assoc 1997; 97:461–462.

28. Martinez-Maestre A, Gonzalez-Cejudo C, Canada-Pulido E. Giant calculus in a female urethral diverticulum. Int Urogynecol J 2000; 11:45–47.

29. Leach GE, Sirls LT, Ganabathi K. L N S C3: a proposed classification system for female urethral diverticula. Neurourol Urodyn 1993; 12:523–531.

30. Hoffman MJ, Adams WE. Recognition and repair of urethral diverticula. A report of 60 cases. Am J Obstet Gynecol 1965; 92:106–111.

31. Ganabathi K, Leach GE, Zimmern PE. Experience with the management of urethral diverticulum in 63 women. J Urol 1994; 152:1445–1452.

32. Faerber GJ. Urethral diverticulectomy and pubovaginal sling for simultaneous treatment of urethral diverticulum and intrinsic sphincter deficiency. Tech Urol 1998; 4:192–197.

33. Jacoby K, Rowbotham RK. Double balloon positive pressure urethrography is a more sensitive test than voiding cystourethrography for diagnosing urethral diverticulum in women. J Urol 1999; 162:2066–2069.

34. Saito S. Usefulness of diagnosis by the urethroscopy under anesthesia and effect of transurethral electrocoagulation in symptomatic female urethral diverticula. J Endourol 2000; 14:455–457.

35. Wang AC, Wang CR. Radiologic diagnosis and surgical treatment of urethral diverticulum in women. J Reprod Med 2000; 45:377–382.

36. Khati NJ, Javitt MC, Schwartz AM. MR imaging of a urethral diverticulum. Radiographics 1998; 18:517–522.

37. Nuremberg P, Zimmern PE. Role of MR imaging with transrectal coil in the evaluation of complex urethral abnormalities. AJR 1997; 169:1335–1338.

38. Juang CM, Wang PH, Yu KJ. Urethral diverticulum presenting with chronic pelvic pain: a case report. Chin Med J (Taipei) 1999; 62:550–553.

39. Shirvani AR, Winters JC. Vaginal leiomyoma presenting as a urethral diverticulum. J Urol 2000; 163:1869.

40. Kohorn EI, Glickman MG. Technical aids in investigation and management of urethral diverticula in the female. Urology 1992; 40:322–325.

41. Fortunato P, Schettini M, Gallucci M. Diagnosis and therapy of the female urethral diverticula. Int Urogynecol J 2001; 12:51–57.

42. Neitlich JD, Foster HE, Glickman MG. Detection of urethral diverticula in women: comparison of a high resolution fast spin echo technique with double balloon urethrography. J Urol 1998; 159:408–411.

43. Blander DS, Rovner ES, Schnall MD. Endoluminal magnetic resonance imaging in the evaluation of urethral diverticula in women. Urology 2001; 57:660–665.

44. Lee TG, Keller FS. Urethral diverticulum: diagnosis by ultrasound. AJR 1977; 128:690–691.

45. Keefe B, Warshauer DM, Tucker MS. Diverticula of the female urethra: diagnosis by endovaginal and transperineal sonography. AJR 1991; 156:1195–1197.

46. Martensson O, Duchek M. Translabial ultrasonography with pulsed colour-Doppler in the diagnosis of female urethral diverticula. Scand J Urol Nephrol 1994; 28:101–104.

47. Lopez Rasines G, Rico Gutierrez M, Abascal Abascal F. Female urethra diverticula: value of transrectal sonography. J Clin Ultrasound 1996; 24:90–92.

48. Vargas-Serrano B, Cortina-Moreno B, Rodriguez-Romero R. Transrectal ultrasonography in the diagnosis of urethral diverticula in women. J Clin Ultrasound 1997; 25:21–28.

49. Siegel CL, Middleton WD, Teefey SA. Sonography of the female urethra. AJR 1998; 170:1269–1274.

50. Chancellor MB, Liu JB, Rivas DA. Intraoperative endo-luminal ultrasound evaluation of urethral diverticula. J Urol 1995; 153:72–75.

51. Gousse AE, Barbaric ZL, Safir MH. Dynamic half Fournier acquisition, single shot turbo spin-echo magnetic resonance imaging for evaluating the female pelvis. J Urol 2000; 164:1606–1613.

52. Seigelman ES, Banner MP, Ramchandani P. Multicoil MR imaging of symptomatic female urethral and periurethral disease. Radiographics 1997; 17:349–365.

53. Blander DS, Broderick GA, Rovner ES. Magnetic resonance imaging of a "saddle bag" urethral diverticulum. Urology 1999; 53:818–819.

54. Hricak H, Secaf E, Buckley DW. Female urethra: MR imaging. Radiology 1991; 178:527–535.

55. Kim B, Hricak H, Tanagho EA. Diagnosis of urethral diverticula in women: value of MR imaging. AJR 1993; 161:809–815.

56. Ramahi AJ, Richardson DA, Ataya KM. Urethral stones in women. A case report. J Reprod Med 1993; 38:743–746.

57. Goldman HB, Mandell BF, Volk EE. Urethral diverticulum: an unusual presentation of Wegener's granulomatosis. J Urol 1999; 161:917–918.

58. Paik SS, Lee JD. Nephrogenic adenoma arising in an urethral diverticulum. Br J Urol 1997; 80:150.

59. Vargas-Serrano B, Rodriguez-Romero R, Burgos F. Nephrogenic adenoma in urethral diverticulum in a woman. J Clin Ultrasound 1994; 22:268–270.

60. Kato H, Ogihara S, Kobayashi Y. Carcinoembryonic antigen positive adenocarcinoma of a female urethral diverticulum: case report and review of the literature. Int J Urol 1998; 5:291–293.

61. Ogihara S, Kato K. Endocrine cell distribution and expression of tissue associated antigens in human female paraurethral duct: possible clue to the origin of urethral diverticular cancer. Int J Urol 2000; 7:10–15.

62. Moran PA, Carey MP, Dwyer PL. Urethral diverticula in pregnancy. Aust N Z Obstet Gynaecol 1998; 38:102–106.

63. Ellik M. Diverticulum of the female urethra: a new method for ablation. J Urol 1957; 77:243–246.

64. Lapides J. Transurethral treatment of urethral diverticula in women. Trans Am Assoc GU Surg 1979; 70:135.

65. Vergunst H, Blom JHM, De Spiegeleer AHVC. Management of female urethral diverticula by transurethral incision. Br J Urol 1996; 77:745–746.

66. Raz S. *Atlas of Transvaginal Surgery. 2nd ed.* Philadelphia: W.B. Saunders, 2002:269–282.
67. Nezu FM, Vasavada SP. Evaluation and management of urethral diverticula. Tech Urol 2001; 7:169–175.
68. Pallapattu G, Vasavada SP, Comiter CV. Repair of urethral diverticulum. In: Raz S, ed. *Atlas of the Urologic Clinics of North America—Vaginal Surgery.* Baltimore: Williams and Wilkins, 2000:61–70.
69. Leach GE. Urethrovaginal fistula repair with martius labial fat pad graft. Urol Clin North Am 1991; 18:409–413.
70. Rovner ES, Banner M, Ramchandani P. Diagnosis and reconstruction of the circumferential urethral diverticulum [abstract 815]. In: Program Abstracts of the American Urological Association Meeting, Anaheim, 2001. J Urol Suppl 2001; 165:196–197.
71. Bass JS, Leach GE. Surgical treatment of concomitant urethral diverticula and stress incontinence. Urol Clin North Am 1991; 18:365–373.
72. Swierzewski SJ, McGuire EJ. Pubovaginal sling for treatment of female stress urinary incontinence complicated by urethral diverticulum. J Urol 1993; 149:1012–1014.
73. Vasavada SP, Comiter CV, Rovner ES. How to prevent complications in vaginal surgery. J Bras Urol 1999; 25:152–160.
74. Moore TD. Diverticula of female urethra with a new approach at surgical excision. J Urol 1952; 68:611–612.

57

Urethral Reconstruction in Women

Jerry G. Blaivas and Adam J. Flisser
Joan and Sanford Weil College of Medicine, Cornell University, New York, New York, U.S.A.

I. INTRODUCTION

Disorders of the female urethra requiring reconstruction are rare. The most common conditions requiring reconstruction are urethrovaginal fistula, urethral diverticulum, stricture, damage from an indwelling catheter, and neoplasm. Surgical injury to the urethra is relatively rare, generally a complication of urethral diverticulectomy or incontinence surgery (1), and considerably less frequent than iatrogenic injury to the bladder or ureter. Urethrovaginal fistulae develop as a consequence of obstetrical trauma, surgical injury during vaginal and pelvic surgical procedures, erosion of synthetic materials placed near the urethra including synthetic pubovaginal slings and vaginal grafts (2,3), neoplasm, and radiotherapy (4). The diagnosis of urethrovaginal fistula is made by history and physical examination in the majority of cases, but in some instances, particularly when there is erosion of a synthetic pubovaginal sling, it is appreciated only at the time of cystoscopy.

Obstetric injuries are rare in industrial countries, but are not uncommon in the developing world, where access to modern obstetric care is comparatively limited. The overwhelming majority of genitourinary fistulae resulting from obstetric etiologies are due to prolonged labor with compression of the fetal head against the undersurface of the pubis, causing pressure necrosis of the bladder neck and urethra (5,6), and resulting in vesicovaginal, vesicouterine, or ureteral fistulae; urethral fistula is relatively rare. Following this, surgical complications from cesarean section for prolonged, obstructed labor, with or without hysterectomy, are the next most common cause of fistula formation (5,7). Rare causes of fistula related to pregnancy include complications from operative vaginal delivery (8) and suture erosions from Shirodkar cerclage (9).

The most common causes of surgical injury to the urethra include urethral diverticulectomy, bladder neck suspension procedures, anterior colporrhaphy, and, much less commonly, vaginal hysterectomy. In our experience, urethral diverticulectomy is a common cause of urethral compromise (10). This most likely results from failure to obtain a tension-free closure of the urethral defect created by excision of the diverticulum. During bladder neck suspension, an unrecognized injury to the bladder or urethra may occur, or an errant suture may result in tissue necrosis and subsequent fistula formation (11). We have also seen several patients who sustained extensive tissue loss after a seemingly simple Kelly plication; pressure necrosis of the urethra may have resulted from plication sutures that were tied too tightly around a urethral catheter. It is more common for long-term indwelling urethral catheters to cause pressure necrosis of the urethra, particularly in patients who are comatose or paralyzed (12,13).

Rarely, a large urethral diverticulum can cause pressure necrosis of the entire musculofascial structure of the urethra, without any obvious signs or symptoms. MRI may reveal the presence of this problem, but in most cases that we have seen the diagnosis was not apparent until the time of surgery, after the diverticulum had been unroofed to expose a markedly attenuated urethral wall; sometimes the urethral wall is composed of nothing more than mucosa.

Pelvic trauma may result in fracture or separation of the symphysis pubis and laceration of the urethra and/or vesical neck (14–16). There may be local invasion of the urethra or bladder neck from carcinoma of vagina or cervix, or there can be extensive fibrosis of the urethra as a consequence of radiation treatment of adjacent cancers (17). In some patients, urethral abnormalities may not be manifest or apparent for months or even years after the precipitating event (4).

Regardless of the cause of urethral damage, the diagnostic and therapeutic challenges to the surgeon are considerable. The goals of surgical correction are to create a continent urethra of appropriate length that permits the volitional, painless, and unobstructed passage of urine. In our experience, these goals can almost always be accomplished with a single operative procedure.

II. DIAGNOSIS

In most patients the diagnosis is apparent at the time of *vaginal examination*, yet we have been surprised to see many patients in whom urinary leakage has been attributed to sphincteric incontinence alone. This observation underscores the dictum that sphincteric incontinence should not be definitively diagnosed unless an episode of incontinence is witnessed by the examiner. A simple test to remove doubt that the urinary leakage is coming from the urethral meatus is to occlude the meatus with a finger and have the patient cough or strain (with a comfortably full bladder) while downward pressure is exerted on the posterior vaginal wall. This maneuver usually allows visualization of vaginal urinary leakage even when the fistula itself cannot be seen clearly.

Cystoscopy and pelvic examination are essential in order to evaluate (a) the extent of the anatomic defect, (b) the possibility of unrecognized secondary fistulae, (c) the pliability of local tissue, (d) the need for securing bulk-ensuring tissue pedicle flaps, (e) the need for concomitant pelvic reconstructive surgery, and (f) the timing of surgery. Coexisting vesicovaginal fistulae are usually apparent at cystoscopic examination. If a vesicovaginal fistula is suspected but not seen at the time of cystoscopy, a *dye test* can be performed by adding Methylene Blue to the cystoscopy fluid. The vagina should then be inspected for signs of urinary leakage while the urethra is occluded with a Foley balloon catheter.

In many patients, *videourodynamic testing* provides important information about urinary incontinence, as well as the presence or absence of urethral obstruction, low bladder compliance, and detrusor instability. Whenever there is surgical or obstetric damage to the urethra, one must have a high index of suspicion that there are concomitant abnormalities such as vesicovaginal or ureterovaginal fistula, ureteral obstruction, low bladder compliance, vesicoureteral reflux, detrusor instability, or intrinsic sphincteric deficiency. In particular, neither a urethrovaginal fistula nor a destroyed distal urethra causes urinary incontinence unless the proximal urethra and vesical neck are also damaged. Sometimes, when the vesical neck remains intact, there may be loss of the entire remaining portion of the distal urethra without any symptoms at all. These lesions are generally discovered incidentally on physical examination and require no treatment unless they are symptomatic. A careful, logically ordered evaluation is thus essential in all patients to determine the underlying pathophysiology of their incontinence.

Owing to the incidence of complicated occult fistulae in patients who have what appears to be simple pathology, we recommend that *intravenous pyelography* be performed in all patients except those in whom it is medically contraindicated. If ureteral injury is suspected, *retrograde pyelography* should be performed, even in patients with a normal-appearing intravenous pyelogram.

Pelvic fractures may cause lower urinary tract symptoms in women due to sphincteric damage, urethrovaginal fistula, or urethral stricture. The first two conditions are usually apparent on physical examination with a full bladder; the last is suggested by a low *flow rate* and confirmed by cystoscopy and videourodynamic testing.

III. INDICATIONS FOR SURGERY

The mere presence of extensive urethral damage is not an indication for surgery. The two main *relative* indications for reconstruction are sphincteric incontinence and urethral obstruction. If there is an associated condition, such as a vesicovaginal fistula, it should be repaired at the same time. When sphincteric incontinence is present preoperatively, we believe that it should be surgically corrected at the time of urethral reconstruction. In general, we prefer to construct a fascial pubovaginal sling (18, Chaikin, 1998) with an interposed free graft of labial fat (10,18–20) between the sling and the reconstructed vesical neck. Others have recommended transvaginal bladder neck suspension in patients with less extensive anatomic damage and incontinence due to urethral hypermobility (21).

Patients with urethral pathology who also suffer from disorders of detrusor function such as impaired detrusor contractility, detrusor instability, or low bladder compliance, in our experience, have improved after successful surgical repair of their urethral pathology. Accordingly, we do not recommend concomitant surgical intervention to treat these conditions at the time of urethral reconstruction. One exception to this rule is low bladder compliance secondary to radiation cystitis: in these patients, the effects of radiation on the bladder and urethra are usually so severe that reconstructive surgery has a limited chance for success. It is usually best to perform continent supravesical urinary diversion in lieu of urethrovesical reconstruction.

IV. TIMING OF SURGERY AND PREOPERATIVE MANAGEMENT

In the past, much controversy surrounded the timing of surgical repair. While for decades it had been taught that surgery should be delayed for 3–6 months or longer to allow adequate time for tissue inflammation and edema to subside, there are abundant recent studies that suggest surgery can be performed safely as soon as the vaginal wound is free of infection and inflammation and the tissues are reasonably pliable (22–29). It is usually possible to perform the surgical repair within 3–6 weeks after the precipitating event; we have performed one reconstruction as early as 7 days after obstetric trauma.

Management of incontinence during this interim period is often a difficult problem, and in some patients Foley catheter drainage is insufficient. If significant leakage occurs with a Foley catheter in place we generally recommend that the catheter be discontinued and the patient be managed with superabsorbent incontinence pads.

V. GENERAL PRINCIPLES OF SURGICAL TECHNIQUE

Urethral reconstruction is technically demanding and requires a considerable degree of experience and skill. In inexperienced hands the risks may be prohibitive, and in some instances, when there is insufficient local tissue for reconstruction, it may be prudent to consider urinary diversion rather than urethral reconstruction. The most important principles of surgical repair include clear visualization and exposure of the operative site; creation of a tension-free, multiple-layered closure; assurance of an adequate blood supply; and adequate bladder drainage. A tension-free closure can usually be accomplished by wide mobilization of surrounding tissue but sometimes requires the use of local pedicle flaps or relaxing incisions in the anterior vaginal wall. These are the same principles that should be employed to prevent urethral damage and fistula formation after urethral diverticulectomy. We regard a urethral diverticulum as if it were a urethrovaginal fistula that has not yet penetrated the vagina, and repair it accordingly.

In a woman with a damaged urethra, the vaginal tissue is often scarred, fibrotic, and ischemic. Careful examination of the vagina is necessary prior to surgery to determine the actual extent of urethral tissue loss and to assess the availability of local tissue for use in the reconstruction. In most instances sufficient anterior or lateral vaginal wall tissue can be mobilized and rolled into a tube or patch graft for urethral reconstruction (6,10,18,20,21,30,31).

After reconstruction of the urethra it is usually advisable to interpose a well-vascularized pedicle flap over the site of the repair. Various sources of tissue have been successfully used, including the labia majora (18,21,32,33, Symmonds, 1928); rectus abdominus muscle (30,34–38); gracilis myocutaneous (10); and perineal artery axial fasciocutaneous (Singapore) flap (39).

To promote healing and prevent postoperative trauma to the repair site, bladder drainage is best accomplished with a large suprapubic catheter placed at the beginning of the procedure. In addition, we recommend the postoperative use of a urethral catheter as a stent. It is crucial that the catheter be fixed to the anterior abdominal wall using adhesive dressings or sutures, in order to prevent tension on the reconstruction while enabling the catheter to maintain urethral patency.

VI. SURGICAL APPROACH

There are three broad approaches to urethral reconstruction: *anterior bladder flaps* (21,40); *posterior bladder flaps* (41); and *vaginal wall flaps* (6,10,20,30,31). These techniques appear to have comparable success with respect to the creation of a neourethra, but continence is achieved in only ~50% of women who undergo anterior or posterior bladder flaps (21,40,41). We believe that vaginal reconstruction with concomitant anti-incontinence surgery is considerably easier, faster, and associated with much less morbidity than the bladder flap operations, and for that reason we have of late found it unnecessary to employ these operations.

VII. RECONSTRUCTIVE TECHNIQUES

There are four basic techniques for urethral reconstruction: *primary closure*; *lateral tube flaps*; *advancement flaps*; and *labia minora pedicle grafts*. In rare instances it may be necessary to consider a myocutaneous flap, but this has never been necessary in our series.

The patient is placed in the dorsal lithotomy position, and cystourethroscopy is performed to assess the relationship of the ureteral orifices to the damaged urethra. If the ureteral orifices are in close proximity to the fistula, ureteral stents are placed and then removed at the end of the case. A percutaneous suprapubic cystotomy tube (at least 14F) is placed and sewn to the anterior abdominal wall unless a pubovaginal sling is planned, in which case this is deferred until the sling has been harvested. A 16F Foley catheter is inserted into the bladder, and the balloon is inflated with enough fluid to hold it securely at the vesical neck.

The choice of incision depends on the amount of tissue loss and the local anatomy. Before incising the vaginal wall for any concurrent procedures, such as pubovaginal sling, it is critical to select the site and shape of the incisions that will be used for urethral reconstruction. Any incisions will irreversibly determine the location and extent of vascularized vaginal tissue available for the repair. For example, if an inverted U-shaped incision is made in the anterior vaginal wall in anticipation of advancing it to cover the reconstruction, that tissue can no longer be used as an advancement flap for urethral reconstruction should that prove necessary. Alternatively, if the surgeon chooses to make two parallel incisions alongside the intended site of the urethra in order to create a tube graft, it is important to be sure that the distance between the two incisions is sufficient so that the flaps can be closed over the entire circumference of the catheter without any tension.

A. Primary Closure

Successful tension-free primary closure is possible for small urethral defects. The defect is circumscribed widely enough so that the edges of the fistula tract can be approximated in the midline without any tension (Fig. 1). We prefer to close the urethra with 3 : 0 or 4 : 0 chromic catgut rather than longer-acting synthetic absorbable sutures because in our experience the latter are subsequently associated with increased dysuria and pain during urethral instrumentation. Since there is usually insufficient urethral wall tissue to allow approximation without narrowing the urethra, it is rarely possible (or necessary) to excise the fistula tract. A second layer of periurethral tissue is approximated as a horizontal layer whenever possible. Only after the repair has been completed is the decision made regarding how to cover the wound. In some instances it is possible to elevate lateral flaps and suture them in the midline over the wound. Alternatively, an inverted U-shaped incision can be advanced. If a Martius labial fat pad graft is needed, it is prepared prior to closure of the wound (Fig. 2). If a pubovaginal sling is necessary, the fat pad graft is placed between the sling and urethra. The vaginal incision is closed with 2 : 0 or 3 : 0 chromic catgut.

B. Advancement Flap

If lateral flaps cannot be mobilized owing to insufficient vaginal tissue lateral to the urethral pathology, it may be possible to repair the urethra and cover the repair with an advancement flap from the vaginal wall cephalad to the damaged site. A U-incision is made in the anterior vaginal wall long enough to be advanced and rotated to form the posterior and lateral walls of a neourethra (Fig. 3). The flap is mobilized with a Metzenbaum scissors, reflected caudally, and sutured in place over the urethral catheter. The resulting defect in the anterior vaginal wall can sometimes be repaired by undermining the lateral and cranial wound edges, but in some instances pedicle flaps may prove necessary.

C. Tube Graft (Fig. 4)

If there is extensive loss of the urethra and sufficient vaginal wall tissue, a rectangular incision can be made wide enough to allow the vaginal wall to be rolled into a tube over a 16F catheter and sewn in the midline without tension. A Martius flap (or other vascularized graft) and pubovaginal sling are usually necessary to promote successful wound healing and continence. The vaginal wall can be closed primarily, or, if there is insufficient tissue for primary closure, it is usually possible to elevate another broad-based vaginal or labia minora pedicle graft to cover the wound. We have found gracilis myocutaneous and rectus pedicle grafts to be unnecessary.

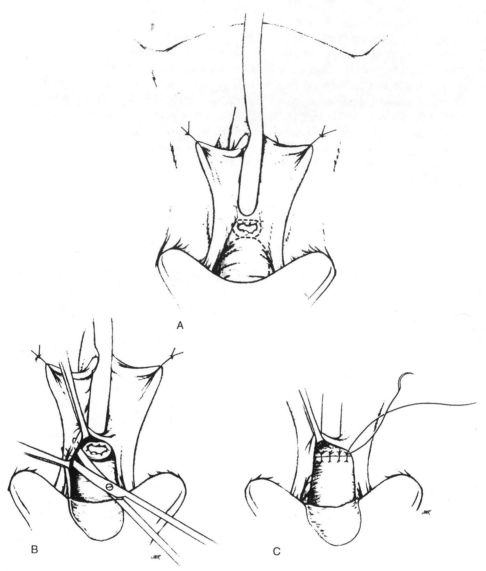

Figure 1   Primary closure of small urethral defect. (A) The small urethral fistula is circumscribed and an inverted "U" incision made. (B) Modified from Blaivas (10) The "U" incision is reflected cranially and laterial flaps created. (C) The fistulae is closed with interrupted 3-0 or 4-0 chromic suture and the U flap closed over the defect.

D.   Labia Minora Pedicle Graft

When there is insufficient local vaginal wall tissue to use for the reconstruction, a labia minora pedicle graft is the next choice. An oval-shaped incision is made in an adjacent hair-free portion of the labia minora as close to the site of the urethra as possible (Fig. 5). The size of the incision should be large enough to roll into a tube around a 16F catheter or to be used as a patch graft over the catheter and allow loose approximation over the catheter. The incision is deepened around the labia and a pedicle graft is raised on an anterior- or posterior-based blood supply. The graft is passed beneath the vaginal wall and rotated so that the mucosal surface forms the inner wall of the reconstructed urethra. In some patients it is not possible to create a tunnel for passage of the graft because of

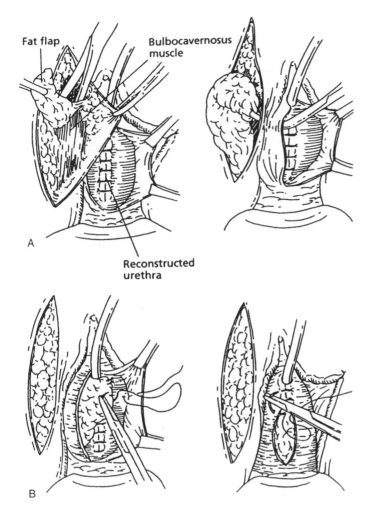

Figure 2 Martius graft. (A) An incision in the labia majora exposes the fat pad, which is freed from its posterior attachments using sharp dissection. A vaginal incision is made in the lateral vaginal wall to provide a passage for the graft. (B) The flap is mobilized through an incision in the lateral vaginal wall and sutured in place over the reconstruction using absorbable suture. The vagina is then closed over the graft. Modified from Rock (48).

extensive scarring, in which case an incision is made in the vaginal wall between the site of the new urethra and the graft. It is usually possible to elevate flaps to cover the graft.

At the conclusion of the reconstructive procedure, the Foley catheter is fixed to the anterior abdominal wall with a gentle loop to insure that undue tension is not placed on the urethra, preventing both traumatic disruption of the repair and pressure necrosis. A Penrose drain should be placed for drainage of the labial harvest sites for the Martius or labia minora flap, if one has been used.

VIII. POSTOPERATIVE CARE

The Penrose drain is removed as soon as there is minimal drainage, usually on the first postoperative day. The urethral wound and catheter are checked frequently to be sure that

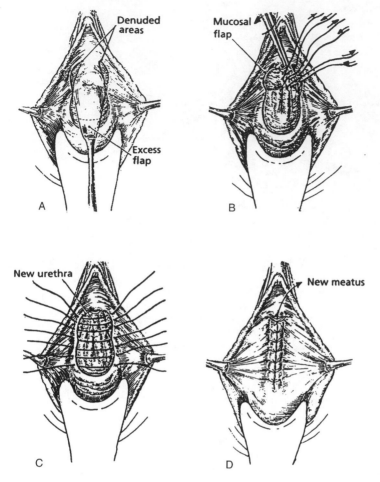

Figure 3 Advancement flap. (A) A U-shaped incision is made in the anterior vaginal wall. (B) The U shaped flap is rotated distally and sutured in place to form the posterior wall of the urethra. (C) The vaginal wall is oversewn using interrupted sutures. (D) The completed repair. Modified from Rock (48).

there is no tension or pressure on the suture line. The urethral catheter is removed as soon as feasible, usually within the first 2–5 days, but always before the patient is discharged from the hospital. A voiding cystourethrogram is performed though the suprapubic catheter on postop day 14. If the patient voids successfully and there is no extravasation, the suprapubic tube is removed. Otherwise, another voiding trial is undertaken 2–4 weeks later.

IX.   ANCILLARY PROCEDURES OFTEN USED WITH URETHRAL RECONSTRUCTION

A.   Pubovaginal Sling (Fig. 6)

A slightly curved transverse lower abdominal incision is made just below the pubic hairline and carried down to the rectus fascia. The surface of the rectus fascia is dissected free of subcutaneous tissue, and a suitable site is selected for excision of the fascial strip that will be used for the sling.

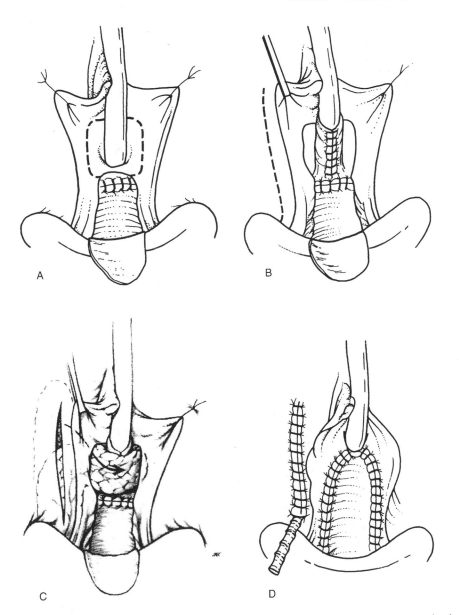

Figure 4 Tube graft. (A) Following mobilization of the vaginal wall, a rectangular incision is made around the urethral meatus. (B) The vaginal wall is rolled into a tubular neourethral over the urethral catheter. (C) Martius graft interposition. (D) The vaginal wall is closed and a Penrose drain is placed in the labial wound. Modified from Blaivas (10).

Two parallel horizontal incisions 2–3 cm apart are made in the midline of the rectus fascia. The incisions are extended superolaterally for the entire width of the wound, following the direction of the fascial fibers. The undersurface of the fascia is freed from muscle and scar. Prior to excising the strip, each end of the fascia is secured with a long 2:0 monofilament nonabsorbable suture using a running horizontal mattress stitch placed at right angles to the direction of the fascial fibers. No attempt is made to mobilize the bladder or vesical neck from above.

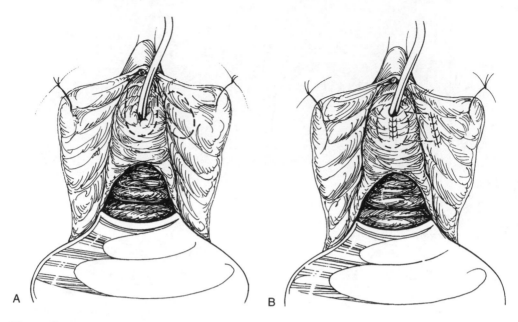

Figure 5 Labia minora flap. (A) An oval-shaped incision is made in the labia minora, which is then reflected medially and sutured over the urethral catheter with chromic suture. (B) The closed labial and urethral operative sites.

Once the appropriate incision for urethral reconstruction has been made in the anterior vaginal wall, the lateral edges of the vaginal wound are grasped with Allis clamps and retracted laterally. The dissection continues just beneath the vaginal epithelium with Metzenbaum scissors pointed in the direction of the patient's ipsilateral shoulder until the periosteum of the pubis or ischium is palpated with the tip of the scissor. During this part of the dissection, it is important to stay as far laterally as possible. This is best accomplished by dissecting with the concavity of the scissors pointing laterally and by exerting constant lateral pressure with the tips of the scissors against the undersurface of the vaginal epithelium. When the periosteum is reached, the endopelvic fascia is perforated and the retropubic space entered. In most instances this is easily accomplished by blunt dissection with the surgeon's index finger. The tip of the finger opposite the nail palpates the periosteum. The bladder and urethra are mobilized medially as the finger advances and perforates the fascia, which frees the vesical neck and proximal urethra from their vaginal attachments. In some instances this dissection must be performed sharply with Metzenbaum scissors.

The surgeon's left index finger is reinserted in the vaginal wound, retracting the vesical neck and bladder medially. The inferior edge of the rectus fascia is grasped with a Kocher clamp, and the right index finger is passed beneath the fascia and slides along the undersurface of the pubis until the two fingers are touching. A long curved clamp (DeBakey) is inserted into the incision and directed to the undersurface of the pubis. The tip of the clamp is pressed against the periosteum and directed toward the index finger that is retracting the vesical neck and bladder medially. In this fashion, the clamp is guided into the vaginal wound. When the tip of the clamp is visible, one end of the long suture, which is attached to the fascial graft, is grasped and pulled into the abdominal wound. The procedure is repeated on the other side. An incision is made in the rectus fascia just above the pubis lateral to the midline on either side just large

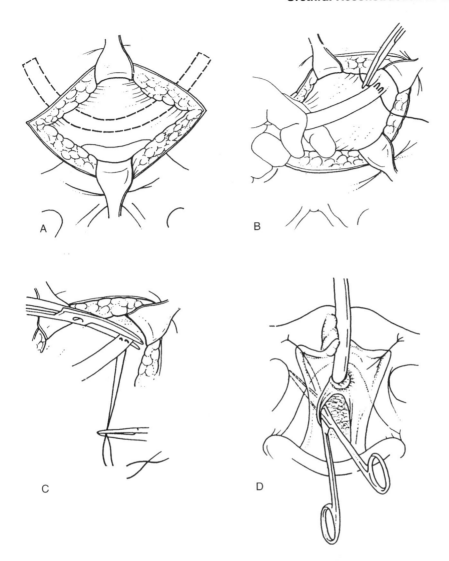

Figure 6   Pubovaginal sling. (A) A Pfannenstiel incision is made exposing the rectus fascia. A 2–3-cm-wide rectus fascial strip is harvested through a Pfannenstiel incision. (B) Prior to harvesting the sling, a 2-0 Prolene suture is placed at the sling margin, securing the end. (C) After the sling is secured with sutures at both ends, the sling is removed. (D) Dissection with a Metzenbaum scissor into the retropubic space opens the avascular plane beneath the vaginal epithelium. Modified from Blaivas (49). *(Continued)*

enough to accept the sling. The long ends of the suture attached to the sling are grasped and pulled through the fascial incisions on either side. The rectus fascia is closed with a running monofilament absorbable 2 : 0 suture. The fascial sling is now positioned from the abdominal wall on one side around the undersurface of the vesical neck and back to the abdominal wall on the other side. At the conclusion of the operation, the long ends of the sling are tied together in the midline over the rectus fascia without any tension at all. The Martius flap is sewn in place between the sling and the reconstructed urethra.

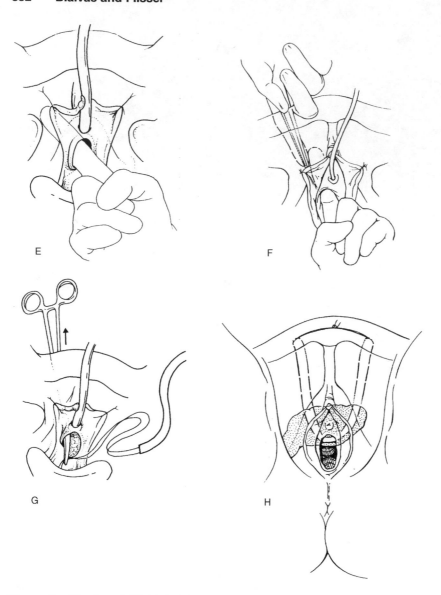

Figure 6   *(Continued)* (E) Digital dissection perforates the retropubic space. (F) Using the vaginal index finger to displace the urethra laterally, a long curved clamp is placed transabdominally onto the lateral aspect of the vaginal finger. (G) The clamp is then threaded into the vagina. (H) The sling is then secured with no tension by tying the sutures superficial to the closed rectus fascia. The sling is placed superficial to the graft, and the vagina is closed directly over the sling.

B.   Martius Flap (Fig. 2)

A vertical incision is made over the labia majora and carried down through Scarpa's fascia. The fat pad is mobilized being careful to preserve the pudendal artery, which arises from the posterior portion of the wound. The fat pad is tunneled underneath the vaginal epithelium and sewn in place over the suture lines of the neourethra. If a single labial fat pad graft does not provide adequate coverage, a second graft may be obtained from the other side or a gracilis, perineal, or rectus pedicle graft may be harvested; in practice, this will rarely be necessary. The pedicle graft is placed between the sling and the reconstructed urethra. The vaginal wall is then closed over the Martius flap.

C. Labia Minora Flap (Fig. 7)

A U-shaped incision is made in the hair-free portion of the labia minora being careful to preserve the posterior and inferior labial blood supply. The fat pad is mobilized and the flap is rotated medially. It may be rotated 180° and used as a patch graft to reconstruct the urethra or left in its anatomic position to cover the vaginal wound.

X. RESULTS

To date there have been few studies concerning reconstruction of the severely damaged urethra (Table 1). Overall, successful anatomic reconstructions were reported in 67–100% of women. Most authors emphasized the need for well-vascularized pedicle flaps to ensure a successful outcome. Continence was achieved in 55–93% after a single operation, and postoperative urethral obstruction was reported in 2–41%. In the great majority of studies, the criteria for incontinence and urethral obstruction were not specified, and, especially in view of lack of follow-up, the results cited above should be considered optimistic. It does seem evident, however, that it is important to perform an anti-incontinence procedure at the same time as the urethral reconstruction. Failure to do so resulted in incontinence rates varying from 50% to 84%. Most reports indicated that secondary procedures to correct incontinence were successful in the majority of patients.

Prior to this report, the largest series of urethral injuries was published by Hamlin and Nicholson (20). All of the women suffered childbirth injuries, and all were quite extensive, usually involving both the urethra and bladder. An excellent anatomic repair was achieved in

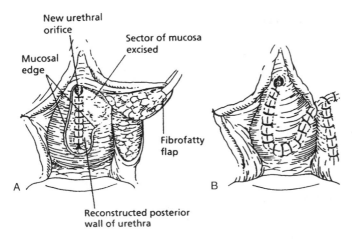

Figure 7 Labia minora flap. (A) A section of the labia minora is mobilized using sharp dissection, and rotated into position to supply the posterior wall of the neourethra. (B) The flap is rotated and the vaginal incisions closed with 3-0 chromic suture.

Table 1 Studies Concerning Reconstruction of Severely Damaged Urethra

Author	Number	Continence (%)	Cure/improved (%)	Anatomic repair	Obstruction (%)
Bruce (34)	6	83	100	100%	0%
Leng (23)	4	75	75	100%	—
Blaivas (10)	49	90	92	96%	2
Tance (42)	34	—	82	82%	—
Elkins (19)	20	50	55	90%	10
Mundy (43)	30	93	—	93%	41
Patel (44)	9	—	78	9/9	0
Morgan, 1978	9	56	89	100%	11
Elkins (30)	6	10	83	67%	17
Hamlin (20)	50	80	84	98%	12
Gray (6)	10	50	50		—
Symmonds (31)	20	65	90	85	—

49 of the 50 women, but eight (16%) had severe incontinence and many more had lesser degrees of incontinence. Incontinence was usually cured after a second procedure.

Elkins et al. (19) reviewed the results of 36 vesicovaginal and/or urethrovaginal fistula repairs performed by American visiting professors in West Africa. All of the vesical neck and urethral fistulas resulted from obstructed labor. In this series, two of 13 proximal urethral fistulas were complicated by "severe stress urinary incontinence" postoperatively. Bazeed et al. (7) reviewed 86 cases of urovaginal fistulae in Egypt, including 13 cases of urethral fistula: two patients had neourethras created, and 11 of 13 were corrected by simple repair, with three failures.

We have operated on 98 women with extensive anatomic vesical neck and urethral defects. The causes of the injury are listed in Table 2. All but one patient underwent a vaginal reconstruction (one patient had a Tanagho anterior bladder flap, which failed). Two patients with squamous cell carcinoma of the distal third of the urethra underwent wide excision and urethral reconstruction with adjacent flaps. We used a Martius flap in all of the remaining patients except one who had a gracilis flap. We have previously published the results of 49 of these women (10). Early in our series, we did not routinely perform concomitant pubovaginal slings, and 50% of the women who underwent a modified Pereyra procedure had persistent sphincteric incontinence; all were subsequently cured by a pubovaginal sling. Three of the remaining women developed sphincteric incontinence; in one patient this was associated with necrosis of the reconstructed urethra. Necrosis of the flap occurred in three patients, one had a previously unrecognized vesicovaginal fistula, and one had urethral obstruction due to the pubovaginal sling. All but one of the failures subsequently underwent reoperation, and all had a successful outcome. No patient required intermittent catheterization, and at 1 year after their last surgery all were dry (except for the one woman who refused reoperation).

XI. BLADDER FLAP TECHNIQUES

We believe that bladder flap reconstructions are almost never necessary in these patients, and the single patient in whom we performed this procedure failed because of refractory detrusor instability; however, these procedures can provide an alternative in patients in whom the extent or location of the urethral pathology discourages a vaginal wall technique.

Table 2 Causes of Urethral Damage in a Case Series of 98 Women

Cause	Number
Transvaginal bladder neck suspension	27
Urethral diverticulectomy	26
Anterior colporraphy	13
Synthetic pubovaginal sling	9
Urethral diverticulum	9
Childbirth	5
Urogenital cancers	5
Trauma	2
Cesarean section	1
Vaginal hysterectomy	1
Total	**98**

Source: Blaivas, 1966.

The basic procedure is depicted in Figure 8 (40). In an extensive series, Elkins et al. (19,21) reported their experience with a Tanagho-like procedure in 20 West African women with extensive urethral damage due to obstructed labor. These patients all had large vesicovaginal fistulas, and because of extensive scarring, were not suitable for vaginal flap techniques. The procedure was performed entirely via a vaginal approach: "The anterior and lateral fistula edges are dissected sharply away from the pubic bone beneath the arch of the pubic ramus, thus entering the retropubic space ... from the vagina ... the anterior bladder wall is dissected free of surrounding tissues to the level of the peritoneal reflection" (21). The anterior bladder was mobilized and a 3 × 3 cm flap was raised and rolled into a tube over a 16F catheter. The new urethra was sutured either to the remaining distal urethra or at the site of the new meatus. The posterior edges of the vesicovaginal fistula were approximated and "fixation sutures (were) placed through the top portion of the neo-urethra to reattach the urethra to the base of the pubic periosteum." In the last three patients a modified Peyrera procedure was performed instead. A Martius fat pad graft was then placed beneath the suture lines.

Eighteen of the 20 women so treated had a satisfactory anatomic repair of the fistula, but four of the 18 had persistent stress incontinence that required further surgery. Two others had refractory detrusor instability or low bladder compliance.

XII. CONCLUSION

Reconstruction of the severely damaged urethra is a technically challenging undertaking that requires considerable surgical expertise. The vast majority of women with traumatic injuries have sufficient vaginal tissue for a vaginal flap reconstruction, and we believe that the vaginal approach offers the best chance for a successful outcome. However, in patients with extensive vaginal scarring from childbirth injuries such as those reported by Elkins, bladder flap techniques may be useful. The most important general principles are (a) adequate exposure of the operative site; (b) careful selection of the vaginal incisions; (c) a tension-free, multiple-layered closure; (d) assurance of an adequate blood supply, through a vascular graft; (e) concomitant pubovaginal sling when anti-incontinence surgery is indicated; (f) adequate bladder drainage; and (g) meticulous attention to catheter care to prevent damage to the repair. Adherence to

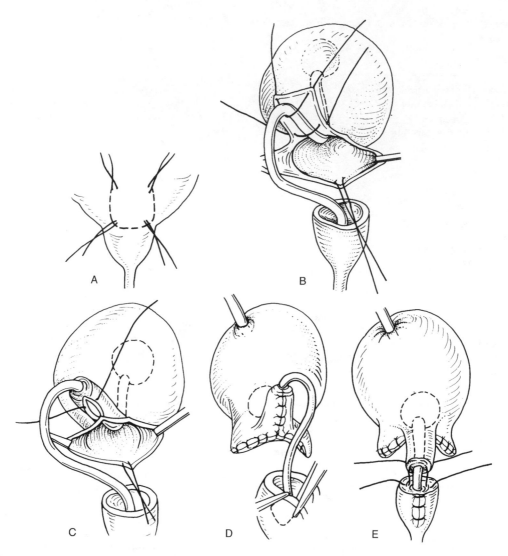

Figure 8 Tanagho procedure. (A) Anterior bladder wall flap is selected, mobilized, and held with suspension sutures. (B) Urethra is transected at site of fistula. (C) The bladder flap is tubularized. (D) The posterior bladder is closed. (E) The neourethra is sutured to the distal urethra.

these principles will substantially increase the chances for a successful reconstruction of the urethra.

REFERENCES

1. Guerriero WG. Operative injury to the urinary tract. Urol Clin North Am 1985; 12(2):339–348.
2. Koelbl H, Stoerer S, Seliger G, Wolters M. Transurethral penetration of a tension-free vaginal tape. Br J Obstet Gynaecol 2001; 108(7):763–765.
3. Madjar S, Tchetgen MB, Van Antwerp A, Abdelmalak J, Rackley RR. Urethral erosion of tension-free vaginal tape. Urology 2002; 59(4):601.

4. Zoubek J, McGuire EJ, Noll F, DeLancey JO. The late occurrence of urinary tract damage in patients successfully treated by radiotherapy for cervical carcinoma. J Urol 1989; 141(6):1347–1349.
5. Danso KA, Martey JOP, Wall LL, Elkins TE. The epidemiology of genitourinary fistulae in Kumasi, Ghana, 1977–1992. Int Urogynecol J 1996; 7:117–120.
6. Gray LA. Urethrovaginal fistulas. Am J Obstet Gynecol 1968; 101:28.
7. Bazeed M, Nabeeh A, El-Kenawy M, Ashamallah A. Urovaginal fistulae: 20 years' experience. Eur Urol 1995; 27:34–38.
8. Tancer ML. Vesicouterine fistula—a review. Obstet Gynecol Surv 1986; 41:743.
9. Golomb J, Ben-Chaim J, Goldwasser B, Korach J, Mashiach S. Conservative treatment of a vesico-cervical fistula resulting from Shirodkar cervical cerclage. J Urol 1993; 149(4):833–834.
10. Blaivas JG. Vaginal flap urethral reconstruction: an alternative to the bladder flap neo-urethra. J Urol 1996; 141:542–545.
11. Dwyer PL, Carey MP, Rosamilia A. Suture injury to the urinary tract in urethral suspension procedures for stress incontinence. Int Urogynecol J 1999; 10:15–21.
12. Chancellor MB, Erhard MH, Kiilholma PJ, Karasick S, Rivas DA. Functional urethral closure with pubovaginal sling for destroyed female urethra after long-term urethral catheterization. Urology 1994; 43(4):499–505.
13. McGuire EJ, Savastano J. Comparative urological outcome in women with spinal cord injury. J Urol 1986; 1335:730–731.
14. Podesta ML, Jordan GH. Pelvic fracture urethral injuries in girls. J Urol 2001; 165:1660–1665.
15. Perry MO, Husmann DA. Urethral injuries in female subjects following pelvic fractures. J Urol 1992; 147:139–143.
16. Armenakis NA, McAninch JW. Anterior urethral trauma. In: McAninch JW, ed. Traumatic and Reconstructive Urology. Philadelphia: W.B. Saunders, 1996:535–550.
17. Boronow RC, Rutledge F. Vesicovaginal fistula, radiation, and gynecologic cancer. Am J Obstet Gynecol 1971; 111:85.
18. Blaivas JG. Female urethral reconstruction. In: Webster G, ed. Reconstructive Urology. Boston: Blackwell Scientific Publications, 1993:873–886.
19. Elkins TE, DeLancey JO, McGuire EJ. The use of modified Martius graft as an adjunctive technique in vesicovaginal and rectovaginal fistula repair. Obstet Gynecol 1990; 75:727–733.
20. Hamlin RHJ, Nicholson EC. Reconstruction of urethra totally destroyed in labor. BMJ 1969; 1:147.
21. Elkins TE, Ghosh TS, Tagoe GA, Stocker R. Transvaginal mobilization and utilization of the anterior bladder wall to repair vesicovaginal fistulas involving the urethra. Obstet Gynecol 1992; 79(3):455–460.
22. Blaivas JG, Heritz DM, Romanzi LJ. Early vs. late repair of vesicovaginal fistulas: vaginal and abdominal approaches. J Urol 1995; 153:1110.
23. Leng WW, Amundsen CL, McGuire EJ. Management of female genitourinary fistulas: transvesical or transvaginal approach? J Urol 1998; 160:1995.
24. Persky L, Herman G, Guerrier K. Nondelay in vesicovaginal fistula repair. Urology 1979; 13:273.
25. Wang Y, Hadley HR. Nondelayed transvaginal repair of high lying vesicovaginal fistulas. J Urol 1990; 144:34.
26. Badenoch DF, Tiptaft RC, Thakar DR, Fowler CG, Blandy JP. Early repair of accidental injury to the ureter or bladder following gynaecological surgery. Br J Urol 1987; 59:516.
27. Cruikshank SH. Early closure of post-hysterectomy vesicovaginal fistulas. South Med J 1988; 81:1525.
28. Raz S, Bregg KJ, Nitti VW, Sussman E. Transvaginal repair of vesicovaginal fistulas using a peritoneal flap. J Urol 1993; 150:56.
29. O'Conor VJ Jr. Repair of vesicovaginal fistula with associated urethral loss. Surg Gynecol Obstet 1978; 146:251.
30. Ellis LR, Hodges CV. Experience with female urethral reconstruction. J Urol 1969; 102:214.
31. Symmonds RE. Loss of the urethral floor with total urinary incontinence: a technique for urethral reconstruction. Am J Obstet Gynecol 1968; 103(3):665–678.

32. Carr LK, Webster GD. Full-thickness cutaneous Martius flaps: a useful technique in female reconstructive urology. Urology 1996; 48:461.
33. Chassagne S, Haab F, Zimmern P. The Martius flap in vaginal surgery: technique and indications. Prog Urol 1997; 7:120.
34. Bruce RG, El-Galley RES, Galloway NTM. Use of rectus abdominis muscle flap for the treatment of complex and refractory urethrovaginal fistulas. J Urol 2000; 163:1212.
35. Fenner GC, Ahn CY, Shaw WW. The use of muscle flaps for coverage of perineal defects. In: Ehrlich RM, Alter GJ, eds. Reconstructive and Plastic Surgery of the External Genitalia: Adult and Pediatric. Philadelphia: W.B. Saunders, 1998:423–435.
36. Tobin GR, Day TG. Vaginal and pelvic reconstruction with distally based rectus abdominis myocutaneous flaps. Plast Reconstr Surg 1988; 81:62.
37. Tobin FR. Pelvic, vaginal and perineal reconstruction in radical pelvic surgery. Surg Oncol Clin North Am 1994; 3:397.
38. Wall LL, Copas P, Galloway NT. Use of pedicled rectus abdominis muscle flap sling in the treatment of complicated stress urinary incontinence. Am J Obstet Gynecol 1996; 175:1460.
39. Zinman L. Use of myocutaneous and muscle interposition flaps in management of radiation-induced vesicovaginal fistula. In: McDougal WS, ed. Difficult Problems in Urologic Surgery. Chicago: Year Book, 1989:143–163.
40. Tanagho EA. Bladder neck reconstruction for total urinary incontinence: 10 years of experience. J Urol 1981; 125:321.
41. Leadbetter GW Jr. Surgical correction of total urinary incontinence. J Urol 1964; 91:261.
42. Tancer ML. A report of thirty-four instances of urethrovaginal and bladder neck fistulas. Surg Gynecol Obstet 1993; 177(1):77–80.
43. Mundy AR. Urethral substitution in women. Br J Urol 1989; 63(1):80–83.
44. Patil U, Waterhouse K, Laungani G. Management of 18 difficult vesicovaginal and urethrovaginal fistulas with modified Ingelman-Sundberg and Martius operations. J Urol 1980; 123:653.
45. Ghoniem GM, Monga M. Modified pubovaginal sling and Martius graft for repair of the recurrent vesicovaginal fistula involving the internal urinary sphincter. Eur Urol 1995; 27:241.
46. Leach GE. Urethrovaginal fistula repair with Martius labial fat pad graft. Urol Clin North Am 1991; 18:409.
47. Webster GD, Sihelnik SA, Stone AR. Urethrovaginal fistula: a review of the surgical management. J Urol 1984; 132:460.
48. Rock JA and Thompson JD, eds. Tc Linde's Operative Gynecology. Philadelphia: JB Lippincott, 1997:1198–1203.
49. Blaivas JG. Pubovaginal Sling Procedure, In: Current Operative Urology, edited by Whitehead ED. JB Lippincott Co., Philadelphia, 93–101, 1990.

58

Radical Cystectomy and Orthotopic Neobladder Substitution in the Female

David A. Ginsberg and John P. Stein
University of Southern California, Los Angeles, California, U.S.A.

I. INTRODUCTION

The primary mode of therapy for muscle-invasive bladder cancer is radical cystectomy and lower urinary tract reconstruction. Over the past several decades numerous advances in chemotherapy, intravesical immunotherapy, and bladder preservation protocols have been identified in the treatment of bladder cancer. However, none of these treatment modalities are able to achieve the survival rates of primary surgical management in the patient with invasive bladder cancer. As we enter the 21st century, urinary diversion after radial cystectomy has reached a new era. The ultimate goal of lower urinary tract reconstruction has become not only a means to divert urine and protect the upper urinary tract, but also to provide patients a continent means to store urine and allow for volitional voiding through the intact native urethra. These advances in urinary diversion have been made in an effort to provide patients a more normal lifestyle and positive self-image following cystectomy. In addition, these advances have lessened the impact of surgery and allowed for a more aggressive approach in patients with higher grade (but less invasive) lesions as well as patients with carcinoma in situ refractory to intravesical therapy.

Transitional cell carcinoma (TCC) of the bladder is the second most common malignancy and cause of death of all genitourinary tumors. Although bladder cancer is more common in men (ratio of 2.7 : 1), it continues to be a considerable source of morbidity and mortality in women. Approximately 75–85% of patients with primary TCC of the bladder present with low grade tumors, superficial tumors. Up to 75% of these superficial tumors recur, but the majority are amenable to repeat transurethral resection and selected administration of intravesical immuno- or chemotherapy as needed (1–3).

However, 20–40% of all patients with transitional cell carcinoma of the bladder will either initially present with, or develop, an invasive carcinoma of the bladder. Invasive bladder cancer includes a spectrum of tumors. Traditionally, tumor invasion of the bladder muscularis has been the primary indication for aggressive surgical therapy. In addition, there is sufficient evidence to suggest that high-grade tumors that invade the lamina propria (T1), superficial bladder tumors with lymphovascular invasion (4,5), and lesions that are associated with carcinoma in situ (6,7) in conjunction with a poor response to repeated transurethral resection and intravesical therapy (8) are also at high risk for progression (3,4,8–13) and warrant an early aggressive management.

Radical cystectomy provides the optimal result with regard to accurate pathologic staging, prevention of local recurrence, and overall survival in both male and female patients. Improvements in medical, surgical, and anesthetic techniques over the past several decades have dramatically decreased the morbidity and mortality associated with radical cystectomy. Prior to 1970, the perioperative complication rate of radical cystectomy was reportedly close to 35%, with a mortality rate of nearly 20%. This has dramatically diminished to a <10% complication rate and 2% mortality rate reported in contemporary series (2).

In addition, efforts have been made to provide an acceptable and functional form of urinary diversion in women without compromise of a sound cancer operation. Two important criteria must be fulfilled when considering any patient for orthotopic urinary diversion. First, under no circumstance must the cancer operation be compromised by the reconstruction at the urethroenteric anastomosis, retained urethra, or surgical margins. Second, the distal urethral sphincteric mechanism must remain intact to provide a continent means of storing urine. If these criteria can safely be maintained, the patient may then be considered an appropriate candidate for orthotopic urinary diversion. We have pathologically demonstrated that the urethra can be safely preserved in the majority of women with transitional cell carcinoma of the bladder (14). Sound pathologic criteria in which to safely select appropriate female candidates for orthotopic reconstruction following cystectomy and has been confirmed by others as well (15). Currently, intraoperative frozen section of the proximal urethra is the most decisive method to determine if a female patient may be an appropriate candidate for orthotopic diversion. It should also be noted that the specific histopathological type of tumor did not preclude orthotopic diversion as long as the aforementioned criteria for orthotopic reconstruction were maintained.

The initial clinical and functional results with this form of diversion in women have been excellent (16–18). Orthotopic urinary diversion most closely resembles the original bladder in both location and function, provides a continent means to store urine, and allows volitional voiding per urethra. This chapter will focus on the technique of radical cystectomy and orthotopic diversion in the female patient with particular emphasis in the surgical preparation of the urethra in women considering orthotopic diversion.

II. DEFINITION

Radical cystectomy (anterior exenteration) in women implies the en bloc removal of the pelvic organs anterior to the rectum. This includes the bladder, urachus, ovaries, Fallopian tubes, uterus, cervix, vaginal cuff, and the anterior pelvic peritoneum. The perivesical fat and pelvic and iliac lymph nodes are also removed en bloc with the specimen. Certain issues regarding the surgical technique of a radical cystectomy in women are critical in order to minimize local recurrence and positive surgical margins, maximize cancer-specific survival, maintain the remaining urethral sphincteric mechanism, and optimize postoperative urinary continence.

III. PREOPERATIVE EVALUATION

The complete evaluation, clinical staging, and decision-making process regarding bladder cancer is beyond the scope of this chapter. Important points for the female patient in whom you are considering orthotopic reconstruction at the time of radical cystectomy include exclusion of tumor involving the anterior vaginal wall and bladder neck. If bimanual exam reveals a deeply invasive posterior lesion with involvement of the anterior vaginal wall, the bladder and tumor mass should be removed en bloc with the anterior vaginal wall. This may require vaginal reconstruction if sexual function is desired postoperatively. In addition, women with tumor involving the anterior vaginal wall are at increased risk of urethral tumor involvement, precluding orthotopic urinary diversion (14).

Furthermore, all women should undergo cystoscopic evaluation of the bladder neck (vesico-urethral junction) as tumor involvement here may also preclude orthotopic reconstruction (14,18). However, we do not recommend routine preoperative biopsy of this region unless there is a significant suspicion for tumor because of the potential risk of injuring the continence mechanism. With a confirmed method to reliably evaluate the proximal urethra (intraopera-tively), we now rely on intraoperative frozen section analysis of the proximal urethra for proper patient selection in women considering orthotopic lower urinary tract reconstruction.

IV. SURGICAL TECHNIQUE

A. Preoperative Preparation

Women undergoing radical cystectomy are admitted the morning prior to surgery for a mechan-ical and antibacterial bowel preparation and intravenous hydration, and to be evaluated and counseled by the enterostomal therapy nurse. A clear liquid diet may be consumed until mid-night, at which time the patient takes nothing per mouth. A standard modified Nichols bowel prep (19) is initiated the morning of admission: 120 mL of Neoloid per mouth at 9:00 AM; 1 g of neomycin per mouth at 10:00 AM, 11:00 AM, 12:00 PM, 1:00 PM, 4:00 PM, 8:00 PM, and 12:00 AM; and 1 g of erythromycin base per mouth at 12:00 PM, 4:00 PM, 8:00 PM, and 12:00 AM. This regimen is well tolerated, obviates the need for enemas, and maintains nutritional and hydrational support. Intravenous crystalloid fluid hydration is begun in the evening prior to surgery, and maintained to ensure an adequate circulating volume as the patient enters the operating room. Intravenous broad-spectrum antibiotics are administered en route to the operating room, providing adequate tissue and circulating levels at the time of incision.

Preoperative evaluation and counseling by the enterostomal therapy nurse is a critical component to the successful care of all patients undergoing cystectomy and urinary diversion. Currently, >85% of female patients requiring cystectomy for bladder cancer undergo orthotopic diversion at our institution (18). Women who are determined to be appropriate candidates for ortho-topic reconstruction are instructed how to catheterize per urethra should it be necessary postopera-tively. Furthermore, all patients are site marked for a cutaneous stoma, instructed in the care of a cutaneous diversion (continent or incontinent form), and instructed in proper catheterization tech-niques should medical or technical factors preclude orthotopic reconstruction. The cutaneous stoma site is determined only after the patient is examined in the supine, sitting, and standing positions.

B. Patient Positioning

The patient is placed in the hyperextended supine position with the iliac crest located just below the fulcrum of the operating table. All female patients considering orthotopic diversion should have their legs placed in the modified frog-leg position, which allows easy access to the vagina (Fig. 1). Care should be taken to ensure that all pressure points are well padded. Reverse Trendelenberg position levels the abdomen parallel with the floor. The vagina is included in the prep as to allow for intraoperative access. After the patient is draped, a 20F Foley catheter is placed in the bladder, and left open to gravity.

C. Incision

A vertical midline incision is made extending from the pubic symphysis to the cephalad aspect of the epigastrium. The incision should be carried lateral to the umbilicus on the contralateral

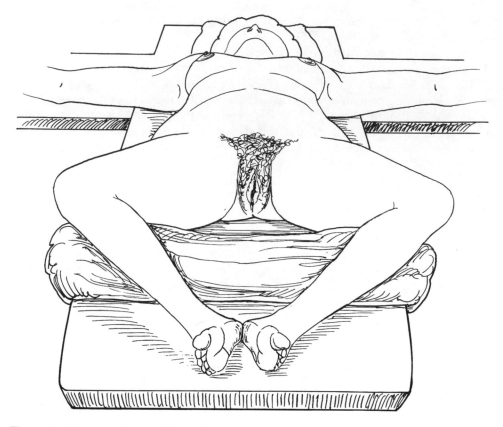

Figure 1   Proper patient positioning for a women undergoing cystectomy. The iliac crest should be located at the break of the table with the patient in the modified frog-leg position. (From Stein JP Skinner DG. Radical cystectomy in women. Atlas Urol Clin 1997; 5(2):37–64.)

side of the marked cutaneous stoma site. The anterior rectus fascia is incised, the rectus muscles are retracted laterally, and the posterior rectus sheath and peritoneum are entered in the superior aspect of the incision. As the peritoneum and posterior fascia are incised inferiorly to the level of the umbilicus, the urachal remnant (median umbilical ligament) is identified, circumscribed, and removed en bloc with the cystectomy specimen (Fig. 2). This maneuver prevents early entry into a high-riding bladder, and ensures complete removal of all bladder remnant tissue. Care is taken to remain medial and avoid injury to the inferior epigastric vessels (lateral umbilical ligaments) that course posterior to the rectus muscles. If the patient has had a previous cystotomy or segmental cystectomy, the cystotomy tract and cutaneous incision should be circumscribed full-thickness and excised en bloc with the bladder specimen. The medial insertion of the rectus muscles attached to the pubic symphysis are then incised, maximizing pelvic exposure throughout the operation.

D.   Abdominal Exploration

A careful systematic intra-abdominal exploration is performed to determine the extent of disease, evaluate for any hepatic metastases, and rule out evidence of gross retroperitoneal adenopathy. The abdominal viscera are palpated to detect any unrelated, concomitant disease. If no contraindications to proceed with surgery exist, all adhesions are incised and freed.

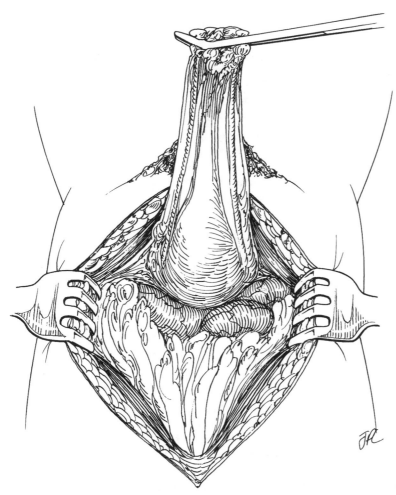

Figure 2   Wide, en bloc excision of urachal remnant with cystectomy specimen. (From Stein JP, Skinner DG. Radical cystectomy in women. Altas Urol Clin 1997; 5(2):37–64.)

E.   Bowel Mobilization

Bowel mobilization starts with the right colon. A large right-angle Richardson retractor elevates the right abdominal wall, and the cecum and ascending colon are then reflected medially to allow incision of the lateral peritoneal reflection along the avascular white line of Toldt. The mesentery to the small bowel is then mobilized off its retroperitoneal attachments cephalad (toward the ligament of Treitz) until the retroperitoneal portion of the duodenum is exposed. Combined sharp and blunt dissection facilitates mobilization of this mesentery along a characteristic avascular fibroareolar plane. This mobilization is critical in setting up the operative field and facilitates proper packing of the intra-abdominal contents into the epigastrium.

The left colon and sigmoid mesentery are then mobilized to the region of the lower pole of the left kidney by incising the peritoneum lateral to the colon along the avascular white line of Toldt. The sigmoid mesentery is then elevated off the sacrum, iliac vessels, and distal aorta up to the origin of the inferior mesenteric artery. This provides a mesenteric window through which the left ureter may pass (without angulation or tension) for later ureteroenteric anastomosis, and also facilitates retraction of the sigmoid mesentery while performing the lymph node dissection.

Care should be taken to dissect along the base of the mesentery, preventing potential injury to the mesenteric blood supply to the colon.

Following mobilization of the bowel, a self-retaining retractor is placed. The right colon and small intestine are carefully packed into the epigastrium with three moist lap pads, followed by a moistened towel rolled to the width of the abdomen. The descending and sigmoid colon are not packed and are left as free as possible, providing the necessary mobility required for the ureteral and pelvic lymph node dissection. Packing of the bowel begins by sweeping the right colon and small bowel under the surgeon's left hand along the right sidewall gutter. A moist open lap pad is then swept with the right hand along the palm of the left hand, under the viscera along the retroperitoneum and sidewall gutter. In similar fashion, the left sidewall gutter is packed. It is often helpful to have the assistant provide counter traction on the descending or sigmoid colon at this time to ensure it is left freely mobile. The central portion of the small bowel is packed with a third lap pad. A moist rolled towel is then positioned horizontally below the lap pads and cephalad to the bifurcation of the aorta. After the bowel has been packed, a wide Deaver retractor is placed with gentle traction on the rolled towel to provide adequate cephalad exposure.

F. Ureteral Dissection

The ureters are most easily identified in the retroperitoneum just cephalad to the common iliac vessels. They are dissected into the deep pelvis several centimeters beyond the iliac vessels and divided between two large hemoclips. A section of the proximal cut ureteral segment (distal to the proximal hemoclip) is then sent for frozen section analysis to ensure the absence of carcinoma in situ or overt tumor. The ureter is then mobilized cephalad and tucked under the rolled towel to prevent inadvertent injury. Frequently, an arterial branch from the common iliac artery or the aorta needs to be divided to provide adequate ureteral mobilization. In addition, the rich vascular supply emanating from the ovarian vessels within the infundibulopelvic ligament should also remain intact and undisturbed. These attachments are an important blood supply to the ureter and help maintain an adequate vascular supply for the ureteroenteric anastomosis at the time of reconstruction. Leaving the proximal hemoclip on the divided ureter during the exenteration allows for hydrostatic ureteral dilation and facilitates the subsequent ureteroenteric anastomosis.

G. Pelvic Lymphadenectomy

A meticulous pelvic lymph node dissection is routinely performed en bloc with radical cystectomy. When performing a salvage procedure following definitive radiation treatment (>5000 rads), a pelvic lymphadenectomy is usually not performed because of the significant risk of iliac vessel and obturator nerve injury (20).

The lymph node dissection is initiated 2 cm above the aortic bifurcation and extends over the inferior vena cava to the genitofemoral nerve, the lateral limits of dissection. The cephalad portions of the lymphatics are ligated with hemoclips to prevent lymphatic leak; the caudal (specimen) side is ligated only when a vessel is encountered. A small anterior tributary vein frequently originates from the vena cava, just above the bifurcation, and should be clipped and divided if identified. At this time the infundibulopelvic ligament and corresponding ovarian vessels are ligated and divided at the pelvic brim.

All fibroareolar and lymphatic tissues are dissected caudally off the aorta, vena cava, and common iliac vessels over the sacral promontory into the deep pelvis. The initial dissection along the common iliac vessels involves skeletonization of the arteries followed by dissection of the left common iliac veins. Lymphatic tissue is then brought medially onto to the sacral promontory and then swept down onto the hollow sweep of the sacrum. At this point, with the combined use of electrocautery and blunt dissection with a Sponge Stick, the lymphatic tissue is pushed down to the presacral region. Significant bleeding from these presacral vessels can occur if not properly controlled. Hemoclips are discouraged in this location as they can be easily dislodged from the anterior surface of the sacrum and result in troublesome bleeding.

Once the proximal portion of the lymph node dissection is completed, a finger is passed from the proximal aspect of dissection, under the pelvic peritoneum (anterior to the iliac vessels), distally toward the femoral canal. The opposite hand can be used to strip the peritoneum from the undersurface of the transversalis fascia. The peritoneum is then divided lateral to the infundibulopelvic ligament. If performed properly, the only structure encountered is the round ligament, which is clipped and divided.

A large right-angled rake retractor (Israel) is then used to elevate the lower abdominal wall to aid in distal exposure in the area of the femoral canal. Tension on the retractor is directed vertically toward the ceiling, with care taken to avoid injury to the inferior epigastric vessels. The distal limits of the dissection are then identified: the circumflex iliac vein crossing anterior to the external iliac artery distally, the genitofemoral nerve laterally, and Cooper's ligament medially. The lymphatics draining the leg, particularly medial to the external iliac vein, are carefully clipped and divided to prevent lymphatic leakage. This includes the lymph node of Cloquet (also known as Rosenmuller), the distal limit of lymphatic dissection at this location. The distal external iliac artery and vein are then circumferentially dissected. At this point in the dissection, an accessory obturator vein (present in 40% of patients), originating from the inferiomedial aspect of the external iliac vein, should be ligated, as inadvertent injury to the vessel can lead to troublesome bleeding.

The subsequent maneuver is to join the proximal and distal dissections and complete the dissection along the iliac vessels. The proximal external iliac artery and vein are skeletonized circumferentially to the origin of the hypogastric artery (Fig. 3). Care should be taken to clip and divide a commonly encountered vessel arising from the lateral aspect of the proximal

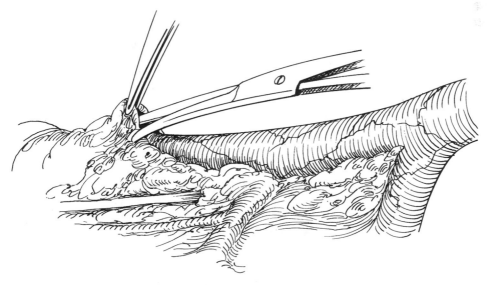

Figure 3   Technique of skeletonizing the external iliac artery and vein. (From Stein JP, Skinner DG. Radical cystectomy in women. Altas Urol Clin 1997; 5(2):37–64.)

external iliac vessels coursing to the psoas muscle. The external iliac vessels are then retracted medially, and the fascia overlying the psoas muscle is incised medial to the genitofemoral nerve. On the left side, branches of the genitofemoral nerve often pursue a more medial course and may be intimately related to the iliac vessels, in which case they are excised.

At this point, the lymphatic tissue surrounding the iliac vessels is composed of a medial and lateral component attached only at the base within the obturator fossa. The lateral lymphatic compartment (freed medially from the vessels and laterally from the psoas) is bluntly swept into the obturator fossa by retracting the iliac vessels medially and passing a small gauze sponge lateral to the vessels along the psoas and pelvic sidewall (Fig. 4A). This sponge should be passed anterior and distal to the hypogastric vein and directed caudally into the obturator fossa. The external iliac vessels are then retracted anteriorly and laterally while the gauze sponge is carefully withdrawn from the obturator fossa with gentle traction using the left hand (Fig. 4B). This maneuver sweeps all lymphatic tissue into the obturator fossa and facilitates identification of the obturator nerve deep to the external iliac vein. The obturator nerve is best identified proximally and carefully dissected free from all lymphatics. The obturator nerve is then retracted laterally along with the iliac vessels (Fig. 5). At this point, the obturator artery and vein can be isolated as they exit the pelvis through the obturator canal. They should be entrapped between the index finger laterally (medial to the obturator nerve) and the middle finger medially of the left hand and then carefully clipped and divided, ensuring that they stay medial to the obturator nerve. The obturator lymph node packet is then swept medially toward the bladder, ligating small tributary vessels and lymphatics from the pelvic sidewall, and removed en bloc with the cystectomy specimen.

H.   Ligation of the Lateral Vascular Pedicle to the Bladder

Following dissection of the obturator fossa and division of the obturator vessels, the lateral vascular pedicle to the bladder is isolated and divided. Isolation of the lateral vascular pedicle is performed with the left hand. Traction is placed on the anterior branches of the hypogastric artery with retraction of the bladder and toward the pelvis. The left index finger is then passed medial to the hypogastric artery and posterior to the anterior visceral branches. The index finger is directed caudally toward the endopelvic fascia, parallel to the sweep of the sacrum, and defines the two major vascular pedicles to the anterior pelvic organs. The lateral pedicle, anterior to the index finger, is composed of the visceral branches of the anterior hypogastric vessel. The posterior pedicle, posterior to the index finger, is composed of the visceral branches between the bladder/vagina, and the rectum.

The lateral pedicle is entrapped between the left index and middle fingers, and traction is applied vertically and caudally. This facilitates skeletonization of the hypogastric artery. The lateral pedicle is then divided between large hemoclips down to the endopelvic fascia, or as far as is technically possible (Fig. 6). With blunt dissection the index finger of the left hand helps identify the lateral pedicle and protects the vagina and rectum with medial displacement. Large right-angle hemoclip appliers and each pair of hemoclips are positioned as far apart as possible to ensure that 0.5–1 cm of tissue projects beyond each clip when the pedicle is divided. This prevents hemoclip dislodgment and unnecessary bleeding. Occasionally, in women with an abundance of pelvic fat, the lateral pedicle may be thick and require division into two manageable pedicles, which can also be suture ligated. The inferior vesicle vein serves as an excellent landmark as the endopelvic fascia is just distal to this structure. It should be emphasized that no dissection be performed along the endopelvic fascia in female patients considering orthotopic reconstruction, which could jeopardize the continence mechanism.

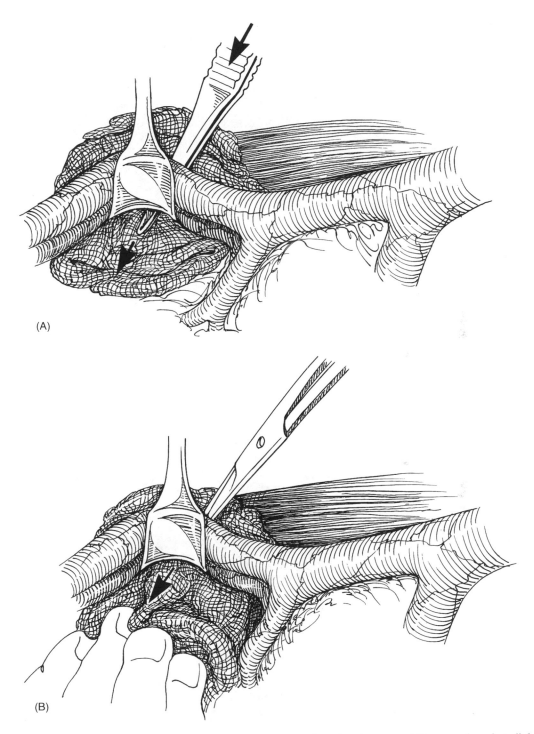

(A)

(B)

Figure 4 (A) Technique of passing a small gauze sponge lateral to the external iliac vessels and medial to the psoas muscle. (B) Technique of withdrawing the gauze sponge with the left hand. This aids in dissecting the obturator fossa. (From Stein JP, Skinner DG. Radical cystectomy in women. Altas Urol Clin 1997; 5(2):37–64.)

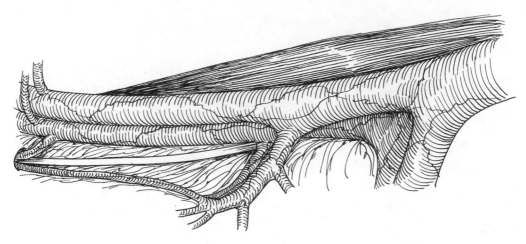

Figure 5   Obturator fossa cleaned. This allows proper identification of the obturator nerve passing deep to the external iliac vein. (From Stein JP, Skinner DG. Radical cystectomy in women. Altas Urol Clin 1997; 5(2):37–64.)

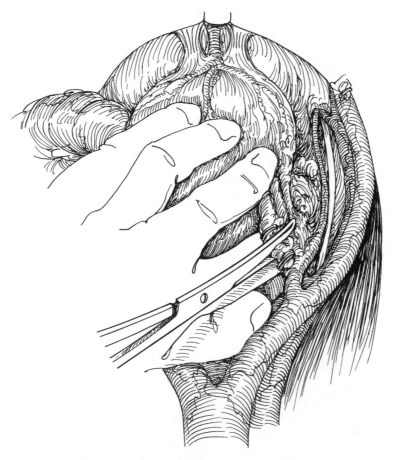

Figure 6   The left hand helps define the right lateral pedicle, extending from the bladder to the hypogastric artery. This vascular pedicle is clipped and divided down to the endopelvic fascia. (From Stein JP, Skinner DG. Radical cystectomy in women. Altas Urol Clin 1997; 5(2):37–64.)

I.   Ligation of the Posterior Pedicle to the Bladder

Following division of the lateral pedicles, the surgeon elevates the bladder anteriorly with a small gauze sponge under the left hand while the assistant retracts on the peritoneum of the recto-sigmoid colon in a cephalad direction, exposing the cul-de-sac (pouch of Douglas) (Fig. 7). This provides excellent exposure to the recess of the cul-de-sac and the peritoneal reflection. The peritoneum lateral to the rectum is incised with the incision extending anteriorly across the cul-de-sac to join the incision on the contralateral side. The peritoneal incision in the cul-de-sac should be made on the rectal side to allow for proper and safe development of Denonvilliers' space between the anterior rectal wall and the posterior sheath of Denonvilliers' fascia. The rectum is swept off the posterior vaginal wall employing a posterior sweeping motion of the fingers. This motion helps to thin and develop the posterior pedicle.

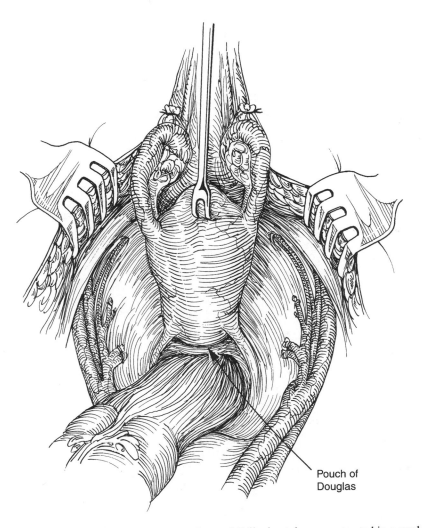

Pouch of
Douglas

Figure 7   The bladder, uterus, ovaries, and Fallopian tubes are retracted in a caudal direction, exposing the pouch of Douglas. (From Stein JP, Skinner DG. Radical cystectomy in women. Altas Urol Clin 1997; 5(2):37–64.)

In the female patient, the posterior pedicles including the cardinal ligaments are divided 4–5 cm beyond the cervix. All tissue is then swept off the lateral aspect of the vagina, and the posterior vagina is incised at the apex just distal to the cervix. Cephalad pressure on a previously placed sponge stick helps to identify the apex of the vagina (Fig. 8). This incision is carried anteriorly along the lateral and anterior vaginal wall, forming a circumferential incision (Fig. 9). The anteriorlateral vaginal wall is then grasped with a curved Kocher clamp to provide traction. This facilitates dissection between the anterior vaginal wall and the bladder specimen. Development of this posterior plane and vascular pedicle is best performed sharply and carried just distal to the vesicourethral junction (Fig. 10). Palpation of the Foley catheter balloon assists in identifying this region. At this point the specimen is only attached at the vesicourethral junction (Fig. 11). This dissection helps maintain a functional vagina which provides pelvic support to the neobladder. The vagina is then closed at the apex and later suspended to the sacrum to maintain adequate vaginal depth and prevent prolapse postoperatively.

Alternatively, in the case of a deeply invasive posterior bladder tumor, the anterior vaginal wall should be removed en bloc with the cystectomy specimen to ensure adequate margins. After dividing the posterior vaginal apex, the lateral vaginal wall subsequently serves as the posterior pedicle, and the anterior vaginal wall remains attached to the posterior bladder specimen. The Foley catheter balloon facilitates identification of the vesicourethral junction as the surgical plane between the vesicourethral junction and the anterior vaginal wall is then developed distally at this location. A 1-cm length of proximal urethra is mobilized while the remaining distal urethra is left intact with the anterior vaginal wall. The vagina may be closed by a clam shell

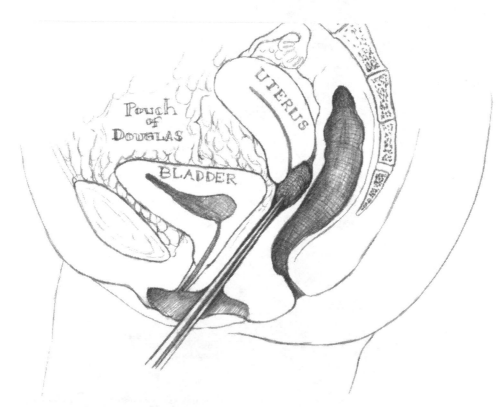

Figure 8   Cephalad pressure on a previously placed sponge stick helps to identify the apex of the vagina prior to making the initial vaginal incision.

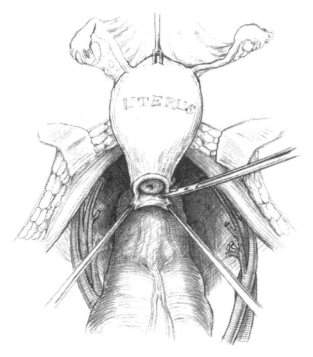

Figure 9   The vaginal incision is carried out circumferentially just distal to the cervix.

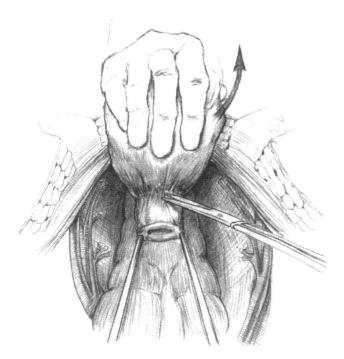

Figure 10   The plane between the anterior vaginal wall and the bladder specimen is sharply dissected. The dissection is facilitated with traction placed at the vaginal wall with Kocher clamps and manually on the bladder.

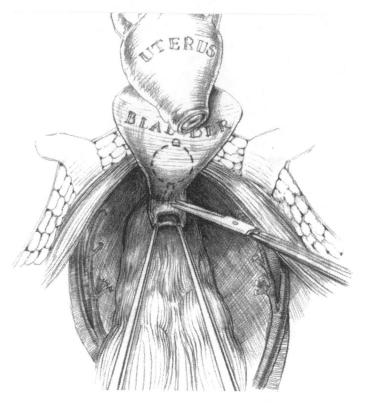

Figure 11   Overhead view of the female pelvis. Palpation of the Foley catheter balloon assists in identifying the distal aspect of the dissection; at this point the specimen is only attached at the vesicourethral junction.

(horizontal) or side-to-side (vertical) technique. Other means of vaginal reconstruction may include a rectus myocutaneous flap, detubularized cylinder of ileum, a peritoneal flap, or an omental flap. We prefer to spare the anterior vaginal wall if orthotopic diversion is planned. This eliminates the need for vaginal reconstruction and helps maintain the complex musculo-fascial support system to the proximal urethra, which may be an important component to the continence mechanism in these women.

An alternative to the standard antegrade approach to the posterior pedicle is a retrograde approach. This should be considered when the proper anatomical plane between the anterior vaginal wall and posterior bladder cannot be easily developed. The urethrovesical junction is identified by palpation of the Foley balloon and the superficial branch of the deep dorsal vein may be identified and ligated. The lateral aspect of the bladder neck and urethra is dissected free to the point where it is easily identified sitting on the anterior aspect of the vagina. The plane between the anterior vaginal wall and posterior bladder is then developed, the bladder neck is elevated off the anterior vaginal wall, and a Satinsky clamp is placed across the bladder neck, allowing division of the urethra just distal to the bladder neck and clamp. With cephalad traction on the specimen, the plane between the bladder and vaginal may be developed, and dissection is continued sharply to the vaginal cuff with lateral attachments between the bladder and vagina clipped as needed.

J. Urethral Preparation

At the terminal stages of the cystectomy, careful preparation of the urethra is critical to avoid injury to the continence mechanism. Minimal dissection should be performed in the region anterior to the urethra. This helps prevents injury to the distal urethral sphincteric mechanism and corresponding innervation, which studies have demonstrated arise from branches off the pudendal nerve that course along the pelvic floor posterior to the levator muscles (21). In addition, the pubourethral suspensory ligaments should be left intact. These ligaments provide support and help maintain an intrapelvic neobladder position, which may also contribute to the continence mechanism in women.

When the posterior dissection is completed (ensuring to dissect just distal to the vesico-urethral junction), a Satinski vascular clamp is placed across the bladder neck. The proximal urethra is divided anteriorly, distal to the bladder neck and clamp. Division of the anterior two-thirds of the urethra exposes the urethral catheter. Six to eight 2-0 polyglycolic acid, anteriorly placed, urethral sutures are then placed equally under direct vision into the urethral mucosa (Fig. 12). The rhabdosphincter, the edge of which acts as a hood overlying the dorsal vein complex, is included in these sutures. This maneuver preserves urinary continence and compresses the dorsal vein complex against the urethra for hemostatic purposes. The urethral catheter is then drawn through the urethrotomy, clamped on the bladder side, and divided. Cephalad traction of the clamped catheter on the bladder side occludes the bladder neck, helps prevents tumor spill from the bladder, and provides exposure to the posterior urethra. Two to four additional sutures are placed in the posterior urethra incorporating the rectourethralis muscle or distal Denonvilliers' fascia. The posterior urethra is then divided, and the specimen

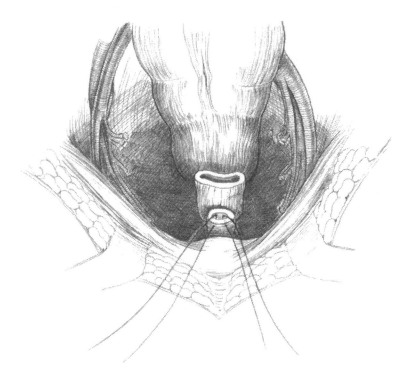

Figure 12   Overhead view of the female pelvis. No anterior dissection has been performed and the initial urethral sutures have been placed.

removed. The urethral sutures are appropriately tagged to identify their location and placed under a towel until the urethroenteric anastomosis is performed. Bleeding from the dorsal vein is usually minimal at this point. If additional hemostasis is required, one or two anterior urethral sutures can be tied to stop the bleeding. Frozen section analysis of the distal urethral margin of the cystectomy specimen is then performed to exclude tumor involvement and confirm appropriateness for orthotopic reconstruction.

Following removal of the cystectomy specimen, the pelvis is irrigated with warm sterile water. The presacral nodal tissue previously swept off the common iliac vessels and sacral promontory into the deep pelvis is collected and sent separately for pathologic evaluation. All nodal tissue in the presciatic notch, anterior to the sciatic nerve, is also sent for histologic analysis. Hemostasis is obtained and the pelvis is packed with a lap pad while attention is directed to the urinary diversion. The pelvis is drained by a 1-inch Penrose drain for 3 weeks, and a large suction hemovac drain for 24 h.

K. Lower Urinary Tract Reconstruction

The various reconstructive techniques (i.e., Kock ileal reservoir, T-pouch) have been described previously and remains standard (22–24). Prior to briefly discussing our present method of lower urinary tract reconstruction several important points need to be stressed for female patients undergoing orthotopic diversion. Appropriate urethral preparation for the urethroenteric anastomosis is essential, and is well described above. After the urethra has been prepared, a well-vascularized omental pedicle graft, based on the left gastroepiploic arthery, is placed between the reconstructed vagina and neobladder. This graft is secured to the levator ani muscles and separates the suture lines of the vagina and neobladder, preventing fistulization (Fig. 13).

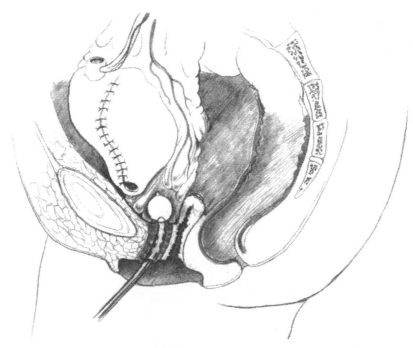

Figure 13 Sagittal section of the female pelvis. Note that a well-vascularized omental graft is placed between the reconstructed vagina and neobladder. The omentum is secured to the levator ani muscles to separate the suture lines and helps prevent fistulization.

Lastly, once the urethroenteric anastomosis is complete the neobladder is secured with a 3-0 polyglycolic acid suture to the inferior aspect of the pubic symphysis. This helps maintains a tension free urethroenteric anastomosis and ensures an intra-abdominal reservoir location.

The primary method by which we now perform lower urinary tract reconstruction is the T-pouch; however, there is no "best" form of lower urinary tract reconstruction, and each surgeon should use what he feels most comfortable with. The terminal portion of the ileum is used to construct the orthotopic T-pouch ileal neobladder. The T-pouch is created from 44 cm of distal ileum placed in an inverted "V" configuration (each limb of the "V" measuring 22 cm), and a proximal 8–10 cm segment of ileum (afferent limb) is used to form the afferent antireflux mechanism. A longer afferent ileal segment (proximal ileum) may be harvested if needed to bridge the gap to a ureter whose length has been shortened/compromised.

The ileum is divided between the afferent ileal segment and the 44-cm segment that will form the reservoir. The mesentery is incised for 2–3 cm, and the segment of mesentery for each piece of bowel is individually maintained. The proximal end of the isolated afferent ileal segment is closed with a running Parker-Kerr suture of 3-0 chromic and a third layer of interrupted 4-0 silk sutures. A standard small bowel anastomosis is performed to reestablish bowel continuity and the mesenteric trap is closed.

The isolated 44-cm ileal segment is then laid out in an inverted "V" configuration (Fig. 14). The antireflux mechanism works as a flap valve with the distal 3–4 cm of the afferent ileal

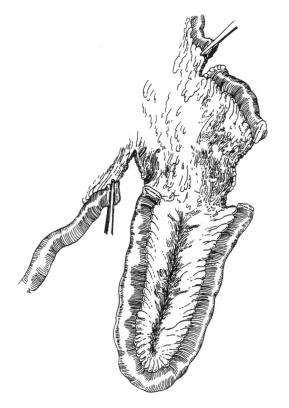

Figure 14   The T-pouch is constructed from an isolated 44-cm ileal segment (laid out in an inverted "V") to form the reservoir and a proximal 8- to 10-cm segment of ileum to form the antireflux limb. (From Ref. 24.)

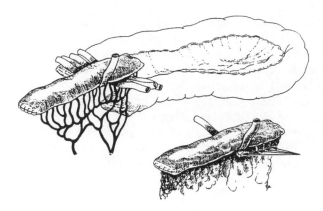

Figure 15   At the distal 3–4 cm of the isolated afferent ileal segment three to four mesenteric windows of Deaver are opened (adjacent to the serosa of the ileum). Small Penrose drains placed through each mesenteric window helps identify this space and facilitates suture passage (see insert with arrows). The distal 3–4 cm of the afferent segment will be anchored into the serosal-lined ileal trough formed by the base of the two adjacent 22-cm ileal segments. (From Ref. 24.)

segment anchored into the serosal-lined ileal trough formed by the base of the two adjacent 22-cm ileal segments. Initially, mesenteric windows of Deaver are opened between the vascular arcades for 3–4 cm proximal to the distal most aspect of the isolated afferent ileal segment (Fig. 15). A series of 3-0 silk sutures (usually two silks per window of Deaver) are then used to approximate the serosa of the two adjacent 22-cm ileal segments at the base of the "V," with each suture passed through the previously opened window of Deaver. Preservation of these arcades (blood vessels) maintains a well-vascularized afferent limb while allowing for appropriate fixation of the afferent limb. Specifically, a silk suture is placed into the seromuscular portion of the bowel (adjacent to the mesentery) at the end of one of the 22-cm ileal segments (Fig. 16A). The suture is then passed through the most proximal window of Deaver in the affer-

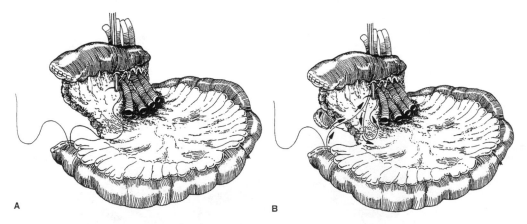

A   B

Figure 16   (A) A series of interrupted silk sutures are use to approximate the serosa of the base of the two adjacent 22-cm ileal segments. (B) After passing the silk suture through the window of Deaver, it is placed in a corresponding site on the adjacent 22-cm ileal segment. This suture will then be brought back through the same window of Deaver and tied down. Maneuvering of the Penrose drains helps facilitate transfer of the suture through the windows of Deaver. (From Ref. 24.)

ent limb, placed in a corresponding seromuscular site of the bowel (next to mesentery) of the adjacent 22-cm ileal segment, and then brought back through the same window of Deaver and tied down (Fig. 16B). This process is repeated through each individual window of Deaver until the distal 3–4 cm of the afferent segment is permanently fixed in the serosal-lined ileal trough. Placement of small (1/4 inch) Penrose drains through each window of Deaver facilitates passage of the silk suture back and forth through the mesentery. The Penrose drains are systematically removed as the afferent limb is fixed within the serosal-lined ileal trough.

Next, the previously anchored portion of the afferent ileal segment (distal 3–4 cm) is tapered on the antimesenteric (anterior) border over a 30F catheter (Fig. 17). Tapering of this portion of the afferent ileal segment reduces the bulk and lumen of the afferent limb, facilitates later coverage of the anchored afferent limb with ileal flaps, and increases the tunnel length-to-lumen diameter ratio allowing for a more effective flap valve mechanism. The remaining portion of the adjacent 22-cm ileal segments are then approximated together with a side-to-side 3-0 polyglycolic acid suture (Fig. 18). Starting at the apex of the "V," the bowel is then opened adjacent to the serosal suture line using electrocautery. This incision is carried upward toward the base where the afferent limb in anchored. At the level of the afferent ostium it is then extended directly lateral to the antimesenteric border of the ileum, and carried upward (cephalad) to the base of the ileal segment (Fig. 19). A similar incision is made on the contralateral 22-cm ileal segment. This incision provides wide flaps of ileum that will ultimately be brought over the tapered afferent ileal segment to create the antireflux mechanism in a flap valve manner (Fig. 20).

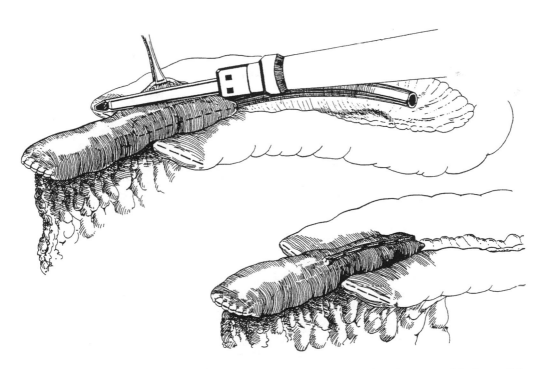

Figure 17 The distal 3- to 4-cm afferent ileal segment, now anchored to the serosa of the base of the adjacent 22-cm ileal segments, is tapered over a 30F catheter on the antimesenteric boarder. This can usually be done with a GIA-55 stapler. (From Ref. 24.)

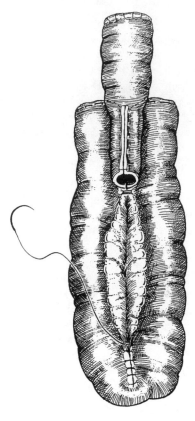

Figure 18   The two 22-cm ileal segments are joined by a running 3-0 polyglycolic acid continuous suture. The suture is placed adjacent to the mesentery and runs from the apex up to the ostium of the afferent ileal segment. Note the formation of the "T" with the horizontal staple lines at the base of each 22-cm ileal segment and the vertical. (From Ref. 24.)

The previously incised ileal mucosa from the apex up to the ostium of the afferent limb is then oversewn with two layers of a running 3-0 polyglycolic acid suture (Fig. 21). An interrupted mucosa-to-mucosa anastomosis is then performed between the ostium of the afferent ileal limb and the incised intestinal ileal flaps with 3-0 polyglycolic acid sutures (Fig. 22). The mucosal edges of the ileal flaps, from both arms of the "V," are then approximated over the tapered portion of the afferent ileal limb (3–4 cm) with a running suture in two layers. This suture line completes the posterior wall of the reservoir and creates the antireflux mechanism (Fig. 23).

The reservoir is then closed by folding the ileum in half in an opposite direction to which it was opened (Fig. 24), and the anterior wall is closed with a running, two-layer 3-0 polyglycolic acid suture (Fig. 25). This anterior suture line is stopped just prior to the end of the right side to allow insertion of an index finger. This is the most mobile and dependent portion of the reservoir and will later be anastomosed to the urethra (Fig. 26).

Once the pouch has been closed, each ureter is spatulated, and a standard, bilateral end-to-side ureteroileal anastomosis is performed using interrupted 4-0 polyglycolic acid suture. These anastomoses are stented with No. 8 infant feeding tubes. A 24F hematuria catheter is placed per

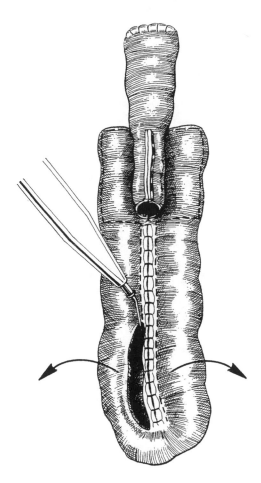

Figure 19 The two 22-cm ileal segments are opened immediately adjacent to the serosal suture line beginning at the apex and carried upward to the ostium of the afferent segment. At the ostium the incision is directed lateral to the antimesenteric boarder and then cephalad to the base. The dashed line depicts the incision line. (From Ref. 24.)

urethra, and the ureteral stents are secured to the end of the urethral catheter with a 3-0 nylon suture, facilitating stent removal. A tension free mucosa-to-mucosa urethroileal anastomosis is performed.

V. POSTOPERATIVE CARE

All patients are monitored in a surgical intensive care unit for at least 24 h or until stable and safe for transfer to the ward. Third-space fluid loss in these patients can be deceivingly large. A combination of crystalloid and colloid fluid replacement is given through the first night after surgery and converted to crystalloid on postoperative day 1. Prophylaxis against stress ulcer is initiated with an H2 blocker. Intravenous broad-spectrum antibiotic are administered and converted to orals with diet progression. Pain control is maintained with an epidural catheter, patient-controlled analgesic system, or a combination of the two. Radiograph evaluation of the diversion is done 3 weeks after surgery and, in the absence of contrast extravasation, results in removal of drainage catheters.

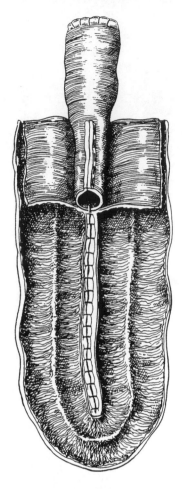

Figure 20 Completing the incision of the bowel. Note the incision provides wide flaps of ileum that can easily be brought over and cover the tapered distal afferent ileal segment to form the antireflux mechanism in a flap-valve technique. (From Ref. 24.)

VI. RESULTS

Results are available in 88 women who have undergone orthotopic lower urinary tract reconstruction with a median age of 67 years (range 31–86 years) and follow-up of 30 months (range 6–117 months).

A. Continence/Voiding Pattern

Of the 88 patients in the study, 81 were evaluated by chart review, and 66 responded to a questionnaire. Results from the chart review revealed 61 (75%) patients dry (34 void spontaneously and 27 intermittently catheterize) and 20 (25%) patients wet (defined as the use of two or more pads a day) postoperatively. The questionnaire revealed similar results, with 52 (78%) patients dry (22 spontaneously void and 30 catheterize) and 14 (22%) patients wet. Twelve patients have undergone secondary procedures for urinary incontinence. Ten patients have undergone one to

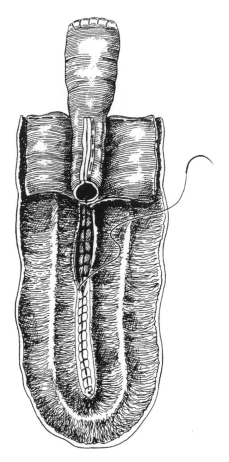

Figure 21   The incised ileal mucosa is oversewn in two layers from the apex to the ostium of the afferent ileal segment. (From Ref. 24.)

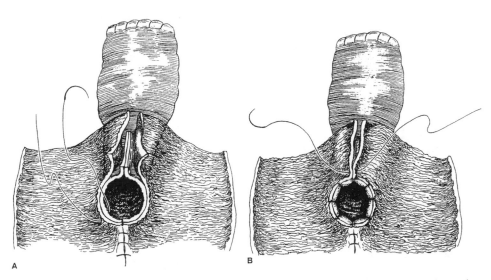

Figure 22   A mucosa-to-mucosa, ileal-to-ileal anastomosis is performed between the ostium of the afferent segment and the edges of the ileal flaps with interrupted 3-0 polyglycolic acid suture. (From Ref. 24.)

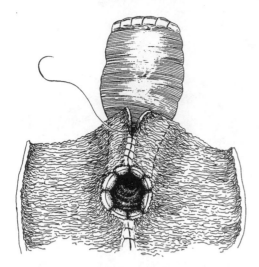

Figure 23   The mucosal edges of the ileal flaps are brought over the tapered distal portion of the afferent ileal segment. This suture line excludes the staple line form the reservoir, completes the posterior suture line and creates the antireflux mechanism. (From Ref. 24.)

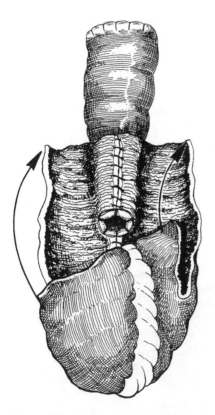

Figure 24   The reservoir is folded and closed in the opposite direction to which it was opened. (From Ref. 24.)

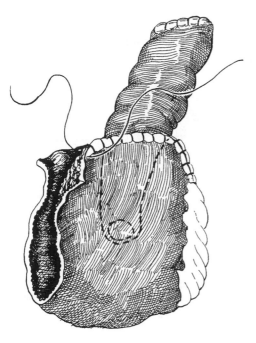

Figure 25 The anterior suture line is completed with two layers of a continuous 3-0 polyglycolic acid suture. The anterior suture line is stopped just short of completion on the right side to the diameter of an index finger, which will be the site of anastomosis to the urethral stump. (From Ref. 24.)

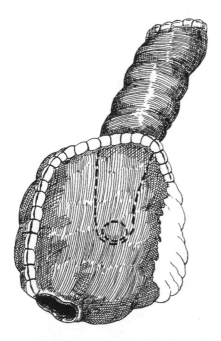

Figure 26 Completion of the T-pouch. The most mobile and dependent portion of the reservoir will be anastomosed to the urethra following the ureteroileal anastomosis. (From Ref. 24.)

four (average 2.8) collagen injections with significant improvement noted in three (30%) and no change in the remaining seven patients. One patient with urinary incontinence underwent conversion to a cutaneous reservoir for a pelvic recurrence and is now dry, and another patient underwent fascial sling with resolution of her leakage.

B. Survival and Recurrence

As of August 1999 there were 75 evaluable patients who underwent cystectomy for TCC of the bladder. Recurrent disease has been identified in 17 patients (23%): six patients with a local/pelvic recurrence (8%), and 11 patients with distant recurrence (11%). There have been 13 deaths secondary to TCC. There have not been any urethral recurrences to date.

C. Complications

Advances in medical, surgical, and anesthetic techniques have reduced morbidity and mortality associated with radical cystectomy. Early complications related to the radical cystectomy are difficult, if not impossible, to separate from complications related to the urinary diversion. Although complications related specifically to female patients requiring cystectomy have rarely been reported (16–18), these complications are comparable to those seen in male patients undergoing the similar procedure.

A total of 21 patients (24%) suffered 24 early complications. Four of these complications required operative management. Two patients returned to the operating room to remove a retained portion of a broken Jackson-Pratt drain, one patient underwent evacuation of a clot after a postoperative bleed 1 day after surgery, and one patient developed a urine leak requiring bilateral percutaneous nephrostomy tube placement. There were two (2.2%) perioperative deaths: one from a pulmonary embolus and one from sepsis.

Late complications were identified in 12 (14%) patients. Six patients were found to have stones in their neobladder which were managed endoscopically. Five patients required operative intervention: three for fistulae (one enterocutaneous, one pouch-bowel and one pouch-vagina), one for a ureteroileal stricture, which ultimately required complete ileal substitution, and one patient with a ventral incisional hernia.

In addition, we have found that age alone does not independently increase the risk of morbidity or mortality from radical cystectomy and should not be a contraindication for definitive surgical therapy for invasive bladder carcinoma (25,26).

VII. DISCUSSION

Although transitional cell carcinoma of the bladder is primarily thought of and seen in men, women also suffer significant morbidity and mortality from this disease. The technique of en bloc radical cystectomy with bilateral pelvic lymphadenectomy has provided superior survival rates with lower pelvic recurrence rates compared to other forms of therapy for invasive bladder cancer (27). Since radical cystectomy has become the primary form of therapy for invasive bladder cancer, emphasis has been directed to the quality-of-life issues, and reconstruction of the genitourinary tract following the ablative surgery. Advances in lower urinary tract reconstruction (particularly women) have increased both patient and physician acceptance of radical cystectomy. One recent report indicated that the option for orthotopic diversion led to an earlier acceptance of cystectomy compared to those offered a cutaneous form of diversion, and that cystectomy improved survival (28). Modern urologic reconstructive techniques now allow for creation of a urinary reservoir (orthotopic neobladder) with similar characteristics to the native bladder: large-capacity, low-pressure, nonrefluxing, continent reservoir that allows volitional voiding per urethra. This eliminates the need for a cutaneous stoma and the need for catheterization, relying on the striated external sphincter for continence. We believe these advances, which allow patients to return to a near normal lifestyle, with a positive self-image, will encourage earlier treatment for invasive bladder tumors when the potential for cure is highest.

The progressive development of urinary diversion has been the result of persistent surgical innovation to improve the treatment and quality of life of patients following cystectomy. This evolution has developed along three distinct paths: an incontinent cutaneous form of diversion (ileal conduit), a continent cutaneous form of diversion (Indiana and Kock pouch), and, most recently, a form of diversion to the intact native urethra (orthotopic neobladder). We firmly believe the orthotopic neobladder represents the most ideal form of urinary diversion available in carefully selected male and female patients. The orthotopic neobladder most closely resembles the original bladder in both location and function. Orthotopic diversion eliminates the need for a cutaneous stoma and its often plagued continence mechanism. Patients retain a more natural voiding pattern which provides a more normal lifestyle and an improved self-image compared to other forms of diversion.

The excellent functional results in 88 women undergoing orthotopic neobladder diversion confirms our initial experience with further follow-up. The majority of women are completely continent (75%). By 6 months most women obtain the maximum degree of continence; however, many of our patients achieve complete continence immediately following removal of their urethral catheter 3 weeks after surgery. We attribute these results to the limited dissection performed anterior to the urethra.

A precise understanding of the continence mechanism in women after orthotopic diversion is still lacking. The multiple factors contributing to the continence mechanism in women undergoing orthotopic diversion likely include the distal urethral sphincteric mechanism and the inherent fascial support of the urethra. Anatomic urethral support is primarily maintained by the condensations of the levator fascia known as the urethropelvic (29) and the pubourethral (30) ligament. The pubourethral ligament attaches at the level of the midurethra and helps maintain the urethra and neobladder in an intra-abdominal position.

The distal urethral sphincteric mechanism is composed of smooth muscle, striated muscle, and spongy tissue. This mechanism is what is primarily responsible for continence in otherwise normal patients with incompetent bladder necks and is identified at the level of the midurethra (31,32). This level of continence has also been identified in fluorourodynamic evaluation of female cystectomy patients with neobladders, and suggests that the distal urethral sphincteric mechanism is the critical component in maintaining urinary continence in these female subjects (33). Passive continence is secondary to the smooth muscle and spongy tissue component of the distal urethral sphincteric mechanism. The striated portion of the sphincter is composed of "fast-twitch" (rapidly contracting muscle responsible for active contraction of the sphincter as well as reflex contractions which are seen with Valsalva-type maneuvers) and "slow-twitch" (responsible for basic urethral tone) muscle, which are positioned extrinsic and intrinsic to the urethral wall, respectively.

Another controversial point in regard to female neobladders relates to the innervation to the sphincteric mechanism in these patients. Although some authors have suggested that a sympathetic nerve-sparing cystectomy is important in maintaining continence in women (16,28,34), we make no attempt to perform a nerve-sparing cystectomy and remove all autonomic sympathetic innervation from just above the aortic bifurcation down to the proximal urethra. In addition, we routinely sacrifice the sympathetic neurovascular bundle coursing along the lateral aspect of the uterus and vagina. This primarily leaves somatic and parasympathetic innervation to the urethral sphincteric mechanism (or sympathetic via pathways that have yet to be identified), which is apparently sufficient as evidenced by the high continence rate in our patients.

We present encouraging clinical and functional data with intermediate follow-up in women undergoing orthotopic lower urinary tract reconstruction following cystectomy for a pelvic malignancy. Orthotopic diversion in women may be performed with few postoperative complications, excellent continence results, a normal voiding pattern, and with high patient acceptance. Although long-term follow-up will be required to define the true risk of urethral recurrence in these women, we feel female subjects considering orthotopic diversion may be safely and appropriately selected using strict pathologic criteria. We have found intraoperative frozen section of the distal surgical margin (proximal urethra) to be the most accurate and reliable method to determine if a woman is an appropriate candidate for orthotopic diversion. Orthotopic reconstruction is a viable option in most male and female patients and signifies another important step forward in the evolution of urinary diversion.

REFERENCES

1. Crawford ED, Davis MA. Nontransitional cell carcinomas of the bladder. In: De Kernian JB, Paulson DF, eds. Genitourinary Cancer Management. Philadelphia: Lea & Febiger, 1987:95–105.
2. Skinner DG, Lieskovsky G. Management of invasive and high-grade bladder cancer. In: Skinner DG, Lieskovsky G, eds. Diagnosis and Management of Genitourinary Cancer. Philadelphia: W.B. Saunders, 1988:295–312.
3. Droller MJ. Individualizing the approach to invasive bladder cancer. Contemp Urol 1990; July/Aug:54–61.
4. Anderstrom C, Johansson S, Nilsson S. The significance of lamina propria invasion on the prognosis of patients with bladder tumors. J Urol 1980; 124:23–26.
5. Malkowicz SB, Nichols P, Lieskovsky G, Boyd SD, Huffman J, Skinner DG. The role of radical cystectomy in the management of high grade superficial bladder cancer (PA, P1, PIS and P2). J Urol 1990; 144:641–645.
6. Prout GR Jr, Griffin PP, Daly JJ, Henery NM. Carcinoma in situ of the urinary bladder with and without associated vesical neoplasms. Cancer 1983; 52:524–532.
7. Utz DC, Farrow DM. Management of carcinoma in situ of the bladder: a case for surgical management. Urol Clin North Am 1980; 7:533–540.
8. Fitzpatrick JM. The natural history of superficial bladder cancer. Semin Urol 1993; 11:127–136.
9. Trasher JB, Crawford ED. Minimally invasive transitional cell carcinoma (T1 and T2). In: Resnick MI, Kursh E, eds. Current Therapy in Genitourinary Surgery. 2nd ed. St. Louis: B.C. Decker, 1992:74–78.
10. Freeman JA, Esrig D, Stein JP, Simoneau AR, Skinner EC, Chen S-C, Groshen S, Lieskovsky G, Boyd SD, Skinner DG. Radical cystectomy for high risk patients with superficial bladder cancer in the era of orthotopic urinary reconstruction. Cancer 1995; 76:833–839.
11. Heney NM, Ahmed S, Flanagan MJ, Frable W, Corder MP, Hafermann MD, Hawkins IR. Superficial bladder cancer: progression and recurrence. J Urol 1983; 130:1083–1086.
12. Dalesio O, Schulman CC, Sylvester R, DePauw M, Robinson M, Denis L, Smith P, Viggiano G. Prognostic factors in superficial bladder tumors. A study of the European Organization for Research on Treatment of Cancer: Genitourinary Tract Cancer Cooperative Group. J Urol 1983; 129:730–733.
13. Herr HW, Jakse G, Sheinfeld J. The T1 bladder tumor. Semin Urol 1990; 8:254–261.
14. Stein JP, Cote RJ, Freeman JA, Esrig D, Elmajian DA, Groshen S, Skinner EC, Boyd SD, Lieskovsky G, Skinner DG. Indications for lower urinary tract reconstruction in women after cystectomy for bladder cancer: a pathological review of female cystectomy specimens. J Urol 1995; 154:1329–1322.
15. Stenzl A, Draxl H, Posch B, Colleselli K, Falk M, Bartsch G. The risk of urethral tumors in female bladder cancer: can the urethra be used for orthotopic reconstruction of the lower urinary tract? J Urol 1995; 153:950–955.

16. Stenzl A, Colleselli K, Poisel S, Feichtinger H, Pontasch H, Bartsch G. Rationale and technique of nerve sparing radical cystectomy before an orthotopic neobladder procedure in women. J Urol 1995; 154:2044–2048.

17. Stein JP, Stenzl A, Esrig D, Freeman JA, Boyd SD, Lieskovsky G, Cote RJ, Bennett C, Colleselli K, Draxl H, Janetschek G, Poisel S, Bartsch G, Skinner DG. Lower urinary tract reconstruction following cystectomy in women using the Kock ileal reservoir with bilateral ureteroileal urethrostomy: initial clinical experience. J Urol 1994; 152:1404–1408.

18. Stein JP, Grossfeld GD, Freeman JA, Esrig D, Ginsberg DA, Cote RJ, Skinner EC, Boyd SD, Lieskovsky G, Skinner DG. Orthotopic lower urinary tract reconstruction in women using the Kock ileal neobladder: updated experience in 34 patients. J Urol 1997; 158(2):400–405.

19. Nichols RL, Broido P, Condon RE, Gorbach SL, Nyhus LM. Effect of preoperative neomycin-erythromycin intestinal preparation on the incidence of infectious complications following colon surgery. Ann Surg 1973; 178:453–462.

20. Crawford ED, Skinner DG. Salvage cystectomy after radiation failure. J Urol 1980; 123:32–34.

21. Colleselli K, Strasser H, Moriggl B, Stenzl A, Poisel S, Bartsch G. Hemi-Kock to the female urethra: anatomical approach to the continence mechanism of the female urethra. J Urol 1994; 151:abstract 1089.

22. Skinner DG, Boyd SD, Lieskovsky G. Technique of continent lower urinary tract reconstruction with Kock pouch urethrostomy following cystectomy. Videotape available from Marketing Communications, 3M Medical-Surgical Division, St. Paul, MN 55144, USA.

23. Boyd SD, Skinner E, Lieskovsky G, Skinner DG. Continent and orthotopic urinary diversion following radical cystectomy. Surg Oncol Clin North Am 1995; 4:277–286.

24. Stein JP, Lieskoksky G, Ginsberg DA, Bochner BH, Skinner DG. The T pouch: an orthotopic ileal neobladder incorporating a serosal lined ileal antireflux technique. J Urol 1998; 159(6):1836–1842.

25. Lerner SP, Skinner E, Skinner DG. Radical cystectomy in regionally advanced bladder cancer. Urol Clin North Am 1992; 19:713–723.

26. Figueroa AJ, Stein JP, Dickinson M, Skinner EC, Thangathurai D, Mikhail MS, Boyd SD, Lieskovsky G, Skinner DG. Radical cystectomy for elderly patients with bladder carcinoma: an updated experience with 404 patients. Cancer 1998; 83:141–147.

27. Wishnow KI, Dmochowski R. Pelvic recurrence after radical cystectomy without preoperative radiation. J Urol 1988; 140:42–43.

28. Hautmann RE, Paiss T, Petriconi R. The ileal neobladder in women: 9 years of experience with 18 patients. J Urol 1996; 155:76–81.

29. Klutke C, Golomb J, Barbaric Z, Raz S. The anatomy of stress incontinence: magnetic resonance imaging of the female bladder neck and urethra. J Urol 1990; 143:563–566.

30. Zacharin RF. The anatomic support of the female urethra. Obstet Gynecol 1968; 21:754–759.

31. Dupont MC, Albo ME, Raz S. A videourodynamic evaluation of bladder neck competence in females. J Urol 1996; 153:abstract 536.

32. Chapple CR, Helm CW, Blease S, Milroy EJ, Rickards D, Osborne JL. Asymptomatic bladder neck incompetence in nulliparous females. Br J Urol 1989; 64:357–359.

33. Grossfeld GD, Stein JP, Bennett CJ, Ginsberg DA, Boyd SD, Lieskovsky G, Skinner DG. Lower urinary tract reconstruction in the female using the Kock ileal reservoir with bilateral ureteroileal urethrostomy: update of continence results and fluorourodynamic findings. Urology 1996; 48:383–388.

34. Cancrini A, De Carli P, Fattahi H, Pompeo V, Cantiani R, Von Heland M. Orthotopic ileal neobladder in female patients after radical cystectomy: 2-year experience. J Urol 1995; 153:956–958.

59
Interstitial Cystitis

Marie-Blanche Tchetgen, Raymond R. Rackley, and Joseph B. Abdelmalak
Cleveland Clinic Foundation, Cleveland, Ohio, U.S.A.

I. INTRODUCTION

Interstitial cystitis (IC) is a poorly understood clinical syndrome characterized by urinary frequency, urgency, and varying degrees of pelvic pain. Although Hunner (1) described bladder ulcerations as early as 1915, and descriptions of submucosal hemorrhages and reduced bladder capacity were attributed to Hand (2) in 1949, the etiology and pathophysiology of the disease remain unclear. Significant research contributions have been made in recent years with the support of the Interstitial Cystitis Association and NIH-NIDDK, but fundamental questions remain.

II. EPIDEMIOLOGY

Epidemiological studies of IC have been scant, slowed by the low frequency of the disease and the lack of a broad consensus regarding the definition of the disease. Criteria established for research purposes by NIDDK have proven to be exceedingly restrictive as up to 60% of patients clinically thought to have the disease would be excluded (3). Recent efforts aimed at better characterizing the epidemiology of IC suggest that the disease may be more prevalent than previously thought (4). The first population-based study aimed at estimating the prevalence of IC was published in 1999. IC-specific questionnaires were completed by participants in two large population based long-term epidemiological studies, the Nurses Health Study (NHS) I and II. A prevalence of confirmed IC cases of 52 per 100,000 in NHS I and 67 per 100,000 in NHS II were reported, much higher than previously reported rates of 18–36 per 100,000 (5,6). Other epidemiological characteristics such as age at onset of symptoms, age at diagnosis, and delay in diagnosis were similar to previous published reports. Mean age at diagnosis was 54.4 in NHS I and 35.8 in NHS II. Mean time from onset of symptoms to diagnosis was 5.3 and 7.1 years, respectively.

The NHS cohorts were limited epidemiologically by the absence of men and children, as well as the lack of racial and ethnic diversity. Current estimates indicate a male-female ratio of approximately 1 : 9 (7), although there is increasing evidence that the disease may be underdiagnosed in men. In a study of 29 men diagnosed with IC over an 8-year period, 14 were initially diagnosed with prostatitis and 11 with BPH, despite the fact that 21 of these men had the classic form of the disease with associated Hunner's ulcers (8). Similarly, the incidence of IC in children may be higher than previously thought, with up to 50% of children with lower urinary tract symptoms suggestive of IC satisfying NIDDK criteria modified for the pediatric population (9). Further longitudinal epidemiological studies are needed in both the adult and pediatric population in order to gain a more comprehensive understanding of the natural history of this disease as well as its impact on quality of life. Evidence gathered so far is consistent with the characterization of this disease as a chronic, often debilitating disease (10); however, little specific information exists which addresses the variability observed in disease presentation. Recently, investigators have proposed the use of a broadened clinical definition of IC, which includes chronic pelvic pain of bladder origin, in an effort to facilitate a more accurate assessment of the prevalence of these symptom complexes in the general population. However, the sensitivity and specificity of such a classification would have to be established before undertaking any longitudinal epidemiological studies (11).

III. ETIOLOGY

Although research advances in recent years suggest that a multifactorial process may be involved in the development of the symptom complex of IC, the exact etiology of the disease remains elusive (Fig. 1). Various theories have been proposed with varying degrees of supporting evidence; however, there is no unifying concept that allows a clear understanding of the pathophysiology of the disease. The dominant theories include:

1. Alterations in urothelial permeability
2. Mastocytosis with release of pro-inflammatory mediators
3. Neural-immune mechanisms
4. Neural plasticity
5. Infectious agents

The hypothesis of increased urothelial permeability was first advanced by Parsons on the basis of studies demonstrating that the glycosaminoglycans (GAG) layer of the bladder formed a

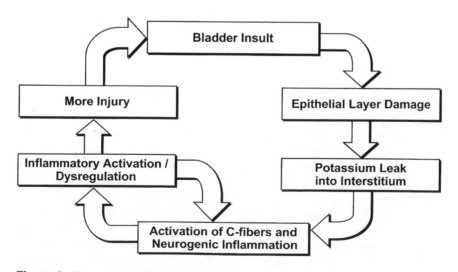

Figure 1   The etiology of interstitial cystitis.

protective barrier preventing urinary solutes from reaching the underlying cell membranes (12). It is proposed that damage to this protective layer allows toxic substances such as urea, calcium, and potassium into the bladder wall, resulting in nerve depolarization with subsequent development of the characteristic symptoms of IC (13). It was further demonstrated that exogenous sulfated polysaccharides such as heparin, pentosan polysulfate, and hyaluronic acid can decrease the movement of urea and potassium chloride across the bladder wall, and improve the symptoms of IC. The potassium chloride test was developed as a "leak test" for the bladder epithelium, to be used in the diagnosis of IC. It is clear, however, that a leaky epithelium is not the sine qua non of IC, as at least 25% patients who satisfy either the NIDDK or clinical definition of the disease have a negative potassium sensitivity test.

Interestingly, patients with a positive test may be more likely to respond to sodium pentosan polysulfate therapy (14). The "leaky" epithelium theory may constitute a piece of the IC puzzle but research evidence to date does not support its consideration as the primary etiological event leading to the clinical presentation of the disease.

Mastocytosis emerged as a potential etiological factor after the presence of mast cells within the bladder wall of IC patients was described (15). Mast cells are found in only about a third of IC patients, and although mast cell activation in this subgroup of IC patients correlates with increased urinary levels of mast cell mediators such as histamine, histamine metabolites (methylhistamines, 1,4-methylimidazole acetic acid), and tryptase (16–18), the diagnostic importance of detrusor mastocytosis largely remains in question. Recent investigations suggest that mast cell degranulation may in fact be one component of a sequence of events involving neurogenic inflammation (19).

Maladaptive neurogenic inflammation has been recently proposed as a mechanism by which the characteristic features of IC may be mediated. Indeed, IC shares many similarities with other chronic visceral pain syndromes thought to be associated with neurogenic inflammation: poor pain localization (pelvic), pain referred to adjacent areas (perineum, suprapubic area, lower back, thighs), and evidence of inflammatory changes of unclear etiology. The evidence suggesting the involvement of neurogenic inflammation in the pathophysiology of IC includes the increased presence of substance P-containing nerve fibers in IC bladder biopsies (20) and increased levels of immunoreactive substance P in the urine of IC patients (21). Substance P is known to induce mast cell degranulation in a dose-dependent fashion (22) and release of histamine, leading to increased vascular permeability and leukocyte migration (23). More direct evidence of a neurogenic process possibly causing IC was presented by Jasmine and colleagues in a model of neurogenic cystitis induced by viral infection of specific neuronal circuits of the rat CNS (24). In these experiments, the abductor caudae dorsalis (ACD) tail muscle was inoculated with the neurotropic pseudorabies virus (PRV), leading to viral infection of the CNS motor neurons which innervate this muscle. Subsequent transsynaptic spread of PRV to the area of the lumbosacral spinal cord, where parasympathetic preganglionic neurons innervating the bladder are located was demonstrated by immunostaining. Approximately 96 h after inoculation, the rats manifested behavioral, macroscopic, and histologic signs of cystitis. PVR immunostaining of the bladder wall was consistently negative, and urine and bladder cultures were also negative for infectious virus. Spinal cord cultures from the ACD-inoculated rats contained infectious virus. Total bladder denervation consistently prevented bladder inflammation after ACD viral inoculation. Based on these observations, the authors proposed that the immune response generated by PRV infection activated adjacent somatic and autonomic central bladder neural circuits, resulting in neurogenically mediated cystitis. Recent studies provide additional evidence supporting the role of mast cells in the genesis of neurogenic cystitis (25): increase in urinary histamine levels precedes the onset of inflammation, normalization of urinary histamine levels parallels a large reduction in the density of granulated mast cells, and pre-emptive mast cell degranulation using a mast cell degranulator compound prior to ACD viral inoculation prevents the development of neurogenic cystitis.

These observations serve as the backdrop for a model of the pathophysiology of IC characterized by three defining stages: (a) centrally mediated neurogenic inflammation involving primary sensory afferents to the bladder which release neuropeptides that in turn induce; (b) mast cell degranulation leading to inflammatory response; and (c) the release of histamine and other mast cell mediators that trigger inflammation (Fig. 2). Ultrastructural analysis of the IC bladder by electron microscopy indicating the presence of mast cells in close proximity to intrinsic nerves in the suburothelium lends further credence to this theoretical model (26). However, the potential cause of such neurogenic inflammation remains unclear, and there is no evidence that a viral infectious process is involved.

CNS Activation (eg: viral infection)
↓
↓

Immune response
↓   *1) Early activation of glia surrounding affected neuron*
↓   *2) Leukocyte invasion*

Release of neuroactive substances
↓   *Cytokines, Nitric oxide*
↓   *↓ Depolarization threshold of neighboring neurons*

Antidromic potentials in central branch
of dorsal root ganglion neurons (dorsal root reflex)
↓
↓

Activation of primary sensory afferents
(C-fibers)
↓   *Blocked by Capsaicin and resiniferatoxin*
↓

Increased peripheral release of pro-inflammatory
neuropeptides
↓   *Substance P*
↓   *↑ Urinary histamine (mast cell degranulation)*

Anomalies of vasculature, epithelial and
subepithelial layers → interstitial cystitis

Figure 2   Proposed model of the pathogenesis of interstitial cystitis.

IV. DIAGNOSIS

The classic clinical presentation of IC is characterized by urinary frequency (≥ 8 times per day), urgency, and pain on bladder filling relieved by voiding. On physical examination, patients may display tenderness of the anterior vaginal wall and bladder base. The disease remains a diagnosis of exclusion because the presenting symptoms are nonspecific and may vary in severity. The diagnosis is based primarily on clinical suspicion, and based on the results of the Interstitial Cystitis Database (ICDB) study, clinicians are discouraged from using the strict NIDDK criteria. Routine urine culture and cytology are necessary to exclude infection or malignancy. Other diagnoses to be ruled out include ureteral or bladder calculi, active genital herpes, urethral diverticulum, chemical cystitis (cyclophosphamide), radiation cystitis, and vaginitis (chalamydia, ureaplasm). If IC is suspected, additional tests may be useful in establishing the diagnosis. These include cystoscopy and hydrodistension under anesthesia, urodynamic evaluation, potassium sensitivity test, urinary markers, and bladder biopsy.

A. Cystoscopy and Hydrodistension

Cystoscopy under anesthesia allows for comfortable and adequate bladder and urethral examination. Hydrodistension is performed by instilling fluid into the bladder under gravity at 80–100 cm of water pressure until the flow slows to a drip or stops altogether. Compression of the urethra around the cystoscope sheath prevents efflux of fluid and ensures an accurate measurement of bladder capacity. According to the NIDDK criteria, distension is held for 1–2 min, although double distension or distension duration up to 10 min have been reported. Upon decompression, the bladder is examined cystoscopically for the presence of glomerulations, which are pinpoint petechial hemorrhages and constitute the most consistent cystoscopic finding in patients with IC (Fig. 3). Glomerulations must be diffuse and present in at least three quadrants of the bladder. Fissures and cracks that bleed after distension may be observed and are suggestive of the classic or ulcer variety of IC. Although the presence of glomerulations has been reported in normal women undergoing tubal ligation, it remains a helpful diagnostic tool in symptomatic patients. Furthermore, hydrodistension may be therapeutic in 20–30% of patients.

B. Urodynamic Evaluation

Urodynamic studies are not routinely recommended in the evaluation of the patient with IC, although some findings make the diagnosis less likely. These include a bladder volume at the first sensation to void >150 cc, maximum bladder capacity >350 cc, and the absence of nocturia on pretesting baseline voiding log.

The presence of involuntary bladder contractions has been reported in ~14% of IC patients (ICDB) and does not exclude a clinical diagnosis of IC. A more stringent research definition of the disease as described by the NIDDK does, however, consider the presence of phasic instability an exclusion criterion.

C. Potassium Sensitivity Test

The potassium chloride test (KCl test) is based on the premise that epithelial permeability dysfunction is the underlying factor which leads to the symptoms of IC. Increased urothelial permeability would allow diffusion of potassium into the submucosal and muscle layers of the bladder, leading to nerve depolarization and possibly neurogenic inflammation. The KCl test was proposed by Parsons as a provocative test aimed at identifying IC patients with epithelial

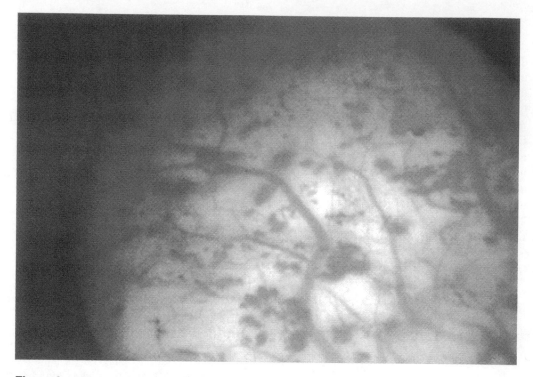

Figure 3 Diffuse glomerulations seen on cystoscopic evaluation of the bladder following hydrodistension.

dysfunction. The test is conducted by instilling a dilute solution of potassium (40 mEq in 100 mL water) in the bladder for 5 min. The degree of urgency and pain is reported on a scale of 0 (none) to 5 (severe), before and after the test. A change in score of ≥ 2 is considered a positive test. The role of the KCl test in the diagnosis of IC remains controversial. It is limited by a poor specificity as falsely positive tests are seen in patients with bladder overactivity, radiation cystitis, and bacterial cystitis. In addition, false-negative tests have been reported in patients with severe disease (13). Furthermore, when positive, the test may cause a significant amount of discomfort and distress to the patient. Despite these limitations, there are data suggesting that the KCl test may identify patients more likely to respond to therapies aimed at restoring urothelial integrity such as sodium pentosan polysulfate and heparin. More studies are needed to further clarify the role of the KCl test.

D. Urine Markers

A number of urine components are reported to be altered in IC patients and as such have been evaluated as possible markers for the disease. The ideal marker should allow discrimination between IC patients and healthy controls with minimal or no overlap and should be predictive of the clinical presence of the disease and should normalize with successful treatment. Most described alterations in IC urinary components relate to one or more of the possible etiologies of IC and show significant overlap between IC and normal controls. Only two markers have been identified that can clearly discriminate between IC patients and normal control groups: glycoprotein-51 (GP-51), and antiproliferative factor (APF).

GP-51 is a glycoprotein produced and secreted by the bladder transitional epithelium of humans and rabbits. Recent studies indicate that decreased levels of GP-51 are found in the bladder and urine of IC patients as compared to controls (27). However, GP-51 discriminates best between IC patients and controls (no overlap in GP-51 urinary levels) when the former meet all NIDDK criteria for the diagnosis of IC (28). Its clinical utility may therefore be as limited as that of the NIDDK criteria.

APF inhibits the proliferation of cultured human bladder epithelial cells by inhibiting the production of heparin-binding epidermal growth factor-like growth factor (HB-EGF). The activity of APF is increased in the urine of IC patients and allows diagnosis of the disease with a sensitivity of 91.4% and a specificity of 90.6%. Increased levels of APF correlate with decreased levels of HB-EGF; therefore both have been evaluated as markers of IC. Urinary levels of APF and HB-EGF have also been used to assess treatment outcome and were found to normalize following cystoscopy and hydrodistension as well as sacral neuromodulation. Importantly, normalization of the levels of these markers correlated with symptomatic relief. These markers are promising but are not yet commercially available. Clearly, additional studies are needed to better characterize the clinical utility of these markers and to understand how they contribute to the pathophysiology of IC.

E. Bladder Biopsy

Bladder biopsy has traditionally played a minimal role in the diagnosis of IC, as the histopathologic features were consistent with inflammation but were characteristically believed to be relatively nonspecific (Fig. 4). Although useful to evaluate suspicious lesions and exclude

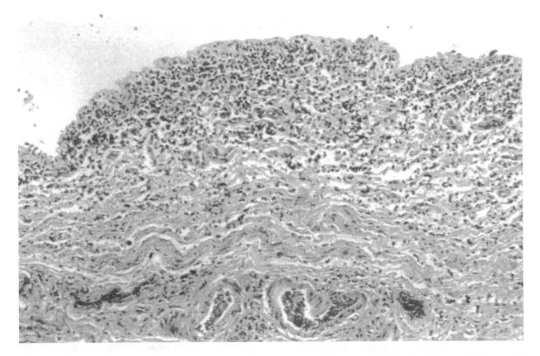

Figure 4   H&E staining revealing nonspecific inflammation of the urothelium and superficial muscle layer.

carcinoma in situ, bladder biopsy is not required to establish the diagnosis of IC. Recent findings, however, suggest that some histopathologic biopsy features may be predictive of specific IC symptoms and in fact may underly the variability observed in IC symptomatology. Indeed, the association between histopathologic features and IC symptoms was investigated using the ICDB cohort population (29), which includes patients clinically diagnosed with IC even if they do not meet the strict NIDDK criteria. Of the 637 patients in the ICDB, 211 consented to bladder biopsy. According to the study protocol, two samples were obtained from the most diseased area of the bladder in the following order of priority: Hunner's ulcer if present; glomerulations if present; normal-appearing posterior bladder wall if neither Hunner's ulcer nor glomerulations were present. In addition a third sample was obtained from the trigone area of the bladder to serve as an internal control. Patients' self-reported symptoms of urgency and pain were recorded on a 10-point Likert scale, and daytime and nighttime frequency were recorded in a 3-day voiding diary. As previously reported, cystoscopic pathology (presence or severity of glomerulations and presence or absence of Hunner's ulcer) was not statistically associated with any specific IC symptom. Select biopsy features, however, were found to be associated with symptoms of nighttime frequency, urinary frequency, and urinary pain when separate multivariable predictive models adjusting for patient characteristics were used for analysis. Specifically, complete loss of urothelium, mastocytosis in the lamina propria, and the presence of granulation tissue in the lamina propria were independently strongly predictive of increased nighttime frequency. Similarly, increasing vascular density in the lamina propria correlated with progressively higher nocturnal frequency. An increase in the percentage of submucosal granulation was associated with increased urgency as well as increased nighttime frequency. Lastly, urinary pain was positively associated with the percentage of mucosa denuded of urothelium and the percentage of submucosal hemorrhage present.

On the basis of these provocative findings, the authors suggest that three biologic processes may be involved in the pathophysiology of IC: loss of the integrity of the urothelium, vascular damage, and mucosal mastocytosis. These findings give credence to some of the existing theories regarding the pathophysiology of the disease and further illustrate the heterogeneity that has made this disease so difficult to characterize. They do little, however, to elucidate the sequence of events that ultimately lead to the development of IC. The relationship between biopsy features and the natural history of the disease or treatment outcome also remains unclear at this time, although long-term follow studies may provide additional insight.

V. TREATMENT

Treatment modalities used in the management of IC are generally directed at one or more of the prevailing theories regarding the etiology of the disease. We propose a treatment algorithm that allows a comprehensive, systematic, and practical approach to the clinical management of this challenging condition (Table 1).

A. Oral Therapy

1. Sodium Pentosan Polysulfate

This is the only FDA-approved drug designated for the treatment of IC. Its mechanism of action is thought to involve correction of defects in the glycosaminoglycan layer of the bladder urothelium. It may possibly act by binding toxic agents in the urine (30). Various clinical studies indicate that 30–40% of patients report a 40–50% improvement in their symptoms. The minimum

Table 1   Practical Approach for the Management
of Interstitial Cystitis

Visit 1
  History and physical examination
  Urine culture, urine cytology, M4 (ureaplasm, chlamydia)
  Vaginal wet prep
  Initiation of oral therapy (for a minimum of 3 months)
    Elmiron
    Elavil or Neurontin if dominant pain component
    Atarax (particularly if allergy prone)
Visit 2
  MRI: rule out urethral diverticulum
  Possible urodynamic testing $\pm$ KCl testing
    If suspect OAB (sensory vs motor urgency)
Visit 3
  Cystoscopy and hydrodistension
  Possible bladder biopsy
Visit 4 (at least 3 months after first visit)
  Continue oral therapy if no side effects
  Intravesical therapy (DMSO, heparin)
  Pelvic floor therapy
  Discuss sacral neuromodulation
Visit 5 (at least 3 months after fourth visit)
  Trial of sacral neuromodulation

---

effective dose is 100 mg TID, although there have been anecdotal reports indicating that higher doses may be more efficacious. Phase IV trials evaluating the efficacy of higher doses (600 mg or 800 mg daily) have not shown a definite difference. Long-term therapy is recommended as it may take 6 months to a year for some patients to experience optimal symptomatic relief.

2.   Antihistamines

Reports of antihistamine use to control the symptoms of IC have been largely anecdotal, and to date, there have been no controlled trials verifying their efficacy. Hydroxyzine (Atarax, Vistaril) is a histamine-1 receptor antagonist that can inhibit neuronal activation of mast cells. It may be effective in atopic IC patients or those with significant mast cells on biopsy. The variability noted in the efficacy of antihistamines may be explained by the previously presented pathophysiologic model in which mast cell degranulation is only one step in the chain of events leading to inflammation and its associated symptoms. Antihistamines may be helpful in preventing symptomatic flares but would be of minimal benefit once the patient is symptomatic. Hydroxyzine is given in doses from 10 to 75 mg at bedtime and it may take up to 3 months to see an improvement in symptoms.

3.   Antidepressants

Antidepressant therapy (TCA, SSRIs) has some efficacy in the treatment of IC largely due to their mode of action as pain neuromodulators. They are prescribed in escalating doses, as the side effects can be prohibitive. Treatment can be initiated early in the course of the disease, particularly if pain is a dominant presenting symptom. Amitryptyline (Elavil) is commonly prescribed in doses beginning at 10 or 25 mg 1 h before bedtime and may be increased up to 75 mg as tolerated. With fluoxetine (Prozac), dosing is started at 20 mg/d and may be increased as needed to 40 mg. Sertraline (Zoloft) is another SSRI that can be used and is well tolerated. Treatment is initiated at 50 mg/d and may be increased to 100 mg. The therapeutic effects of antidepressants are multifactorial: they improve sleep and as a result decrease nocturia; they have a neuromodulating effect by increasing pain thresholds; they elevate mood; and they have an anticholinergic effect on the bladder and thus may improve frequency by controlling instability.

4. Gabapentin (Neurontin)

This is an antiseizure medication that is used increasingly in the management of chronic pain. It is thought to have a neuromodulating effect by increasing pain thresholds and may be useful in IC patients in whom pain is a dominant symptom (31).

5. Anticholinergics, Antispasmotics

Patients with mild symptoms or coexisting bladder instability may get relief with the use of these agents, but in the face of moderated to severe symptoms, they appear to have little efficacy.

B. Intravesical Therapy

1. Dimethyl Sulfoxide

DMSO is an organic solvent with anti-inflammatory, analgesic, and muscle-relaxant effect. It also has collagen dissolution effects, which raises the issue of possible fibrosis developing with long-term use of DMSO, and could be the underlying factor leading to progressive resistance characteristically seen after several cycles of therapy. A review of the published experience with DMSO in over 300 treated patients indicates a favorable response in a significant number of patients with minimal associated morbidity (32). It remains a mainstay of therapy and can be used in combination with hydrocortisone, heparin, and sodium bicarbonate to enhance its effect.

2. Heparin

Chronic intravesical instillation of heparin has been reported to have clinical efficacy in IC patients (33). It consists of daily instillations of 10,000–20,000 units in 10 cc saline. Time lag to symptomatic relief varies between 2 and 6 months, with the best results seen after 1–2 years of treatment. The mechanism of action is likely similar to that of sodium pentosan polysulfate, as heparin has also been shown to reverse epithelial "leaks."

3. Bacillus Calmete-Guerin (BCG)

A randomized, prospective, double-blind, placebo-controlled trial evaluating the efficacy of intravesical BCG in the treatment of IC noted a 60% BCG response rate compared to a 27% placebo response rate at a mean follow-up of 8 months (34). Outcome measures using a validated IC survey indicated a 63% improvement in IC symptomatology. The mechanism of action of BCG in this setting is poorly understood but is thought to be immune mediated. Phase III studies confirming the clinical efficacy of BCG therapy in the management of IC are lacking.

C. Muscle Manipulation and Sacral Neurostimulation

Physical therapy aimed at the pelvic floor musculature can have a therapeutic effect in some IC patients. This is based on the premise that a dysfunctional pelvic floor may be the initiating event ultimately leading to bladder wall neurogenic inflammation and that increased pelvic floor tension may be both a source of pain as well as a trigger for neurogenic inflammation via antidromic reflexes (35). Ten IC patients underwent myofascial manual therapy that consisted of transvaginal one-finger compression and lateral traction of the periurethral tissues and pubourethralis muscle against the symphysis pubis followed by posterior traction via the vagina, and isometric contractions of the pubovaginalis muscle. Seven of the 10 patients reported moderate to marked improvement (51–99% improvement) in their symptoms at a mean follow-up of 19 months. Patients with urgency-frequency syndrome (which many believe is a milder form of IC) with or without pain also responded favorably to this form of therapy, with 83% reporting marked to moderate improvement or complete resolution of symptoms (35). Transvaginal Theile massage in IC patients has also yielded encouraging results, with 90% of patients showing short-term improvement in their symptoms (36).

Sacral neurogenic stimulation with the use of the Interstim device has recently been applied to IC patients with promising results. A recent multicenter clinical trial evaluated the clinical benefit of sacral neuromodulation in 22 IC patients and reported a significant decrease in urinary frequency and pain as well as a significant improvement in IC symptom and problem index score in 60% of the patients (O'Leary-Sant IC symptom and problem index) (37). As other investigators have reported similar findings (38,39), sacral neuromodulation is increasingly considered in patients whose symptoms are refractory to oral or intravesical therapics, and in whom a cystectomy with urinary diversion would otherwise be the next best treatment option. The mechanism of action of this form of neuromodulation is unclear but likely fits within the paradigm of IC as a neurogenically mediated cystitis. Interestingly, normalization of two previously described urinary markers of IC, heparin-binding epidermal growth factor (HB-EGF) and antiproliferative factor (APF), was associated with symptomatic relief in IC patients treated with sacral neurostimulation (40).

D. Surgical Treatment

1. Cystoscopy and Hydrodistension

As alluded to earlier in the chapter, cystoscopy and hydrodistension may have a therapeutic effect in some patients, inducing symptom resolution for a period of 4–12 months in up to 60% of patients. The mechanism of symptomatic improvement is not clear, although there is evidence that the stretch stimulus of hydrodistension increases HB-EGF and reduces APF activity in urine up to 2 weeks after distension (41).

2. Cystectomy and Urinary Diversion

Bladder removal remains a treatment option of last resort for patients whose symptoms are refractory to less invasive forms of treatment. Most patients are symptom free after simple cystectomy or supratrigonal cystectomy with enterocystoplasty, although persistent pelvic pain has been reported in a few patients (42).

E. Treatment Outcome

There is a lack of outcome studies in the literature when it comes to the various treatments available for the management of IC, mostly due to the paucity of valid outcome measures.

The O'Leary-Sant IC symptom index was recently validated in a randomized double-blind clinical study evaluating the therapeutic effect of higher dosing of sodium pentosan polysulfate, and proved to be a reliable and responsive measure of clinical improvement. There is clearly a need for randomized controlled studies that critically evaluate the outcome of each of the many IC treatments, and the ICSI is a useful outcome instrument that, if used uniformly, would facilitate comparisons between studies.

VI. THE FUTURE

The primary issue to be addressed in the near future remains elucidating the pathophysiology of IC. Theories abound, but unifying concepts are sketchy at best. The role of neurogenic inflammation is being actively investigated and has added a new dimension of neural-directed therapies to the treatment armamentarium, though more long-term studies are needed to confirm early promising results. Other potential therapies such as Montelukast (a cysteinyl leukotriene D4 receptor antagonist), capsaicin/resiniferatoxin (C-fiber neurotoxins), and quercetin (a bioflavonoid) also need to be further evaluated in larger randomized placebo-controlled trials.

REFERENCES

1. Hunner GL. A rare type of bladder ulcer in women. Report of cases. J Boston Med Surg 1915; 172:660–665.
2. Hand J. Interstitial cystitis. Report of 223 cases. J Urol 1949; 61:291.
3. Hanno PM, Landis JR, Matthews-Cook Y. The diagnosis of interstitial cystitis revisited: lessons learned from the national institutes of health interstitial cystitis database study. J Urol 1999; 161(2):1–8.
4. Curhan GC, Speizer FE, Hunter DJ. Epidemiology of interstitial cystitis: a population based study. J Urol 1999; 161(2):549–552.
5. Oravisto K. Epidemiology of interstitial cystitis: 1. In: Hanno P, Staskin D, Krane R, Wein A, eds. Interstitial Cystitis. New York: Springer-Verlag, 1990:25.
6. Held P, Hanno P, Wein A. Epidemiology of interstitial cystitis: 2. In: Hanno P, Staskin D, Krane R, Wein A, eds. Interstitial Cystitis. New York: Springer-Verlag, 1990:29.
7. Jones CA, Nyberg L. Epidemiology of interstitial cystitis. Urology 1997; 49(suppl 5A):2–9.
8. Novicki DE, Larson TR, Swanson SK. Interstitial cystitis in men. Urology 1998; 52:621–624.
9. Schuster GA. Interstitial cystitis in children: not a rare entity. Urology 2001; 57(suppl 6A):107.
10. Propert KJ, Schaeffer AJ, Bresinger CM. A prospective study of interstitial cystitis: results of longitudinal follow-up of the interstitial cystitis database cohort. J Urol 2000; 163:1434–1439.
11. Kusek JW, Nyberg LM. The epidemiology of interstitial cystitis: is it time to expand our definition? Urology 2001; 57(6 suppl 1):95–99.
12. Parsons CL. Interstitial cystitis. Clinical manifestations and diagnostic criteria in over 200 cases. Neurourol Urodyn 1990; 9(3):241–250.
13. Parsons CL, Greenberger M, Gabal L. The role of urinary potassium in the pathogenesis and diagnosis of interstitial cystitis. J Urol 1998; 159:1862–1867.
14. Teichman JM, Nielsen-Omeis BJ. Potassium leak test predicts outcome in interstitial cystitis. J Urol 1999; 161:1791–1794.
15. Larsen S, Thompson SA, Hald T. Mast cells in interstitial cystitis. Br J Urol 1982; 54:283–286.
16. Yun SK, Laub DJ, Weese DL. Stimulated release of urine histamine in interstitial cystitis. J Urol 1992; 148:1145–1148.
17. El-Mansoury M, Boucher W, Sant GR. Increased urine histamine and methylhistamine in interstitial cystitis. J Urol 1994; 152:350–353.

18. Holm-Bentzen M, Sondergaard I, Hald T. Urinary excretion of a metabolite of histamine (1,4 methyl-imidazole-acetic-acid) in a painful bladder disease. Br J Urol 1987; 60:39–42.
19. Theoharides TC, Pang X, Letourneau R. Interstitial cystitis: a neuroimmunoendocrine disorder. Ann NY Acad Sci 1998; 840:619.
20. Pang X, Marchand J, Sant GR. Increased number of substance P positive nerve fibers in interstitial cystitis. Br J Urol 1995; 75(6):744–750.
21. Kream RM, Carr DB. Interstitial cystitis: a complex visceral pain syndrome. Pain Forum 1999; 8:139–145.
22. Suzuki H, Miura S, Liu YY. Substance P induces degranulation of mast cells and leukocyte adhesion to venular endothelium. Peptides 1995; 16:1447.
23. Bjorling DE, Jerde TJ, Zine MJ. Mast cells mediate the severity of experimental cystitis in mice. J Urol 1999; 162:231.
24. Jasmin L, Janni G, Manz HJ. Activation of CNS circuits producing a neurogenic cystitis: evidence for centrally induced peripheral inflammation. J Neurosci 1998; 18(23):10016–10029.
25. Jasmine L, Janni G, O'Hara PT. CNS induced neurogenic cystitis is associated with bladder mast cell degranulation in the rat. J Urol 2000; 164(3):852–855.
26. Elbadawi A. Interstitial cystitis: a critique of current concepts with a new proposal for pathologic diagnosis and pathogenesis. Urology 1999; 53(1):239.
27. Byrne DS, Sedor JF, Estojak J. The urinary glycoprotein GP-51 as a clinical marker for interstitial cystitis. J Urol 1999; 161:1786–1790.
28. Moskowitz MO, Byrne DS, Callahan HJ. Decreased expression of a glycoprotein component of bladder surface mucin (GP-51) in interstitial cystitis. J Urol 1994; 151:343–345.
29. Tomaszewski JE, Landis JR, Russack V. Biopsy features are associated with primary symptoms in interstitial cystitis: results from the interstitial cystitis database study. Urology 2001; 57(suppl 6A):67–81.
30. Sadhukhan PC, Tchetgen BM, Rackley RR. Sodium pentosan polysulfate reduces urothelial responses to inflammatory stimuli via an indirect mechanism. J Urol 2002; 168:289–292.
31. Sasaki K, Smith CP, Chuang YC. Oral gabapentin (neurontin) treatment of refractory genitourinary tract pain. Tech Urol 2001; 7(1):47–49.
32. Parkin J, Shea C, Sant GR. Intravesical dimethyl sulfoxide (DMSO) for interstitial cystitis: a practical approach. Urology 1997; 49(5A suppl):105–107.
33. Parsons CL, Housley T, Schmidt JD. Treatment of interstitial cystitis with intravesical heparin. Br J Urol 1994; 73:504–507.
34. Peters K, Diokno A, Steinert B. The efficacy of intravesical Tice strain bacillus Calmette-Guerin in the treatment of interstitial cystitis: a double blind, prospective, placebo-controlled trial. J Urol 1997; 157(6):2090–2094.
35. Weiss J. Pelvic floor myofascial trigger points: manual therapy for interstitial cystitis and the urgency-frequency syndrome. J Urol 2001; 166(6):2226–2231.
36. Holzberg A, Kellog-Spadt S, Lukban J. Evaluation of transvaginal theile massage as a therapeutic intervention for women with interstitial cystitis. Urology 2001; 57(6 suppl 1):120.
37. Whitmore KE, Lukban JC, Payne CK. Sacral neuromodulation in patients with interstitial cystitis: a multicenter clinical trial. J Urol 2001; 165(5 suppl):69.
38. Paszkiewicz EJ, Siegel SW, Kirkpatrick C. Sacral nerve stimulation in patients with chronic, intractable pelvic pain. Urology 2001; 57(6 suppl 1):124.
39. Caraballo R, Bologna RA, Lukban J. Sacral nerve stimulation as a treatment for urge incontinence and associated pelvic floor disorders at a pelvic floor center: a follow-up study. Urology 2001; 57(6 suppl 1):121.
40. Chai TC, Zang C, Warren JW. Percutaneous sacral third nerve root neurostimulation improves symptoms and normalizes urinary HB-EGF levels and antiproliferative activity in patients with interstitial cystitis. Urology 2001; 57(1):207.
41. Chai TC, Ahang CO, Shoenfelt JL. Bladder stretch alters urinary heparin-binding epidermal growth factor and antiproliferative factor in patients with interstitial cystitis. J Urol 2000; 163(5):1440–1444.
42. Van Ophoven A, Oberpenning F, Hertle L. Long-term results of trigone-preserving orthotopic substitution enterocystoplasty for interstitial cystitis. J Urol 2002; 167(2 Pt 1):603–607.

60
Chronic Pelvic Pain in Interstitial Cystitis

James Chivian Lukban
Urogynecology Associates of Colorado, Denver, Colorado, U.S.A.

Kristene E. Whitmore
Graduate Hospital, Philadelphia, Pennsylvania, U.S.A.

I. INTRODUCTION

Interstitial cystitis (IC) is a clinical condition of multifactorial etiology characterized by urinary frequency, urgency, debilitating episodic bladder discomfort, and the potential for the development of chronic pelvic pain (CPP). In a multicenter, observational study designed to evaluate the treated history of IC, 379 of 424 patients (94%) reported the presence of pain, with 24% of those suffering from severe discomfort (1). In a survey of 374 patients performed to characterize the natural history of IC, 96% of respondents overall reported pain, with 54% of subjects describing their discomfort as severe or excruciating (2). Of respondents with symptoms for >15 years, 99% reported pain, with 62% reporting the presence of severe or excruciating discomfort. Pelvic pain has been found to be a preponderant, durable, and potentially debilitating component of IC symptomatology. This chapter will consider the etiology and treatment of CPP in patients with IC.

II. ETIOLOGY OF CHRONIC PELVIC PAIN IN INTERSTITIAL CYSTITIS

Contributing mechanisms to IC etiopathogenesis include, but are not limited to, a deficient or dysfunctional glycosaminoglycan layer, altered urothelial permeability, mastocytosis, "toxic urine," and autoimmunity (3–7). One common element contributing to IC symptomatology, independent of etiology, is the presence of chronic inflammatory changes within the bladder wall. Prolonged bladder epithelial inflammation leads to persistent peripheral afferent stimulation, and the potential for the development of reduced nociceptive thresholds, neuronal hypersensitivity and spontaneous neuronal activity within the central nervous system (CNS). This phenomenon is termed central sensitization, and is an important mechanism in the evolution of centrally derived CPP.

Patients with IC have also the potential to exhibit neurogenic pelvic floor muscle spasm (high-tone pelvic floor dysfunction), which may add to the generation of CPP. Pelvic muscle spasm in patients with IC occurs, in theory, as a result of centrally mediated sacral somatic efferent activity following sacral afferent barrage. Nociceptive impulses created by a spastic pelvic floor may also perpetuate IC pathology through the indirect trigger of antidromic (retrograde) transmission along visceral afferent C fibers with resultant neurogenic bladder inflammation.

III. CENTRALLY DERIVED CHRONIC PELVIC PAIN

The bladder wall contains parasympathetic afferents in the form of lightly myelinated Aδ fibers and unmyelinated C fibers, possessing predominantly mechanosensitive (tension) and chemosensitive (nociception) properties, respectively (8). Upon bladder filling, Aδ fibers respond to physiologic, low-threshold intravesical pressure, while C fibers are typically silent. Unmyelinated bladder afferents exhibit impulse transmission following chemical irritation and may display ongoing activity even after irritant removal (9). Significant inflammation of the bladder epithelium may also provide chemosensitive afferents the ability to adopt a mechanosensitive capacity, firing in response to low-threshold intravesical pressure (9,10). Such novel mechanosensitivity is thought to be mediated by nerve growth factor, as has been suggested in experimental rodent models (11). Myelinated mechanosensitive afferents may undergo a similar reactive change and develop chemosensitive properties, responding to urinary toxins and inflammatory mediators (12). Postinflammation C-fiber activation and peripheral afferent change play an important role in the creation of visceral pain, as physiologic bladder filling and epithelial exposure to mildly noxious stimuli may result in a significant afferent barrage.

Chronic nociceptive input from the periphery as mediated by the presynaptic release of neuropeptides (e.g., substance P) and excitatory amino acids (e.g., glutamate) can establish long-standing functional changes within the CNS essential to the development of central sensitization (13). As substance P (SP)-laden C fibers bombard sacral dorsal horn cells, postsynaptic upregulation of SP receptors (NK1 receptors) may occur (14). Upregulation following long-term somatic stimulation has been observed, with evidence supporting similar changes in response to chronic visceral inflammation having recently been reported (14,15). Ishigooka et al. studied NK1 receptor immunoreactivity in the lumbosacral dorsal horn cells of 12 female rats following cyclophosphamide-induced bladder inflammation. Significant increases in postsynaptic NK1 receptor staining intensity, consistent with enhanced neuronal receptor expression, was observed in bladder-specific spinal segments L_6–S_1. It has also been postulated that repetitive dorsal horn cell depolarization, as triggered by SP, relieves a voltage dependent Mg^{2+} block of postsynaptic glutamate receptors (NMDA receptors) (13,16). Both the upregulation of NK1 receptors and the increased availability of NMDA receptors following chronic afferent nociceptive input increase the total number of postsynaptic sites for neurotransmission. Such events may result in lower nociceptive thresholds and postsynaptic hypersensitivity, consistent with a state of central sensitization.

In an electrophysiologic study of postinflammation CNS changes in rats, McMahon observed the behavior of dorsal horn cells in L_6 and S_1 following turpentine and mustard oil–induced bladder inflammation (10). An evaluation of 14 postsynaptic neurons revealed progressive increases in response to subsequent electrical stimulation in eight dorsal horn cells (57%) and spontaneous activity in 10 (71%). These findings provide further evidence for the development of central sensitization in response to significant visceral insults. The durability of these changes, however, is not known, with some advocating the essential need for continued peripheral input in the maintenance of central sensitization (17,18).

IV. NEUROGENIC PELVIC FLOOR MUSCLE SPASM

A. Anatomy of the Pelvic Floor

The pelvic floor contains layers of connective tissue and muscle that provide support to the pelvic viscera. The urethra, vagina, and rectum are attached to the pelvic sidewalls by the endopelvic fascia (vesico vaginal adventitia), penetrating the pelvic floor at the urogenital hiatus.

Immediately beneath the endopelvic fascia is the pelvic floor musculature (PFM). It is composed of the puborectalis, levator ani (pubococcygeus and iliococcygeus), and coccygeus muscles. The puborectalis originates from the pubis and runs posteriorly to join its contralateral muscle behind the anorectal junction, forming a U-shaped sling. The pubococcygeus muscle emanates from the pubis, traveling posteromedially to insert on the superior surface of the coccyx and the anococcygeal raphe. The iliococcygeus arises from the arcus tendineus levator ani, running posteromedially to insert on the coccyx and anococcygeal raphe. The coccygeus muscle originates from the ischial spine and sacrospinous ligament, inserting onto the lateral coccyx and lower sacrum. Beneath the PFM is the perineal membrane, which together with the PFM defines the pelvic floor. The perineal membrane is a triangular sheet of dense fibromuscular tissue spanning the anterior half of the pelvic outlet. Its attachments include the urethra, vagina, and perineal body medially, and the inferior ischiopubic rami laterally (19).

B.   Innervation of the Pelvic Floor and Bladder

The nerve supply to the pelvic floor and bladder is of somatic and autonomic origin respectively. Somatic fibers from S_2-S_4 form the pudendal nerve, which supplies the perineal surface of the PFM. Sacral nerve root branches also innervate the pelvic floor directly through fibers traveling to the visceral surface of the PFM. Parasympathetic innervation of the bladder begins with preganglionic fibers emanating from S_2-S_4 and ends in the postganglionic muscarinic receptors of the bladder wall. Sympathetic innervation arises from $T_{10}-L_2$, with postganglionic fibers traveling to beta-adrenergic receptors in the smooth muscle of the bladder wall, and alpha-adrenergic receptors in the smooth muscle of the bladder neck and proximal urethra (20).

C.   Normal Pelvic Floor Function

The PFM performs an important role in tonic support of the pelvic viscera. Such support is provided by a preponderance of type I (slow-twitch) fibers within the PFM. In the maintenance of urinary continence, tonic muscular forces are provided by the external striated urethral sphincter (composed of the intramural striated sphincter and the periurethral levator ani musculature) and are important in effecting adequate urethral support. In addition, a minority population of type II (fast-twitch) fibers within the levator ani musculature provides a mechanism for active periurethral muscular contraction at the time of provocative increases in intra-abdominal pressure (21). Less perceptible tonic increases in the PFM occur during bladder filling as part of a sacral spinal mechanism known as the guarding reflex whereby parasympathetic impulses triggered by vesical distension lead to somatic efferent stimulation of the PFM and the external striated urethral sphincter (20).

D.   High-Tone Pelvic Floor Dysfunction

High-tone PFD refers to the clinical condition of hypertonic, spastic PFM with resultant impairment of muscle isolation, contraction, and relaxation. Manifestations include voiding dysfunction, urinary frequency, urinary urgency, pelvic pain, painful bowel movements, and impaired rectal evacuation. High-tone PFD, as a chronic, painful clinical condition, was introduced in the colorectal literature, having been reported as any one of the following clinical entities: coccygodynia; tension myalgia of the pelvic floor; coccygeus-levator spasm syndrome; levator syndrome; and levator ani spasm syndrome.

Thiele described coccygodynia in 1937 as an entity not only characterized by pain localized to the coccyx, but as a syndrome also noteworthy for the presence of levator ani and coccygeus muscle spasm (22). In his original communication, 64 of 69 patients with coccygeal pain were found to have spastic PFM on rectal examination. Work published by the same author in 1963 further characterized coccygodynia based on a review of 324 case records (23). Patient symptoms included pain localized to the lower sacrum and coccyx, often exacerbated by prolonged sitting. Few of his patients, however, exhibited tenderness of the coccyx upon direct palpation or manipulation, a finding consistent with pain born of PFM spasm, and not of primary sacrococcygeal pathology. Common etiologic factors included anal infection and chronic trauma as identified in 178 (55%) and 106 (33%) patients, respectively. Anal infection was thought to cause reflex PFM spasm through lymphatic drainage of organism-laden lymph. Chronic trauma included poor sitting posture and extended vehicle rides.

Sinaki et al. employed the term tension myalgia of the pelvic floor to describe a sample of 94 patients with spastic, tender PFM (24). Common symptoms included low back pain in 82% and a "heavy feeling in the pelvis" in 64%, with the appearance of symptom aggravation in 88% of patients following prolonged sitting. Pelvic floor muscle spasm was attributed to habit contraction of the pelvic floor in addition to a component of hypochondriasis.

Paradis and Marganoff used the term coccygeus-levator spasm syndrome to characterize 92 patients with pelvic floor spasm and "rectal" pain (25). Patients were found to be particularly tender at muscular sites adjacent to the ischial spines and coccyx, with a suggestion by the authors of a more significant involvement of musculofascial, ligamentous, and tendinous structures than of the muscles themselves. Neither infection nor trauma was identified in his patients as an etiologic factor, with the attribution of disease presence to psychoneurosis.

Grant et al. employed the term levator syndrome to describe a sample of 316 patients exhibiting PFM spasm and tenderness (26). The predominant symptom was that of rectal discomfort. The etiology of levator syndrome was reported as unknown.

All of the syndromes as presented above represent a similar clinical condition characterized by tender, spastic PFM manifesting as pain localized to the coccyx and lower sacrum, rectal pain, or generalized pelvic discomfort. Etiologic factors as reported are varied and include infection, chronic sacrococcygeal trauma from poor posture or prolonged sitting, and hypochondriasis or hysteria. A definitive cause of high-tone PFD as encountered in patients with IC has not been established and is most likely the result of several coexisting factors.

E. High-Tone Pelvic Floor Dysfunction in Patients with Interstitial Cystitis

In 1973, Lilius et al. published a thoughtful study on the prevalence of levator spasm in patients with IC (27). As many of their patients complained of pain not only in the area of the bladder but also in the regions of the sacrum, coccyx, and anus, they investigated the presence of concomitant PFM spasm. Twenty-five of 31 patients (81%) with IC were found to have spasm and tenderness of the levator ani musculature, which they termed levator ani spasm syndrome. Lilius and coworkers postulated that frequent restraint of urine led to sustained PFM spasm, and in cases of more severe bladder disease, high-tone pelvic floor musculature was thought to appear in response to afferent autonomic pain impulses from the bladder wall. The researchers also assigned importance to poor sitting or working posture as contributing factors to the development of levator ani spasm syndrome. Their excellent clinical observations, which have since been supported by Schmidt and Vapnek (28) and Moldwin and Mendelowitz (29), suggest both a neurologic and musculoskeletal etiology to the development of high-tone pelvic floor dysfunction in patients with IC.

One speculative possibility in the neurogenic development of high-tone PFD is that the afferent "bombardment" seen in patients with IC may enhance and sustain the guarding reflex which manifests as pelvic floor hypertonus. This concept has been alluded to previously by Chancellor (30). A significant musculoskeletal component to high-tone PFD has been suggested by several authors. Thiele (23), Sinaki et al. (24), and Lilius et al. (27) have associated PFM spasm with poor posture and prolonged sitting. The "typical pelvic pain posture" as described by Baker, characterized by exaggerated lumber lordosis, anterior pelvic tilt, and thoracic kyphosis, has been implicated in the subsequent development of sacroiliac pathology (31). As the sacroiliac joint moves, however slightly, through upslip, downslip, or torsion, the PFM to which it is attached is also subject to dynamic change (32). Muscles that are stretched or compressed are prevented from maintaining a normal resting tone and are prone to trigger point formation and hypertonicity (31). Pelvic floor dysfunction is also thought to appear in reaction to overflexion of the coccyx while sitting with incorrect posture (23). Spasm in these cases may be the result of a change in tension of the PFM to which the coccyx is attached (23). The presence of sacroiliac dysfunction with or without a contribution of poor posture may reasonably serve as a trigger for the development of high-tone PFD. It is likely that the degree of high-tone PFD encountered in IC represents the sum of both neurologic and musculoskeletal components (33). Of interest is the report of lateral sacral shift in an unknown number of patients with coccygeus spasm (34).

V. ANTIDROMIC NEUROINFLAMMATION

Painful pelvic floor musculature may perpetuate bladder pathology through the induction of CNS-mediated antidromic impulse transmission along visceral bladder afferents with resultant neurogenic inflammation. Experimental evidence for centrally mediated neurogenic bladder inflammation was reported by Pinter and Szolcsanyi, who created an animal model to prove antidromic transmission through capsaicin-sensitive afferents (C fibers) to the bladder following CNS stimulation (35). Electrical stimulation of the lumbosacral dorsal nerve roots in anesthetized rats resulted in significant plasma extravasation as quantified by the accumulation of Evans Blue tracer in bladder tissue. Extravasation indicative of neurogenic bladder inflammation was significantly reduced following the functional inactivation of visceral bladder afferents through pretreatment with capsaicin.

Jasmin et al. employed the neurotropic pseudorabies virus (PRV) to illustrate the appearance of immune-mediated hemorrhagic cystitis following sacral somatic inoculation (36,37). Following injection of PRV into the abductor caudae dorsalis (ACD) tail muscle of the rat, behavioral and histologic evidence of cystitis appeared 84 h postinjection. A specific sacral somatic fiber—dorsal horn cell—bladder afferent (C-fiber) circuit was suggested, as systemic examination of other abdominopelvic viscera revealed the absence of postinoculation inflammation. Additionally, selective peripheral and central denervation prevented the appearance of cystitis. These researchers theorized that sacral somatic neurons within the dorsal horn have the capacity to trigger neighboring visceral afferent neurons, resulting in antidromic C-fiber impulse transmission with subsequent neurogenic bladder inflammation. In additional work by the same investigators, local neuroinflammation as a mast cell–mediated event was proved as a significant reduction in the number of microscopically visible mast cells (consistent with degranulation) was detected in the bladder wall post-PRV inoculation (37). Additionally, pre-emptive mast cell degranulation with the mast cell degranulator, compound 48/80, resulted in the absence of cystitis.

Clinical evidence of antidromic bladder neuroinflammation following pelvic floor muscle spasm was offered by Weiss, who noted moderate to marked symptom improvement in 35 of 42 patients (83%) with urgency-frequency syndrome and similar improvement in seven of

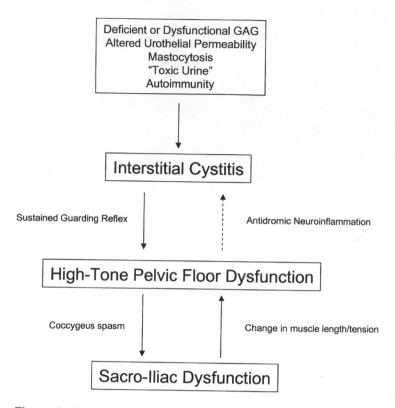

Figure 1 Proposed mechanism for concomitant IC and PFD.

10 patients with IC following internal pelvic floor myofascial trigger point massage (38). A proposed mechanism for concomitant IC and PFD is presented in Figure 1.

VI. TREATMENT OF CENTRALLY DERIVED CHRONIC PELVIC PAIN

A. Opioids

Pain relief from the administration of opioids occurs in part through the activation of opioid receptors in the periaqueductal gray (PAG) of the midbrain, with descending inhibitory impulses providing pain relief by raising nociceptive thresholds within dorsal horn cells. Inhibitory control from the PAG is transmitted through the rostral ventromedial medulla and the dorsal lateral funiculi with spinal nociceptive inhibition mediated by serotonin, norepinephrine, and acetylcholine (39).

In patients with severe pelvic pain from interstitial cystitis, narcotics are added to the treatment regimen. We typically employ short-acting oxycodone or hydrocodone for significant episodic discomfort. Long-acting formulations of oxycodone or morphine serve a role in the treatment of severe persistent pelvic pain, and are administered in conjunction with immediate-release opioids for breakthrough discomfort. The quantification of immediate-release drug consumption daily is used to titrate an appropriate dose of long-acting narcotic (40). We begin with an initial regimen of long-acting, controlled-release oxycodone at a dose of 10 mg BID, and titrate as appropriate. Opioids may be used in conjunction with other oral IC agents, with both hydroxyzine and amitriptyline exhibiting the ability to potentiate narcotic pain relief (40).

B. Amitriptyline

Tricyclic antidepressants have been employed as analgesic agents in nonurologic populations, with clinical benefit proved in patients with postherpetic neuralgia, diabetic peripheral
neuropathy, and chronic low back pain (41–43). Its use in those with IC has more recently
been reported (44,45). The mechanism of tricyclics in alleviating pain is thought to result
from the inhibition of serotonin and noradrenaline reuptake (46). Its analgesic benefit is thought
to be independent of its effect on mood (42).

Hanno et al. evaluated 20 IC patients treated with amitriptyline employing an initial dose
of 25 mg at bedtime, with increases to 50 mg and 75 mg in weeks 2 and 3, respectively (44).
Treatment resulted in a significant decrease in daytime frequency (average minutes between
voids: pretreatment, 62.8; posttreatment, 117) and in pain as rated on a 1 to 10 scale (mean
value: pretreatment, 6.1; posttreatment, 3.3). Eleven of 19 patients reported an improvement
in urinary urgency. Kirkemo et al. evaluated 30 IC patients administered 25–75 mg of amitriptyline nightly (45). Patients were issued questionnaires and voiding diaries to assess symptom
improvement. Ninety percent reported subjective improvement at 2 months. A 50% reduction
in frequency and nocturia was reported in those with a maximum cystometric capacity under
anesthesia >450 cc. In patients with a bladder capacity <450 cc, despite persistent frequency,
an improvement in suprapubic pain was reported.

Initial doses of amitriptyline should begin with 10 mg at bedtime. Increases to 25 mg,
50 mg, and 75 mg at 2- and 3-week intervals may follow with a maximum dose of 150 mg
recommended. Dry mouth and sedation are typically the two most common side effects (41,42).

C. Gabapentin

Gabapentin is an anticonvulsant medication with proven effectiveness in neuropathic pain syndromes (47,48). It has been employed more recently as an agent in the treatment of pain in those
with IC. Its mechanism of action has not been completely elucidated. Gabapentin is a structural
analog to gamma-aminobutyric acid (GABA); however, it does not stimulate GABA receptors,
nor does it alter GABA reuptake (49). In two case studies reported by Hansen, IC patients taking
1600 mg gabapentin daily (one for 6 weeks and one for an undefined period of time) exhibited a
substantial improvement in pain, with a concomitant decrease in narcotic use (50). Sasaki et al.
recently reported data on 21 patients with refractory genitourinary pain treated with gabapentin
(51). A mean dose of 1200 mg daily (range 300–2100 mg) was administered over a 6-month
period. Pain severity was evaluated by a 1 to 5 subjective severity index and a 10-cm visual
analog scale. Ten of 21 patients reported subjective improvement in pain, with five out of
eight patients diagnosed with IC reporting benefit.

Dosing may begin with 100 mg at bedtime, with increases in increments of 100 mg every
3–7 days as tolerated. In our practice, we begin with dosing at bedtime followed by the addition
of medication in the morning, and then at midday as warranted. Doses up to 3600 mg daily have
been administered, with dizziness and somnolence noted to be the most common side effects
(47,48).

D. Additional Therapeutic Considerations

1. Resiniferatoxin

Resiniferatoxin is an ultrapotent vanilloid receptor agonist which functions through C-fiber
desensitization following intravesical instillation. Sensory stimulation by this agent has been
found to occur without the intense noxious excitation as encountered with the instillation of

capsaicin (52). A randomized, placebo-controlled study of resiniferatoxin in the treatment of hypersensitive disorders of the bladder was performed by Lazzeri et al. (53). Eighteen IC patients with a mean disease duration of 16.9 months were evaluated through a voiding pattern assessment and pain scale. After a single treatment, patients receiving resiniferatoxin were noted to exhibit a significant reduction in frequency and pain at a 30-day follow-up with loss of significant pain relief at 90 days. A dose of 10 nM of resiniferatoxin was employed with no reported neurotoxic effects. Four of the patients receiving drug complained of a transient light warm or burning sensation at the suprapubic or urethral level. The efficacy of intravesical C-fiber desensitization in the treatment of centrally derived pain is unknown, and completion recently of a pilot RCT showed no clinical benefit.

2. Sacral Neuromodulation

Sacral nerve root stimulation has shown promise as a therapeutic modality in patients with IC. Its mechanism of pain relief is thought to involve stimulation of sacral somatic afferents with competitive inhibition of slow C-fiber transmission to the CNS (54,55). This theory is based on the cutaneous "gate control" theory of pain in which large diameter fibers inhibit transmission of small diameter fibers to higher centers (56).

Several recent studies have evaluated sacral nerve root stimulation in patients with pelvic pain and the apparent absence of pelvic floor muscle spasm. Maher et al. prospectively evaluated 15 consecutive IC patients with a mean disease duration of 5.2 years who underwent a 7-to-10-day trial of percutaneous third nerve root stimulation (57). Evaluation was in the form of voiding diary, pain score (0 to 10), and quality-of-life questionnaire. Test stimulation resulted in statistically significant improvements in mean daytime frequency (decrease from 20 to 10 voids per day), nocturia (decrease from six to two voids per night), mean voided volume (increase from 90 to 143 cc), and mean bladder pain (decrease from 8.9 to 2.4). The quality-of-life variables of general health, social health, and bodily pain also exhibited significant improvement.

The efficacy of sacral nerve stimulation following permanent implantation in patients with chronic intractable pelvic pain of a median duration of three years was considered by Siegel et al. (58). Ten patients following successful percutaneous sacral nerve root stimulation were implanted with a neuroprosthetic device, with lead placement in sacral foramen 3 or 4 in eight and two cases, respectively. The permanent implant was found to decrease the severity, number of hours (total duration of pain per week), and "rate of pain," with six of 10 patients reporting a significant improvement in overall pelvic pain symptomatology (median follow-up of 19 months). No serious device complications were reported. A total of 27 adverse events were listed, with the three most common found to be local wound complications (6 cases), change in pain location (4), and implant site pain (4). The long-term benefit of sacral neuromodulation in the treatment of centrally derived pain is unknown. As patients in the aforementioned studies had symptoms of pelvic pain measured in years, it is likely that some possessed centrally derived pain. Such patients in theory may receive therapeutic benefit from the elimination of peripheral contributions to dorsal horn cells which possess hypersensitivity and low nociceptive thresholds. A summary of therapeutic measures for the treatment of IC patients with central sensitization is offered in Table 1.

3. Surgical Therapy

Major surgical therapy is the final therapeutic option for patients with IC, of whom only 10% may have disease severity appropriate for such intervention (59). Procedures including subtrigonal or supratrigonal cystectomy with substitution cystolplasty are typically employed, with success rates ranging from 25% to 100% (60). Urinary diversion with or without cystectomy may be

Table 1   Therapy for Centrally Derived Chronic Pelvic Pain

Agent	Proposed mechanism of action	Initial dosage
Opioids (oxycodone)	Stimulation of opioid receptors in midbrain periaqueductal gray	5 hrs 4–6 PRN (immediate release) 10 mg BID (long acting)
Amitriptyline	Inhibition of serotonin and norepinephrine reuptake	10 mg at bedtime
Gabapentin	Unknown	100 mg at bedtime
Resiniferatoxin	Desensitization of C fibers	Single treatment
Sacral neuromodulation	Inhibition of C-fiber transmission to CNS	Test stimulation

indicated following failure of substitution cystoplasty, or in patients who are inappropriate candidates for orthotopic substitution (e.g., severe stress incontinence or inability to catheterize via urethra due to exacerbation of symptoms) (60). Despite technically appropriate surgical intervention, patients may still suffer from persistent discomfort. In a report of four patients (three with IC and one with voiding dysfunction) with severe intractable pelvic pain despite cystectomy, hysterectomy, and bilateral salpingo-oophorectomy, Baskin et al. suggested the presence of central sensitization or untreated pelvic floor dysfunction as potential contributors to persistent symptomatology (61). Appropriate preoperative workup in IC patients prior to embarking upon surgical therapy should thus include not only an appropriate genitourinary and gynecologic assessment, but an evaluation of the pelvic floor, a visit to a pain specialist (to rule out psychogenic pain and/or central sensitization), and a thorough psychological assessment.

VII.   TREATMENT OF HIGH-TONE PELVIC FLOOR DYSFUNCTION

A.   Physical Therapy

Patients identified with high-tone PFD are subsequently sent to a physical therapist for assessment to identify sacroiliac malalignment, also known as sacroiliac dysfunction. Evaluation in brief includes a specific assessment of the following: pelvic alignment; lumbar and hip active and passive range of motion; strength and flexibility of the spinal and pelvic stabilizers; and tenderness and spasm of the pelvic supportive musculature. Typical manual therapy techniques employed in the correction of sacroiliac dysfunction, if identified, include myofascial release, joint mobilization, muscle energy, strengthening, stretching, neuromuscular reeducation, and instruction in an extensive home exercise program. The speculative logic in correcting sacroiliac dysfunction in patients with high-tone PFD is such that if sacroiliac alignment is restored, normal tension to the PFM returns, allowing for the resolution of a high-tone state.

In a pilot study of 16 patients with high-tone PFD, sacroiliac dysfunction, and IC, manual physical therapy was performed to assess the benefit of such treatment in reducing IC symptoms (frequency, urgency, nocturia, pain) as measured by the O'Leary-Sant Symptom Index (62). Dyspareunia was also evaluated in these patients employing the "sex life" question as taken from the Modified Oswestry Disability Scale. A comparison of pre- and posttreatment Modified Oswestry scores revealed an improvement in dyspareunia in 15 (94%) patients. A comparison of pre- and posttreatment O'Leary-Sant scores also showed improvement in 15 (94%) subjects. Schroeder reported the use of an undefined regimen of physical therapy in a pediatric and adolescent population in which 20 of 21 patients with musculoskeletal pelvic pain were success-fully treated (63).

B. Thiele Massage

Following sacroiliac realignment, patients are reassessed by digital exam and perineometry. If PFM spasm persists as either diffuse or localized hypertonicity, subjects undergo a regimen of Thiele massage. In his original description of this technique, Thiele reported a personal series of 31 cases of coccygodynia and PFM spasm in which 19 (61.3%) were cured and 17 (35.5%) were improved (undefined criteria) following transrectal massage (22). The author combined his data with those taken from eight other proctologists employing the same technique, and reported a 93.7% cured and improved rate in a total of 80 patients. Treatment consisted of an average of 11 treatments over an average of 11 weeks.

Weiss recently reported the use of PFM trigger point massage in 45 women and seven men with "urgency-frequency syndrome" of whom 10 fulfilled undefined cystoscopic IC criteria (38). Following one to two visits per week for 8–12 weeks, seven of 10 IC patients exhibited >50% improvement in overall symptoms.

In our practice, we perform Thiele massage transvaginally as this is more comfortable for our patients. In performing this technique, pressure is applied to the PFM fibers longitudinally from origin to insertion. Ten to 15 sweeps of maximally tolerated pressure are performed on each side followed by myofascial massage (10–15 sec of sustained pressure) to tender points. Patients are treated once or twice a week for a duration of 6–8 weeks, less frequently than prac-ticed by Thiele, who applied therapy every day for 5–6 days then every other day for 7–10 days as an initial course.

C. Pelvic Floor Muscle Exercises and Biofeedback

Patients with persistent high-tone PFD despite manual physical therapy and Thiele massage may benefit from PFME and BF. In a study of 60 patients with intractable rectal pain, 70% of whom were diagnosed with either levator spasm or coccygodynia, Ger performed BF on 14 subjects employing rectal EMG (64). Following a minimum of six weekly 30- to 60-min sessions, pain relief was rated as excellent or good (undefined) in six (43%) patients at a mean follow-up of 15 months. Heah prospectively treated 16 patients with levator ani syndrome with biofeed-back employing a rectal manometric balloon (65). A significant improvement in pain was achieved with scores recorded on a 0-to-10 linear analog scale (median pain score before BF, 8; median pain score after BF, 2). All patients exhibited nontender musculature posttherapy. The theory behind BF in the treatment of high-tone PFD is that of achieving conscious control over PFM contraction and relaxation, thus breaking the cycle of spasm.

D. Electrical Stimulation

The use of electrogalvanic stimulation (EGS) in patients with levator syndrome was first described by Sohn (66). Seventy-two patients were treated with EGS at 80 Hz to a point of mild discomfort for a duration of 1 h/d for three sessions over a 3-to-10 day period. Fifty (69%) patients rated treatment as excellent (complete pain relief), and 15 (21%) rated therapy as good (pain resolution with <3 recurrences in the 6–30 month follow-up). The mechanism of pain relief in these patients was reported as muscle fatigue following sustained contractions in addition to motoneuron suppression. Other investigators have reported the use of EGS in patients with levator syndrome reporting variable results with excellent or good improvement ranging from 43% to 91% (67–70). Electrical stimulation in patients with high-tone PFD is delivered with the same intention as EGS in creating muscle fatigue with resultant relaxation; however, ES employs low-voltage alternating current whereas EGS employs high-voltage direct current (71). Electrical stimulation may be provided for patients with high-tone PFD at the time of BF therapy.

Administration of anogenital electrical stimulation involves the use of an intravaginal or intrarectal probe with delivery of current to the pudendal nerve or its branches. Electrical stimulation in the treatment of PFD employs a frequency of 50 Hz (or higher) to ensure PFM contraction and resultant fatigue. Therapy may be performed in combination with PFM exercises and biofeedback in the form of weekly 23-min sessions over 6 weeks. Each session begins with 4 min of biofeedback during which time the patient is asked to offer PFM contractions for 5 sec followed by 10-sec intervals of relaxation. Anogenital stimulation is then applied for 15 min followed by four additional minutes of PFM exercises with biofeedback. Patients with high-tone PFD may maintain PFM fitness with a home device.

E. Pharmacologic Therapy

Several authors have reported success in the treatment of high-tone PFD with diazepam. Grant reported the use of this medication in conjunction with heat and transrectal massage, with 68% of patients reporting good (symptom relief by three or fewer massage treatments) results (26). In a smaller series of six females with external sphincter spasm, sustained relief from urgency, suprapubic discomfort, and voiding dysfunction was achieved following a 2-to-6-month course of diazepam taken in doses of 2–6 mg/d (72).

We have had anecdotal success with tizanidine hydrochloride in relieving high-tone PFD. As it is a centrally acting α-adrenergic agonist, it should be used with caution in patients taking other centrally acting agents. We usually begin with a low dose of 2 mg/d and titrate as appropriate.

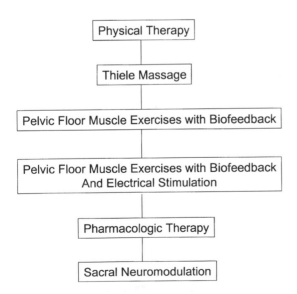

Figure 2 Treatment of high-tone pelvic floor dysfunction.

F. Sacral Neuromodulation

Subacute sacral nerve stimulation in 26 subjects with pelvic pain (with or without PFD) was reported by Everaert et al. (73). Following unilateral percutaneous nerve evaluation of S_3 for a maximum of 4 weeks, 16 patients exhibited significant pain relief as defined by $\geq 50\%$ improvement on visual analog scale. All responders exhibited pain related to urodynamically defined pelvic floor dysfunction. The mechanism of action of sacral neuromodulation in the relief of painful pelvic floor muscle spasm may involve the aforementioned gate theory, with inhibition of impulse transmission to the sacral spinal cord interneurons from which somatic efferents to the pelvic floor emanate (54,74).

G. Treatment Algorithm for High-Tone Pelvic Floor Dysfunction

High-tone pelvic floor dysfunction is treated initially with manual physical therapy performed in an effort to restore sacroiliac and sacrococcygeal alignment, with resultant relief from abnormal muscular tension. Thiele massage is initiated if the PFM exhibits persistent hypertonus despite appropriate bony alignment. Pelvic floor muscle exercise, biofeedback, and electrical stimulation then provide a mechanism to achieve maximal PFM contraction and relaxation in the restoration of normal muscular function. Pharmacologic therapy may be used as adjunctive therapy in patients with high-tone PFD. Sacral neuromodulation testing may be considered in patients with pain born of PFD refractory to other therapy. The treatment algorithm for PFD is represented in Figure 2.

VIII. CONCLUSION

Pain can become the most debilitating symptom in a patient with long-standing IC. A better understanding of the etiology of CPP in this population is essential to improve treatment and restore quality of life. We propose the derivation of CPP in IC to be the product of centrally induced changes (with or without the need for a measure of peripheral nociceptive input) in addition to neurogenic pelvic floor muscle spasm. Evidence for central sensitization has been well established in the pain literature. Experimental proof supporting generation of PFD from nociceptive afferent barrage and dynamic changes in the bony pelvis is less well established. Additionally, antidromic neuroinflammation in the perpetuation of bladder pathology is an investigational consideration.

Clinically, we employ therapy to control centrally derived pain and maintain a high index of suspicion for the presence of concomitant PFD in patients with IC. We eagerly treat the pelvic floor in appropriate candidates, as any degree of therapeutic benefit achieved in a patient with chronic debilitating discomfort outweighs the attendant risks of such therapy.

REFERENCES

1. Simon LJ, Landis R, Erickson DR, Nyberg LM, ICDB Study Group. The Interstitial Cystitis Database Study: concepts and preliminary baseline descriptive statistics. Urology 1997; 49(suppl 5A):64–75.
2. Koziol JA, Clark DC, Gittes RF, Tan EM. The natural history of interstitial cystitis: a survey of 374 patients. J Urol 1993; 149:465–469.
3. Parsons CL, Lilly JD, Stein P. Epithelial dysfunction in nonbacterial cystitis (interstitial cystitis). J Urol 1991; 145:732–735.

4. Erickson DR, Sheykhnazari M, Ordille S, Bhavanandan VP. Increased urinary hyaluronic acid and interstitial cystitis. J Urol 1998; 160:1282–1284.

5. Sant GR, Theoharides TC. The role of the mast cell in interstitial cystitis. Urol Clin North Am 1994; 21:41–53.

6. Keay S, Zhang CO, Hise MK, Hebel JR, Jacobs SC, Gordon D, Whitmore K, Bodison S, Gordon N, Warren JW. A diagnostic in vitro urine assay for interstitial cystitis. Urology 1998; 52:974–978.

7. Ochs RL, Tan EM. Autoimmunity and interstitial cystitis. In: Sant GR, ed. Interstitial Cystitis. Philadelphia: Lippincott-Raven, 1997:47–52.

8. De Groat WC. A neurologic basis for the overactive bladder. Urology 1997; 50(suppl 6A):36–52.

9. Habler HJ, Janig W, Koltzenburg M. Activation of unmyelinated afferent fibres by mechanical stimuli and inflammation of the urinary bladder of the cat. J Physiol 1990; 425:545–562.

10. McMahon SB. Neuronal and behavioural consequences of chemical inflammation of rat urinary bladder. Agents Actions 1988; 25:231–233.

11. Dmitrieva N, McMahon SB. Sensitisation of visceral afferents by nerve growth factor in the adult rat. Pain 1996; 66:87–97.

12. Habler HJ, Janig W, Koltzenburg M. Receptive properties of myelinated primary afferents innervating the inflamed urinary bladder of the cat. J Neurophysiol 1993; 69:395–405.

13. Coderre TJ, Katz J, Vaccarino AL, Melzack R. Contribution of central neuroplasticity to pathological pain: review of clinical and experimental evidence. Pain 1993; 32:259–285.

14. Ishigooka M, Zerman DH, Doggweiler R, Schmidt RA, Hashimoto T, Nakada T. Spinal NK1 receptor is upregulated after chronic bladder irritation. Pain 2001; 93:43–50.

15. Abbadie C, Trafton J, Liu H, Mantyh PW, Basbaum AI. Inflammation increases the distribution of dorsal horn neurons that internalize the neurokinin-1 receptor in response to noxious and non-noxious stimulation. J Neurosci 1997; 17:8049–8060.

16. McMahon SB, Lewin GR, Wall PD. Central hyperexcitability triggered by noxious inputs. Curr Opin Neurobiol 1993; 3:602–610.

17. Koltzenburg M, Torebjork HE, Wahrin LK. Nociceptor modulated central sensitization causes mechanical hyperalgesia in acute chemogenic and chronic neuropathic pain. Brain 1994; 117:579–591.

18. Coderre TJ, Katz J. Peripheral and central hyperexcitability: differential signs and symptoms in persistent pain. Behav Brain Sci 1997; 20:404–419.

19. DeLancey JOL. Surgical anatomy of the female pelvis. In: Rock JA, Thompson JD, eds. TeLinde's Operative Gynecology, ed 8. Philadelphia: Lippincott-Raven, 1997:63–93.

20. Steers WD. Physiology and pharmacology of the bladder and urethra. In: Walsh PC, Retig AB, Vaughan ED, Wein AJ, eds. Campbell's Urology, ed 7. Philadelphia: W.B. Saunders, 1998:870–915.

21. Gosling JA, Dixon JS, Critchley HOD, Thompson S. A comparative study of the human external sphincter and periurethral levator ani muscles. Br J Urol 1981; 53:35–41.

22. Thiele GH. Coccygodynia and pain in the superior gluteal region. JAMA 1937; 109:1271–1275.

23. Thiele GH. Coccygodynia: cause and treatment. Dis Colon Rectum 1963; 6:422–436.

24. Sinaki M, Merritt JL, Stillwell GK. Tension myalgia of the pelvic floor. Mayo Clin Proc 1977; 52:717–722.

25. Paradis H, Marganoff H. Rectal pain of extrarectal origin. Dis Colon Rectum 1969; 12:306–312.

26. Grant SR, Salati EP, Rubin RJ. Levator syndrome: an analysis of 316 cases. Dis Colon Rectum 1975; 18:16–163.

27. Lilius HG, Oravisto KJ, Valtonen EJ. Origin of pain in interstitial cystitis. Scand J Urol Nephrol 1973; 7:150–152.

28. Schmidt RA, Vapnek JM. Pelvic floor behavior and interstitial cystitis. Semin Urol 1991; 9:154–159.

29. Moldwin RM, Mendelowitz F. Pelvic floor dysfunction and interstitial cystitis. J Urol 1994; 151(suppl):285A.

30. Das AK, White MD, Longhurst PA. Sacral nerve stimulation for the management of voiding dysfunction. Rev Urol 2000; 1:43–60.

31. Baker PK. Musculoskeletal origins of chronic pelvic pain. Obstet Gynecol Clin North Am 1993; 20:719–741.

32. Woerman AL. Evaluation and treatment of dysfunction in the lumber-pelvic-hip complex. In: Donatelli R, Wooden MJ, eds. Orthopaedic Physical Therapy, ed 1. New York: Churchill Livingstone, 1989:403–483.

33. Messelink EJ. The overactive bladder and the role of the pelvic floor muscles BJU Int 1999; 83(suppl 2):31–35.

34. TichyM,MalbohanIM,OtahalM,ChalupovaM.Pelvicfloormusclesinfluencethelumbosacralregion.Third InterdisciplinaryWorldCongressonLowBackandPelvicPain,Vienna,November1998.

35. Pinter E, Szolcsanyi J. Plasma extravasation in the skin and pelvic organs evoked by antidromic stimulation of the lumbosacral dorsal roots of the rat. Neuroscience 1995; 68:603–614.

36. Jasmin L, Janni G, Manz HJ, Rabkin SD. Activation of CNS circuits producing a neurogenic cystitis: evidence for centrally induced peripheral inflammation. J Neurosci 1998; 18:10016–101029.

37. Jasmin L, Janni G, Ohara PT, Rabkin SD. CNS induced neurogenic cystitis is associated with bladder mast cell degranulation in the rat. J Urol 2000; 164:852–855.

38. Weiss JM. Pelvic floor myofascial trigger points: manual therapy for interstitial cystitis and the urgency-frequency syndrome. J Urol 2001; 166:2226–2231.

39. Urban MO, Gebhart GF. Central mechanisms of pain. Med Clin North Am 1999; 83:585–596.

40. Brookoff D. The causes and treatment of pain in interstitial cystitis. In: Sant GR, ed. Interstitial Cystitis. Philadelphia: Lippincott-Raven, 1997:177–192.

41. Watson CP, Evans RJ, Reed K, Merskey H, Goldsmith L, Warsh J. Amitriptyline versus placebo in postherpetic neuralgia. Neurology 1982; 32:671–673.

42. Max MB, Culnane M, Schafer SC, Gravely RH, Walther DJ, Smoller B, Dubner R. Amitriptyline relieves diabetic neuropathy pain in patients with normal or depressed mood. Neurology 1987; 37:589–596.

43. Pheasant H, Bursk A, Goldfarb J, Azen SP, Weiss JN, Borelli L. Amitriptyline and chronic low back pain. A randomized double-blind crossover study. Spine 1983; 8:552–557.

44. Hanno PM, Buehler J, Wein AJ. Use of amitriptyline in the treatment of interstitial cystitis. J Urol 1989; 141:846–848.

45. Kirkemo AK, Miles BJ, Peters JM. Use of amitriptyline in interstitial cystitis (abstract). J Urol 1990; 143(suppl):279A.

46. Pontari MA, Hanno P. Oral therapies for interstitial cystitis. In: Sant GR, ed. Interstitial Cystitis. Philadelphia: Lippincott-Raven, 1997:173–176.

47. Rowbotham M, Harden N, Stacey B, Bernstein P, Magnus-Miller L, Gabapentin Postherpetic Neuralgia Study Group. Gabapentin for the treatment of postherpetic neuralgia. A randomized controlled trial. JAMA 1998; 280:1837–1842.

48. Backonja M, Beydoun A, Edwards KR, Schwartz SL, Fonesca V, Hes M, LaMoreaux L, Garofalo E, Gabapentin Diabetic Neuropathy Study Group. Gabapentin for the symptomatic treatment of painful neuropathy in patients with diabetes mellitus. JAMA 1998; 280:1831–1836.

49. Gabapentin. Physicians' Desk Reference, 2000:2269–2271.

50. Hansen HC. Interstitial cystitis and the potential role of gabapentin. South Med J 2000; 93:238–242.

51. Sasaki K, Smith CP, Chuang YC, Lee JY, Kim JC, Chancellor MB. Oral gabapentin (Neurontin) treatment of refractory genitourinary tract pain. Tech Urol 2001; 7:47–49.

52. Avelino A, Cruz F, Ciombra A. Intravesical resiniferatoxin desensitizes rat bladder sensory fibres without causing intense noxious excitation. A c-fos study. Eur J Pharmacol 1999; 378:17–22.

53. Lazzeri M, Beneforti P, Spinelli M, Zanollo A, Barbagli G, Turini D. Intravesical resiniferatoxin for the treatment of hypersensitive disorder: a randomized placebo controlled study. J Urol 2000; 164:676–679.

54. Chancellor MB, Chartier-Kastler EJ. Principles of sacral nerve stimulation (SNS) for the treatment of bladder and urethral sphincter dysfunctions. Neuromodulation 2000; 3:15–26.

55. Shaker H, Wang Y, Loung D, Balbaa L, Fehlings MG, Hassouna MM. Role of C-afferent fibers in the mechanism of action of sacral nerve root neuromodulation in chronic spinal cord injury. BJU Int 2000; 85:905–910.

56. Melzack R, Wall PD. Pain mechanisms: a new theory. Science 1965; 150:971–979.

57. Maher CF, Carey MP, Dwyer PL, Schluter PL. Percutaneous sacral nerve root neuromodulation for intractable interstitial cystitis. J Urol 2001; 165:884–886.

58. Siegel S, Paszkiewicz E, Kirkpatrick C, Hinkel B, Oleson K. Sacral nerve stimulation in patients with chronic intractable pelvic pain. J Urol 2001; 166:1742–1745.

59. Webster GD, Galloway N. Surgical treatment of interstitial cystitis. Indications, techniques, and results. Urology 1987; 29:34–39.

60. Hohenfellner M, Linn J, Hampel C, Thuroff JW. Surgical treatment of interstitial cystitis. In: Sant GR, ed. Interstitial Cystitis. Philadelphia: Lippincott-Raven, 1997:223–233.

61. Baskin LS, Tanagho EA. Pelvic pain without pelvic organs. J Urol 1992; 147:683–686.

62. Lukban J, Whitmore K, Kellog-Spadt S, Bologna R, Lesher A, Fletcher E. The effect of manual physical therapy in patients diagnosed with interstitial cystitis, high-tone pelvic floor dysfunction, and sacroiliac dysfunction (abstract). Urology 2001; 57(suppl 6A):121.

63. Schroeder B, Sanfilippo JS, Hertweck P. Musculoskeletal pelvic pain in a pediatric and adolescent gynecology practice. J Pediatr Adolesc Gynecol 2001; 13:90.

64. Ger GC, Wexner SD, Jorge JMN, Lee E, Amaranath LA, Heymen S, Nogueras JJ, Jagleman DG. Evaluation and treatment of chronic intractable rectal pain—a frustrating endeavor. Dis Colon Rectum 1993; 36:139–145.

65. Heah SM, Ho YH, Tan M, Tan M, Leong AFPK. Biofeedback is effective treatment for levator ani syndrome. Dis Colon Rectum 1997; 40:187–189.

66. Sohn N, Weinstein MA, Robbins RD. The levator syndrome and its treatment with high-voltage electrogalvanic stimulation. Am J Surg 1982; 144:580–582.

67. Nicosia JF, Abcarian H. Levator syndrome: a treatment that works. Dis Colon Rectum 1985; 28:406–408.

68. Oliver GC, Rubin RJ, Salvati EP, Eisenstat TE. Electrogalvanic stimulation in the treatment of levator syndrome. Dis Colon Rectum 1985; 28:662–663.

69. Billingham RP, Isler JT, Friend WG, Hostetler J. Treatment of levator syndrome using high-voltage galvanic stimulation. Dis Colon Rectum 1987; 30:584–587.

70. Hull TL, Milson JW, Church J, Oakley J, Lavery I, Fazio V. Electrogalvanic stimulation for levator syndrome: how effective is it in the long term? Dis Colon Rectum 1993; 36:731–733.

71. Lampe G. Transcutaneous electrical nerve stimulation. In: O'Sullivan SB, Schmitz TJ, eds. Physical Rehabilitation: Assessment and Treatment, ed 2. Philadelphia: E.A. Davis, 1988:647–665.

72. Kaplan WE, Firlit CF, Schoenberg HW. The female urethral syndrome: external sphincter spasm as etiology. J Urol 1980; 124:48–49.

73. Everaert K, Devulder J, De Muynck M, Stockham S, Depaepe H, De Looze D, van Buyten J, Oosterlink W. The pain cycle: implications for the diagnosis and treatment of pelvic pain syndromes. Int Urogynecol J 2001; 12:9–14.

74. Everaert K, Plancke H, Lefevere F, Oosterlink W. The urodynamic evaluation of neuromodulation in patients with voiding dysfunction. BJU Int 1997; 79:702–707.

61

Fecal Incontinence

Tracy Hull
Cleveland Clinic Foundation, Cleveland, Ohio, U.S.A.

I. INTRODUCTION

Fecal incontinence, although not a life-threatening condition, can be a life-altering problem. The symptoms range from minor soiling to gross loss of stool. For some with this problem, the fear of soilage prevents them from functioning outside their homes and away from a toilet. The inclusion of a chapter on this subject in a book devoted to anterior pelvic organ problems is appropriate as the pelvic floor is viewed more as a single entity due to shared innervation and muscular support. The common etiology leading to most urogenital dysfunction is the same for fecal incontinence: namely, childbirth. At our institution, we found that a third of women presenting to the urogynecologist for urinary incontinence also had fecal incontinence (1). Similarly, Tetzcher et al. found that 18% of women who had a previous obstetric anal sphincter disruption had both urinary and fecal incontinence (2). Therefore, women presenting to the urogynecologist frequently have combined problems.

II. PREVALENCE

The true incidence of fecal incontinence is unknown. Factors that lead to an inaccurate estimation of how many people are afflicted with this problem include the lack of a standard and accepted definition for severity and frequency; reluctance of patients to discuss it with health care providers; lack of awareness of the problem and treatment options by health care providers; and the wide variety of populations sampled when calculating the incidence (3). The prevalence has been estimated in the general population by an English postal survey to be 1.7/1000 women aged 15–64 and 13.3/1000 women over 65 years of age (4). A study of patients visiting primary care doctors or gastroenterologists in Illinois found the prevalence of fecal incontinence to be 18.4% (5). One-third of symptomatic patients had not discussed their problem with their doctor. Similarly in a Swiss study 5.6% of women in a general outpatient clinic had incontinence, but only 20% reported symptoms to their medical practitioner (6). In a random telephone survey in Wisconsin, 2.2% had fecal incontinence (7). In this study one-third were >65 years old and 63% were women. A recent British study reported that 2% of the population has fecal incontinence and it afflicts 7% of those over 65 years (8). Therefore an accurate assessment of the number of people afflicted with this problem is not clear. It is safe to say that it is probably underestimated and a significant issue.

III. ETIOLOGY

As stated in the introduction, the most common etiology is childbirth during a vaginal delivery. After review of 11 studies, Sultan found fecal incontinence after an obstetric injury to be 20–50% with a median follow-up of 6–12 months (9). In his landmark study, Sultan found that 35% of primiparous women had a sphincter defect after a vaginal delivery, and 44% of multiparous (10). Others have found the incidence of anal sphincter defects to be 7–34% for primiparous women and 12–37% for multiparous (11–13). Therefore, a significant group of women will have a sphincter defect after a vaginal delivery. Not all these women have incontinence initially. Normal aging may influence problems in older women. Until long-term prospective data are collected, the actual influence of a remote childbirth disruption of the sphincter complex versus natural aging will not be known.

Additional causes of fecal incontinence include surgical sphincter damage (i.e., hemorrhoidectomy or sphincterotomy), irradiation, trauma, congenital abnormalities, rectal prolapse, bowel tumors, inflammation, neurologic conditions (i.e., diabetes, dementia, multiple sclerosis), and others (i.e., diarrhea, scleroderma).

IV. EVALUATION

A comprehensive history is the first step in evaluating these patients. This includes questions about the duration and frequency of incontinence. Additionally, the quality of the stool that is lost and the ability to control flatus are elucidated. The use of pads in fecal urgency is questioned. Effect on the patient's quality of life is important to determine for optimal treatment options. Owing to its frequent coexistence, questions about urinary incontinence should be asked.

A past obstetric and surgical history along with other medical problems is obtained to give clues regarding etiology. Some medications can contribute to fecal incontinence by producing loose stools, and therefore all medicines and their side effects are reviewed.

On physical exam, looking at the undergarments for soiling and the perineum for scarring or anal gapping is the initial step. The anus should be visualized while the patient is asked to strain and squeeze to view muscle movement. This should be repeated with a finger in the anus to assess sphincter movement. It is important to distinguish puborectalis contraction from external sphincter contraction. Stool retained in the rectum or fecal impaction is noted.

Visualization of the distal large bowel with proctoscopy or a flexible sigmoidoscopy will rule out any rectal abnormalities predisposing to incontinence. If the diagnosis is still in question, a 100-cc tap water enema can be administered. If the patient can hold this, her fecal incontinence is probably not significant.

V. DIAGNOSTIC TESTING

Objective testing may be beneficial to determine the degree of impairment. It is not mandatory for an uncomplicated sphincter disruption, but may be needed for redo procedures or those that do not appear straightforward.

Anorectal manometry reflects pressures that are generated by the anal sphincters. The internal anal sphincter is the primary determinant of the resting pressures. The external anal sphincter primarily determines the squeeze pressures. There are many types of catheters available to do these measurements, but most are water perfused with four or eight radial port channels. The length of the anal canal can also be determined as the distance of increased pressure from the rectum to the outer skin. Additionally, rectal compliance (which is responsible for the degree of urgency to evacuate) can be calculated. The amount of air inserted in a balloon until the patient first senses it and the maximal tolerated volume are measured. The rectal compliance can be calculated from this. It is the rectal capacity (maximum tolerated volume minus the first sensation) divided by gradient pressure. The sensation of urgency has been correlated with rectal compliance (14). Thus, patients with a low compliance may have difficulty waiting to defecate and thus have severe urgency, which may be misinterpreted or contribute to fecal incontinence.

Traditionally, needle electromyography (EMG) was used to evaluate the striated muscle of the anorectum. Cutaneous surface electrodes placed in pairs at the anal orifice were developed because of the pain from EMG. They may be inaccurate owing to electrical activity of adjacent large muscles such as the gluteus (15). However, this has not been a uniform finding, and surface EMG has been found to be accurate and comparable to needle EMG (16). Currently, EMG has been replaced by anal ultrasound (17), which is much more accurate at delineating defects and differentiating scar from muscle. However, EMG still has a place in evaluating neuromuscular integrity.

Pudendal nerve terminal motor latency is the length of time needed after the pudendal nerve is stimulated at the ischial spine, until the sphincter muscle contracts. A prolonged pudendal nerve motor latency has been shown by some to decrease success after sphincter repair (18,19).

Endoanal ultrasonography has emerged as a preferred tool to map the sphincters. The internal anal sphincter appears as a hypoechoic circular band that is best visualized in the mid-anal canal. The external sphincter is thicker and of mixed echogenicity (Fig. 1). Correlation of

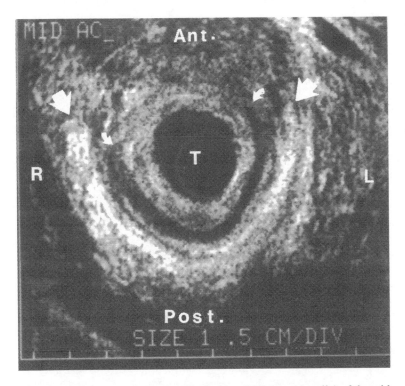

Figure 1   This is an anal sphincter ultrasound (done transanally) of the mid anal canal. This is a woman who has fecal incontinence 10 years after the birth of her last baby. The probe of the transducer is faintly seen in the center. The internal anal sphincter is the black hypoechoic circle, which has an anterior defect. The ends are shown with the small arrows. The external anal sphincter (with mixed echogenicity) also has an anterior defect. The ends of the muscle are shown with the fat arrows. ANT, anterior; POST, posterior; R, right; L, left; T, transducer in lumen of anal canal.

preoperative detected lesions with intraoperative findings is high, close to 100% in two studies (20,21). However, Sentovich et al. found that even though the accuracy correlated 100% with intraoperative findings, transanal ultrasound falsely showed a sphincter injury in 5–25% of nulliparous women (22). Recent innovations to improve preoperative sphincter visualization include three-dimensional anal ultrasound and magnetic resonance imaging (MRI) with endo-anal receiver coil (23). One study suggests that endoanal ultrasound and endoanal MRI are equivalent in diagnosing external anal sphincter injury, but MRI is inferior at diagnosing internal anal sphincter defects (24).

Defecography is not routinely used to evaluate fecal incontinence unless defecation dysfunction exists. The study is done looking for rectal prolapse or internal intussusception.

VI. NONSURGICAL TREATMENT

All treatment of fecal incontinence starts with optimization of any medical condition (such as proctitis). Diarrhea should be evaluated and aggressively treated (25). Sometimes treating diarrhea will eliminate fecal incontinence. Some commercial bulking agents such as Metamucil, Citrucel, or Konsyl improve the consistency of stool and improve incontinence. In one prospective randomized study, patients using psyllium had 50% fewer episodes of incontinent stools over controls due to improvement in stool consistency (26). Agents such as loperamide (Imodium) and diphenoxylate hydrochloride with atropine (Lomotil) are used for patients with diarrhea of no obvious etiology. Similarly, patients with constipation and overflow incontinence require aggressive enemas or laxatives to keep the rectum empty.

More recently, amitriptyline (20 mg at bedtime) may improve fecal incontinence (27). It is felt that this agent works by decreasing the amplitude and frequency of rectal motor complexes. This leads to firmer stools.

There are multiple barrier creams on the market today. Aggressive protection of the anal skin with these agents is needed to protect skin from excoriation. Some patients benefit from an enema program, which washes out the rectum to prevent stool loss. Special cone-tipped catheters can be used for patients with poor tone and difficulty administering an enema.

Biofeedback involves providing patients visual (and occasionally auditory) feedback about contraction of the external sphincter. Many methods and forms exist. A popular method involves placing a balloon in the rectum to simulate stool and measuring anal sphincter contraction with a separate balloon in the anal canal, or by an anal plug, or by perianal surface electrodes. Patients are encouraged when the proper sphincter response is made. The goal is to increase sphincter strength and to teach patients to respond to smaller volumes of material in the rectum. A recently published study looked at 46 studies from the English literature where biofeedback was used to treat fecal incontinence in adults (28). After biofeedback 49% were said to be cured of their fecal incontinence, and 72% were cured or improved. The limitations of this study were that methods of biofeedback varied and few studies used controls. Also, no standard tool was used to assess outcome. However, the authors felt that their results suggest that biofeedback helps the majority of patients. In another review of articles published on biofeedback, comparing coordination training (coordination of pelvic floor muscle contraction with the sensation of rectal filling) with strength training (like kegels), the success rate was ~70% for both (29). Biofeedback requires a dedicated, caring therapist to teach and encourage the biofeedback. Patients must be alert and extremely motivated. Multiple sessions are usually required. Long-term results do not seem to diminish with time (30,31). One interesting application was the use of biofeedback in patients who did not have functional improvement after "successful" sphincteroplasty. These patients were found to improve after biofeedback (32).

VII. SURGICAL TREATMENT

A. Sphincteroplasty

The most common surgical procedure is directed at repair of the muscle. The most common type of repair is after an obstetric injury, and thus an anterior repair is performed. A few are performed to repair defects from anorectal surgery. Attempts are usually made to repair obstetric injury at the time of occurrence; thus, this repair is done in a delayed fashion when the original repair at childbirth has failed. Originally the ends were reapproximated end to end. Currently, the scar is divided but retained, and an overlapping repair as described by Parks and McPartlin is performed (33). Patients can be positioned in the lithotomy or prone position. The surgery can be done under regional or general anesthesia. I prefer a full bowel preparation; however, some only administer enemas in the preoperative area. I also prefer perioperative antibiotics continuing for several days after the procedure. A curvilinear incision is made over the perineal body. To avoid injury to the pudendal nerve, the arc of the incision should not extend to the extreme posterior lateral position. The dissection is deepened and carried laterally into the ischiorectal fat. Since the medial border of the ischiorectal fossa is the external sphincter muscle, it is identified in this area. The same procedure is carried out on the other side (Fig. 2). Then the midline scar is divided and further elucidation of the ends is done (Fig. 3). If both the internal and external sphincters are injured, sometimes leaving them intact as a unit facilitates repair. If only the external sphincter is injured, then the internal is not mobilized.

The levator ani muscle may be plicated at this point using No. 0 or 2-0 delayed absorbable sutures. The vagina should be checked after the plication to ensure that no ridge or narrowing was created. The sphincter complex is next overlapped and approximated using 2-0 polyglactin

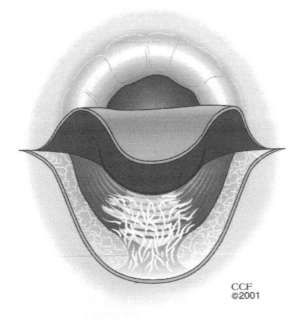

CCF
©2001

Figure 2 This is a schematic in the prone position. A semicircular incision is made over the perineal body. The muscle is identified with a scar in the anterior midline. (Reprinted with permission of the Cleveland Clinic Foundation, Cleveland, OH.)

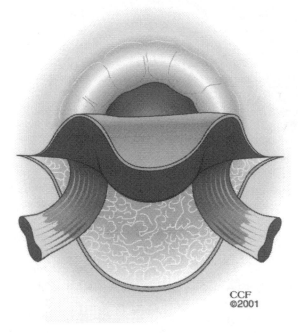

Figure 3 The scar is divided in the middle, leaving scar on the ends of the muscle. The ends are further dissected. (Reprinted with permission of the Cleveland Clinic Foundation, Cleveland, OH.)

mattress sutures. Approximately three or four sutures are placed on each side (Fig. 4). During the procedure irrigation of the wound is carried out with antibiotic solution. The skin edges are reapproximated (Fig. 5). Sometimes it must be closed in a V-Y fashion owing to tension from lengthening the perineal body. I usually leave the middle open to facilitate drainage of any fluid collection.

Postoperatively I prefer 2 days of IV antibiotics and withhold oral intake. I do not use sitz baths due to the tendency to macerate tissue. However, showers are permitted. I also do not use constipating agents. At discharge one of the most important points is to ensure that patients do not get constipated. I prefer to use a bulking fiber agent along with an ounce of mineral oil each morning for the first 2 weeks. Also, if the patient has not had a bowel movement by postoperative day 4, milk of magnesia 1 ounce twice daily is advised until there is a bowel movement.

The use of a diverting stoma is reserved for redo procedures, complicated repairs (such as a cloaca), and patients with concomitant inflammatory bowel disease or diarrhea. Not all of these patients require a stoma, and its use does not guarantee success; the question is therefore left up to the surgeon's discretion.

Table 1 shows the success rates for this repair in a number of recent studies. Unfortunately, it appears that long-term results are not as optimistic as once thought. Other treatment options are therefore considered for those who fail.

B.   Gluteal Muscle Transposition

This was popular 8–10 years ago, but has now been replaced by other techniques. Similarly, the posterior anal imbrication (*Park's postanal repair*) has also been nearly abandoned as has the *Thiersch encirclement procedure*.

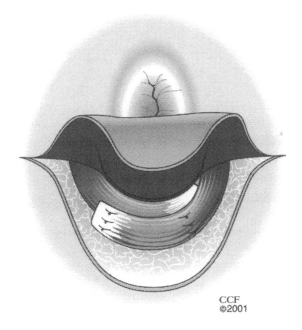

Figure 4 An overlapping repair is done taking advantage of the strength of the scar versus the muscle belly. The sutures go through the scar and anchor it to the opposite muscle with mattress sutures. (Reprinted with permission of the Cleveland Clinic Foundation, Cleveland, OH.)

The *stimulated gracillis transposition* and encirclement around the anus emerged as a promising treatment option over the past 15 years. Even though this remains in the armamentarium of incontinence surgeons in Canada and Europe, the stimulator is no longer available in the United States. This procedure has a steep learning curve with a high morbidity rate. The gracilis muscle is mobilized from the inner thigh, preserving the neurovascular bundle proximally. The tendon of insertion is divided at the knee. The muscle is wrapped around the anus and the tendon is sewn to the opposite ischial tuberosity. An electrical stimulator is placed at an optimal site on the abdomen, and leads are tunneled from the stimulator to the muscle. The leads are positioned in the proximal aspect of the nerve.

The results of a multicenter study showed that 74% had adverse events (infection, muscle wrap problems, pain, device problems, and other problems) with 40% requiring one or more operations to treat complications (39). Successful results (50% reduction in incontinence episodes) were obtained in 57% of patients at 18 months.

C. Artificial Anal Sphincter

This has emerged as the newest accepted option for patients with intractable fecal incontinence. American Medical Systems, Minnetonka, MN, has modified the device used in urinary incontinence for fecal incontinence. It consists of three parts: an inflatable cuff which surrounds the anus; a central pump positioned in the labia for women and the scrotum for men; and a regulating balloon in the space of Retzius (Fig. 6). When a patient needs to defecate, the central pump is pumped, which forces the fluid into the regulating balloon. Then over the next 8 min, the fluid gradually returns to the cuff which surrounds the anus to occlude the opening. Problems with the

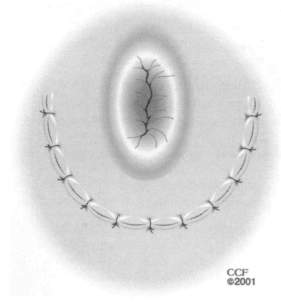

Figure 5   The skin is reapproximated. (Reprinted with permission of the Cleveland Clinic Foundation, Cleveland, OH.)

procedure include infection, erosion, mechanical failure, and difficult evacuation. Complications range from 23% to 67% (40–43). The results of 33 patients being implanted at an experienced European center revealed that 83% of patients had an activated device at a minimum of 6 months' follow-up (44). Good to excellent results were obtained in 75% of these patients.

VIII.   NEW INVESTIGATIONAL TREATMENTS

The internal anal sphincter contracts in response to adrenergic stimulation. *Phenylephrine* is an alpha$_1$ adrenergic agonist. It has been shown to increase resting pressure when applied topically (45). Carapeti et al. applied 10% cream to patients with an intact sphincter and fecal

Table 1   Success Rates of Sphincteroplasty[a]

	N	Excellent	Good	Fair	Poor	Mean follow-up
Yugoslavia (34)	53	47%	23%	21%	9%	?
Miami (35)	22	74%	6%	14%	6%	20 mos
France (36)	74	28%	23%	—49	%—[b]	40 mos
St. Marks, U.K. (37)	38	0	11%	—89	%—[b]	77 mos
CCF, Ohio (38)	48	14%	30%	—56	%—[b]	63 mos

[a]Excellent = no incontinence; good = incontinence to gas only; fair = incontinence to gas and liquid stool; poor = incontinence to solid stool.
[b]Combined fair and poor into one group.

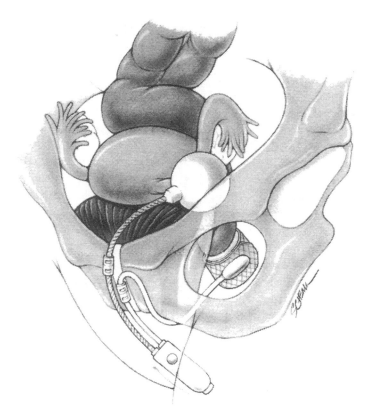

Figure 6   This is the artificial bowel sphincter implanted in a woman. The cuff is seen encircling the anus. The pump would be in the labia. A reservoir balloon sits in the space of Retzius anterior to the bladder. (Reprinted with permission of American Medical Systems, Inc., Minnetonka, MN.)

incontinence in a double-blind crossover study (46). Six of 18 in the treatment arm and two of 18 in the placebo crossover arm had more than 75% subjective improvement. They concluded that further studies are needed to determine the exact subgroup of patients, which would respond.

Radiofrequency energy delivered to a target temperature of 85°C for 1 min 23–32 times in the anal canal has been shown to be safe and effective. In a poster presentation at the American Society of Colorectal Surgeons meeting, there was significant improvement at 12 months in all parameters tested (47). The exact mechanism for this improvement is unknown.

Another new treatment is *sacral spinal nerve stimulation*. Originally, attempts were made to stimulate the muscle directly in patients with intact but functionally suboptimal sphincters. However, infection, migration, and fibrotic reactions led to failure. Based on a urology model, the site for electrostimulation was shifted to the peripheral nerve supply at the level of the sacral spinal nerves. The level of the sacral nerve is chosen (S2, S3, or S4) by passing a percutaneous electrode through the sacral foramen and stimulating each sacral nerve (at the S2, S3, or S4 level). The sacral nerve is chosen based on maximal contraction of the pelvic floor and minimal affect on the lower extremities (48). It is usually S3. The patient then undergoes stimulation with temporary electrodes and an external generator. If their fecal incontinence improves, a permanent generator and leads are implanted. Thus far, results from Europe in small groups of patients show incontinence improves in most patients through increased striated anal sphincter function (48–50).

Finally, for patients who have failed or who are not candidates for other surgical repairs, a *stoma* may improve their quality of life. It may allow patients the opportunity to leave home, attend work, and enjoy social functions. However, patients deserve evaluation at a center that specializes in all options of evaluating and treating fecal incontinence before a stoma is felt to be the final treatment option.

IX. CONCLUSION

Fecal incontinence is a complicated problem. The choice of treatment depends of the etiology of incontinence, the sphincter anatomy, and the impact of incontinence on the patient's quality of life. Usually nonsurgical treatment is the first choice. It is important to treat diarrhea first and be alert to anal skin problems. The best surgical option is a sphincter repair in a patient with an isolated anterior defect and otherwise good muscle function. In the past 10 years, many new treatments have been developed for patients with fecal incontinence that has not responded to traditional therapies. Considerable enthusiasm has been directed toward these new treatments, many of which are still in the preliminary stages.

REFERENCES

1. Jackson SL, Weber AM, Hull TL, Mitchinson AR, Walters MD. Fecal incontinence in women with urinary incontinence and pelvic organ prolapse. Obstet Gynecol 1997; 89:423–427.
2. Tetzscher T, Sorensen M, Lose G, Christiansen J. Anal and urinary incontinence in women with obstetric anal sphincter ruptures. Br J Obstet Gynaecol 1996; 103:1034–1040.
3. Varma MG, Madoff RD. Fecal incontinence. Clin Colon Rectal Surg 2001; 14:253–263.
4. Thomas TM, Egan M, Walgrove A, Meade TW. The prevalence of faecal and double incontinence. Community Med 1984; 6:216–220.
5. Johanson JF, Lafferty J. Epidemiology of fecal incontinence: the silent affliction. Am J Gastroenterol 1996; 91:33–36.
6. Faltin DL, Sangalli MR, Curtin F, Morabia A, Weil A. Prevalence of anal incontinence and other anorectal symptoms in women. Int Urogynecol J 2001; 12:117–120.
7. Nelson R, Norton N, Cautley E, Furner S. Community-based prevalence of anal incontinence. JAMA 1995; 274:559–561.
8. Francombe J, Carter PS, Hershman MJ. The aetiology and epidemiology of faecal incontinence. Hosp Med (Lond) 2001; 62:529–532.
9. Sultan AH. Anal incontinence after childbirth. Curr Opin Obstet Gynecol 1997; 9:320–324.
10. Sultan AH, Kamm MA, Hudson CN, Thomas JM, Bartram CI. Anal-sphincter disruption during vaginal delivery. N Engl J Med 1993; 329:1905–1911.
11. Zetterstrom J, Mellgren A, Jensen LL, Wong WD, Kim DG, Lowry AC, Madoff RD, Congilosi SM. Effect of delivery on anal sphincter morphology and function. Dis Colon Rectum 1999; 42:1253–1260.
12. Fynes M, Donnelly V, Behan M, O'Connell PR, O'Herlihy C. Effect of second vaginal delivery, on anorectal physiology and faecal continence: a prospective study. Lancet 1999; 353:983–986.
13. Varma A, Gunn J, Gardiner A, Lindow SW, Duthie GS. Obstetric anal sphincter injury. Prospective evaluation of incidence. Dis Colon Rectum 1999; 42:1537–1543.
14. Salvioli B, Bharucha AE, Rath-Harvey D, Pemberton JH, Phillips SF. Rectal compliance, capacity, and rectoanal sensation in fecal incontinence. Am J Gastroenterol 2001; 96:2158–2168.
15. O'Donnell P, Beck C, Doyle R, Eubanks C. Surface electrodes in perineal electromyography. Urology 1988; 34:375–379.

16. Gee AS, Jones RS, Durdey P. On-line quantitative analysis of surface electromyography of the pelvic floor in patients with faecal incontinence. Br J Surg 2000; 87:814–818.

17. Tjandra JJ, Milsom JW, Schroeder T, Fazio VW. Endoluminal ultrasound is preferable to electromyography in mapping anal sphincter defects. Dis Colon Rectum 1993; 36:689–692.

18. Sangwan YP, Coller JA, Barret RC, Murray JJ, Roberts PL, Schoetz DJ. Unilateral pudendal neuropathy: significance and implications. Dis Colon Rectum 1996; 39:249–251.

19. Gilliland R, Altomare DF, Moreira H Jr, Oliveira L, Gilliland JE, Wexner SD. Pudendal neuropathy is predictive of failure following anterior overlapping sphincteroplasty. Dis Colon Rectum 1998; 41:1516–1522.

20. Deen KI, Kumar D, Williams JG, Olliff J, Keighley MR. Anal sphincter defects: correlation between endoanal ultrasound and surgery. Ann Surg 1993; 218:201–205.

21. Sultan AH, Kamm MA, Talbot IC, Nicholls RJ, Bartram CE. Anal endosonography for identifying external sphincter defects confirmed histologically. Br J Surg 1994; 81:463–465.

22. Sentovich SM, Wong WD, Blatchford GJ. Accuracy and reliability of transanal ultrasound for anterior anal sphincter injury. Dis Colon Rectum 1998; 41:1000–1004.

23. De Souza NM, Puni R, Zbar A, Gidlerdale DJ, Coutts GA, Krausz T. MR imaging of the anal sphincter in multiparous women using an endoanal coil: correlation with in vitro anatomy and appearance in fecal incontinence. AJR 1996; 167:1465–1471.

24. Malouf AJ, Williams AB, Halligan S, Bartram CI, Khillon S, Kamm MA. Prospective assessment of accuracy of endoanal MR imaging and endosonography in patients with fecal incontinence. AJR 2000; 175:741–745.

25. Soffer EE, Hull T. Fecal incontinence: a practical approach to evaluation and treatment. Am J Gastroenterol 2000; 95:1873–1880.

26. Bliss DZ, Jung HJ, Savik K, Lowry A, Lemoine M, Jensen L, Werner C, Schaffer K. Supplementation with dietary fiber improves fecal incontinence. Nurs Res 2001; 50:203–213.

27. Santoro GA, Eitan BZ, Pryde A, Bartolo DC. Open dose study of low-dose amitriptyline in the treatment of patients with idiopathic fecal incontinence. Dis Colon Rectum 2000; 43:1676–1681.

28. Norton C, Kamm MA. Anal sphincter biofeedback and pelvic floor exercises for faecal incontinence in adults—a systematic review. Alim Pharmacol Ther 2001; 15:1147–1154.

29. Heymen S, Jones KR, Ringel Y, Scarlett Y, Whitehead WE. Biofeedback treatment of fecal incontinence: a critical review. Dis Colon Rectum 2001; 44:728–736.

30. Ench P, Daublin G, Lubke HJ, Strohmeyer G. Long-term efficacy of biofeedback training for fecal incontinence. Dis Colon Rectum 1994; 37:997–1001.

31. Ryn AK, Morren GL, Hallbook O, Sjodahl R. Long-term results of electromyographic biofeedback training for fecal incontinence. Dis Colon Rectum 2000; 43:1262–1266.

32. Jensen LL, Lowry AC. Biofeedback improves functional outcome after sphincteroplasty. Dis Colon Rectum 1997; 40:197–2000.

33. Parks AG, McPartlin JF. Late repair of injuries of the anal sphincter. Proc R Soc Med 1971; 64:1187–1189.

34. Barisic G, Krivokapic Z, Markovic V, Popovic M, Saranovic D, Marsavelska A. The role of overlapping sphincteroplasty in traumatic fecal incontinence. Acta Chir Yugoslav 2000; 47(suppl 1):37–41.

35. Salom E, Penalver M, Estape R, Pietro P, Angioli R. The treatment of fecal incontinence after traumatic vaginal delivery: overlapping sphincteroplasty, internal anal sphincter imbrication, levatorplasty, culdoplasty, and perineorrhaphy. Obstet Gynecol 2001; 97:S51.

36. Karoui S, Leroi AM, Koning E, Menard JF, Michot F, Denis P. Results of sphincteroplasty in 86 patients with anal incontinence. Dis Colon Rectum 2000; 43:813–820.

37. Malouf AJ, Norton CS, Engel AF, Nicholls RJ, Kamm MA. Long-term results of overlapping anterior anal-sphincter repair for obstetric trauma. Lancet 2000; 355:260–265.

38. Halverson A, Hull TL. Long term outcome of overlapping anal sphincter repair. Dis Colon Rectum 2002; 45:345–348.

39. Baeten CG, Bailey HR, Belliveau P, Berg E, Buie WD, Burnstein MJ, Christiansen J, Coller JA, Galandiuk S, LaFontaine LJ, Lange J, Madoff RD, Matzel KE, Pahlman L, Parc R, Reilly JC, Seccia M, Thorson AG, Vernava AM 3rd, Wexner S. Safety and efficacy of dynamic gracilloplasty

for fecal incontinence: report of a prospective, mulicenter trial. Dynamic Graciloplasty Therapy Study Group. Dis Colon Rectum 2000; 43:743–751.

40. Wong WD, Jensen LL, Bartolo DC, Rothenberger DA. Artificial anal sphincter. Dis Colon Rectum 1996; 39:1345–1351.

41. Savoye G, Leroi AM, Denis P, Michot F. Manometric assessment of an artificial bowel sphincter. Br J Surg 2000; 87:586–589.

42. Vaisey CJ, Kamm MA, Gold DM, Bartram CI, Halligan S, Nicholls RJ. Clinical, physiological, and radiological study of the new purpose-designed artificial bowel sphincter. Lancet 1998; 352:105–109.

43. Lehur P-A, Michot F, Denis P, Grise P, Leborgne J, Teniere P, Buzelin J-M. Results of artificial sphincter in severe anal incontinence: report of 14 consecutive implantations. Dis Colon Rectum 1996; 39:1352–1355.

44. Lehur PA, Roig JV, Diunslaeger M. Artificial anal sphincter: prospective clinical and manometric evaluation. Dis Colon Rectum 2000; 43:1100–1106.

45. Cheetham MJ, Kamm MA, Phillips RK. Topical phenylephrine increases anal canal resting pressures in patients with faecal incontinence. Gut 2001; 48:356–359.

46. Carapeti EA, Kamm MA, Phillips RK. Randomized controlled trial of topical phenylephrine in the treatment of faecal incontinence. Br J Surg 2000; 87:38–42.

47. Takahashi T, Garcia-Osogobio S, Valdovinos MA, Mass W, Jimenez R, Jauregui JL, Bobadilla J, Belmonte C, Edelstein PS, Utley DS. Radiofrequency energy delivery for the treatment of fecal incontinence. American Society of Colon and Rectal Surgeons meeting. Poster presentation 32, San Diego, CA, June 2–7, 2001.

48. Matzel KE, Stadelmaier U, Hohenfellner M, Hohenberger W. Chronic sacral spinal nerve stimulation for fecal incontinence: long-term results with foramen and cuff electrodes. Dis Colon Rectum 2001; 44:59–66.

49. Ganio E, Ratto C, Masin A, Luc AR, Doglietto GB, Dodi G, Ripetti V, Arullani A, Frascio M, BertiRiboli E, Landolfi V, DelGenio A, Altomare DF, Memeo V, Bertapelle P, Carone R, Spinelli M, Zanollo A, Spreafico L, Giardiello G, De Seta F. Neuromodulation for fecal incontinence: outcome in 16 patients with definitive implant. The initial Italian Sacral Neurostimulation Group (GINS) experience. Dis Colon Rectum 2001; 44:965–970.

50. Malouf AJ, Vaizey CJ, Nicholls RJ, Kamm MA. Permanent sacral nerve stimulation for fecal incontinence. Ann Surg 2000; 232:143–148.

Index